EMERGENCY MEDICINE
AN APPROACH TO CLINICAL PROBLEM-SOLVING

Glenn C. Hamilton, M.D., M.S.M.
Professor and Chair,
Department of Emergency Medicine,
Wright State University School of Medicine,
Dayton, Ohio

Arthur B. Sanders, M.D., M.H.A.
Professor,
Department of Emergency Medicine,
University of Arizona School of Medicine,
Tuscon,Arizona

Gary R. Strange, M.D.
Professor and Head,
Department of Emergency Medicine,
University of Illinois;
Chief of Emergency Service,
University of Illinois Medical Center,
Chicago, Illinois

Alexander T. Trott, M.D.
Professor of Emergency Medicine,
University of Cincinnati College of Medicine;
Associate Chief of Staff,
University of Cincinnati Medical Center;
Vice President, System Quality,
The Health Alliance,
Cincinnati, Ohio

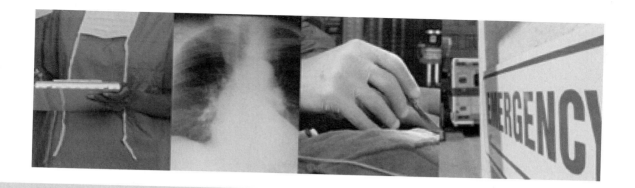

EMERGENCY MEDICINE
An Approach to Clinical Problem-Solving

SECOND EDITION

SAUNDERS
An Imprint of Elsevier Science

SAUNDERS
An Imprint of Elsevier Science

The Curtis Center
Independence Square West
Philadelphia, Pennsylvania 19106

NOTICE

Emergency Medicine is an ever-changing field. Standard safety precautions must be followed, but as new research and clinical experience broaden our knowledge, changes in treatment and drug therapy may become necessary or appropriate. Readers are advised to check the most current product information provided by the manufacturer of each drug to be administered to verify the recommended dose, the method and duration of administration, and contraindications. It is the responsibility of the treating physician, relying on experience and knowledge of the patient, to determine dosages and the best treatment for each individual patient. Neither the Publisher nor the editor assume any liability for any injury and/or damage to persons or property arising from this publication.

THE PUBLISHER

Library of Congress Cataloging-in-Publication Data

Emergency medicine: an approach to clinical problem-solving /
Glenn C. Hamilton [et al.].—2nd ed.
p. cm.
Includes bibliographical references and index.
ISBN 0–7216–9278–8
1. Emergency medicine. I. Hamilton, Glenn C.
RC86.7 .E5783 2003 616.02′5—dc21

2002—021840

Acquisitions Editor: Judy Fletcher
Developmental Editor: Heather Krehling
Publishing Services Manager: Frank Polizzano
Project Manager: Marian A. Bellus
Book Designer: Karen O'Keefe Owens

EMERGENCY MEDICINE: An Approach to Clinical Problem-Solving, 2/e

ISBN 07216-9278-8

Printed in the United States of America

Last digit is the print number: 9   8   7   6   5   4   3   2   1

Dedication

To Lynda as we approach 30 years together, for her sustained support and continued ability to make life interesting. To James, Kate and Liz who are choosing their own life paths on their terms, from a proud father. To the EM faculty, 200+ EM residents and 2000+ medical students at Wright State with whom I've had the privilege and pleasure to teach and learn from over the last 20+ years.

G.C.H.

To Debra, Louis, and Noah—thanks for your love and support. To all the students who have taught me so much, thank you.

A.B.S.

To my wife, Sarah, and daughters, Jackie and Betsy, for their support and patience through the years. And to all the students and residents at the University of Illinois whose feedback we so greatly appreciate.

G.R.S.

To my children Alexandra, Jacqueline, Buffy, and Hays, a talented, wondrous, and loving bunch of ragamuffins, and to my wife, Jennifer, the wise and marvelous architect of the life we all enjoy.

A.T.T.

Contributors

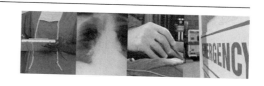

William Ahrens, MD
Associate Professor and Director of Pediatric Emergency Medicine, University of Illinois, Chicago, Illinois
Dehydration

Nicholas Benson, MD
Professor and Chair, Department of Emergency Medicine, Brody School of Medicine, East Carolina University; Chief of Emergency Services, University Health System of Eastern Carolina, Greenville, North Carolina
Earache

Jennifer M. Bocock, MD
Faculty Development Fellow, Wright State University School of Medicine, Department of Emergency Medicine, Dayton, Ohio
Approach to HIV in the Emergency Department; Psychobehavioral Disorders; Acute Dyspnea; Acute Pelvic Pain

James Brown, MD
Assistant Professor and Program Director, Department of Emergency Medicine, Wright State University School of Medicine, Dayton, Ohio
Head and Neck Trauma

E. Bradshaw Bunney, MD
Associate Professor of Emergency Medicine, University of Illinois, Chicago, Illinois
Hypothermia

Rhodessa Capulong, MD, FACEP
Clinical Instructor, University of Illinois College of Medicine, Chicago; Attending Physician, Emergency Department, MacNeal Hospital and Medical Center, Berwyn, Illinois
Anaphylaxis

Lisa Chan, MD
Assistant Residency Director, University of Arizona, Tucson, Arizona
Epistaxis

Todd J. Crocco, MD
Assistant Professor, Director of Clinical Research Emergency Medicine, West Virginia University, Morgantown, West Virginia
Acute Diarrhea

Natalie M. Cullen, MD
Assistant Professor, Department of Emergency Medicine, Wright State University, Dayton; Attending Physician, Kettering Medical Center, Kettering, Ohio
Alcohol Intoxication

Stephen W. Dailey, MD
Primary Care Sports Physician, Wellington Orthopaedics, Cincinnati, Ohio
Lower Extremity Injury

Virgil Davis
Department of Emergency Medicine, University of Arizona Health Sciences Center, Tucson, Arizona
Headache

Scott A. Doak, MD
Assistant Clinical Professor, Department of Emergency Medicine, Wright State University School of Medicine, Dayton, Ohio
Airway Management; Wound Care

Valerie Dobiesz, MD, FACEP
Associate Residency Director, University of Illinois Emergency Medicine Program, University of Illinois; Clinical Associate Professor, University of Illinois Hospital, Chicago, Illinois
Closed Injuries of the Upper Extremity

Wesley Eilbert, MD, FACEP
Clinical Associate Professor, Department of Emergency Medicine, University of Illinois College of Medicine; Director of Undergraduate Education, Department of Emergency Medicine, Mercy Hospital and Medical Center, Chicago, Illinois
Febrile Adults

Matthew L. Emerick, MD, FACEP
Staff Emergency Physician, Singing River Hospital System, Pascagoula, Mississippi
Acute Abdominal Pain; Acute Gastrointestinal Bleeding

Gregory J. Fermann, MD
Assistant Professor, Department of Emergency Medicine, College of Medicine, University of Cincinnati; Clinical Director, Center for Emergency Care, University Hospital, Inc., Cincinnati, Ohio
Abdominal Trauma

Carl M. Ferraro, MD
Clinical Associate Professor, Department of Emergency Medicine, Univercity of Illinois; Mercy Hospital and Medical Center, Chicago, Illinois
Diabetes

Denis J. Fitzgerald, MD
Assistant Professor, Department of Emergency Medicine, University of Cincinnati, Cincinnati, Ohio
Approach to HIV in the Emergency Department

Melissa Gillespie, MD
Clinical Assistant Professor, University of Illinois; Associate Attending Physician in Emergency Medicine, Advocate Illinois Masonic Medical Center, Chicago, Illinois
Open Injuries to the Hand

Robert A. Girmann, MD
Medical Director, Wayne Hospital Emergency Department, Greenville, Ohio
Acute Gastrointestinal Bleeding

John A. Guisto, MD
Associate Professor of Clinical Emergency Medicine, University of Arizona; Clinical Director, Emergency Department, University Medical Center, Tucson, Arizona
Heat Illness

Glenn C. Hamilton, MD
Professor and Chair, Department of Emergency Medicine, Wright State University, Dayton, Ohio
Introduction to Emergency Medicine; Chest Pain; Acute Metabolic Acidosis and Metabolic Alkalosis

Mary Kay Hinkebein, MD
Emergency Physician, Peninsula Emergency Physicians, Hampton, Virginia; Medical Director, Tidewater Community College; Medical Advisor, Virginia Beach Volunteer Rescue Squad, Virginia Beach, Virginia
The Red Painful Eye

Teresita Hogan, MD
Clinical Associate Professor, Department of Emergency Medicine, University of Illinois; Residency Director, Resurrection Medical Center, Chicago, Illinois
Domestic Violence

Courtney Hopkins, MD
Clinical Instructor, University Hospital, Cincinnati, Ohio
Vaginal Bleeding

David S. Howes, MD
Associate Professor of Clinical Medicine (Emergency Medicine); Residency Director, Department of Emergency Medicine, University of Chicago, Chicago, Illinois
The Red, Painful Eye

Karel Isely, MD
Emergency Physician, St. Joseph's Hospital, St. Paul, Minnesota
Psychobehavioral Disorders

Timothy G. Janz, MD
Associate Professor, Department of Emergency Medicine, Pulmonary/Critical Care Division, Department of Internal Medicine, Wright State University School of Medicine, Dayton, Ohio
Cardiopulmonary Cerebral Resuscitation; Chest Pain; Syncope

Steven Joyce
Professor, Department of Surgery, Division of Emergency Medicine, University of Utah; University of Utah Hospitals and Clinics Emergency Medical Services Department, Salt Lake City, Utah
Epistaxis

Thomas Krisanda, MD
Attending Physician, Department of Emergency Medicine, York Hospital, York, Pennsylvania
Vaginal Bleeding

Kevin W. Kulow, MD
Instructor, Department of Emergency Medicine, Wright State University, Dayton, Ohio; USAF Staff Physician and EMS Director, Wright - Patterson Medical Center, Fairborn, Ohio
Penetrating Trauma

Shawna Langstaff, MD
Medical Director, Paramedic Programs, Pike's Peak Community College; Emergency Department Physician, Penrose-St. Francis Hospital, Colorado Springs, Colorado
Seizures

Patricia Lee, MD
Clinical Associate Professor, EA University of Illinois College of Medicine, Department of Emergency Medicine; Medical Director, Illinois Masonic Medical Center, Chicago, Illinois
Sickle Cell Disease

Ray Legenza, MD
Medical Director, Emergency Services, Keesler Air Force Base, Biloxi, Mississippi
Head and Neck Trauma

Elizabeth A. Lindberg, MD
Associate Professor, Department of Emergency Medicine, Section of Urgent Care, University of Arizona College of Medicine; Clinical Director of Urgent Care, Department of Emergency Medicine, Section of Urgent Care, University Medical Center, Tucson, Arizona
Acute Sore Throat

Sharon Malone, MD
Emergency Medicine Physician, Texoma Medical Center, Denison, Texas
Chest Pain

Joseph J. Moellman, MD
Assistant Professor, Emergency Medicine, University of Cincinnati; Associate Medical Director, Jewish Hospital of Kenwood, Cincinnati, Ohio
Acute Pelvic Pain

Teresita Morales-Yurik, MD
Emergency Medicine Department Staff, Med Central Health System, Mansfield, Ohio
Stridor

Elif E. Oker, MD
Assistant Professor of Clinical Emergency Medicine, University of Illinois at Chicago; Attending Physician, University of Chicago Medical Center, Chicago, Illinois
Shock

T. J. Rittenberry, MD
Associate Professor of Clinical Emergency Medicine, Associate Residency Director, University of Illinois at Chicago; Director of Emergency Medical Education, Illinois Masonic Medical Center, Chicago, Illinois
Lower Extremity Injury

Ronald M. Salik, MD, FACEP
Assistant Professor, Department of Emergency Medicine, University of Arizona; Director of Children's Emergency Care, Tucson Medical Center, Tucson, Arizona
Earache

Arthur B. Sanders, MD, MHA
Professor, Department of Emergency Medicine, University of Arizona School of Medicine Tucson, Arizona
Hypertension; The Swollen and Painful Joint; Stroke

Steve Sigrist, MD
Emergency Physician, Licking Memorial Hospital, Newark, Ohio
Wheezing

Jonathan I. Singer, MD
Professor of Emergency Medicine and Pediatrics; Vice Chair and Associate Program Director, Department of Emergency Medicine, Wright State University School of Medicine; Staff Physician, Children's Medical Center, Dayton, Ohio
Febrile Infants; Dehydration

Edward P. Sloan, MD
Assistant Professor of Emergency Medicine, University of Illinois, Chicago, Chicago, Illinois
Lower Extremity Injury

Sidney Starkman, MD
Assistant Professor of Medicine/Emergency Medicine and Neurology, University of California, Los Angeles, School of Medicine; Director, UCLA Emergency Medicine Residency Program, UCLA Medical Center, Los Angeles, California
Altered Mental Status

Gary R. Strange, MD
Professor and Head, Department of Emergency Medicine, University of Illinois; Chief of Emergency Medicine, University of Illinois Medical Center, Chicago, Illinois
Diabetes; Stridor

Alexander T. Trott, MD
Professor of Emergency Medicine, University of Cincinnati College of Medicine; Associate Chief of Staff, University of Cincinnati Medical Center; Vice President, System Quality, The Health Alliance, Cincinnati, Ohio
Rash; Approach to HIV in the Emergency Department; Chest Trauma

Dennis T. Uehara, MD
Clinical Associate Professor, Department of Emergency Medicine, University of Illinois, Rockford, Rockford, Illinois
Open Injuries to the Hand

Jonathan Van Zile, MD
Assistant Professor of Emergency Medicine, University of Ohio; Residency Director, Emergency Medicine and Internal Medicine, The Jewish Hospital, Cincinnati, Ohio
Acute Abdominal Pain

Douglas Ward, MD
Emergency Physician, St Mary's Hospital, Decatur, Illinois
Syncope

John M. Wightman, MD
Director, Education Division, Department of
Military and Emergency Medicine, Uniformed
Services University, Bethesda, Maryland
*Multiple Blunt Trauma; Penetrating
Trauma*

Robert Wilson, MD
Emergency Physician, Sanford, North Carolina
The Poisoned Patient

Leslie Wolf, MD, FACMT
Associate Editor, Living Longer Health Courier;
Vice President, Living Longer Operations, Proscan
Imaging, Cincinnati, Ohio
The Poisoned Patient; Wheezing

Mark D. Wright, MD
Assistant Professor, Department of Emergency
Medicine, University of Cincinnati, Cincinnati,
Ohio
Acute Low Back Pain

Stewart D. Wright, MD
Assistant Professor, Department of Emergency
Medicine, University of Cincinnati School of
Medicine Cincinnati, Ohio
Altered Mental Status

Steve Yamaguchi, MD
Emergency Department Medical Director,
Mercy Fairfield Hospital, Fairfield, Ohio
Acute Dyspnea

Preface

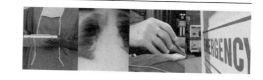

Eleven years is a long time between editions by any standard. This fact is acknowledged as a means of apology to a number of medical student educators who politely, but persistently, wondered aloud if a second edition would ever appear. The reasons for straying from the standard scheme of a 4- to 5-year cycle are myriad, but can best be stated as "life intervenes." I'm relieved the distractions subsided, and the editors persevered to create this edition, while establishing a firm basis for the next.

This book is written for medical students rotating on an emergency medicine clerkship or selective, PGY-I EM residents, and residents from other services spending their one to two months with us. Anyone else can read it, as the common thread for the readership is singular. How do emergency physicians efficiently approach a patient with an undifferentiated presenting complaint or finding and discover its cause or causes, while clinically multi-tasking in the realms of stabilization, evaluation, treatment, and disposition?

The book offers a course of study in this multi-layered approach to the 40 or more most common patient presentations in our specialty. It is not a comprehensive text, a bedside manual, a procedure guide, or an EM peripheral brain; it was never meant to be. It is a compilation of best evidence and clinical experience organized to guide students in the way emergency physicians think and care for their patients.

So what did we learn, and therefore incorporate over these years while contemplating the second edition? First, the basic principles of the emergency medicine approach stand up well over time. The initial phases of disease recognition and stabilization haven't changed significantly. The real advances have been in evaluation (especially imaging), and treatment. Second, the first edition was too big, and too expensive for its intended audience. Therefore, this text's page count is reduced, chapters down from 64 to 49, a soft cover applied, and the price reduced accordingly. Third, the chapter structure well represented the parallel processing of emergency medicine in a sequential manner, but some areas were redundant or excessive for the readership. Therefore, the Pre Hospital Care information was deleted or moved into Initial Approach and Stabilization, the Documentation section was removed, and the often confusing multiple case examples integrated throughout each chapter were, for the most part, consolidated as a single case example with commentary at the end of the chapter. Fourth, new principles to guide educators have appeared over this last decade. The most important has been Evidence-Based Medicine. Where available and appropriate the current "best evidence" has been and will continue to be incorporated into the text. A new section, Uncertain Diagnoses, has been added. This topic was intermittently explored previously, but now is discussed in each chapter. Uncertainty is a common theme in our practice, and the opportunity to regroup, rethink, or refer is worth an extra paragraph when all the diagnostic effort comes to naught.

Finally, the book continues to be the centerpiece of a successful and time-tested curriculum, built around case discussions and clinical supervision guidelines. They incorporate 20 chapters of the text, those considered by the WSU faculty to be most appropriate for a 4-week training experience in emergency medicine. A Student Workbook and Faculty Instructor Guide are now in their 5th edition and available to establish or supplement curricular plans in any Emergency Department. These are available directly from the Department of Emergency Medicine, Wright State University School of Medicine.

Thus concludes the Preface, always written at the end of the labor. The text is leaner, not meaner, and still in keeping with the lessons learned from the maturation of our specialty over the last 10 years. From the editors and me, it's nice to be back. Opinions, comments, and even the rare compliment are appreciated — at *glenn.hamilton@wright.edu*. (an address that had no relevance the first time around!)

GLENN C. HAMILTON, MD
SEPTEMBER, 2002

Acknowledgments

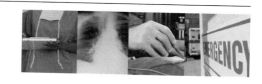

Judy Fletcher and Heather Krehling, transitioned through Saunders to Harcourt to Elsevier while waiting for this Second Edition to appear. Once it did, their efficiency was remarkable. Drs. Sanders, Strange, and Trott kept the faith through several false starts and a prolonged promise of completion. The Wright State Emergency Medicine faculty produced timely drafts and remained committed in the face of multiple revisions. Jennifer Bocock, MD, our first Faculty Development Fellow, tackled data gathering and editing with an enthusiasm and talent that assured the final block of chapters would be finished. The Word Processing Center at Wright State University SOM, Diane Ebert and Sandy Rieder who maintained the multiple revisions and kept the tables aligned, always with a rapid turnaround. The support staff in the Department of Emergency Medicine who represent the best of individuals and their collective efficiency. They took this challenge as they approach all others, with a positive "can do" attitude, and the wise knowledge that their efforts reach beyond the confines of the department offices. Linda Stanchina, who coordinated all these materials while transcribing many of them; Shirley Foreman, who always was there to transcribe, edit, and maintain the flow; Anne Carlisle, who unraveled the mysteries of Word to create tables, charts, and algorithms from scribbled notes; Sandy Scarborough who made sure it said what it meant, transcribed and kept the previous chapters supplied to residents and students alike, Lynn DeWine who transcribed notes, mastered revisions and memorized all the Fed Ex contacts, Alaine White, who transcribed and was always available for the next task. A great team, without whom there would be no book.

GLENN C. HAMILTON

I would like to acknowledge Alicia Gonzales and Janice Martinez for their help in preparation of the manuscripts.

ARTHUR B. SANDERS

In Chicago: Many thanks to the office staffs in our hospitals. At the University of Illinois: Zenobia Chaney-Watson, Brenda Fuller-Colar and Bailet Wright. At Illinois Masonic Medical Center: Sharon Thovsen and Rose Sturgill-Bradford. At Mercy Hospital and Medical Center: Julie Mendez. At Resurrection Medical Center: Denise Toriani.

GARY R. STRANGE

I want to acknowledge Angela Wilson who provided all my manuscript and administrative support for my portion of the book.

ALEXANDER T. TROTT

An additional acknowledgement belongs to each of the authors who contributed to the first edition. Each of these individuals was asked to write a chapter in a format that had never been tried before and each made a substantial effort toward the quality and success of this text. More than 10 years later, many of these authors' contributions remain in this text and well demonstrate the timelessness of a well-thought-out, approach to addressing an undifferentiated chief complaint. Our professional and personal thanks to each of you for your enduring endeavors.

Contents

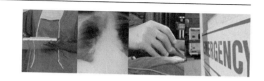

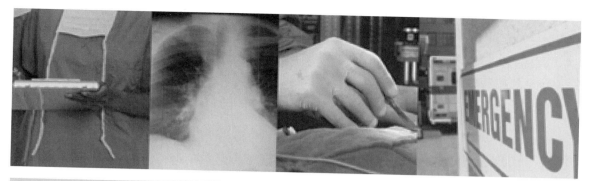

ORIENTATION TO EMERGENCY MEDICINE

CHAPTER 1

Introduction to Emergency Medicine

GLENN C. HAMILTON

As a third-year medical student entering the emergency room for the first time in 1971, my initial impression was, "This is where the action is! But I don't think I'd want to live here!" Surely, thousands of students, residents, and attending physicians had similar thoughts. The emergency room was at the bottom of the medical prestige ladder. The students, interns, and residents usually taught and supervised themselves. Many patients were delivered by modified hearses run by the mortuary. Over the past 3 decades, the primary goal of emergency medicine as a specialty has been to fulfill the trust placed in its hands by the now millions of people who present themselves for care. The ill, injured, poor, lost, intoxicated, and confused all needed a place to go where physicians and nurses were trained to treat them in the best manner possible, 24 hours a day, 365 days a year. What changed their fate and fulfilled our goal is that thousands of physicians *have* chosen to "live" in the emergency department and to make it their place of specialty practice. Beginning in 1968 with the formation of the American College of Emergency Physicians, emergency medicine has grown as a clinical specialty and academic discipline in concert with the increasing public demand for competent and compassionate emergency care. This growth has had several milestones:

1970: The first emergency medicine residency program was established at the University of Cincinnati.

1973: The Emergency Medical Services Act authorized the establishment and expansion of emergency medical services system and research.

1975: The American Medical Association House of Delegates approved a permanent Section on Emergency Medicine and accepted standards for emergency medicine residencies.

1979: Emergency medicine was recognized as the twenty-third medical specialty by the American Medical Association and the American Board of Medical Specialties. Certification examinations began the following year. The American Board of Emergency Medicine was convened as a modified conjoint board with required representation by several other specialties.

1982: Special requirements for emergency medicine residency training programs were approved by the Accreditation Council for Graduate Medical Education. Almost 50 programs were reviewed.

1989: Primary board status was granted by the American Board of Medical Specialties.

2000: Sixty academic departments and 125 residency programs were actively training thousands of medical students, and over 1200 emergency medicine residents. Emergency medicine had ranked in the top three specialty choices of medical students for nearly a decade.

Each of these steps has contributed to validating the credentials and rewarding the commitment of the thousands of individuals who make up the "emergency medical care team" serving in the United States and throughout the world. The health care "safety net" in this country has been defined and secured by the specialty of emergency medicine.

Table 1–1 lists the vital statistics of the specialty in the United States comparing 1990 with 2000. As an essential component of the health care structure in this country, emergency medicine continues to be a core subject in the training of medical students, a highly valued residency training experience, and a satisfying career for thousands of physicians.

This chapter is written to introduce the reader to the scope of emergency medicine practice, the principles of care behind the practice, and the basis for the problem-solving approach used in this book. In addition, a number of "pearls from practice" supplied by the authors are listed. Sharing the practice principles guiding our clinicians is another way of conveying the character of emergency physicians and their specialty.

SCOPE OF PRACTICE IN EMERGENCY MEDICINE

In 1975, the House of Delegates of the American Medical Association defined the emergency physician as a physician trained to engage in:

TABLE 1–1. US Emergency Medicine Statistical and Historical Profile—1990/2000

Emergency Physicians	23,000/32,020
Total emergency physicians (in clinical practice)	13,360/21,000
Members of American College of Emergency Physicians	8332/17,300
Diplomates of American Board of Emergency Medicine	1600/5000
Members of Society for Academic Emergency Medicine	
Emergency Medicine Residencies	
Emergency medicine residency programs approved by Residency Review Committee/	
Emergency Medicine (RRC/EM)	80/126
Average annual number of graduates (approximate)	450/1150
Total residents currently in training in RRC/EM-approved programs	1629/3700
Emergency Nurses	
Total emergency nurses (approximate)	85,000/89,300
Nurses certified by the Board of Certification for Emergency Nurses	17,180/26,000
Emergency Medical Providers (includes first responders, basic intermediate paramedics)	434,498/815,000
Emergency Departments	
Hospital-based emergency departments (approximate)	5600/3900
Emergency department visits	87 million/108 million
Ambulance Services	12,000/17,000

Modified from Emergency Medicine Statistical Profile, American College of Emergency Physicians, Dallas, Texas, February 2002, with permission.

1. The immediate initial recognition, evaluation, care, and disposition of patients with acute illness and injury.
2. The administration, research, and teaching of all aspects of emergency medical care.
3. The direction of the patient to sources of follow-up care, in or out of the hospital as may be required.
4. The provision when requested of emergency, but not continuing, care to in-hospital patients.
5. The management of the emergency medical system for the provision of prehospital emergency care.

Six years later, a "Definition of Emergency Medicine" was developed by the American College of Emergency Physicians and endorsed by the three other organizations representing residents in training and academic emergency physicians. This definition has had several iterations; the most recent dates from 2001 and states:

Emergency medicine is the medical specialty with the principal mission of evaluating, managing, treating, and preventing unexpected illness and injury. It encompasses a unique body of knowledge, reflected in "The Model of the Clinical Practice of Emergency Medicine." Clinical emergency medicine may be practiced in emergency departments, urgent care clinics, and other settings. The clinical practice of emergency medicine encompasses the initial evaluation, treatment, and disposition of any person at any time for any symptom, event, or disorder deemed by the person—or someone acting on his or her behalf—to require expeditious medical, surgical, or psychiatric attention.

Emergency medicine provides valuable clinical and administrative services to the health care delivery system, including care for individuals who lack other access to health care, prehospital care planning and medical control, and patient-care coordination—across venues and among providers. Consequently, emergency medicine serves as America's health care safety net. Emergency physicians develop a deep understanding of health care systems and are uniquely positioned to plan, implement, and evaluate them.

The critical word in this definition is "emergency," and it must be clarified. *Emergency* is defined by the perception of the patient who comes or the people who bring the patient to the emergency department. Over 70% of emergency patients believe they need medical care within 2 hours of their decision to seek help. Therefore, the patient defines the "emergency" regardless of the ultimate nature of the illness or injury. Although discrepancies may exist between what the patient believes is emergent and how that concern is perceived by the emergency physician, many problems need 24 to 48 hours or more of evaluation and treatment before they are retrospectively determined to be "emergent" or not. This gap between the patient's perception, the emergency physician's perception, and the time delay before the reality of the hazard is revealed is often a source of frustration and anger. This difficult situation may influence the emergency physician's relationship with the patient, the admitting physician, family members of the patient, and the insurance system involved in reimbursing the transaction. Accepting the contextual nature of the term *emergency* will help the reader to understand the specialty more fully.

In addition to the acute care of the ill or injured patient, the specialty has evolved to include added responsibilities in the following areas:

- *Administration.* Management of the medical and administrative aspects of the emergency services system is included in this category (e.g., public education about services, 911 telephone access, and emergency department categorization).
- *Disaster planning and management for both natural and man-made events.* The events of September 11, 2001, changed the way we think about bioterrorism and weapons of mass destruction. Emergency medicine is at the forefront of surveillance and response in these difficult times.
- *Toxicology.* This includes poison center development and improved means of recognition of environmental hazards.
- *Health care services research.* Problems in society and in our health care delivery system are often noted first in the emergency department. For example, problems of the homeless, hospital closures, and the drug "wars" have manifested themselves as increasing numbers of patients with higher acuity of illness crowding into the emergency department—with no place else to go. As the front line of medicine, emergency medicine has a special obligation to ensure access to quality health care for all patients and communicate problems in this access to the rest of organized medicine when they occur.
- *Education.* The emergency department has always been a popular training site. The shift of care and training to outpatient and ambulatory settings has made it an even more valuable asset.
- *Preventive medicine.* Only a brief exposure to the practice of emergency medicine will generate an interest in improving and enforcing the laws regarding seat belt use, driving while intoxicated, or job-related safety. The specialty has an important public health role in monitoring and recognizing significant health patterns and problems in the populations it serves.
- *Basic and clinical research.* The scientific rationale for the efficacy of resuscitative interventions is an essential element in expanding the academic base of the specialty. The past 20 years have brought significant advances in trauma care, cardiac and cerebrovascular disease intervention, pediatric and elderly care, imaging techniques, use of technology, integration of evidence-based medicine, and advances in human immunodeficiency virus infection, cancer, and transplant patient care. Emergency medicine has served its academic purpose and continues to expand its influence in research.

The future holds bright promise for the scope of practice available in emergency medicine. Pediatric emergency care, trauma care, aerospace medicine, sports medicine, critical care medicine, industrial medicine, clinical epidemiology, and quality assurance have benefited and will continue to gain from the ideas and energy of emergency physicians.

Emergency medicine is a specialty that was created to fulfill the needs of ill and injured people. It arrived at a time when both the general population and a select group of physicians recognized its importance. It remains a clinical specialty serving all those who find themselves seeking its care, competence, and advocacy.

PRINCIPLES OF EMERGENCY CARE

The nature of clinical emergency medicine has been briefly described. In this section, 12 principles guiding the decisions made in practice are examined. "Guiding principles" is a carefully chosen description. Emergency medicine should not be identified with or practiced by "cook-book" or algorithmic thinking. The patients rarely follow the recipe and often do not cooperate at the branch points. Emergency medicine is best practiced by following *heuristics,* that is, incomplete guidelines that lead to new knowledge or discovery.

These 12 principles are well-tested guides to ensure the highest quality practice of this specialty. By adopting and practicing them, the emergency physician can deliver patient-directed and humane care while enjoying a satisfying and respected career.

1. Is a Life-Threatening Process Causing the Patient's Complaint?

This is always the first question asked by the emergency physician. Emergency medicine is primarily a *complaint-oriented* rather than a *disease-specific* specialty. Its emphasis rests on anticipating and recognizing a life-threatening *process,* rather than seeking the diagnosis. This is an important difference between emergency medicine and other specialties. A patient with severe substernal chest pain is first considered as having a life-threatening problem with the potential for hypoxia, hypoperfusion, or dysrhythmia, rather than as having a myocardial infarction. Anticipation of life-threatening problems focuses the physician's attention on both the underlying pathophysiology and the influence of time on the presentations and outcome of dynamic disease processes. The goal is simply to think about and plan to prevent "bad things" from happening or progressing in the patient.

2. What Must Be Done To Stabilize the Patient?

Stabilizing a patient may require the direct intervention in a life-threatening process or an intervention that *anticipates* a critical problem developing. In a patient with chest pain, a cardiac monitor and an intravenous line are placed in anticipation of a dysrhythmia and the need for medications or volume repletion. These steps demonstrate the emergency physician's awareness of the potential hazards of the pathologic processes associated with the presenting symptoms, not the diagnosis. They represent actions performed to monitor the course of the process while preparations are made to intervene quickly if necessary.

3. Beyond the Life-Threatening Process, What Are the Most Serious Disorders (Highest Potential Morbidity) That Are Consistent with the Patient's Presentation?

The emergency physician approaches a problem by considering the most serious disease consistent with the patient complaint and working to exclude it. "Thinking the worst" is a reversal of the assessment sequence in many specialties. In emergency medicine, the "worst comes first." Only after these concerns have been ruled out are the more benign processes considered.

This principle is even more important when it is placed in the context of the patient population seen in the emergency department. The majority of patients are strangers to the physician, a significant proportion may be intoxicated, and many are brought by others rather than coming of their own volition. Confronted with an array of fragmented histories, masked physical findings, and emotional overlay, it is imperative for the emergency physician to maintain the highest level of suspicion for serious disease.

4. Is More Than One Active Pathologic Process Present?

A single diagnosis is not always possible or appropriate. The emergency physician must maintain an open and continually probing approach that is the hallmark of the effective clinician. Always thinking "Is that all there is?" encourages the physician to consider alternative diagnoses and seek additional information from the patient, other sources, or response to therapy. The time for assessment is usually brief, and it is essential to resist the tendency to rapidly narrow the underlying possibilities. An example is the driver involved in a motor vehicle accident who is hypotensive. The hypotension may be the result of the trauma, but it may also have been the cause. Hypotension after a motor vehicle accident is very likely to be secondary to blood loss, but the possibility of anaphylaxis, myocardial failure, or distributive shock from a drug overdose must be considered.

5. Would a Diagnostic-Therapeutic Trial Serve in This Case?

One of the emergency physician's important tools is a stabilizing therapy that also gives diagnostic information. This information may be precise or may just help differentiate the seriously ill patient from others. Glucose, thiamine, and naloxone given to the unconscious patient are examples of this "diagnostic-therapeutic" concept. Judicious fluid boluses to improve a patient's hemodynamic status are another. Integrating therapy and diagnosis is especially valuable in the time-dependent setting that usually begins with undifferentiated illness. Seeking new *diagnostic-therapeutic* tests or maneuvers and determining where they can be applied is an important role of the emergency physician.

6. Is a Diagnosis Possible or Even Necessary?

One of the most difficult aspects of emergency medicine is becoming comfortable with uncertainty regarding an exact diagnosis before important decisions are made. This principle has been discussed in terms of stabilization. It also applies throughout the steps of care in the emergency department, especially during disposition decisions. Knowing when to stop an assessment or treatment is as important as knowing when to persist. Many common complaints such as chest or abdominal pain remain undiagnosed at the time the patient leaves the emergency department. Other serious problems may require early disposition to sites outside of the department without a precise diagnosis being made (e.g., obvious penetrating trauma to the abdomen).

7. Is Hospitalization Appropriate? If So, Where?

The "bottom line" decision for the emergency physician is whether the patient is admitted to the hospital or discharged from the emergency department. In many cases, once the patient's condition has been recognized as requiring hospitalization and stabilization has begun, much of the emergency physician's clinical work is accomplished. Still, there are other reasons for continued care. It may be necessary to benefit the admitting physician, to maintain one's clinical acumen, or because the hospital staff do not have an available inpatient bed.

Risk stratification is an important concept in emergency medicine. It delineates different groups of patients with varied potential for a specific diagnosis. Within these groups, treatment and disposition decisions may vary. Acute coronary syndrome (ACS) patients may require immediate medication and transfer to the catheterization unit, or observation and cardiac stress testing. The choices depend on the emergency physician's ability to classify (stratify) the patient's chances of having ACS and which form of the disease may be present.

8. If the Patient Is To Be Discharged, Is the Disposition Adequate?

The most difficult patients cared for by the emergency physician are the ones who are discharged. This is doubly true for those who leave without a clear diagnosis. Unfortunately, in a limited and often first-time assessment, the data available may be insufficient for a disease process to be identified or understood. Despite their wishes, both patients and physicians must recognize that all important information is not available immediately. To ensure optimal care, an appropriate discharge disposition should include the patient's basic understanding of (1) the underlying problem that caused him or her to seek emergency care, (2) the evaluation and treatment given in the emergency department, (3) when and with whom follow-up is planned, and (4) criteria by which the patient can judge whether a return for further assessment is necessary.

9. In Working with Admitting or Primary Physicians, Has the Concept of "Our" Patient Been Well Established?

Emergency physicians have a unique relationship with other physicians. They serve as the "always available" consultant and specialist in common and catastrophic diseases. Combining the historical knowledge of the primary physician or specialist with the emergency physician's information obtained from the patient's bedside can offer the best of acute care. Emergency physicians are the gatekeepers of one of the major access routes into the medical system. Their relationship with other physicians is always based on the concept of "our" patient. It must be a healthy relationship—one based on mutual trust and respect.

10. Does the Chart Reflect the Full Extent of Evaluation and Treatment Given in the Emergency Department?

The medicolegal cliché "If it isn't charted, it didn't happen" is generally true. Part of the experience in emergency medicine is learning to write or dictate accurate, useful information in limited time and space. The importance of developing patterns of recording the right information efficiently cannot be overstated.

11. Have the Patient's Expectations, Voiced and Unvoiced, Been Met?

The emergency physician must often look beyond the words of a complaint to sense the patient's fears and concerns about being in the emergency department: "Am I going to die?" "Is it cancer?" "Will there be a scar?" and "Can you relieve my pain?" are questions to be anticipated and answered. The hidden potential for suicide or the reality of child abuse must also be uncovered during a brief interview within an often harried environment. This skill demands a sensitivity, awareness, and ability to concentrate on many clues during the physician-patient exchange. Only training and a commitment to clinical excellence in this setting allow these skills to develop fully.

Every patient assessed in the emergency department is given something. It may be an explanation, a referral, or a specific therapeutic regimen. Each patient has a requirement, and the emergency physician makes an attempt to fulfill it, if it is legitimate and reasonable. If the requirement cannot be met, an explanation in layperson's terms is necessary. For example, parents may ask for a skull radiograph for their asymptomatic child's head contusion. This expectation is addressed by discussing the lack of indications, the hazards of radiation, and the expense. On occasion, when reason fails, obtaining the films may be appropriate. The key is to ensure the cooperation of the parents so they will comply with the more important follow-up observation and return visit, if necessary.

12. Are the Resources Available To Allow the Full Range of Emergency Services To Be Efficiently Administered?

The emergency physician has a role in maintaining the equipment and staffing of the department at the highest level of quality. Trends and breakthroughs are monitored in the literature. Equipment and supplies representing real advances in patient care are purchased. The education and skills development of the staff are maintained. Developing a viable and continuous quality assurance program for physicians and staff, maintaining a relationship with attending physicians to facilitate patient care, and actively participating in the affairs of the hospital and medical services in the community are all necessary to contribute to the overall quality of medicine.

An important correlate of this principle is the recognition of what the emergency department team cannot do. It cannot be all things to all people. It should not be thought of as a walk-in clinic when other facilities are nearby and available, a storage depot for patients waiting to be admitted, or an extended critical care unit on demand. To serve its purpose, the emergency department must be dedicated first to the critically ill and injured patient. Because this degree of severity is not always realized immediately, no one is turned away without an appropriate assessment. This service is essential to the community, and it must not be abused.

THE APPROACH TO CLINICAL PROBLEM-SOLVING IN THE TEXT

The process of clinical problem-solving begins with the acquisition of a fundamental body of knowledge, including anatomy and physiology as well as the pathology and epidemiology of disease patterns. The clinician uses this knowledge base to address specific patient complaints. The emergency physician is particularly concerned with conditions that may result in morbidity or mortality if not immediately addressed. The secondary concern is the common or serious diseases that may be the cause of the patient's complaint.

In the typical sequence of care, anticipating the emergent condition is the focus of emergency medicine in the prehospital and initial stabilization period. After initial stabilization, the emergency physician applies the knowledge of disease processes to direct specific data gathering from the patient and other sources. This complaint-directed assessment in a time-limited framework is not a simple task. The data gathered are added to the understanding of the pathophysiology of diseases to develop a rational set of guidelines regarding the further assessment, treatment, and disposition of each patient. These decisions are made in the context of the inexact science of clinical medicine. It is not improbable for the same patient to present in different emergency departments with the same history and physical findings and be treated differently at each hospital. There are few totally right answers in clinical medicine. There *are* wrong interpretations, priorities, and actions that violate the scientific basis of practice or the accepted principle of "first, do no harm, and second, do some good."

An element of problem-solving is the discipline of decision analysis. This quantitative science attempts to attach actual probabilities to the various options available at decision points. When given the probabilities of various alternatives, the clinician can then choose the most likely alternative. Unfortunately, this discipline is relatively new in emergency medicine. In most circumstances, the emergency physician does not have sufficient information to reliably calculate probabilities at every decision point for each disease process. The specialty, therefore, continues to rely on judgments about the probabilities of various decision alternatives based on experience, the scientific literature, and data gathered from the patient. In situations where probability analysis is available and valuable, the information is integrated into this text.

Another element in clinical problem-solving involves the subjective factors of the patient, the setting, and the treating physician. The patient who is particularly uncooperative or has poor social support may need a more extensive evaluation than the responsible patient who will follow up with his or her primary physician. The new "alternative health care delivery" setting can make a difference in how a problem is solved. A "managed care" plan representative may refuse admission for a patient that the emergency physician believes may benefit from inpatient care. This may result in other dispositions, such as home health care, being sought. Although not always acknowledged, the emergency physician's personality and experience can influence the approach to clinical problem-solving. A physician who has been affected by the malpractice environment may practice more defensive and expensive medicine than the physician who is more comfortable with uncertainty. One clinician believes that if a 1% chance exists that the patient with a headache has a subarachnoid hemorrhage, a diagnostic computed tomographic head scan is indicated. Another physician may accept a 5% or 0.5% probability before ordering the same test.

Despite all these influences, a decision about a particular problem still must be made in a timely manner. These decisions are often made with incomplete information and a changing clinical pattern. For example, a β-agonist aerosol treatment may be ordered to relieve a patient's symptoms of severe dyspnea and wheezing. Later in the assessment, it is determined that the patient does not have a pulmonary source of the symptoms but has congestive heart failure from an acute myocardial infarction. Was the aerosol order a wrong decision? The emergency physician must accept the fact that many decisions made in emergent or urgent circumstances are not optimal. Each patient is different and presents with unique diagnostic challenges. Decisions must be accepted and integrated into the next decision. Understanding the approach to problem solving and how decisions are reached is one element in the maturation of a specialist in emergency care.

This textbook is designed to reflect the thinking process of the emergency physician confronted by a patient with an undifferentiated clinical complaint. It represents the most common sequence of events followed in caring for emergency patients. Although the chapters are written in a sequential format, it is assumed that in many situations stabilization, evaluation, diagnosis, and thoughts about disposition must proceed simultaneously. The organization of the book's major headings is similar to that used in the Model of Clinical Practice of Emergency Medicine published by the American Board of Emergency Medicine and the American College of Emergency Physicians. This listing covers the full range of clinical and administrative subjects included in the specialty. This text is not an exhaustive listing of all these presentations but represents the major complaints encountered in most clinical practices.

Most chapters begin with a specific complaint or presentation, and most have a similar structure. One chapter presents laboratory findings (e.g., acid-base disturbances). In this chapter the format is modified to give the laboratory values before the preliminary differential diagnosis. To facilitate the reader's understanding of the chapter format used, each chapter heading is explained briefly. Statements made in these paragraphs are applicable to all designated chapter sections in this book.

Cases

Problem cases are introduced at the beginning and then elaborated upon at the end of the chapter as a means of reinforcing the material presented in each chapter. The author's comments on the case management are presented in *italics* at various points in the presentation of the patient's problem. These cases are supplemental to the text.

Introduction

The introductory paragraphs are written to supply the basic information necessary to help solve the clinical problem. First, the important basic scientific data necessary to make a set of decisions are given. These include pertinent anatomy, physiology, and pathophysiology. Second, the importance of the presenting complaint to emergency medicine is discussed. Clinical epidemiologic data are useful to provide context for the incidence, significance, and outcome of the patient's complaint and some of the diseases that cause it.

Initial Approach and Stabilization

During the first 5 to 15 minutes of care, many of the most important decisions for the patient are made. The heading *Priority Diagnoses* represents the most significant (and potentially frequent) disease states to consider early in the course of care. The next section describes the *Rapid Assessment* directed toward the vital areas of airway, breathing, circulation, and others. The *Early Intervention* actions are also discussed. This care is often closely integrated with the activities pursued during the prehospital care period, and the two are considered complementary.

As part of this initial approach, the emergency physician first determines whether the patient is "sick" and rapidly confirms or excludes the presence of catastrophic disease. Second, the physician must stabilize the patient's vital signs, while anticipating the complications the underlying disease process may manifest. Third, the physician needs to address relief of the patient's acute symptoms. Although this is not always possible or advisable at this stage, the relief of suffering is central to the values of medical practice. To do so, medication is not always necessary. A brief commentary about early clinical impressions, especially thoughts on serious problems that are *not* present, can do much to lessen the patient's fears. The simple phrase "We are here to help you feel better" can help build trust and decrease anxiety. It also helps establish the patient's confidence regarding the competency of the entire department team.

Clinical Assessment

The history is a directed exploration of the presenting complaint. A full history and physical examination are generally not warranted in the emergency department. Each chapter supplies the reader with the elements of data gathering appropriate to the specific complaint and why they are pertinent.

Certain historical elements appear repeatedly to maintain chapter autonomy and to stress their importance. These include allergies, medications, and pertinent past medical history. The need to obtain information from many sources is emphasized in a number of chapters. It is easy to allow one's data-gathering efforts to remain trapped behind the automatic doors of the emergency department. Information is always gained and the patient's statements corroborated by discussions with friends, family, witnesses, and primary physicians. Communicating with contacts in the waiting room can provide information while alleviating their often escalating concerns.

The physical examination commonly begins with a reassessment of the primary survey. This is followed by a more thorough, but often directed, examination emphasizing the organ systems involved in the chief complaint. Selected diagnostic maneuvers, such as orthostatic vital signs and oculovestibular testing (cold caloric testing), may be included in this section. When possible, the value of specific findings in determining serious problems and data on the limits of a variety of physical findings are given.

As in most clinical presentations, the combination of the history and physical examination results in a reasonable diagnosis or recognition of serious disease in the vast majority of patients.

Clinical Reasoning

After data gathering, the emergency physician usually has sufficient information to answer specific key questions that will establish a preliminary differential diagnosis, prioritize concerns about serious illness, and guide management decisions. In this section, the bridge between emergency medicine and the more traditional specialties is established. The focus is first on life-threatening disease: How has the patient progressed with stabilizing efforts? Are any unrecognized life-threatening processes present? If so, what organ systems do they involve? What is the major diagnostic possibility within these organ systems? Second, attention is directed toward identifying the less urgent and common causes of the patient's signs or symptoms. Again, the findings are weighed against a series of differential diagnostic categories and a preliminary list of possible causes is developed.

Each question is asked, answered, and repeated throughout the remainder of the patient's stay. This serial and comparative analysis is the core of the problem-solving process in the emergency department.

In the text, the common and catastrophic causes of the condition are discussed in either a table or a paragraph. This information is given to more clearly define the characteristics of specific diseases, thereby allowing better comparisons with the patient's findings.

Diagnostic Adjuncts

The preliminary differential diagnosis guides the selection of diagnostic studies. In most cases, the tests are chosen as confirmatory evidence of a specific disease or to rule out a serious process. Occasionally, the test makes the diagnosis or, at least, must be available before a differential pathway is rational. This section covers the topics of laboratory studies, radiologic imaging, electrocardiography, and other tests. These are the "tools of the trade" that support the initial clinical impressions. Suggestions are made about when to order diagnostic adjuncts, how they may be interpreted, and, once interpreted, how valuable this information is in identifying a specific disease process.

The emergency physician plays an important role in cost control through test selection. Knowing when a battery versus a single test is indicated is an important skill. Because clinical judgment is influenced by a variety of factors, including cost, the physician must be aware of the relative costs of the commonly ordered tests in the emergency department. These are listed in Table 1–2. A conscious effort to limit the number of ancillary tests ordered, within the constraints of high-quality medicine, is the responsibility of all physicians. Unfortunately, this positive goal is often offset by the present medicolegal environment in this country, summarized by the phrase, "When things go wrong, no one thanks you for saving them money." Cost awareness remains an important area to be mastered in clinical emergency medicine.

Expanded Differential Diagnosis

After ancillary testing, additional or more specific diagnoses may be made. A definitive diagnosis may not be available or necessary, but an improved "working" diagnosis can guide management and disposition decisions. It is common not to have a precise diagnosis at the time of disposition. For example, in up to 40% of patients presenting with undifferentiated abdominal pain, the cause remains undiagnosed when the patient leaves the emergency department. In many cases it is more important to have a clear idea of what is *not* going on than it is to have a precise diagnosis.

TABLE 1–2. Cost Ranges for Diagnostic Adjuncts Commonly Ordered in the Emergency Department—2001

	Range (in $)
Laboratory Tests*	
Chemistry	
Alkaline phosphatase	9.00–12.00
Amylase	12.00–18.00
Arterial blood gas	75.00–112.00
Aspartate aminotransferase	9.00–12.00
Bilirubin, total	7.50–15.00
Blood urea nitrogen	9.00–15.00
Calcium	7.50–10.50
Creatinine phosphokinase (CPK)	9.00–19.50
CPK MB fraction	37.00–52.00
Creatinine	13.00–18.00
Electrolyte panel (sodium, potassium, chloride, bicarbonate)	37.00–52.00
Glucose	13.00–18.00
Human chorionic gonadotropin, β-subunit	21.00–27.00
Lactate dehydrogenase (LDH)	9.00–12.00
LDH isoenzymes	37.00–60.00
Lactic acid	27.00–39.00
Hepatitis B surface antigen	19.00–33.00
Heterophil antibody, monospot	12.50–15.00
Human immunodeficiency virus	22.50–45.00
Osmolality, serum	22.50–30.00
Osmolality, urine	22.50–30.00
Potassium	6.75–13.50
Sodium	10.50–15.00
Toxicology	
Screen (EMIT)	67.50–90.00
Comprehensive (routine)	120.00–150.00
VDRL	8.25–21.00
Urinalysis (dipstick and microscopic)	15.00–22.50
Urine chemistry (sodium/potassium)	13.50–36.00 each
Hematology	
Complete blood cell count and differential	37.50–45.00
Hemoglobin/hematocrit	18.00–22.50
Platelet count	7.50–12.00
Partial thromboplastin time	12.00–22.00
Prothrombin time	9.75–12.00
Peripheral smear	22.50–30.00
Bacteriology	
Blood culture	60.00–75.00
Gonococcus culture	37.50–52.50
Gram stain	12.00–18.00
Chlamydia culture	67.50–82.50
Streptococcus screen	30.00–37.50
Throat culture	60.00–75.00
Urine culture	60.00–75.00
Radiologic Imaging†‡	
Plain Films	
Skull series	120.00–135.00
Cervical spine series	112.50–127.50
Lateral only	52.50–67.50
Posteroanterior and lateral chest	90.00–105.00

Continued on following page

TABLE 1–2. Cost Ranges for Diagnostic Adjuncts Commonly Ordered in the Emergency Department—2001 *Continued*

	Range (in $)
Portable anteroposterior chest	165.00–180.00
Abdominal series (four views)	135.00–150.00
Anteroposterior pelvis	75.00–90.00
Lumbosacral spine series	135.00–150.00
Upper extremity	
Shoulder	82.50–97.50
Humerus	67.50–82.50
Elbow	67.50–82.50
Forearm	67.50–82.50
Wrist	67.50–82.50
Hand	67.50–82.50
Lower extremity	
Hip (with pelvis)	120.00–135.00
Femur	105.00–120.00
Knee	67.50–82.50
Tibia/fibula	97.50–112.50
Ankle	67.50–82.50
Foot	67.50–82.50
Soft tissue of neck	67.50–82.50
Foreign body, soft tissue	82.50–97.50
Facial series	97.50–120.00
Contrast Enhanced	
Esophagus (barium swallow)	120.00–135.00
Urethrogram	135.00–150.00
Cystogram	225.00–247.50
Intravenous pyelogram	210.00–240.00
Computerized Tomography	
Head (nonenhanced)	375.00–450.00
Chest	390.00–420.00
Abdomen (nonenhanced)	375.00–450.00
Cervical spine	397.50–427.50
Nuclear Medicine	
Lung scan	390.00–420.00
Testicular scan	112.50–150.00
Angiography	
Aortic arch	712.50–795.00
Ultrasound	
Pelvis	180.00–210.00
Abdomen (visceral)	210.00–240.00
Electrocardiography†	
12-lead electrocardiogram	60.00–90.00

*Many hospital laboratories add a $5 to $10 STAT surcharge because the tests are ordered from the emergency department.
†The charge for interpretation is not included.
‡Portable radiographs have a $50 to $70 added charge.
EMIT, enzyme-multiplied immunoassay technique.

Overattention to seeking the definitive cause can promote inefficiency and divert effectiveness in the emergency department.

Principles of Management

This text assumes that treatment is the natural outcome of the problem-solving process that includes all the information preceding it. Its emphasis is on the general principles of assessment and management for a presenting complaint. A secondary listing of specific therapies is given for specific diseases. The purpose is to give the reader an overview of what needs to be done and a limited number of details about selected problems. Clinical guidelines and management algorithms are presented as available and appropriate.

Uncertain Diagnosis

Emergency physicians are frequently faced with uncertainty regarding their clinical diagnosis. Guidelines and opinions are offered on further assessment and disposition decisions in common situations.

Special Considerations

In most complaints, age, pregnancy, or an immunosuppressed condition is a complicating factor. This section gives additional information about pediatric, elderly, and other at-risk populations that may influence the evaluation, diagnosis, and treatment of the patient. This material is considered supplemental to the problem-solving process up to the disposition. It is a means of including important "risk factors" not always viewed as contributing to the patient's illness or injury.

Disposition and Follow-up

Disposition and follow-up plans are often the most difficult components of problem resolution. Even when admission is obviously needed, decisions remain about the appropriateness of critical care monitoring, the need for surgical intervention, and other problems. Discharge from the emergency department has its own set of risks for both the patient and the physician. Because of this difficulty, useful guidelines for admission to the hospital, admission to the critical care unit, continued observation, obtaining consultation, and discharge are part of the emergency medicine literature. Each chapter lists guidelines intended to aid these decisions.

Patients admitted to the hospital are under the care of their attending or primary physician. No recommendations for admitting orders are given because, with rare exceptions, this is not the task of the emergency physician. Writing these orders extends liability, assumes more complete knowledge of the patient than may be correct, and may create a sense of complacency on the part of the admitting physician.

Discharging patients is a complex process often overlooked by individuals new to emergency medicine. It is a time when the most important influence on following care instructions is established. All discharge procedures are initiated by the physician and reinforced by the nursing staff. The information is given to the patient and to individuals responsible for further care. The discharge instructions include

1. A summary of findings.
2. A brief description of the problem from the physician's perspective. This is linked to the reason for the patient's coming to the emergency department.
3. Treatment plans, including medications, possible hazards, and, optimally, their approximate cost.
4. Queries of the patient or family members as to whether they have other questions and a brief quiz to make sure they understand the instructions.
5. Plans for the follow-up care after leaving the emergency department. Reasons for returning to the department are also given.

All of this information is supported in writing. Preprinted materials written in the lay public's terminology are very helpful.

Discharged patients should contact their primary physician within 24 to 48 hours of being seen in the emergency department. They may not need an appointment, but all are instructed to call their physician's office to give notice of their emergency care and a statement of their present conditions.

In high-risk situations or by the patient's own request, the primary physician is contacted near the time of discharge, and the responsibility for ensuring follow-up is shared between the physician and patient. In these situations, determining a specific appointment date and time increases the patient's compliance by 40% to 50%.

Final Points

This section lists the important points made in each chapter. It is a means of quick review or a way of presenting the "highlights" of problem-solving given in the chapter. Each of these sections is well worth remembering.

Bibliography

Emergency medicine remains a maturing academic science. The student of the specialty should have a familiarity with the literature that contributes to its growth. Each chapter has a list of useful texts and journal articles pertinent to the subject. In addition, the following texts are considered standard references for the specialty:

1. Roberts JR, Hedges JR: Clinical Procedures in Emergency Medicine, 3rd ed. Philadelphia, WB Saunders, 1998.
2. Marx J, Hockberger B, Walls R, et al: Rosen's Emergency Medicine: Concepts and Clinical Practice, 5th ed. St. Louis, CV Mosby, 2002.
3. Tintinalli JE, Kelen G, Stapczynski S: Emergency Medicine: A Comprehensive Study Guide, 5th ed. New York, McGraw-Hill, 2000.
4. Fleischer FR, Ludwig S, Henretig FM: Textbook of Pediatric Emergency Medicine, 4th ed. Baltimore, Williams & Wilkins, 2000.
5. Harwood-Nuss L, Wolfson AB: The Clinical Practice of Emergency Medicine, 4th ed. London, Lippincott Williams & Wilkins, 2001.

CLINICAL PEARLS

The practice and art of this specialty is like that of any other medical specialty. It is learned over time, patient by patient. The "sixth sense" used to identify serious illness is an acquired skill. The patient who manifests seizures as a sign of hemodynamic collapse from a ruptured ectopic pregnancy, the child abuser who brings his infant to the emergency department and then attempts to sign out quickly, the surviving accident victim who was trying to commit suicide but now fears and desires discovery—all these patients and thousands more demand the learned patience, perception, and understanding that a trained, experienced emergency physician can offer.

The following is a list of selected clinical pearls gathered from the authors of this text.* Many apply every day to care in the emergency department. Many will stand the test of time; others will be forgotten as research proves them obsolete. At the present time, they offer an insight into the hazards and rewards of the specialty. Reviewing them before each tour of duty is a worthwhile exercise. Although many others are worth learning, these are some of the best.

- *The New Job*
  - Respect is earned.

---

* A personal note of appreciation to Richard Feldman, MD, who supplied many of these pearls.

- Befriend, through a show of respect, your nursing staff.
- *Maximizing Patient Satisfaction with Your Care*
  - Listen first. A physician interrupts a patient every 18 seconds; in emergency medicine it is every 10 seconds.
  - Avoid medical jargon.
  - Briefly describe the planned management plan. Patients who know what is happening are more willing to wait and are more trusting.
  - Learn how to tell a patient you do not know what is wrong.
  - Let the patient know he or she is always welcome to return.
- *Minimizing Patient Dissatisfaction*
  - One hour feels like 3 hours behind a curtain.
  - Give the patient an estimate of the time needed to complete the evaluation. Significant delays require an honest accounting.
  - When you leave, say when you will be back, and do it.
  - Call patients at home 24 to 48 hours later, especially those with headache, chest pain, and abdominal pain. They will like it, and your clinical judgment will get a reality test.
- *You Are the Patient's Advocate*
  - If you must err, err on the side of helping the patient.
  - Respect the patient's need for privacy.
  - Always consider the "costs" of your interventions.
  - Do not negotiate any medically important decision with a patient with an altered sensorium, particularly if it is caused by alcohol or other substance abuse.
  - If a patient is a source of potential harm to himself/herself or others, or cannot take care of himself/herself, the patient must stay for observation or admission.
  - Physical restraint may be necessary and appropriate to protect the patient or emergency department staff.
  - Do not discharge a now "sobered" patient who has recovered from acute alcoholism without performing a repeat history and physical examination.
  - Anxiety, attention-seeking behavior, and hysteria are diagnoses of exclusion.
- *Cultural Awareness*
  - Actively study cultural differences. The more you know, the more effective you will be.
  - Your background and heritage will be different from many of the people you see. Protect yourself and them from early judgments based on your values.

- "Dark humor" about others' language, lifestyle, and behavior is a coping mechanism with dangerous potential for establishing bias.
- *Clinical Judgment*
  - "Badness" is how we think, what we pursue. It is rare to go wrong by first searching for "badness."
  - When the clinical impression does not fit with the history, physical examination results, or laboratory evaluation, STOP! Rethink and expand services of data gathering and the differential diagnosis.
  - If the patient acutely cannot walk, he or she cannot go home.
  - If the ancillary data do not fit the clinical picture, reconfirm the accuracy of the data before making treatment and disposition decisions.
  - If you seriously consider a specific diagnosis when working through a differential diagnosis, then you should rule it out with the appropriate tests.
  - "If you do not know what to do—do nothing." Observe the patient *closely* for the evolution of the disease process instead of gambling on a marginally indicated therapeutic intervention.
  - *Always* assume that females of childbearing age might be pregnant, and act accordingly.
  - The patient who returns to the emergency department on an unscheduled basis is first assumed to be at high risk for a serious illness. This is your chance to get it right!
  - Abnormal vital signs must be repeated and explained.
  - A patient who will not look at you during the history and physical examination is usually either depressed or manipulative. Almost never is such a person shy.
  - Patients usually have one major medical problem for each decade of life after the age of 60.
  - Never completely "trust" a young child, an elderly patient, an alcoholic, or a drug abuser. That is, corroborate the history and carefully interpret the physical findings for each of these patients.
  - Listen closely to the suggestions of patients and their families about what is wrong and how they should be treated.
- *Specific Clinical Situations*
  - During the winter months, if the whole family has "the flu," be sure to consider carbon monoxide poisoning.
  - Ask what *caused* the trauma in the patient you are treating. Trauma is often considered the *only* problem and not potentially the *result* of another problem.
  - Consider the diagnosis of ruptured (or expanding) abdominal aortic aneurysm in all patients older than 60 years old who appear to have renal colic.
  - Since the eye is to see, record its acuity!
  - Always confirm a field or bedside glucose oxidase strip reading in the emergency department with a blood glucose level.
  - Multiple drug allergies often correlate highly with functional or psychogenic complaints.
  - Chest pain radiating below the umbilicus or above the maxilla is seldom cardiac in origin.
  - All patients with right lower quadrant pain have appendicitis until it has been proved otherwise.
  - It is best to confirm, with β-human chorionic gonadotropin testing, the statement "she said she couldn't be pregnant."
- *The Pediatric Encounter*
  - Speak to children in language they can understand.
  - Allow the parent(s) to stay in the room. Observing the child's interaction with the parents is an important part of the evaluation.
  - Children are rarely hypochondriacs.
  - Examine neurovascular and motor integrity before focusing on the injured area.
- *Communicating with the Attending or Consulting Physician*
  - Confirm admission or discharge with the primary physician before committing yourself to the patient.
  - When in doubt, a second opinion to confirm a clinical impression is always appropriate.
- *Avoid Supporting the Legal Profession*
  - Do not think you are going to win just because you are in the "right."
  - Protect yourself by protecting the patient.
  - A printed form never saved anyone.
  - One of the most hazardous moments in emergency medicine is "signing out" patients to a colleague at the end of one's shift. A complete and accurate exchange of information and impressions is necessary.
  - Document as thoroughly and clearly as you can. Read your dictations.
- *Destroying Your Credibility*
  - Subvert the call schedule or be chronically late.
  - Yell at someone.
  - Give an opinion before looking at the patient.
  - Treat a number, not the patient.
  - "You lie, you die."
- *Your Mental Health*
  - Every physician has moments of self-doubt.
  - There is always a disposition.
  - When you find yourself becoming angry with a patient ("positive personal hypertension sign") during history taking, you must step

away momentarily. The patient may be malingering and withholding or providing misleading information, or you may be fatigued or have lost your perspective on your role. In any case, the emotion and its origin must not be allowed to influence or impair your judgment.

- If possible, take a break (e.g., lunch) during each shift.
- Balance your life. Emergency medicine practice and knowledge is an expanding universe. There is always another patient, always another article. You must pick and choose, then do something else.
- Burnout is not from the hours or patients. It is from unmet expectations because we did not know what expectations to set.
- Teach something to someone.
- *Do's*
  - Meet every patient turned over to you at the change of shift.
  - Order soft tissue radiographs to rule out suspected soft tissue foreign bodies.
  - Respond to complaints by private attending physicians immediately to avoid irreparable damage. Just because they're angry, doesn't mean they're right.

- Always see and interpret the diagnostic studies you have ordered.
- *Don't's*
  - Never say: "There is nothing wrong with you."
  - Do not expect a patient to remember verbal information.
  - Do not try to "weasel out" of accepting responsibility when you blew it—admit the error, apologize, and get on with life.

Bibliography

American College of Physicians: Standards for Residency Training Program in Emergency Medicine, as approved by the American Medical Association House of Delegates on June 17, 1975.

Definition of emergency medicine. Ann Emerg Med 2001; 38:616.

Hamilton GC: Emergency medicine: Where to from here? Emerg Med 1999; 11:229–233.

Hamilton GC, Lumpkin JR, Tomlanovich MC, et al: Special Committee on the Core Content Revision: Emergency medicine core content. Ann Emerg Med 1986; 15:853–862.

Hockberger RS, Binder LS, Graber MA, et al: The model of clinical practice of emergency medicine. Ann Emerg Med; 2001; 37:745–770.

Rosen P: The biology of emergency medicine. J Am Coll Emerg Phys 1979; 8:58–61.

CHAPTER 2

Airway Management

SCOTT A. DOAK

CASE *Study*

An 8-year-old girl presents after falling from a second-story window onto her head while escaping from a house fire. She is hypertensive, bradycardiac, poorly responsive, and spontaneously breathing at a rate of 14 breaths per minute.

INTRODUCTION

Airway assessment and management have priority over all other aspects of resuscitation in the critically ill or injured patient. Airway management is the "A" in the **ABC** mnemonic (**A**irway, **B**reathing, **C**irculation) used to prioritize the care of critically ill or injured patients. Proper airway management saves more lives than any other single intervention accomplished in emergency medicine.

The most common error in airway management is failure to anticipate the need for active intervention in patients at high risk for airway obstruction or respiratory insufficiency. This group includes patients with decreased levels of consciousness, cardiorespiratory disease, head and neck disorders, and major traumatic injury.

Despite the importance of anticipating the need for airway management, there are a few important exceptions to the rule that airway management has first priority: (1) The patient with ventricular fibrillation or pulseless ventricular tachycardia should be immediately defibrillated before cardiopulmonary resuscitation (CPR) or intubation if the rescuer is alone and has immediate access to a monitor-defibrillator; (2) An immediate solitary precordial thump is recommended in the pulseless patient with a witnessed cardiac arrest, before CPR and intubation, if a monitor-defibrillator is not immediately available; and (3), Immediate defibrillation, before CPR and intubation, is recommended in a pulseless patient if a defibrillator is available without a monitor.

First aid, including the Heimlich maneuver (subdiaphragmatic abdominal thrusts), chest thrusts, and finger sweeps, is not covered in this chapter. It is discussed in *Standards and Guidelines for Cardiopulmonary Resuscitation and Emergency Cardiac Care*, which is part of the Advanced Cardiac Life Support course published by the American Heart Association.

Epidemiology

The National Emergency Airway Registry represents a prospective observational study of over 6300 cases. Data gathered in the year 2000 noted rapid sequence intubation (RSI) was the most frequently used (75%) and most successful means (98%) of endotracheal intubation. Esophageal intubation occurred in up to 4% of cases, although early recognition was the rule. Blind nasotracheal intubation was attempted in about 5% of cases, with a success rate of 86%, using up to three attempts. Complications, including epistaxis and emesis, were more common in this approach. Less than 1% of intubation attempts required cricothyrotomy.

Airway Anatomy

An understanding of basic airway anatomy is essential for successful airway management. The pertinent structures are reviewed here.

The nasal cavity provides access to the upper airway. Its inferomedial aspect is the safest route for passage of a nasotracheal tube. The nasal turbinates and paranasal sinus ostia occupy lateral positions in the nasal cavities and are sites of potential complications. During intubation, the turbinates can be lacerated, fractured, or avulsed. Once the endotracheal tube is in place, the paranasal sinus ostia may be occluded, resulting in sinus blockage and infection.

The oropharynx begins below the posterior opening of the nasal passage just beyond the soft palate. Entry into this area may stimulate the protective gag reflex mediated by the glossopharyngeal and vagus nerves (cranial nerves IX and X). The laryngopharynx (hypopharynx) extends from the vallecula to the true vocal cords and includes the piriform recesses (piriform sinuses) just superolateral to the thyroid cartilage (Fig. 2–1A). The epiglottis serves to cover and protect the

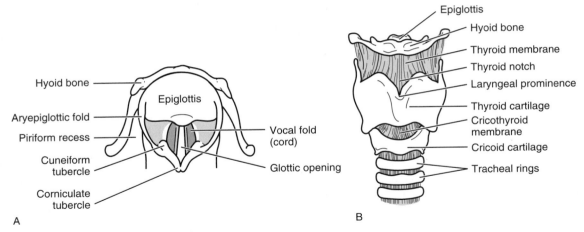

FIGURE 2–1 • Larynx. *A,* View from above. *B,* Anterior view.

glottic opening. The thyroid cartilage forms the laryngeal prominence and thyroid notch. Between the thyroid and cricoid cartilages is the cricothyroid membrane (see Fig. 2-1*B*). It is an important access site in emergency surgical airway management. The cricoid cartilage is the only circumferential cartilage of the airway and provides structural stability. If this cartilage is cut or fractured, that stability can be endangered. Below the cricoid cartilage, the cervical trachea is deep and is partially covered by the thyroid gland and other vascular structures. It is near the cupola of the lungs, and its posterior membranous portion is adjacent to the esophagus.

Indications for Airway Management

Airway management is not simply the passage of an endotracheal tube. It is a series of steps ranging from simple interventions such as repositioning the patient's head and neck and supplying supplemental oxygen to an emergent cricothyrotomy. Regardless of what intervention is indicated, the general indications for airway management are as follows:

- Secure and maintain *Patency* (e.g., evolving laryngeal edema)
- *Protection*—two components
  - Anticipate aspiration (e.g., altered mental status, loss of gag reflex).
  - Search for associated conditions (e.g., cervical spine fracture).
- *Oxygenation* (e.g., pneumonia)
- *Ventilation* (e.g., exacerbation of chronic obstructive pulmonary disease)
- *Treatment*
  - Treat associated conditions (e.g., medications per endotracheal tube).
  - Suction or raise secretions.

There are numerous reasons for definitive airway management. The two most common are securing patency and establishing protection. The most critical is intubating the patient for protection from potential aspiration. Macroaspiration of acidic gastric contents carries a mortality approaching 30%.

Any patient in whom the ability to protect the airway is in question should have prompt endotracheal intubation. Patients in this category may include intoxicated patients, patients who have overdosed, and patients with head injuries. Caution should be exercised when testing the gag reflex of a patient to assess airway protective reflexes. The presence of a gag reflex does not always imply the ability to protect the airway and, conversely, the absence of a gag reflex does not imply that the patient cannot protect the airway. Moreover, occasionally this technique may induce vomiting in a patient who may have inadequate airway reflexes.

Another condition for which airway protection may be required is in patients who are uncooperative because of intoxication, head injury, or pain. These patients can place themselves at risk by either interfering with their own timely medical or surgical care or specifically causing themselves harm, such as flailing around when they have an unstable cervical spine fracture.

Hypoxic patients will benefit from airway management. Improved availability of F_{IO_2} and positive-pressure ventilation each improve oxygenation in nearly all forms of hypoxia. Respiratory distress in a patient with acute asthma or an exacerbation of chronic obstructive pulmonary disease will commonly result in hypercarbia from inadequate ventilation. Although the lungs may still be poorly compliant, positive-pressure ventilation will significantly improve ventilation, especially in patients who are fatigued.

Administration of the following drugs through an endotracheal tube is effective when an intravenous line is not available: **N**arcan, **A**tropine, **V**ersed (midazolam), **E**pinephrine, and **L**idocaine. A useful mnemonic for remembering this list is **NAVEL**. Airway management, especially endotracheal intubation, can facilitate a patient's ability to manage secretions. Nebulization and suction are both part of this care.

Finally, there are reasons to prophylactically intubate a patient to avoid what is considered impending harm. Examples of this include a patient with evolving laryngeal edema, the uncooperative overdosed patient who requires gastric lavage, and a patient with a flail chest who may ultimately require ventilatory support.

The caveat, "WHEN IN DOUBT, INTUBATE" is a basic guide in airway management.

INITIAL APPROACH AND STABILIZATION

Failure to secure the airway in a timely manner is the most common fatal error in airway management. The fundamentals of airway assessment and management are the same in the prehospital setting and in the emergency department. An assessment of the airway and breathing status is performed in every patient. The goal is to determine whether the airway is patent and protected and whether breathing is present and adequate. A standardized interventional approach will allow the care provider to recognize the patient with a subtle deficit and apply systematic measures to support airway protection, patency, oxygenation, and ventilation. The following six sections can be considered as a stepwise approach to the evaluation and support of a patient's airway. Although the need for definitive airway management (e.g., endotracheal intubation) may become apparent at any time during this progression, one or more of these steps may prove adequate for a given patient's airway support.

Assessment of Airway and Breathing

The primary survey of airway and breathing is completed in 10 to 15 seconds and consists of inspection, palpation, and auscultation.

Inspection includes observing the patient's mental status, respiratory rate, and breathing effort. If the patient is responsive, talking spontaneously, and speaking clearly and comfortably, there is seldom a need for airway management beyond supplemental oxygen. A tongue blade may be used to assist in the inspection of the mouth and posterior pharynx for

blood, vomitus, or foreign bodies if the patient is unable to cooperate. If there is any suspicion the patient's airway reflexes are impaired, assessing the patient's ability to swallow his own saliva or manage a small amount of water are useful screens of airway protective capability. Testing for a gag reflex is most often done in patients who are unable to cooperate with swallowing, owing to an altered (usually depressed) level of consciousness. It is gently accomplished, to avoid inducing emesis with the tongue blade. In the unconscious patient, the presence or absence of a gag reflex may be the deciding factor that motivates the physician toward definitive airway management. Patient tolerance of an oropharyngeal airway or laryngoscopy certifies the need for endotracheal intubation. However, there are special circumstances, such as narcotics-induced respiratory depression, that may be rapidly reversed with naloxone (Narcan), obviating the need for definitive airway management.

Palpation includes feeling for tracheal deviation and for chest deformities, bony crepitance, or subcutaneous emphysema. Placing a hand or ear near the patient's mouth and nares provides a crude assessment of air motion.

Auscultation begins with listening to the patient speak and assessing the voice quality. Noisy breathing suggests partial airway obstruction and mandates further inspection. Hoarseness signifies a laryngeal pathologic process. Both hemithoraces are auscultated in the midaxillary line for symmetry of breath sounds.

If the airway and breathing are intact, supplemental oxygen is supplied to any critically ill patient. If airway patency or protection is in jeopardy, the health care provider must intervene immediately.

Manual Airway Opening Maneuvers

The most common cause of airway obstruction is laxity of the tongue and other supporting muscles accompanying a decreased level of consciousness. This allows the tongue to fall posteriorly and obstruct the oropharynx, or the epiglottis to fall posteroinferiorly and obstruct the glottic opening. Regardless of the cause, a manual airway opening maneuver is indicated in any patient with partial or complete airway obstruction.

The most effective manual airway opening maneuvers are the chin-lift and the jaw-thrust maneuvers (Fig. 2–2*A* and *B*). Each may be attempted successively or in combination. In the setting of trauma with the potential for cervical spine injury, the chin-lift maneuver should be avoided because it involves significant neck extension.

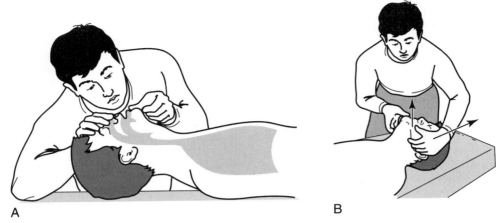

A   B

FIGURE 2–2 • Chin-lift maneuver: *A*, Chin-lift. *B*, Jaw-thrust.

Suction

A functioning large-bore, large-volume suction device is important in any airway management procedure. There are many types of suction tips. The Yankauer suction tip is usually the best choice because it has the largest bore and allows rapid clearance of fluids and particulate matter (e.g., vomitus) from the oropharynx.

Oxygen

Immediately after the airway is opened and the oropharynx is suctioned, supplemental oxygen is administered. Table 2–1 lists the most common oxygen delivery systems and the approximate percentages of oxygen they can deliver. More precise measurements of oxygen levels are made by oximetry testing. Oxygen is always administered before more definitive airway management procedures.

Ventilation

The patient who has inadequate respiratory effort after the airway is opened and supplemental oxy-

TABLE 2–1. Supplemental Oxygen Delivery Systems

System	O_2 Percentage	Advantages	Disadvantages
Nasal cannula	Each 2 L/min increase in flow raises the FIO_2 3–4%	Comfortable at 6–8 L/min	Intolerable and impractical at >8–10 L/min. Exact FIO_2 uncertain because it varies with respiratory rate and depth
Simple and partial rebreather masks	60% at 10 L/min	Higher FIO_2	May promote CO_2 retention at lower flow rates
Venturi mask, Ventimask	24% or 28% at 4 L/min	Fairly exact FIO_2 control Excellent for COPD with chronic CO_2 retention	Poorly humidified
	31% at 6 L/min 35% or 40% at 8 L/min 50% at 10 L/min		
Reservoir/Nonrebreathing mask	90% at 15 L/min	High FIO_2 for severe hypoxia and CO poisoning	Oxygen toxicity a small concern in emergency department
Bag-valve mask	Almost 100% at 15 L/min	High FIO_2 for severe hypoxia and CO poisoning Ventilatory assistance	Mechanical device between patient and physician Variable operator skills
Manually triggered oxygen-powered breathing device (OPBD)	100% with 40 L/min	Highest FIO_2 Ventilatory assistance	Contraindicated in children because of barotrauma Can be dangerous if inexperienced operator

FIO_2, fraction of inspired oxygen; CO, carbon monoxide

gen supplied needs positive-pressure ventilation. This can be initiated with mouth-to-mouth or mouth-to-mask ventilation, but when the equipment is available, bag-valve mask ventilation with supplemental oxygen is preferable. The mask should be the proper size for the patient's face and have an inflatable cuff to facilitate a tight seal. Because it is difficult for one person to hold the mask tightly on the face, a jaw-thrust maneuver is performed and the bag is squeezed; two people are often needed to use the bag-valve mask method effectively. In adult patients, trained emergency care personnel can use a mask incorporating an oxygen-powered breathing device, which releases oxygen under pressure when a button on the mask is pushed.

Temporizing Airway Management Devices

There are numerous circumstances in which partial or temporary control of an airway is indicated when formal endotracheal intubation is not immediately attainable and airway maneuvers are inadequate. Familiarity with these various devices, detailed in Table 2–2, is essential.

Although manual airway opening maneuvers require no equipment, they do require the constant involvement of one rescuer. To overcome this disadvantage, a nasopharyngeal airway or oropharyngeal airway can be used to hold the tongue away from the posterior wall of the pharynx (Fig. 2–3).

Insertion of a nasopharyngeal airway is indicated in patients who "snore" because of a partial airway obstruction and in patients with tightly clenched teeth. This device is placed through a lubricated naris and bypasses the soft palate. It does not always reach a level in the oropharynx that ensures protection from blockage by the tongue. It is better tolerated than an oropharyngeal airway, and its major usefulness is in patients who are intoxicated or somewhat sedated, but not to the point that they require definitive airway management.

The oropharyngeal airway can be inserted with the concave side down, with a tongue blade depressing the tongue during insertion of the airway, or concave side up, followed by 180-degree

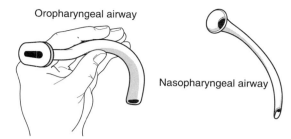

FIGURE 2–3 • Simple artificial airways.

rotation when the flange is at the lips. The latter method is not recommended in children, because of their relatively large tongues and the potential for further obstruction of the pharynx by pushing the tongue posteriorly. Contraindications to insertion of the oropharyngeal airway include tightly clenched teeth and intolerance of the airway as evidenced by gagging. Patients who tolerate an oropharyngeal airway without gagging are demonstrating they *cannot adequately protect their airway* and require more definitive airway management. Before definitive airway management, an oral airway can be useful to control the upper airway soft tissue during manual bagging. After orotracheal intubation, the oropharyngeal airway is used to prevent biting and occlusion of the endotracheal tube.

Another temporizing measure is the laryngeal mask airway (Fig. 2–4A). A laryngeal mask airway is a tool that has a larger-diameter tube affixed to an inflatable oval end piece. The end piece is angled such that when the device is blindly placed down into the hypopharynx, the oval cup seals around the laryngeal opening, including the epiglottis. When the cuff of the laryngeal mask airway is inflated, a seal is established, allowing for ventilation through the tube. The laryngeal mask airway does not protect against aspiration and thus is not definitive airway management. The intubating LMA (ILMA) is modified to allow an endotracheal tube to be passed through the lumen of the laryngeal mask airway into the trachea (Fig. 2-4B). Initial studies have demonstrated excellent success in the emergency department.

The esophageal-tracheal Combitube (ETC) is another airway rescue device. It is a dual lumen tube that is usually blindly inserted into the pharynx. When advanced, it lodges in the esophagus almost 99% of the time. Ventilation is through one of the coded tubes. The large balloon is inflated in the oropharynx.

Another temporizing measure is transtracheal jet ventilation. Transtracheal jet ventilation is useful more as a rescue method when endotracheal intubation is not possible or has failed. It is

---

TABLE 2–2. Selected Temporizing Airway Management Devices

Nasopharyngeal airway
Oropharyngeal airway
Laryngeal mask airway
Transtracheal jet ventilation

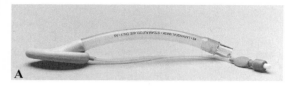

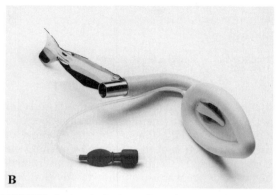

FIGURE 2–4 • *A*, Laryngeal mask airway (LMA). *B*, Intubating LMA. (*A*, from Marx J, et al: Rosen's Emergency Medicine: Concepts and Clinical Practice, 5/e. St. Louis, Mosby, 2001; *B*, Courtesy of LMA North America, Inc, San Diego.)

accomplished by puncturing the cricothyroid membrane with a No. 14 gauge or larger Angiocath in a caudad direction. Positive-pressure oxygenation is delivered from wall oxygen by means of a stopcock or intermittent pressure regulator. The patient passively exhales through the upper airway. This method affords adequate oxygenation but inadequate ventilation over 30 to 60 minutes. Therefore, it is only a temporizing airway procedure. It may be helpful in pediatric patients younger than the age of 8 because emergency cricothyrotomy is contraindicated below this age.

There are a number of alternate temporizing airway support measures that are not discussed in this text. They include the esophageal obturator airway (EOA), the esophageal gastric tube airway (EGTA), and the pharyngotracheal lumen airway (PTLA). These devices are still occasionally used by prehospital personnel, but they have become increasingly rare in modern emergency airway management.

CLINICAL ASSESSMENT

History

Because of the emergent nature of airway management, no history may be necessary before initiating definitive airway care. In cases in which urgent rather than emergent airway intervention is required, a brief history should focus on the follow-

ing areas: **A**llergies, **M**edications, **P**ast medical history (as it pertains to the emergent airway presentation), **L**ast meal, and **E**vents of the recent illness. These historical points are easily recalled with the mnemonic **AMPLE**. Historical questioning is not done if the patient's respiratory status may decompensate during the questioning or because of the stress caused by the patient's answering.

Physical Examination

As with history taking, the physical examination should not either delay definitive treatment or cause undue stress to a patient with tentative respiratory status. Physical examination is focused on the evaluation of the adequacy of airway and breathing as detailed in the previous section as well as the evaluation of the patient's external upper airway anatomy. This evaluation of upper airway anatomy is used to predict the ease of intubation and is discussed in more detail in the following section.

CLINICAL REASONING

Once the determination has been made that the patient requires a definitive airway, that is, endotracheal intubation, numerous anatomic and clinical factors need to be evaluated to achieve a high level of success while minimizing the risk to the patient. The most common definitive airway management techniques are detailed in Table 2–3.

The immediate method reflects a patient who is deeply comatose, obtunded, or fully arrested in whom there is no resistance to direct laryngoscopy and intubation. The oral awake method, a variation of the immediate method, involves judicious anxiolysis coupled with topical anesthesia of the oropharynx and tongue to allow direct laryngoscopy and intubation in an awake and cooperative patient. This method is most useful when anatomic or clinical conditions exist that preclude the safety of neuromuscular blockade.

Rapid sequence intubation (RSI) integrates the simultaneous administration of a rapid-acting general anesthetic and neuromuscular blocking agent to achieve optimal intubating conditions in less than 1 minute. It is most useful in patients who

TABLE 2–3. Definitive Airway Management Techniques

Immediate
Oral awake
Rapid Sequence Intubation (RSI)
Nasotracheal
Cricothyrotomy

have a higher risk of aspiration (e.g., full stomach) or in whom the stress of intubation may exacerbate an alternate condition, such as increased intracranial pressure or myocardial ischemia.

Nasotracheal intubation is a technique in which the endotracheal tube is passed through a naris into the trachea in a conscious, upright, breathing patient. It is most useful in patients without intravenous access and in patients in whom neuromuscular blockade carries significant risk. Cricothyrotomy is a surgical approach establishing an alternative access to the trachea. It may be used in patients with facial/laryngeal trauma or laryngeal edema or if other methods fail.

It is prudent to spend a moment, if time permits, to critically evaluate a number of questions before taking action. These will direct the physician toward the best course of action to secure a definitive airway as detailed in Figure 2–5.

How much time do the patient and I have?

Emergency physicians are frequently presented with patients who are apneic or fully arrested. These patients will benefit most from immediate intubation. An apneic or arrested patient is not a candidate for nasotracheal intubation because spontaneous respirations are required for tube placement.

Oxygenation will be impaired by the delay it takes to establish intravenous access, evaluate the airway, and proceed with a more time-consuming RSI. For these patients, immediate orotracheal intubation is the procedure of choice. In the patient in respiratory extremis who has no intravenous access, timely control of the airway with endotracheal intubation may be superior to delaying airway control and risking respiratory arrest by preparing for RSI.

HOW DIFFICULT WILL IT BE TO INTUBATE THIS PATIENT?

Most potential problems can be predicted in patients who will be difficult to intubate with a brief, focused examination of the external upper airway anatomy and associated clinical factors. These predictors are listed in Table 2–4. Patients with short necks, as well as younger children, have a larynx that is superior relative to the oropharynx. This makes visualizing the glottis more difficult because there is more of an acute angle to overcome during direct laryngoscopy. When an attempt is being made to visualize the glottis, the tongue must be moved out of the way. If a patient has either a large tongue, such as a patient with Down's syndrome, or has a small jaw, for example, micrognathia, the tongue is relatively large

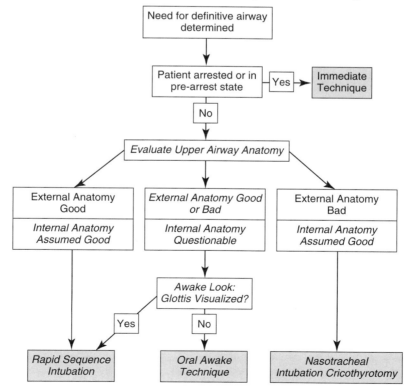

FIGURE 2–5 • Decision making regarding initial method of airway control.

TABLE 2–4. Factors Predictive of a Difficult Airway

Anatomic	Clinical
Short neck	Cervical spine immobilization
Children	Blood, vomit, or secretions in
Big tongue	the airway
Small jaw	Airway edema
Poor neck extension	Facial trauma
Prominent upper incisors	Laryngeal trauma
Bearded patients	Combative patients

compared with the floor of the mouth and is difficult to move or compress to visualize the glottis. Neck extension is important to align the oral and pharyngeal planes. Patients with poor neck extension, such as those with rheumatoid arthritis, are more challenging to treat with direct laryngoscopy. Similarly, patients with prominent upper incisors or poor mouth opening will offer a smaller oral opening through which one can manipulate the laryngoscope and attempt direct laryngoscopy. Patients with beards may be problematic if intubation is not successful and bag-valve-mouth-mask ventilation is required. It is more difficult to achieve a mask-to-face seal in the bearded individual.

A number of clinical parameters also impact the ability to pass an orotracheal tube. Orotracheal intubation is more challenging in a trauma patient who requires cervical spine immobilization. The head must remain in a neutral position without extension of the neck until the cervical spine has been cleared. Success rates of orotracheal intubation in this circumstance are very high when a second operator provides manual in-line stabilization. Any alteration of the normal internal anatomy of the mouth, oropharynx, hypopharynx, or larynx, for example, secondary to facial trauma or airway edema, will negatively impact one's ability to identify landmarks and successfully intubate a patient. Additionally, a patient who is combative because of hypoxia, head injury, or intoxication will be more challenging if this behavior is not controlled before the intubation attempt.

Despite this long list of factors affecting the ability to intubate, the experienced emergency physician can assess a patient's status in approximately 15 seconds. The clinical factors such as cervical spine immobilization, emesis, and facial trauma are immediately obvious. The external anatomic factors can be assessed by examining three anatomic relationships in rapid succession. The first is to determine the Mallampati score. The patient is asked to open the mouth, or he or

she is assisted if unable to do so, and the view into the oropharynx is evaluated as detailed in Figure 2–6. Mallampati class I and class II oral airways are predictive of a very high success rate with orotracheal intubation.

The second anatomic relationship to assess is the thyromental distance. This is the distance from the thyroid notch to the mentum. A thyromental distance of 6 cm or greater is predictive of a successful intubation. For most practitioners, 6 cm can be approximated by the width of the second through fourth digits at the level of the distal interphalangeal joint. The third component to evaluate is neck extension. As the three fingers are placed to measure the thyromental distance, the other hand can be placed on the occiput and the patient's neck can be extended if the cervical spine has not been immobilized. A 30-degree neck extension reliably implies the ability to align the oral and pharyngeal axes for visualization of the glottis. Thus, the patient's anatomy can be rapidly evaluated and the potentially difficult airway can be anticipated by looking in the patient's mouth and assessing the Mallampati classification, rapidly followed by measuring the thyromental distance with one hand, while the neck is extended.

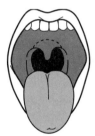

Class I: soft palate, uvula, fauces, pillars visible

No difficulty

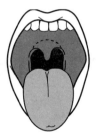

Class II: soft palate, uvula, fauces visible

No difficulty

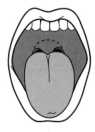

Class III: soft palate, base of uvula visible

Moderate difficulty

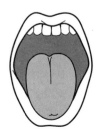

Class IV: hard palate only visible

Severe difficulty

FIGURE 2–6 • Modified Mallampati classification (four classes).

The final group of clinical conditions that impact the predicted ease of intubation relate to the patient's internal airway anatomy. All these elements can distort the airway anatomy and increase the difficulty of endotracheal intubation. They include airway edema from thermal burns, angioedema or anaphylaxis, penetrating neck trauma, foreign bodies, and various infectious processes such as epiglottitis and retropharyngeal abscesses. These factors are not directly visualized but rather are anticipated by the clinical presentation of the patient. For example, patients with thermal burns of the head and neck, stridor from any cause, or penetrating neck injuries should all be considered to have distorted internal anatomy until proven otherwise. These, and the aforementioned items, will all impact the physician's decisions about the most successful and safest method of intubation.

How might I harm this patient?

Endotracheal intubation is associated with a number of complications. These may be caused by the procedure itself, the physiologic changes associated with intubation, and the physiologic effects of medications used to assist in intubation (Table 2–5).

The most dramatic complication encountered in endotracheal intubation is the inability to intubate the patient. Of course, this sustains the ongoing risk the patient was already exposed to. The critical element is not the inability to pass the tube but the inability to subsequently oxygenate and ventilate the patient with a bag-valve mask. With appropriate assessment of the anatomic and clinical risk factors for the difficult airway mentioned earlier, this problem has become exceedingly rare.

Esophageal intubation occurs occasionally even with direct visualization and in the most skilled hands. In this situation, the unparalyzed, breathing patient may still provide their own sustaining, albeit inadequate oxygenation and ventilation. Esophageal intubation does provide a substantial stimulus for emesis with potential esophageal perforation and/or aspiration. Appropriate confirmatory techniques of endotracheal tube placement will minimize, but not completely prevent, these risks.

The most commonly lethal complication associated with endotracheal intubation is aspiration. Aspiration of a macroscopic amount of acidic gastric contents is associated with a mortality approaching 30%. It is incumbent on the physician to take any steps necessary to prevent its occurrence.

A rare complication of nasotracheal intubation is passage of the endotracheal tube through the fractured roof of the nasal cavity into the cranial vault. Intracranial intubation has been described in only a handful of cases that have involved severe midfacial trauma, basilar skull fractures, and, specifically, fractures of the cribriform plate. Evidence is gathering that, with proper technique, nasotracheal intubation in this patient population is safe and effective. However, if presented with this scenario, alternative approaches to nasotracheal intubation are considered first.

Significant cervical spine motion has been observed in all forms of endotracheal intubation, including cricothyrotomy. Therefore, the risk of disruption of an unstable cervical spine fracture in a trauma patient is a true concern. This complication, fortunately, is rare and does not impact the decision on the route of endotracheal intubation because all routes cause a similar degree of cervical spine motion and proper in-line immobilization does limit this movement.

Direct laryngoscopy and endotracheal intubation may lead to an elevation of intracranial and intragastric pressures. These pressure shifts can lead to brain herniation in the patient with a closed-head injury or to herniation of abdominal contents into the chest in the patient with a ruptured diaphragm. Additionally, fasciculations associated with the use of succinylcholine can lead to similar pressure changes. Care must be taken in these patient populations to mitigate these pressure responses before intubation.

Direct laryngoscopy and endotracheal intubation are associated with a hypertensive and tachycardic response in the majority of adult patients. These hemodynamic changes increase myocardial oxygen demand with the increased myocardial work of tachycardia coupled with the increased afterload of hypertension. Additionally, tachycardia decreases the time the heart is in diastole and decreases coronary filling time leading to decreased myocardial oxygen supply. This combination of increased myocardial oxygen demand and decreased myocardial oxygen supply can

---

TABLE 2–5. Harm Associated with Endotracheal Intubation

Anatomic injury from procedure (e.g., vocal cord, epiglottis)
Inability to intubate the trachea
Esophageal intubation
Aspiration
Intracranial intubation
Cervical spine injury
Increased intracranial pressure
Increased intragastric pressure
Hemodynamic changes
    Hypertension
    Tachycardia
    Bradycardia (Primarily pediatric)
    Hypotension (often medication related)

theoretically convert myocardial ischemia to myocardial infarction or expand an evolving infarct.

Children and young adults with high vagal tone may have a bradycardic response to airway manipulation. This should be anticipated and atropine used prophylactically or at least be immediately available. Finally, several of the general anesthetics used to optimize intubating conditions have the side effect of hypotension, especially in a volume-depleted patient. This should be anticipated as well. Drugs should be chosen judiciously, and intravenous access should be established and reliable.

What is the Operator's level of comfort with the procedure?

This question is more applicable to the relative novice at airway management. Successful intubation is more likely when the operator uses the most comfortable technique. However, the physician knowledgeable in airway management should be well versed with all methods of intubation, various laryngoscope blades, medications involved, and positional manipulations.

AIRWAY MANAGEMENT PRINCIPLES

Initial Preparation

The first step and the key to success in endotracheal intubation is proper preparation, as detailed in Table 2–6. Equipment malfunction should be anticipated, and redundancy is the key when preparing to intubate. The first step is to evaluate the patient's airway as discussed previously. Cardiac and pulse oximetry monitoring should be in place, and reliable intravenous access should be established. Yankauer suction should be tested and immediately available to the operator. Most physicians choose to tuck the suction tip underneath the mattress of the stretcher by the patient's head.

A bag-valve mask of the appropriate size for the patient should be available and tested as well.

TABLE 2–6. Preparation for Endotracheal Intubation

Evaluate airway anatomy
Cardiac monitor is placed
Continuous pulse oximetry
Intravenous access (or two)
Yankauer suction (tested)
Bag-valve mask (correct size)
Laryngoscopes (several and tested)
Endotracheal tubes (several and tested)
10-mL syringe available to inflate balloon
Drugs (drawn up and ready)
Patient positioning

Laryngoscopes of different sizes with different blades must be available, and more than one should be tested because the bulbs tend to burn out at the most inopportune times. Similarly, several endotracheal tubes of different sizes should be available and their balloon cuffs should be checked ahead of time. Optimally, one tube is styletted, lubricated, and ready to use. If RSI is planned, all of the medications anticipated should be drawn up, labeled, and ready. Moreover, medications that may be needed, such as atropine, must be immediately available. Additionally, if a nasotracheal intubation is planned, a topical anesthetic and vasoconstrictor are instilled into both nares during the preparatory stage.

Finally, the patient is positioned in such a way as to maximize the opportunity to visualize the glottis if planning an orotracheal intubation or is positioned to maximize tracheal placement of the tube if the nasotracheal route is planned. For orotracheal intubation, the oral, pharyngeal, and laryngeal axes must be aligned to maximize visualization of the glottis. This is achieved by a combination of neck extension and head elevation. This position, called the "sniffing position," simulates the position of the head and neck that is used when one sniffs a flower. A common error is neglecting to elevate the head, which is best achieved by placing 1 to 2 inches of towels beneath the patient's head. To maximize comfort of the operator, the bed is elevated so that the practitioner need not stoop over during the procedure. For nasotracheal intubation, the patient is also placed in the "sniffing position" but is often seated upright.

AIRWAY MANAGEMENT: SPECIFIC TECHNIQUES

Immediate Technique

This technique is reserved for patients who are deeply comatose or in respiratory arrest. In these circumstances, it is necessary to secure the airway as rapidly as possible. Advantages of this technique are its rapidity and technical ease. A completely comatose patient generally allows considerably more manipulation of the upper airway tissues. The potential disadvantages are twofold. First, if the patient's obtundation is caused by elevated intracranial pressure, the stress of intubation may exacerbate this pressure and lead to herniation. If the patient is not as deeply comatose as expected, emesis can result during airway manipulation. This results in a high risk of aspiration, because comatose patients generally have poor airway reflexes.

Oral Awake Technique

Oral awake intubation is a method by which a judicious amount of intravenous sedative or anxiolytic is given to a cooperative, awake, and breathing patient, followed by topical anesthesia of the oropharynx and tongue. This should allow an operator to perform a direct laryngoscopy, visualize the glottis, and place an endotracheal tube. The primary advantage of this technique is that it preserves airway reflexes and spontaneous respirations in the patient. In other words, if intubation is unable to be done, the patient may be no worse off than before the procedure was attempted. Emesis during airway manipulation is less of a problem because the patient's airway reflexes are intact. It is most useful for patients in whom questionable internal anatomy exists, such as laryngeal edema and retropharyngeal abscess. These are situations in which paralysis confers greater risk. The primary disadvantages of this technique are that it can be quite uncomfortable for the patient and may be, by far, the most stressful of all techniques to both the physician and patient. Caution is exercised in patients with intracranial or cardiac disorders because stress responses associated with this technique could cause harm. Caution is also exercised regarding the degree of sedation given to the patient. The purpose of sedation in the oral awake technique is limited to providing anxiolysis and relaxation of the patient and not to impair airway reflexes.

RAPID SEQUENCE INTUBATION (RSI)

RSI is the rapid induction of general anesthesia and neuromuscular blockade before endotracheal intubation and positive-pressure ventilation are provided. It is used primarily in patients who are awake and breathing and who may not have adequate airway reflexes. It is used in patients in whom the external upper airway examination is predictive of a high success rate of intubation and in whom no suspicion of internal anatomic distortion exists. Limiting its use to this patient population maximizes benefit and minimizes risk. Its main advantages are that it provides optimal intubating conditions while minimizing the risk of aspiration during the procedure.

A conscious alert patient with intact airway reflexes has minimal risk of aspiration. Similarly, a patient who is completely sedated and paralyzed has a relatively small aspiration risk because paralysis prohibits active emesis. However, there is a window of about 45 seconds as a patient undergoes RSI when the patient is partially sedated, but not yet completely paralyzed, and able to vomit and potentially aspirate. This vulnerable time is the reason why RSI drugs used for induction and paralysis have a rapid onset. It is also the reason why positive-pressure ventilation is not provided before intubation because distention of the stomach will increase the risk of emesis during this critical period. Slower-acting agents such as benzodiazepines or narcotics are not recommended as induction agents. Similarly, slower-acting and longer-lasting competitive neuromuscular blocking agents such as vecuronium and related nondepolarizing agents are less commonly used. This may change as newer agents are developed.

The main contraindication to RSI is the questionable status of the patient's upper airway anatomy (both external and internal). RSI should not be used in the majority of patients in whom assessment of the airway anatomy does not predict ease of intubation. This circumstance could result in the purposeful removal of a patient's spontaneous respirations and airway reflexes with an inability to secure a definitive airway. Specific consideration should be given to the use of RSI in patients who present with a closed-head injury or myocardial ischemia because it is the least stressful technique for these tenuous situations. Moreover, a patient with a full stomach, who is representative of the majority of emergency department patients, carries a higher aspiration risk and would benefit from RSI.

The technique of RSI can be thought of as several separate steps. These steps, the six "*Ps*," are listed and detailed below in Table 2–7.

Preparation. Preparation for intubation was discussed in detail earlier in this chapter, and the major steps are listed in Table 2–6. Preparation for RSI does not significantly differ from that previously discussed. The physician's mandate is to anticipate all reasonable complications and potential side effects of the patient's impending treatment.

Preoxygenation. One of the goals of RSI is to secure endotracheal placement before positive-pressure ventilation. It is imperative to preoxygenate the patient as much as possible to increase the time before desaturation. Optimally, 5 minutes of preoxygenation is allowed, which is sufficient time for nitrogen washout from the lungs. If 5 minutes is not available owing to the clinical situation, four vital capacity breaths of 100% oxygen will

TABLE 2–7. The Six "*Ps*" of RSI

Preparation
Preoxygenation
Pretreatment
Paralysis (with induction)
Placement of the tube
Postintubation management

increase the FIO_2 within the lungs to about 70%. In normal subjects, 5 minutes of preoxygenation will allow an average of 8 minutes of apnea before the saturation drops below 90%! In ill patients, this time frame is reduced to about 4 minutes. For this reason, preoxygenation is a critical step if time permits.

Pretreatment. There are clinical scenarios (Table 2–8) in which pretreatment is beneficial. The first is in the pediatric patient. Pediatric patients and young adults with high vagal tone have an exaggerated vagal response to laryngeal manipulation and to succinylcholine administration. This bradycardia can lead to hemodynamic instability at times, but it can be controlled by pretreatment with atropine. It is recommended that all children 5 years old or younger be pretreated with 0.02 mg/kg of atropine during the pretreatment phase of RSI. The minimum dose should be 0.1 mg because doses less than this may cause a paradoxical bradycardia. The maximum dose is 1 mg. It is further recommended that, in older children and young adults, atropine be readily available and administrated if bradycardia occurs.

Pretreatment also is vital in patients with a closed-head injury or ruptured diaphragm. The elevation of intracranial or intragastric pressure associated with direct laryngoscopy and intubation may worsen their condition. The depolarizing muscle relaxant succinylcholine directly depolarizes all motor endplates, simultaneously causing fasciculations and a rise in these pressures. Premedication with vecuronium, administered in the dose of 0.01 mg/kg, can prevent these pressure rises. Furthermore, intracranial pressure is elevated during direct laryngoscopy and intubation both by means of a direct response elevating intracranial pressure and a hemodynamic response to intubation leading to an elevation in the mean arterial pressure and, thus, the intracranial pressure. The direct elevation in intracranial pressure may be controlled with lidocaine premedication in the dose of 1.5 mg/kg. The hemodynamic mechanism increas-

ing intracranial pressure can be controlled by pretreatment with fentanyl in the dose of 3 µg/kg.

Laryngeal manipulation and endotracheal intubation causes a direct bronchospastic reflex in all patients. Therefore, patients with tenuous respiratory status caused by reversible airway disease are at risk for precipitous decompensation. Administration of lidocaine, in the dose of 1.5 mg/kg, can partially mitigate this bronchospastic response. Ketamine (1.5 mg/kg), as the anesthetic agent, has bronchodilatory properties, and may be used in patients with significant reactive airway disease.

The final group of patients are those with myocardial ischemia or infarction who require airway intervention. The hemodynamic response, as mentioned earlier, is that of hypertension and tachycardia. Because the hemodynamic changes can negatively impact these patients, fentanyl, in the dose of 3 µg/kg, is administered to blunt this hemodynamic reflex.

Paralysis (with Induction). With rare exception, neuromuscular blockade in RSI is achieved using succinylcholine. Succinylcholine is used because it has the fastest onset to achieve muscle relaxation, reducing the patient's vulnerable window to approximately 45 seconds. None of the nondepolarizing agents, including the newer products, are as fast as succinylcholine. It is administered in the dose of 1.5 mg/kg in adults and 2.0 mg/kg in pediatric patients. Succinylcholine can cause bradycardia in pediatric patients and elevation in intracranial and intragastric pressures. Premedication can prevent these side effects. Succinylcholine also has been associated with prolonged paralysis in patients with pseudocholinesterase deficiency (1:2,500) and with malignant hyperthermia (1:10,000). These complications are far less harmful than the alternative of expanding the patient's vulnerable window by using a nondepolarizing muscle relaxant with a longer time of onset.

Succinylcholine use can also result in hyperkalemia. In healthy patients, a therapeutic dosage

TABLE 2–8. Pretreatment in Rapid Sequence Intubation

	Pediatric	Elevated ICP	Elevated IGP	Bronchospasm	Cardiac Ischemia
Atropine (mg/kg)	0.02 (min 0.1 mg)	—	—	—	—
Vecuronium (mg/kg)	—	0.01	0.01	—	—
Lidocaine (mg/kg)	—	1.5	—	1.5	—
Fentanyl (µg/kg)	—	3.0 (slowly)	—	—	3.0
Ketamine (mg/kg)	—	—	—	1.5	—

ICP, intracranial pressure; IGP, intragastric pressure.

administration leads to a serum potassium rise of about 0.5 mEq/dL. Patients with denervating conditions, large body surface area burns, or crush injuries can have an exaggerated rise in serum potassium level. However, these patient populations are at risk for an exaggerated rise in serum potassium level only during 1 week to 6 months after onset of the condition. Patients with renal failure, or hyperkalemia of any cause, may rarely suffer cardiac complications from the moderate rise of 0.5 mEq/dL. In patients who fit these criteria, a nondepolarizing muscle relaxant, such as vecuronium, is selected. The time of onset for vecuronium, 2 to 5 minutes, can be shortened by increasing the dose from 0.1 mg/kg to 0.2 to 0.3 mg/kg, which provides an onset of 1 to 2 minutes. However, the use of vecuronium introduces the additional risk of prolonged paralysis. Succinylcholine has a duration of 5 to 10 minutes, whereas vecuronium has a duration of 20 to 30 minutes with the regular dose and 30 to 60 minutes with the larger dose. If intubation, for whatever reason, is unsuccessful, the patient will be apneic for considerably longer if a nondepolarizing neuromuscular blocking agent is used.

Neuromuscular blockade leads to the relaxation of the lower esophageal sphincter. A significant degree of passive reflux can lead to aspiration before securing the airway. For this reason, cricoid pressure, known as the *Sellick maneuver*, is instituted at the time of neuromuscular paralysis. Because the cricoid is a circular structure, pressure on the anterior cricoid will occlude the esophagus posteriorly and prevent passive reflux. This maneuver is maintained until the endotracheal tube is confirmed to be in the correct place. If active vomiting occurs, the Sellick maneuver is stopped to prevent the possibility of esophageal rupture. Additionally, if vecuronium is used during the pretreatment phase, cricoid pressure is applied at that time. The "defasciculating dose" of vecuronium can cause lower esophageal sphincter relaxation.

Simultaneously with neuromuscular blockade, an induction agent is given. As mentioned previously, the only induction agents used in RSI are general anesthetics. Benzodiazepines and narcotics play no role. Common induction agents used are listed in Table 2–9. All of the induction agents discussed have similar pharmacokinetics to succinylcholine. They have an onset of less than 1 minute and a duration of 5 to 10 minutes. They are highly lipophilic and redistribute throughout the body rapidly. Their other advantage over benzodiazepines and narcotics is their reliable dose-response relationships, which allow a reasonably consistent and predictable anesthesia.

TABLE 2–9. Common Induction Agents

Barbiturates
    Sodium pentothal (Thiopental)
    Methohexital (Brevital)
Nonbarbiturate Sedative-Hypnotics
    Etomidate (Amidate)
    Propofol (Diprivan)
Dissociative Anesthetic
    Ketamine

Sodium pentothal, a barbiturate, historically has been the most common induction agent used. Its advantages include a decrease in intracranial and intragastric pressure. Its drawbacks include histamine release–induced bronchospasm and cardiodepression-induced hypotension. It is specifically helpful in patients in whom intracranial and intragastric pressure are a concern. Patients with acute bronchospasm should not be given sodium pentothal, and caution is advised in patients with a history of chronic obstructive pulmonary disease or asthma. Its use should be avoided in patients who are hypotensive or in those considered to be hypovolemic. Its cardiodepressant and hypotensive effects are exaggerated by volume depletion. Methohexital is another barbiturate with similar effects to sodium pentothal.

Etomidate, a nonbarbiturate sedative-hypnotic, has recently replaced sodium pentothal as the most popular induction agent in RSI. It is administered in the dose of 0.3 mg/kg and also decreases intracranial and intragastric pressures. It does not induce histamine release or exacerbate bronchospastic disease and does not cause hypotension, even in volume-depleted patients. Etomidate use causes virtually no change in heart rate or blood pressure. Its only disadvantages are myoclonus and adrenal suppression. The effect of myoclonus in RSI is insignificant because the drug is always combined with neuromuscular blockade. A single dose of etomidate will decrease cortisol levels for months. However, longitudinal studies have failed to show this change to be associated with any morbidity or mortality in this patient population. Etomidate is an excellent induction choice for patients with elevated intracranial pressure, myocardial ischemia, hypotension, or volume depletion. Propofol, another nonbarbiturate sedative-hypnotic, has similar effects to etomidate. It is rarely used in the emergency setting because it is suspended in a lipid vehicle that requires refrigeration.

Ketamine, a dissociative anesthetic, has a similar chemical structure to phencyclidine. Rather than producing sedation or hypnosis, it produces a dissociative state. The patient, if not paralyzed, continues to breath spontaneously with the eyes open but remains unresponsive to external stimuli. It is given in the dose of 1.5 to 2.0 mg/kg. Its primary advantages and disadvantages are the result of an associated catecholamine release that causes hypertension, tachycardia, and bronchodilation. This is a disadvantage in the patient with a head injury or myocardial ischemia. However, the resultant bronchodilation may be quite beneficial to patients with reversible airway disease. Its primary use is in young asthmatics. Caution is urged when it is considered in the older bronchospastic population. Many of these older patients may have potential myocardial ischemia secondary to ongoing hypoxia or a noncritical lesion that may be exposed if they are subjected to a "ketamine stress test." Other side effects include laryngospasm, which is not an issue in RSI due to paralysis, and a dysphoric emergence reaction, which occurs as the anesthetic effect wanes. Usually after intubation the patient is sedated, obviating any concern for an emergence reaction.

Placement of the Tube. Considerable anxiety may be associated with the period of time between induction/neuromuscular blockade and the moment when the patient is ready to be intubated. It is difficult to observe a patient while he or she becomes apneic, not bag him or her, and not attempt intubation until a safe amount of time has passed. Attempts to intubate someone before complete neuromuscular blockade is dangerous because this is the period of time during which the airway reflexes have been compromised by the induction agent yet the person is not completely paralyzed and is still able to vomit. It is better to wait a few moments too long than to begin too soon. If the patient has not been pre-medicated with vecuronium, the cessation of fasciculations will be an indicator that the patient is ready to be intubated. Different areas of the body stop fasciculating at different times, and it is generally taught that the toes and the lips are the last muscles to fasciculate. It is common to grasp the mandible and test its laxity after fasciculations have ceased to confirm full muscle relaxation. The patient is then orotracheally intubated under direct laryngoscopy, as illustrated in Figure 2–7 and described in Table 2–10.

Because the appropriately preoxygenated patient will not desaturate for 3 to 5 minutes, the clinician has the opportunity for several attempts at orotracheal intubation before the risk of desaturation, let alone permanent injury, is a concern. This time period is shorter in patients who were unable to be maximally preoxygenated because of clinical factors and in pediatric patients who tend to desaturate more quickly. Some practitioners suggest the operator should hold his or her breath while intubating and when he or she needs to breathe, the patient should be ventilated. This practice underestimates the amount of time a well-preoxygenated patient will hold oxygen saturation and serves to add to the anxiety and discomfort of the operator. It is preferable to have an assistant announce the time, in 30-second intervals, or to listen to the sound of the pulse oximetry unit. As the saturation begins to drop, the pulse oximetry unit will progressively emit lower tones, which indicates desaturation is occurring. In experienced hands, the average time to pass an endotracheal tube is approximately 20 seconds. This affords plenty of time for failed attempts or esophageal intubations to be corrected. Additional attempts may require different laryngoscope

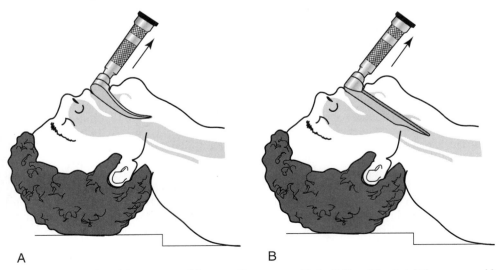

A   B

FIGURE 2–7 • Orotracheal intubation. *A,* Use of the curved laryngoscope blade. *B,* Use of the straight laryngoscope blade.

TABLE 2–10. Technique of Orotracheal Intubation

1. The two main types of blades are straight (e.g., Miller) and curved (e.g., MacIntosh). Most adults can be intubated using a size 3 blade, although some physicians prefer the guideline "the larger the better." Assemble the laryngoscope and blade, checking the light and making sure that the bulb is screwed in tightly and will not fall off during the procedure. Fiberoptic laryngoscopes obviate this last concern.
2. Select an endotracheal tube of the proper size. Average sizes are 7.5–8.5 mm for men and 7.0–8.0 mm for women.
3. Using a 10-mL syringe, inflate the cuff on the tube until it is taut and palpate it to check for leaks. Then deflate it completely. The ventilator adaptor on the proximal end of the tube is twisted and pressed firmly onto the tube.
4. It is best to use a malleable wire stylet, placed so that the distal end of the stylet is 1 cm proximal to the tip of the endotracheal tube. The stylet adds rigidity and allows the tube to be curved to facilitate passage.
5. Unless there is a concern about cervical spine injury, the patient's head is raised 1 to 2 inches, extended on the neck, and the neck is slightly flexed in relation to the trunk. This "sniffing position" allows optimal visualization of the vocal cords.
6. Preferably, an assistant stands to the physician's right, holding suction and the endotracheal tube in one hand and using the other hand to depress the cricoid cartilage posteriorly at the proper time. Cricoid pressure occludes the esophagus and decreases the risk of regurgitation and aspiration. It also positions the glottis for easier viewing during laryngoscopy.
7. The laryngoscope is held in the left hand, and the patient's mouth is opened with the right hand by pushing the superior teeth rostrally with the index finger and the inferior teeth caudally with the thumb. The laryngoscope blade is inserted on the far right side of the patient's mouth, and the blade is used to sweep the tongue to the left, out of the field of view. Suction is used as necessary to clear the oropharynx.
8. The tip of the blade is advanced along the dorsal surface of the tongue, looking for the epiglottis. When a curved blade is used, the tip is positioned in the vallecula anterior to the epiglottis and lifted, thus lifting the epiglottis and exposing the glottic opening (see Fig. 2–6A). The blade is not used as a lever, which can damage teeth. With a straight blade, the tip of the blade is placed posterior to the epiglottis and lifted to expose the vocal cords (see Fig. 2–6B).
9. When the vocal cords are clearly seen, the endotracheal tube tip is passed through the vocal cords until the proximal end of the cuff is 2 cm beyond the cords. The laryngoscope and stylet are removed, and the balloon cuff is inflated with 5–10 mL of air.
10. In most adults, the tube will be properly positioned when the 22-cm mark is at the patient's teeth, yielding the TT-TT mnemonic (tip-to-teeth, twenty-two).
11. The tube should be fixed to the upper lip with tape or tied with a ribbon that completely encircles the head. It should never be secured to the lower lip because the mobility of the mandible allows too much movement of the tube.
12. Tube placement is confirmed as soon as possible.

blades or different-sized endotracheal tubes. In the event that intubation is unsuccessful and oxygen saturation drops below 90%, the patient is ventilated with a bag-valve mask several times until the saturation returns to normal before reattempting intubation.

In the event that a patient is unable to be intubated or ventilated by bag-valve mask, emergency cricothyrotomy is the procedure of choice. If the patient cannot be intubated but can be ventilated, this is considered a failed airway and there are a number of other procedural techniques to establish a nondefinitive or definitive airway. An intubating laryngeal mask airway, esophageal-tracheal Combitube, and transtracheal jet ventilation have been mentioned. A detailed discussion of alternative definitive approaches, which are listed in Table 2–11, is beyond the scope of this text. Please refer to Table 2–12 to review the timing of the various steps of RSI.

Postintubation Management. Confirmation of tube placement, administering additional sedative agents, and considering long-acting neuromuscular blocking agents are all part of postintubation management.

Nasotracheal Technique

The nasotracheal route of endotracheal intubation is a time-honored method that has been less fre-

TABLE 2–11. Rescue Techniques for the Failed Airway

Nondefinitive

Laryngeal mask airway
Transtracheal jet ventilation

Definitive

Lighted stylet
Retrograde intubation
Bullard laryngoscope
Fiberoptic intubation
Digital intubation
Cricothyrotomy
Intubating laryngeal mask airway
[Esophageal-tracheal Combitube]

quently used, because of the increased popularity of RSI. It is a technique with a high degree of success and a reasonable complication rate. It is a required skill of any practicing emergency physician, because there are a number of clinical circumstances in which it may represent the only reasonable method of securing a timely airway short of a cricothyrotomy. The technique of nasotracheal intubation is outlined in Table 2–13.

Because air movement is required to guide the endotracheal tube, the nasotracheal technique cannot be performed on an apneic patient. This

TABLE 2–12. Timing of Steps for Rapid Sequence Intubation

Time (min)	Step
Early	Preparation
−5:00	Preoxygenation
−3:00	Pretreatment
	Cricoid pressure (if pretreated with vecuronium)
−1:00	Paralysis
	Induction
	Cricoid pressure (if not pretreated with vecuronium)
0:00	Intubate (witness passage through vocal cords)
+0:05 sec	[Confirm endotracheal tube placement]
+1.00–2.00	Begin ventilation and postintubation management

represents the only absolute contraindication. There are a number of relative contraindications detailed in Table 2–14. The rare but theoretical possibility of intracranial intubation in a patient with a cribriform plate, basilar skull, and/or midfacial fracture has been discussed previously. Although mild epistaxis is common and inconsequential, a patient with a hemostatic disorder, such as platelet inhibition, anticoagulant use, or liver disease, may have massive epistaxis. This may require active intervention and an alternative approach to airway management.

Any patient with the potential for having altered internal airway anatomy should not be intubated nasotracheally unless absolutely necessary. This group includes patients with inhalational injuries, anaphylaxis with laryngospasm or laryngeal edema, epiglottitis, parapharyngeal or retropharyngeal abscesses, upper airway foreign bodies, or penetrating neck injuries that may involve the upper airway.

TABLE 2–13. Technique of Nasotracheal Intubation

1. As with oral intubation, proper preparation is crucial. There are important differences between oral and nasotracheal intubation.
   a. A stylet is not used in nasotracheal intubation.
   b. The endotracheal tube is 0.5–1.0 mm smaller in diameter.
   c. The tube may be tied into a loose knot and left for a minute to increase its curvature.
   d. Optimally, the nares are sprayed with a topical anesthetic and a vasoconstrictor such as cocaine or a combination of phenylephrine and lidocaine.
   e. The outside of the tube is lubricated lightly with water-soluble lubricant.
   f. The more patent naris is selected after inspection.
2. During the intubation attempt, an oxygen mask or other source of high-flow oxygen is held near the mouth.
3. Intubation is begun by rotating the tube so that the distal bevel is flat against the nasal septum. The tube is gently slid posteriorly along the inferomedial aspect of the nasal cavity. It is during this part of the procedure that significant epistaxis can be produced. Therefore, advance the tube slowly and gently past any resistance. If resistance is firm against slight pressure, pull the tube out and try the other naris. When the tip of the tube passes the posterior choana into the oropharynx just above the soft palate, the resistance will decrease.
4. After the tube passes the posterior choana, the physician should position his or her ear directly over the endotracheal tube adaptor so that air passing through the tube can be heard and felt. Breath sounds become louder as the tip of the tube approaches the glottic opening. Advance the tube to the loudest point. Auditory devices are also used to identify this juncture.
5. When the patient inspires, move the tube swiftly but gently forward 2–4 cm. The glottis and vocal cords are open during inspiration, and the tube should advance without significant resistance. As the tube passes into the trachea, the patient will often cough, and a rush of air will come out of the tube. Other material may be coughed out, so one must be aware which way the proximal end is directed.
6. If the tip of the endotracheal tube has not entered the trachea, it will usually be in one of four places: in the esophagus, just above the cords, in a piriform sinus, or in the vallecula. If the patient is not intubated successfully on the initial attempt, the physician should continue to supply oxygen, assess the location of the endotracheal tip, and take corrective measures.
   a. Esophagus: All air motion through the tube will cease. Withdraw the tube until loud breath sounds are heard. Apply more cricoid pressure to occlude the esophagus and displace the larynx posteriorly. If neck motion is not contraindicated, the neck can be extended. The tube is than readvanced.
   b. Rostral to the cords: laryngospasm may be blocking passage of the tube. Position the tube just on the cords and maintain very gentle pressure until the patient takes a deep breath. If the patient's ventilation is compromised by the laryngospasm, the tube should be removed and the patient ventilated with bag-valve mask.
   c. Piriform sinus: Location of the tube in the piriform sinus often causes a visible or palpable bulge superolateral to the thyroid cartilage. This condition can be corrected by slightly withdrawing and rotating the tube tip away from the bulge. If neck motion is not prohibited the patient's head can also be rotated toward the side of the bulge. The tube is readvanced.
   d. Vallecula: This location is rare. It causes a visible or palpable bulge superior to the hyoid bone. Gentle anterior traction is applied on the larynx. If neck motion is not contraindicated, the neck is flexed. The tube is advanced. If these measures fail, a tube with less curvature can be used.
7. After the tube enters the trachea, the cuff is inflated and tube placement confirmed. Because of the increased risk of esophageal intubation with this blind technique, it is important to check tube placement carefully.

TABLE 2–14. Contraindications to Nasotracheal Intubation

Absolute

Apnea

Relative

Midface/basilar skull fractures
Hemostatic disorder
Potentially altered internal airway anatomy
    Inhalation injury
    Angioedema/anaphylaxis
    Penetrating neck injury
Impaired airway reflexes
Closed-head injury
Myocardial ischemia

Another relative contraindication is the absence of adequate airway reflexes. As with all other methods of intubation in the unparalyzed patient, nasotracheal intubation can cause emesis before securing the airway. Thus, the risk of aspiration in a patient without adequate reflexes is present. Moreover, if the nasotracheal tube is not immediately withdrawn, when retching occurs, the tip of the endotracheal tube can interfere with the normal closure of the epiglottis and other airway reflexes, increasing the risk of aspiration.

Occasionally, nasal turbinates can be torn, fractured, or avulsed during passage of the tube. However, these complications are usually related to improper technique.

There is evidence to suggest that long-term use of a nasotracheal tube impairs the drainage of the paranasal sinuses and increases the risk of sinusitis. Also, because the nasotracheal tube is of a smaller diameter, it may be more difficult to manage weaning in the intensive care unit. These issues are best left to the intensivist. A nasotracheal tube can be changed to an orotracheal tube in the controlled setting of the intensive care unit at any time. These issues should not enter into the decision making of how to secure the emergency airway.

Finally, the nasotracheal route of intubation is more stressful to the patient and results in more exaggerated rises in intracranial pressure, heart rate, and blood pressure. It should be avoided, whenever possible, in patients with closed-head injuries or myocardial ischemia.

Clinical circumstances in which nasotracheal intubation offers a significant advantage generally revolve around the patient who has questionable external airway anatomy. RSI is contraindicated in such a situation. If there is no reason to believe the internal anatomy is abnormal, nasotracheal intubation offers an excellent alternative. If a patient's internal anatomy is questionable secondary to inhalation injury or the like, the oral awake method would be preferable.

Cricothyrotomy

Cricothyrotomy is indicated for definitive airway control when all nonsurgical methods have failed or are contraindicated. The procedure of cricothyrotomy is described in Table 2–15 and illustrated in Figure 2–8. It is relatively contraindicated in patients with bleeding diatheses, an infectious laryngeal pathologic process, and laryngotracheal or cervical tracheal disruption. Only relative contraindications exist because it is the airway procedure of last resort.

Immediate complications include bleeding, subcutaneous emphysema, esophageal laceration, laceration of the neurovascular structures in the carotid sheath, tube misplacement (anterior to the trachea), fracture or dislocation of the thyroid or cricoid cartilages, asphyxia, and death. Problems developing later include cellulitis, subglottic granulations, cuff site granulomas, and cuff site strictures. It is avoided in children younger than 8 years old because of the small size of the cricothyroid membrane and a high incidence of complications.

Emergency tracheostomy is technically difficult, is time consuming, and is best performed by a surgeon experienced in the procedure. Its only indication in the emergency setting is when there is a penetrating disruption of the trachea at or below the cricothyroid membrane. In these circumstances, it is not safe to attempt to pass an endotracheal tube or to perform a cricothyrotomy from above the injury.

Confirmation of Endotracheal Tube Placement

As mentioned previously, there is minimal immediate risk associated with the intubation of the esophagus. Rather, it is the failure to recognize such a misplacement that leads to ischemic brain injury and/or death. The best predictor of endotracheal rather than esophageal intubation is actually visualizing the tube going through the cords during orotracheal intubation. In the awake patient, successful tracheal intubation will result in the patient no longer being able to speak and generally will be associated with a vigorous cough reflex with pronounced air movement through the tube. In a patient who is sedated, is poorly responsive, or has been paralyzed for intubation, confirmation of tube placement may be more challenging.

There are numerous observations, techniques, and devices that aid the physician in confirmation of tube placement. These are listed in Table 2–16.

TABLE 2–15. The Technique of Cricothyrotomy

1. Locate the cricothyroid membrane.
2. Make a midline longitudinal incision 3 to 4 cm over the cricothyroid membrane.
3. Stabilize the larynx with the nondominant hand in one of two ways:
   a. By grasping the larynx between the thumb and middle finger
   b. By using a tracheal hook inserted in the cephalad portion of the cricothyroid membrane and hooking the thyroid cartilage.
4. Make a transverse incision in the caudal portion of the cricothyroid membrane (Fig. 2–7A). This avoids involvement of the cricothyroid arteries in the cephalad portion of the cricothyroid membrane.
5. Curved Mayo scissors or a hemostat is inserted beside the scalpel and spread horizontally to widen the space (Fig. 2–7B)
6. The tracheostomy tube is then placed between the blades of the Mayo scissors or the hemostat (Fig. 2–7C). The curved tip is pointed caudad. The placement should not be forced, but proceed gently because loss of control of the larynx can be disastrous. Appropriate-sized Shiley tracheostomy tubes are a No. 6 for an adult male, a No. 5 for an adult female, and a No. 4 for any patient with an edematous airway. If a tracheostomy tube is not available, an endotracheal tube can be substituted. The endotracheal tube can be used as is, or it can be shortened. To shorten an endotracheal tube, the adaptor cap is removed and the tube is cut with attention paid not to disrupt the cuff inflation tube.
7. The cuff is then inflated.
8. Tube placement is confirmed in the usual manner.

TABLE 2–16. Methods to Confirm Endotracheal Tube Placement

Potentially Unreliable	Preferred
Chest auscultation	Pulse oximetry
Epigastric auscultation	End-tidal CO_2
Chest movement	Esophageal detector device
Tube condensation	Direct laryngoscopy
Bag compliance	
Cuff palpation	
Exhaled tidal volumes	
Chest radiograph	

Auscultation of the chest is an unreliable method. In 15% of esophageal intubations, ventilation of the stomach will produce deceiving "breath sounds" with chest auscultation. Epigastric auscultation after esophageal intubation will usually, but not always, detect gurgling sounds when ventilating the stomach. This is somewhat more reliable than chest auscultation and should be performed first after intubation followed by chest auscultation. Watching the chest rise and fall with ventilation and looking for condensation in the tube during exhalation are suggestive, but not confirmatory, of tracheal intubation. Similarly, tracheal intubation is suggested by greater compliance of the bag-valve mask while bagging the patient because it is much more difficult to bag the stomach. This also proves to be an unreliable finding. The cuff of the endotracheal tube can be palpated in the patient's neck; however, this does not discern a cuff within the trachea from a cuff within the esophagus. It merely predicts the depth to which the cuff has been placed. If the trachea has been intubated, the exhaled tidal volume should be similar to the inhaled tidal volume. If the stomach is being ventilated, the esophagus tends to collapse on expiration and the "exhaled" tidal volumes are less than the "inhaled" tidal volumes. However, equal inhaled and exhaled tidal volumes are not confirmatory of tracheal placement of the tube either. Contrary to popular belief, even the chest radiograph is not completely confirmatory of endotracheal placement of the tube. The esophagus is very close to the trachea, and on a single anteroposterior view of the chest the two structures may be superimposed.

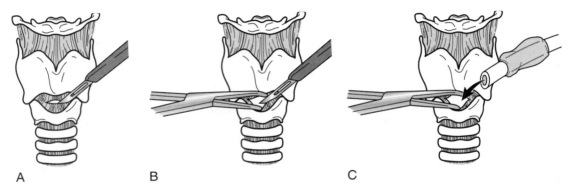

A   B   C

FIGURE 2–8 • *A* to *C*, Method of cricothyrotomy.

Fortunately, more reliable methods are available. In the paralyzed or apneic patient, pulse oximetry is quite reliable. If the oxygen saturation remains high in these patients beyond the period of time afforded by hyperventilation, one can conclude tracheal placement of the tube. However, in the spontaneously breathing patient, it can create a false sense of security because the spontaneous respirations may be supporting the oxygen saturation. For this reason, pulse oximetry is added to one of two other methods for confirming endotracheal tube placement.

The first method is end-tidal CO_2 detection. If CO_2 is consistently returned during exhalation, it can be assumed that the trachea has been intubated. CO_2 detection can be achieved by an expensive digital waveform machine or by the simple addition of a calorimetric end-tidal CO_2 detector placed between the endotracheal tube and the bag. This detector changes colors when exposed to CO_2 and will pulse yellow to purple with inspiration and expiration if the trachea has been intubated.

The other method, the esophageal detector device, relies on the anatomic differences between the trachea and the esophagus to determine tube placement. It resembles a large bulb syringe or turkey baster that is placed over the end of the endotracheal tube in a collapsed form. When released, it will fill quickly if within the rigid and open trachea. However, it will remain collapsed or relatively collapsed if the tip of the tube rests within the floppy, nonrigid esophagus.

The prudent physician will take full advantage of all these confirmatory techniques to ensure correct tube placement. Although visualizing the tube passing through the cords should be confirmatory, endotracheal tubes are readily displaced during patient movement or tube taping. A rather obvious, but all too often omitted, technique is to take another look. If doubt exists regarding tube placement, direct laryngoscopy and revisualizing that the tube is passing through the cords is most helpful.

DIFFERENTIAL DIAGNOSIS

Although an understanding of the pathophysiologic cause of respiratory distress is important in the management of the critically ill patient, initial assessment and stabilization do not depend on the differential diagnosis (see Chapter 37, Acute Dyspnea). Contemplating the cause of respiratory failure rather than intervening immediately can be a fatal error.

DIAGNOSTIC ADJUNCTS

In the emergency department most indications for airway management appear during the primary survey. The airway must be stabilized immediately before determining arterial blood gas levels, taking radiographs, or performing other diagnostic adjuncts. These studies are often ordered after the fact and are an important part of the patient's further management.

Occasionally, adjunctive data are part of the decision process during which definitive management of a patient's airway is selected in a "semi-elective" manner. This situation most commonly occurs in patients with reversible airways disease (asthma) or chronic obstructive pulmonary disease. Guidelines for ordering these tests and using them to make airway management decisions are delineated in Chapters 37, Acute Dyspnea, and 38, Wheezing.

UNCERTAIN DIAGNOSIS

Appropriate airway management has little to do with accurate diagnosis. The only "diagnosis" that needs to be made is whether a patient requires temporizing or definitive airway management (endotracheal intubation). Far more harm will come to the patient who is managed less aggressively. **WHEN IN DOUBT, INTUBATE!**

SPECIAL CONSIDERATIONS

Pediatric Patients

The pediatric airway is more prone to obstruction because it is of a smaller caliber, its opening is surrounded by aggregates of lymphoid tissue, and a child has a relatively large tongue. Table 2–17 outlines the major differences between the adult and pediatric airway. Children may become bradycardiac during intubation, so premedication with atropine is recommended for children 5 years of age and younger.

The appropriate size of endotracheal tube can be estimated by the size of the patient's little finger, by the size of the patient's naris, or by using the following formula:

ET tube diameter (mm) = 4 + 1/4 (age in years)

It is far more accurate and reliable to use the formula because the other anatomic relationships vary widely in individual patients. Premature newborns take a 2.5- to 3.0-mm endotracheal tube, term newborns take a 3.0- to 3.5-mm endotracheal tube, and infants (younger than 1 year old) need a 3.5- to 4.0-mm endotracheal tube. Laryngoscope blade types and sizes vary with age

TABLE 2–17. Pediatric Versus Adult Airway Anatomy and Management

Category	Adult	Pediatric
Airway caliber	Larger	Smaller
Airway resistance	Lesser	Greater
Mucosa and submucosa	More adherent and less fragile	Looser and more fragile
Lymphoid tissue	Less prominent	Prominent
Hyoid bone	Far from larynx	Close to larynx
Epiglottis	More pliable, less prominent	Stiffer, more prominent, U-shaped
Pharyngolaryngeal angle	Less acute	More acute
Larynx	Relatively caudal and posterior	Relatively rostral and anterior
Laryngeal prominence	Apparent or palpable	More obscure
Cricothyroid membrane	Palpable	More obscure (not palpable in infants)
Narrowest portion of airway	Glottis	Subglottic (cricoid cartilage)
Flexion at the cervicothoracic junction used in the sniffing position	Requires flat object under occiput	Naturally present in infants due to relatively large heads
Laryngoscope blade	Curved or straight	Straight in infants younger than 2 years old; straight or curved in infants older than 2 years old
Endotracheal tube	Cuffed	Uncuffed if child is younger than 10 years old
Cricothyrotomy	Appropriate	Very difficult and relatively contraindicated

as well. A size 0 straight blade is used for premature newborns, and a size 1 straight blade is used for term newborns and infants through approximately 2 years of age. After age 2, a size 2 straight or curved blade may be used; and after age 12, a size 3 straight or curved blade is appropriate.

Blind nasotracheal intubation is not recommended in infants or children because of the small tube size and low success rate. The relatively anterosuperior position of the larynx and the sharp pharyngolaryngeal angle contribute to the poor frequency of success. There is also a greater risk of bleeding and avulsion of the large, friable adenoids and the loose fragile mucosa with nasotracheal intubation in infants and children. Transtracheal jet ventilation is preferred to cricothyrotomy in children because cricothyrotomy is difficult and carries an increased complication rate in pediatric patients.

DISPOSITION

Patients who require definitive airway management in the prehospital setting or the emergency department usually require admission to an intensive care unit. A possible exception is the patient who presents with decreased mental status from intoxication with alcohol or another short-acting central nervous system depressant, is intubated for gastric lavage, and awakens in the emergency department. If the emergency department is staffed to allow prolonged observation, such a patient may be extubated and then observed for at least 6 to 8 hours for deterioration of mental status

or signs of airway complications, such as laryngeal edema or aspiration. It is extremely rare to discharge a patient who has required active airway management.

All intubated patients must have their airway reassessed before transfer from the emergency department. Because endotracheal tubes frequently move during transport, tube placement must be confirmed before and after moving any patient (e.g., stretcher to bed).

FINAL POINTS

- Airway assessment and management have priority over all other aspects of resuscitation and, when performed well, save more lives than any other single intervention.
- Manual airway maneuvers (chin-lift, jaw-thrust), basic airway devices (nasopharyngeal airway, oropharyngeal airway) and bag-valve masks can be used to rapidly temporize oxygenation and ventilation while preparation for definitive airway intervention is accomplished or its need is determined.
- Establishing airway patency and protection, while securing oxygenation and ventilation are the primary reasons for airway management. The ability to medicate through an endotracheal tube and suction secretions are other important reasons.
- Unless immediate intubation is required, appropriate thought is necessary before determining the method of airway control. The potential risks and benefits of the various techniques (RSI, oral awake, nasotracheal) should

be considered as they apply to each individual patient.

- The oral awake method should be considered in all patients in whom internal airway anatomy is questionable.
- RSI is not attempted unless a patient's external (and anticipated internal) anatomy is highly predictive of successful intubation.
- Nasotracheal intubation is most helpful when external anatomy predictors are poor but internal anatomy is expected to be good.

- Confirmation of endotracheal tube placement is best accomplished by combining continuous oxygen saturation monitoring with either the esophageal detector device or an end-tidal CO_2 measurement.
- When doubt exists as to whether definitive airway intervention is indicated, the correct decision invariably will be the more aggressive. (When in doubt, intubate.)

CASE *Study*

The 8-year-old who fell while escaping a house fire arrived at the emergency department, fully immobilized, on a 100% non-rebreather mask. Two large-bore peripheral intravenous lines had been established, and she was spontaneously breathing with an oxygen saturation of 100%. She only responded to painful stimuli and had no gag reflex.

Because of her altered mental status and the absence of a gag reflex, she clearly required a definitive airway to protect against aspiration. However, she was spontaneously oxygenating and ventilating and the "immediate technique" of airway control was not indicated. Therefore, a moment was taken to consider the optimal approach to the control of her airway.

She was hypertensive and bradycardiac. Examination of her head and neck found that she had considerable contusion and abrasion of her left temple. Her right pupil was normal, but her left pupil was dilated and sluggish to react. She had no evidence of facial burns, singeing of facial hair, oropharyngeal burns, or carbonaceous sputum.

She had suffered a head injury. There was concern that she may have intracranial hypertension and be at increased risk during the process of intubation. Her pupillary findings and the fact that she was hypertensive and bradycardiac (Cushing's response) indicated that she was suffering from significant elevated intracranial pressure and was beginning to herniate. It was decided that RSI would be the safest way to intubate her because it would mitigate a significant rise in intracranial pressure during the procedure. Her external airway anatomy was evaluated and was found to be predictive of successful intubation. However, because questionable internal anatomy (airway burns in this case) is a contraindication to the use of RSI, care was taken to ensure no evidence of facial or oropharyngeal burns existed.

She was preoxygenated with 100% oxygen for 3 minutes while equipment was assembled and checked. Preoxygenation continued as she was premedicated with lidocaine, fentanyl, and vecuronium. Atropine was brought to the bedside. These premedication drugs were allowed to circulate for 2 minutes, induction was performed, and she was paralyzed with etomidate and succinylcholine.

She was preoxygenated a total of 5 minutes to maximize her apneic desaturation time, and the premedication was given 2 minutes before induction to ensure adequate circulation. Lidocaine was used to blunt the direct intracranial pressure response to intubation, fentanyl was used to blunt the hemodynamic intracranial response to intubation, and vecuronium was used to prevent fasciculation-induced intracranial hypertension. Atropine was made immediately available because children in this age-group occasionally have a dramatic bradycardiac response to laryngoscopy. Etomidate was selected as the induction agent because it does not elevate intracranial pressure, and succinylcholine was used to minimize the window of partial paralysis because emesis during this time period would undoubtedly result in significant aspiration.

No fasciculations occurred, and the patient was allowed to become apneic without positive-pressure ventilation. One minute after induction the physician checked the laxity of her jaw and laryngoscopy proceeded. She was then intubated with a No. 3 curved blade and a 6.0-mm endotracheal tube.

Because she had received vecuronium, fasciculations were not expected. Positive-pressure ventilation was avoided to minimize the risk of inducing emesis during partial paralysis. A 6.0-mm tube was chosen according to the equation 4 + 1/4 (age).

Continued on following page

Intubation was confirmed by visualization of the tube going through the cords, a persistent high oxygen saturation, end-tidal CO_2 detector, and, eventually, a chest radiograph. Immediately after intubation, she was paralyzed and completely sedated with vecuronium and midazolam.

Several methods were used to confirm placement of the tube because any single method can be misleading. She was promptly sedated and paralyzed so that she would not awaken, cough on the tube, and suffer a secondary increase in intracranial pressure.

Computed tomography of the head confirmed a left epidural hematoma as her most significant intracranial injury, and she was transferred to the operating room for definitive treatment. Endotracheal tube placement was checked before and after transfer. Her epidural hematoma was drained, and she was extubated the following morning in the intensive care unit. She was eventually discharged from the hospital and experienced a complete recovery.

Bibliography

TEXTS

Dailey RH, Simon B, Young GP, Stewart ED: The Airway: Emergency Management. St. Louis, Mosby–Yearbook, 1992.

Roberts J: Clinical Management of the Airway. Philadelphia, WB Saunders, 1994.

Walls R: Manual of Emergency Airway Management. Philadelphia, Lippincott Williams & Wilkins, 2000.

JOURNAL ARTICLES

Effros RM, Jacobs ER, Schapira RM, Biller J: Response of the lungs to aspiration. Am J Med 2000; 108(Suppl 4a):15S–19S.

Falk JL, Sayre MR: Confirmation of airway placement. Prehosp Emerg Care 1999; 3:273–278.

Gerardi MJ, Sacchetti AD, Cantor RM, et al: Rapid-sequence intubation of the pediatric patient. Pediatric Emergency Medicine Committee of the American College of Emergency Physicians. Ann Emerg Med 1996; 18:55–74.

Kharasch M, Graff J: Emergency management of the airway. Crit Care Clin 1995; 11:53–66.

Orebaugh SL: Succinylcholine: Adverse effects and alternatives in emergency medicine. Am J Emerg 1999; 17:715–721.

Orebaugh SL: Difficult airway management in the emergency department. J Emerg Med 2002; 22:31–48.

Reardon RF, Martel M: The intubating laryngeal mask airway: suggestions for use in the emergency department. Acad Emerg Med 2001; 8:833–838.

Silber SH: Rapid sequence intubation in adults with elevated intracranial pressure: A survey of emergency medicine residency programs. Am J Emerg Med 1997; 15:263–267.

Simon B, Young GP: Emergency airway management. Acad Emerg Med 1994; 1:154–157.

Tobias JD: Airway management for pediatric emergencies. Pediatr Ann 1996; 25:317–320.

Tobias JD: The laryngeal mask airway: A review for the emergency physician. Pediatr Emerg Care 1996; 12:370–373.

Walls RM: Management of the difficult airway in the trauma patient. Emerg Med Clin North Am 1998; 16:45–61.

Walls RM, Gurr DE, Kulkarni RG, et al: 6294 emergency department intubations: second report of the ongoing National Emergency Airway Registry (NEAR) II Study. Ann Emerg Med 2000; 36:551.

CHAPTER 3

Cardiopulmonary Cerebral Resuscitation

TIMOTHY G. JANZ

CASE *Study*

A 60-year-old man with a past history of angina developed severe substernal chest pain associated with dyspnea and diaphoresis. He asked his wife to call the rescue squad. When the paramedics arrived 10 minutes later he was unresponsive, pulseless, and apneic.

INTRODUCTION

The emergency physician must be prepared to treat cardiac arrest in an organized manner. Well-accepted principles have been established through the Basic and Advanced Cardiac Life Support (BLS and ACLS) programs developed by the American Heart Association. The goal of these programs is to save hearts and minds "too good to die."

Cardiopulmonary arrest is the preterminal event in more than 600,000 "out-of-hospital" deaths in the United States. More than 200,000 people in the United States die annually of coronary heart disease before they reach a hospital. Although cardiopulmonary cerebral resuscitation (CPCR) of all cardiac arrest patients is not possible or ethical, a number of patients may return to a normal life if they are treated quickly and correctly. Most cardiac arrest patients seen in the emergency department are victims of "sudden cardiac death." This is usually an ischemia- or dysrhythmia-based event that occurs with little or no prodrome. Before the widespread use of external cardiopulmonary resuscitation (CPR) and the development of emergency medical services, such an event frequently resulted in death.

The "chain of survival" represents four closely linked steps that improve the arrest victim's chance for survival. They are rapid access (911 system/hospital code team), rapid CPR (bystander/medical professional training), rapid defibrillation (automatic external defibrillators, implantable defibrillators), and rapid advanced care (airway management and medications).

Currently, 15% to 30% of all sudden cardiac death patients are resuscitated in the field or the emergency department. Ten percent to 15% of these patients are discharged from the hospital functionally intact. After initial resuscitation, central nervous system impairment remains the greatest cause of morbidity and mortality. The public's expectations of survival after CPR are unrealistic in terms of successful recovery.

The most important factor determining the chance of survival to discharge is the time that elapses from cardiac arrest until restoration of adequate perfusion. Basic CPR started within 4 minutes can result in a survival rate of up to 40% as opposed to a 6% survival rate if it is delayed to 8 minutes. Early advanced cardiac life support, particularly the ability to defibrillate, has a similar influence on outcome. Rates of survival to hospital discharge of up to 70% have been reported for patients who receive their first defibrillation within 3 minutes of collapse.

The many pathophysiologic causes of cardiac arrest can be divided into three general categories. These categories may be linked to one another, and each should be considered while CPCR is being initiated. Ischemic cardiovascular disease remains the most common cause in adults by far.

1. Electrical or conduction failure
   a. Primary dysrhythmia
   b. Electrocution
2. Decrease in myocardial oxygen/substrate delivery
   a. Decreased flow (e.g., coronary artery thrombosis, cardiac tamponade, tension pneumothorax, pulmonary embolus, hypovolemia)
   b. Decreased oxygen content (e.g., low hemoglobin, hypoxemia, drowning, asphyxia, airway obstruction)
   c. Hypoglycemia
3. Myocardial toxicity
   a. Electrolyte abnormalities (e.g., hyperkalemia or hypokalemia, hypocalcemia)
   b. Drug-induced (e.g., tricyclic antidepressant, propranolol, digitalis)

The most common dysrhythmia presenting as prehospital cardiac arrest is ventricular fibrillation. It occurs in one half of the cases, followed in frequency by bradysystole/asystole, pulseless electrical activity, and ventricular tachycardia. Ventricular tachycardia has the best prognosis (Table 3–1).

Neurologic sequelae in cardiac arrest survivors also correlate with the length of arrest. Recovery of good neurologic function becomes increasingly less likely with longer arrest time (more than 6 minutes) and CPR time (more than 30 minutes).

A major concern in current treatment is the marginal cerebral and coronary blood flow provided by standard external CPR techniques. It averages 15% to 20% of normal cardiac output. Even under optimal conditions, cardiac output and cerebral blood flow are usually less than 30% of normal. With prolonged CPR, this flow may decrease to near zero.

INITIAL APPROACH AND STABILIZATION

The cardiac arrest patient in the emergency department is initially managed by a team approach. The team may include physicians, nurses, electrocardiography and radiology technicians, and respiratory therapy personnel. Members of the team and supplies are mobilized to provide immediate and continued ACLS therapy when the patient arrives.

Prehospital Care

Because the opportunity for successful resuscitation is time dependent, intervening at the scene may be lifesaving. The extent of therapy depends on the training level of responders. Defibrillation, endotracheal airway management, intravenous access, and use of cardiac drugs are part of the paramedic on-scene capability. Faster emergency medical services response is associated with better outcomes. Basic life support, by bystanders or emergency medical technicians, even simple chest compressions alone, has demonstrated benefit in increased survival and quality of life at 1 year. When ventricular fibrillation is discovered, early defibrillation by prehospital care responders

at the scene is the most important priority. Emergency medical technicians having the ability to defibrillate and nonparamedic personnel using automatic defibrillators may allow the widespread use of early defibrillation. Automatic external defibrillators have demonstrated similar effectiveness as standard defibrillators. They are sophisticated, computerized devices that are able to reliably analyze the cardiac rhythm and, when appropriate, deliver defibrillatory countershocks.

Beyond the initial therapy, field care is limited by the need for rapid transport to the hospital. The emergency physician should expect the following information to be given during the initial contact with prehospital care providers:

1. Status of the airway—is the patient intubated or not?
2. Vital signs including presence of pulse or blood pressure
3. Cardiac rhythm determined by cardiac monitor or "quick look" paddles
4. Therapy given and response to therapy
5. Other significant findings: skin color, pupillary size and reflexes, mental or motor status
6. Briefly, events preceding arrest that may give a clue to the cause
7. Estimated time the patient was pulseless and apneic and the time of resuscitation. Was the patient's collapse witnessed?
8. Estimated time of arrival

Treatment orders are given depending on this information. Prehospital personnel are encouraged to follow BLS or ACLS protocols for cardiac arrest while rapidly transporting the patient to the emergency department. The emergency department staff is notified of the anticipated arrival.

Preparation

Once notified of an incoming cardiac arrest patient, the staff prepares immediately. Equipment and supplies for (1) airway management, (2) defibrillation, (3) cardiac drugs, and (4) intravenous access are readied in the resuscitation area. Establishing a "team approach" mindset in those participating in the resuscitation greatly facilitates a quiet, efficient, well-run "code." Individual assignments are made before the patient's arrival, such as airway management and chest compression. One physician is designated as the team leader, who directs, monitors, and oversees the resuscitation.

A "code" or "crash" cart containing most drugs and supplies is brought to the bedside (Table 3–2). In addition to airway equipment and emergency drugs, this cart contains intravenous

---

TABLE 3–1. Prognosis of Presenting Cardiac Arrest Rhythms

Rhythm	Predicted Survival to Hospital Discharge
Ventricular tachycardia	66%–76%
Ventricular fibrillation	10%–25%
Asystole and pulseless electrical activity	0%–2%

TABLE 3–2. Standard Elements in Crash Cart Airway Equipment at Bedside

Equipment and Supplies

Endotracheal tubes—multiple sizes from 6.0 to 9.0 mm internal diameter	Lubricating gel
Laryngoscope with curved and straight blades	Tape for securing tube
Stylet	Lidocaine (topical)
Oxygen—high-flow	Oral and nasal airways
Ambu bag and mask	Needle cricothyrotomy setup
Suction with dental tip	Cricothyrotomy setup

Emergency Drugs (standard packaging)

Adenosine (syringe), 6 mg	Lidocaine (syringe), 100 mg/5 mL
Atropine (syringe), 1 g/10 mL	Lidocaine (bag), 2 g/500 mL
Amiodarone (vial), 150 mg	Magnesium sulfate
Bretylium (ampule), 500 mg	Midazolam (vial), 2 mg or 10 mg/2 mL
Calcium chloride (syringe), 1 g/10 mL	Naloxone (ampule), 0.4 mg/1 mL
Dextrose 50% (syringe)	Phenytoin (vial), 100 mg/2 mL
Diazepam (vial), 10 mg/2 mL	Procainamide, 1000 mg/10 mL
Dopamine (bag), 500 mg/250 mL	Sodium bicarbonate, 50 mEq/50 mL
Dobutamine (bag), 400 mg/250 mL	Normal saline, 30-mL vial
Diphenhydramine, 50 mg/1 mL	Vasopressin, 40 IU/mL
Epinephrine (syringe), 1 mg/10 mL	Verapamil, 5 mg/2 mL
Furosemide (vial), 100 mg	Norepinephrine, 4 mg/ampule
Heparin flush (vial), 100 mg/5 mL	Nitroglycerin, 50 mg/250 mL
Isoproterenol (ampule), 1 mg	

---

catheters and supplies, needles, syringes, blood gas kits, pericardiocentesis needles, and electrocardiographic and transcutaneous pacemaker pads.

Airway. Airway management equipment is made available at the bedside. Oxygen tubing is attached to the oxygen wall outlet on one end, and the Ambu bag is attached on the other end. The endotracheal tube is prepared, the balloon tested, a stylet placed in the tube, and the laryngoscope checked. The Ambu bag and mask are placed at the head of the bed with high-flow oxygen turned on. Suction equipment is turned on, and the suction tip is placed at the head of the bed.

Defibrillation. The defibrillator is turned on at the bedside; contact pads or paste is made readily available. Cardiac monitoring with the defibrillator display monitor allows rapid selection of defibrillation, cardioversion, or external pacing. Special large pads (8 to 10 cm) are applied on the anterior and posterior thorax if external pacing is necessary.

Cardiac Drugs. Selected emergency and cardiac drugs are identified on the "code" cart (see Table 3–2). Drug dosing guidelines including concentrations for mixing continuous intravenous infusions must be memorized or readily available.

Intravenous Access. Peripheral and central intravenous lines and materials are prepared. Optimally, during cardiac arrest, drugs are given centrally. Several studies have demonstrated that drugs appear centrally faster and reach higher peak levels when they are administered through a central line compared with a peripheral line. This advantage is tempered by the time delay and difficulties often encountered in obtaining central access.

Radiology, electrocardiography, and respiratory therapy personnel are notified. In a trauma-related cardiac arrest, the surgery department and the blood bank are also notified.

While anticipating the patient's arrival, the priority diagnosis noted earlier must be reviewed. Is this potentially electrical or conduction failure, a decrease in myocardial oxygen or substrate delivery, or myocardial toxicity? A broad differential diagnosis must be maintained. Following the mechanics, algorithms, and patterns of CPR are essential, but they must be combined with a continued search for the underlying cause.

On Arrival

First, the cardiac rhythm is determined from the cardiac monitor or the "quick-look" option through the defibrillator paddles. If the patient's rhythm is ventricular fibrillation or pulseless ventricular tachycardia, immediate defibrillation is performed. The sooner the defibrillation, the better the chance of survival. Three shocks are sequenced in rapid order at 200 J, 300 J, or 360 J, depending on the rhythm response to defibrillation. Conducting gel or pads are important to deliver maximum electricity to an arrested heart.

If the patient is pulseless, external cardiac massage is begun. If a spontaneous pulse is palpable, a blood pressure measurement is obtained. The pulse is continuously checked, and chest compressions are reinstituted if a spontaneous pulse is lost. Use of a portable Doppler device may add to the accuracy of pulse detection. A spontaneously pumping heart generating a palpable pulse supplies better perfusion than external CPR.

If the patient is not intubated, the oropharynx is suctioned of debris, the airway is opened using a jaw-thrust maneuver, and the lungs are ventilated with 100% oxygen by bag-mask or mouth-to-mask techniques. Noting the anterior chest wall rise and listening for symmetric breath sounds checks the effectiveness of the ventilatory effort.

The patient is orotracheally intubated if initial defibrillation attempts fail or if the patient has an unprotected airway. Rapid sequence intubation (RSI) techniques are applied as necessary and appropriate. The laryngeal mask airway (LMA), intubating LMA (ILMA), or esophageal-tracheal combitube may be useful in the patients with a difficult or failed airway (see Chapter 2, Airway Management). If the patient was intubated in the field, location of the endotracheal tube must be confirmed. The endotracheal tube can dislodge into the esophagus or right mainstem bronchus during transport. To confirm tube placement, breath sounds are auscultated over both lung fields and the stomach. The chest wall is observed for symmetric expansion during ventilation. Esophageal detection with bulb or syringe aspiration is recommended in pulseless patients. If proper endotracheal tube placement is in question, tube placement between the vocal cords is visualized with the laryngoscope. Adequacy of the airway and ventilation is assessed serially throughout the resuscitation. In patients presenting with a pulse, tube placement may be assessed by end-tidal CO_2 measurement. The physician should be familiar with the known pitfalls of field resuscitation (e.g., right mainstem bronchial intubation, esophageal intubation, and rib fractures resulting in tension pneumothorax or hemothorax). Checking for these complications is an important part of the initial assessment after ACLS has been initiated in the field.

CLINICAL ASSESSMENT

Once the airway, pulse, blood pressure, and cardiac rhythm are addressed, a brief history is taken (if possible) and the physical examination is completed.

History

The initial source of the history is usually the rescue personnel. The following questions are asked:

1. What were the *events surrounding* the *cardiac arrest?* Was it witnessed or unwitnessed?
2. What was the *estimated time since* the *arrest* and initiating CPR?
3. What was the *estimated duration* of *CPR?*
4. What was the *initial rhythm?*
5. What *airway intervention* was performed?
6. Was *defibrillation* performed? If so, how many times and at what energy level?
7. What *drug therapy* was given?
8. Was *restoration* of *blood pressure* or *pulse* achieved? Even temporarily?
9. What has been the *mental status* of the patient *throughout* the resuscitation?
10. What is the *past medical history* including medical problems, medications, and allergies?
11. Are there prescriptions, physician cards, or *medical identification* bracelets available?

Answers to these questions will assist in determining any reversible causes and the need for additional therapy.

The physician should be notified when the patient's family arrives. Family members need to have their fears addressed, and they can supply valuable information concerning the patient's past problems and the events preceding the cardiac arrest. If it is not possible for the senior physician to leave the bedside, another medical person should talk briefly with the family. During this first contact it is necessary to communicate the critical nature of the patient's problem and establish the basis for the next visit after the resuscitative effort.

Physical Examination

Once CPR is begun, the physical examination is brief and has two objectives. The first is to find signs suggesting or indicating the cause of the cardiac arrest. A careful observation of the patient may provide additional clues to the patient's pre-arrest medical problems. For example, the presence of an arteriovenous fistula may suggest renal failure with complicating hyperkalemia. The second objective is to assess the effectiveness of cardiac arrest therapy and possible complications. Table 3–3 outlines the directed physical examination during cardiac arrest. This examination is repeated every 5 to 10 minutes throughout the

TABLE 3–3. Directed Physical Examination during Cardiac Arrest

Physical Examination	Abnormalities with Possible Diagnoses/Comments
General appearance	Pallor; evidence of trauma or blood loss, emaciation, or tumor
	Hypovolemic arrest
	Possible cancer patient
Vital signs	Serial assessment of heart rate, pulse (consider Doppler), respiratory effort, and, early in care, core temperature
Airway	Secretions, vomitus or blood, stridor, resistance to ventilation
	Airway obstruction leading to respiratory arrest or hypoxia, tension pneumothorax
Neck	Distended neck veins, deviated trachea
	Cardiac tamponade, tension pneumothorax
Lungs	Unilateral breath sounds, rales, bronchi, wheezing

resuscitation effort, or as indicated by a change in patient status or a new intervention.

CLINICAL REASONING

Two questions need to be addressed in any cardiopulmonary arrest situation.

What Is the Immediate Rhythm Disturbance Associated with the Cardiopulmonary Arrest?

Establishing the rhythm disturbance is critical for administering appropriate care. The most frequently found initial rhythms are ventricular fibrillation (45%), asystole (30%), and pulseless electrical activity (10%). Although basic life support is instituted in all arrests, definitive treatment differs according to the rhythm disturbance present. An excellent example is the classic "sine wave" ECG pattern associated with significant hyperkalemia. This pattern requires specific treatment (calcium) that would usually not be given if the rhythm were not recognized. Knowledge of the rhythm may also be helpful in determining the origin of the arrest. For instance, pulseless electrical activity often has a different cause than a bradydysrhythmia.

What Is the Most Likely Underlying Cause of the Cardiopulmonary Arrest?

Of the estimated 1000 cardiac arrests that occur per day in the United States, approximately half are cardiovascular in origin. Underlying ischemic heart disease accounts for two thirds of these arrests. Another major cause of cardiopulmonary arrest is hypoxia, which results in dysrhythmias, myocardial ischemia, and eventual infarction. Hypoxia may be the result of alveolar hypoventilation, upper airway obstruction, or any severe

parenchymal lung disease. Lethal dysrhythmias are also associated with severe acid-base disorders, electrolyte abnormalities, hypoglycemia, and drugs or toxins (Table 3–4).

DIAGNOSTIC ADJUNCTS

Electrocardiogram

The electrocardiogram (ECG) and cardiac monitoring are the most useful tests performed in patients with cardiac arrest. Continuous electrocardiographic monitoring is maintained during the resuscitation. Lead II or a modified V_1 lead is usually used to identify the underlying rhythm disturbance. A 12-lead ECG is mandatory after all successful resuscitations.

Acute myocardial infarction occurs in an estimated 20% of patients with cardiac arrest and may manifest as ST segment elevation, inverted T waves, or Q waves. The ECG can be useful in patients with noncardiac causes of cardiac arrest as well. For example, prominent U waves are often associated with hypokalemia, and large peaked T waves, prolonged PR intervals and QRS complexes, loss of P waves, and a sine wave configuration of the QRS complex are associated with significant hyperkalemia. Findings compatible with hyperkalemia should suggest a presumptive diagnosis of renal failure.

On rare occasions, ventricular fibrillation can present in some leads with small undulations or may even masquerade as asystole. In apparent asystole, more than one lead is interpreted to exclude the presence of fine ventricular fibrillation.

Laboratory Studies

Arterial Blood Gases. Arterial blood gas measurements are obtained as quickly as possible in an arrest situation and are used to monitor the patient's oxygenation and acid-base status. Although arterial blood gases are preferred,

TABLE 3–4. Common Causes of Cardiopulmonary Arrest

Immediate Cause	Associated Disease	Comments
Cardiac etiology	Ischemic heart disease, cardiomyopathies, hypertensive heart disease, valvular heart disease, intrinsic rhythm disturbances, circulatory shock or hypovolemia	Two thirds of cardiopulmonary arrests from primary cardiac disorders are due to ischemic heart disease; acute myocardial infarction accounts for only 25% of cardiac-related arrests; 20% of ischemic heart disease patients will have cardiac arrest as their initial presentation; circulatory shock and hypovolemia are always included in the differential diagnosis of pulseless electrical activity.
Alveolar hypoventilation	Central nervous system disease, head trauma, neuromuscular disease (e.g., Guillain-Barré syndrome, myasthenia gravis), drugs (narcotics, sedatives), metabolic encephalopathies (e.g., hepatic, uremic)	Any pulmonary disease is capable of causing a cardiopulmonary arrest; however, the common denominator is severe hypoxemia.
Upper airway obstruction	Foreign body, infection, trauma, neoplasm	The most common causes of upper airway obstruction in adults are foreign body aspiration and neoplasms; in children, foreign body aspiration and infection (epiglottitis/croup) are the most common causes.
Lung disease	Asthma, chronic obstructive pulmonary disease, pneumonia, pulmonary edema, pulmonary embolus, combinations	Primary lung disease, chronic obstructive pulmonary disease, and pneumonia are the most common causes of pulmonary origin cardiac arrest.
Electrolyte/glucose abnormalities	Hypokalemia, hyperkalemia, hypomagnesemia, hypocalcemia, hyper/hypoglycemia	Ventricular dysrhythmias are the most frequent rhythm disturbances associated with electrolyte abnormalities; renal failure is often associated with hyperkalemia or hypocalcemia and is prone to ventricular dysrhythmias.
Drugs and toxins	Digitalis, antidysrhythmics (e.g., quinidine, procainamide, encainide, flecainide); tricyclic antidepressants, cocaine, carbon monoxide	The most common drugs associated with lethal dysrhythmias are cardiovascular agents. Especially common are digitalis toxicity and quinidine. Currently, cocaine is the drug most commonly associated with life-threatening rhythm disorders.
Other	Lightning or electrical injuries, drowning or near-drowning, autonomic dysfunction, hypothermia	These are unusual causes of cardiopulmonary arrest. The clinical setting often suggests their involvement.

venous blood gases obtained during external cardiac compression can also be useful as a rough approximation of acid-base balance but not oxygenation. The role of arterial pH determination has been questioned because it does not seem to predict the degree of tissue acidosis or the success of resuscitation efforts. In addition, $PaCO_2$ may not be a good representation of tissue or cellular carbon dioxide levels. Central venous or mixed venous blood samples may correlate better with tissue pH and carbon dioxide levels and may be better predictors of the resuscitation outcome. At present, arterial blood gas analysis continues to be part of the serial monitoring of resuscitation efforts during a cardiac arrest situation.

Electrolytes/Glucose. The serum potassium level is valuable to measure early in the arrest.

Although it is usually determined from serum, it can be measured from plasma. Plasma levels do not require clot formation; and if the determination is prearranged with the laboratory, the turn-around time is less than 5 minutes. A plasma potassium level requires a heparinized blood sample (green top tube). It is 0.35 to 0.5 mEq/L lower than a serum potassium level and is more accurate. Plasma potassium is not affected by potassium release during platelet activation and clot formation and is most useful in the setting of severe thrombocytosis. A serum potassium level can also be determined from arterial blood samples; however, it may be as much as 1.1 mEq/L lower than that from a venous sample. The presence of hyperkalemia and presumptive renal failure warrants specific therapy and determining serum creatinine and blood urea nitrogen levels. Bedside blood glucose test strip measurement is generally performed early in the resuscitation.

Toxicology Studies and Drug Levels. If the situation dictates, toxicology studies or serum concentrations of therapeutic agents may be useful in making a presumptive diagnosis. However, results may take hours to days to complete and cannot be relied on during the arrest.

Radiographic Imaging

Chest radiographs can be useful in establishing a definitive diagnosis in a patient with cardiac arrest associated with a respiratory disease and in confirming the placement of the endotracheal tube and central venous catheter. Because of the time involved in acquiring chest radiographs, they are not useful in the immediate resuscitation period and are rarely used to diagnose acute tension pneumothorax or cardiac tamponade before instituting treatment. Optimally, these diagnoses are based on physical assessment and response to intervention rather than on radiographic studies.

Ultrasonography may have benefit in the cardiac arrest patient. In the patient with pulseless electric activity, it can rapidly diagnose pericardial tamponade, assess ventricular filling, and determine cardiac contractile activity. It may be useful in differentiating asystole from ventricular fibrillation. The value of ultrasound is ultimately dependent on the skill of the operator.

EXPANDED DIFFERENTIAL DIAGNOSIS

After the initial rhythm disturbance is identified and the history, physical assessment, and basic diagnostic studies are completed, a more definitive diagnosis can be determined. The history is often very useful in establishing a presumptive cause. The past medical history and a listing of current medications from the family or paramedics can support or suggest an underlying disease process (Table 3–5). For instance, a past history of hypertension, diabetes mellitus, and hypercholesterolemia or the use of nitrates, β blockers, or calcium channel blockers should raise the suspicion of ischemic heart disease as the underlying cause of the arrest. Severe hypoxia of pulmonary origin resulting in cardiac arrest is usually associated with serious or advanced lung disease. Hypokalemia, hyperkalemia, hypomagnesemia, and hypocalcemia can each result in ventricular dysrhythmias. A clinical situation in which ventricular dysrhythmias are particularly likely to occur is renal failure associated with hyperkalemia and hypocalcemia.

Nontraumatic cardiac arrest in a young or middle-aged individual always raises the suspicion of drug ingestion until another cause has been proved. Cocaine is a common drug of abuse that can induce hypertension, acute myocardial ischemia or infarction, and various cardiac dysrhythmias, including ventricular tachycardia, ventricular fibrillation, and asystole (see Chapter 15, The Poisoned Patient).

PRINCIPLES OF MANAGEMENT

Management of cardiac arrest is centered on five principles. A sixth principle will apply if the resuscitation attempt is unsuccessful.

Principle I: The Underlying Cardiac Arrest Rhythm Determines the Initial Therapy

In 2000 the American Heart Association updated the suggested guidelines and algorithms for the therapy of cardiac arrest rhythms. Initial drug therapy is dependent on the underlying cardiac rhythm.

Ventricular fibrillation remains the most common underlying rhythm of cardiac arrest. The goal of therapy is to convert ventricular fibrillation (or pulseless ventricular tachycardia) rapidly to a stable and perfusing cardiac rhythm. Survivability from ventricular fibrillation decreases 7% to 10% per minute of delay in defibrillation. The conversion is done with electrical defibrillation because ventricular fibrillation rarely, if ever, spontaneously converts. Only after initial defibrillation attempts fail is epinephrine, and possibly vasopressin, administered and the patient's airway definitively managed (Fig. 3–1). In shock-resistant ventricular fibrillation, several drugs may be administered to convert the rhythm. Amiodarone has shown some improved survival rates compared with lidocaine usage in several studies. Countershock of ventricular fibrillation that results in asystole or pulseless electrical activity has as poor a prognosis as an initial asystole or pulseless electrical activity rhythm.

The clinical presentation of ventricular tachycardia varies from a hemodynamically stable rhythm to a pulseless "cardiac arrest" rhythm. The urgency of treatment is established based on the patient's mental status, pulse, and blood pressure (Fig. 3–2).

Bradydysrhythmias leading to asystole have a uniformly poor prognosis. Efforts to reestablish a spontaneous rhythm focus on the use of epinephrine, atropine, and adequate oxygenation. Atropine may enhance sinus node automaticity and atrioventricular conduction through its

---

TABLE 3–5. Expanded Differential Diagnosis of Cardiopulmonary Arrest

---

Cardiovascular Causes

Intrinsic dysrhythmias
Ventricular
Bradydysrhythmias
Sinus arrest
Second- or third-degree atrioventricular block
Ischemic heart disease
Angina
Myocardial infarction
Silent ischemia
Cardiomyopathies or congestive heart failure
Valvular heart disease

Hypertensive heart disease
Congenital heart disease
Circulatory shock/hypovolemia (hemorrhagic)
Gastrointestinal bleeding
Trauma
Anaphylaxis
Sepsis
Cardiogenic shock
Cardiac tamponade
Hypomagnesemia

Respiratory Causes

Tension pneumothorax
Pulmonary embolism
Hypoxia
Upper airway obstruction
Any serious parenchymal lung disease
Cor pulmonale

Severe acid-base abnormality
Thyroid disease
Thyroid storm
Myxedema coma

Metabolic Causes

Electrolyte abnormality
Hypokalemia
Hyperkalemia
Hyper/Hypoglycemia
Toxins
Drug overdose
Tricyclic antidepressants
Stimulants
Cocaine
Phencyclidine (PCP)
Amphetamines
Antihistamines
Central nervous system depressants

Cardiac medications
  Digitalis
  Antidysrhythmics
  Quinidine
  Procainamide
  Encainide
  Flecainide
  Beta blockers
  Calcium channel blockers
  Beta agonists or inotropic agents
  Catecholamines
  Amrinone

Other Causes

Lightning or electrical injuries
Drowning or near-drowning
Trauma

Autonomic dysfunction
Hypothermia

---

vagolytic activity. With the availability of external pacers, early pacing of patients with bradydysrhythmias can be accomplished in the prehospital setting. However, attempts to electrically pace patients presenting in asystole have had uniformly dismal results (Fig. 3–3).

Many disease processes present as pulseless electrical activity (Fig. 3–4). This rhythm has cardiac electrical activity without mechanical pumping, that is, a rhythm without a pulse (Table 3–6). Its prognosis is usually poor, with a 1% to 4% rate of survival to hospital discharge. Although most cardiopulmonary arrest is related to severe hypoxemia and subsequent lethal dysrhythmias, pulseless electrical activity may have one of four unique origins. Hypovolemic shock may present as cardiac arrest (hemorrhage secondary to gastroin-

testinal bleeding or trauma is the most common cause). Cardiac tamponade is often associated with hemorrhagic pericardial effusions related to trauma, neoplasms, uremia, or blood dyscrasias. Tension pneumothorax is typically traumatic or iatrogenic in origin (e.g., central line insertion, rib fracture during chest compression). Finally, large pulmonary embolus obstructing more than 50% to 60% of the pulmonary blood flow may present as pulseless electrical activity. In parallel with treating the rhythm, initial efforts in pulseless electrical activity are directed toward finding a reversible cause.

Therefore, in the setting of pulseless electrical activity, some therapeutic maneuvers may be diagnostic. Tension pneumothorax can be treated and diagnosed by a needle thoracostomy followed

Text continued on page 51

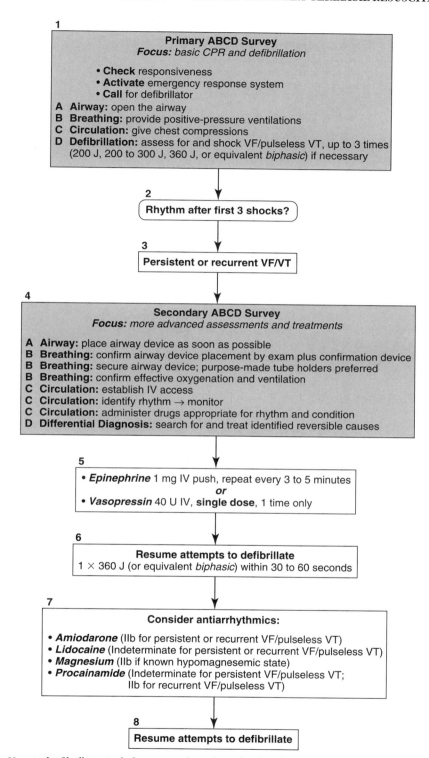

FIGURE 3–1 • Ventricular fibrillation/pulseless ventricular tachycardia algorithm. (Reproduced with permission from ACLS Provider Manual. ©2001, Copyright American Heart Association.)

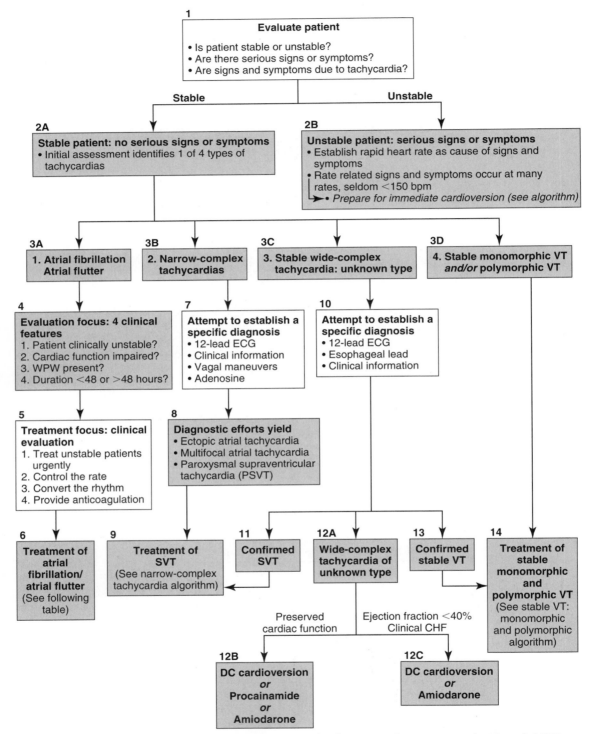

FIGURE 3–2 • The tachycardias: overview algorithm. (Reproduced with permission from ACLS Provider Manuarl. ©2001, Copyright American Heart Association.)

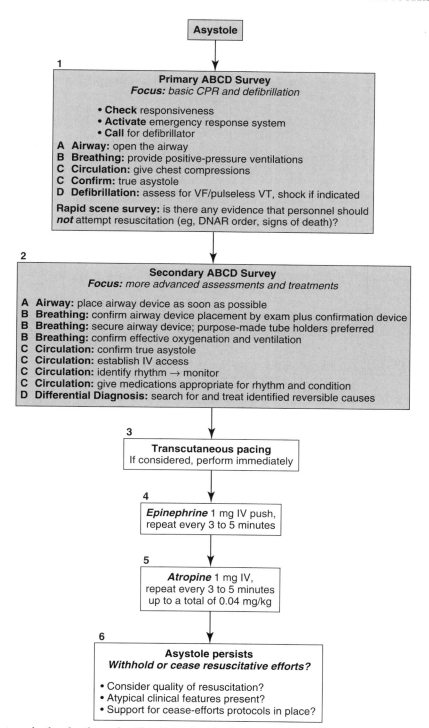

FIGURE 3–3 • Asystole: the silent heart algorithm.(Reproduced with permission from ACLS Provider Manual. ©2001, Copyright American Heart Association.)

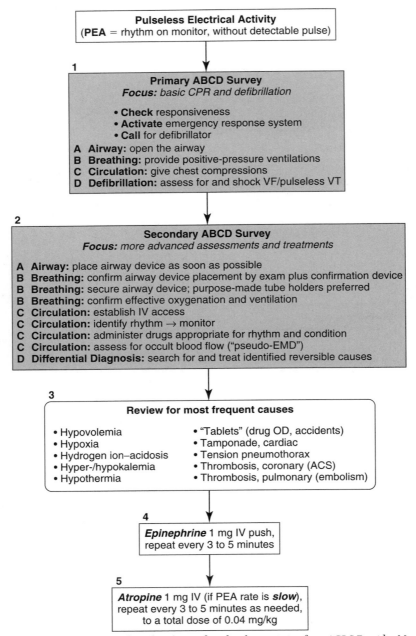

FIGURE 3–4 • Pulseless electrical activity algorithm. (Reproduced with permission from ACLS Provider Manual. ©2001, Copyright American Heart Association.)

TABLE 3–6. Differential Diagnosis of Pulseless Electrical Activity

Hypovolemic shock	Anaphylactic factors
Hemorrhagic causes	Toxigenic factors
Adrenal crisis	Dissecting thoracic aneurysm
Severe dehydration	Thoracic or abdominal aneurysm rupture
Obstructive shock	Severe hypoxia or acidosis
Pericardial tamponade	Cardiogenic shock
Massive pulmonary embolus	Severe left ventricular dysfunction
Tension pneumothorax	Left ventricular rupture
Distributive shock	Papillary muscle rupture
Septic factors	

by insertion of a chest tube. A 16- or 18-gauge needle is inserted into the anterior second or third intercostal space of the involved hemithorax. A rush of air from the needle on insertion is diagnostic of tension pneumothorax. The immediate treatment of cardiac tamponade is pericardiocentesis. Blood aspirated from the pericardial space is usually defibrinated and clots poorly. In addition, the removal of 10 to 20 mL of pericardial fluid may be associated with significant improvement in the cardiovascular status. This improved cardiac function directly related to pericardiocentesis is very suggestive of cardiac tamponade. A fluid challenge (e.g., bolus therapy of 300 to 500 mL normal saline) is also warranted in pulseless electrical activity. The development of palpable pulses after fluid administration strongly suggests hypovolemia as the underlying cause.

Principle II: Adequate Ventilation Rather Than Bicarbonate Is Critical for Early Acid-Base Management

Measurement of mixed venous gases probably reflects the tissue and cellular acid-base state better than arterial blood gases. Typically, they show a respiratory acidosis rather than a metabolic acidosis as the primary acid-base disorder early in cardiac arrest. Elevated $PaCO_2$ levels may worsen intracellular acidosis and cause further depression of myocardial and cerebral function. The administration of sodium bicarbonate may exacerbate the problem, owing to additional carbon dioxide being liberated when the hydrogen ions are buffered. Sodium bicarbonate administration may cause other detrimental effects, including hyperosmolality, hypernatremia, and a left shift of the oxyhemoglobin dissociation curve. Consequently, current recommendations place their emphasis on alveolar ventilation to control acidemia. Sodium bicarbonate administration may be indicated in hyperkalemia, prolonged arrest states, preexisting metabolic acidosis, and certain toxic states (i.e., tricyclic antidepressant overdose). End-tidal CO_2 monitors are recommended to indicate the adequacy of CPR and the likelihood of a successful resuscitation.

Principle III: To Perfuse the Heart, an Arteriovenous Pressure Gradient Must Exist Across the Heart

Perfusion of the heart depends on the coronary perfusion pressure. Experimentally, this pressure has been approximated as the mean arterial diastolic pressure minus the mean right atrial pressure. Animal studies suggest that a certain minimal coronary perfusion pressure is necessary to successfully resuscitate the fibrillating heart.

During cardiac arrest, external cardiac compression and the use of vasoconstrictive agents (e.g., epinephrine and vasopressin) facilitate both pressure and perfusion. It is the alpha effects of epinephrine that account for the potentially improved perfusion seen during CPR. During CPR the vasopressor activity seems to prevent vascular collapse, particularly of the intrathoracic vessels. In addition, vasoconstriction causes shunting of blood flow from less essential vascular beds.

Principle IV: The Cardiac Rhythm Can Frequently Change During Resuscitation

Throughout the resuscitation attempt there may be numerous dysrhythmias requiring intervention. After initial therapy, the cardiac rhythm must be continuously observed. After successful defibrillation, the patient's rhythm may degenerate back into ventricular fibrillation. If the patient is closely monitored, immediate repeat defibrillation has an improved chance of conversion. Bradydysrhythmias and heart blocks often occur during CPR (Fig. 3–5). Again, close cardiac monitoring is essential to guide therapy to prevent further ischemic injury. Degeneration of the cardiac rhythm to asystole is an ominous sign associated with a very poor recovery rate.

Principle V: An Organized Approach to Postresuscitative Care Is Indicated in All Cardiac Arrest Patients Who Are Successfully Resuscitated

The ideal resuscitation attempt results in an awake, responsive, and spontaneously breathing patient. More often, the patient is hemodynamically unstable, requires ventilatory support, and has an altered mental status. Correctly managing the immediate postresuscitative period is critical to the patient's survival.

Initial Assessment

All successfully resuscitated patients require a thorough repeat physical examination. In addition, ancillary studies usually include a 12-lead ECG, chest radiograph, arterial blood gas analysis, cardiac enzymes, electrolyte and renal panel, complete blood cell count, and determination of drug levels if appropriate. Particular attention is directed toward adequate oxygenation and ventilation, correcting existing acid-base and electrolyte abnormalities, and careful cardiovascular

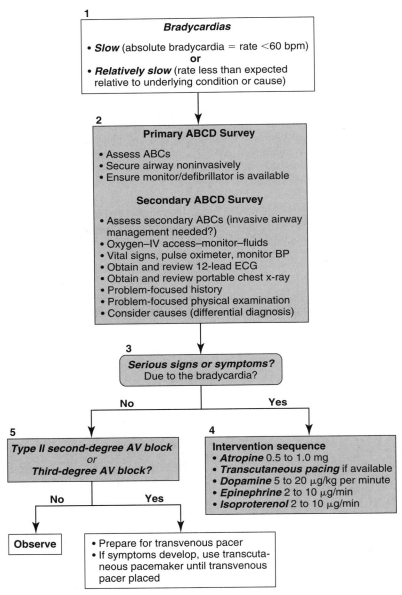

1

Bradycardias

• ***Slow*** (absolute bradycardia = rate <60 bpm)
or
• ***Relatively slow*** (rate less than expected relative to underlying condition or cause)

2

Primary ABCD Survey

• Assess ABCs
• Secure airway noninvasively
• Ensure monitor/defibrillator is available

Secondary ABCD Survey

• Assess secondary ABCs (invasive airway management needed?)
• Oxygen–IV access–monitor–fluids
• Vital signs, pulse oximeter, monitor BP
• Obtain and review 12-lead ECG
• Obtain and review portable chest x-ray
• Problem-focused history
• Problem-focused physical examination
• Consider causes (differential diagnosis)

3

Serious signs or symptoms?
Due to the bradycardia?

No   **Yes**

5

Type II second-degree AV block
or
Third-degree AV block?

4

Intervention sequence
• ***Atropine*** 0.5 to 1.0 mg
• ***Transcutaneous pacing*** if available
• ***Dopamine*** 5 to 20 μg/kg per minute
• ***Epinephrine*** 2 to 10 μg/min
• ***Isoproterenol*** 2 to 10 μg/min

No   **Yes**

Observe

• Prepare for transvenous pacer
• If symptoms develop, use transcutaneous pacemaker until transvenous pacer placed

FIGURE 3–5 • Bradycardia algorithm. (Reproduced with permission from ACLS Provider Manual. ©2001, Copyright American Heart Association.)

monitoring. Physical examination, end-tidal CO_2 monitoring, or air-aspiration devices reconfirm endotracheal tube placement. A chest radiograph is obtained to assess position of the endotracheal tube relative to the carina and evaluate for lung disease. Mechanical ventilation is initiated, if required. Adequacy of oxygenation can be determined with pulse oximetry, and ventilation is best assessed with frequent arterial blood gas determinations.

Dysrhythmia Management

Because dysrhythmias are a major cause of recurring cardiac arrest, continuous ECG monitoring and the standard 12-lead ECG are critical elements in postresuscitative care. All patients resuscitated from cardiac arrest caused by ventricular tachycardia or ventricular fibrillation are maintained on continuous antidysrhythmic therapy for a minimum of 24 to 36 hours.

Abnormal cardiac rhythms in the postresuscitation period are not uncommon. These may be bradydysrhythmias or tachydysrhythmias. Regardless of the abnormal rhythm, the approach to the patient remains the same. The presence of a pulse is sought. It the patient is pulseless, cardiopulmonary resuscitation is initiated. If a pulse is present, the blood pressure is determined. In addition to blood pressure, other signs and symptoms of cardiac stability are sought, such as chest pain, dyspnea, altered mental status, abnormal heart sounds, or abnormal lung sounds. The stability of the patient determines the approach to treatment. (See the bradycardia algorithm in Figure 3–5 and the tachycardia algorithm in Figure 3–2.)

If the initial arrest rhythm was ventricular fibrillation or tachycardia, parenteral antidysrhythmic medication (lidocaine or amiodarone) is usually administered prophylactically.

Hemodynamic Monitoring

Special attention is given to closely monitoring the status and stability of the cardiovascular system. Close attention to the patient's blood pressure and pulse rate is essential. Hypotension in the postresuscitation period is common and often requires the use of vasopressors (e.g., dopamine or norepinephrine). Although blood pressure control is very important, blood pressure is not necessarily a good indicator of cardiac function. Patients who remain hemodynamically unstable or vasopressor dependent may require invasive hemodynamic monitoring (i.e., intra-arterial catheterization and a pulmonary artery flow-directed catheter). Invasive hemodynamic monitoring can precisely and continuously assess the intravascular fluid status and cardiac function. The ability to accurately determine the pulmonary artery pressure, pulmonary artery wedge pressure, cardiac output, and systemic vascular resistance offers the physician more precise guidance in fluid administration as well as diuretic, vasopressor, inotropic, and vasodilator therapies.

Cerebral Resuscitation

Current research suggests some neuronal function may be preserved after 30 to 60 minutes of total anoxia. Unfortunately, a significant amount of brain damage may occur as blood flow is *reestablished* after resuscitation. This effect is called *reperfusion injury* and involves complex pathophysiologic processes combining hypoperfusion, local tissue acidosis, cytotoxic cerebral edema, mitochondrial dysfunction, and toxic oxygen free radical generation. In addition to the complex biochemical milieu established with anoxia and reperfusion, the immediate postresuscitation period is associated with reduced cerebral blood flow despite adequate systemic blood pressure. This response appears to be related to the vasoconstriction of the cerebral vasculature. Evidence suggests that abnormal calcium ion influx into the neuron may play a major role in reperfusion injury. A variety of therapeutic modalities have been suggested to reduce cerebral damage in the postresuscitation period. These include barbiturates, calcium channel blockers, oxygen free radical scavengers, phenytoin, prostaglandin inhibitors, hemodilution, hypothermia, and chelating agents. Much of this work remains experimental, but some important basic principles are included in Table 3–7. Mild hypothermia (32°C to 34°C) for 24 hours post cardiac arrest has shown some promise in improving neurologic outcome at 6 months after the event.

The most clinically relevant therapy is maintenance of an adequate systemic blood pressure and oxygenation. Cerebral anoxia is associated with loss of cerebral autoregulation, and cerebral blood flow is directly dependent on mean arterial pressure. Therefore, maintenance of adequate blood pressure and oxygenation is paramount during the postresuscitative period.

Principle VI: When to Stop CPR is a Difficult Decision; Some Guidelines Are Necessary

Resuscitative efforts beyond 30 minutes without a return of spontaneous circulation have a very poor prognosis. Exceptions include patients who are hypothermic, have been immersed in cold water, and may have overdosed, especially on barbiturates. A patient with intermittent ventricular fibrillation or ventricular tachycardia should continue to have prolonged resuscitation. Ultimately, quality of life projections remain critical in determining whether to continue CPR.

Patients with unwitnessed arrest, rhythms such as bradycardia, asystole or pulseless electrical activity, and pulselessness after 10 minutes generally do not survive. An attempt should be made to time cessation of CPR with family awareness of the events and the decision to stop resuscitative efforts.

SPECIAL CONSIDERATIONS
Pediatric Patients

Sudden death in a young person is rare. After the first year and through the third decade, the most

---

TABLE 3–7. Guidelines for Cerebral Stabilization During the Postresuscitation Period

---

Cardiovascular stabilization
Cellular or neuronal stabilization
Maintain normal blood pressure (mean arterial pressure = 70–90 mm Hg)
Normalize blood volume (CVP = 10–15 cm H_2O)
Use invasive hemodynamic monitoring in unstable states
Maintain adequate oxygen-carrying capacity (hemoglobin = 10–12 g/dL) and saturation ($SaO_2 >94\%$)
Elevate head of bed 10 to 30 degrees
Avoid hyperthermia (temperature > 100°F or 38°C)
Control or avoid seizures (diazepam, phenytoin, and barbiturates)
Metabolic stabilization (glucose, electrolytes)
Immobilization (neuromuscular paralysis), as needed
Sedation, as needed
Maintain:
    $PaO_2 \geq 80$–100 mm Hg (avoid pulmonary end-expiratory pressure)
    $PaCO_2 = 30$–35 mm Hg
    pH = 7.35–7.45
    Glucose = 100–250 mg/dL
    Serum osmolality = 280–320 mOsm/kg
Avoid hypoproteinemia (albumin <3.0 g/dL)
Medications to consider (primarily experimental):
    Calcium channel blockers (lidoflazine, nimodipine, flunarizine)*
    Toxic oxygen radical scavengers (superoxide dismutase, dimethyl sulfoxide, tocopherols)*
    Chelating agents (deferoxamine)*
    Prostaglandin inhibition (indomethacin)*
    Suppression of lactic acid production (dichloroacetate)*
    Amino acid antagonists*

Diagnostic Considerations:

Computed tomography
    Mass lesions
    Intracerebral hemorrhage
    Subarachnoid hemorrhage
Lumbar puncture
    Meningitis
    Subarachnoid hemorrhage
Electroencephalogram
    Subclinical seizure activity
Cerebral perfusion scan
    Certify brain death

---

*Experimental treatment.

---

common cardiac causes are myocarditis, hypertrophic cardiomyopathy, coronary artery disease or congenital anomalies, mitral valve prolapse, and aortic dissection. Several disorders may be identified in advance. Commotio cordia is a documented phenomenon of sudden death in young athletes caused by blunt nonpenetrating impact of modest intensity to the left chest. It has been witnessed in baseball, football, and hockey. The mechanism is thought to be the mechanical impact of the vulnerable portion of the cardiac conduction cycle resulting in heart block or ventricular fibrillation. Prevention through protection is essential, because the prognosis is generally poor.

Adult cardiopulmonary arrest is most commonly caused by cardiac disease. Pediatric arrest is more often the result of acute respiratory failure.

Attention to airway control and breathing is paramount in resuscitating the child. The approach to airway control and artificial ventilation is the same as that used in adults. Pediatric endotracheal intubation requires the same manipulative techniques on the part of the physician and adds requirements of calculation skills. The size in millimeters of the uncuffed endotracheal tube is based on age: 4 + age (years)/4. The depth of endotracheal tube placement is calculated at three times the size of the tube. To facilitate intubation, Miller size 0 blades are used in the newborn period, Miller size 1 blades are used until the child is 2 to 3 years old, and Miller size 2 blades are used after age 3. Intravenous access techniques for fluid and medications are appropriate in patients older than 6 years of age.

Another major difference in pediatric resuscitation concerns defibrillation and drug dosage based on the patient's weight. In the unusual circumstance that pediatric cardiopulmonary arrest requires defibrillation, the initial setting of the defibrillator is 2 J/kg and 4 J/kg if the initial defibrillation attempt is unsuccessful. Epinephrine, sodium bicarbonate, lidocaine, and bretylium are given in the same weight-adjusted doses as those used for adults. However, atropine is given as 0.02 mg/kg/dose and is repeated, but the dose must not exceed a total of 1 mg in the child (Table 3–8). In an arrest situation calculation errors can be reduced by the use of an emergency length-based system (Broselow tape). The tape provides correct drug dose amounts and proper-sized equipment that facilitate a resuscitative effort.

Elderly Patients

Two thirds of the sudden death victims in the United States are older than 65 years of age. Age has been demonstrated as a significant influence on patient, family, and physician attitudes about resuscitation efforts. There is evidence that age alone does not predict a poor outcome. Decisions to initiate or withhold resuscitation for cardiac arrest in the elderly should be based on patient preferences, disease prognosis, and the likelihood of success. This likelihood is negatively influenced by acute myocardial infarction precipitating the arrest, bradysystole or pulseless electrical activity as the initial rhythm, prior function status, or the presence of comorbid disease before the cardiac arrest.

Most elderly survivors of cardiac arrest do not have significant neurologic or functional impairment. Most return to pre-arrest activities.

Trauma Patients

The most common sources of traumatic arrest are hypovolemia, tension pneumothorax, and cardiac tamponade. Trauma patients who are unresponsive to vigorous fluid resuscitation require open thoracotomy, cardiac massage, and surgical intervention. Cardiac arrests caused by blunt chest or abdominal trauma continue to have a dismal outcome despite early and appropriate intervention (see Chapters 43, Abdominal Trauma, and 44, Chest Trauma).

Pregnant Patients

Prior to 24 weeks' gestation, survival of the fetus in a pregnant woman with cardiac arrest is unlikely and resuscitative measures are directed toward the mother. Resuscitation from cardiopulmonary arrest in a pregnant woman occurring after 24 weeks' gestation is directed to both the mother and the fetus. Standard resuscitation techniques are applied in the pregnant patient without modification, including pharmacologic therapy. In the more than 24 weeks' setting, if standard resuscitative therapy is not successful after 4 to 5 minutes of cardiac arrest, immediate cesarean section is considered.

Electrocution Patients

Cardiopulmonary arrest secondary to electric shock, especially from alternating current, is most commonly associated with ventricular fibrillation. Arrest secondary to lightning injury is often caused by asystole or accompanying respiratory arrest. Resuscitation is initiated with these underlying causes in mind.

Do Not Resuscitate Orders

Considerable controversy surrounds the legal and ethical aspects of deciding when not to resuscitate a patient. Not all patients who suffer a cardiopulmonary arrest need resuscitative care. Severely debilitated patients or those with known terminal disease (e.g., metastatic cancer, severe dementia, end-stage cardiac disease) may not be candidates for resuscitation. Patients have a right to die with dignity; therefore, patients who request no

---

TABLE 3–8. Drug Dosing for Pediatric CPR°

Drug	How Supplied or Prepared	Dose
NaHCO	1 mEq/mL	1–2 mEq (1–2 mL)/kg
Epinephrine	0.1 mg/mL (1:10,000 solution)	0.01 mg (0.1 mL)/kg
Atropine	0.1 mg/mL	0.02 mg (0.2 mL)/kg
Isoproterenol	1.5 mg/250 mL (6 µg/mL)	0.1–1.0 µg (1–10 mL)/kg/min
Calcium chloride	100 mg/mL (10% solution)	20 mg (0.2 mL)/kg
Lidocaine	10–20 mg/mL (1–2% solution)	1 mg (0.1 mL)/kg
Lidocaine infusion	300 mg (15 mL of 2% solution)/250 mL (1200 µg/mL)	20 µg (1 mL)/kg/hr
Dopamine	150 mg (3.75 mL)/250 mL (600 µg/mL)	100 µg (1 mL)/kg/min

°Broselow tape may be helpful.

life-sustaining measures should not be resuscitated. A thin line often separates the legal ramifications of no resuscitation from the patient's right to die with dignity. A "living will" or written physician order that is available at the time of cardiopulmonary arrest may represent adequate documentation not to resuscitate. However, because the issue is far from resolved, the emergency physician should always err on the side of active resuscitation if any doubt exists about the patient's "do not resuscitate" status.

Implantable Cardioverter Defibrillators

Implantable cardioverter defibrillators (ICDs) improve survival in a subset of cardiovascular risk patients. Most have coronary artery disease, a low (<30%) ejection fraction, and ventricular dysrhythmias refractory to medical therapy. ICDs are increasing in usage, and more than 60,000 patients were given ICDs in 2000. They have evolved to having sensing, pacing, atrial ventricular defibrillation, rhythm recording, and playback capabilities. ICDs can malfunction with a wide range of complications, including failure to deliver or inappropriate/ineffective therapy. As an implanted "foreign body," they also have non–function-related complications, including infection, thromboembolic disease, and significant psychological impact. Most patients who present with ICDs will have been shocked. They require careful assessment, electrocardiography and monitoring, an "interrogation" of the ICD via telemetry, and cardiology consultation.

DISPOSITION

Before transfer to the intensive or coronary care unit, the patient should be as stable as possible. Orders may be written for maintenance of intravenous infusions (e.g., lidocaine, dopamine), for ventilator settings (e.g., rate, mode, tidal volume), and for supplemental oxygen. The physician who will be caring for the patient in the coronary care unit is contacted and the case discussed in as much detail as possible. The patient's family is briefed in detail about the progress and continued critical status of the patient. One or two family members may accompany the patient to the intensive care unit, depending on the patient's condition and hospital policy.

Death in the Emergency Department

Seventy percent to 80% of cardiopulmonary arrest patients will not be successfully resuscitated. One of the most difficult responsibilities of a physician is informing the family and relatives of the death of a loved one. Even though no standard approach works in every case, a few guidelines are worth remembering (Table 3–9). Informing the family is best done in a private room with the assistance of a member of the clergy or a social worker. After introducing oneself to the family, the physician should sit with the family and address the member closest to the patient. A brief summary of the events that have taken place can be a good introduction, preparing the family for the fatal outcome. When informing the family, one should be as direct as possible and should use terms such as *died* and *dead,* avoiding vague terms such as *passed on* or *no longer with us.* It is also important to allow a brief period of immediate grieving and to answer any questions that the family may have. If the family wishes to view the deceased, one should inform the nurses and allow time for preparation of the body.

FINAL POINTS

- Cardiopulmonary resuscitation is the true life or death emergency. Successful resuscitation depends on rapidly identifying the cardiac arrest victim and promptly instituting basic life support maneuvers. Once basic life support has been established, recognition of the rhythm disturbance is necessary, and advanced cardiac life support is begun.
- The best survival results in cardiac arrest victims occur with early recognition and defibrillation of patients with ventricular fibrillation or pulseless ventricular tachycardia.
- Prognosis in patients with pulseless electrical activity is very poor unless a reversible cause can be identified and corrected.
- The best preparation for treating cardiopulmonary arrest is familiarity with and ability to recognize and treat lethal cardiac rhythms. This subject is best summarized in the American Heart Association's Standards for Advanced Cardiac Life Support (Emergency Cardiovascular Care Committee, 2000).
- Although all patients in cardiopulmonary arrest are candidates for resuscitation, not all need to be resuscitated. The patient who is "dead on arrival," one who does not desire life-support measures, or the patient with documented "terminal" disease should not be resuscitated.

TABLE 3–9. Guidelines for Informing the Family of an Unexpected Death

Preparation

Have the family gather in a private room/area. Optimally, the family will be updated as to ongoing efforts, if any. Social services or the clergy are contacted. Prepare yourself for this important and difficult duty.

Notification

Step into the room and quietly gain control of the scene. Do not respond to quick questioning such as, "Is he dead?" Introduce yourself, and determine who is present. Address the closest relative or the one who looks the most composed.

Sit down, if possible. Unless the situation is a hostile circumstance, move away from the door and physically join the group.

Briefly, in less than 30 seconds, relate the circumstance as you know it. Give the status of activity in the emergency department up until the cessation of resuscitative efforts. Then describe the present situation that the patient is dead. If you use other terminology, it may need to be repeated or clarified.

Grief Response

Anticipate a grief response and give physical comfort if you are comfortable in doing so, but do not move away.

After the initial response has lasted 30 to 60 seconds, ask the least emotional or closest person to the deceased a question about his or her knowledge of the events preceding the arrest. This usually stops or lessens the grieving in the group.

Talk with them about the history. Reassure them there was no pain involved (unless this is obviously not so); support the emergency medical services and other physicians. If major problems in the quality of care exist, do not address them at this time. If asked, simply state that more information must be gathered. If appropriate, reassure family and friends that they did everything they could. This is important to decrease their potential guilt, and assist their grieving process.

Concluding the Process

At this time, enlist the aid of the clergy or the social service, if present. You should be preparing to leave.

Once completely standing, explain your tasks of notifying the coroner, private physician, and so on. This introduces the work you must leave to do. Also, direct questions concerning burial arrangements to the clergy or social service.

As part of your closure to the first visit, inquire about the potential for an autopsy and transplantation. Don't press this issue at this juncture. Ask if they want to view the body and make sure all arrangements are made before they do.

Let them know you will return to answer any questions after your discussions with the coroner and the private physician.

Express your sorrow for their loss, and scan the group for those who might need further support.

Make every effort to speak with them again after talking with the coroner or private physician. Discuss the autopsy and transplantation request in more depth. Know the law and the hospital procedures (e.g., who pays for the autopsy if not requested by the coroner). Have the appropriate paperwork readily available and know how to complete it.

Viewing the Body

Express your sympathy and allow the interested individuals to view the body (no more than two at a time). Make sure the body is prepared, and a staff member accompanies the family. The staff member must be empathetic and have some familiarity with the care of the patient.

Departure

Direct the social service personnel to follow up on individuals who seem to need further support and with the person closest to the deceased. Make sure this person has a reasonable support system.

Do not prescribe sedatives or sleeping medications to group members without having them register.

At some point, arrange a debriefing session both medically and emotionally with the emergency department nursing staff and others involved. This is difficult to arrange but worthwhile.

Modified from Hamilton GC: Sudden death in the ED: Telling the living. Ann Emerg Med 1988; 17:382.

CASE*Study*

A 60-year-old man with a past history of angina developed severe substernal chest pain associated with dyspnea and diaphoresis. He asked his wife to call the rescue squad. When the paramedics arrived 10 minutes later, he was unresponsive, pulseless, and apneic.

Basic life support was initiated, and a "quick look" with the monitor paddles showed ventricular fibrillation. Three successive countershocks with 200, 300, and 360 J failed to defibrillate the heart. The patient was orotracheally intubated. Bag ventilation with oxygen and chest compressions were continued. Repeated attempts to establish an intravenous line were unsuccessful. Radio contact was made with the base hospital. The paramedics were instructed to give 2 mg of 1:10,000 epinephrine (10 mL) through the endotracheal tube, continue CPR, and transport the patient to the hospital as rapidly as possible.

Once ventricular fibrillation is noted, immediate defibrillation becomes the top priority. As was done in this case, three successive shocks with increasing joules is recommended. Endotracheal drug administration is relatively unique to emergency medical care. Absorption of selected drugs is rapid, without pulmonary sequelae. In the right circumstances, use of this route may be lifesaving. Other drugs that may be administered by this route are naloxone, atropine, lidocaine, and midazolam (Versed).

The rescue personnel arrived in the emergency department 6 minutes after their last radio contact. The patient was noted to have symmetric chest expansion and bilateral breath sounds during ventilation. No palpable carotid or femoral pulse was noted. Chest compressions were continued. The cardiac monitor showed ventricular fibrillation. The patient was successfully defibrillated after two 360-J countershocks. The post-defibrillation rhythm was complete third-degree heart block at a rate of 40 beats per minute. The systolic blood pressure was 70 mm Hg. An intravenous line was established.

In both the emergency department and the prehospital setting, defibrillation is not delayed until after intravenous access is established. Placement of the endotracheal tube was correctly done. A well-functioning resuscitation team will accomplish all of the early essential elements almost simultaneously.

Paramedics related the 60-year-old patient had a prior history of myocardial infarction. His medications included furosemide, digoxin, potassium replacement, and nitroglycerin. Reassessment of the patient's physical condition revealed absent breath sounds on the left side with asymmetric chest expansion. The endotracheal tube was pulled back 2 to 3 cm, and equal breath sounds were heard.

Right mainstem bronchus intubation is the most common cause of asymmetric breath sounds during cardiac arrest. It can easily evolve during the resuscitation effort despite the endotracheal tube being "secured." The history and use of medications support a cardiac origin for this arrest.

Applying the previously presented questions to this case shows that ventricular fibrillation was the immediate rhythm disturbance responsible for the arrest state. From the limited history available, the immediate cause of the arrest was probably a cardiac disturbance secondary to ischemic heart disease; however, noncardiac etiologies should remain in the differential diagnosis.

The use of quick-look paddle electrodes allowed the paramedics to identify the presence of ventricular fibrillation rapidly and institute treatment immediately. The history, physical examination, and ECG rhythm monitoring are the most useful evaluative tools during cardiopulmonary arrest.

When the cardiac monitor was rechecked, the patient was found to be in complete heart block with a heart rate of 40 beats per minute. Blood pressure was 60 mm Hg, palpable. A total of 3 mg atropine was administered intravenously without any change in heart rate or rhythm. A transcutaneous external pacemaker was applied. The patient was paced at a rate of 70 beats per minute. Blood pressure improved to 100/60 mm Hg.

After defibrillation, various dysrhythmias may occur and require therapy. Cardiac monitoring is usually the best means of recognizing these changes in rhythm. The use of a transcutaneous external pacer, as in this case, is indicated for patients with hemodynamically significant bradydysrhythmias.

The patient was placed on an amiodarone infusion and maintained on the external transcutaneous pacemaker. Once in the coronary care unit, the transcutaneous pacemaker was discontinued. Results of laboratory studies including arterial blood gases, electrolytes, glucose, and complete blood cell count were within normal limits. The patient's blood pressure and mental status improved over several hours. The patient required a permanent pacemaker and had an otherwise uneventful hospital course. He returned home with a moderate degree of neurologic impairment.

Bibliography

TEXT

Emergency Cardiovascular Care Committee, Guidelines 2000 for Cardiopulmonary Resuscitation and Emergency Cardiovascular Care, American Heart Association, 2000.

JOURNAL ARTICLES/INTERNET

Dorian P, Cass D, Schwartz G, et al: Amiodarone as compared with lidocaine for shock-resistant ventricular fibrillation. N Engl J Med 2002; 346:884–890.

Eisenberg MS, Mengert TJ: Cardiac resuscitation. N Engl J Med 2001; 344:1304–1313.

Eisenberg MS: Is it time for over-the-counter defibrillation? JAMA 2000; 284:1435–1441

Hallstrom A, Cobb L, Johnson E, et al: Cardiopulmonary resuscitation by chest compression alone or with mouth-to-mouth ventilation. N Engl J Med 2000; 342:1546–1553.

Hypothermia After Cardiac Arrest Study Group: Mild hypothermia to improve the neurologic outcome after cardiac arrest. NEJM 2002; 346:549–556.

Myerburg RJ, Kessler KM, Castellanos A: Sudden cardiac death: Structure, function, and time-dependence of risk. Circulation 1992; 85(Suppl I):I2–I10.

Nichol G, Stiell IG, Hebert P, et al: What is the quality of life for survivors of cardiac arrest? A prospective study. Acad Emerg Med 1999; 6:95–102.

Pepe PE, Abramson NS, Brown CC: ACLS—does it really work? Ann Emerg Med 1994; 23:1037–1041.

Robertson S: Cardiopulmonary cerebral resuscitation—present and future perspectives. Acta Anesthesiol Scand 1999 43:526–535.

Safar P: Cerebral resuscitation after cardiac arrest: Research initiatives and future directions. Ann Emerg Med 1993; 22:324–349.

Soo LH, Gray D, Young T, et al: Resuscitation from out-of-hospital cardiac arrest: Is survival dependent on who is available at the scene? Heart 1999; 81:47–52.

Takata TS, Page RL, Joglar JA: Automated external defibrillators: technical considerations and clinical promise. Ann Intern Med 2001; 135:990–998.

Tiffany BR, Pollack CV: Dying on Arrival: The first 15 minutes caring for the moribund patient. Emerg Med Pract 2000; (2):1–20.

Tilden FF, Spirko BA: The implantable cardioverter defibrillator: Technology, complications, and emergency management. EM Reports 1998; 19:163–172.

Tresch DD, Thakur RK: Cardiopulmonary resuscitation in the elderly. Emerg Med Clin North Am 1998; 16:649–663.

van Walraven C, Forester AJ, Parish DC: Validation of a clinical decision aid to discontinue in-hospital cardiac arrest resuscitation. JAMA 2001; 285:1602–1606.

Learn CPR. Available at http://www.learncpr.org (University of Washington). Emergency Cardiac Care. Available at www.cpr-ecc.org (American Heart Association).

CHAPTER 4

SHOCK

ELIF E. ÖKER

CASE_Study_

A 75-year-old man presents to the emergency department with a chief complaint of feeling weak and dizzy for 2 days. He had symptoms of persistent vomiting and diarrhea for several days. He has not urinated for the past 12 hours. At triage, the patient is noted to be hypotensive and tachycardic.

INTRODUCTION

Shock is an acute circulatory dysfunction resulting in tissue hypoperfusion wherein tissue blood flow is unable to meet metabolic demands. When untreated, shock results in end-organ compromise and ultimately end-organ failure. Hypoperfusion triggers a series of compensatory events that help to maintain blood flow to vital organs. Initially, a catecholamine surge causes an increase in cardiac output and peripheral vasoconstriction, shifting blood flow to the brain and myocardium. The renin-angiotensin system and vasopressin are stimulated to regulate salt and water retention. As compensatory mechanisms fail, myocardial perfusion and cardiac output decline. Inadequately perfused cells shift to anaerobic metabolism, resulting in lactic acid production. Tissue acidosis produces vasodilation and worsening hypotension. Clinically, these late changes are manifested as mental status abnormalities, oliguria, and diminished peripheral pulses. Extremities may be cool and clammy, secondary to peripheral vasoconstriction, or warm, owing to dilatation. At some point, the process reaches an irreversible stage and the patient does not respond to therapeutic interventions. Death results from multisystem organ failure.

Shock is classified in several ways. For the purposes of this discussion, we will consider four types of shock (Table 4–1):

- Hypovolemic shock
- Cardiogenic shock
- Distributive (vasodilatory) shock
- Obstructive shock

Hypovolemic shock is the most common type and results from the loss of circulatory volume. The most common causes of hypovolemic shock are hemorrhage and dehydration. The treatment of hypovolemic shock centers on intravascular volume expansion, using intravenous fluids or blood products.

Cardiogenic shock is caused by myocardial dysfunction. The most common cause of cardiogenic shock is myocardial infarction, occurring in 5% to 10% of cases. Treatment of cardiogenic shock is based on optimization of circulatory volume with intravenous fluids followed by inotropic (pump) assistance and myocardial reperfusion. The maintenance of adequate tissue perfusion often requires the use of vasopressors. Careful hemodynamic monitoring is usually required.

In _distributive_ or _vasodilatory shock_, vascular dilatation occurs in response to the release of a variety of mediators and cytokines (e.g., nitric oxide), causing a large decrease in systemic vascular resistance. A hyperdynamic state occurs, with an increase in heart rate and cardiac output to compensate for these changes. Sepsis is the most frequent cause of this type of shock.

Obstructive shock represents either actual or pressure gradient–based blockages of blood flow leading into or out of the heart. These are often reversible causes of shock or pulseless electrical activity (see Chapter 3, Cardiopulmonary Cerebral Resuscitation) and include acute cardiac tamponade, tension pneumothorax, and massive pulmonary embolism.

Independent of etiology, the most common problem addressed in the emergency department is volume loss leading to circulatory compromise and vital organ dysfunction.

INITIAL APPROACH AND STABILIZATION

All patients with signs or symptoms of shock require immediate attention. The physician must first address the clinical consequences of shock, often without being sure of the underlying cause(s). Initial stabilization occurs simultaneously with taking a history and performing a

TABLE 4–1. Types of Shock

Hypovolemic	Cardiogenic	Distributive (Vasodilatory)	Obstructive
Hemorrhagic	Pump failure	Sepsis	Acute pericardial
Trauma	Acute myocardial infarction	Anaphylaxis	tamponade
Gastrointestinal bleeding	Cardiomyopathy	Neurogenic	Massive pulmonary
Ruptured aortic aneurysm	Myocarditis	Toxins	embolus
Ruptured aortic dissection	Ruptured chordae tendinae	Cyanide	Tension pneumothorax
Pregnancy-related bleeding	Ruptured ventricular septum	Carbon monoxide	May manifest as pulseless
Severe dehydration	Papillary muscle dysfunction	Prolonged severe hypotension	electric activity
Gastroenteritis	Prosthetic valve dysfunction	from other causes of shock	
Diabetic ketoacidosis	Acute aortic insufficiency		
Adrenal crisis	Toxins		
Burns/severe dermatitis	Myocardial contusion		
	Rate problems		
	Bradycardia		
	Tachycardia		

physical examination. The information obtained often allows one of the four major categories of shock to be considered, and specific treatment then can be initiated.

Rapid Assessment

What Is the Patient's General Appearance?

Patients in shock will often appear pale or dusky, and their skin may be diaphoretic. A notable exception is the patient in septic shock, who may have pink, warm extremities caused by vasodilatation.

Is the Patient Alert and Oriented?

Mental status changes are the neurologic and organ manifestation of hypoperfusion, hypoxia, hypoglycemia, and/or central nervous system pathology. If alert, most patients in shock are anxious and verbalizing their distress.

What Are the Patient's Vital Signs? Is the Patient Having Difficulty Breathing?

Blood Pressure. Blood pressure may be difficult to measure or monitor in a patient with severe shock. Invasive monitoring or Doppler-assisted measurements may be necessary. A mean arterial pressure less than 70–80 mm Hg indicates a circulatory shock state. Mean arterial pressure equals the diastolic pressure plus one third of the pulse pressure (difference between systolic and diastolic pressure). Pulses are generally palpable down to the following pressures: radial artery, 80 mm Hg; carotid artery, 70 mm Hg; femoral artery, 60 mm Hg. Hypertensive patients may have "shock" states with blood pressure levels that would be considered normal in the general population.

Heart Rate. The heart rate is usually accelerated; tachycardia is more than 100 beats per minute. The patient's response may be influenced by age, medication, and disease.

Respiratory Rate. Respiratory distress can present as dyspnea, tachypnea, or bradypnea. Tachypnea is most common and represents a nonspecific response to the stress of shock; it is potentially a result of respiratory compensation for metabolic acidosis. Hypoxia may be subtle, and early pulse oximetry monitoring is important, recognizing its limitations in peripheral hypoperfusion states.

Early Intervention

Airway

If the patient is unable to maintain a patent and protected airway, active airway management is essential. The need for intubation and mechanical ventilation must be determined. Even patients without respiratory distress may require intubation if they are unable to maintain their airway and avoid aspiration. Work of breathing can be markedly reduced by mechanical ventilation, benefiting the seriously ill patient in shock who may have little physiologic reserve.

Breathing

Supplemental oxygen is provided, and the patient's rate and work of breathing are continuously assessed. Oxygenation is commonly monitored using pulse oximetry; however, in advanced stages of shock, peripheral perfusion may be too poor for accurate measurements. Arterial blood gas analysis is often performed to assess the patient's ventilation, oxygenation, and acid-base status.

Oxygen is provided by means of a nasal cannula or face mask. A nasal cannula provides low flow oxygen with variable oxygen delivery. Each 2 L/min increase in supplemental oxygen increases the F_{IO_2} by 3% to 4%. At 6 L/min, the nasal cannula delivers approximately 34% oxygen. Flow rates greater than 10 L/min may excessively dry the nasal mucosa. A simple face mask delivers oxygen at variable concentrations, up to 40% F_{IO_2}. Non-rebreather masks supply a constant flow of oxygen at concentrations exceeding 60%. At 10 L/min, essentially 70% to 80% oxygen is delivered. The non-rebreather mask is a useful oxygen delivery device for the severely ill patient in shock.

Circulation

Two or more large-bore (16-gauge or larger) intravenous lines should be established and blood drawn for laboratory analysis. Bedside glucose and hemoglobin measurements are determined (if available). An initial bolus of 1 to 2 L of intravenous fluid in the adult is administered over 20 to 30 minutes, provided there is no evidence of fluid overload. Faster rates may be necessary in extreme circumstances. Cautious fluid administration, with 200- to 300-mL boluses of isotonic crystalloid solution, is indicated if cardiogenic shock is suggested. Continuous monitoring for improvement in vital signs or signs of fluid overload is essential and includes mental status, vital signs, and general appearance. Continuous cardiac monitoring and pulse oximetry is also part of the assessment. The lungs are examined for rales to assess potential fluid overload.

Patients who exhibit inadequate response require additional fluid. Vasopressor support is initiated only after the patient is adequately hydrated and there is still inadequate response of the blood pressure and other perfusion parameters.

Specific Intervention (Related to Shock Type)

Hemorrhagic. In cases of hemorrhagic shock, external sources of bleeding are controlled. Internal sources are actively pursued. These may include gastrointestinal, thoracic, abdominal, and retroperitoneal sites. Pelvic and long-bone injuries are notorious for multiple sites of internal blood loss. Early blood replacement therapy is initiated based on severity of initial presentation or lack of response to intravenous fluid.

Obstructive. Especially in cases of penetrating trauma to the chest, cardiac tamponade must be considered, with pericardiocentesis used for diagnostic and therapeutic purposes (see Chapter 44, Chest Trauma).

Tension pneumothorax is also a cause of shock in patients with blunt or penetrating thoracic trauma or in those who are receiving positive-pressure ventilation. Needle thoracostomy is first indicated, immediately followed by tube thoracostomy.

Distributive. Vasodilating shock may require large fluid volumes. In anaphylaxis, epinephrine (0.01 mg/kg) has a unique treatment role (see Chapter 12, Anaphylaxis). Sepsis-associated, neurogenic, and drug-associated vasodilatation each have their own specific therapies.

Cardiogenic Shock. Initial therapy may be directed toward chronotropic (rate-related) causes or inotropic (pump-related) causes. The vital signs and cardiopulmonary examination are useful in discriminating between the two causes.

CLINICAL ASSESSMENT

History

Once immediate life-threatening conditions are addressed, a detailed history is sought. History-taking and treatment usually occur simultaneously. Information is obtained from family members, paramedics, and others who may be familiar with the case, especially when the patient is unable to provide detailed information.

The physician should obtain an overview of the patient's complaint. The chief complaint and events preceding the patient's arrival at the hospital are often major clues to the etiology of the problem. Past medical history, medications, and allergies are also explored.

Key questions include

- What *event* triggered the emergency department visit?
- How *long* has the patient been *ill*?
- Has there been a *change* in *symptoms*? For example, pain may change in location, quality, or duration and symptoms such as weakness or dizziness may be progressive or intermittent.
- Is the patient potentially immunocompromised? Age, diabetes, steroid use, chemotherapy, or HIV may impair the patient's ability to resist or manifest clinical findings of infection.
- Does anything make the *symptoms improve* or *worsen*?
- Does the patient have *previous medical problems* or *allergies*? What medications (including nonprescription and homeopathic forms) are taken? Has anything similar occurred previously?

- A brief *review of systems*, tailored to the chief complaint, is helpful. Patients in early stages of shock may complain of thirst, but this sensation is often blunted in elderly patients. Pulmonary, genitourinary, and central nervous systems are generally high-yield systems.

Physical Examination

The physical examination should be thorough but guided by the history. Special attention should be paid to the vital signs and physical appearance for indication of the presence of shock and degree of compensation. In addition, a careful head-to-toe examination of the patient may provide clues to the etiology when the cause is uncertain. Components of the examination as related to shock are listed in Table 4–2.

General Appearance

The appearance of the patient provides important clues to the severity of the condition. Is the patient awake or somnolent? Is the patient easily arousable and following commands? If the patient is communicative, assessment of the mental status includes questions about the patient's orientation to person, place, and time. The skin is assessed for rashes or signs of trauma. Anaphylactic shock may be associated with urticaria or angioedema, whereas septic shock may be associated with petechial or purpuric rashes. Scars may help to piece together some aspects of the past medical and surgical history.

Vital Signs

Regardless of the cause, the patient in advanced stages of shock will exhibit tachypnea and hypotension. Tachycardia is an early finding and is present in most cases; however, bradycardia may be present in the setting of cardiogenic shock resulting from untreated bradydys-rhythmias. Bradycardia may also result from vagal influences or from medication use, such as β-adrenergic blocking agents in which the patient may be unable to mount a tachycardic response.

Tachypnea may be caused by a pulmonary pathologic process or may be present as a compensatory reaction to metabolic acidosis. Unexplained tachypnea may be an early manifestation of sepsis.

Hypotension is a late manifestation of shock. The goal should be to detect early signs of impending shock and to initiate treatment before the patient becomes hypotensive. A narrow pulse pressure (the difference between the systolic and diastolic blood pressures) may be an early sign of volume contraction. Assessment of the pulse rate and blood pressure in the supine position, followed by repeat assessment in the upright position (orthostatic assessment), is another way to test for early evidence of volume contraction or blood loss. If the patient becomes severely symptomatic on attempting to sit up or stand, the test is considered positive and is not pursued further. Asymptomatic patients should be allowed to stay in the upright (standing or sitting with legs dangling) position for 1 to 2 minutes before the vital signs are rechecked. An increase in the pulse rate of 20 to 30 beats, or a decrease in the systolic blood pressure by 20%, is considered a positive result. Although a positive finding on orthostatic evaluation may be helpful, a negative result does not rule out volume depletion. Orthostatic testing is not a sensitive or specific indicator when used in isolation from other clinical findings.

Abnormalities of body temperature are most commonly associated with septic shock, manifested as abnormally high or low measurements of core temperature.

Secondary Survey (Head-to-Toe Examination)

The reader is referred to Table 4–2.

CLINICAL REASONING

After stabilization and initial assessment of the patient, the physician must formulate a differential diagnosis. The following questions are considered.

Is the Patient in Shock?

Does the patient show clinical evidence of inadequate tissue perfusion? Signs of inadequate perfusion include skin and mental status changes, diminished urine output, and cardiovascular instability. Especially in young, healthy patients, compensation for acute stress (such as blood loss), with tachycardia and peripheral vessel constriction, results in maintenance of blood flow to essential organs such as the heart and brain. As a result, patients in compensated shock appear relatively well on cursory examination. These patients will soon reach a limit of compensation and their condition may suddenly deteriorate if the shock goes unrecognized and without treatment. In decompensated cases, hypotension develops, tachycardia is usually present, but bradycardia does *not* rule out shock.

TABLE 4–2. Components of the Physical Examination in Shock

Area of Examination	Component	Significance in the Setting of Shock
Vital signs	Temperature	Temperature ≥38°C or <36°C consistent with sepsis.
	Pulse rate	Tachycardia is a common compensatory response.
		Tachydysrhythmias or bradydysrhythmias may cause shock.
	Respiratory rate	Tachypnea may indicate respiratory compromise or be a compensatory response to metabolic acidosis.
	Blood pressure	Hypotension is the final common pathway regardless of etiology and is usually a late finding.
General appearance	Skin	Pale, dusky or diaphoretic in uncompensated shock.
		Warm and pink in early phase of septic shock.
	Mental status	Alert, anxious, ill-appearing followed by obtundation.
		Obtundation may be caused by many toxins that also result in hypotension.
Head	Inspection, palpation	Head injury is an important component of multisystem trauma.
Eyes	Pupils	Miosis or mydriasis may be caused by toxins, which also lead to shock owing to cardiac rate or pump effects.
Neck	Inspection, palpation	Tracheal displacement ± subcutaneous emphysema suggests tension pneumothorax.
		Distended neck veins may be present with cardiogenic shock or cardiac tamponade.
		Tenderness and deformity of the cervical spine may be found with cervical spine trauma and neurogenic shock.
Chest and lungs	Palpation, auscultation	Chest wall tenderness, wounds, contusion, or deformity are consistent with trauma that can result in tension pneumothorax, cardiac tamponade, or aortic rupture.
		Unilateral diminished breath sounds are consistent with pneumothorax or hemothorax.
		Rales suggest infection or pulmonary congestion consistent with sepsis or cardiogenic shock.
		Stridor may be present with upper airway edema and wheezing may be present with bronchospasm as manifestations of anaphylaxis.
Heart	Auscultation	Tachycardia is common, but bradycardia can be found due to vagal influences, drug effects, or bradydysrhythmias.
		New murmurs suggest the possibility of acute aortic insufficiency, ruptured chordae tendinae, or ruptured intraventricular septum.
		Muffled heart sounds are consistent with cardiac tamponade.
Abdomen	Inspection, palpation	Abdominal distention may be due to intraperitoneal blood, third-spacing of fluid, or bowel distention with ileus.
		Tenderness may be found with trauma, infection, or ruptured abdominal aneurysm. Pulsatile mass suggests aortic aneurysm.
Pelvis	Speculum and bimanual examination	Pelvic tenderness is consistent with pelvic infection or ruptured ectopic pregnancy.
		Bleeding in the third trimester of pregnancy can rapidly lead to shock (speculum examination contraindicated).
		Postpartum bleeding may lead to shock.
Rectal examination	Digital with check for occult blood	Tenderness is consistent with pelvic or intra-abdominal infection.
		Gastrointestinal bleeding sufficient to cause shock is common and may not always be obvious at the time of initial evaluation.
Extremities/bony pelvis	Inspection, palpation	Bleeding into the thigh or pelvis after fracture can be sufficient to lead to shock.
		Diminished pulses expected in most types of shock. If noted in the lower extremities only, consistent with ruptured aortic aneurysm.
Neurologic	Motor, sensory, and reflexes	Focal deficits are consistent with cervical spine injury, cord injury, and neurogenic shock.
Skin	Rashes	Urticaria or angioedema may be present in anaphylaxis.
		Petechial or purpuric rashes are consistent with bacterial infection and septic shock.

What Type of Shock Is Present?

Once the presence of impending or established shock is determined, and the patient stabilized, the differential diagnosis of shock is reexplored (see Table 4–1). Is the underlying cause hypovolemic, obstructive, cardiogenic, or a form of distributive (vasodilatory) shock?

Hypovolemic shock is caused by either acute hemorrhage or severe dehydration. *Hemorrhagic shock* is most commonly caused by blunt or penetrating trauma, with external or internal bleeding. Gastrointestinal bleeding from peptic ulcers or esophageal varices is another common cause. Less common and more difficult to recognize and treat is internal hemorrhage from major vascular catastrophes, such as ruptured aortic aneurysm.

Severe dehydration also may result in shock as a result of external or internal fluid losses. Gastroenteritis with vomiting and diarrhea is a major cause of shock and death in the pediatric population worldwide. Although less common as a cause of death in the United States, gastroenteritis is still a common cause of significant dehydration that can progress to shock if not properly treated. Diabetic ketoacidosis can cause hypovolemic shock secondary to the osmotic diuresis that occurs in association with continued glycosuria. A similar osmotic diuresis occurs in patients with adrenal crisis, with sodium and fluid loss associated with the mineralocorticoid deficit. Burns and severe cases of dermatitis cause external fluid losses sufficient to result in shock. Fluid sequestration in the peritoneal cavity (third-spacing) secondary to inflammation or trauma also causes circulatory system depletion.

Hypotension in the presence of chest pain or other cardiac symptoms suggests *cardiogenic shock*. Hypotension associated with cardiac dysrhythmias, both fast and slow, may also be considered a form of cardiogenic shock. The most common form of cardiogenic shock is that caused by acute myocardial infarction, with massive (>40%) myocardial dysfunction. Cardiac output is decreased, and pulmonary edema is common.

Obstructive shock was discussed previously in the section "Initial Approach and Stabilization."

The major forms of *distributive* or *vasodilatory* shock are septic, anaphylactic, and neurogenic shock. All result in systemic vasodilatation and, ultimately, hypotension. Patients with *sepsis* may be febrile or occasionally hypothermic. A history of recent infection is often present. A rash may be associated, such as erythroderma in toxic shock syndrome or petechiae and purpura in meningo-coccemia. Septic shock results from the release of toxins associated with invading microorganisms and the inflammatory response to them. In the early phase, septic shock is characterized by a hyperdynamic phase in which the cardiac output is high and the pulse pressure is widened. Pulses are bounding, and the skin is pink and warm. If untreated, this early phase progresses with end-organ damage similar to other forms of decompensated shock. This progression may be rapid and must be anticipated. A "cold" shock state typically occurs late in the process, distinguishing this from other shock types.

Anaphylactic patients may present in respiratory distress from bronchospasm or upper airway edema and may demonstrate generalized urticaria and edema as a result of exposure to an allergen. Profound vasodilatation and increased vascular permeability result in hypotension.

Neurogenic shock develops as a result of loss of sympathetic cardiovascular tone, usually in association with spinal cord injury. Marked vasodilatation results in systemic hypotension, with or without tachycardia.

DIAGNOSTIC ADJUNCTS

Shock is a clinical diagnosis, but many diagnostic adjuncts are useful in establishing the etiology and monitoring the response to treatment.

Bedside Tests

Blood Glucose. A glucose oxidase reagent test can provide a quick and accurate check for hypoglycemia or hyperglycemia, allowing early assessment for the presence of diabetic ketoacidosis, which may be associated with hypovolemic shock, or hypoglycemia, which may be present with adrenal failure.

Hemoglobin/Hematocrit. Severe anemia associated with blood loss may be detected by a rapid hemoglobin test or hematocrit determination. A normal value does not however rule out hemorrhage, because a patient may still have a normal hemoglobin value when blood loss has been acute.

Gastric/Stool Hemoglobin. Hemoccult testing of rectal or gastric specimens provides evidence of gastrointestinal blood loss.

Urinary Flow. Indwelling urinary catheterization provides useful information about urine output and end-organ perfusion. Monitoring changes in urine output can help direct resuscitation efforts. For patients with normal renal function, urine output of 0.05 to 1.0 mL/kg/hr indicates adequate hydration.

Laboratory Studies

Lactic Acid. Most laboratory studies are not useful in the diagnosis of shock, but they may be useful to confirm the etiology of the condition. A significant exception is arterial or venous lactic acid levels. This level is one of the most sensitive and specific means of confirming global tissue hypoperfusion.

Complete Blood Cell Count (CBC). Leukocytosis or leukopenia denotes infection in cases in which sepsis is suggested, although leukocytosis also occurs with the stress of shock alone. Serum hemoglobin may provide evidence of blood loss (anemia) or volume loss (hemoconcentration).

Arterial Blood Gas Analysis. Regardless of the cause of shock, inadequate tissue perfusion will lead to anaerobic metabolism and the production of lactic acid. Arterial pH and serum bicarbonate levels will be low. Both measures should improve as appropriate treatment is provided. Hypoxemia or hypercarbia may be found in patients with inadequate ventilation or when a pulmonary pathologic process prevents adequate gas exchange.

Serum Electrolytes. Fluid losses sufficient to cause shock may also be associated with electrolyte abnormalities. Potassium depletion is common with vomiting, diarrhea, and diabetic ketoacidosis. Sodium loss associated with the osmotic diuresis of adrenal crisis leads to hyponatremia. The serum bicarbonate level will be low in all cases of uncompensated shock, secondary to associated metabolic acidosis. Calculation of the anion gap [serum sodium − (serum chloride + serum bicarbonate)] will show a gap in excess of the normal range, indicating excess anion presence. Patients receiving large amounts of intravenous fluid have the potential for developing electrolyte abnormalities and should be closely monitored.

Renal Function. Blood urea nitrogen and serum creatinine levels are usually measured with the serum electrolytes. The blood urea nitrogen value will be elevated in cases of severe dehydration and in cases of gastrointestinal bleeding. Its origin is breakdown of blood in the gastrointestinal tract (a protein load) and absorption of urea into the blood. Serum creatinine is a more specific measure of renal function. Elevation in the setting of shock may signify acute renal insufficiency or acute tubular necrosis, resulting from inadequate perfusion of the kidney.

Blood Glucose. Bedside glucose testing is usually confirmed by measurement in the laboratory.

Urinalysis. The urine specific gravity is elevated (>1.020) when there is significant dehydration or blood loss. The onset of proteinuria or hematuria during the course of shock may signify the development of acute tubular necrosis. White blood cells and bacteria on microscopic evaluation of the urine or leukocyte esterase on dipstick testing suggest urinary infection. The urine is a common source for infection that leads to septic shock, especially in elderly patients and in those with indwelling urinary catheters.

Cultures. Cultures of the blood, urine, sputum, and other suspected sites of infection may identify the causative organism of sepsis and guide future antibiotic choices. Culture results are not available in the acute setting, and diagnostic and treatment decisions must initially be broad based to cover likely pathogens for the suspected infection.

Radiologic Imaging

Plain Films. A chest radiograph may provide evidence of pneumonia (contributing to systemic infection and septic shock) or pulmonary edema (a component of cardiogenic shock). A chest radiograph may also show pneumothorax. Tension pneumothorax is a life-threatening problem that should be diagnosed on clinical grounds and treated immediately.

If the patient is hemodynamically unstable, a portable supine anteroposterior view of the chest should be obtained, rather than the routine views that are obtained in the upright position. A reverse Trendelenburg film (upward angling of head of stretcher) may help define a chest pathologic process.

Computed Tomography. Patients who have incurred major trauma will often need to undergo extensive imaging, including plain films of the cervical spine, pelvis, and any injured extremities. Computed tomography of the head, thorax, and abdomen is often needed to rule out injury.

Ultrasonography. Portable ultrasonography is a valuable tool that can be quickly performed at the bedside and is now commonly used for patients with unstable conditions who cannot leave the main treatment area to undergo extensive imaging procedures. Abdominal aortic aneurysm, ectopic pregnancy, or free fuid in the peritoneal space may be diagnosed with ultrasound. Transesophageal echocardiography is a specialized ultrasound technique that is very helpful in diagnosing aortic dissection and cardiac tamponade. Echocardiography can aid the clinician in assessing left ventricular function, and thereby differentiating hypovolemia from cardiogenic shock in the hypotensive patient. Research has demonstrated a use for these approaches in the emergency department.

The history and physical examination of the patient determines the need for other imaging. Patients in shock with abdominal pain, back or flank pain, abdominal distention, pulsatile mass, or diminished lower extremity pulses need evaluation for the presence of a ruptured abdominal aneurysm. Unstable patients with this symptom-complex should be taken directly to the operating room for exploration and probable aortic repair. Stable patients may undergo diagnostic testing, which may include cross-table lateral views of the abdomen, ultrasonography, and computed tomography of the abdomen.

Electrocardiogram

A 12-lead electrocardiogram may provide evidence of cardiac ischemia, infarction, or dysrhythmias as the cause of cardiogenic shock. Either of these findings may also be present as a complication of the stress of shock of any type. Electrical alternans, suggestive of cardiac tamponade, is present when P, QRS, and T wave complexes alternate between low and high voltage.

PRINCIPLES OF MANAGEMENT

Shock and impending shock are true emergencies and require rapid diagnosis and treatment to avoid morbidity and mortality. Initial stabilization with airway management and volume resuscitation is directed at providing ventilation, oxygenation, and tissue perfusion. The initial goals are to treat the underlying disease, begin to reverse the shock state, and bring the MAP into the perfusion range for essential organs, usually 80 to 90 mm Hg. Rapid return of the patient's vital signs to baseline values is rarely necessary and may result in over treatment.

Specific Management

After initial stabilization, specific management is tailored to the type of shock and the patient's response to early interventions.

Vasopressor Support

Patients with transient, minimal, or no response to fluid challenges may require the use of vasopressors.

Dopamine is a precursor to norepinephrine. It exerts a dose-dependent effect on dopamine, β-adrenergic, and α-adrenergic receptors. Dopamine infusion is initiated when mean arterial pressures are less than 90 mm Hg in the presence of signs of decreased perfusion and adequate fluid status. Renal dose dopamine, 2 to 3 μg/kg/min, results in vasodilatation of splanchnic, coronary, and renal vasculature secondary to action at dopamine receptors. At 3 to 5 μg/kg/min, β_1-receptor stimulation causes increased cardiac contractility. At 5 to 10 μg/kg/min, α_1-adrenergic receptor stimulation results in increased mean arterial pressure (peripheral vasoconstriction), tachycardia, and decreased renal blood flow. At higher doses, α-adrenergic effects predominate. The resulting increases in afterload may compromise cardiac output.

Dobutamine, given in doses of 2 to 20 μg/kg/min, is a synthetic catecholamine with β_1 (cardiac), β_2 (peripheral), and α_1 (peripheral) adrenergic effects. Dobutamine primarily increases cardiac contractility without a significant increase in heart rate and also causes systemic vasodilatation. Dobutamine is indicated when the mean arterial pressure is greater than 90 mm Hg and there is clinical evidence of hypoperfusion, with adequate fluid status. Adverse effects are seen at higher doses, including tachycardia and dysrhythmias.

Norepinephrine, given in doses of 0.5 to 30 μg/min, is used to treat shock refractory to other catecholamines. Norepinephrine is a naturally occurring catecholamine with α- and β-adrenergic effects. It increases cardiac contractility (β_1) and peripheral vasoconstriction (α) and is useful in settings with low systemic vascular resistance, such as sepsis.

Hemorrhagic Shock

Central to the management of hemorrhagic shock is control of bleeding and volume replacement with blood component therapy (Fig. 4–1). Control of hemorrhage may be as simple as applying direct external pressure or as complex as surgical intervention. The goal of blood component therapy is to restore oxygen-carrying capacity. Hemoglobin levels less than 7 g/dL require transfusion, whereas those above 10 g/dL usually do not. In cases in which the hemoglobin level is between 7 and 10 g/dL, the patient's physiologic condition determines the need for transfusion. Packed red blood cells, a concentrated suspension of red blood cells after the separation of plasma from whole blood, is the blood component of choice. Massive transfusions (greater than 1.5 times the patients blood volume) may result in a coagulopathic state, requiring the transfusion of platelets or fresh frozen plasma. Blood component therapy has an increased risk of infectious

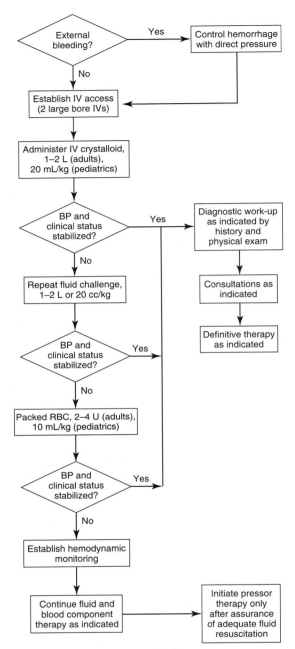

FIGURE 4–1 • Hemorrhagic shock resuscitation.

disease transmission, and unnecessary use of blood components should be avoided. Platelets and fresh frozen plasma are indicated when coagulopathy develops, demonstrated clinically by spontaneous bleeding from wounds, puncture or surgical sites, or mucous membranes. Significant bleeding from thrombocytopenia alone rarely occurs at platelet counts above 20,000/mm^3.

Cardiogenic Shock

Cardiogenic shock is usually the combination of hypotension and pulmonary edema (Fig. 4–2). The most common cause of cardiogenic shock is acute myocardial infarction, with resultant pump failure. In general, this occurs when more than 40% of the myocardium is damaged. Sinus tachycardia is often seen as the failing left ventricle compensates for diminishing stroke volume. As cardiac output falls, hypotension develops, left ventricular filling pressures rise, and pulmonary congestion develops.

In cardiogenic shock, administration of intravenous fluids must be balanced against the risk of inciting or worsening fluid overload and pulmonary edema. If the lungs are clear, cautious administration of crystalloid at the rate of 200 to 300 mL over 10 to 20 minutes may provide needed volume expansion without inducing pulmonary edema. Fluid administration in the setting of cardiogenic shock is best gauged with invasive hemodynamic monitoring. If pulmonary capillary wedge pressure monitoring is available, crystalloid may be administered until the pulmonary capillary wedge pressure rises to 18 mm Hg and as the patient's condition allows.

The usual initial approach to the patient with left ventricular failure includes diuresis with loop diuretics (e.g., furosemide), followed by preload and afterload reduction with intravenous nitrates. Furosemide is administered in a dose of 0.5 to 1.0 mg/kg IV. Nitroglycerin infusion is started at 10 μg/min and titrated to effect (diuresis and pressure changes). Neither of these modalities is typically used if the patient is already hypotensive (systolic blood pressure < 100 mm Hg), although cautious use of low doses of furosemide may be initiated.

If the systolic blood pressure is more than 90 mm Hg, dobutamine may be started at 2 μg/kg/min, with titration as needed to a maximum of 20 μg/kg/min. Dobutamine increases cardiac output and leads to reduced peripheral vascular resistance. This results in lower myocardial oxygen demand than is seen with dopamine or norepinephrine. If the systolic blood pressure is less than 90 mm Hg, dopamine should be started at a rate of 5 μg/kg/min and titrated up until the pressure responds or a maximum of 20 μg/kg/min is reached. Once the systolic pressure is above 90 mm Hg, dobutamine may be used simultaneously with dopamine and the dopamine dose can be titrated downward. If there is inadequate response to the maximum dose of dopamine, norepinephrine is added, beginning at 2 μg/min and

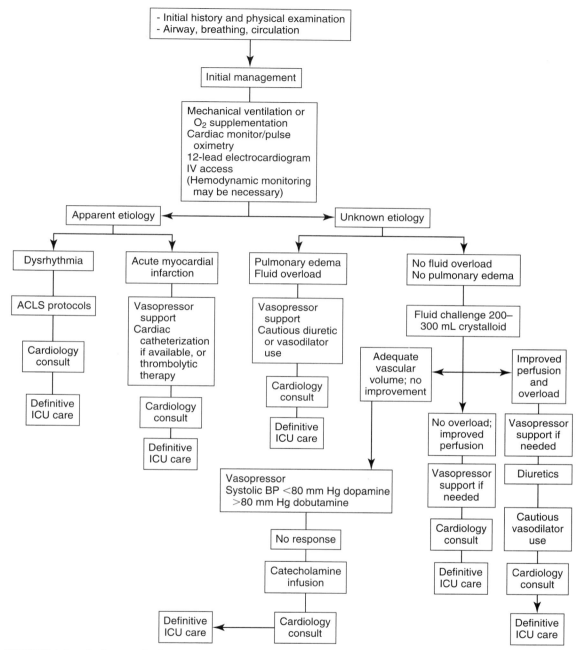

FIGURE 4–2 • Cardiogenic shock.

titrated up (to a maximum of 30 μg/min) until the systolic pressure improves. Intra-aortic balloon counterpulsation may be used in refractory cases and is especially helpful as a bridging device for patients who are candidates for coronary artery bypass grafting.

The use of thrombolytic therapy for patients with myocardial infarction with cardiogenic shock remains controversial and has not been shown to consistently improve outcome. Percutaneous transluminal coronary angioplasty has been shown to reduce mortality rates in these patients and is widely advocated. Thrombolytic therapy may be cautiously used in situations in which percutaneous transluminal coronary angioplasty is not available.

Anaphylactic Shock

Hypotension associated with an anaphylactic reaction is treated with intravenous fluids and vasopressors. Additionally, epinephrine (0.2 to 0.5 mL of 1:1000 in adults) is given subcutaneously to counteract mediator-induced vasodilatation and bronchospasm. Intravenous epinephrine and a continuous infusion may be necessary in extreme cases. Antihistamines (H_1 and H_2 blocking agents) and corticosteroids may be useful. For a more complete discussion, see Chapter 12, Anaphylaxis.

Septic Shock

The treatment of septic shock requires airway management, antibiotics, intravenous fluids, and vasopressor therapy (Fig. 4–3). Specimens for all appropriate cultures must be obtained immediately and appropriate intravenous antibiotics initiated promptly. The setting in which the infection developed and the patient's specific symptom-complex are typically all that is available to help define the source of infection and the likely pathogen. This information also guides selection of the most appropriate antibiotics. Broad-spectrum antibiotic coverage, with at least two antibiotics, is typically indicated (Table 4–3). Other modalities are being assessed to treat septic shock. Recombinant human activated protein C increases fibrinolysis and inhibits tumor necrosis factor, and has been approved for use in combination with standard therapy. Other anti-inflammatory agents, including autocoids and cytokines, are being researched.

UNCERTAIN DIAGNOSIS

The initial approach to the patient in shock is essentially the same, regardless of the cause. As airway, breathing, and circulation are being evaluated and stabilized, the possible causes related to each area are considered. Failure to recognize tension pneumothorax or cardiac tamponade and to provide lifesaving treatment leads to failure of other interventions. A common mistake is failure to give sufficient fluid to resuscitate the severely hypovolemic patient. Pressors will work poorly or not at all in patients with ongoing intravascular depletion. When the diagnosis remains unclear, the clinician can ask, "Have any elements of the history or physical examination been missed? Have there been changes in the examination that reveal the source of shock?" A careful head-to-toe reexamination may reveal clues that were initially missed, and additional information from care providers, emergency medical services personnel, or family members may be helpful.

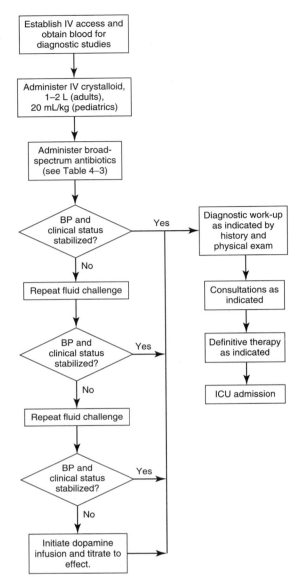

FIGURE 4–3 • Septic shock resuscitation.

It may be useful to repeat certain diagnostic tests. A second electrocardiogram may demonstrate an evolving myocardial infarction, or another hemoglobin or hematocrit determination may demonstrate blood loss even though the initial levels were normal.

Consultation with an intensivist or surgeon may help clarify the etiology, and a patient in shock requires admission to an intensive care unit. The goal in the emergency department is to provide initial stabilization and aggressive hemodynamic support to a critically ill patient. At times, despite aggressive efforts, the cause of shock may

TABLE 4–3. Initial Antibiotic Therapy for Empirical Treatment of Patients in Septic Shock

Classification of Patient	Antibiotics of Choice, Dose	Alternatives, Dose
Community-acquired infection of urinary tract origin	Cefotaxime, 2 g, or ceftizoxime, 2 g, or ceftriaxone, 2 g	Piperacillin, 3 g, or ticarcillin, 3 g, or ciprofloxacin, 400 mg (and gentamicin,* 2 mg/kg)
Community-acquired infection with source above the diaphragm and not associated with aspiration	Ceftizoxime, 2 g, or cefoperazone, 2 g (and gentamicin,* 2 mg/kg)	Ticarcillin/clavulanate, 6.2 g, or ampicillin/sulbactam, 3 g, or imipenem/cilastatin, 1 g (and gentamicin,* 2 mg/kg)
Community-acquired infection with source below diaphragm or associated with aspiration	Ceftizoxime, 2 g, or cefoperazone, 2 g, *and* metronidazole, 15 mg/kg, or clindamycin, 900 mg (gentamicin,* 2 mg/kg)	Ticarcillin/clavulanate, 6.2 g, or ampicillin/sulbactam, 3 g, or imipenem/cilastatin, 1 g (and gentamicin,* 2 mg/kg)
Hospital- or nursing home–acquired infections in immunocompetent hosts	Ceftazidime, 2 g, or cefoperazone, 2 g (and metronidazole, 15 mg/kg, or clindamycin, 900 mg, if source below the diaphragm or aspiration is a concern)	Ticarcillin/clavulanate, 3 g, or ampicillin/sulbactam, 3 g, or imipenem/cilastatin, 1 g *and* Gentamicin,* 2 mg/kg
Neutropenic patients (ANC < 1000/mm^3)	Ticarcillin, 3 g, or piperacillin, 3 g, or imipenem/cilastatin, 1 g *and* Gentamicin,* 2 mg/kg	Ceftazidime, 2 g, or cefoperazone, 2 g, *and* Gentamicin,* 2 mg/kg, or aztreonam, 2 g, or ciprofloxacin, 400 mg
Intravenous drug abusers	Nafcillin, 1.5 g, or vancomycin, 500 mg *and* Gentamicin,* 2 mg/kg	Ceftizoxime, 2 mg, or cefotaxime, 2 g, or ceftriaxone, 2 g (and vancomycin, 500 mg)
Patients with indwelling vascular catheters	Nafcillin, 1.5 g, or vancomycin, 500 mg *and* Gentamicin,* 2 mg/kg	Ceftazidime, 2 g, or cefoperazone, 2 g

* Alternatives are tobramycin, 2 mg/kg, and amikacin, 5 mg/kg.
ANC, absolute neutrophil count.

not be determined until the pathologic process evolves or further diagnostic evaluation is completed in the intensive care unit.

SPECIAL CONSIDERATIONS

Pediatric Patients

Worldwide, the most common cause of shock in the pediatric age group is dehydration secondary to infectious gastroenteritis (see Chapter 28, Dehydration). In the United States, hemorrhagic shock (secondary to trauma) replaces dehydration as the major cause of death. As in adults, the treatment of shock is aggressive and follows the same principles of rapid evaluation and stabilization.

Key points in the evaluation of children in shock include

- Normal vital signs vary with each pediatric age group. Immediate access to reference material defining what is normal for the age of the patient is essential (see Ch 26: The Febrile Infant). The Broselow tape is a length-based system for determining normal vital signs, correct medication dosages, and equipment sizes for children.
- Important elements of the pediatric history include information on birth history, birth weight, immunizations, feeding patterns, developmental milestones, and any medical conditions.
- Children have very strong compensatory mechanisms and may appear reasonably stable in the early stages of shock; however, when compensation mechanisms fail, children's conditions deteriorate very rapidly.
- Fluid resuscitation with crystalloid is administered as a 20 mL/kg bolus, infused as rapidly as possible. If there is no improvement after the first bolus, a second bolus is given. Most children in hypovolemic shock will respond to 40 mL/kg. If a third bolus is required, the child may require hemodynamic monitoring, which is used to guide further fluid administration and pressor therapy.
- Parental observations and concerns should be noted and given significant consideration during patient evaluation and management.

Elderly Patients

Certain problems that lead to shock are significantly more common in older patients. The frail elderly patient (especially those who are institutionalized) is more susceptible to a variety of infectious diseases. The presence of an indwelling bladder catheter is a major predisposing factor. Localized infections rapidly develop into systemic sepsis, secondary to impairment of immune defenses, with septic shock the result. An aggressive approach to management, with early institution of appropriate broad-spectrum antibiotics, is indicated.

Severe cardiac failure and cardiogenic shock are more common in elderly patients, as are the catastrophic sequelae of vascular disease (aortic dissection and rupture of aortic aneurysms). The diagnosis of acute myocardial infarction is often more difficult in elderly patients with nonspecific complaints or the lack of typical complaints associated with cardiac ischemia. The management of the elderly patient with both severe congestive heart failure and cardiogenic shock is very complicated and requires guidance with invasive hemodynamic monitoring.

Thoracic or abdominal vascular catastrophes have high mortality rates and require aggressive resuscitation, prompt diagnostic evaluation, and surgical intervention. Ruptured abdominal aneurysm in the elderly may have few abdominal findings to assist with the diagnosis, and a very high level of suspicion is required. All elderly patients with even vague complaints of abdominal, flank, testicular or lower back pain are considered candidates to be evaluated for the presence of a leaking or ruptured aortic aneurysm.

Regardless of the underlying process, elderly patients frequently present with nonspecific complaints and have limited ability to tolerate hemodynamic derangements or aggressive attempts at their correction. Underlying renal or cardiac disease will severely limit the ability of an elderly patient to tolerate large, rapidly administered fluid volumes. Smaller boluses of crystalloid (100 to 250 mL) followed by frequent reassessment are necessary when treating shock in this population. An aggressive approach and prompt intervention are essential to improve the outcome in elderly patients.

DISPOSITION AND FOLLOW-UP

Patients in shock require admission to an intensive care unit. Depending on the cause of the shock, emergency surgery may be indicated. The etiology of shock dictates the appropriate consultations and type of intensive care needed, but when it is unclear, both medical and surgical consultation may be needed.

FINAL POINTS

- Shock is a life-threatening diagnosis that requires early identification and treatment.
- Aggressive measures should be directed at securing the airway and supporting the breathing and circulation and perfusion.
- The vital signs and response to treatment should be frequently assessed. Changes in mental status, urine output, and work of breathing are indices of therapeutic response.
- The history and physical examination should focus on determining the possible etiology of shock.
- Shock is a clinical diagnosis. Few diagnostic adjuncts will help identify the presence of shock, but they may assist in monitoring response to therapeutic interventions.

CASE *Study*

The patient was a 75-year-old man who appeared fatigued and listless. He had been ill for several days. He reported having vomiting, diarrhea, and abdominal pain. Vital signs were systolic blood pressure of 80 mm Hg, pulse rate of 130 beats per minute, respiratory rate of 25 breaths per minute and labored, and an oral temperature of 98.6°F (37°C). He had no urine output for 12 hours. He had no known allergies and took no prescription medication. His past medical history was unknown.

On physical examination, his mucous membranes were dry. His chest was clear to auscultation, and his heart sounds were regular, tachycardic, and without murmur or gallop. His abdomen was diffusely tender and slightly distended, and minimal bowel sounds were present. He had no edema or cyanosis. There were diminished pulses in the lower extremities.

At the bedside, pulse oximetry revealed an oxygen saturation of 98% on room air, the cardiac monitor demonstrated sinus tachycardia, the bedside hemoglobin level was 16 g/dL, the bedside glucose value was 100 mg/dL, and an initial 12-lead electrocardiogram was only significant for sinus tachycardia.

A brief history and physical examination was sufficient to begin treatment. The patient was tachycardic and hypotensive and in shock. The examination revealed dehydration. At this point, the most likely cause for the shock appeared to be dehydration caused by gastroenteritis. The patient required intravenous hydration, cardiac monitoring, and oxygen.

After 2 L of normal saline was instilled, the patient's systolic blood pressure remained at 80 mm Hg and his heart rate was 120 beats per minute. The patient had not urinated, and a Foley catheter was placed with 50 mL of dark urine obtained. A third liter of normal saline was started.

There should be concern about the amount and rate of fluid administration because of the patient's age and unknown past history. The original diagnosis of dehydration secondary to gastroenteritis should be questioned and a search made for other causes of shock.

The patient's lungs remained clear on repeat auscultation, and a repeat electrocardiogram was also unchanged. During a second examination, the physician did a rectal examination, remarkable for black, tarry stool that was Hemoccult positive. A detailed interview with a family member revealed that the patient was diagnosed with an ulcer 1 year ago and had been noncompliant with his medication. He had no history of cardiac disease.

The fluids were continued and blood was ordered for transfusion. A gastroenterologist and surgeon were consulted, and the patient was admitted to the intensive care unit. A repeat hemoglobin value taken in the intensive care unit was 8 g/dL. Hemodynamic status slowly improved after blood transfusion.

Elderly patients may be unable to give detailed and accurate histories, and physical findings may be very nonspecific. Confirmation of history, by interviewing family members or caregivers, and careful, complete examination is necessary to ensure that accurate data are collected and a reasonable differential diagnosis list is generated.

Bibliography

TEXTS

American College of Surgeons: Advanced Trauma Life Support Course for Physicians. Chicago, American College of Surgeons, 1997.

Brillman JC, Quyenzer RW (eds): Infectious Disease in Emergency Medicine, 2nd ed. Philadelphia, Lippincott–Raven, 1998.

JOURNAL ARTICLES

Activated protein C (Xigris) for severe sepsis. Med Lett Drugs Ther 2002; 44:17–18.

Bamberger DM, Gurley MB: Microbial etiology and clinical characteristics of distributive shock. Clin Infect Dis 1994; 18:726–730.

Bone RC, Balk RA, Cerra FB, et al: Definitions for sepsis and organ failure: Guidelines for the use of innovative therapies and sepsis. The ACCP/SCCM Consensus Conference Committee. American College of Chest Physicians/Society of Critical Care Medicine. Chest 1992; 101:1644–1655.

Checchia PA, Dietrich A, Perkid RM, et al: Current concepts in the recognition and management of pediatric cardiogenic shock and congestive heart failure. Pediatr Emerg Med Reports 2000; 5:41–60.

Ferguson KL, Brown L: Bacteremia and sepsis. Emerg Med Clin North Am 1994; 14:185–195.

Healey MA, Samphire J, Hoyt DB, et al: Irreversible shock is not irreversible: A new model of massive hemorrhage and resuscitation. J Trauma 2001; 50:826–834.

Hollenberg SM, Kavinsky CJ, Parrielo JE: Cardiogenic shock. Ann Intern Med 1999; 131:47–59.

Landry DW, Oliver JA: The pathogenesis of vasodilatory shock. N Engl J Med 2001; 345:588–595.

Marik PE, Varon J: The hemodynamic derangements in sepsis: Implications for treatment strategies. Chest 1998; 114:854–860.

McGee S, Abernethy WB, Simel DL: The rational clinical examination. Is this patient hypovolemic? JAMA 1999; 281:1022–1029.

McNutt S, Denninghoff KR, Terndrug T: Shock: Rapid recognition and appropriate ED intervention. Emerg Med Pract 2000; 2(8):1–24.

Perkin RM: Current concepts in the recognition and management of pediatric hypovolemic and septic shock. Pediatr Emerg Med Rep 1999; 4(10):95–114.

Rodgers KG: Cardiovascular shock. Emerg Med Clin North Am 1995; 13:793–811.

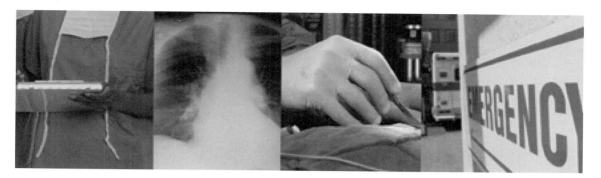

ABDOMINAL AND GASTROINTESTINAL DISORDERS

CHAPTER 5

Acute Abdominal Pain

JONATHAN VAN ZILE

MATTHEW L. EMERICK

CASE_Study_

A 72-year-old man was brought to the emergency department by paramedics for mid-epigastric and right flank pain that started suddenly while he was eating at a restaurant. Witnesses stated the patient "Fainted" and slumped forward.

INTRODUCTION

The patient presenting to the emergency department with acute abdominal pain is one of the most common as well as difficult challenges confronting the emergency physician. Four percent to 8% of all emergency department patients have the chief complaint of abdominal pain. Only 50% of those patients will have a clear diagnosis after assessments in the emergency department.

Abdominal pain is often vague and ill defined and requires a thorough understanding of abdominal organ pathophysiology, as well as a gentle and thoughtful approach to the patient. Also, nonabdominal disease may cause abdominal complaints that can complicate a patient's evaluation. Newer technology has certainly helped with more accurate diagnosis and disposition, but it should not supplant a detailed history and physical examination. Fifteen percent to 30% of patients with acute abdominal pain will require a surgical procedure. This percentage increases in the elderly. The most common disorder requiring surgical intervention remains appendicitis. It continues to be the most commonly misdiagnosed abdominal disease. Pediatric and elderly patients with abdominal pain have unique clinical characteristics that make them especially challenging to evaluate and properly diagnose.

Neuroanatomy of Pain Transmission

Determining the exact etiology of a patient's abdominal pain is difficult, owing to the vague types of pain perceived by the patient early in the course of disease. As the disorder progresses, the patient's symptoms often become more defined. To better understand the nature of abdominal pain, a basic knowledge of the gastrointestinal nervous system is necessary.

Clinically, there are three anatomic types of abdominal pain. These are visceral, somatic, and referred pain. Visceral pain is generated by stretch receptors located in the walls and capsules of hollow organs (i.e., gallbladder and intestines) and solid organs (i.e., spleen and liver). Distention, inflammation, and/or ischemia stimulate these receptors. They transmit impulses via unmyelinated fibers that enter the spinal cord bilaterally, and are perceived in the midline. Visceral pain is felt in the epigastrium or periumbilical or suprapubic area and is usually described as dull, achy, and cramping. Autonomic responses accompany visceral pain, causing pallor, diaphoresis, nausea, and vomiting. There are visceral pain location patterns that suggest certain organ groups. Pain originating from the stomach, gallbladder, liver, duodenum, and pancreas localizes to the epigastric area. Pain from the appendix, small bowel, and cecum usually localizes to the periumbilical area, and pain originating from the kidneys, ureter, bladder, colon, uterus, and ovaries localizes to the suprapubic area.

Somatic pain is initiated by pain receptors located in the parietal peritoneum surrounding or adjacent to the abdominal organs. Because the parietal peritoneum is not part of the organ it surrounds, it is usually involved later in the course of disease. Parietal-origin peritoneal pain is transmitted by myelinated afferent fibers to specific dorsal root ganglia on the same side and dermatome level as the origin of the pain. This type of pain is usually described as sharp, discrete, and localized. It is responsible for the physical findings of tenderness to palpation, guarding, and rebound. Somatic tenderness in a certain specific abdominal quadrant can narrow the differential diagnosis (Fig. 5–1).

Referred pain is discomfort perceived at a cutaneous site distant from the diseased organ (Fig. 5–2). These cutaneous areas and the diseased organ have overlapping pain transmission pathways. For example, visceral afferents from

DIFFERENTIAL DIAGNOSIS OF ACUTE ABDOMINAL PAIN BY LOCATION

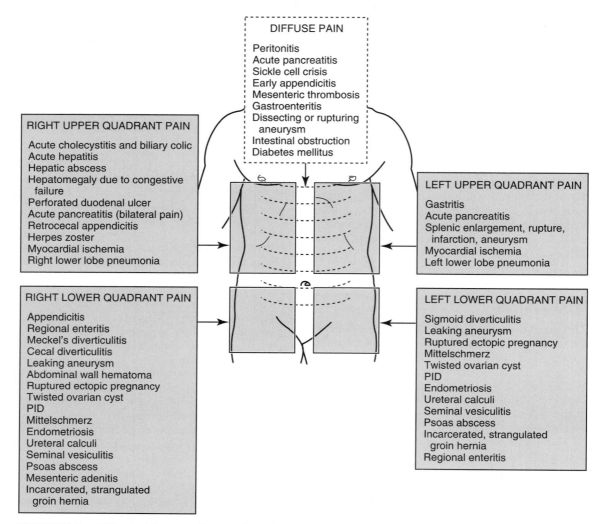

FIGURE 5–1 • Differential diagnosis of acute abdominal pain by location. (From Wagner DK: Approaches to the patient with acute abdominal pain. Curr Topics [a program of the Medical College of Pennsylvania] 1:3, 1978. Used by permission.)

the diaphragm enter the spinal cord at C3–C5. Pain from the diaphragm caused by irritation by free air, blood, or inflammation may be referred to the dermatomal distribution of C3–C5 (the lateral neck and posterior shoulder). The diseased organ refers pain to the ipsilateral cutaneous site (i.e., a ruptured spleen causes left shoulder pain). Extra-abdominal organs can produce referred pain to the abdomen by a similar mechanism.

INITIAL APPROACH AND STABILIZATION

The majority of patients who present to the emergency department with nontraumatic abdominal

pain arrive ambulatory; therefore, skillful triage is mandatory to recognize patients with potential life-threatening or organ-threatening problems.

Priority Diagnoses

The emergency physician must consider the following life-threatening conditions to ensure the safety of the patient:

- Vascular catastrophes: leaking/ruptured abdominal aneurysm or mesenteric ischemia/infarct

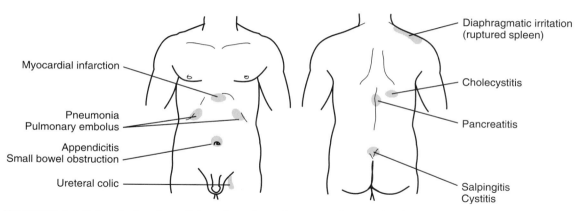

FIGURE 5–2 • Referred pain patterns. Pain or discomfort in these areas often provides clues to underlying disease process. (From Trott AT: Acute abdominal pain. In Rosen P, Markovchick VJ, Barkin RM, et al [eds]: Emergency Medicine: Concepts and Clinical Practice. St. Louis, CV Mosby, 1988.)

- Acute myocardial infarction or ischemia (with referred pain to the epigastric area)
- Ruptured ectopic pregnancy
- Perforated viscus
- Intestinal obstruction
- Acute hemorrhagic pancreatitis
- Esophageal rupture

Risk factors associated with more acutely ill patients include the following:

- Extremes of age. Causes of abdominal pain in the elderly (age > 65) are more likely to be diseases requiring surgical treatment, a vascular catastrophe, ischemic heart disease, or sepsis. Infants (age < 2) are unable to communicate their history or degree of pain and become dehydrated and septic sooner than adults. Vital signs in these groups often do not accurately reflect their degree of illness.
- Any abnormal vital sign
- Severe pain of rapid onset
- Signs of dehydration
- Skin pallor and diaphoresis (visceral pain signs)

Rapid Assessment

A brief medical history from the patient or family includes previous history of abdominal surgery, heart disease, vascular disease, pregnancy, peptic ulcer, diverticulitis, pancreatitis, or human immunodeficiency virus infection. The potential of allergies and the date of the last menstrual period are addressed.

The primary examination includes the patient's general appearance, level of consciousness, skin condition, cardiopulmonary auscultation, and an abdominal examination. The abdominal examination is focused on bowel sounds, areas of tenderness, guarding, and assessment for peritoneal signs. A rectal examination is important to assess for local tenderness, rectal tone, and prostate size, and to obtain stool for blood.

Early Intervention

If the initial assessment is consistent with a suspected underlying etiology, the following actions are performed.

1. The patient is placed on a cardiac monitor and a rhythm strip is obtained. In elderly patients or those at risk for cardiovascular disease, a complete electrocardiogram is obtained.
2. An intravenous line running isotonic crystalloid is initiated. For patients with hemodynamic instability, intravenous access with two large-bore catheters is accomplished. For the hypotensive patient, an initial bolus of 250 to 500 mL over 10 to 20 minutes is given and vital signs are rechecked. Elderly patients are initially given 100- to 250-mL boluses, whereas younger patients without underlying cardiovascular disease may be given 500 to 1000 mL initially. Higher rates may be necessary.
3. Supplemental O_2 at 2 to 4 L/min by nasal cannula or mask is started, and pulse oximetry results monitored.
4. A nasogastric tube is placed early in the course of care for patients with persistent vomiting, gastrointestinal bleeding, suspected bowel obstruction, suspected severe pancreatitis, or hemodynamic instability.
5. A urinary catheter may be therapeutic in relieving bladder obstruction. It is more often a diagnostic aid to obtain urine for a urinalysis and monitor the patient's output.
6. Blood and urine samples are obtained for analysis. Initially, one purple-, one blue-, and two red-topped tubes are sufficient.

7. Analgesics may be withheld until the initial assessment, with emphasis on the abdominal examination, is completed. Early dosing may be necessary to allow patient cooperation.

8. Early surgical consultation is essential for unstable patients or those suspected to have the previously noted priority diagnoses.

CLINICAL ASSESSMENT

The history and physical examination must be methodical and thorough, because abdominal pain is a common symptom that can arise from numerous intra- and extra-abdominal organs. After the initial stabilization, a complete assessment is necessary, not only to arrive at a diagnosis but also to re-assess the overall status of the patient. It is essential to understand the dynamic nature of pain progression and avoid hasty judgments based on a single examination. Unless the patient presents with a catastrophic condition, repeated abdominal examinations over time will often reveal the nature of the pain. Descriptive terms, such as "sharp," "stabbing," and "achy," must be clarified and mutually understood. Unclear language is a significant source of diagnostic error. Often a careful chronologic approach, with timing based around meals, work, or sleep patterns, can unravel a complex abdominal pain history.

Pain History

Onset. Rapid onset of severe pain is more consistent with a vascular catastrophe, passage of a ureteral or gallbladder stone, torsion of the testis or ovary, or rupture of a hollow viscus, ovarian cyst, or ectopic pregnancy. Slower, insidious onset is more typical of an inflammatory process such as appendicitis or cholecystitis.

Duration and Pattern of Change. Patients with pain less than 24 hours in duration or that is steadily increasing in intensity are at greater risk for surgical conditions. Constant pain has a worse diagnostic outcome.

Character of Pain. Pain that is dull, achy, or crampy is more likely to be visceral. Pain that is sharp or stabbing is more likely peritoneal or somatic. Crampy pain that comes in waves is associated with obstruction of a viscus, whereas severe, tearing back pain is classic for a dissecting aneurysm.

Severity. The patient's quantification of pain is notoriously unreliable. In general, nonspecific abdominal pain is less severe than pain of surgical conditions, but there is considerable individual variation. Assigning a 1–10 pain scale rating does allow a standard for monitoring response to treat-

ment and communication with consultants. Severe epigastric or midabdominal pain out of proportion to physical findings is classic for mesenteric ischemia or pancreatitis.

Location. The location of abdominal pain can vary with time, especially as the pain progresses from a visceral to a somatic origin. Periumbilical pain that migrates to the right lower quadrant is classic for appendicitis. Epigastric pain localizing during a period of several hours to the right upper quadrant is characteristic of cholecystitis.

Radiation. Given the pain patterns already discussed, involvement of certain organs can be implicated based on the radiating pattern of the pain (see Fig. 5–2).

Aggravating or Alleviating Factors. What makes the pain better or worse? Movement, such as hitting bumps on the ride to the hospital or even walking, aggravates parietal peritoneal pain. This finding is particularly supportive of the diagnosis of pelvic inflammatory disease or appendicitis. Eating usually relieves ulcer pain, whereas biliary colic is made worse by eating fatty foods (usually 1 to 4 hours after eating a meal). The pain of pancreatitis is alleviated by a curled-up posture (fetal position), whereas frequent movement or writhing pain is typical of renal colic.

Prior Pain History. After careful questioning, patients with cholecystitis will reveal having had similar pains in the recent past. The pain of ulcers, pancreatitis, diverticulitis, and renal colic tends to recur.

Pain Treatment. A patient's self-treatment provides insight into the patient's medical sophistication. The response to treatment may help measure the severity and evolution of the pain.

Associated Symptoms

Nausea and Vomiting. Almost any kind of visceral abdominal pain will elicit nausea with or without vomiting. The presence of vomiting is less useful for determining the diagnosis than for assessing severity of the patient's illness, potential dehydration, or the eventual ability of the patient to manage care at home. Excessive vomiting should raise the suspicion of bowel obstruction or pancreatitis, whereas the lack of vomiting is common in uterine or ovarian disorders. The temporal relationship of pain to the vomiting is an important piece of information. Pain present before vomiting is more likely to be caused by a disorder that will require surgery. Vomiting before abdominal pain is more likely caused by gastroenteritis or another disorder that will not require surgery.

Urgency to Defecate. This symptom may suggest intra-abdominal bleeding or purulent material in the cul-de-sac. It is thought to be caused by inflammation and irritation in the rectosigmoid area. It has been reported in ectopic pregnancy, abdominal aortic aneurysm, retroperitoneal hematoma, and omental vessel hemorrhage.

Anorexia. Intra-abdominal inflammation usually causes loss or decrease in appetite. Anorexia is a consistent, but not invariable, finding in patients with appendicitis.

Change in Bowel Habits. The presence of diarrhea with vomiting is almost always associated with gastroenteritis, but diarrhea may occur with pancreatitis, diverticulitis, and occasionally appendicitis. The reporting of blood in the stool is always an important finding to be explained promptly. Constipation with difficulty in passing stool or gas may be secondary to ileus or mechanical obstruction.

Genitourinary Symptoms. Dysuria, urgency, and frequency are hallmarks for cystitis. They can be found with inflammatory conditions adjacent to the bladder such as salpingitis, diverticulitis, or appendicitis. These conditions can cause sterile pyuria (white blood cells [WBCs] in the urine without bacteria). Hematuria with associated pain is generally specific to the urinary tract and can indicate renal colic, prostatitis, or cystitis.

Extra-abdominal Symptoms. Because life-threatening conditions such as myocardial infarction, pneumonia, or pulmonary embolus can present as abdominal pain, a complete review of symptoms is necessary to discover these and other extra-abdominal disorders.

Past Medical History

Medical Illness. Patients with diabetes, heart disease, lung disease, liver disease, hypertension, or renal disease are at increased risk for certain abdominal disorders and may require specialized stabilization, treatment, and surgical preparation. Hypertension is associated with abdominal aneurysm. Atrial fibrillation may cause mesenteric ischemia.

Medications. Corticosteroids and other immunosuppressants can significantly alter the patient's response to abdominal pathology. Pain is often less severe, peritoneal findings can be absent in the presence of perforation, fever can be absent, and WBC counts can be lower. Many antibiotics, especially erythromycin and tetracycline, can cause gastrointestinal discomfort and diarrhea. Laxatives, narcotics, and psychotropic medication may alter intestinal motility and can cause abdominal pain. Aspirin and nonsteroidal anti-inflammatory agents are frequent causes of

gastritis, peptic ulcer disease, and associated gastrointestinal bleeding.

Past Surgery. Prior abdominal surgery is a common cause of peritoneal adhesions and subsequent bowel obstruction. Also, prior abdominal surgery, depending on the procedure, can eliminate certain diagnoses, such as appendicitis and cholecystitis.

Menstrual History. A complete menstrual history is essential, especially in evaluating lower abdominal pain in female patients. A history of salpingitis, intrauterine devices, tubal ligation, or previous ectopic pregnancy increases the risk of ectopic pregnancy.

Habits. Alcohol history is important and may be minimized by the patient. Asking a family member may elicit a better estimate of a patient's suspected alcohol history. Alcohol abuse predisposes a patient to ulcers, gastritis, hepatitis, and pancreatitis. Laxative abuse is associated with diverticular disease and cecal volvulus.

Psychiatric Disorders. A psychiatric history can be important in the patient with abdominal pain. Patients with chronic undifferentiated abdominal pain, often with many visits to an emergency department, can have a coexisting psychiatric illness.

Family History. Associated family history may occur in inflammatory bowel disease, diverticulitis, cholecystitis, and abdominal aortic aneurysm. Brothers are often affected in the latter.

Physical Examination

A reliable physical examination requires a thorough, systematic approach and a cooperative patient. A calm, reassuring manner will often alleviate the patient's anxiety and make the examination more meaningful. It is almost certain a single examination will be inadequate to fully appreciate and properly interpret the abdominal findings. Reexamination and interval observation of the patient will greatly enhance the likelihood of arriving at the correct diagnosis or assessment. The accuracy of the physical examination findings, when compared with the final diagnosis, ranges between 55% and 65%.

The primary goals are to determine whether a "surgical" abdomen is present (rebound tenderness, involuntary guarding, and/or distention), or to localize the disease process to a specific abdominal area by determining the maximal area of tenderness. In addition, the physician assesses the patient's general medical condition and evaluates the requirement for stabilization and specific interventions.

The major components of the physical examination for the patient with abdominal pain include the following:

General Appearance

The patient's color and demeanor are important initial observations. Pale, diaphoretic, and motionless patients are generally more acutely ill and more likely to have a local or diffuse peritoneal involvement. Agitated, writhing patients are more likely to have visceral causes of abdominal pain, such as renal or biliary colic, mesenteric ischemia, or nonspecific abdominal pain. Advanced age is associated with increased risk of serious pathology.

Vital Signs

Temperature. Temperature is neither a sensitive nor a specific indicator of abdominal disease or patient condition. Patients with appendicitis often have a low-grade fever, less than 101°F (38.3°C). At least one third of appendicitis patients are afebrile. Patients with high temperatures, greater than 102°F (38.9°C), often have serious but nonsurgical conditions such as salpingitis, pyelonephritis, or bacterial enteritis. In elderly or immunosuppressed patients an absence of fever is common, even with serious and surgical conditions. These patients may have a lower basal temperature; thus a temperature of 99°F (37.2°C) may be significant.

Blood Pressure and Pulse Rate. These vital signs are helpful in gauging the severity of the disease process and potential for blood or fluid loss. In patients with poor intake, vomiting, diarrhea, or significant signs of dehydration, supine and orthostatic blood pressures and pulse rates can assist in determining the degree of volume depletion and the need for fluid replacement. A rise in the pulse rate of 20 to 30 beats per minute or a fall in the systolic blood pressure of 20 to 30 mm Hg measured at least 1 minute after standing indicates significant volume loss. Orthostatic values are obtained in patients without baseline hypotension or tachycardia. The changes in heart rate may be blunted by medications, including β blockers and calcium channel blockers.

Respiratory Rate. The respiratory rate can be indicative of severe illness. Pneumonia, pulmonary embolism, myocardial infarction, sepsis, or acidosis secondary to hypoperfusion can raise the respiratory rate. Resting tachypnea (>20 breaths per minute) in a patient who is not clearly anxious warrants careful assessment.

Extra-abdominal Examination. Before examining the abdomen, the physician examines pertinent extra-abdominal areas. Gentle, first contact with an "uninvolved" site can help put the patient at ease. The heart and lungs are examined for disease as well as to assess the cardiopulmonary status of the patient. The patient's flanks are percussed to elicit tenderness if present. The male external genitalia can harbor the cause (e.g., testicular torsion) of abdominal pain. The peripheral pulses are palpated, and skin and mucous membranes are assessed for signs of dehydration, hypoperfusion, or jaundice.

Abdominal Examination

Inspection. Distention, asymmetry, prior surgery, masses, ecchymoses, pregnancy, or cutaneous signs of portal hypertension may be detected with inspection.

Auscultation. Auscultation is carried out before deep palpation to avoid a potential increase in bowel sounds. Decreased bowel sounds are heard in peritonitis and other inflammatory processes that slow peristalsis and lead to ileus. Increased bowel sounds can be heard in patients with nonspecific abdominal pain and gastroenteritis. Bowel obstruction classically produces high-pitched sounds and rushes. In general, bowel sounds vary widely for any given cause of abdominal pain and are of little diagnostic value.

Percussion. Gentle percussion in all four abdominal quadrants can localize the site of pain initially. Percussing the abdomen can often provide information about the size of certain organs and the cause of abdominal distention, whether gas (bowel obstruction), liquid (ascites), or solid (enlarged liver). It may be useful for detecting an overdistended bladder.

Palpation. Most of the time and effort in the abdominal examination is spent on palpation. At this point, the patient needs to be the most cooperative and at ease. Asking the patient to flex the legs at the hips and knees may relax the abdominal musculature. It is important to note the patient's facial expressions during palpation. A grimace is usually more significant than the statement, "It hurts."

A crucial distinction between pain and tenderness has to be made for the patient before and during palpation. When trying to elicit true tenderness, the patient might give an inappropriate affirmative answer to the question, "Does this hurt?," when in fact the area in question is not tender. By carefully seeking "tenderness," the chances of identifying a diseased organ are greatly increased.

Palpation is started as far away as possible from the perceived location of the pain. The epigastrium, suprapubic area, and all four quadrants are slowly and gently palpated systematically, ending at the perceived area of maximum pain. Palpation is gentle but firm. Gradual increases of pressure while palpating are better tolerated than a single movement. Deep palpation is often limited by the patient's pain tolerance. In abdominal pain of visceral origin, localization of tenderness is less likely. With somatic involvement, localization of true tenderness is possible.

Additional Associated Findings

Muscular Signs. Guarding is the reflex contraction of the abdominal wall musculature in response to palpation or underlying peritoneal irritation. It can be voluntary or involuntary. Voluntary guarding is less significant in predicting surgical disease and may be a response to anxiety or a rushed examination. Reassurance and gentle palpation can usually resolve it. Involuntary abdominal muscle spasm is elicited by asking the patient to take a deep breath while firm pressure is held on a tender area. If spasm is not relieved, involuntary guarding is present. If the muscles relax, voluntary guarding is present and deeper palpation is made possible. Increased tenderness to palpation with contracted abdominal muscles (e.g., patient lifting head or legs) has a high correlation with pain of abdominal wall origin.

Rebound Tenderness. Rebound is classically the hallmark of peritoneal irritation, although it may be present in up to 25% of patients with nonspecific abdominal pain and absent in up to 50% of patients with appendicitis. It is elicited by slow, gentle, deep palpation of the tender area followed by abrupt, but discreet withdrawal of the examiner's hand. Optimally, the patient is distracted by conversation. Often, this procedure is not necessary because rebound can be elicited by having the patient cough, thumping the examiner's hand against the patient's heel, or percussion of the tender area. When the rebound maneuver is performed in a nontender area and tenderness is elicited in the painful area in question, peritoneal involvement is likely at the site of the disease. Rebound or its absence is less diagnostic in the elderly population.

Special Techniques

Iliopsoas and Obturator Signs. The iliopsoas sign is performed by having the patient flex the thigh against resistance created by the examiner. The obturator sign is performed with the hip in the flexed position and then internally and externally rotated. Pain elicited by these maneuvers is suggestive of an overlying inflammatory disease such as appendicitis, diverticulitis, or pelvic

inflammatory disease. It is seen in less than 10% of patients with appendicitis.

Murphy's Sign. The physician palpates deeply in the right upper quadrant and asks the patient to take a deep breath. Abrupt cessation of inspiration caused by pain is suggestive of cholecystitis, hepatitis, or other right upper quadrant abnormalities.

Fist Percussion. Gently percussing the costovertebral angles of the back with a fist elicits tenderness in patients with pyelonephritis or obstructive uropathy.

Rovsing's Sign. In cases of appendicitis, tenderness is elicited over McBurney's point by performing the rebound maneuver on the left side of the abdomen. This is noted in only 5% of patients.

Related Examinations

Vascular. In elderly patients with known arterial vascular disease, the abdominal aorta and femoral pulses are palpated. Gently palpating the aorta from both sides with the fingers in the nonobese patient can provide an estimate of the aortic diameter. The presence of palpable *lateral* aortic pulsations is suggestive of aortic aneurysm. Auscultation for abdominal bruits can be performed. They are often present in young, healthy people.

Hernial and Genital. The groin areas are inspected and palpated for direct and indirect hernias. Unrecognized hernias can progress to bowel obstruction. External genitalia are examined and the testes palpated.

Rectal. This examination is necessary in the search for melena, blood, masses, and prostate tenderness or enlargement. It is important in diagnosis and is not to be deferred. Rectal tenderness is a sign of appendicitis, salpingitis, or any process that allows inflammatory fluid to collect in the pelvic cul-de-sac. It occurs in less than 50% of cases of appendicitis and is not specific to any cause of lower abdominal disease.

Pelvic. All women of childbearing age with abdominal pain require a pelvic examination as well as a test for pregnancy. Cervical appearance, cervical motion tenderness, uterine size, and adnexal size and tenderness are all assessed. As with the rectal examination, cervical motion tenderness may be elicited by inflammatory fluid in the cul-de-sac.

Bedside Tests

Pregnancy testing and dipstick urinalysis in the emergency department may be more cost effective and provide rapid diagnosis and management for selected patients. Bedside systems are becoming more prevalent and can test for WBC count, amylase, and electrolytes.

Bedside ultrasonography has become a very useful adjunct for patients with abdominal pain. The emergency medicine physician proficient in the use of ultrasonography can make more definitive diagnoses in the area of biliary colic, ovarian cysts, ectopic pregnancy, renal colic, and abdominal aneurysm (ultrasonography is not diagnostic for a leaking aneurysm). User inexperience, patient obesity, and bowel gas may limit the effectiveness of abdominal ultrasonography. For this reason, formal training is recommended for emergency physicians.

CLINICAL REASONING

Throughout the care of a patient with abdominal pain, the emergency physician proceeds in a logical, stepwise manner toward the diagnosis, treatment, and disposition. The algorithm provides a framework on which to make decisions at key points in the patient's care (Fig. 5–3). Urgency for action rests on determining whether the patient falls into three general states.

Is the Patient Hemodynamically Unstable, or Are There Any Signs, Symptoms, or Findings for Life-threatening Disease?

If this is the case, the emergency physician proceeds as outlined earlier for initial stabilization. Even though life-threatening causes of abdominal pain do not occur frequently, they always take the highest priority. The important clinical findings in life-threatening, intra-abdominal causes of acute abdominal pain, including myocardial infarction, pulmonary embolus, and lobar pneumonia, are summarized in Table 5–1.

Is the Pain Acute, and Is There a Potential Surgical Cause for the Pain?

Severe pain accompanied by localized tenderness with peritoneal findings is the hallmark of serious and possibly surgical disease. Usually the pain will have been acute in onset, and there will be accompanying abnormal vital signs or laboratory test results to support the suspicion of a disease that requires surgical intervention. Early surgical consultation is indicated for these patients.

As Is the Case for Most Patients, Does the Patient Have Abdominal Pain Without a Clear Initial Cause or Any Instability or Indication for Surgery?

In this case, the full range of diagnostics are available. Reexamining the patient, over a period of time, is the mainstay of this assessment.

Would the Patient Benefit from Symptomatic Relief?

Rehydration, antiemetics, and gastric decompression by nasogastric tubing may be helpful in relieving patient symptoms while diagnostic evaluation proceeds. Judicious analgesics have been demonstrated *not* to impair the assessment of patients with acute abdominal pain and should not be withheld.

DIAGNOSTIC ADJUNCTS

These studies are selected to support the diagnosis suggested by clinical findings, and assess the underlying condition and stability of the patient. Overreliance on diagnostic adjuncts is to be avoided. Ultimately, there is no substitute for the clinical examination and, specifically, the abdominal examination.

Laboratory Studies

Complete Blood Cell Count. This study is often ordered in cases of abdominal pain presenting to the emergency department. It is a nonspecific test with little diagnostic value and may be considered a potentially misleading study. The WBC count, differential, or absolute neutrophil count is not the deciding factor for determining whether a patient has a surgical abdomen or a serious abdominal disorder.

There is a less than 20% chance the WBC count will impact clinical decision making in patients with possible acute appendicitis. From 10% to 60% of patients with surgically proven appendicitis have an initially normal WBC count. In appendicitis, pelvic inflammatory disease, and cholecystitis, WBC counts are often higher for complications, such as perforation, peritonitis, fulminant pancreatitis, or sepsis. Still, elevated WBC counts are seen in 40% of patients with gastroenteritis and 30% of patients with abdominal pain of unknown etiol-

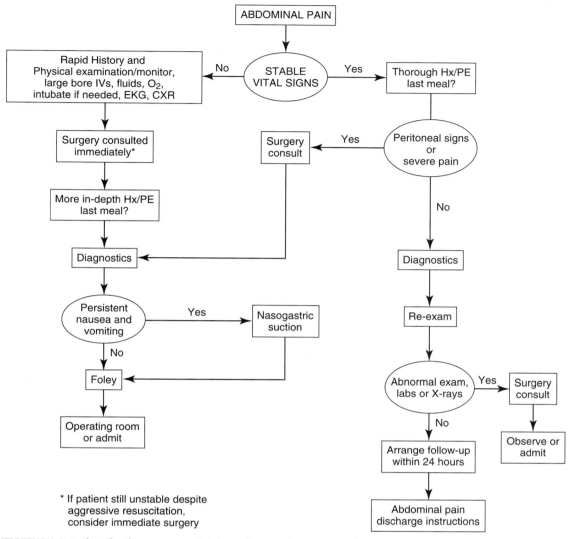

FIGURE 5–3 • Algorithm for assessment of abdominal pain in the emergency department.

ogy. An elevated WBC count reveals only 50% of severe abdominal pathology. In geriatric or immunosuppressed patients, the WBC count may be low or normal.

The hemoglobin-hematocrit is important for patients with suspected hemorrhage, dehydration, or anemia. If an acute hemorrhage is suspected, as in a patient with a ruptured ectopic pregnancy or leaking aortic aneurysm, the initial hemoglobin-hematocrit level may be unchanged but will provide a baseline from which to estimate blood loss over time. If chronic bleeding from a gastrointestinal or genitourinary source is suggested, the initial hemoglobin-hematocrit reading will help estimate the degree of blood loss.

Amylase-Lipase. The serum amylase value is neither sensitive nor specific in the diagnosis of

pancreatitis. It may be elevated in peptic ulcer disease, small bowel obstruction or ischemia, common duct stone, ectopic pregnancy, renal failure, alcoholic intoxication, or facial trauma (salivary amylase). As many as 20% of patients with proven pancreatitis may present with a normal amylase value. An elevated amylase level does often indicate serious abdominal pathologic processes. Lipase is more specific and sensitive for pancreatitis than amylase. Lipase rises in acute pancreatitis as early as amylase and stays elevated for longer periods of time. The amylase value may be normal with chronic pancreatitis, whereas the lipase level is usually elevated. Small elevations of either enzyme do not necessarily indicate disease. Elevations of two to three times normal are more specific for true pancreatic inflammation.

TABLE 5–1. Potential Life-Threatening Causes of Abdominal Pain

	Epidemiology	Etiology	Presentation	Physical Examination	Useful Tests
Ruptured or Leaking Abdominal Aortic Aneurysm	Incidence increases with advancing age. More frequent in men. Risk factors include HTN, DM, smoking, COPD, and CAD.	Atherosclerosis in over 95%. Intimal dissection causes aortic dilatation and creation of a false lumen. Leakage or rupture causes shock.	Patient often asymptomatic until rupture. Acute epigastric and back pain often associated with or followed by syncope or signs of shock. Pain may radiate to back, groin, or testes.	Vital signs may be normal (in 70% of patients) to severely hypotensive. Palpation of a pulsatile mass is usually possible in aneurysms 5.0 cm or greater. If suspected, the examination should not be relied on only. CT or US usually indicated. Bruits or inequality of femoral pulses are an inconsistent finding.	Abdominal plain films abnormal in 80% of cases. Lateral abdominal film may be helpful. Ultrasound can define diameter and length but limited by obesity and gas. Spiral CT test of choice if patient is stable.
Perforated Viscus	Incidence increases with advancing age. History of peptic ulcer disease or diverticular disease common. History of NSAID use common. The longer the time between perforation and diagnosis, the higher the mortality rate.	Often a duodenal ulcer that erodes through the serosa. Colonic diverticula, large bowel, small bowel, and gallbladder perforations are rare. Spillage of bowel contents causes peritonitis.	Acute onset of epigastric pain is common. Vomiting occurs in 50%. Fever may be present later. Pain may localize with omental walling off of peritonitis. Elderly patients may have minimal pain.	Fever, usually low grade, is common; higher fever occurs with time. Tachycardia is common. Shock may be present with bleeding or sepsis. Abdominal examination often reveals distention, diffuse guarding, and rebound. A "boardlike" abdomen is noted in later stages. Bowel sounds are decreased.	WBC count is usually elevated due to peritonitis. Amylase level may be elevated as well. LFT results are variable. Upright view of radiographs reveals free air in 70% to 80% of cases with perforated ulcers. CT identifies free air and may give more information.
Acute Pancreatitis	Peak age in adulthood. Rare in childhood and elderly. Male preponderance. Alcohol abuse and biliary tract disease.	Alcohol, gallstones, hyperlipidemia, hypercalcemia, or endoscopic retrograde pancreatography causes pancreatic damage, saponification, and necrosis. ARDS, sepsis, hemorrhage, and renal failure are secondary.	Acute onset of epigastric pain radiating to the back. Nausea and vomiting common. Pain out of proportion to physical examination findings. Adequate volume repletion is important in the initial therapy.	Low-grade fever common. Patient may be hypotensive or tachypneic. Some epigastric tenderness usually present. Because it is a retroperitoneal organ, guarding or rebound is not present unless severe.	Lipase is test of choice. Amylase level 3 times normal is more specific for diagnosis. US may show edema or pseudocyst. CT may show abscesses, necrosis, hemorrhage, or pseudocysts. CT is ordered if severe acute pancreatitis is suspected.

Intestinal Obstruction	Adhesions, carcinoma, hernias, abscesses, volvulus, and infarction occur. Obstruction leads to vomiting, third spacing of fluid, strangulation, and necrosis of bowel. Peaks in infancy with advancing age. More common with history of previous abdominal surgery.	Crampy diffuse abdominal pain associated with vomiting.	Vitals signs usually normal unless dehydration or bowel strangulation has occurred. Abdominal distention, hyperactive bowel sounds, and diffuse tenderness occur. Local peritoneal signs indicate strangulation.	WBC count may indicate strangulation if elevated. Electrolytes may be abnormal if associated with vomiting or prolonged symptoms. Abdominal films are useful for identifying level of obstruction. US or CT rarely needed to make diagnosis.
Mesenteric Ischemia	Occurs most often in elderly people with CV disease, CHF, cardiac dysrhythmias, DM, sepsis, and dehydration. Responsible for 1 of 1000 hospital admissions. Mortality is 70%. Mesenteric venous thrombosis is associated with hypercoagulable states, hematologic disorders, intraperitoneal inflammation, and trauma. Twenty percent to 30% of lesions are nonocclusive. The causes of ischemia are multifactorial, including transient hypotension in the presence of preexisting atherosclerotic lesion. The arterial occlusive causes (65%) are secondary to emboli (75%) or acute arterial thrombosis (25%).	Severe pain that is acute and colicky and starts in periumbilical region and then becomes diffuse is suggestive of SMA embolus. Vomiting and diarrhea are often associated. SMA thrombosis is usually more gradual in onset. Patient may have history of abdominal angina, weight loss, or diarrhea. Mesenteric vein thrombosis evident with progressive onset of pain. Patient may have venous thrombosis history.	Early examination results can be remarkably benign in the presence of severe ischemia. Bowel sounds often still present. Rectal examination is important because mild bleeding with positive guaiac stools can be present.	Often a pronounced leukocytosis is present. Elevations of amylase and creatine phosphokinase levels are seen. Metabolic acidosis due to lactic acidemia is often noted with infarction. Plain films are of limited benefit. CT with contrast, MRI, and angiography are accurate to varying degrees. Angiography is best for arterial causes.

ARDS, adult respiratory disease syndrome; CAD, coronary artery disease; CHF, congestive heart failure; COPD, chronic obstructive pulmonary disease; CT, computed tomography; CV, cardiovascular; DM, diabetes mellitus; HTN, hypertension; LFT, liver function tests; MRI, magnetic resonance imaging; NSAID, nonsteroidal anti-inflammatory drug; SMA, superior mesenteric artery; US, ultrasound; WBC, white blood cell.

Liver Function Tests. These tests are not routinely ordered for screening. They are best used if the clinical history or physical suggests hepatic or biliary disease. Elevations in the alkaline phosphatase and bilirubin levels are consistent with biliary tract disease or common bile duct obstruction. Elevations of the serum levels of the aminotransferases (arginine [AST] and alanine [ALT]) are consistent with hepatitis.

Serum Chemistries. Electrolytes and blood urea nitrogen (BUN)–creatinine are useful in patients with poor intake, vomiting, or signs of dehydration. Potassium levels are often low after severe vomiting and diarrhea. A low bicarbonate level may be associated with an anion gap acidosis, as noted in sepsis, mesenteric ischemia, or diabetic ketoacidosis. A high BUN:creatinine ratio is a good indicator of sustained volume depletion, or blood retained in the intestinal lumen.

Urinalysis. The urinalysis is interpreted with caution in patients with abdominal pain, because many nonurinary conditions may be associated with abnormal urine. Generally, more than 10 WBCs per high-power field, bacteria, or positive nitrite or positive leukocyte esterase determination in a clean-catch urine sample are findings consistent with a urinary tract infection. Red blood cells in the urine can be seen with infection, tumor, trauma, or stone. Inflammatory conditions, such as appendicitis, adjacent to the ureter or bladder, can cause a sterile pyuria, blood, or bacteriuria in up to 20% to 30% of patients without actual urinary tract infection. Premature attribution of a patient's abdominal pain to a urinary tract infection must be avoided. Gross hematuria may be seen in abdominal aortic aneurysm (30%) and may delay the diagnosis while a urinary etiology is evaluated.

Pregnancy Tests. Any woman of childbearing age presenting with abdominal pain should have a qualitative test for pregnancy. Serum and urine tests are highly sensitive to the low levels of human chorionic gonadotropin (hCG) of early pregnancy. A positive test in a patient with abdominal pain requires ectopic pregnancy be considered and ruled out. A serum quantitative hCG test and ultrasonography are performed in consultation with an obstetrician or gynecologist (See Chapter 39; Acute Pelvic Pain).

Other Laboratory Studies. Creatinine phosphokinase, lactate, and serum inorganic phosphate levels may be elevated in mesenteric ischemia or infarction. Lactate levels have been shown to be 100% sensitive and 42% specific for mesenteric ischemia. Also, serum inorganic phosphate levels may be elevated in 80% of patients with intestinal infarction. Unfortunately, if these tests are abnormal in the presence of intestinal vascular compromise, it may be prognostically too late for the patient.

Radiologic Imaging

Traditionally, obtaining a flat and upright radiologic view of the abdomen was routine in accessing the patient with abdominal pain. With the improvement of ultrasound and computed tomography (CT) techniques, plain radiographs have become less useful. They have specific value if perforated viscus (free air), bowel obstruction, foreign body, and, more rarely, bowel ischemia are suggested.

Chest Radiograph. An upright chest radiograph can help diagnose pneumonia, pleural effusion, and other pulmonary causes of abdominal pain. It is the best view for free intraperitoneal air from a perforated viscus and is capable of detecting as little as 5 mL of air.

Abdominal Radiograph. An abdominal series usually consists of flat and erect views of the abdomen as well as a posteroanterior chest view. If the patient is unable to stand, an abdominal left lateral decubitus film is obtained to rule out free air and to evaluate air-fluid levels. Abdominal films are usually of low yield for patients with abdominal pain. It has not been shown to be of benefit in diagnosing appendicitis. Radiographic findings that either confirm or reveal the cause of pain occur in only 10% to 38% of cases. Of these, only 10% will actually alter the diagnosis or management plan. Radiographic signs most commonly sought are dilated loops of small or large bowel (i.e., volvulus or small bowel obstruction), air-fluid levels, abnormal calcifications in the urinary tract system or vascular calcifications outside of their usual anatomic location (i.e., aortic aneurysm), free air under the diaphragm, and gallstones.

Ultrasonography. Ultrasound imaging has become the diagnostic test of choice for right upper quadrant pain and suspected pelvic causes of abdominal pain. If immediately available, it can rapidly secure the diagnosis of abdominal aneurysm. Ultrasound can show multiple organ systems, including the biliary tract, pancreas, kidneys, aorta, uterus, and ovaries. The sensitivity of ultrasound in the detection of gallstones approaches 94% to 100%. Other conditions commonly detected by ultrasound include biliary obstruction, aortic aneurysm, pancreatic pseudocysts, ureteral obstruction, and intrauterine versus ectopic pregnancy. In experienced hands, ultrasonography can detect appendicitis with a high degree of accuracy.

Computed Tomography. The spiral or helical abdominal CT scan provides excellent visualization of retroperitoneal organs, solid organs, and the abdominal aorta. CT scans identify free air in the peritoneal space. A spiral CT is the test of choice for suspected leaking or ruptured abdominal aneurysm. In patients with right lower quadrant abdominal pain, CT has shown to be very sensitive and specific for appendicitis. Accuracy rates have exceeded 95%. Oral and rectal contrast media increase the sensitivity and specificity of the scan and allow better visualization of the bowel and appendix. In patients with an unclear etiology for their abdominal pain, CT scans make a diagnosis in 95% of cases and lead to a change in the treatment plan in 30% of cases. Abdominal CT has become a major diagnostic tool for emergency physicians and represents a significant advance in clinical care. The patient must be sufficiently stable to be transferred out of the emergency department. Unstable patients are at increased risk in the radiology suite.

Nuclear Medicine. Hepatobiliary scintigraphy with technetium-99m–radiolabeled imaging agents is useful in the diagnosis of cholecystitis, especially when ultrasound cannot confirm gallstones or inflammation. Nonfilling of the gallbladder is consistent with a stone obstructing the cystic duct. The level of bilirubin does not affect the test. Also, a bleeding scan is useful for identifying the site of a gastrointestinal hemorrhage (>0.1 mL/min).

Angiography. This diagnostic procedure is usually reserved for patients with suspected mesenteric ischemia or gastrointestinal bleeding (a bleeding rate of >0.5 mL/min will usually result in a positive test). This procedure is also useful for diagnosis of a leaking aortic aneurysm; however, spiral CT is the initial test of choice.

Electrocardiogram

As previously discussed, myocardial ischemia can be referred to the upper abdomen; therefore, an electrocardiogram is indicated for most adult patients (especially those older than 40 years old) with upper abdominal pain and a nontender abdomen. An electrocardiogram is also indicated for elderly and unstable patients.

EXPANDED DIFFERENTIAL DIAGNOSIS

After performing the clinical assessment, interpreting the radiologic and laboratory studies, and observing the patient, a refined differential diagnosis can be formulated for the catastrophic (see Table 5–1) and common (Table 5–2) causes of abdominal pain.

PRINCIPLES OF MANAGEMENT

For patients with acute abdominal disorders, the main treatment goals are to stabilize vital functions, replete volume loss, control emesis and gastric emptying, relieve pain, and administer antibiotics as necessary. In patients with surgical disorders, the emergency physician can best serve the patient by preparing the patient for surgery.

Volume Repletion

Intravenous access with volume repletion is indicated for patients with demonstrable changes in their vital signs, dry mucous membranes, or a history of significant vomiting or diarrhea. An intravenous line is also indicated for patients who need to avoid oral intake before surgical intervention. The usual choice of intravenous solution is an isotonic crystalloid. The degree of hypovolemia, the cardiovascular status of the patient, and the response of the vital signs to the initial therapy determine the rate and amount of volume repletion. If the patient is actively bleeding or judged to have a life threat, two large-bore intravenous lines are started in addition to other measures, such as oxygen supplementation and cardiovascular monitoring.

Gastric Emptying

Nasogastric suction is indication for patients with persistent vomiting, suspected ileus, or bowel obstruction. In addition, nasogastric suction is indicated for patients requiring surgery.

Control of Emesis

Antiemetics are used with caution in any patient with abdominal pain. They can be useful for patients with gastroenteritis, gastritis, renal colic, or conditions in which nausea and vomiting are prominent. Antiemetics do not alter pain sensation but can make a patient lethargic, drowsy, and confused. This effect is more common in very young and elderly patients. Commonly used parenteral or rectal antiemetics are promethazine (Phenergan) and prochlorperazine (Compazine).

Pain Relief

Recent studies show opiate analgesics do not hinder the surgeon's diagnosis or management. The diagnosis may be aided by enhanced patient

TABLE 5–2. Common Causes of Abdominal Pain

	Epidemiology	Etiology	Presentation	Physical Examination	Useful Tests
Acute Appendicitis	Peak age: adolescence and young adulthood. Less common in children and elderly. Higher perforation rate in women, children, and elderly. Mortality rate is 0.1% but increased to 2% to 6% with perforation.	Appendiceal lumen obstruction leads to swelling, ischemia, infection, and perforation.	Epigastric or periumbilical pain migrates to RLQ over 8–12 hours (50%–60%). Later presentations associated with higher perforation rates. Pain, low-grade fever (15%), and anorexia (80%) common; vomiting less common (50%–70%).	Mean temperature 100.5°F (38°C). Higher temperature associated with perforation. RLQ tenderness (90%–95%) with rebound (40%–70%) in majority of cases. Rectal tenderness in up to 30%.	Leukocyte count usually elevated or may show left shift. Urine may show sterile pyuria. C-reactive proteins sensitive, but accuracy varies. CT is sensitive and specific. US may have use in women with RLQ pain.
Biliary Tract Disease	Peak age: 35–60. Rare in patients younger than 20. Female-to-male ratio of 3:1. Risk factors include multiparity, obesity, alcohol intake, and birth control pills.	Passage of gallstones causes biliary colic. Impaction of a stone in cystic duct or common duct causes cholecystitis or cholangitis.	Crampy RUQ pain radiates to right subscapular area. Prior history of pain is common. Longer duration of pain favors diagnosis of cholecystitis or cholangitis.	Temperature normal in biliary colic and elevated in cholecystitis and cholangitis. RUQ tenderness, rebound, and jaundice (less common) may be present.	WBC count elevated in cholecystitis and cholangitis. Amylase and liver function tests may help differentiate this from gastritis or ulcer disease. US shows anatomy, stones, or duct dilatation. Hepatobiliary scintigraphy diagnoses gallbladder function.
Ureteral Colic	Average age: 30–40. Men primarily affected. Prior history or family history of stones is common.	Family history, gout, *Proteus* species infections. Renal tubular acidosis and cystinuria lead to stone formation.	Acute onset of flank pain radiating to groin. Nausea, vomiting, and pallor are common. Patient usually writhing in pain, or unable to remain in single position.	Vital signs usually normal. Tenderness on CVA percussion with benign abdominal examination.	Urinalysis usually shows hematuria. Intravenous pyelography is the mainstay of diagnosis. Helical or spiral CT may be more appropriate in older patients or patients with elevated renal functions. US ± KUB with fluid bolus useful diagnostically.
Diverticulitis of the Colon	Incidence increases with advancing age; occurs in males more than females. Recurrences are common. Often called "left-sided" appendicitis.	Colonic diverticula become infected or perforated or cause local colitis. Obstruction, peritonitis, abscesses, and fistulas result from infection or swelling.	Common to have change in stool frequency or consistency. Left lower quadrant pain is common. Associated fever, nausea/ vomiting, rectal bleed may be seen.	Fever usually low grade. Left lower quadrant pain without rebound is common. Stools may be heme positive.	Most testing usually normal. Plain films may show obstruction or mass effect. Barium enema is often diagnostic.
	Occur in all age groups. Peak at age 50. Men affected twice that of women. Severe bleeding or perforation in less than 1% of patients.	May be associated with *Helicobacter pylori* infection. Risk factors include COPD, NSAID use, and tobacco and alcohol use.	Nonradiating epigastric pain that starts 1 to 3 hours after eating and is relieved by food or antacids . Pain frequently awakens . patient at night.	Epigastric tenderness without rebound or guarding. Perforation or bleeding leads to more severe clinical findings.	Uncomplicated cases are treated with antacids or H₂ blockers before invasive studies are contemplated. Gastroduodenoscopy is valuable in diagnosis and

					biopsy. Valuable in diagnosing *H. pylori*. Also blood test for *H. pylori*. US, barium enema, or CT with contrast medium may have diagnostic benefit.
Acute Gastroenteritis	Usually viral	Common diagnosis. Seasonal. Most common misdiagnosis of appendicitis. May be seen in multiple family members.	Pain usually poorly localized. Intermittent, crampy diffuse pain. Diarrhea is key element in diagnosis, usually large volume, watery. Nausea and vomiting usually begin before pain. Sense of increased peristalsis may be noted.	Abdominal examination usually nonspecific without peritoneal signs. Watery diarrhea or no stool noted on rectal examination. Fever is usually present.	Usually symptomatic care with antiemetics and volume repletion. Key is not using this diagnosis and missing more serious disease.
Nonspecific Abdominal Pain	Unknown	More common in persons of young and middle age, women of childbearing years, those of low social class, and those with psychiatric disorders. Up to 10% of patients older than 50 years of age prove to have intra-abdominal cancer.	Variable but tends to be chronic or recurrent.	Variable but no peritoneal signs.	Variable and can often be done on an outpatient basis.

COPD, chronic obstructive pulmonary disease; CVA, costovertebral angle; KUB, kidney, ureter, bladder; LFT, liver function tests; LLQ, left lower quadrant; NSAID, nonsteroidal anti-inflammatory drug; RLQ, right lower quadrant; RUQ, right upper quadrant; US, ultrasound.

cooperation. If judicious narcotic analgesics are used (morphine sulfate, 1 to 2 mg per dosage), their effects can be reversed using naloxone (Narcan). An alternate strategy is to use an anxiolytic medication (e.g., hydroxyzine [Vistaril]) intramuscularly, which should relieve some of the anxiety surrounding the pain but not alter the surgical consultant's examination. Giving narcotic pain relief is best done after consultation with the surgeon, even if by phone, before the bedside visit by that surgeon. Withholding analgesics is no longer necessary or recommended in the patient with acute abdominal pain.

Antibiotics

Occasionally in the emergency department it is necessary to give antibiotics to patients with abdominal pain complicated by peritonitis, perforation of a viscus, or presumed sepsis from an abdominal source. Abdominal infections can be caused by gram-positive, gram-negative, and anaerobic organisms. These infections are usually polymicrobial. The initial dose administered in the emergency department is wide spectrum, and often guided by the consultant's preferences. Ampicillin/sulbactam (Unasyn), ticarcillin with clavulanic acid (Timentin), or clindamycin plus gentamicin (for patients sensitive to β-lactam agents) provide initial coverage for infections with an abdominal source.

UNCERTAIN DIAGNOSIS

Uncertainty of diagnosis is common in patients with abdominal pain. Follow-up studies show that 40% to 50% of all patients with this complaint will have resolution without a clear diagnosis. This conclusion comes in spite of intense diagnostic efforts, including exploratory laparotomy in some cases. The following are steps to be considered when faced with this eventuality:

- **Observation:** Most cases with an uncertain course are not unstable or life-threatening. Observation up to 6 hours is appropriate in the acute care setting. This period allows for multiple reexaminations. In cases of appendicitis, or another operable condition, the abdomen will "declare" itself. Just as important, this period allows the physician to observe the demeanor of the patient. Patients without a significant cause of their pain tend to get restless, ask for drink and food, and, in general, improve to the point of discharge. Patients with a significant cause tend to remain quiet, appear ill, and do not query regarding discharge.

- **Review nonabdominal causes and dangerous "mimics":** Many nonabdominal conditions cause abdominal discomfort. Reconsidering these conditions and repeating with selected examinations and diagnostic adjuncts may be necessary. In elderly patients, a "silent" myocardial infarction can present in this manner. Lower lobe pneumonia has led to an occasional unnecessary laparotomy. Table 5–3 lists the serious causes of abdominal pain and their common misdiagnoses.

- **Consider uncommon and systemic causes:** When the diagnosis remains elusive, it is useful to consider uncommon causes. Sickle cell disease, diabetes, acute porphyria, and preeruption herpes zoster are examples of uncommon causes of abdominal pain.

- **Observation/Consultation:** Ultimately, when the diagnosis is unclear and it is not prudent to discharge the patient, the emergency physician can observe or consult an admitting physician, usually a surgeon or gastroenterologist. If the patient is observed, a consultation in the emergency department should be considered. Consultation is carried out in a timely manner to ensure the best care of the patient.

SPECIAL CONSIDERATIONS

Pediatric Patients

In pediatric patients with abdominal pain, an important part of the evaluation is to relieve fear and anxiety. Because the history in a very young patient may not be reliable and parents can only provide part of the story, carefully observing the patient's behavior and repeated examination of the abdomen over time is necessary. Causes of abdominal pain in children differ from adult causes. In this age group, abdominal pain is usually medically related (50% to 60%), such as gastroenteritis, constipation, urinary tract infection, viral illness, streptococcal pharyngitis, viral pharyngitis, pneumonia, and otitis media. In 5% to 10% of patients the cause (usually appendicitis) will require surgical intervention, and in 30% of cases the cause is not found.

Appendicitis remains a commonly misdiagnosed entity in children. It is initially missed in up to 60% of children younger than 6 years old. Acute gastroenteritis is the most common misdiagnosis. In younger children with appendicitis, the chances of perforation are significantly increased (up to 50%) compared with adults. In children with suspected appendicitis, a WBC count of over $13,000/mm^3$ or a temperature of over 102°F (38.9°C) is consistent with a perforated

TABLE 5–3. In Uncertain Diagnosis, Consider the Dangerous Mimics in Abdominal Pain

True Diagnosis	Initial Misdiagnosis
Appendicitis	Gastroenteritis, pelvic inflammatory disease, urinary tract infection
Ruptured abdominal aortic aneurysm	Renal colic, diverticulitis, lumbar strain
Ectopic pregnancy	Pelvic inflammatory disease, urinary tract infection, corpus luteum cyst
Diverticulitis	Constipation, gastroenteritis, pyelonephritis
Perforated viscus	Peptic ulcer disease, pancreatitis, nonspecific abdominal pain
Bowel obstruction	Constipation, gastroenteritis, nonspecific abdominal pain
Mesenteric ischemia	Gastroenteritis, constipation, ileus, small bowel obstruction
Incarcerated or strangulated hernia	Ileus or small bowel obstruction
Shock of sepsis from perforation, bleeding, abdominal infection (in elderly)	Urosepsis or pneumonia (in elderly)

appendix. The peak incidence for appendicitis is 9 to 12 years old. Inclusion of ultrasonography and CT in evaluating the pediatric patient suspected of having appendicitis is increasing the yield and decreasing the cost of care. Accuracies approaching 100% have been documented.

For a child with bowel obstruction, intussusception, hernia, and volvulus are most likely to be the cause. Other obstructing diseases unique to children include pyloric stenosis, midgut volvulus, and Hirschsprung's disease.

Children are often undertreated with analgesics in the emergency department. The same principles of analgesic use in abdominal pain for adults apply to children. Pain reduction does not adversely affect the examination or ability to identify surgical conditions.

Pregnant Patients

Intrauterine pregnancy, especially in the third trimester, makes the diagnosis of patients with abdominal pain more problematic. Because of uterine growth, the location of the appendix is shifted posterior and toward the right upper quadrant, altering somatic pain and physical findings from the classic findings. Rebound tenderness and guarding may be lost as findings. True tenderness of the pregnant abdomen consistently present on repeat examinations cannot be dismissed until the cause is determined. Early ultrasonography, followed by CT if negative results, has demonstrated benefit in these patients.

AIDS Patients

Patients with AIDS frequently present to the emergency department with gastrointestinal disorders. Abdominal pain associated with diarrhea can be caused by an enteropathic organism such as *Salmonella, Shigella, Campylobacter, Giardia,* cytomegalovirus, *Cryptosporidium,* and *Mycobacterium avium-intracellulare.* Pain without diarrhea may be secondary to AIDS cholangiopathy. AIDS patients also may present with acalculous or calculous cholecystitis. Portal lymphadenopathy due to AIDS-related neoplasms or infections may cause biliary obstruction. Esophagitis is very common in AIDS patients and is primarily caused by *Candida* or herpes simplex virus.

Elderly Patients

As a rule, elderly patients with abdominal pain are more likely to have surgical causes than younger patients. Conversely, they present with fewer disease-specific symptoms and signs. Physical examination findings do not reliably predict or exclude serious disease. Elderly patients tend to have higher pain tolerance and stay away from health care facilities longer than younger patients. They have lower WBC counts and temperatures than young adults given the same disease process. Signs such as guarding and rebound are often not present in the presence of peritoneal inflammation. In addition, their premorbid medical illnesses and medications complicate the diagnosis and management.

Elderly patients are more likely to have cholecystitis, malignancy, bowel obstruction, diverticulitis, peptic ulcer disease, and vascular disorders. Nonspecific pain is much less common. Special attention is directed to potential vascular catastrophes because of their high morbidity and mortality. Ruptured or leaking abdominal aortic aneurysm should be considered in all elderly patients with abdominal pain. It is the primary working diagnosis in all abdominal pain patients with hypotension, low back or flank pain, and/or a pulsatile abdominal mass. The other major vascular disorder that carries a high mortality rate in the elderly is mesenteric ischemia. Atherosclerotic disease of the superior mesenteric artery may cause "intestinal angina," consisting of postprandial abdominal pain, early satiety, and weight loss. Occlusive disease secondary to emboli or thrombosis, or poor blood flow secondary to hypotension, may cause bowel ischemia or infarction. Patients classically present with pain out of proportion to their physical findings. Associated findings include nausea, vomiting, diarrhea, and hematochezia. Laboratory tests and plain films of the abdomen are helpful but not diagnostic, especially early in the disease process. Patients with underlying cardiac disease (atrial fibrillation, cardiomyopathies) are predisposed to mesenteric ischemia. Early angiography or abdominal CT is the test of choice to confirm the diagnosis. Early surgical consultation is imperative for these vascular disorders.

A liberal policy of admission or observation with aggressive use of diagnostic adjuncts is necessary. In one study, 50% of patients were admitted and 22% of that group required surgery or inpatient procedures. The most common abdominal diagnoses included infection, mechanical-obstructive disorders, and malignancy. Hypotension, advanced age, and abnormal tests projected worse outcomes.

DISPOSITION AND FOLLOW-UP

Immediate Surgical Consultation

Patients who present with unstable hemodynamics require immediate surgical consultation. In otherwise stable patients, localized or diffuse peritoneal signs ("surgical abdomen") or a suspected vascular disorder deserve an immediate surgical consultation as well. As soon as any surgical condition is suspected, it is best to initiate a consultation. The necessary diagnostic tests and imaging studies can be carried out concurrently. In patients with clear findings of a leaking or ruptured abdominal aneurysm, time may be wasted performing a confirmatory computed tomogram or aortogram. Activation of the surgical team and opening an operating room, particularly during off hours, takes time, and unnecessary delays can be deleterious to the patient. The four most common surgically treatable causes of abdominal pain are acute appendicitis, intestinal obstruction, perforated viscus, and acute cholecystitis.

Emergency Department Clinical Decision Units (Observation)

Patients with mild or equivocal abdominal tenderness on examination, and who have no laboratory or radiographic findings indicative of a potential surgical cause of disease, are often observed in the emergency department for a period of up to 6 hours. Preferably the *same* physician follows the patient and performs and documents serial examinations. Repeated diagnostic adjuncts (e.g., ultrasonography) may be helpful. This strategy of observation allows the clinical situation to clarify itself and usually provides a disposition for the patient. Often these patients will have complete resolution of their pain and can be discharged.

Discharge and Follow-Up

Patients with the subjective complaint of abdominal pain, no accompanying tenderness, and a negative evaluation may also be observed for a period of time. If their condition does not become worse, they can be discharged with very specific instructions. They are placed on a clear liquid diet, and clearly communicated follow-up is arranged within 24 hours. The patients are instructed to return if increasing pain, fever, vomiting, abdominal swelling, fainting, or blood in emesis or stools develops. Narcotic pain relief is avoided. In spite of the difficulty in accurately diagnosing abdominal pain in emergency department patients, studies show few errors of disposition are made. However, occasionally a patient is sent home who subsequently returns with a cause of that pain that will require surgery. The most common diagnosis on return visit is acute appendicitis or intestinal obstruction.

FINAL POINTS

- Abdominal pain remains one of the most challenging presenting complaints in emergency medicine. Despite the best and most intense diagnostic efforts, only 50% to 60% of patients presenting with this complaint are assigned a diagnosis.
- Abdominal pain is a common symptom of the large number of varied organs that reside within the abdominal cavity. Often the pain will remain visceral in nature and therefore will not progress to a more somatic component.
- Emergency physicians must recognize the 10% to 20% of patients whose pain is caused by a disorder that requires surgical intervention.
- The physician's most important diagnostic tools are the history and repeated physical examination.
- Laboratory and other ancillary diagnostic procedures are of limited value in the patient with abdominal pain. Ultrasonography and abdominal CT scanning have provided more answers and may help greatly with disposition. It cannot supersede the physician's clinical judgment in regard to a particular patient.
- Patients who do not have an obvious diagnosis are observed, and repeat examinations are performed.
- The potential for serious outcome and sequelae always exists as part of this complex presenting complaint. **"When in doubt, don't send them out!"**

CASE *Study*

The 72-year-old man with acute epigastric and flank pain with a brief loss of consciousness arrived by ambulance pale and diaphoretic with a pulse of 100 beats per minute, blood pressure of 170/100 mm Hg, and respiration of 18 breaths per minute. He complained of severe right flank pain, nausea, and vomiting. The paramedics had started a line and placed the patient on 100% O_2 by mask. They reported a brief history including that the patient had a remote history of kidney stones. The emergency department was very busy with all the monitored beds full, and the charge nurse placed the patient in an unmonitored bed.

When the emergency department is busy, and beds are full, patients with potentially unstable conditions can be placed in a routine care bed. This bed assignment can, on occasion, mislead the caregivers to believe that the patient is stable. In this case, the busy physician gave orders consistent with a kidney stone. He had not yet "laid hands on."

The nurse assigned to the patient documented the patient's past medical history, vital signs, and O_2 saturation of 96% on room air by pulse oximetry. The patient had a long history of hypertension, previous coronary artery bypass graft, and one kidney stone 30 years previous. After a verbal report from the nurse, the physician ordered ketorolac (Toradol), 30 mg, and Phenergan IV and told the nurse to obtain urine for a dipstick for blood analysis and urinalysis, a renal panel, a complete blood cell count, and an abdominal radiograph.

Although this patient arrived with stable but abnormal vital signs, he had many risk factors that should have alerted the staff to a potentially life-threatening problem. The patient's age, history of hypertension, and history of other atherosclerotic disease are risk factors for an aneurysm.

The nurse reported the dipstick test in the emergency department as negative. Also, the physician looked at the abdominal radiograph and noted no obvious kidney stones but did note an abnormal calcified curved line over the lower lumbar spine area. The nurse reported that vital signs now show the patient's blood pressure to

be 80 mm Hg systolic and his pulse to be 120 beats per minute. The patient was lethargic but arousable. The patient was transported immediately to the resuscitation area. The physician ordered 100% O_2 by non-rebreather mask, two large-bore intravenous lines, a cardiac monitor, and a fluid bolus of 500 mL of normal saline. The physician palpated a pulsatile abdominal mass.

At this point, the physician has to make rapid and appropriate decisions with regard to stabilization, further testing, and consultation. Some emergency departments have immediately available blood that can be administered for shock, whereas continued crystalloid or albumin-based solutions are the only immediate options in other emergency departments. Bedside, "quick-look" ultrasonography would rapidly confirm the diagnosis. It is a skill that emergency physicians are becoming trained in. CT would be ideal, but the information gained has to be weighed against the time it takes to obtain versus the need to get the patient to the operating room. In all cases of suspected aneurysm, surgical consultation must be obtained immediately. If a qualified surgeon is not available, then transport, under resuscitation, by air or ground, needs to be arranged.

A call was made to the on-call vascular surgeon. Blood was sent to the laboratory for immediate type and crossmatch. The emergency physician, who was trained in ultrasound for emergency use, confirmed that an aneurysm of 8 cm in diameter was located just below the renal arteries. When the surgeon was alerted to this finding and because of the continuing instability of the patient, the surgeon decided to save time by going straight to the operating room and wait for the patient there. On arrival of the patient, the surgical team was gowned, gloved, and ready to go. On anesthetic induction of the patient, a successful aneurysmectomy with graft placement was carried out. The patient had an uneventful recovery.

Not all cases go this well. Time awareness, aggressive management, and early surgical consultation are the essential ingredients. The mortality rate of a ruptured abdominal aortic aneurysm may approach 90%.

Bibliography

TEXT

Silen W: Cope's Early Diagnosis of the Acute Abdomen, 20th ed. New York, Oxford University Press, 2000.

JOURNAL ARTICLES

Bonancini M: Hepatobiliary complications in patients with HIV infection. Am J Med 1992; 92:404.

Brewer RJ, Golden F, Hitch D, et al: Abdominal pain: An analysis of 1000 consecutive cases in a university emergency room. Am J Surg 1976; 131:219.

Colucciello SA, Lukens TW, Morgan DL: Assessing abdominal pain in adults: A rational, cost-effective and evidence-based strategy. Emerg Med Pract 1999; 1:1.

Gallagher EJ, Bijur PE, Latimer C, et al: Reliability and validity of a Visual Analog Scale for acute abdominal pain in the emergency department. Am J Emerg Med 2002; 20:287.

Garcia Pena BM, Mandl KD, Kraus SI, et al: Effect of computed tomography on patient management and costs in children with suspected appendicitis. Pediatrics 1999; 104:440.

Gupta H: Advances in imaging of the acute abdomen. Surg Clin North Am 1997; 77:1245.

Gwydd LK: The diagnosis of acute appendicitis: clinical assessment versus computed tomography evaluation. J Emerg Med 2001; 21:119.

Hals G, Larson JL: Acute appendicitis: Meeting the challenge of diagnosis in the ED. Emerg Med Rep 1999; 20(8):72.

Horwitz BJ, Fisher RS: The irritable bowel syndrome. N Engl J Med 2001; 344:1846.

Kim MK, Strait RT, Sato TT, et al: A randomized clinical trial of analgesia in children with acute abdominal pain. Acad Emerg Med 2002; 9:281.

Lederle EA, Simel DL: Does this patient have an abdominal aortic aneurysm? JAMA 1999; 281:77.

Lukens TW, Emerman C, Effron D: The natural history and clinical findings in undifferentiated abdominal pain. Ann Emerg Med 1993; 22:690.

Marco CA, Schoenfeld CN, Keyl PM, et al: Abdominal pain in geriatric emergency patients: Variables associated with adverse outcomes. Acad Emerg Med 1998; 5:1163.

Pace S, Burke TF: Intravenous morphine for early pain relief in patients with acute abdominal pain. Acad Emerg Med 1996; 3:1086.

Powers RD, Guertler AT: Abdominal pain in the ED: Stability and change over 20 years. Am J Emerg Med 1995; 13:301.

Reynolds SL, Jaffe DM: Diagnosing abdominal pain in a pediatric emergency department. Pediatr Emerg Care 1992; 8:126.

Smith FC, Grimshaw GM, Paterson IS, et al: Ultrasonographic screening for abdominal aortic aneurysm in an urban community. Br J Surg 1993; 80:1406.

Snyder BK, Hayden SR: Accuracy of leukocyte count in the diagnosis of acute appendicitis. Ann Emerg Med 1999; 33:565.

Wagner JM, McKinney WP, Carpenter JL: Does this patient have appendicitis? JAMA 1996; 276:1588.

CHAPTER 6

Acute Gastrointestinal Bleeding

ROBERT A. GIRMANN

MATTHEW L. EMERICK

CASE *Study*

The rescue squad was called to the home of a 50-year-old man 10 minutes after he vomited a large amount of bright red blood. He complained of nausea and persistent epigastric pain.

INTRODUCTION

Gastrointestinal (GI) bleeding is a common problem encountered in the emergency department. The annual incidence of lower GI bleeding is estimated to be between 20 and 27 cases per 100,000 persons, and the incidence of upper GI bleeding is estimated between 100 and 150 cases per 100,000 persons. GI bleeding may be seen in any age group, but it is most commonly encountered during the fifth through eighth decades of life. Most deaths caused by GI bleeding occur in patients older than 60 years of age. As today's patient population increases in age, GI bleeding will continue to be a frequently encountered problem. Up to 80% of GI bleeding stops spontaneously. Despite this fact, the overall mortality of admitted patients with GI bleeding has not changed significantly in the past 40 years and remains 8% to 10%.

GI bleeding is divided into upper GI (UGI) bleeding and lower GI (LGI) bleeding. UGI bleeding is bleeding that occurs proximal to the ligament of Treitz (the anatomic junction of the duodenum and jejunum). LGI bleeding originates distal to the ligament of Treitz. UGI bleeding is more common than LGI bleeding, and UGI bleeding occurs twice as often in men as women.

Hematemesis is the vomiting of blood, "bright red" or otherwise. The "coffee grounds" material often seen with UGI bleeding is partially digested whole blood. *Hematochezia* is the passage of bright red bloody stools or frank blood from the rectum. This is opposed to the black tarry malodorous stools of *melena*, which often represent a UGI source of bleeding. Melena occurs when more than 150 mL of blood traverses the GI tract over a prolonged time

(>8 to 12 hours). Maroon, burgundy, or "currant jelly" stools are simply descriptive terms for stools that contain partially metabolized hemoglobin. The color of the stool, whether bright red or densely black, is dependent on the rate of bleeding and the time the blood has spent in passing through the intestines. Therefore, color alone does not necessarily localize the site of hemorrhage. Although most cases of hematochezia are from LGI bleeding, frank hematochezia may be the result of a UGI hemorrhage.

UGI bleeding presenting as hematemesis is usually caused by a breakdown of the mucosal and vascular integrity of the esophagus, stomach, or duodenum. Melena is usually the result of non–massive UGI hemorrhage. The blood is digested during its transit through the gut. Common causes of UGI bleeding include peptic ulcer disease, erosive gastritis, esophageal varices, and Mallory-Weiss tears.

LGI bleeding that manifests as hematochezia or nonmelenic stool is commonly caused by hemorrhoids, diverticula, angiodysplasia, carcinoma, UGI hemorrhage, and infectious or inflammatory bowel conditions. Its origin is similar to that of UGI bleeding, although vascular causes are more common than mucosal damage.

Most cases of acute GI bleeding are first encountered in the emergency department, where the knowledge and expertise of the emergency physician can mean the difference between life and death. Even after thorough evaluations, no source of bleeding is found in up to 10% of patients.

INITIAL APPROACH AND STABILIZATION

Patients with acute GI hemorrhage who arrive by ambulance are taken immediately to a monitored bed for assessment. Ambulatory patients who give a history of GI bleeding are rapidly triaged and assigned to an area appropriate for their clinical status.

Priority Diagnoses

Peptic ulcer disease, gastric erosions, and esophageal varices account for almost 75% of adult patients presenting with UGI bleeding. Approximately 80% of LGI bleeding is caused by diverticulosis or angiodysplasia.

Rapid Assessment

A brief history is obtained and relevant questions are asked about the nature, duration, and amount of bleeding. One must determine if bright red blood coming from the mouth or nose is true hematemesis of GI origin or another source, such as hemoptysis or a severe case of epistaxis. Also, questions are asked about possible causes of the hemorrhage, such as alcohol, medications (e.g., nonsteroidal anti-inflammatory drugs [NSAIDs]), varices, or liver disease. A brief overview of previous GI disorders or other complicating conditions (e.g., heart disease, pulmonary disorders, or abdominal surgeries like aortic grafting) is obtained. Patients with abdominal aortic grafts should be considered at risk for aortoenteric fistula. Early surgical consultation is recommended.

The vital signs are obtained and compared with the prehospital vital signs. If the patient is not hypotensive, orthostatic vital signs ("tilt test") may be taken. The blood pressure and pulse are recorded after the patient has been supine for at least 3 minutes. The patient is then asked to sit or stand for a minimum of 1 minute, and the blood pressure and pulse are recorded again. Positive orthostatic changes are indicated by a pulse rate rise of more than 20 to 30 beats per minute, a systolic blood pressure drop of more than 20 to 30 mm Hg, or a diastolic pressure drop of 10 mm Hg or more. The patient is warned to mention the onset of lightheadedness and is watched for signs of presyncope. If symptoms occur, the patient is quickly returned to the supine position. A "positive" test result may indicate an intravascular volume loss of 20% or more. It may be influenced by a number of factors, including age, autonomic status of the patient, and medications (e.g., β-blocking agents). Assessing orthostatic changes has significant limitations and may or may not reflect true volume status.

The level of consciousness, the adequacy of respirations, and the cardiovascular status of the patient are assessed. The patient is observed for the stigmata of chronic alcohol use or advanced liver disease such as spider angiomas, gynecomastia, jaundice, or palmar erythema. The abdomen is examined for distention, tenderness, and organomegaly. A rectal examination is performed, and any stool or mucus is tested for blood. Early stool sample testing (Hematest) is a quick means of establishing the diagnosis in the patient without obvious hemorrhage.

Early Intervention

In the initial stabilization of the patient with GI bleeding the basic principles of resuscitation are followed.

Airway/Oxygen. Oxygen through a nasal cannula or mask is administered at an initial rate of 4 to 6 L/min. The airway is protected by whatever interventions are required. Because the patient may be obtunded or vomiting with risk of aspirating, endotracheal intubation may be necessary depending on the patient's ability to protect the airway.

Monitor. Monitoring is established with a pulse oximeter and a cardiac monitor. An electrocardiogram is taken early if there is associated chest pain, dysrhythmia, the patient is older than age 50 years, or acute myocardial ischemia is suspected.

Initial Volume Resuscitation. One or two large-bore (14 to 16 gauge) intravenous catheters are inserted peripherally if there is any suspicion or obvious evidence of significant blood loss. If the patient is hypotensive or in shock, a crystalloid bolus of 10 to 20 mL/kg is infused rapidly. This may be repeated up to 30 mL/kg. The patient who remains unstable after this initial fluid infusion should be given blood products. The degree of acute hemorrhage is estimated by simple clinical parameters, and the volume replacement amount is adjusted accordingly (Table 6–1; see Chapter 4, Shock). Blood products are usually administered after the responses to the initial crystalloid bolus have been assessed.

Blood Product Transfusion. Blood transfusion therapy is directed toward the restoration of diminished oxygen-carrying capacity, coagulation factors, or platelet function. This topic is addressed in Chapter 4, Shock, and will be briefly summarized here. Blood component therapy helps obviate these clinical problems and treats the specific hematologic deficit. Packed red blood cells (RBCs) can restore the body's need for oxygen transport while reducing the risk of a plasma-related mismatch reaction. The acutely hemorrhaging patient needs RBCs most; therefore packed RBCs are the blood components of choice to transfuse. Fresh frozen plasma (FFP) may be given later if the prothrombin or partial thromboplastin time (PT/PTT) values are prolonged, indicating possible depletion of coagulative factors. Patients with advanced liver disease who are actively hemorrhaging will often need factor replacement with FFP because of their factor-depleted hypocoagulable state. Platelet transfusion may be indicated in patients with thrombocytopenia or if platelet dysfunction (e.g., with recent aspirin or NSAID use) is suspected.

TABLE 6–1. Estimated Fluid and Blood Requirements for Acute Blood Loss* (Based on Initial Presentation of the Patient)

	Class I	Class II	Class III	Class IV
Blood loss (mL)	Up to 750	750–1500	1500–2000	2000 or more
Blood loss (% blood volume)	Up to 15%	15%–30%	30%–40%	40% or more
Pulse rate (beats per minute)	<100	>100	>120	≥140
Blood pressure	Normal	Normal	Decreased	Decreased
Pulse pressure (mm Hg)	Normal or increased	Decreased	Decreased	Decreased
Capillary blanch test	Normal	Positive	Positive	Positive
Respiratory rate (breaths per minute)	14–20	20–30	30–40	>35
Urine output (mL/hr)	30 or more	20–30	5–15	Negligible
CNS–mental status	Slightly anxious	Mildly anxious	Anxious and confused	Confused, lethargic
Fluid replacement (3:1 rule)†	Crystalloid	Crystalloid	Crystalloid + blood	Crystalloid + blood

*For a 70-kg male.
†Multiply estimated blood loss by 3 to get estimated crystalloid replacement.
Adapted from American College of Surgeons Committee on Trauma: Advanced Trauma Life Support. American College of Surgeons, 1988.

Patients who require large volumes of replacement therapy should receive warmed blood to prevent decreases in body temperature.

Initial Laboratory Studies. Blood samples should be obtained immediately and initial laboratory studies requested. These may include a complete blood cell count, coagulation studies (PT, PTT, and platelet count), electrolytes, blood urea nitrogen (BUN), creatinine, liver function tests, and type and screen for 4 to 6 units of blood. Type and crossmatch is ordered if it is obvious that blood products will be necessary.

Patient Comfort. During the dramatic presentation of active GI bleeding, it is important to talk with the patient and family, explain briefly what is being done, and attempt to reduce their anxiety. The intensity of an aggressive resuscitation in the emergency department (and the possible ambulance ride to the hospital) can be overwhelming.

CLINICAL ASSESSMENT

A careful history and physical examination often define the source and extent of GI bleeding. If the patient is unable to give a detailed history, useful information is frequently available from the accompanying friends or family, rescue squad, old records, or primary physician. The extent of the history and physical examination is tempered by the stability of the patient's condition. The more unstable the patient's condition, the more focused and expedient the clinical assessment.

History

The history is essential but has demonstrated limited usefulness in predicting the source or severity of the hemorrhage. Slightly more than half the patients with a known bleeding site present with bleeding from the same site.

Onset/Duration of Bleeding. *When did the bleeding begin?* Because of the dramatic presentation of most acute GI bleeding, the time of onset is easily noted by the patient. Did the onset occur before or after vomiting? Was it of gradual or rapid onset? About 50% of patients present with hematemesis. Duration of bleeding may be difficult to assess. Slower hemorrhages allow more time for hemodynamic compensation, and even with low hemoglobin levels, these patients may manifest few physical findings of hemodynamic instability.

Nature of Bleeding. *Where is the site of blood loss? Is there melenic stool currently?* Black stool may persist for several days after cessation of bleeding. *Is the stool bright red or maroon?* This is most often caused by rectal disorders (e.g., hemorrhoids). A thorough assessment is necessary to diagnose more serious causes.

Blood Loss. *Can the amount of blood loss be estimated?* Patients usually overestimate the amount of loss, but a gross estimate is helpful.

Syncope. *Is there a history of syncope or near-syncope associated with this bleeding event?* Obviously, this is a serious symptom.

Related Past History. *Has there been a past history of similar events?* Many patients with UGI bleeding have an easily identified cause (e.g., liver disease, peptic ulcer disease, varices, or the use of NSAIDs, salicylates, or ethanol). Stress remains a comorbid factor in peptic ulcer disease.

Extragastrointestinal Sources. *Has there been bleeding in or from the mouth or nose? Is there a pulmonary source of bleeding?*

Abdominal Pain. *Is there abdominal pain? What is its character?* Bleeding can be either painless or associated with the pain of the underlying condition. Peptic ulcer disease ranging from gastritis to penetrating ulcer is typically painful in advance of the hemorrhage. Symptoms that occur during defecation can point toward the cause of LGI bleeding.

Extra-abdominal Symptoms. *Are there associated symptoms such as chest pain, dizziness, or shortness of breath?* Hemodynamic compromise can result in poor myocardial or cerebral perfusion. One percent to 2% of UGI hemorrhages are associated with myocardial infarction, which is often "silent." Almost 20% of patients present with nonspecific complaints such as fatigue or weakness.

Family History. *Is there a family history of bleeding disorders, gastric cancer, colon cancer, or peptic ulcer disease?*

Physical Examination

Just as the history of the present illness is stimulated by the chief complaint, the physical examination is guided by clues from the history. Its goals are to assess the severity of bleeding, determine how the patient is tolerating the insult, and search for clues to the source. Serial examinations are beneficial in these patients because of potentially rapid changes in the patient's status.

General Appearance. How does the patient present initially? What is the patient's mental status? How is the patient tolerating the event? Is there diaphoresis, pallor, cyanosis, or jaundice? Are there any stigmata of liver disease or purpura and petechiae such as occur with a blood dyscrasia?

Vital Signs. In the euvolemic patient, the blood pressure and pulse in the upright position *may* approximate the values occurring when the patient is supine. An intravascular volume loss of up to 20% to 30% can occur without causing a measurable difference in the comparative blood pressures, particularly in the pediatric population. Clinicians may be falsely reassured by misleading vital signs that the blood volume is adequate. Normal vital signs do not exclude significant hemorrhage, and postural changes in vital signs may occur in individuals who are not bleeding. Because pulse rate changes occur before blood pressure declines, a persistent tachycardia or a significant increase in pulse rate with orthostatic testing may herald hypovolemia. The limited value of orthostatic vital signs is discussed in the section "Initial Approach and Stabilization."

Patients presenting with vital signs consistent with volume loss do not require orthostatic testing for confirmation.

Head and Neck. The nose and mouth are examined for sources of recent or active bleeding. Is there evidence of recent trauma or surgery? Is there an infectious or inflammatory condition in the oropharynx? The conjunctiva should be checked for pallor or jaundice.

Chest and Cardiac Examination. The male chest is inspected for gynecomastia, which can occur in liver disease. The lungs are examined for signs of possible aspiration. The heart is examined to assess any dysrhythmia that might be induced by hypoxemia or ischemia.

Abdomen. The abdomen is inspected for distention and the presence of any abnormal skin findings such as abdominal wall varices (caput medusae). Bowel sounds are auscultated, although both hyperactive and hypoactive sounds are common. The presence of arterial bruits is actively sought. The abdomen is palpated for hepatosplenomegaly, possible abdominal aneurysms or thrills, hernias, or other masses. Tenderness on palpation is localized, and the presence of guarding or rebound is noted. The latter may indicate increased risk of a surgical emergency. Percussion techniques can help to identify the presence of ascites.

Rectum. The perianal area and rectum are examined to check for anal, perianal, or rectal pathologic processes as well as the presence of blood in the stool. Testing for occult hemoglobin is necessary in essentially all patients. The absence of black, maroon, or red stool does not exclude the diagnosis of GI bleeding.

Bedside Testing

Examination for Occult Blood. Testing for occult blood in the stool or vomitus is based on the peroxidase activity of hemoglobin. It results in a reagent changing to a blue color when present. Normal blood loss in the alimentary tract is 2 to 2.5 mL of blood/day. The Hemoccult card (GlaxoSmithKline, Philadelphia) is a guaiac-impregnated filter paper that tests positive if there is a GI blood loss of 5 to 10 mL/day. This amount corresponds to 5 to 10 mg of hemoglobin per gram of stool. The Hemoccult card is 95% sensitive if there is 20 mg of hemoglobin per gram of stool. False-negative results can occur if the bleeding is intermittent. False-positive results occur in up to 12% of samples. Peroxidase-containing foods such as bananas, turnips, and broccoli can cause false-positive test results. Iodine, red fruits, and red meats also can cause a false-positive result. Ingested iron and bismuth may darken the stool color mimicking melena, but they will not cause a positive result in the Hemoccult test. False-negative results can be caused by the ingestion of magnesium-containing antacids or ascorbic acid. A similar card for testing gastric contents for blood is called the Gastroccult card. It is designed to compensate for the acidity of the gastric contents when analyzing for blood. Positive testing for hemoglobin may persist for 1 to 2 weeks after GI bleeding.

Nasogastric Aspirate and Lavage. The placement of a nasogastric (NG) tube either can be part of the management process or used as a diagnostic aid. If the patient's vomitus is positive for hemoglobin, an NG tube is not necessary. In patients without obvious GI hemorrhage, the nasogastric aspirate and lavage fluid can be tested for hemoglobin (Gastroccult test). After assessment of the gastric aspirate, the NG tube can be removed in most patients. Readily available endoscopy has replaced the NG tube in many hospital settings. If blood is present, gastric lavage may serve as preparatory for endoscopy. It does not reduce blood loss in patients with UGI bleeding. Normal temperature water or saline is recommended.

CLINICAL REASONING

The initial clinical information guides management decisions by establishing the condition of the patient and allowing a preliminary formulation of a differential diagnosis. Key questions influencing these decisions are presented next.

What Is the Severity of Blood Loss and How Is the Patient Tolerating It?

Is there clinical evidence of hypoperfusion of vital organs, namely, "shock"? The initial estimates of blood loss (see Table 6–1) are reassessed in the context of more information and the patient's response to treatment.

Is True Gastrointestinal Bleeding Occurring?

Food, tobacco products, or medication may be mistaken for blood in vomitus or stool (e.g., black stools from a recent ingestion of iron supplement tablets). Swallowed blood from epistaxis or oropharyngeal bleeding can be mistaken for GI bleeding. A careful ear, nose, and throat history and examination should resolve the issue.

If Gastrointestinal Blood Is Present, Is It Upper or Lower in Origin?

If the patient presents with what appears to be an upper source of GI bleeding (coffee-ground emesis or hematemesis), and an extraintestinal source has been ruled out (e.g., hemoptysis, epistaxis), the bleeding is then presumed to be UGI in origin. If, on the other hand, the bleeding appears to be lower (e.g., melena, hematochezia), then a gastric aspirate is performed as a screening tool to rule out an upper source of bleeding. Hemorrhage from below the ligament of Treitz rarely appears in the stomach. Localizing the bleeding site is important in terms of immediate and subsequent therapy, possible causes, and prognosis. Tables 6–2 and 6–3 list the common and uncommon causes of UGI and LGI bleeding, respectively. Brisk UGI bleeding may be the cause of LGI hematochezia.

How Rapid Is the Blood Loss?

Rate of blood loss can be estimated by the time of onset and the clinical status of the patient. Early

TABLE 6–2. Causes of Upper Gastrointestinal Bleeding

Common	Uncommon
Epistaxis and oral bleeding	Aortoenteric fistula
Duodenitis	Boerhaave's syndrome
Duodenal ulcer	Blood dyscrasias
Esophageal/gastric varices	Carcinoma, leiomyoma
Esophagitis	Mallory-Weiss lesions
Gastric ulcer	Vascular anomalies
Gastritis/erosions	Arteriovenous malformations
	Hereditary telangiectasia
	Angiodysplasia

TABLE 6–3. Causes of Lower Gastrointestinal Bleeding

Common	Uncommon
Angiodysplasia	Aortoenteric fistula
Anal fissures	Blood dyscrasias
Carcinoma	Meckel's diverticulum
Colonic diverticula	Mesenteric ischemia
Hemorrhoids	
Infectious diarrhea with invasive agents	
Inflammatory bowel disease	
Inflammatory proctitis	
Upper gastrointestinal bleeding (peptic ulcer, gastritis, varices)	

endoscopy is the best method to accurately determine the rate of blood loss. Esophageal varices and a rapidly bleeding duodenal or gastric ulcer are the most common causes of massive UGI bleeding. A bleeding colonic diverticulum is the most common cause of significant LGI bleeding.

Is There the Possibility of a Hemostatic Disorder?

It is important to consider the integrity of the hemostatic system as well as the mucosa while gathering data from the patient. A history of alcohol abuse, advanced liver disease, aspirin or NSAID use, and subsequent effects on platelet function and mucosal integrity may explain persistent hemorrhage. Hemostatic disorders involving platelet numbers and function (e.g., disseminated intravascular coagulation, von Willebrand's disease) may present as mucosal bleeding with GI bleeding.

DIAGNOSTIC ADJUNCTS

Laboratory Studies

Laboratory testing can assist in assessing the severity of hemorrhage, the physiologic tolerance and compensation for the hemorrhage, and the general metabolic condition of the patient. Tests are usually ordered early in the course of evaluating a patient with an acute GI hemorrhage. In patients with severe bleeding, all of the following tests are requested.

Hemoglobin/Hematocrit. Acute recent hemorrhage may not present as anemia. The hemoglobin level or hematocrit alone is a poor estimate of blood volume because it takes several hours for the body to mobilize extravascular fluid to compensate for an acute blood loss. In the case of aggressive crystalloid resuscitation, the hemoglobin and hematocrit will equilibrate much faster. When the decision is made to transfuse the critically ill patient, the optimal hematocrit with respect to oxygen-carrying capacity and viscosity has been reported to be 33%. Patients with hemoglobin levels of 7 g/dL or less (<21% hematocrit) are considered candidates for blood replacement therapy. Hemodynamic status, patient age, patient tolerance, and underlying disorders are important factors in this decision.

White Blood Cell Count and Differential. A mild leukocytosis may be evident during active bleeding. A very high WBC count, more than 25,000 cells/mm^3 with a "leukemoid" reaction on peripheral smear, may be seen in patients with cancer of GI origin.

An elevated WBC may be one of the few clues to a patient with mesenteric ischemia, although it has poor specificity.

Electrolytes. The most useful values are the bicarbonate concentration and the anion gap. The bicarbonate level may decrease secondary to lactic acidosis from tissue ischemia or from another cause of metabolic acidosis, such as salicylism. The anion gap will increase. The sodium, potassium, and chloride concentrations usually are not significantly changed with hemorrhage but may reflect medication use or underlying disease states.

Blood Urea Nitrogen and Creatinine. The BUN and creatinine are indirect measures of renal function. A high BUN:creatinine ratio (normal, 10:1) may signify severe dehydration or digested blood protein absorbed through the GI tract. A BUN:creatinine ratio greater than or equal to 35 in patients without renal failure is suggestive of upper GI bleeding, whereas a ratio less than 35 is not helpful. A low BUN may occur in patients with hepatic failure.

Blood Glucose. Blood glucose levels tend to be higher than normal during massive bleeding caused by glycogen breakdown secondary to the increased circulating levels of the "stress hormones" epinephrine and glucagon.

Coagulation Studies. Prolonged prothrombin and partial thromboplastin times can suggest severe liver disease, vitamin K deficiency, oral anticoagulant therapy, or a primary coagulation disorder. Both values begin to increase when the coagulation factor levels fall below 40% of normal. This occurs after the liver loses 85% to 90% of its functional ability to produce coagulation factors.

Platelets. A platelet count is not a measure of platelet function. The count may be decreased because of the effects of ethanol, splenomegaly, or disseminated intravascular coagulation. The most common drugs that impair platelet function are aspirin and the NSAIDs, such as ibuprofen. Serial counts are performed if platelet counts are low (e.g., >50,000/mm^3). Special testing (aggregometry) is necessary to assess platelet function.

Arterial Blood Gases. Measurement of arterial blood gases is useful indirectly in evaluating the efficacy of cardiac output in hypovolemic shock and the metabolic acidemia that occurs secondary to hypoperfusion. The Pao$_2$ measures the dissolved oxygen in the blood rather than the oxygen content. Oxygen content more accurately represents the patient's oxygenation status.

Liver Function Tests. These tests are helpful in recognizing the patient with preexisting hepatic disease.

Ammonia. The ammonia level may be indicative of hepatic encephalopathy secondary to severe acute or chronic liver disease.

Lactic Acid. An elevated lactic acid level helps confirm the origin of a metabolic acidosis and is usually elevated in patients with hypoperfusion and, specifically, acute mesenteric ischemia. A normal lactate level decreases the possibility of this diagnosis.

Electrocardiogram

An ECG is indicated in any patient with hemorrhage resulting in unstable vital signs, especially those older than 50 years of age. Significant blood loss can unmask occult ischemia and increase the chance for a new dysrhythmia. As noted previously, an acute myocardial infarction occurs in 1% to 2% of all patients with UGI bleeding, often without symptoms.

Radiologic Imaging

Chest Radiograph. A chest radiograph is part of the assessment of patients being considered for admission to the hospital. Aspiration of blood is possible, and other sources of pulmonary pathologic processes are sought. Free air in the peritoneum is best seen on this view.

Abdominal Radiograph. Plain abdominal radiographs in the supine and upright positions are only indicated if perforation with free peritoneal air or mesenteric ischemia, with subsequent "thumb printing," is suspected. GI hemorrhage alone is not an indication for plain abdominal radiographs.

Barium Contrast Radiographs. This study was once the mainstay for the detection of peptic ulcer disease and colonic lesions such as neoplasms and diverticula. It has largely been replaced today by endoscopic intervention. Barium studies do not detect mucosal lesions as well as upper and lower GI endoscopy. Prior use of barium may obscure the endoscopic view. Only 70% to 80% of duodenal ulcers detectable through an endoscope are localized by barium studies.

Angiography. Angiography is considered by many as the procedure of choice for either massive or continuous LGI bleeding or when other diagnostic modalities have failed to reveal a source of bleeding. Angiography is a good diagnostic tool and can be used for therapeutic interventions. These include the administration of vasopressin or embolization of bleeding vessels with Gelfoam or autologous clots. For angiography to localize the site of hemorrhage, bleeding must be occurring at a rate of 0.5 to 1.0 mL/min.

Currently, angiography is only required in about 1% of the cases of UGI bleeding because of the effectiveness of localizing the site of bleeding with endoscopy. This modality is more commonly used in LGI bleeding.

Radionuclide Imaging. Radionuclide imaging is primarily used in the evaluation of stable patients with bleeding distal to the ligament of Treitz. Imaging with labeled red cells tagged with technetium 99m sulfur or ^{99m}Tc pertechnetate allows the detection of blood loss at a minimal rate of 0.1 mL/min. Scanning with ^{99m}Tc pertechnetate allows for repeat scanning in 24 to 36 hours to detect intermittent bleeding. Radionuclide scanning is often used to screen patients before angiography is instituted. This reduces the incidence of negative angiograms and also allows for more selective angiography, thus reducing radiation and dye load.

Other Adjuncts

Type and Screen/Cross. The completeness of crossmatch of red cells is varied depending on the urgency of need for blood replacement. Type O-negative blood is considered a "universal donor" and can be administered immediately without crossmatch. The Rh factor is important for women of childbearing age but not for men. Therefore, O-positive blood can be given to males. In type-specific blood, which can be available in 10 to 15 minutes, the ABO and Rh groups are matched. Type-specific blood has a very low incidence of major transfusion reactions. A full crossmatch takes 30 to 45 minutes. In the patient requiring replacement therapy, type and crossmatch is requested for at least 4 to 6 units of packed RBCs.

Gastric Intubation. If significant GI bleeding is suspected but not obvious, or a patient presents with lower GI bleeding (melena, hematochezia), a nasogastric tube may be placed and the gastric aspirate tested for hemoglobin. This is to rule out an upper GI source for the bleeding and may be superseded by readily available endoscopy. There is no evidence that gastric tube placement aggravates hemorrhage from esophageal or gastric varices or from a Mallory-Weiss tear. The aspirate is considered normal if the fluid is blood free (Gastroccult negative) and bile tinged. This finding implies that the stomach and duodenum contain no intraluminal blood and assumes that bleeding distal to the ligament of Treitz does not move retrograde. A negative gastric aspirate does not totally rule out UGI bleeding. Up to 25% of patients with duodenal bleeding can have a negative gastric aspirate secondary to failure of blood to flow retrograde past the pylorus.

If test results are positive or if the patient presents with obvious UGI bleeding (hematemesis, coffee-ground emesis), the stomach may be lavaged with water or isotonic crystalloid that has been warmed to room temperature. This is done until the aspirate returns clear. The lavage is mainly to evacuate the stomach contents for future endoscopy and to prevent further blood-induced emesis. Ideally, the stomach is lavaged with a large Ewald orogastric tube with the patient in the left-lateral decubitus position. The lavage fluid (in 200- to 300-mL aliquots) should be introduced and removed by gravity. The Ewald tube allows the evacuation of large clots, while the gravity drainage saves the stomach from mucosal injury from suction. If the irrigant fails to clear with repeated lavage, it means that the bleeding source is active and emergent endoscopy is indicated.

Upper Gastrointestinal Endoscopy. Early endoscopy is the most accurate method for identifying the site and source of UGI bleeding. It has been established as the diagnostic "gold standard" for UGI bleeding and can identify a lesion in 80% to 90% of cases. Not only is endoscopy effective in diagnosing, but it has also become an effective modality through which definitive therapeutic interventions can be attempted. Endoscopic intervention has a greater than 90% rate of effective hemostasis on the first attempt. Methods used include endoscopic laser, multipolar electrocoagulation, injection therapy, hemoclipping, and ligation. The rate of recurrent bleeding is 15% to 20%.

Anoscopy and Sigmoidoscopy. Direct visualization techniques are more readily available and useful in finding many common sources of bleeding. Anal and distal rectal lesions may be seen with an anoscope, a procedure available in the emergency department. Sigmoidoscopy is used to detect rectal and sigmoid colon lesions. It is a procedure performed by a consultant, usually outside the emergency department. Blood coming from above the scope may be from a proximal bleeding source or may be from retrograde movement of blood into the proximal colon.

Colonoscopy. Like endoscopy in UGI bleeding, colonoscopy has become the diagnostic modality of choice for LGI bleeding. As alluded to earlier, colonoscopy has generally replaced barium enema for diagnostic evaluation of lower GI bleeding. In severe LGI bleeding, urgent colonoscopy or diagnostic angiography is the diagnostic modality of choice.

Angiograph. Angiography is used in less than 1% of patients with UGI bleeding. It is more commonly applied in LGI bleeding and can identify the bleeding site in almost half the patients. If the bleeding vessel is located, vasopressin or arterial embolization may be accomplished through an arterial catheter. Active bleeding increases the diagnostic benefit but also increases the risk of moving the patient into the radiology suite.

EXPANDED DIFFERENTIAL DIAGNOSIS

The actual anatomic site of GI bleeding may not be determined in the emergency department, but the differential diagnosis is often narrowed to a few choices. The most common causes of UGI bleeding include peptic ulcer disease, gastric erosions (6% to 30%), and esophageal varices (8% to 16%). Other less common causes include Mallory-Weiss tears, aortoenteric fistulas, Boerhaave's syndrome, carcinoma, and vascular anomalies. The most common causes of LGI bleeding include diverticulosis, angiodysplasia, neoplasm, mesenteric ischemia, hemorrhoids, and inflammatory bowel disease.

Upper Gastrointestinal Bleeding

Peptic Ulceration

Peptic ulcers result from the breakdown of the mucosa of the stomach or duodenum. Peptic ulceration is the most common cause of UGI bleeding, accounting for 50% to 80% of cases. Of these cases, two thirds occur from the duodenum and one third arise from a gastric site. Twenty percent to 30% of patients with documented ulcers will have significant bleeding at some point during the disease. Bleeding from a peptic ulcer may occur at any age but is approximately five times more common after the age of 50. The characteristic history of persistent aching or burning pain usually precedes the bleeding episode. Occasionally, hemorrhage is the initial manifestation of the disease. This is often seen in elderly patients. Duodenal ulcers are two to three times more common in males than females and have a prevalence in the population estimated to be 6% to 15%. Predisposing factors for peptic ulcer disease include use of NSAIDs, alcohol, excessive acid production, *Helicobacter pylori,* heredity (it is three times more common in first-degree relatives), blood group O, and cigarette smoking. A history of salicylate ingestion before the onset of bleeding is elicited in approximately 50% of patients with UGI bleeding associated with peptic ulcer disease. The importance of stress and other psychological factors remains controversial.

The majority of patients with duodenal ulcer present with burning or gnawing epigastric pain that occurs 1 to 3 hours after eating. This pain is usually accompanied by tenderness in the epigastrium or just to the right of that location. Changes in the character of the pain can herald the onset of complications. Acute onset and persistent pain suggest perforation, particularly if peritoneal signs develop.

Erosive gastritis (small, circumscribed, mucosal defects that do not penetrate the muscularis mucosa) is responsible for 10% to 15% of cases of GI bleeding. Predisposing factors include indiscreet use of ethanol and NSAIDs, prolonged corticosteroid use, and severe underlying disease with associated stress (e.g., major trauma, burns, and head injury). The clinical presentation of gastritis is often indistinguishable from that of duodenal ulcer, although consumption of food tends to make the pain better in patients with gastritis and worse in those with peptic ulcer disease. The diagnosis of this disease is based on the clinical setting, characteristic predisposing factors, and confirmation by endoscopy.

Varices

Some of the most catastrophic and difficult-to-manage upper GI hemorrhages are seen in patients with esophagogastric varices. Varices are spontaneous venous dilatations of portosystemic collateral vessels that develop from portal hypertension. These occur most often in the esophagus and proximal stomach. Bleeding from varices is often abrupt and massive. One third of all cases of massive UGI bleeding are caused by varices. One third of patients with cirrhosis will bleed from varices, and the overall mortality rate is 30%, which is much higher than the 8% to 10% mortality rate for all UGI bleeding. Of these 30%, two thirds will die within 1 year of presentation. Clinical clues supporting varices as the source of bleeding include the stigmata of advanced liver disease with portal hypertension (e.g., ascites), enlarged abdominal wall veins, splenomegaly, and hemorrhoids. Unfortunately, up to 50% of patients with known varices have bleeding episodes from gastritis or peptic ulcer disease, and endoscopy is necessary to confirm the source of hemorrhage. Endoscopic therapy consists of variceal band ligation or injection sclerotherapy and has successfully controlled active bleeding in up to 90% of patients, while reducing the frequency and severity of rebleeding. Pharmacologic therapy with nitroglycerin, vasopressin or analogues, and somatostatin or analogues (octreotide, vapreotide) are considered in any patient with suspected varices.

Importantly, up to two thirds of patients with an acute bleed from varices rebleed within the first several weeks after the initial episode. Secondary prophylaxis is an important part of planned long-term therapy.

Mallory-Weiss Tear

A relatively uncommon but dramatic cause of UGI bleeding is a Mallory-Weiss tear of the esophagus. This is a partial-thickness longitudinal laceration of the gastroesophageal junction that is usually caused by violent vomiting, coughing, or retching. Risk factors that may predispose a patient to this include alcohol use, hiatal hernia, or underlying esophagitis. The abrupt onset of significant hemorrhage soon after such an episode is characteristic. The bleeding usually resolves with conservative management, but occasionally it can be life-threatening. Endoscopic procedures have demonstrated benefit in these cases. Occasionally after vomiting or retching, a complete rupture of the esophagus (Boerhaave's syndrome) can occur with leakage of gastric contents into the mediastinum and chest. This is a catastrophic event with a poor prognosis, requiring early surgical consultation.

Aortoenteric Fistula

A rare but catastrophic cause of UGI bleeding results from erosion of an aortic aneurysm or a aortic graft into the distal duodenum. The classic presentation is a "herald" hemorrhage that occurs and stops spontaneously hours or occasionally weeks before the exsanguinating hemorrhage. This entity is usually seen months to years after the actual surgery. In patients with a history of an abdominal aortic aneurysm repair and GI bleeding, the cause is an aortoenteric fistula until proven otherwise. These patients require aggressive resuscitation and must be moved immediately to the operating suite.

Lower Gastrointestinal Bleeding

Anorectal Sources

Anorectal problems, most commonly internal and external hemorrhoids, are the most frequent cause of LGI bleeding. Other sources include fissures, fistulas, foreign bodies, and infectious proctitis. Hemorrhoids result from increased hydrostatic pressure in the portal venous system. Straining at stool is by far the most common cause of such increased pressure, followed by pregnancy and portal venous hypertension. The bleeding of hemorrhoids presents as bright red blood on toilet paper or red streaking of stool. If present at all, pain symptoms range from mild anal discomfort to the severe pain of thrombosis. The diagnosis of hemorrhoids can be made by inspection and digital examination. Anoscopy is confirmatory for internal hemorrhoids. Even in patients who have known hemorrhoids, new-onset LGI bleeding often is caused by other lesions.

Diverticulosis

Diverticular disease is generally seen in older patients and is the most common cause of massive LGI bleeding. Diverticula are found in 20% to 50% of Americans older than the age of 50 and in 70% of patients aged 75 to 80 years. They occur most commonly in the sigmoid and descending colon. Despite this, the preponderance of bleeding diverticula occur on the right side of the colon. Diverticula are found at the sites of penetration of nutrient vessels in the colonic wall. Bleeding is much less common than irritation and inflammation (diverticulitis) and results from the erosion of a small vessel in the diverticular sac by a fecalith. The bleeding is usually painless and self-limited. Significant bleeding requires angiography for diagnosis and localization of the bleeding site.

Angiodysplasia

Angiodysplasia is a lesion occurring predominantly in the cecum and right colon. Like diverticular disease, it is common and affects people older than the age of 50. After diverticulosis, angiodysplasia is the second most common cause of major LGI bleeding. Hypertension and aortic stenosis are associated conditions, but the pathogenesis of these lesions is not known. Patients bleeding from an arteriovenous malformation may have either melena (23%) or hematochezia (54%). The most accurate method of diagnosing angiodysplasia is selective mesenteric angiography, although occasionally colonoscopy can identify the lesions. The sensitivity of colonoscopy is 80%, with a 90% specificity.

Mesenteric Ischemia

Mesenteric ischemia is seen in patients (often elderly) who have peripheral atherosclerotic vascular disease, cardiac dysrhythmia, or any condition predisposing to thrombus formation and embolization (e.g., congestive heart failure, atrial fibrillation, or oral contraceptive use). The ischemia evolves from a low-flow state or frank occlusion of a mesenteric vessel secondary to thrombus or emboli. Clinically, patients with mesenteric ischemia often have severe abdominal pain out of proportion to their relatively benign examination. A leukocytosis (greater than $10,000/mm^3$) is almost always present. A characteristic laboratory finding in about 50% of these patients is a significant anion-gap metabolic acidosis secondary to lactic acid production. However, an elevated lactate level is seen in over 90% of patients with mesenteric ischemia. A leukocytosis (and usually an elevated lactate level) may be the only abnormal findings in elderly or obtunded patients. Plain abdominal films may show the classic "thumbprinting" lesion of the colon. This represents edema in the ischemic intestinal wall. Bleeding occurs from ischemic-necrotic sloughing of intestinal mucosa. The mortality in mesenteric ischemia is high, up to 70%, regardless of the exact cause.

Cancer

Adenocarcinoma is the most common malignancy of the colorectal region. It is a relatively uncommon cause of major LGI bleeding. Early symptoms are often vague and include malaise, change in bowel habits, weight loss, and anemia. Rectal bleeding is likely to be noticed by 70% of patients who have left-sided lesions, whereas fewer than 25% of patients with right-sided lesions have that complaint. Pain is an unusual symptom of colonic cancer in its early stages. Diagnosis is made by colonoscopy or barium enema.

Other Causes of Bleeding

There are many other causes of LGI bleeding. Inflammatory bowel disease has its peak incidence in the second and third decades of life. It presents as abdominal cramping, weight loss, and a varying degree of bloody diarrhea. Infections that cause diarrhea can also cause LGI bleeding. A history of travel to endemic areas, eating suspect foods, or variant sexual practices is explored as appropriate. Other less common causes of LGI bleeding include blood dyscrasias and Meckel's diverticulum in pediatric patients.

PRINCIPLES OF MANAGEMENT
General Approach

The main objectives of emergency department management are to correct volume losses and prevent hemodynamic instability. Eighty percent to 90% of GI hemorrhage is self-limited and ceases spontaneously within 24 to 48 hours.

General support includes oxygen, volume replacement with isotonic crystalloid, and blood component transfusions as indicated. The goal is always to anticipate the possible needs of the patient rather than to react to a series of acute problems or complications. Most bleeding will not require advanced treatment techniques in the emergency department.

If the GI hemorrhage is persistently active or associated with hemodynamic instability, it is essential to seek early consultation with a gastroenterologist or surgeon.

Figures 6–1 and 6–2 provide structured clinical approaches to the management of UGI bleeding and LGI bleeding.

Specific Therapies

Upper Gastrointestinal Bleeding

Gastric Lavage. Lavage is performed selectively as already mentioned under "Diagnostic Adjuncts."

Esophagogastroduodenoscopy. Once the bleeding has been stabilized, endoscopy can be performed to visualize the bleeding source. If the bleeding is located, a variety of transendoscopic therapies can be used to treat it. These include needle sclerotherapy for esophageal varices, direct application of medication (ethanol, epinephrine, or sodium tetradecyl sulfate) to the bleeding site, laser photocoagulation, banding of varices, and thermal contact of bleeding sites.

Somatostatin and Octreotide Infusions. Somatostatin is a naturally occurring polypeptide that lowers portal venous pressure by inducing splanchnic vasoconstriction and decreases gastric acid secretion. Octreotide is a synthetic analogue of somatostatin with similar hemodynamic properties but a longer duration of action. Both medications have shown limited effectiveness for short-term control of variceal bleeding. They have been considered as the drugs of choice for treatment of acute variceal bleeding, although further studies are necessary. Other studies have supported their use in combination with endoscopic sclerotherapy or endoscopic band ligation for controlling and reducing the incidence of rebleeding of varices.

Vasopressin Infusion. Vasopressin is a potent, nonselective vasoconstrictor with effects on the splanchnic bed. Infusion of vasopressin, following the angiographic demonstration of the UGI bleeding site, has been successful in controlling bleeding from esophageal varices, severe erosive gastritis, and uncontrolled stress ulcers. It is most commonly used to treat massive variceal hemorrhage. Because of the risk of end-organ ischemia, vasopressin should be used with caution in patients with coronary artery or other vascular diseases. Vasopressin should only be used when endoscopy is unavailable and the patient is exsanguinating. The concomitant use of nitroglycerin with vasopressin has been shown to reduce the systemic adverse affects of vasopressin while maintaining splanchnic vasoconstriction.

Esophageal Tamponade. Massive UGI bleeding from varices not controlled by pharmacotherapy or endoscopic therapy may be temporarily controlled with a Sengstaken-Blakemore tube. This device can be passed orogastrically and the two balloons inflated to provide a pressure tamponade of the varices. There is a large intragastric balloon, which is inflated first, and another esophageal balloon with a single suction port at the distal tip in the stomach. It is usually left in place 12 to 24 hours. Complications are common (15%) and include esophageal rupture and pharyngeal blockage with asphyxiation from the esophageal portion of the balloon. The Edlich-Minnesota modification of the Sengstaken-Blakemore tube provides proximal esophageal suction, thereby minimizing the risk of aspiration. With improved endoscopic diagnostic techniques and other modes of therapy, balloon tamponade is not used as often as previously. Although use of these tubes is less successful than use of other modalities, they can provide control of bleeding in up to 80% of cases.

Histamine-2 Antagonists/Proton Pump Inhibitors. Histamine antagonists are thought to decrease bleeding by blocking acidity in the stomach and constricting vessels at the bleeding site, thereby decreasing the "force" of bleeding. H_2 antagonists, proton pump inhibitors, and antacids are used more for prevention than for stopping active bleeding. The use of H_2 blockers and proton pump inhibitors may reduce the rate of rebleeding and subsequent death in patients with acute bleeding from gastric ulcers.

Surgical Intervention. Surgical intervention is the final option in treating UGI hemorrhage. Most esophageal bleeding episodes are treated nonoperatively. In other sites (stomach and duodenum), massive bleeding, continued bleeding, and rebleeding are the usual indications for surgery. In patients with a gastric ulcer, a visible bleeding vessel is associated with a rebleeding rate of over 50%. The need for operative intervention is also about 50%. Emergent surgical indications include free perforation into the peritoneal cavity and massive bleeding unresponsive to medical or endoscopic treatment.

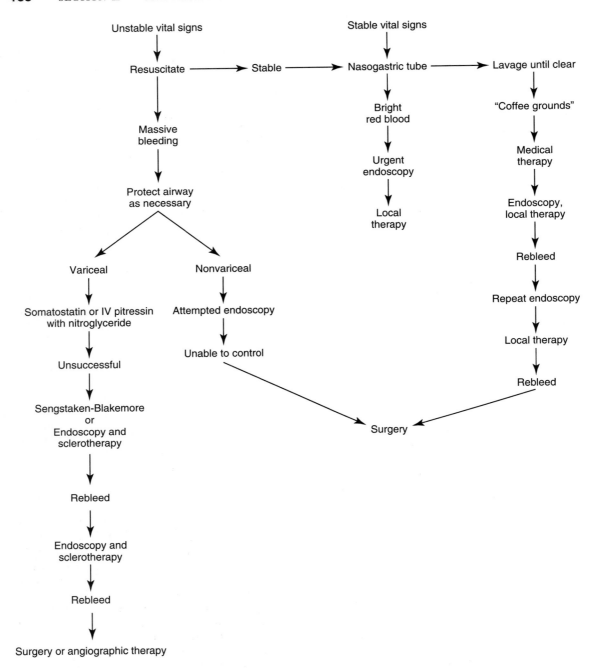

FIGURE 6–1 • Management approach to upper gastrointestinal bleeding.

Lower Gastrointestinal Bleeding

Colonoscopy. Like endoscopy for UGI bleeding, colonoscopy affords the same advantages both in locating the site of bleeding and in therapeutic interventions. It has become the interventional modality of choice in LGI bleeding. Urgent colonoscopy combined with active interventions (epinephrine injection, bipolar coagulation) may prevent recurrent bleeding and the need for surgery in lower GI bleeding of diverticular origin.

Arteriography. If anoscopy, sigmoidoscopy, or colonoscopy cannot identify the source of the LGI bleeding or if continuous bleeding prevents

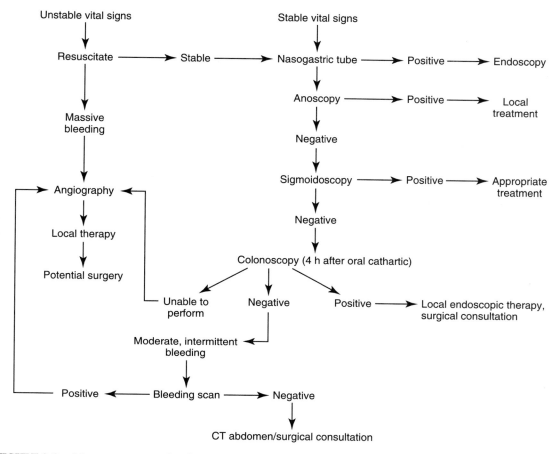

FIGURE 6–2 • Management approach to lower gastrointestinal bleeding.

endoscopy, selective arteriography is used to detect the bleeding site. For this procedure to be used, the bleeding rate from the site must exceed 0.5 to 1 mL/min; if bleeding is intermittent, the test may be falsely negative. Arteriography is necessary for the evaluation of areas not amenable to endoscopy or in the difficult circumstance of a suspected stable aortoenteric fistula. Selected vessel angiography can also be used for the infusion of vasopressin or embolization.

Vasopressin Infusion. Vasopressin is used for its vasoconstrictor action. Direct vasopressin infusion by selective catheterization of the mesenteric arteries has not been shown to be more effective in reducing hemorrhage than intravenous systemic vasopressin alone.

Surgical Intervention. The indications for urgent interventional surgery in cases of LGI bleeding are similar to those for UGI causes. If medical support does not stabilize the patient's condition, operative control of the bleeding site is

the only recourse. Of sources of LGI bleeding, diverticular disease is the most likely to cause heavy bleeding and rebleeding. Severe bleeding requiring a transfusion of more than 4 units of packed RBCs is associated with an operative rate of close to 60%. In patients with other lesions, such as an aortoenteric fistula, the need for early surgical control of hemorrhage is clear if the diagnosis is made in time.

UNCERTAIN DIAGNOSIS

The presence or absence of blood coming from the GI tract can be ascertained in the emergency department. The location of the blood loss is often not known at the time of disposition from the emergency department. These patients are essentially all admitted for further evaluation. Occult GI bleeding is commonly caused by vascular ectasia of the small bowel. Patient referral and a complete GI assessment can identify the sites of hemorrhage in more than 90% of patients.

SPECIAL CONSIDERATIONS

Pediatric Patients

The evaluation of GI bleeding in the pediatric population is often complicated by communication limitations between the physician and the patient. The history given by the parent or guardian and the physical examination assume primary importance. Associated symptoms such as pain, irritability, changes in normal activity and feeding, vomiting, diarrhea, or altered stools can accompany a wide range of potential diagnoses. Information about a term or premature birth, any perinatal complications, or a history of similar familial disorders must be known.

In children, esophagitis, gastritis, and peptic ulcer disease are the most common causes of UGI bleeding; as causes of LGI bleeding, infectious colitis and inflammatory bowel disease are noted most often. Vomiting with evidence of UGI or LGI bleeding suggests a bowel obstruction with possible hemorrhage from injured or ischemic intestinal mucosa.

LGI bleeding can be caused by a colonic polyp, intussusception, or Meckel's diverticulum. Intestinal polyposis may be an inherited familial condition. Intussusception is characterized by progressively more frequent episodes of abdominal colic with apparently normal intervals in between. It is the most common cause of intestinal obstruction in children aged 2 months to 6 years. The classic finding of "currant jelly stool" with intussusception is a late finding that implies bowel mucosal damage. Meckel's diverticulum is a remnant of the omphalomesenteric duct found near the terminal ileum. It can contain ectopic rests of acid-producing gastric mucosa in about 50% of cases. These can erode the intestinal mucosa and induce bleeding. This entity can be seen at any age but is most commonly seen in the first 2 years of life. The most common presentation is painless rectal bleeding. It also can mimic the presentation of appendicitis and is associated with a higher risk of intestinal obstruction.

In the neonatal or young infant period, congenital malrotation of the gut with a midgut volvulus can present as acute hemorrhage. Emergent surgery is needed to prevent massive intestinal gangrene. Another neonatal condition, although very rare, is portal hypertension with bleeding esophageal varices secondary to congenital hepatobiliary disease or extrahepatic portal vein thrombosis.

Noncongenital causes of pediatric GI bleeding must always be considered as well, such as the possibility of nonaccidental trauma or sexual abuse, foreign body ingestions, or toxic ingestion (e.g., massive iron overdose).

Management of pediatric patients generally follows adult guidelines except for the amount of fluid used in volume resuscitation. Isotonic crystalloid is the initial fluid of choice, and 20 mL/kg is the standard initiating volume for repletion. Early consultation with the appropriate specialists in pediatric gastroenterology, pediatric surgery, and radiology is vital for appropriate diagnostic testing and definitive treatment.

DISPOSITION AND FOLLOW-UP

Almost all patients with significant UGI or LGI bleeding are admitted to the hospital. Patients are admitted to critical care units if their condition remains unstable in the emergency department, their bleeding persists, hemorrhage is massive, they are at high risk for complications, or they have other concomitant acute medical problems, such as coronary ischemia.

Admission

Any person who has significant UGI or LGI bleeding with abnormal vital signs is admitted for observation and diagnosis even if the person is young and otherwise healthy. If the patient has a preexisting anemia, a new hemorrhage may compromise an already reduced hemodynamic reserve. Any patient with a significant degree of blood loss demonstrable by vomiting, gastric lavage, or stool analysis in the emergency department is admitted.

Risk stratification methods are being applied to identify where in the hospital the patient may be placed for optimum care. Most of these decisions are made after endoscopy and, therefore, are more the concerns of the surgeon and gastroenterologist than the emergency physician. One interesting high-risk complication patient classification method with potential benefit in the emergency department is

B—bleeding, ongoing
L—low systolic blood pressure (<100 mm Hg)
E—elevated prothrombin time (>1.2 times control)
E—erratic mental status
D—disease, unstable comorbid conditions

These patients are routinely admitted to monitored intensive care unit settings.

Discharge

Patients who can safely be discharged home with self-care instructions include the following:

- Those healthy patients with minimal UGI bleeding that has ceased, for example, following an episode of gastritis
- Those with simple uncomplicated fissures and hemorrhoids
- Elderly people with occult blood in the stool without discernible disease requiring admission

These patients should all have normal, stable vital signs, no new orthostatic changes, anemia, or blood dyscrasias, and no other serious complicating associated conditions. Follow-up with a primary care physician or gastroenterologist is arranged within 1 to 3 days. Education about the possible cause of their disorder, and specific means of avoiding it (e.g., avoiding aspirin, NSAIDs), is important before discharge.

FINAL POINTS

- Patients with GI bleeding, whether upper or lower, require expedient stabilization and frequent reassessments. Anticipate; don't wait for a catastrophe to occur.
- The most common causes of frank UGI bleeding include peptic ulcer disease, erosive gastritis, and varices.
- The most common causes of massive LGI bleeding include diverticulosis and angiodysplasia.
- Despite the advances made in diagnosis and therapy, the mortality rate for UGI bleeding remains 8% to 10%.
- Because of the variable rate of transit time through the GI tract, the color of the stool is not reliable in determining the site of the bleeding.
- The initial hemoglobin value is a poor indicator of the quantity of blood lost.
- Endoscopy, both UGI and LGI, is the mainstay of emergent diagnosis and therapy.

CASE *Study*

The rescue squad was called to the home of a 50-year-old man who had vomited a large amount of bright red blood. On arrival at the patient's home, the rescue squad found him lying on the bathroom floor. He was alert but pale and diaphoretic. There was bloody vomitus in the toilet bowl. His blood pressure was 80/50 mm Hg, pulse was 130 beats per minute, and respirations were 24 breaths per minute. The patient stated the episode came on suddenly after 1 to 2 days of persistent abdominal pain. He was noted to be confused and anxious. His airway was patent and protected, breath sounds were equal, and the abdomen was tender but soft. Oxygen at 4 L/min was given by nasal cannula. He was transported to the ambulance, equipment to start an intravenous line was readied, and a radio call was placed to the hospital.

The squad acted quickly to assess the patient while simultaneously initiating stabilization. Only the essential historical information was collected, and the physical examination was limited to examination of the airway, chest, heart, and abdomen. Transport was the first priority, and intravenous access procedures were performed while in transit. The rescue squad successfully established one large-bore intravenous line; and because of the obvious hemorrhage, along with the patient's hypotensive/hypoperfused state, 1 L of isotonic crystalloid was infused rapidly.

After arrival in the emergency department, the patient's repeat vital signs were blood pressure of 90/60 mm Hg, pulse of 120 beats per minute, and respirations of 20 breaths per minute. He was less confused and anxious but still pale and diaphoretic. The 1 L of fluid had been given.

Based on the vital signs, appearance, and signs of poor peripheral perfusion, the patient had a class III (30% to 40%) blood loss and required further crystalloid and potential blood infusion (see Table 6–1). A second large-bore intravenous line was established, the crystalloid was maintained at high flow, and blood type and crossmatch for 4 units was requested.

After a careful history and physical examination, it was apparent this patient had several risk factors for severe GI bleeding. He was a heavy alcohol abuser and took aspirin regularly for his "hangovers." He had some stigmata of advanced liver disease, including spider angiomas, splenomegaly, and enlarged abdominal veins.

Although no definitive diagnosis could be reached at this point, it was evident that this patient had active blood loss, was tolerating the loss poorly, and had at least a UGI source of blood loss. Considering his underlying ethanol abuse, the likely causes of hemorrhage include bleeding

Continued on following page

esophageal varices, erosive gastritis, and duodenal ulcer. All are capable of causing life-threatening hemorrhage. His aspirin use, especially within the last week, increased his risk for serious mucosal bleeding because of induced platelet dysfunction.

The laboratory results showed a hemoglobin and hematocrit of 8.0 g and 24%. The electrolyte measurements were normal except for a bicarbonate level of 20 mEq/L and potassium level of 5.5 mEq/L. The platelet count was 92,000/mm³, and the PT was 3 seconds over control.

This patient has had a major loss of blood. The metabolic acidemia was probably related to hypoperfusion. Other possible causes for the acidemia (e.g., salicylism or ischemic bowel) should be considered. The platelet count and PT may have been abnormal because of severe liver disease or early disseminated intravascular coagulation. A peripheral smear looking for broken cells (schizocytes) might point to disseminated intravascular coagulation.

Gastric lavage was performed until clear fluid was returned in preparation for endoscopy. In addition, an H_2 blocker was administered intravenously. Subsequently, the patient's bleeding ceased after 30 minutes. The patient was given 4 L of isotonic crystalloid and 3 units of type-specific packed red cells to reverse the hypovolemia and hypoperfusion. The blood pressure returned to 110/80 mm Hg, pulse to 90 beats per minute, and respirations to 18 breaths per minute.

A consultant was contacted early in the care of this patient, because early endoscopy was planned. Also, octreotide or vasopressin infusion were being considered if the patient's bleeding did not stop with conservative therapy and blood product replacement. Considering the patient's history of alcoholism and probable liver disease, vitamin K supplementation would be warranted.

After lavage and stabilization, the patient was ready for esophagogastroduodenoscopy.

Because of the patient's significant hemorrhage requiring blood transfusion, he was admitted to an intensive care unit. Endoscopy found severe erosive gastritis.

Bibliography

TEXTS

Bockus H (ed): Gastroenterology, 5th ed. Philadelphia, WB Saunders, 1994.

Yamada T (ed): Textbook of Gastroenterology, 3rd ed. Philadelphia, Lippincott-Raven, 1999.

JOURNAL ARTICLES

Bono MJ: Lower gastrointestinal tract bleeding. Emerg Med Clin North Am 1996; 14:547–556.

Chalasani N, Clark WS, Wilcox CM: Blood urea nitrogen-to-creatinine concentration in gastrointestinal bleeding: A reappraisal. Am J Gastroenterol 1997; 92:1796.

Gotzche PC: Somatostatin or octreotide for acute bleeding oesophageal varices. The Cochrane Library. Oxford, 2000, Issue 2.

Jensen DM, Machicado GA: Colonoscopy for diagnosis and treatment of severe diverticular hemorrhage. N Engl J Med 2000; 342:78–82.

Johnson SE, Ignatoff WB: Lower gastrointestinal bleeding in the elderly population. Geriatr Emerg Med Rep 2002; 1–12.

Kollef MH, O'Brien JD, Zuckerman GR, et al: BLEED: A classification tool to predict outcomes in patients with acute upper and lower gastrointestinal hemorrhage. Crit Care Med 1997; 25:1125–1132.

Lee JG, Turnipseed S, et al: Endoscopy-based triage significantly reduces hospitalization rates and costs of treating upper GI bleeding: A, randomized controlled trial. Gastrointest Endosc 1999; 50:755–761.

Lewis JD, Brown A, Localio AR, et al: Initial evaluation of rectal bleeding in young persons: a cost-effectiveness analysis. Ann Intern Med 2002; 136: 99–110.

McGuirk TD, Coyle WJ: Upper gastrointestinal tract bleeding. Emerg Med Clin North Am 1996; 14:523–545.

Peter DJ, Dougherty JM: Evaluation of the patient with gastrointestinal bleeding: An evidence based approach. Emerg Med Clin North Am 1999; 17:239–261.

Sharara AI, Rockey DC: Gastroesophageal variceal hemorrhage. N Engl J Med 2001; 345:669–679.

Terdiman JP: Update on upper gastrointestinal bleeding: Basing treatment decisions on patients' risk level. Postgrad Med 1998; 103:43–47, 51–52, 58–59.

Van Dam J, Brugge WR: Endoscopy of the upper gastrointestinal tract. N Engl J Med 1999; 341:1738–1748.

Zuccaro GR: Management of the adult patient with acute lower gastrointestinal bleeding. Am J Gastroenterol 1998; 93:1202–1208.

Zuckerman GR, Prakash C: Acute lower intestinal bleeding: I. Clinical presentation and diagnosis. Gastrointest Endosc 1998; 48:606–617.

Zuckerman GR, Prakash C: Acute lower intestinal bleeding: II. Etiology, therapy, and outcomes. Gastrointest Endosc 1999; 49:228–238.

CHAPTER 7

Acute Diarrhea

TODD J. CROCCO

CASE *Study*

A 22-year-old woman presented to the emergency department with diarrhea, abdominal pain, and nausea and vomiting for 2 days. The symptoms started with the nausea, followed by brief vomiting, then frequent, loose bowel movements accompanied by severe lower abdominal cramping. She became progressively weak and was advised to go to the emergency department after talking to her primary physician.

INTRODUCTION

Epidemiology

Diarrhea is defined as an increase in stool weight or volume to greater than 200 g/day. The term also describes stools that are loose or watery or bowel movements of greater frequency than three per day. Acute diarrhea is differentiated from chronic diarrhea by the duration of symptoms. If the symptom duration is less than 4 weeks, the physician should consider this acute diarrhea. Beyond a 4-week duration, the symptoms are termed persistent or chronic.

Diarrheal illnesses cause enormous morbidity and mortality worldwide. Enteric disease is responsible for over 3 million infant deaths in the world every year. In some developing countries, diarrhea is the leading cause of childhood death. In the United States, it is estimated that 100 million cases of acute diarrhea affect adults. Diarrhea accounts for 5% to 7% of outpatient visits to physicians and is second only to the common cold as a source of days lost from school or work. Annually, approximately 250,000 hospital admissions and 8 million health care visits are diarrhea related. Diarrhea is responsible for up to 10,000 deaths in the United States each year.

Physiology

Normally, the small intestine performs the majority of intestinal fluid absorption. A typical daily fluid load of 9 L is reduced to 1 L by the small intestine. The large intestine performs the remaining absorptive process, thereby transforming a fluid stool into solid form and a fluid loss of less than 100 mL/day. Disruption of the absorptive and secretory processes that occur in both the small and large bowel may result in diarrhea.

Diarrhea can occur as a result of osmotic, inflammatory, secretory, or altered motility causes. Osmotic diarrhea results from an increase of unabsorbable or poorly absorbable molecules within the intestinal lumen. This results in fluid retention within the intestine, leading to diarrhea. Lactulose, disaccharide malabsorption, and laxatives can create osmotic diarrhea. Inflammatory diarrhea occurs when the intestinal mucosa is inflamed such that normal fluid absorption and secretion is interrupted. Infectious agents such as *Shigella*, *Salmonella*, and *Giardia* may cause an inflammatory diarrhea. Secretory diarrhea exists when there is an increased amount of intestinal fluid secretion relative to fluid absorption. Bacterial toxins, such as those produced by *Vibrio cholerae* and toxigenic *Escherichia coli*, may cause a secretory diarrhea without any histologic injury to the intestinal mucosa. Finally, disorders of intestinal motility can also precipitate diarrhea as seen in patients with irritable bowel syndrome, intestinal resection, or intestinal fistulas.

It is important for the emergency physician to have a sound understanding of acute diarrheal illnesses because of their frequency of occurrence and diversity of cause. Furthermore, diarrhea remains a common, life-threatening illness in regions of the world where emergency medicine practitioners confront it routinely.

INITIAL APPROACH AND STABILIZATION

Priority Diagnoses

Dysentery is diarrhea accompanied by blood and purulent material. It may be caused by bacterial infection or inflammatory bowel disease. Any patient with complaints consistent with dysentery should be viewed as seriously ill. Also, hemodynamic instability with or without abdominal peritoneal findings is also indicative of serious illness.

Rapid Assessment

The initial approach to the patient with acute diarrhea includes a rapid assessment of hemodynamic stability. Depending on the volume and duration of diarrhea, patients may manifest evidence of dehydration or even shock. The following information is quickly obtained:

1. Duration of the diarrhea.
2. Severity of the diarrhea. How many stools per day? How large are the stools?
3. Appearance and odor of the stools. Is blood, pus, or mucus present? Are the stools dark? Are the stools green (or any other color)? Are the stools greasy or foul smelling?
4. Presence or absence of fever.
5. Presence or absence of vomiting. Has there been any blood in the vomitus? How often does vomiting occur and is it related to eating?
6. Presence or absence of abdominal pain. Is the pain constant or intermittent? How severe is the pain? Is the pain relieved with bowel movements or vomiting? Did the pain precede the nausea, vomiting, or diarrhea?
7. It is important to carefully assess the patient's vital signs.
8. A thorough abdominal examination is mandatory. This may allow the physician to determine whether the diarrhea is caused by an illness requiring surgical intervention. In addition to the abdominal examination, a rectal examination should also be performed. This may suggest the cause of the patient's diarrhea. The presence of fistulas and/or fissures may reflect inflammatory bowel disease. Palpation of hard stool suggests the possibility of fecal impaction or Hirschsprung's disease. Stool color should be noted, and the presence or absence of blood (gross and occult) should be determined.

Early Intervention

If the patient's condition is stable, then progression to an expanded history and physical is appropriate. If the patient's condition is unstable, then fluid resuscitation should be implemented at once. In the adult, volume resuscitation should include 20 to 30 mL/kg of isotonic crystalloid solution. In the pediatric population, 20 mL/kg boluses of isotonic crystalloid are initiated. The need for additional therapy during the stabilization phase is unusual but may be necessary in the elderly and pediatric populations. These two age-groups have less physiologic reserve than most adults and may experience more rapid hemodynamic decompensation with volume loss.

CLINICAL ASSESSMENT

Most patients with diarrhea are not in imminent danger and can undergo a more thorough history and physical examination.

History

Historical details will often influence the physician's differential diagnosis and direct the emergency physician to important aspects of the physical examination. Furthermore, ordering of laboratory studies may be heavily influenced by a patient's historical information.

The emergency physician should recognize many patients may feel uncomfortable discussing the topic of diarrhea. Patients will often desire private and confidential discussions on this matter. Additionally, patient pain and discomfort may obstruct the patient's ability to offer an accurate history. As in all patient encounters, it is important to be patient and sympathetic toward the patient's condition.

Characteristics of the Diarrhea

Onset and Duration. The time course of symptom onset and duration is important to discern. If, for instance, the patient reports the sudden onset of diarrhea within a few hours of eating or drinking, then food poisoning may be strongly considered as the cause. If, however, the diarrhea has been slow in onset and persistent for many weeks, then, by definition, the patient has chronic diarrhea and the differential diagnoses are substantially different.

Severity. The patient is asked about the frequency of stools and the volume of fluid expelled. Colonic infection is usually associated with a pattern of many small stools, whereas more proximal enteric infection usually causes fewer, large volume stools. Symptom severity also offers early guidance in deciding which patients may require aggressive intervention.

Appearance. The patient is also asked about the color, odor, and consistency of the stools. Questions about color primarily focus on bright red blood or dark melenic stools. The presence of blood or mucus indicates a violation of the intestinal mucosa, which may occur with ulceration, invasive infectious agents, inflammatory bowel disease, bowel ischemia, and neoplasms. Malodorous stools that float may occur in patients with intestinal malabsorption.

Factors That Relieve or Worsen the Diarrhea

The effect of eating or drinking may improve or worsen the diarrhea. Diarrhea that is worse after ingesting milk products may indicate lactose intolerance. The ingestion of alcohol or medications of many varieties may also exacerbate diarrhea. Conversely, patients may observe that abstinence from alcohol, milk products, or other foods improves their symptoms.

Previous History of Diarrhea

Patients with an acute exacerbation of a chronic illness may describe their symptoms as identical to a previous episode. Patients with pancreatic insufficiency, celiac sprue, inflammatory bowel disease, hyperthyroidism or hypothyroidism, and numerous other conditions may experience acute flares of their illness for a variety of reasons. The importance of asking about any similar history of diarrhea is underscored by the fact that diarrhea-causing chronic illnesses can be easily forgotten in the acute setting. Stress-related episodes should be explored.

Associated Symptoms

Fever. The presence of fever suggests an invasive organism may be causing the patient's symptoms. *Shigella, Salmonella, Campylobacter,* and other infectious agents may penetrate the intestinal mucosa and invade the bloodstream, thereby inducing fever within the host. This finding is not exclusive to infectious causes. There are numerous systemic or extraintestinal illnesses that can also produce diarrhea and fever.

Vomiting. Vomiting can occur in association with diarrhea secondary to a variety of illnesses. The presence of vomiting implies proximal small bowel involvement. Partial bowel obstruction, gastroenteritis, or food poisoning may cause vomiting and diarrhea together. The presence of vomiting should alert the physician to the possibility of even greater fluid losses and the potential inability to accomplish oral rehydration.

Pain. The location and character of pain can be helpful to the physician. Pain secondary to colonic involvement is usually located in the lower quadrants or back, whereas small bowel involvement usually causes periumbilical pain. It is important to determine whether the pain is constant, intermittent, or colicky. Constant pain is more suggestive of a disorder that will require surgical treatment, whereas colicky or cramping pain is typical of self-limited acute diarrhea. An intermittent pain that is exacerbated with eating may represent intestinal ischemia in an older patient.

Weight Loss. Weight loss suggests prolonged disease or malabsorption. If the patient's symptoms are of extended duration, gastrointestinal carcinoma should be considered.

Constipation. Diarrhea alternating with constipation suggests an obstructing colonic mass lesion. Irritable bowel syndrome can also cause this symptom.

Flatulence. Flatulence and bloating are common in patients with malabsorption syndromes or parasitic infections.

Risk Factors

Recent Travel. The patient is asked about any recent travel, especially to developing countries. Depending on the location of travel, the physician may be able to select a potential infectious source. Contaminated water or improperly prepared foods are more commonly consumed in developing countries. Traveler's diarrhea is most often caused by enterotoxigenic *Escherichia coli.* Outdoor enthusiasts may become infected with *Giardia lamblia* from drinking stream or lake water. A patient's symptoms usually start within 5 days of arrival to the region, but some parasitic infections may incubate for 1 to 3 weeks. Infectious sources can be bacterial, viral, or parasitic.

Recent Ingestions. Identifying any unusual or unsafe ingestions may also help discern the cause of diarrhea. Unsafe ingestions, for example, may include foods with high protein content (ham, egg salad, potato salad) that are left uncovered during a warm day. The sudden onset of vomiting and diarrhea after this type of ingestion suggests food poisoning secondary to *Staphylococcus aureus* (custards) or *Bacillus cereus* (fried rice). If other individuals consumed the same foods or beverages, it is important to find out if they are experiencing similar symptoms. Food poisoning is considered when symptoms begin 1 to 6 hours after eating high-risk foods.

Sexual Orientation. In the setting of acute diarrhea, an individual's sexual orientation and sexual practices may offer the explanation for the symptomatology. Individuals who engage in fecal-oral contact may acquire pathogens such as *Shigella, Salmonella, Campylobacter,* and others. In addition, receptive anal intercourse may expose the patient to *Neisseria gonorrhoeae, Chlamydia* *trachomatis,* herpes simplex virus, or other sexually acquired infectious agents.

Immunocompromise. If the patient has never been tested for human immunodeficiency virus infection or does not know the results of such a test, then potential risk factors for this viral infection should be investigated. The immunocompromised state (CD4 < 200/ mm^3) exposes patients to a host of unusual infections that may precipitate diarrhea. Infection with *Microsporidium, Cryptosporidium,* cytomegalovirus, *Mycobacterium avium-intracellulare,* and other agents may be more seriously considered in light of a patient's immune status. Immunocompromised states also exist in patients on chemotherapy, those taking high doses of corticosteroids, diabetics, and transplant recipients.

Exposure and Environment. Does the patient work with animals, in a day-care center, or in a closed institution such as a prison? For public health reasons, the patient is questioned about being a food handler.

Past Medical History

Illnesses. As previously mentioned, patients may present to the emergency department with the complaint of acute diarrhea secondary to an exacerbation of a chronic illness. Obtaining a thorough past medical history will help determine whether a previous illness is actually responsible for a patient's acute symptomatology. Lactose intolerance, inflammatory bowel disease, adrenal insufficiency, and diverticulitis are just a few diseases that may have remissions punctuated by exacerbations.

Medications. Patients taking a course of antibiotics may develop acute diarrhea. It is particularly common among patients taking multiple or prolonged antibiotics. Ampicillin, clindamycin, and cephalosporins are notorious for causing this type of diarrhea. *Clostridium difficile* may be a causative organism as a consequence of the altered bowel flora. Discontinuation of the offending drug(s) and implementation of oral vancomycin or metronidazole usually provides resolution. Questions about over-the-counter and herbal medicines may be useful. Patients can be taking castor beans or cassia senna, both potent motility agents, without being aware of it.

Allergies. It is always important to determine a patient's known allergies. In some cases, patients may report an allergy to a specific medication when, in fact, it is a side effect of the drug.

Physical Examination

Although a complete physical examination may be indicated in some cases, for the most part the examination can be focused on key sites and components.

Vital Signs. The hemodynamic status of the patient can vary from outright shock to minimal volume contraction. Vital signs in the normal range should be repeated for orthostatic changes. A fall in systolic pressure of 20 to 30 mm Hg or a rise in pulse of 20 to 30 beats per minute, which may be accompanied by symptoms of presyncope, is suggestive of significant volume loss.

General Appearance. The patient should be observed for dry mucous membranes, pallor, decreased skin turgor, sunken eyes, and diminished mental status. Any of these may reflect diminished intravascular fluid volume. *Salmonella typhi, Shigella,* and *Campylobacter* have an increased association with altered mental status.

Abdominal Examination. A careful abdominal examination may reveal masses, pain, rebound, guarding, or distention. Bowel sounds are auscultated. Coupled with the patient's historical features, a thorough abdominal examination may suggest the etiology. In most cases of infectious (particularly viral) diarrhea, the examination is largely unremarkable. Although the patient may complain of abdominal cramping, significant tenderness is often absent. Exceptions include infection with *Campylobacter* or *Yersinia.* These infections can mimic mesenteric adenitis or appendicitis, potentially leading to a laparotomy. Differential diagnostic details of the abdominal examination are outlined in Chapter 5, Abdominal Pain.

Rectal Examination. A rectal examination is an important part of assessing the complaint of diarrhea. It is particularly important in those individuals with associated abdominal pain. Rectal examination should include inspection (for fistulas and fissures), palpation (for masses or tenderness), prostate assessment, and stool testing (for gross/occult blood and stool color). A patient with a complaint of diarrhea may have melenic stools associated with gastrointestinal bleeding. Elderly or bedridden patients may have "overflow" diarrhea from a fecal impaction. The rectal examination can also provide a sample for fecal leukocyte determination.

CLINICAL REASONING

During the evaluation of the patient, the historical details and physical findings should guide the physician through a decision algorithm. Based on this clinical information, the emergency physician can then order appropriate laboratory studies to assist in the decision-making process. Figure 7-1 summarizes a treatment algorithm for patients with acute diarrhea. There are several critical questions to be answered when caring for the patient with acute diarrhea.

Is the Patient Hemodynamically Stable?

A patient's hemodynamic status is evaluated immediately on patient arrival. As with any patient presenting to an emergency department, initial assessment of airway, breathing, and circulation is mandatory. Resuscitative measures should be instituted without delay in those patients found to have any abnormalities in their primary assessment.

How Severe Are the Patient's Symptoms?

If the patient is determined to be hemodynamically stable, it is then prudent to ascertain the severity of the symptoms. Mild diarrhea without

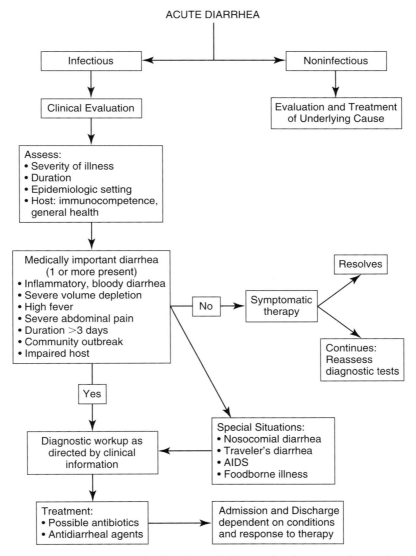

FIGURE 7–1 • Approach to patient with acute diarrhea. The goal of the initial evaluation is to distinguish medically important diarrhea from benign self-limited diarrhea. By focusing on four categories of information—the severity of illness, the duration of diarrhea, the setting in which diarrhea was obtained, and the state of host defenses and immunity—the clinician can decide which patients require additional investigation and treatment. (From Aranda-Michel J, Giannella RA: Acute diarrhea: A practical review. Am J Med 1999; 106:674, with permission.)

associated symptomatology may be amenable to oral rehydration without any further workup. However, severe diarrhea associated with vomiting may require intravenous fluid rehydration, antiemetics, and electrolyte repletion.

Are the Patient's Symptoms Consistent with an Illness That May Require Surgery?

Patients presenting with acute diarrhea associated with abdominal pain, rebound, and guarding may have an underlying illness requiring surgical intervention. Appendicitis, diverticulitis, and intestinal ischemia may all precipitate emergency department visits for diarrhea. Surgical intervention may be necessary for any of these causes. Diarrhea may occur secondary to a disease that requires surgical treatment.

Is the Patient's Diarrhea Most Consistent with Inflammatory or Noninflammatory Causes? Is There Blood or Mucus in the Stool?

Patients with bloody or mucus-laden stools, fever, and abdominal pain are at risk for inflammatory diarrhea (dysentery) (Table 7–1). It is often caused by pathogens that invade the intestinal mucosa. It is important to obtain a stool culture and tests for ova and parasites in these patients. Antimicrobial therapy may be initiated in some patients. Illnesses that need to be treated surgically may also present as a similar clinical picture and should be considered in these patients. Noninflammatory diarrhea occurs secondary to toxins released by intestinal pathogens. Cholera is an example of

TABLE 7–1. Clinical Characteristics of Inflammatory vs. Noninflammatory Causes of Diarrhea

Characteristic	Inflammatory	Noninflammatory
Onset	Gradual, rarely sudden	Sudden
Fever	Present	Absent
Abdominal pain	Common, severe	Less common, mild
Systemic symptoms: Nausea, vomiting, headache, myalgias	Common	Uncommon
Abdominal tenderness	Prominent	Minimal
Fecal leukocytes	Present	Absent
Hemoglobin	Present	Absent

Adapted from Bitterman R: Acute gastroenteritis and constipation. In Rosen P, Barkin RM, et al (eds): Emergency Medicine: Concepts and Clinical Practice, 3rd ed. St. Louis, Mosby–Year Book, 1992, p 1537.

toxin-mediated diarrhea. The diarrhea is usually rapid in onset, is nonbloody, and can be associated with vomiting. Fluid rehydration and symptomatic therapy is administered.

In What Setting Did the Diarrhea Occur?

Traveler's diarrhea can come from a variety of sources, and often may be serious in nature. Multiple cases involving a family or school class is typically viral. An isolated case of diarrhea in an elderly person may represent a change in medication, or dosage, fecal impaction, or underlying disease.

What Is the Patient's Immunologic Competency?

AIDS is notorious for opportunistic infections that cause diarrhea. A sexual history is essential in most cases. In addition to the disease, medications used for treatment also can cause gastrointestinal symptoms. Diabetes can impair host defenses, alter motility, and precede vascular lesions.

DIAGNOSTIC ADJUNCTS
Laboratory Studies

Patients with mild episodes of acute diarrhea do not require laboratory evaluation. The clinical assessment often provides adequate information for determining the patient's disposition. Furthermore, most cases of acute diarrhea are self-limiting. If the patient is immunosuppressed, reports persistent symptoms of moderate to severe diarrhea, or demonstrates systemic toxicity, significant dehydration, or bloody diarrhea, then laboratory investigation is usually warranted. The elderly and very young populations may also benefit from further laboratory evaluation.

Complete Blood Cell Count and Differential. In most patients with diarrhea, the complete blood cell count is not particularly helpful. It can, however, reveal the presence of leukocytosis or anemia in a patient. The complete blood cell count may be more useful in the elderly and very young patient populations as a nonspecific marker of disease severity.

Electrolytes. Serum electrolyte determination can be useful in those patients with severe or prolonged diarrhea, evidence of dehydration, or electrolyte abnormalities. Diarrheal stool has a bicarbonate concentration twice that of plasma. Additionally, potassium losses are substantial in patients with diarrhea. Sodium and chloride content of diarrheal stools are less than that found in plasma. Consequently, electrolyte abnormalities may include hypokalemia and hypernatremia. A metabolic acidosis may also exist secondary to the bicarbonate losses.

Renal Function. Determination of blood urea nitrogen and creatinine is appropriate in those patients with moderate to severe volume loss. The blood urea nitrogen increases out of proportion to the creatinine value in the setting of dehydration. These two laboratory values are inexpensive and reliable methods of quantifying renal function.

Stool Microscopy. Sending a stool sample for microscopic evaluation can reveal the presence or absence of polymorphonuclear leukocytes by using Wright's or methylene blue stains. Stool microscopy may be ordered in patients with suspected inflammatory origins of their diarrhea. Normally the stool does not contain leukocytes, and their presence indicates colonic inflammation. Invasive organisms frequently cause acute diarrhea associated with stool leukocytes, but other disease processes (e.g., inflammatory bowel disease) may also cause colonic inflammation. Noninvasive enteric pathogens that cause acute diarrhea through a toxigenic process do not result in stool leukocytes. Similarly, diarrhea caused by viruses and parasites usually does not contain fecal leukocytes. In the United States, about 80% of diarrheal illnesses in which fecal leukocytes are found are caused by *Shigella, Salmonella,* and *Campylobacter.* The sensitivity of the test is about 50% for most pathogens. *Shigella* may be as high as 75% sensitivity. Patients with polymorphonuclear leukocytes in their stool should undergo further diagnostic evaluation, including stool culture.

Stool Culture. Obtaining a stool culture can be very helpful in determining the cause of a patient's diarrhea. Optimally, it is performed within 30 minutes of stool passage. A culture should be considered if any of the following indications exist: fever, diarrhea of more than 2 weeks duration (not previously treated with antibiotics), bloody stools (or stools found to have occult blood), suspicion of *Escherichia coli* 0157:H7 infection, or polymorphonuclear leukocytes found on stool microscopy. In bacterial causes, two separate cultures have a 99% detection rate. Most stool cultures test for *Shigella, Salmonella,* and *Campylobacter.* If a parasitic source for the patient's diarrhea is suggested, the stool sample should be specifically examined for ova and parasites. Several stool samples may be needed to identify these pathogens. Finally, stool should be sent for *Clostridium difficile* toxin assay in those patients whose diarrhea was preceded by antibiotic therapy.

Other Studies. In some circumstances, additional tests will be needed for complete evaluation of a patient's acute diarrhea. Many of these tests will need to be performed or followed up on an outpatient basis. Therefore, arranging for close patient follow-up is important in the emergency department management of acute diarrhea, just like so many other clinical situations. Additional studies may include sigmoidoscopy; biopsy; serum albumin, folate, vitamin B_{12}, and iron studies; and thyroid function tests. A sigmoidoscopy may be especially helpful if pseudomembranous colitis or inflammatory bowel disease is suspected.

Radiologic Imaging

Abdominal Plain Films. Plain film radiography is rarely indicated in patients with diarrhea. It can be useful when partial bowel obstruction, toxic megacolon, or bowel perforation is suggested. Occasionally, overflow stool incontinence cannot be differentiated from diarrhea in the elderly or institutionalized patient. A plain film of the abdomen will demonstrate large amounts of stool in the colon.

EXPANDED DIFFERENTIAL DIAGNOSIS

It is important for the emergency physician to recognize the wide array of potential causes that may be responsible for a patient's acute diarrhea (Table 7–2). Infectious causes are most common, and an expanded list is given in Table 7–3. Patients may present with first-time manifestations of a chronic illness, such as ulcerative colitis, colon cancer, or hyperthyroidism. Therefore, emergency physicians should never disregard chronic causes of diarrhea simply due to a symptom time course of less than 2 weeks. Irritable bowel syndrome is often diagnosed to explain recurrent symptoms. It is not a diagnosis that can be adequately made in the emergency department. Patients suspected of having this chronic and problematic disorder should be referred to a primary care physician or gastroenterologist for a complete assessment.

PRINCIPLES OF MANAGEMENT

The emergency department management of patients with acute diarrhea includes five main objectives: rehydration, symptomatic therapy, prevention of spread, possible antibiotic therapy, and dietary discretion.

TABLE 7–2. Expanded Differential Diagnosis of Acute and Chronic Diarrhea

---

Acute Diarrhea

Infectious
   Bacterial
      Salmonella
      Shigella
      Campylobacter
      Escherichia coli 0157:H7
      Staphylococcus aureus
      Clostridium perfringens
      Bacillus cereus
      Yersinia enterocolitica
   Viral
      Norwalk agent/rotavirus
      Vibrio species
   Protozoal
      Giardia lamblia
      Entamoeba histolytica
   Ova and parasites
      Cryptosporidium
      Mycobacterium
Medications
   Broad-spectrum antibiotics
   Sorbitol-containing elixirs
   Magnesium- and phosphate-containing antacids
   Antiarrhythmics (e.g., guanidine)
   Antineoplastics
   Antihypertensives
   Osmotically active agents
   Laxatives
   Prokinetic agents
   Anti-inflammatory agents (e.g., colchicine)
Enteral feeding tube nutrition
   Infusion rate
   Position of feeding tube
   Tonicity of formula
   Formula contamination
Gastrointestinal disorders
   Appendicitis
   Partial bowel obstruction
   Ischemic bowel
   Initial attack of ulcerative colitis and Crohn's disease
   Diverticulitis
   Pseudomembranous colitis
Other
   Excessive alcohol ingestion
   Dietary indiscretion
      Mushrooms
      Unripened fruit
      Bran
      Fiber
      Fructose
      Herbal medicines
   Heavy metal poisoning
   Nongastrointestinal causes
   Otitis media
   Salpingitis/tubo-ovarian abscess

Chronic Diarrhea

Osmotic diarrhea
   Malabsorption syndrome
   Maldigestion syndromes
Secretory diarrhea
   Cystic fibrosis
   Carcinoid

Zollinger-Ellison syndrome (gastrinoma)
Pancreatic cholera (VIPoma)
Neoplasm (colonic and villous adenoma)
Stimulant or laxative abuse
Bile salt malabsorption
Mucosal inflammation
Crohn's disease
Ulcerative colitis
Lymphocytic colitis
Collagenous colitis
Radiation enteritis
Motor disorders
Irritable bowel syndrome
Endocrine disorders
Diabetic diarrhea
Adrenal insufficiency
Hyperthyroidism
Hypothyroidism
Addison's disease
Surgical procedures
Obstruction
Gastrectomy
Pyloroplasty
Vagotomy
Antrectomy
Small bowel resection
Infiltrative disorders
Lymphoma
Scleroderma

Rehydration

Table 7–4 lists the electrolyte composition of several intravenous and oral solutions used to treat diarrhea.

Oral. Either the oral or intravenous route can accomplish rehydration in the emergency setting. The oral route is the preferred method because it avoids potential complications associated with intravenous cannulation. Furthermore, oral rehydration has been very successful in reducing mortality rates from diarrhea in developing countries. The fluid choice should be a carbohydrate-containing (glucose or cereal-based) solution to improve water absorption. The presence of an organic cotransport molecule such as glucose improves water and electrolyte absorption without increasing intraluminal osmolarity. Coupled transport of sodium and water across the intestinal membrane is linked to an organic molecule. This transport mechanism remains intact during enterotoxigenic illnesses. In the United States, there are several commercially available solutions, including Pedialyte, Lytren, and Rehydralyte. If the patient is capable of tolerating oral fluids, this is the preferred method for rehydration. Rice-based oral rehydration solutions have demonstrated effectiveness in reducing stool output in patients with cholera.

Intravenous. In patients with severe dehydration, shock, altered level of consciousness, or inability to tolerate oral fluids, intravenous rehydration is necessary. Isotonic crystalloid solution is utilized in these situations. Potassium chloride can be added to these crystalloid solutions, as necessary. Depending on the patient's degree of volume depletion, several liters of crystalloid may be necessary to restore adequate intravascular volume. In children, 20 mL/kg normal saline boluses should be provided for initial resuscitation. The patient's electrolyte status is monitored during intravenous rehydration, as necessary.

Symptomatic Therapy

Patients with diarrhea often request antimotility agents. These agents also may be requested if nausea and vomiting are present. Antimotility agents, such as loperamide (Imodium), may have some benefit in controlling severe symptoms. The concern of retaining infectious pathogens with these agents has been overstated. They can be used safely for 1 or 2 days and thereafter under the supervision of the primary physician. Opiate derivatives, diphenoxylate (Lomotil), or codeine-containing compounds are effective but should be reserved for more extreme cases. Careful

TABLE 7–3. Characteristics of Diarrhea Caused by Infectious Agents

Agent	Features
Invasive Agents	
Campylobacter jejuni	Fecal-oral spread, culture must be requested
	Occurs in wet, warm months
Shigella	Highly infectious
	Person-to-person spread
	>50 WBC/high-power field in stool
Salmonella	Common source of epidemic, easily isolated in culture
	Antibiotics used in those with septicemia or the immunocompromised or young. May present as fever (92%) with bradycardia (40%), headache (65%), confusion (20%)
Invasive *Escherichia coli*	Rare in United States
	Mimics *Shigella* infection
	Mimics appendicitis
Yersinia enterocolitica	Antibiotics can be used selectively in those with septicemia, immunocompromised status, or focal extraintestinal infection. May mimic appendicitis
	Common in Japan
Vibrio parahemolyticus	Shellfish contaminant
	Associated with antibiotic use
Clostridium difficile	Severe illness
	Workup may include sigmoidoscopy, cytotoxin assay
Toxin producers (Food poisoning)	
Staphylococcus	1–6 hr incubation period
	Self-limited, <24 hours
	Emesis predominant; culture food or vomitus
	Toxin in food is identified
Clostridium perfringens	6–24 hr incubation period
	Self-limited (24–48 hr)
	Incriminated food is cultured
Vibrio cholera	Occurs in Near, Middle, Far East
	Raw oysters
	Common in travelers
Toxigenic *E. coli*	Self-limited (1 week)
Bacillus cereus	Emetic (1–6 hours) and diarrheal (6–24 hours) forms
	Culture foods (fried rice) or stool
	Self-limited (12–24 hr)
Virus	
Rotavirus	Occurs in young children in winter months
	Lasts less than 5 days
Norwalk agent	Diagnose with Rotazyme
	Family outbreaks
	Lasts less than 36 hours
Parasites	
Giardia lamblia	2–3 wk incubation period
	Malabsorption, flatulence, abdominal cramping/bloating, prolonged symptoms
Entamoeba histolytica	Low-grade fever
	Bloody stool
	Up to 3-wk incubation period
Cryptosporidium	Immunocompromised status
	Special request needed for stain

monitoring is necessary when these medications are prescribed. Anticholinergic agents are not effective and can cause unpleasant side effects. Bismuth subsalicylate (Pepto-Bismol) promotes intestinal water and sodium reabsorption, inactivates enterotoxins, and has an antibacterial effect. This agent, as well as loperamide, is available over the counter but should be taken under the direction of a physician in cases of severe diarrhea. Antiemetics, such as promethazine (Phenergan) or prochlorperazine (Compazine), are effective and can be parenterally administered initially and then per rectum as necessary as diarrheal symptoms subside.

TABLE 7–4. Fluids Used to Treat Diarrhea

Intravenous Fluids for Maintenance After NS boluses

To: 1 liter of 5% dextrose and half normal saline (adult)
or
1 liter of 5% dextrose and 25% normal saline (child)
Add: 50 mEq $NaHCO_3$ (1 amp)
      and
      10 to 20 mEq KCl
This provides per liter:

	Adult	Child
Na (mEq)	125	87
Cl (mEq)	85–95	47–57
HCO_3 (mEq)	50	50
K (mEq)	10–20	10–20
Dextrose (gm)	50	50

Oral Fluids

	World Health Org. Soln.	Rehydralyte	Pedialyte RS	Lytren	Pedialyte	Infalyte	Gatorade
Na (mEq/L)	90	75	75	50	45	50	21
K (mEq/L)	20	20	20	25	20	20	2.5
Cl (mEq/L)	80	65	50	45	35	40	11
HCO_3 (mEq/L)	30	30	30	30	30	30	0
Sugar (g/L)	20	25	25	20	25	20	60

Prevention of Spread

Patients, families, and caregivers must be educated about the necessity of strict personal hygiene. Because infectious causes of diarrhea are spread by means of the fecal-oral route, proper hygiene can be immensely helpful in limiting the spread of infection. Public health officials should be notified of unanticipated (e.g., outside of flu season) outbreaks of diarrhea in the community. Children should be removed from school or day-care centers during their illness. Health care personnel with diarrhea should avoid close patient contact, and all physicians should wash their hands thoroughly between patient encounters. Finally, close contacts of infected individuals should be notified about their exposure.

Antibiotic Therapy

Most cases of acute diarrhea are self-limited and do not require antibiotic therapy. In some cases, antibiotics are initiated empirically. In general, antibiotics therapy can be considered in any patient with diarrhea who has fever, stool leukocytes, Hemoccult-positive stools, diarrhea duration of more than 3 days, or traveler's diarrhea. The fluoroquinolones are considered the drugs of choice and can shorten the duration of traveler's diarrhea. Because resistance is increasing in some areas, the role of fluoroquinolone therapy in acute diarrhea continues to evolve. A conservative approach is recommended. Other antibiotics can be used based on culture results or the physician's clinical suspicion (Table 7–5).

With the exception of giardiasis, antibiotics should be withheld in cases of suspected intestinal parasitic infection until laboratory confirmation is established. Patients who have had diarrhea for 2 weeks or longer, and in whom infection with *Giardia* is suspected, can be started on antimicrobial therapy. In patients with moderate illness or when antibiotics are not clearly indicated, a stool culture can assist the decision. At follow-up, if the patient is not improving and the culture is positive for a susceptible agent, antibiotics can be started at that time.

Probiotics, such as *Lactobacillus*, have demonstrated limited benefit in children presenting with post antibiotic diarrhea (most commonly amoxicillin).

Dietary Discretion

Although potentially obvious, it is important for the clinician to advise the adult patient of dietary

TABLE 7–5. Antibiotic Treatment of Choice for Bacteria or Parasite-Induced Diarrhea

Condition/Pathogen	Antibiotic Choice
Traveler's diarrhea	Fluoroquinolones (norfloxacin, ciprofloxacin)
	TMP-SMX, rifaximin
Cholera	Tetracycline
	Furazolidone, fluoroquinolones
Shigellosis	Ciprofloxacin, ampicillin
	TMP-SMX, ceftriaxone
Campylobacter jejuni	Erythromycin
	Ciprofloxacin
Salmonellosis (invasive)	Ciprofloxacin, ampicillin
	TMP-SMX
Typhoid fever	TMP-SMX
	Ampicillin
	Chloramphenicol
	Ciprofloxacin
Aeromonas, Plesiomonas	TMP-SMX
Yersinia enterocolitica	TMP-SMX
Clostridium difficile	Metronidazole or vancomycin (oral)
Entamoeba histolytica	
Asymptomatic	Diiodohydroxyquinoline or paromomycin
Diarrhea	Metronidazole plus diiodohydroxyquinoline
Giardia lamblia	Metronidazole
	Mepacrine
	Furazolidone (children)
Cryptosporidium	Spiramycin
	Paromomycin (only in severe diarrhea or the immunocompromised)
Microsporum, Cyclospora	No antibiotic
Isospora	TMP-SMX (in AIDS patients)

TMP-SMX, trimethoprim-sulfamethoxazole.

discretion during the first few days of acute diarrhea. A graduated diet moving from clear to full liquids, then including solids, can decrease cramping and stool frequencies.

UNCERTAIN DIAGNOSIS

An uncertain diagnosis is common after assessment in the emergency department. Rehydration, symptomatic relief, and evaluating for acute serious underlying causes are the responsibility of the emergency physician. Additionally, arranging appropriate follow-up and clear instructions for care are the best means by which the uncertain causes of diarrhea are addressed.

SPECIAL CONSIDERATIONS

When discussing acute diarrhea, there are three population groups that deserve special mention: the pediatric population, the elderly, and the immunosuppressed. Among these three groups, the possible causes of acute diarrhea are diverse and the management strategy for each is often intensive.

Pediatric Patients

The management of children with acute diarrhea has undergone substantial changes in recent years. Although pediatric mortality from diarrhea in the United States is lower than in most other regions of the world, diarrhea still has a significant impact on pediatric morbidity and hospitalization. More than 200,000 children up to age 5 years are hospitalized annually for diarrheal illnesses in the United States. The optimal management of pediatric patients with acute diarrhea includes the following:

Rehydration. An appropriate oral solution for rapid rehydration and maintenance of hydration is used. Glucose-based and cereal-based solutions optimize intestinal water absorption. Cereal-based solutions offer the added benefit of reduced diarrhea volume and duration. Although there are currently no commercially available cereal-based solutions, the World Health Organization has developed a glucose-based oral rehydration solution that has been found to be safe and effective in children with diarrhea of all causes. Children with severe dehydration or shock should receive intravenous fluids (isotonic crystalloid) followed by oral rehydration therapy.

Refeeding. The traditional approach of feeding children a clear liquid diet and gradually returning to a normal diet has been shown to have a negative impact on nutritional status and prolong the course of diarrhea. Early administration of a mixed diet, particularly one rich in carbohydrates, may reduce diarrhea duration and severity. Furthermore, breast feeding should be encouraged to continue because it, too, may reduce diarrhea duration and severity. During the early refeeding process, children should be observed for evidence of lactose intolerance. If such symptoms appear, then dietary changes can be made.

Antibiotics. Antimicrobial therapy can be instituted in patients with identified (or strongly suspected) bacterial or parasitic pathogens. The patient's age should be considered when choosing antimicrobial agents, and age restrictions or limitations should be observed.

Elderly Patients

The evaluation of acute diarrhea can be difficult in the elderly population. Historical details are sometimes less forthcoming, and physical examination findings can be deceiving. For example, elderly patients who live alone or have no primary caregiver may have difficulty recounting the development of their symptoms. Associated symptoms and prior medical history may also be challenging to discern. The physical examination may be difficult to interpret owing to altered mental states (e.g., dementia), comorbid illnesses, or decreased perception of pain. Furthermore, the elderly population, in general, is at risk for several serious causes of acute diarrhea, including partial bowel obstruction, ischemic bowel, diverticulitis, and neoplasms. Generally, older persons have a higher rate of diseases that require surgical treatment.

As a consequence of the impaired clinical assessment and possibility of significant illness, laboratory tests, radiologic evaluation, surgical consultation, and hospital admission are more common in this age-group than in their younger cohorts. The elderly can also have a reduced ability to tolerate dehydration and an inability to care for themselves through outpatient management.

Immunosuppressed Patients

Acute diarrhea is a common symptom in the AIDS population and causes significant morbidity and mortality. Among patients with AIDS it is a more common symptom in homosexual males (80%) than heterosexual men with intravenous drug abuse history (60%). In some instances, the onset of diarrhea may be the first symptom of the patient's undiagnosed human immunodeficiency virus infection. Not only are AIDS patients susceptible to the same enteric pathogens that immunocompetent patients acquire, but a host of opportunistic pathogens may induce diarrhea as well. These include viral, bacterial, fungal, and protozoal agents such as cytomegalovirus, *Cryptosporidium* species, *Mycobacterium avium-intracellulare*, and *Isospora belli*. In addition to infectious causes, AIDS patients can have diarrhea caused by medications, worsening lactose intolerance with disease progression, and malabsorption disorders. The diarrhea may be associated with nausea, vomiting, abdominal pain, and hematochezia.

A more aggressive diagnostic workup is pursued in AIDS patients because an identifiable etiology frequently can be found. It is important to obtain a stool culture in these patients and start with empirical antibiotic therapy (usually a fluoroquinolone). The nonopportunistic bacterial, viral, and parasitic infections are considered first, followed by the opportunistic infectious agents just mentioned. The stool should be tested for the presence of *Clostridium difficile* toxin.

Patients with immunosuppression for other reasons (e.g., chemotherapy, transplant recipients) are managed in similar fashion. The principles of rehydration, maintenance of hydration, and close follow-up apply to all immunosuppressed populations.

Patients with Traveler's Diarrhea

Up to 60% of travelers in developing nations have diarrhea. Enterotoxigenic *Escherichia coli*, *Campylobacter, Shigella,* and *Salmonella* account for the majority of bacterial pathogens. Symptoms last 4 days on average. Standard avoidance procedures are helpful in preventing diarrhea, and prophylaxis is generally not necessary. Mild to moderately severe cases may be treated with an antispasmodic and an antibiotic as necessary. Fluoroquinolones are generally selected, but resistance to these agents has been increasing. Children and pregnant women may consider azithromycin. In severe cases, with associated blood or mucus, early antibiotics, aggressive hydration, and proper medical care are essential. Rifaximine, a nonabsorbed antimicrobial, has demonstrated good tolerance and a decrease in the number of unformed stools in the first 24 hours of treatment. It is another new agent with potential benefit in the battle against the increasing resistance of enteropathogens.

DISPOSITION AND FOLLOW-UP

Consultation

A surgical consultation is occasionally warranted. Patients with acute diarrhea caused by diseases that will require surgical treatment usually have associated abdominal pain, abdominal distention, rebound, or guarding. No patient is discharged in which a diagnosis of a disease that may mandate surgery is entertained until a surgical consultation is obtained, especially at the extremes of age.

If the patient has immunosuppression, it is useful to consult an infectious disease specialist for recommendations regarding antibiotic coverage, follow-up, and further diagnostic testing.

Observation

A period of observation in the emergency department can be vital to determining patient disposition. During this time, the emergency physician should pay particular attention to the patient's ability to tolerate oral fluids, frequency of diarrhea, and resolution of associated symptoms. The observation period often requires several hours and repeated examinations.

Admission

The emergency physician should consider admitting the following patients for inpatient care:

1. Patients with severe dehydration or shock not responsive to intravenous rehydration
2. Very young or very old patients with severe illness
3. Patients in whom the possibility of disease requiring surgery cannot be reasonably eliminated
4. Patients whose symptoms do not respond to emergency department interventions
5. Patients with severe, underlying comorbid illnesses

The benefits of hospitalization for patients with acute diarrhea include the following:

1. Intravenous rehydration with ongoing monitoring of electrolytes
2. Further investigation regarding etiology of diarrhea
3. Management of complications from severe dehydration, shock, and comorbid illnesses
4. Education of patient, family, or caregivers

Discharge and Follow-up

Patients may be candidates for outpatient management in the following circumstances:

1. The patient is hemodynamically stable without evidence of orthostasis or oliguria.
2. The patient is tolerating oral rehydration (without nausea or vomiting) and has an oral intake that exceeds gastrointestinal losses.
3. No evidence of severe electrolyte abnormality exists.
4. There is reasonable exclusion of underlying disease that requires surgery as the cause of diarrhea.
5. The patient has arrangement for outpatient follow-up in 24 to 48 hours as deemed necessary by the emergency physician.

Emergency physicians should provide clear, detailed recommendations regarding appropriate care as an outpatient and instructions that describe when to seek medical reevaluation. Patients to be managed as outpatients should understand the following key points:

1. It is important to continue oral hydration at home for at least 24 hours.
2. All medications (antibiotics, antiemetics, and antimotility agents) should be taken only as directed.
3. The patient should return for reevaluation if abdominal pain or severe vomiting occurs.
4. Follow-up with their primary physician should be as scheduled, or planned, if no improvement is noted beyond 48 hours.
5. Patients whose condition has not improved can be managed as follows: if a stool culture has been performed and the patient has been discharged without antibiotics, the patient can be started on antibiotics if a bacterial source is identified.
6. Strict hygiene should be maintained and close contacts who may have been exposed to a pathogen should be notified.
7. Parents of children should understand the importance of early refeeding. Dietary discretion is directed toward adults.

FINAL POINTS

- An immediate assessment of the hemodynamic stability of all patients with acute diarrhea is required. It is assumed that significant dehydration has occurred, even in patients with adequate vital signs.
- Abdominal and rectal examinations are part of the evaluation of the patient with acute diarrhea.

- Diarrhea due to invasive pathogens (dysentery) is associated with fever, bloody or mucus-laden stools, abdominal cramping, and fecal leukocytes.
- Early refeeding of children with acute diarrhea is not only safe but also improves nutritional status when compared with the "clear liquid diet" only.
- The specific cause of diarrhea is usually not found during the emergency department assessment. Management is directed primarily toward rehydration and symptomatic relief.
- Breast feeding should continue through the course of a diarrheal illness.

- Patients with acute diarrhea should be evaluated for possible causes of their illness that involve disease that may require surgical treatment.
- Antimicrobial therapy should be considered in patients with diarrhea with fever, bloody stools, or fecal leukocytes.
- Stool cultures should be obtained only in those patients suspected of having diarrhea caused by invasive pathogens.
- Chronic illnesses may present as acute diarrhea.

CASE*Study*

A 22-year-old woman with a 2-day history of diarrhea and abdominal pain had severe lower abdominal cramping and progressive weakness. On arrival at the emergency department, the patient appeared acutely ill. She was placed directly in a monitored bed, and her history was confirmed. Vital signs included blood pressure of 110/50 mm Hg, heart rate of 100 beats per minute, respiratory rate of 16 breaths per minute, and temperature of 101.6°F (39°C). The nurse attempted orthostatic blood pressure and pulse readings, but after a few moments of standing the patient became dizzy and weak. The pulse rate rose to 130 beats per minute, and the systolic pressure fell to 90 mm Hg. The nurse placed a large-bore intravenous line and began an infusion with normal saline. The emergency physician was called to the bedside.

Initial recognition of sick and potentially unstable patients as they come to the emergency department is a critical skill and function of the nursing staff. Most emergency departments have triage protocols and criteria designed to identify these patients and initiate appropriate rapid evaluation and stabilization. Obtaining orthostatic vital signs in this patient has some risk. Results may be equivocal, and she already was manifesting signs of hypovolemia. If the decision is made to do orthostatics in this type of patient, starting from a sitting position with the legs dangling may give the same result with less risk.

The patient had been at a barbecue 2 days before becoming sick. She had eaten chicken that appeared slightly pink in the center. She also ate potato salad and baked beans. The diarrhea was loose and watery but did not

appear bloody to the patient. The patient was otherwise healthy and had never been to an emergency department before. On physical examination, the mucous membranes were slightly dry. Heart and lung examinations were unremarkable. Her abdomen was diffusely, but mildly, tender. Bowel sounds were present, and there were no signs of peritoneal irritation. A rectal examination was positive for occult blood, Therefore, a stool specimen was sent for fecal leukocytes and culture.

The key finding in the history is that the food she had eaten might not have been fully cooked. Poultry is notorious for carrying non-typhoid Salmonella species. The presence of occult blood indicates that the offending organism is invasive. A key finding is that the abdomen is only mildly and diffusely tender. Even in cases of obvious infectious diarrhea, the physician needs to maintain a healthy suspicion of abdominal disease that will require surgical treatment. This potential of invasive bacteria prompts the ordering of the stool test for fecal leukocytes and culture. Without blood in the stool, these tests are generally not requested.

After the rapid infusion of 2 L of normal saline, vital signs were repeated. The resting pulse was 90 beats per minute, and the supine blood pressure was 120/70 mm Hg. The patient said she felt better but still very weak. Urinary output had not yet begun. A third liter of saline was hung, and a rapid infusion rate was maintained.

In a young, healthy patient, with normal cardiovascular function, aggressive rehydration is well tolerated. Because the patient has ceased vomiting,

Continued on following page

there is no need for antiemetics. Keeping the patient comfortable during fluid infusion is all that is required. The patient can be relied on to void and does not require an indwelling urinary catheter.

The stool specimen was positive for fecal leukocytes. After 4 L of fluid, the patient no longer had orthostatic changes and felt much better. The abdominal cramping was lessened as well. The patient was given clear fluids to drink and tolerated them well. At this point, the patient was ready for discharge. The patient was instructed to continue clear fluids for 24 hours and then try light solids such as toast. An appointment was arranged to follow up with her primary physician in 48 hours. No antibiotics were prescribed.

The finding of fecal leukocytes confirms an invasive organism as the cause of the diarrhea. Several clues point to a Salmonella species.

The poultry exposure is the most compelling clue. This case has features of invasiveness (occult blood and fecal leukocytes) as well as toxin exposure (watery diarrhea). Salmonella can be both invasive as well as produce enterotoxins. Because this patient had improved in the emergency department, antibiotics were not prescribed. Most cases of bacterial diarrhea will resolve with conservative measures.

At her follow-up appointment with her primary physician, the patient reported a marked reduction in diarrheal stools and cramping. She was able to eat soup and other light foods. The stool culture confirmed a nontyphoid *Salmonella* organism. Because the patient was doing well, no antibiotics were indicated and the patient was advised to gradually increase her diet as tolerated. She was advised not to return to work until her symptoms ceased and her stools returned to normal.

Bibliography

JOURNAL ARTICLES

Cook GC: Diarrhoeal disease: a world-wide problem. Journal of the Royal Society of Medicine 1998; 91:192–194.

Diskin A, Khan A: Gastroenteritis. emedicine: Emergency Medicine (Internet text).

Dupont HL: Guidelines on acute infectious diarrhea in adults. Am J Gastroenterol 1997; 92(11):1962–1975.

Framm SR, Soave R: Agents of diarrhea. Medical Clinics of North America 1997; 81(2):427–443.

Hogan DE: The emergency department approach to diarrhea. Emerg Med Clin North Am 1996; 14(4):673–694.

Mathan VI: Diarrhoeal diseases. British Medical Bulletin 1998; 54(2):407–419.

McNeely WS, Dupont HL, et al: Occult blood versus fecal leukocytes in the diagnosis of bacterial diarrhea: A study of U.S. travelers to Mexico and Mexican children. Am J Trop Med Hyg 1996; 55:430–433.

Meyers A: Modern management of acute diarrhea and dehydration in children. Am Fam Physician 1995; 51(5): 1103–1115.

Plevris JN, Hayes PC: Investigation and management of acute diarrhoea. British Journal of Hospital Medicine 1996; 56(11):569–573.

Reisdorff EJ, Pflug VJ: Infectious Diarrhea: Beyond Supportive Care. EM Reports 1996; 17(14):141–150.

Ryan ET, Kain KC: Health Advice and Immunizations for Travelers. NEJM 2000; 342:1716–1724.

Sabol VK, Friedenberg FK: Diarrhea. AACN Clinical Issues 1997; 8(3):425–436.

Sullivan PB: Nutritional management of acute diarrhea. Nutrition 1998; 14(10): 758–762.

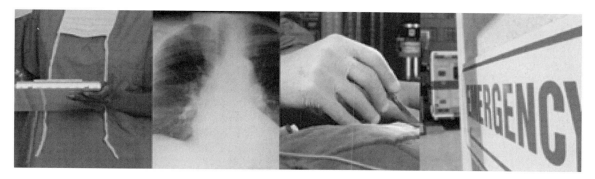

CARDIOVASCULAR DISORDERS

CHAPTER 8

Chest Pain

GLENN C. HAMILTON
SHARON MALONE
TIMOTHY G. JANZ

CASE *Study*

The rescue squad brought a 73-year-old woman to the emergency department. She complained of lower chest and epigastric discomfort persisting for 12 hours. The discomfort was described as "indigestion." She noted slight nausea and increased belching since it began.

INTRODUCTION

Discomfort in the chest is derived from many separate anatomic structures. It is described not only as pain but also "pressure," "burning," "ache," or "choking." Many thoracic structures are innervated by sensory fibers from the spinal cord segments C2 to T5 and the tenth (X) cranial nerve. All may be involved in the sensation of "pain in the chest." This broad innervation accounts for the referral of pain from intrathoracic structures to the jaw, arm, shoulder, or back. Superficial pain is easier to localize than visceral pain. The origin of visceral pain correlates poorly with the site where it is perceived.

Myocardial ischemia exists when impaired coronary flow causes an inadequate oxygen supply to meet the requirements of the myocardium. Ischemia is influenced by each element: coronary flow, oxygen supply, and tissue demand. It is the central problem in angina, unstable angina, and myocardial infarction (MI).

Although its incidence is declining, American men have a 20% chance of manifesting coronary artery disease (CAD) in their lifetime. It causes chest pain and other symptoms in more than 10 million persons in the United States. The incidence of CAD is increasing in women and is the leading cause of death in women in the United States. Cardiovascular disease has the dual hazard of being both common and potentially catastrophic. CAD accounts for over 500,000 deaths per year in the United States. Still, over the past 30 years overall mortality has decreased 40%.

Chest pain constitutes 5% to 6% of chief complaints in the emergency department. Of the 6 million patients assessed for acute chest pain, almost 900,000 develop an acute MI. Ischemic heart disease (IHD) accounts for 10% to 30% of all undifferentiated chest pain cases presenting to the emergency department. Therefore, despite other diagnostic concerns, determining the potential for the cardiovascular origin of acute chest pain is a primary goal. Three to 5 percent of patients with acute MI are discharged undiagnosed from the emergency department. Most of these are younger patients (<50 years) with atypical presenting complaints. Missed acute MI represents more than 20% of all emergency medical malpractice settlements. Still, the cost of care for those patients unnecessarily admitted for cardiac care exceeds $3 billion annually.

Defining the cause of acute chest pain is difficult for the following reasons:

- The patient's ability to describe the symptoms can greatly influence the outcome of the evaluation.
- The patient's presentation style may alter the physician's approach.
- The severity of the pain correlates poorly with its life-threatening potential.
- There is little correlation between the location of the pain and its source.
- More than one disease process may cause the pain.
- Because of the broad innervation, a number of different pathologic processes in a variety of organs may present in a similar manner.
- The situation is dynamic. *At any time in the evaluative process, the patient may require rapid therapeutic intervention for increased pain, dysrhythmia, shock, or cardiac arrest.*

In many cases, an extensive evaluation is the only means of making a correct diagnosis. Yet in caring for a patient with chest pain, the emergency physician must differentiate rapidly between potentially catastrophic disease and benign illness, determine the probability of IHD, anticipate management, and proceed to disposition. The data-gathering and observation skills necessary to diagnose and manage chest pain correctly are developed by serial exposure and close follow-up of these patients.

INITIAL APPROACH AND STABILIZATION

With few exceptions, such as superficial chest wall pain caused by injury, *all* patients with chest pain are brought immediately into the acute care area of the emergency department and are seen by a physician. The physician must anticipate the need to manage the airway, correct dysrhythmias, stabilize hypotension, and provide pain relief at any time.

Priority Diagnoses

The priority diagnoses represent the six catastrophic causes of acute chest pain:

1. Acute myocardial infarction
2. Unstable angina
3. Thoracic aortic aneurysm with dissection
4. Pulmonary embolism
5. Tension pneumothorax
6. Esophageal rupture

Rapid Assessment

The initial assessment and stabilization includes the following information:

1. What is the location, severity, character, radiation, and duration of the pain? What causes and relieves it? Is there a relationship with activity such as exercise, cold, and sexual activity? Is drug use implicated in the pain?
2. Are there associated symptoms, such as diaphoresis or shortness of breath?
3. What is the medical history? Is there a known history of coronary artery disease, hypertension, or diabetes mellitus?
4. Vital signs are taken and compared with values from the prehospital setting.
5. The patient is undressed. A rapid physical assessment is done. Attention is directed to the level of consciousness, pain tolerance, skin color, and auscultation of heart and lungs. Any cardiac murmurs or pulmonary rales are noted, which may suggest left ventricular insufficiency and a cardiac inability to tolerate aggressive volume repletion.
6. A 12-lead electrocardiogram (ECG) is often appropriate at this juncture. With the advent of myocardial salvage therapies, the appearance of "classic" MI changes on the ECG significantly directs the management plan in the emergency department.

Early Intervention

1. Cardiac monitoring is established and a rhythm strip is recorded. Supplemental oxygen is given, and an intravenous line is placed or the established access is checked.
2. Pain may be often relieved with oxygen and reassurance. Sublingual nitroglycerin (NTG, tablet or aerosol, 0.3 or 0.4 mg q5 to 15 minutes × 3) may be given for relief, if IHD is seriously considered. Optimally, before NTG administration, an intravenous line is established and blood pressure is measured. Caution is exercised and hypotension anticipated if the systolic blood pressure is less than 110 mm Hg. Repeat blood pressure readings are taken 2 to 3 minutes after the NTG dose. Stronger analgesics, such as nalbuphine (Nubain) or morphine sulfate, may be necessary to control pain early in the course of care.
3. Aspirin is given to any patient without a known bleeding disorder who has suspected unstable angina or an acute MI.

The clinical appearance of the patient may require more definitive treatment to supersede or proceed concomitantly with the preliminary assessment. The clinical "sixth sense" of the experienced emergency nurse and physician is useful in assessing the severity of illness of each patient.

CLINICAL ASSESSMENT

History

A careful history is the most important factor in the assessment of the patient with acute chest pain. It is of particular value in identifying patients who are at high risk for potentially catastrophic illness.

The physician must appreciate the psychologic impact the pain, emergency setting, and interview have on the patient. When confronted by a complex or confusing history, calm reassurance and directing the history to a chronologic sequencing of the event will provide a structure for the patient's recollection. The history is guided but not led. Key historical points include the following:

Characteristics of the Pain

Character or Quality of Pain. The patient is asked to describe the "discomfort" rather than the "pain." Patients may deny "pain" but admit to a "squeezing" or "choking" feeling. The words "heaviness," "pressure," or "crushing" may describe the sensation. "Burning" pain is problematic because it has the same frequency of association with MI as with upper gastrointestinal disorders. The symptoms are first assumed to be cardiac in origin. Other descriptive terms less typical of cardiac pain are "stabbing" and "sharp." These words are often used to describe the severity of pain rather than the character. The meaning of each word must be mutually understood.

Onset. Circumstances and pattern of onset are important. Were there any episodes of discomfort before this episode? Was it related to exercise, sexual activity, stress, or did it occur after a meal?

Severity. Severity may be measured against the "worst pain" the patient has previously experienced. A 1 to 10 pain severity scale may help the patient be more precise. Although severity of pain does not always relate to life-threatening potential, it remains important among factors that suggest IHD.

Site and Radiation. The patient is asked whether the pain is centrally or laterally located in the thorax. Whether it "goes anywhere else" is important to ascertain, but prompting the patient with a list of possible referral sites is avoided. The clinical pattern of chest pain radiation increases the probability of MI. Radiation into both arms increases the likelihood seven times, right shoulder three times, and left shoulder two times, as opposed to patients without radiation. Pain localized with one finger is usually not angina pectoris.

Duration and Pattern of Pain. The total time of the episode, the length of individual episodes of discomfort, and the varying degree of symptoms are details of importance. Recent change in any of these symptoms is important to ascertain. Angina pectoris usually lasts 2 to 5 minutes and is relieved with rest. Unstable angina may last 10 minutes or more and can occur at rest.

Factors That Relieve or Worsen the Pain. The influence of time of day, meals, exercise, with smoking or in heavy traffic (carbon monoxide), emotional stress, cold exposure, reaching or stretching, deep inspiration, and cough on increasing or decreasing the pain can help to differentiate superficial from visceral pain and ischemic cardiac pain from pain of other origins. The search is for predictable relationships with circumstances that increase myocardial oxygen demand or decrease the supply. Pleuritic and positional pain are less indicative of IHD. Response to therapy can give useful information about the source of pain, the patient's perception of pain, and the patient's medical sophistication.

Previous History of Pain. How does this pain compare to previous episodes or a prior documented MI or angina? Pain that is similar to previous pain associated with IHD is *very* suggestive of cardiac origin. However, pain that is different from previous episodes does not exclude IHD.

Associated Symptoms. Other symptoms may suggest a visceral origin for the pain.

1. *Diaphoresis.* "Sweating" is an important symptom that is often associated with a serious pathologic process. It must be differentiated from the sensation of being "warm" or "flushed."
2. *Dyspnea.* "Shortness of breath" is the subjective sensation of working harder to breathe associated with decreased lung compliance. It must be differentiated from hyperventilation and anxiety.
3. *Dizziness or syncope.* "Dizziness" is the term used for symptoms ranging from "lightheadedness" to true vertigo. Syncope, a true loss of consciousness with or without chest pain, requires patient admission for evaluation.
4. *Nausea, vomiting, belching.* All these symptoms can be nonspecific responses to deep pain. Belching is further explored in context of the pain episode and response to therapy. It has a unique association with inferior myocardial ischemia or infarction.

Risk Factors

Identifying risk factors has not been found to increase the diagnostic accuracy of chest pain assessment. They do influence the physician's judgment of the probability of IHD. Factors that correlate with IHD include the following:

1. **Age.** The incidence of coronary artery disease in the general population increases with each decade: 30 to 39 years (8%), 40 to 49 years (24%), 50 to 59 years (44%), and 60 to 69 years (56%).
2. **Male sex.** Risk is increased in men, particularly in the younger age groups. Postmenopausal females without hormone replacement therapy have the same risk level as males.
3. **Hypertension.** This is especially a risk in elderly patients with moderate to severe levels of hypertension or with target organ damage. Hypertension is also a risk factor for dissecting aneurysm.
4. **Diabetes mellitus.** The risk for CAD is two times control in diabetic men and three times control in diabetic women.
5. **Cigarette smoking.** Only 2 pack-years or more are required to be a risk factor. This is a significant risk factor at *three times controls or more*, depending on the number of pack-years.
6. **Known history of arteriosclerotic vascular disease.**

7. **Lipids.** Increased total serum cholesterol or increased low-density lipoprotein cholesterol is a risk factor.
8. **Family history of IHD.** Has IHD occurred in female family members younger than 65 years or in males younger than 55 years?
9. **Oral contraceptives in women older than 35 years.** This is especially true if higher estrogen doses were taken.

Other factors less well correlated with IHD but supportive of suspicion include

1. Sedentary versus active lifestyle
2. Stress level
3. Obesity
4. Type A personality
5. Gout

Past Medical History

1. **Known history of CAD, IHD, or acute MI.** Almost 50% of patients without previous angina will develop it within 1 year after MI.
2. **Surgical/trauma history.** The physician should explore the details of any surgery and inquire about previous chest or neck trauma.
3. **Medications.** Information about medications—what, why, how faithfully taken, and perceived side effects—offers insight into the patient's understanding of illness and compliance with treatment.
4. **Allergies**, especially to medications, are always important to determine.

Two actions are automatic to maximize efficiency early during care. First, the patient's old chart is ordered. The chart can clarify a confusing history, supply a comparison ECG, list a complex and poorly recalled medical regimen, and reveal a supporting or an unconsidered prior diagnosis (e.g., drug-seeking behavior). Second, supplemental corroborating information is sought by talking with family, friends, and the patient's private physician. These data also assist in assessing the patient's living circumstances and support systems.

Physical Examination

The physical examination may complement the history but is not often a deciding factor in the diagnosis of acute chest pain. It can supply important information when guided by a few principles:

1. The history directs the emphasis of the examination.
2. The *vital signs* and *general appearance* are the most important determinants in separating deep visceral from superficial pain. How the patient is tolerating the pathophysiologic process may be reflected in vital signs.
3. The examination should seek evidence supporting the presence of atherosclerotic vascular disease.
4. Evidence of myocardial ischemia is most often found when the pain is present. Changes include diastolic blood pressure elevation, S_3 or S_4, and papillary muscle dysfunction murmur (mitral insufficiency).
5. Specific evidence of catastrophic illness is sought first, such as unequal pulses (aortic dissection) or hyperresonance on chest percussion (pneumothorax); then the examiner moves on to more subtle findings or less serious diagnoses.

The important components of the physical examination are listed in Table 8–1.

Bedside Tests

Bedside tests have limited benefit differentiating the site of chest pain. *None is diagnostic*, but each may direct attention toward an organ system.

1. **Pulmonary system.** Intentional hyperventilation for 1 to 3 minutes may reproduce psychogenic central pain or consistently aggravate pleuritic pain.
2. **Gastrointestinal system.** Antacids may be used, and if pain is relieved, may suggest an esophageal origin of the pain. The "GI cocktail" (Mylanta, 30 mL, and viscous lidocaine [Xylocaine], 10 mL, with or without Donnatal, 10 mL) is a test for which sensitivity and specificity are unknown. The use of this test is avoided as long as a cardiac origin is considered.
3. **Cardiac system.** When the history is suggestive but not convincing for angina pectoris, a trial of NTG resulting in the complete relief of pain in less than 3 minutes increases the probability of IHD. This test is not diagnostic of any disease. It produces false-positive results in 20% of patients, presumably owing to placebo effect or esophageal relaxation.

CLINICAL REASONING

Simultaneously with the initial stabilization of the patient and data gathering, the physician develops decision priorities and forms a preliminary differential diagnosis by answering several questions.

TABLE 8–1. Important Components of the Physical Examination in Acute Chest Pain

Area of Examination	Important Components	Comments
Vital signs	Heart rate/pulse	Tachycardia (>95 beats/per minute) is common, vagal response to visceral pain may result in bradycardia (<60 beats/per minute). Assess symmetry and quality of pulses.
	Blood pressure	Often elevated secondary to increased sympathetic tone. Hypotension is always a serious sign.
	Respiratory rate	Tachypnea is one of the earliest signs of shock and is a common response to pain.
	Fever	Suggests infectious or inflammatory process
General appearance	Position, movement, color, diaphoresis	Rough gauge of "distress," although interpretation is complicated by patient pain tolerance or denial
Eyes	External—xanthelasma	All indications of atherosclerotic status
	Iris—arcus senilis	
	Fundus—arteriovenous nicking and thickening of capillary wall ("copper wiring")	
Neck	Inspection, palpation, auscultation	Check position of trachea and jugular venous distention. Palpate the carotid pulse for rate and quality. Crepitant subcutaneous emphysema may be noted. Auscultate for bruits and for referred aortic stenosis murmur.
Chest wall	Palpation	Superficial, reproducible and localized pain is one of the few findings helpful in ruling out visceral disease. Still, up to 5% of patients with documented myocardial infarction have this finding. Subcutaneous emphysema may be noted.
Lungs	Percussion	Particularly useful in pulmonary effusion and pneumothorax
	Auscultation	Listen for signs of consolidation, rales, wheezes
Cardiac	Palpation	Feel for size and lateral shift of apex, which suggests higher return. Paradoxical S_2 can be present as a result of left ventricular hypertrophy. Rocking motion at left sternal margin may be due to akinetic myocardium.
		Examination while pain is present yields a higher return. Paradoxical S_2 can be present as a result of transient left ventricular dysfunction during ischemia. Listen for S_3 and S_4 heart sounds and mitral insufficiency murmur due to papillary muscle dysfunction. Pericardial rubs heard best with the patient sitting up and leaning forward
Abdomen	Auscultation	Rectal and pelvic examinations are not deferred if history suggests origin of pain related to these areas.
Extremities	Inspection, auscultation, percussion, palpation	Ask patient to reach or stretch and observe pain response to motion. Note edema, signs of circulatory insufficiency, or thrombophlebitis
Neurologic	Altered sensation, motor function	Assess the cervical spine and dermatomes that radiate to the chest (C2 to T5).

Which Pattern (Location/Character) Does the Patient's Complaint Best Fit: Central, Lateral Pleuritic, Lateral Nonpleuritic?

Categorizing the patient complaint in this way quickly divides the diagnostic pursuit into high probability (central) and lower probability (lateral) locations for acute visceral pathology. This scheme is not without potential sources of error; for example, both pneumothorax and pulmonary embolism may present as lateral or lateral pleuritic pain. It is useful as a *beginning* and can be modified as experience with the patient and in the practice of emergency medicine develops.

If the Pattern is Central, Is There a Potentially Catastrophic Disease Requiring Immediate Intervention?

Unless the pain is obviously superficial and totally reproducible by palpation, the historical features of the pain or discomfort and the physical examination must be compared with the typical and atypical presentations of six immediately life-threatening diseases (Table 8–2): *MI, unstable angina, aortic dissection, pulmonary embolism, tension pneumothorax, and esophageal rupture.* Any patient *presenting in shock with chest pain* has one of these six emergent problems until proved otherwise.

Is an Acute Coronary Syndrome (ACS) Present?

Acute coronary syndrome includes acute MI and unstable angina. Acute MI is often subdivided on the presence or absence of ST segment elevation on the electrocardiogram. This distinction is important because it potentially alters the emergent treatment of acute coronary syndrome. Classification of acute coronary syndrome is often based on history, physical examination, findings on the ECG, and cardiac enzyme determination (Table 8–3).

If Catastrophic Disease Is not Present, Is There a Continued Risk of Acute Coronary Syndrome?

ACS is common, often subtle, dynamic, possibly lethal, and generally treatable. To determine its presence, the physician reviews the history. Several algorithms for chest pain have been published, and each adds a weighted value to the elements of the history. Although none has demonstrated superiority over the others, these algorithms may be beneficial for the new clinician. An example is given in Figure 8–1.

If the Risk of Acute Coronary Syndrome Is Low, What Other Possibilities for the Symptoms Are Logical?

If the discomfort is central but does not appear to be catastrophic or ischemic, the organ system approach outlined in the section on "Expanded Differential Diagnosis" is followed. The possibility of serious illness is continually reviewed in the patient with acute central chest pain or discomfort.

If the pain is of the lateral pleuritic pattern, it usually originates from the pleura or elements of the chest wall. The most important concerns at this time are whether pulmonary embolism or pneumothorax is present and whether the patient data are correlated with the information given in Table 8–2. If the risk of embolism is high (e.g., in pregnant patients or those with recent surgery or distal thrombophlebitis) or if the physical examination raises suspicion, the assessment proceeds with arterial blood gas analysis, D-dimer testing, chest radiography, spiral CT and/or a ventilation-perfusion lung scan. Pneumothorax is considered next. It is confirmed by radiography unless circumstances warrant immediate intervention. Other diagnoses such as infection, rib fracture, muscle injury, or muscle spasm are considered after embolism and pneumothorax are ruled out.

Lateral nonpleuritic pain as an isolated symptom is usually not life threatening. It commonly represents pain of musculoskeletal, neurologic, or psychogenic origin. Its evaluation becomes part of the organ system approach described in "Expanded Differential Diagnosis."

DIAGNOSTIC ADJUNCTS

Electrocardiogram

A 12-lead ECG is performed on most adult patients presenting with acute chest pain. Patients with lateral pleuritic or lateral nonpleuritic pain often do not need an ECG. Many patients with known CAD have a normal resting ECG. The test remains popular among physicians and patients; and, despite its limitations, it is a cost-effective and predictive tool in assessing chest pain. Its critical role remains as the most commonly used test to decide on reperfusion therapy in acute coronary syndrome. The ECG changes in three types of ACS are listed in Table 8–4. If the results are positive, the probability of ischemia in patients with equivocal histories is increased. In patients

TABLE 8–2. Causes and Differentiation of Potentially Catastrophic Illness Presenting with Central Chest Pain or Discomfort

	Pain History	Associated Symptoms	Supporting History	Prevalence in Emergency Department	Physical Examination	Useful Tests	Atypical or Additional Aspects
Myocardial infarction	Discomfort is usually moderately severe to severe and rapid in onset. May be more "pressure" than pain. Usually retrosternal, may radiate to neck, jaw, both arms, and sides of chest (left more than right). Lasts more than 15–30 min and is unrelieved by nitroglycerin	Diaphoresis, nausea, vomiting, dyspnea	May be precipitated by emotional stress or exertion. Prodromal pain pattern often elicited. Previous history of MI or angina. Over 40 years old, positive risk factors, and male sex increase possibility.	Common	Patients are anxious, restless, uncomfortable, and may be confused. Blood pressure is usually elevated but normotension and hypotension are seen. The heart rate is usually increased, but bradycardia can be noted. Patients may be diaphoretic and show peripheral poor perfusion. There are no diagnostic examination findings for MI although S_3 and S_4 heart sounds and mitral regurgitant murmur are supportive.	ECG changes (new Q waves or ST segment T wave changes) occur in 80% of patients. Use of cardiac enzymes (CPK-MB, troponin) in selected populations (e.g., elderly, patients presenting late in course) has demonstrated benefit.	Pain may present as "indigestion" or "unable to describe." Other atypical presentations include altered mental status, cerebrovascular accident, angina pattern without extended pain, and severe fatigue. Elderly may present with weakness, congestive heart failure, or chest tightness. Twenty-five percent of nonfatal MIs are unrecognized by patient. The pain may have resolved by the time of evaluation.
Unstable angina	Changes in pattern of preexisting angina with more severe, prolonged, or frequent pain (crescendo angina). Pain usually lasts > 10 min. Angina at rest lasting 15–20 minutes or new-onset angina (duration less than 2 months) with minimal exertion. Pattern of pain change important in gauging risk for acute MI. Unpredictable responses to nitroglycerin and rest	Often minimal May have mild diaphoresis, nausea, dyspnea with pain	Not clearly related for precipitating factors May be a decrease in amount of physical activity that initiates pain. Previous history of MI or angina. Over 40 years old, presence of risk factors, and male sex increase probability.	Common	Nonspecific findings of a transient nature; may have similar cardiac findings as in MI.	Often no ECG or enzyme changes	May be pain free at presentation. Full history is essential. Fewer than 15% of patients hospitalized for unstable angina go on to acute MI. Variant angina (Prinzmetal's) has episodic pain, at rest, often severe, with prominent ST segment elevation. May respond to nitroglycerin. May manifest similarly to non-Q wave infarction.
Aortic dissection	Ninety percent of patients have rapid-onset severe chest pain that is maximal at beginning. Radiates anteriorly in chest to the back interscapular area or into abdomen. Pain often migrates with a "tearing" sensation	Neurologic complications of stroke, peripheral neuropathy, paresis or paraplegia, abdominal and extremity ischemia possible	Median age is 59 years. History of hypertension in 70%–90% of patients. 3:1 ratio males to females; Marfan's syndrome and bicuspid aortic congenital valves have increased incidence. 24% die in 1 day, 50% in 1 week.	Rare	Often poorly perfused peripherally but with elevated BP. In 50–60% of cases there is asymmetric decrease or absence of peripheral pulses. Fifty percent of proximal dissections cause aortic insufficiency. Other vascular occlusions: coronary (1–2%), mesentery, renal, spinal cord.	ECG usually shows left ventricular hypertrophy, nonspecific changes. Chest film shows abnormal aortic silhouette (90%). Aortic angiography has diagnostic accuracy of 95%–99%.	It is rare for patient to present pain free. May present with neurologic complications. Physical examination findings may be minimal. Dissection into coronary arteries can mimic MI. Ascending aortic aneurysms are approached more surgically. *Continued on following page*

137

TABLE 8–2. Causes and Differentiation of Potentially Catastrophic Illness Presenting with Central Chest Pain or Discomfort *Continued*

	Pain History	Associated Symptoms	Supporting History	Prevalence in Emergency Department	Physical Examination	Useful Tests	Atypical or Additional Aspects
					New-onset pericardial friction rub or aortic insufficiency murmur supportive of diagnosis.	Ultrasound, CT, MRI most useful in screening.	Descending are generally managed medically.
Pulmonary Embolism	Pain is more often lateral-pleuritic. Central pain is more consistent with massive embolus. Abrupt in onset and maximal at beginning	Dyspnea and apprehension play a prominent role, often more than pain. Cough accompanies about half the cases. Hemoptysis occurs in less than 20%. Angina-like pain may occur in 5%.	Usually some period of immobilization has occurred, (e.g., immobile, without previous history) Pregnancy, oral contraceptives, heart disease, thrombophlebitis, and previous embolus are all risk factors	Rare in ambulatory patients	Patients are anxious and have a respiratory rate over 16 breaths per minute. Tachycardia, inspiratory rales, and an increased pulmonic second sound are common. Fever, phlebitis, and diaphoresis are seen in 30%–40% of patients. Wheezes and peripheral cyanosis are less common	Arterial blood gases show Po_2 <80 mm Hg in 90%. ~15% of pulmonary embolisms have normal $(A-a)o_2$. Chest film is usually normal, although up to 40% show some volume loss, oligemia, or signs of consolidation. Lung perfusion scan rules out, if negative and low probability. Spinal CT improving yield. Angiogram definitive.	Patients may present with dyspnea with or without bronchospasm. Severe abdominal pain can be the primary complaint. Acute mortality rate is 10%. Emboli usually from lower extremities above knee, prostate/pelvis venous plexus, right side of heart.
Pneumothorax	Pain is usually acute and maximal at onset. Most often lateral-pleuritic, but central pain can occur in large pneumothoraces.	Dyspnea has a prominent role. Hypotension and altered mental states occur in tension pneumothorax.	Chest trauma, previous episode, or asthenic body type	Infrequent	Decreased breath sounds, increased resonance on percussion. Elevated pressure in neck veins and tracheal deviation occur in tension pneumothorax.	Chest film definitive. Inspiratory and expiratory films may enhance contrast between air and lung parenchyma. Tension pneumothorax should be diagnosed on physical examination.	May be subtle in COPD, asthma, cystic fibrosis. Can be complicated by pneumomediastinum
Esophageal rupture	Pain is usually preceded by vomiting and is abrupt in onset. Pain is persistent and unrelieved, localized along the esophagus, and increased by swallowing and neck flexion.	Diaphoresis, dyspnea (late), shock	Older individual with known gastrointestinal problems. History of violent emesis, foreign body, caustic ingestion, or blunt trauma	Rare	Signs of lung consolidation and subcutaneous emphysema may be present.	Chest film usually has mediastinal air, a left-sided pleural effusion, pneumothorax, or a widened mediastinum. pH of pleural effusion is < 6.0. Diagnosis supported by water-soluble contrast esophagogram or esophagoscopy	Patient may present in shock state. This entity is often considered late in differential diagnostic process.

COPD, chronic obstructive pulmonary disease; CT, computed tomography; MI, myocardial infarction; MRI, magnetic resonance imaging.

TABLE 8-3. Classification of Acute Coronary Syndromes

Category	History	Physical Examination	ECG	Cardiac Enzymes
I. STEMI (ST Elevation MI)	Chest pain typical of angina; history of coronary artery disease; chest pain similar to previous ACS	Hypotension, pulmonary rales, diaphoresis, transient mitral regurgitation, S_3, S_4	ST segment elevation; new bundle branch block	Elevated CK-MB and/or troponin
II. UA/NSTEMI (Unstable Angina/Non–ST Elevation MI)	Same as category I	Same as category I	ST segment depression and/or T wave inversion	Elevated troponin; normal CK-MB (UA)
III. Probable ACS	Chest pain typical of angina; age > 70 years; diabetes mellitus; extracardiac vascular disease; at least 2 risk factors (hypertension, smoking, hypercholesterolemia)	Often noncontributory	Nonspecific ST/T wave changes	Normal
IV. Possible ACS	Typical chest pain without diabetes mellitus or risk factors; atypical chest pain with diabetes mellitus or at least 2 risk factors (hypertension, smoking, hypercholesterolemia)	Often noncontributory	No ST/T wave changes	Normal
V. Non–coronary artery disease process	Atypical chest pain; no risk factors or diabetes mellitus	Often noncontributory; may be diagnostic (friction rub, reproducible chest pain, Hamman's crunch, etc.)	Not contributory or suggestive of non-CAD process	Normal

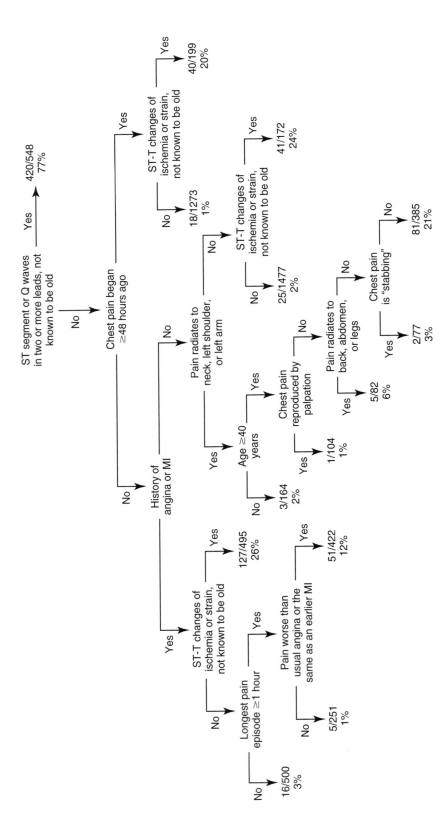

FIGURE 8–1 • Prospectively validated multivariate algorithm for the prediction of a patient's risk of acute myocardial infarction (AMI) on the basis of emergency department data. Low risk of AMI ≤7%. High risk of AMI > 7%. Values for each subgroup are the number of patients with AMI, divided by the total number of patients in each subgroup. The Chest Pain Study enrolled 6149 patients. (From Lee TH, Juarez G, Cook EF, et al: Ruling out myocardial infarction. N Engl J Med 1991; 324:1240.)

TABLE 8–4. ECG Findings in Acute Coronary Syndrome

Classic myocardial infarction	Q waves ≥ 0.04 second duration. ST segment depression (greater than 1 mm) or ST segment elevation (greater than 1 mm) is seen, depending on the degree and location of ischemia. ST-T wave segments are usually convex or flat in acute myocardial infarction.
Subendocardial infarction	Persistent T-wave inversion and ST segment depression occur in several limb or precordial leads.
Unstable anginal pain	Most often has no ECG changes. Elevation or depression ST segments may be seen. Symmetric inversion of T waves

Note: Conduction abnormalities and blocks also may be seen in infarct and ischemia.

who present to the emergency department with chest pain from acute MI, 50% to 80% have an initial ECG that is not diagnostic. For all patients with acute MI regardless of duration of symptoms, more than half had new ST segment/T wave changes suggestive of acute MI or acute myocardial ischemia.

Current equipment technology allows the real-time monitoring of 12-lead ECG with comparison of various criteria (ST segment/T waves) over time. Such monitoring can establish changes in ECG morphology that are highly suggestive of ongoing myocardial ischemia. The actual contribution of this technology to diagnosing acute MI remains under study. The use of 15-lead ECG has been shown to increase the sensitivity for diagnosis of acute MI by demonstrating abnormalities in the three extra leads, especially right ventricular infarction. Noncardiologists may not be familiar with interpreting these leads, and further assessment is necessary in the emergency department. Prehospital 12-lead ECG technology is clinically practical. Prehospital identification of thrombolysis candidates can significantly reduce time to treatment. This time savings is perceived as beneficial to the patient.

The ECG is best for "ruling in" MI. A single emergency department ECG in a patient with "classic" changes of MI shows false-positive results in only 2.3% of patients. Therefore, classic changes are highly specific, and finding them nearly establishes the diagnosis, even in a patient with a weak history for MI. Myocardial salvage therapy is considered when these changes are found. Classic changes of MI on ECG are rare in cases of nonischemic chest pain.

Problems occur when a single ECG tracing is used to rule out MI. Twenty percent of ECGs in patients diagnosed as having MIs are read as normal in the emergency department. The ECG is often "overread," looking for subtle changes that may or may not represent ACS. Comparison with previous ECGs may improve the yield of positive results and increases the physician's propensity to admit the patient. **The absence of classic ECG findings alone does not significantly alter the probability of MI if the history is highly suggestive**. For example, in a patient with a history that is 90% probable for MI, the probability would be increased to 99.5% if the ECG showed the classic changes of MI, but if the ECG did not show such changes, the probability of infarction would decrease only to 80%. Negative ECG results in patients with histories showing a low probability for MI may lower the chances but do not remove MI as a possible cause.

Radiologic Imaging

The results of the history and physical examination direct the radiographic assessment. Posteroanterior and lateral chest radiographs are most useful for diagnosing cardiac- and pulmonary-related pain and for assessing congestive heart failure. Patients with undiagnosed central chest pain are not sent to the radiology department. An anteroposterior upright portable film is an adequate screening view for serious pathologic processes. Inspiratory-expiratory films may be beneficial in patients with suspected pneumothorax. Tables 8–2 and 8–5 list the characteristic findings in specific problems. In patients with IHD only, most radiographs are interpreted as normal.

Cervical or thoracic spine films may be taken if nerve compression is suspected. Abdominal films usually yield few results but may be considered if an abdominal pathologic process is suspected. Most organs in the upper abdominal quadrants can produce pain that is referred to the chest. Gallbladder disease and peptic ulcer disease are particularly common sources of such pain.

Other imaging or contrast techniques have not played a major role in emergency department diagnosis. Two exceptions are the use of CT imaging in patients with suspected dissecting aneurysm and technetium-99m (^{99m}Tc) lung scans in patients with suspected pulmonary embolism. Imaging combined with ECG and laboratory testing may be helpful in selected patients with equivocal histories. ^{99m}Tc pyrophosphate myocardial scanning is both sensitive and specific for myocardial damage but not clinically useful for 24 to 36 hours after the

TABLE 8–5. Other Chest Pain Syndromes and Common Causes by Organ System

	Typical Pain Pattern of Organ System	Diagnosis	Supporting History	Physical Examination	Test (Diagnostic and Exclusionary)	Comments
Cardiac nonischemic	Dull, aching recurrent pain unrelated to exercises or meals. Or it may be a sharp, stabbing pleuritic-type pain that does not change with chest wall motion. May be severe. Not relieved by nitroglycerin.	Pericarditis; be aware tamponade is a rare complication.	Pain is often worse when supine but improves sitting up. Often preceded by viral illness or underlying disease (SLE or uremia). Associated dyspnea or diaphoresis	Friction rub may be heard, often fleeting, position dependent (50% patients).	ECG pattern typical for ST segment elevation across the precordial leads. Erythrocyte sedimentation rate may be elevated.	More common in 20 to 50-year olds. May have associated tachycardias, ventricular dysrhythmias. Idiopathic most common (80%) treated with aspirin, NSAID.
		Mitral valve prolapse	Women often with long history of undiagnosed chest pain. May have associated symptoms such as palpitations, sharp chest pain	Often mid to late systolic mitral regurgitant murmur with or without click	Echocardiogram diagnostic, ECG may show extrasystoles, ST-T wave changes	Approximately 5% of young women in United States
		Hypertropic cardiomyopathy/ aortic stenosis	Symptoms usually with exertion	Usually exercise-induced characteristic murmur	Echocardiogram diagnostic of hypertropic cardiomyopathy	HC associated with sudden death. Bicuspid valve may need surgical replacement.
Pulmonary	Peripheral pleuritic pain pattern, sharp, stabbing with respiratory variations. Dyspnea often more prominent complaint	Upper airway tracheobronchitis	Associated viral illness and cough, usually minimally productive. Low-grade fever	Ear, nose, and throat may be involved; lungs–upper airway, Rhonchi and possible wheezes	Examination and history usually are sufficient, unless sputum examination is desired	Very common
		Lower airway pneumonia	Fever, cough often productive; general malaise	Patient is ill-looking. Fever is common. Lung sounds consistent with early pneumonitis or consolidation.	Sputum examination and chest film diagnostic. Cultures necessary to be specific	Atypical causes on the rise
		Pleurisy	May follow viral infection. Localized laterally	Rarely, rub is heard on auscultation. Chest wall usually not tender. Fever is rare	No other tests, chest film usually not helpful unless effusion is noted	Coxsackievirus B causes unique severe spasmodic pain–pleurodynia
Gastrointestinal	Dull, deep aching with occasional severe increases in degree. Long history of recurrence. May be "burning" or "pressure." Occasionally associated with bad taste or burning in hypopharynx particularly after ingesting alcohol or spicy food	Esophagitis	"Heartburn," worse bending over or supine. Improves with antacids	No typical findings except epigastric discomfort	Definitive tests: esophagoscopy, biopsy, or acid stimulation test. Not available in the emergency department	Very common differential diagnostic concern in emergency department.

	Esophageal spasm	Constricting chest pain often occurring at time of swallowing. Long recurrent history. May be associated with hot or cold foods or drink or pills	No typical findings except epigastric discomfort	Barium swallow may assist. Definitive tests: manometry with stimulation not readily available.	Responds to "GI cocktail" and nitroglycerin. Usually short-lived. Often responds in emergency department
	Peptic ulcer disease, gastritis	Persistent, recurrent aching pain or burning. May relate to meals. Often some improvement after antacids	No typical findings except epigastric discomfort	May see response to antacid trial. Esophagoscopy and contrast not readily available	Assess recent ethanol use, aspirin use, and situational stress. Review previous history of peptic ulcer disease.
Musculoskeletal	Costochondritis Xiphoiditis	May be sharp or dull. Usually persistent and changes with chest wall movement (deep breaths) and upper torso movement. May last 1–2 hours, and occur post exercise. Younger patient, previous history Similar to costochondritis, located at xiphoid	Often chest wall tenderness, seldom swelling or redness	ECG negative, may not be required. Pain may decrease with local anesthetic injected at "trigger" point	Very common differential consideration. Requires analgesia and reassurance. Do not settle on this diagnosis too quickly
Psychogenic	Hyperventilation	Usually substernal pressure or lateral "cardiac apex" discomfort associated with considerable concern or anxiety Associated breathlessness, occasional circumoral and distal extremity tingling. If nitroglycerin used, slow to impact.	Difficult to determine on physical examination	May ask patient to hyperventilate to re-create pain. Confirmation with ABGs. ECG may show T-wave inversion that reverses after pain episode	Usually occurs in younger population. They respond well to reassurance and short-term anxiolytics. Do not settle on this diagnosis too quickly
	Situational stress	History of hyperventilation, anxiety or panic disorder. May have fear of imminent death.	As above	As above	As above

ABGs, arterial blood gases; MRI = magnetic resonance imaging; NSAID, nonsteroidal anti-inflammatory drug; SLE, systemic lupus erythematosus.

onset of pain. ^{99m}Tc sestamibi is one of the newer radioisotopes being studied for emergency department evaluation of acute chest pain. It does not redistribute over time and can be given during the acute pain episode, allowing images to be obtained later. The value of the study is directly related to image quality and the experience of the radiologist. Its use is currently experimental in the emergency department.

Emergency coronary arteriography is becoming more readily available as myocardial salvage techniques become more established.

Echocardiography can be used to evaluate myocardial wall motion, wall and septum thickness, and the presence of pericardial fluid. It cannot distinguish between old and new wall motion abnormalities. It can be technically difficult, and subtle to interpret, but is gradually becoming more available in the emergency department.

Laboratory Studies

Creatine Kinase. The combination of the history, findings of the ECG, and serial cardiac enzyme determinations, particularly creatine kinase (CK) with or without fractionation, is the basis for the diagnosis of MI. Therefore, CK measurements would logically serve as a useful tool in evaluating acute chest pain. Unfractionated CK levels have not proved useful because CK comes from a variety of sources. In contrast, 98% of the MB isoenzyme of fractionated CK arises from within myocardial muscle. CK-MB levels have demonstrated variable diagnostic capability in identifying myocardial ischemia as the source of acute chest pain. At present, CK-MB levels may be drawn in patients at high risk (e.g., elderly or diabetic patients) who have equivocal histories and ECG results. The duration since the onset of pain should be greater than 3 hours. The value of these enzyme levels is in observing their change over time. Therefore, a normal first level can be followed by a repeat level in 3 to 4 hours. No studies have established the validity of using CK-MB levels to make disposition decisions.

Troponin Complex. Troponin is located on the thin filament of striated muscle fibers and regulates muscle contraction. It is a myocardial-specific complex consisting of three subunits with different functions:

1. Troponin T binds the troponin complex to tropomyosin molecules.
2. Troponin I is an inhibiting protein that prevents muscle contraction in the absence of calcium and troponin C.
3. Troponin C has four binding sites for calcium. The fundamental role of the complex is

regulation of calcium-mediated muscle contraction.

The time of observed increase for troponin T and troponin I are essentially the same as that of CK-MB, but they persist for 4 to 7 days longer than CK-MB. Troponin I has demonstrated substantial usefulness in the assessment of acute MI. It may replace CK-MB as the current "standard" cardiac enzyme measurement. The presence of troponin I and troponin T in the peripheral circulation has been associated with increased mortality risk. Troponin is more sensitive (fewer false-negative results) but less specific (more false-positive results) than CK-MB in the diagnosis of acute MI.

Other Cardiac Enzymes. Lactate dehydrogenase level with or without isoenzymes and aspartate aminotransferase value may be diagnostic in the patient arriving 24 hours after a chest pain episode.

Serum Myoglobin. Myoglobin is a heme protein present in all muscle tissue in a single form. It is attractive as an indicator of myocardial injury because levels can be elevated in the serum 1 to 2 hours after injury. It is a sensitive but nonspecific marker of acute myocardial injury. Myoglobin can be detected in more than two thirds of patients with acute myocardial ischemia at 3 hours and in almost all these patients at 6 hours after the onset of pain. Although a significant number of studies have addressed the sensitivity and specificity of myoglobin, the definition of a positive test is inconsistent and is not routinely available.

Other Studies. In preparing for hospital admission, these laboratory studies are commonly ordered: complete blood cell count; arterial blood gas analysis; determination of electrolytes, blood urea nitrogen, and creatinine; and hemostasis studies. Most are baseline assessments rather than specific assessments for acute chest pain. Recent studies suggest an elevated white blood cell count on admission is a predictor of a higher 30-day mortality.

EXPANDED DIFFERENTIAL DIAGNOSIS

Once the clinical examination, laboratory test results, response to therapy, and observation data are available, the physician can reassess the preliminary differential diagnosis based on the presence of central or lateral pain. One must confirm or resolve any persistent concerns about the presence of the six catastrophic diseases or the potential for acute coronary syndromes.

Beyond this point, the physician may approach the problem by matching the patient data with patterns typical of organ systems and with common diseases within those systems (see Table 8–5). In order of frequency, central pain may arise from chest wall structures, psychogenic factors, esophagus, nonischemic myocardium, pericardium, or lung. Lateral pain usually originates in the chest wall, psychogenic factors, or lung.

It is serial experience and follow-up of patients that allow the trained emergency physician to weigh the multiple bits of data and, despite a vague atypical history or lack of supporting data, reach a correct disposition, if not diagnosis. There is no reason to order multiple laboratory tests and hope for a "shotgun" diagnosis. The level of uncertainty is not reduced in most cases.

PRINCIPLES OF MANAGEMENT

General Principles

The underlying principle of management is the same as that for the initial diagnosis: **always anticipate the worst possible diagnosis**. In patients with acute chest pain, initial management is guided by anticipating four major complications. The majority of patients with pain, discomfort, or associated signs and symptoms of a suspicious nature should receive:

1. Oxygen to prevent *hypoxia*, commonly from ventilation-perfusion mismatch.
2. An ECG to seek *dysrhythmias*. Most dysrhythmias are ventricular in origin, and they are treated with antidysrhythmic medication or electrical conversion or both.
3. An intravenous line or heparin lock for possible *hypotension* and drug administration. The origin of hypotension is usually cardiac pump failure or hypovolemia or a combination of the two. They are first treated with volume repletion and then inotropic or chronotropic agents once adequate volume is restored.
4. Analgesia to relieve *suffering* and *stress*. The drug is selected after assessing the nature of the pain, patient tolerance, and the suspicion or probability of catastrophic disease.

Specific Principles

The six potentially catastrophic diseases have specific therapies.

Acute Coronary Syndromes (Acute MI or Unstable Angina)

Goals in stabilizing suggested acute MI and unstable angina or new-onset angina include to relieve pain, anxiety, and ischemia and to decrease the risk of acute MI and sudden death. The following are implemented:

1. Supplemental oxygen, to improve the oxygen supply-demand imbalance
2. Intravenous access for fluid and medication administration
3. Intravenous narcotic analgesia, as necessary: small doses (1 to 4 mg) and frequent dosage (every 5 to 15 minutes) of morphine sulfate is the treatment of choice in patients without hypersensitivity. The dose is adjusted in the context of patient tolerance, cardiac hemodynamics, and side effects of the medication (e.g., nausea, sedation, atrioventricular block).
4. Aspirin administration for platelet inhibition.
5. Treatment of ventricular dysrhythmia is initially accomplished with defibrillation for ventricular fibrillation and/or lidocaine for less critical rhythms. The dose is adjusted for age, the presence of liver disease or congestive heart failure, and patient symptoms related to administration. Prophylactic lidocaine in acute MI is not recommended.
6. Anticipation of major complications, as noted under General Principles.
7. Intravenous magnesium is used specifically in patients with ventricular dysrhythmias, prolonged QT interval, or hypertension not responding to usual therapy.
8. After further assessment, the patient can be classified as having stable angina, unstable angina, acute MI, or nondiagnostic ECG. The acute coronary syndrome groups and current approaches in management are outlined in Figure 8–2.

Aortic Dissection

Therapy is directed toward decreasing the "pulse" of the pressure wave to impede progression of the dissection. This goal is accomplished initially by achieving controlled hypotension and suppressed myocardial contractility using sodium nitroprusside and β-adrenergic blockade. Early surgical consultation is critical when this diagnosis is strongly considered. The preferred imaging sequence is chest computed tomography in advance of aortography. This may not be possible in severe cases.

Pulmonary Embolism

Because the majority of pulmonary emboli are thrombotic in origin, initial therapy is intravenous heparin. The goal is to prevent the next embolus, not "dissolve" the current one. Therapy

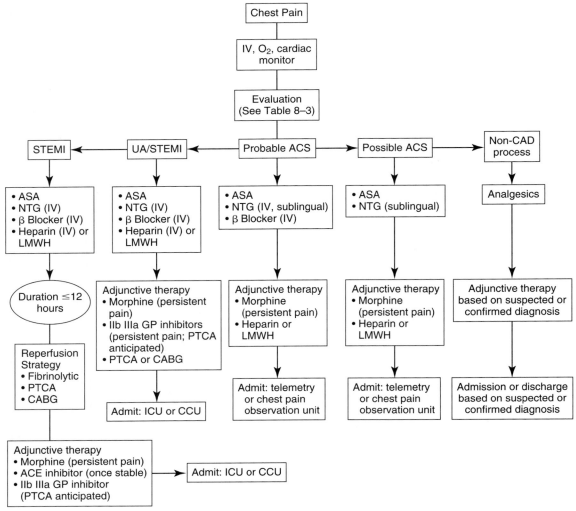

FIGURE 8–2 • Chest pain treatment algorithm. STEMI, ST segment elevation myocardial infarction; UA, unstable angina; ACS, acute coronary syndrome; CAD, coronary artery disease; ASA, aspirin; NTG, nitroglycerin; LMWH, low-molecular-weight heparin; GP, glycoprotein; PTCA, percutaneous transluminal coronary angioplasty; CABG, coronary artery bypass graft; ACE, angiotensin-converting enzyme; ICU, intensive care unit; CCU, coronary care unit.

is started immediately if there is a strong suspicion of embolism based on clinical data, arterial blood gas measurements, or chest radiograph or lung scan interpretation. The goals of therapy are to inhibit the growth of thromboembolism, promote clot resolution, and prevent recurrence. Thrombolytic therapy may be considered in circumstances of massive embolism and hypotension.

Tension Pneumothorax

Rapid decompression with needle thoracostomy can be lifesaving. The goal is to decrease the intrapleural pressure below that of the right ven-

tricular filling pressure, allowing blood to return to the heart. A thoracostomy tube is inserted after the initial needle decompression. Tension pneumothorax is a clinical diagnosis. Patients usually present in cardiopulmonary distress with tracheal deviation, jugulovenous distention, and decreased breath sounds with hyperresonance on the affected side.

Esophageal Rupture

Early diagnosis and treatment of accompanying hypotension are important stabilizing efforts while waiting for the surgeon. Antibiotics are given only after discussion with the consultant.

UNCERTAIN DIAGNOSIS

What is done with the patient in whom the diagnosis remains elusive?

This point is often reached in patients with chest pain. An approach to this clinical dilemma is essential. A great deal of information has been assembled, a number of diagnoses have been considered, and the patient has survived to the present. The following steps will help resolve the disposition:

1. Reassess the information. Has the patient's history been fully explored? Have all sources of information been used? Would other or repeat (e.g. ECG, CK-MB, troponin I) tests supply useful data?
2. Reassess the patient and support system. Is there a reason the patient may not be telling the truth or giving only part of the story? Does the patient have significant stoicism or denial? How medically sophisticated are the patient and supporting individuals? Will they be compliant with medication regimens and plans for follow-up?
3. Have the diagnostic possibilities been reviewed and a decision made on at least an organ system as the most likely site of pain?
4. Importantly, the case is discussed with the patient's primary physician, if available. The diagnostic process and concerns are often shared with a colleague. *Decisions of importance are not made in a vacuum.*
5. Additional observation is appropriate. The added time must be part of a formulated plan for treatment and disposition. This may include stress testing, ultrasound, nuclear scanning, reexamination, and data review.
6. Enlist the consultative opinion of a potentially admitting cardiologist. Difficult decisions "up close" may be easier from a new perspective.
7. If doubt remains, admit the patient for "rule out" MI. Sufficient time has been spent, and there is always another patient.

SPECIAL CONSIDERATIONS

Pediatric Patients

Previously healthy children younger than 14 years old who present with acute chest pain without a history of trauma and without significant physical findings generally do not have serious disease. A precise history is obtained from the child, if possible. Parents often incorporate their own concerns into the story but may not share their main concern about "heart problems." Musculoskeletal syndromes, hyperventilation, and functional problems are common causes. They present as either short-lived localized stabbing pain or a dull persistent "chest ache" in a child who is otherwise normal. Lateral pleuritic pain is associated with viral illnesses (e.g., pleurodynia, pneumonitis). An ECG and additional laboratory studies are usually not indicated but are often requested by parents.

Organic diseases causing acute chest pain in the pediatric population may include the following:

1. Pain of cardiac origin: pericarditis, hypertrophic cardiomyopathy, mitral valve prolapse, aortic stenosis, pulmonary stenosis, anomalous coronary vessels
2. Pain of esophageal origin: strictures, esophagitis
3. Pain of toxic origin: alcohol, cocaine
4. Pain of hematologic or oncologic origin: leukemia, sickle cell anemia, neuroblastoma
5. Pain of metabolic origin: diabetes mellitus, hyperlipoproteinemia syndromes

Elderly Patients

The sources of acute chest pain in elderly patients do not differ significantly from those in the general adult population. Unfortunately, the presentation of serious IHD is often atypical. "Classic" chest pain may be elicited in only 30% of elderly patients with MI, and IHD may present without chest discomfort at all. Instead of pain, the presenting complaint may be sudden progressive dyspnea, abdominal or epigastric fullness, extreme fatigue, confusion, or syncope. The associated symptom of diaphoresis is significantly less common in the elderly. Because the history may be misleading or difficult to obtain, ancillary testing takes on more significance in this population. ECG changes may be more difficult to interpret, because of a longer history of ischemic problems. Isolated cardiac enzyme changes do not make the diagnosis in the emergency department, although repeat CPK-MB or troponin I levels may have benefit.

The emergency physician must be aware of the increased risk of silent atypical MI in the elderly. Suspicion of MI is always raised when elderly patients are in a medically stressful situation, such as occurs with general anesthesia, hypotensive states, hypoxia, systemic infection, or anemia. Even after timely diagnosis, elderly patients with MI have mortality rates (30% to 40%) double those of their younger counterparts. They also have more post-MI complications, including heart block, cardiogenic shock, myocardial rupture, and pulmonary edema.

Diabetic Patients

Patients with diabetes mellitus, type 1 or 2, are at high risk for IHD. They have a dual problem of early atherosclerosis and the atypical pattern of chest pain similar to that seen in the geriatric population.

Cocaine Users

Cocaine increases the release of catecholamines from central and peripheral stores and blocks reuptake of both epinephrine and norepinephrine, resulting in sympathomimetic stimulation of the central nervous system, heart, and vascular smooth muscle. As a result, cocaine reduces coronary artery caliber and coronary blood flow. Cocaine prolongs the PR interval and QT duration and results in ventricular tachycardia. Evidence exists implicating cocaine in platelet aggregation and atherosclerosis.

Because β blockers may increase the α-adrenergic stimulation caused by cocaine, they are not used in acute chest pain caused by cocaine. Nitroglycerin and benzodiazepine are the first line of treatment in cocaine-induced chest pain.

Women with Chest Pain

Women are evaluated and treated for cardiac diseases less frequently than men with similar symptoms. They account for 29% of all patients with IHD. Atypical pain is more common in women. They have a higher prevalence of less common causes of ischemia (e.g., vasospastic) and nonischemic chest pain (e.g., mitral valve prolapse). They have a lower prevalence of angiographically demonstrated coronary disease in all forms of chest pain. Women are more likely to have anginal pain during rest, sleep, or mental stress. In acute MI, symptoms of nausea, vomiting, fatigue, dyspnea, and neck, jaw or shoulder pain are more common. Postmenopausal women, without hormone replacement therapy, have a risk factor for IHD similar to males. Other important positive risk factors in women include family history, central obesity, and "high stress, low control" situations. No specific diagnostic adjunct has yielded additional diagnostic accuracy. Generally, women have fewer positive findings in all testing. Women are more likely to have a non–Q-wave infarction, but they have a higher postinfarction mortality than men. Recent studies have found eligible women with acute MI are less likely than men to receive thrombolytic, β blocker, and aspirin therapy. This gender bias must be recognized and remedied.

DISPOSITION AND FOLLOW-UP

Disposition plans usually progress in concert with patient evaluation. Most plans are formulated at the time of the initial stabilization and preliminary differential diagnosis and revolve around the following questions.

Is There a High Probability of Catastrophic Disease?

Disposition is admission with appropriate treatment as necessary.

Is There a High Probability of Acute Coronary Syndrome?

This diagnosis is based on the *history*. It may be supported by the physical examination, laboratory test results, response to therapy, and observation. The disposition includes therapy and admission unless there are unique reasons to decide otherwise (e.g., stable angina patient in for a prescription refill or another problem).

The disposition process may be facilitated in the future by computer-based predictive instruments. Presently, these probability generators are most useful for training. One system increased the physician's diagnostic accuracy from 83% to 91%, decreased the cardiac care unit admissions from 23% to 14%, and did not increase the 3% inappropriate discharge rate. Another computer protocol reduced the admission of patients without infarction to intensive care by 11.5% without jeopardizing the patients who required intensive care. These programs are an adjunct, not a replacement, for a careful history and a physician's experience.

The possibility of ACS, concerns about its progression and sequelae, and the lack of definitive tests for identifying its presence are sources of tremendous stress on the decision-making capabilities of the emergency physician. About 90% of all patients evaluated in an emergency department and found to have an MI are appropriately admitted to the intensive care unit. Another 7% are brought into the hospital, and 3% or less are discharged. Only 20% to 30% of all patients admitted to the intensive care unit with acute chest pain prove to have an MI. Therefore, another disposition issue must be resolved.

If a Patient Is Admitted, Are There Guidelines for Choosing Between Intensive Care and Intermediate Care?

The ECG in the emergency department can help stratify risk across the spectrum of acute coronary syndromes. An ECG interpreted as "normal" during the initial evaluation in the emergency department correlates with a 0.6% chance of a serious hospital complication. An "abnormal" ECG result correlates with a 14% chance. Therefore, patients with a normal ECG who are admitted as "rule-out" MI are considered for admission to an intermediate care area with telemetry and trained nursing staff. The 30-day risk of death or myocardial reinfarction was increased in patients with ST segment elevation, depression, or both on the initial ECG. Other studies suggest that, in patients with acute MI, a normal or nonspecific initial ECG relates to a lower but clinically significant chance of morbidity or death compared with those patients with classic ECG changes.Patients diagnosed as having unstable angina rather than MI may also fall into a low-risk group for complications. Admission to an intermediate care unit may be appropriate for them as well. In general, the coronary care unit is reserved for patients with a moderate to high probability of acute MI.

Planning for Discharge

If ACS and other serious disorders are ruled out, the patient's pain status is briefly reassessed. If the patient is without disabling pain and is clinically stable, plans are made for discharge. The care given is documented, and a sentence is included about serious disorders considered ruled out and the organ system considered as the site of pain. An analgesic or other useful medications (e.g., antacids) are prescribed. The findings are discussed with the patient and family, and mention is made of the "serious problems" that are considered unlikely. Given sufficient information to decrease their anxiety, most people understand all the answers cannot be supplied in a limited time frame.

It is critical to arrange close follow-up for patients being discharged with the complaint of acute chest pain, whether the diagnosis has been made or not. Optimally, both the emergency physician and the primary physician or consultant participate in follow-up activities. A discussion on current medication and possible addition of preventive medication (e.g., aspirin) is important. Any patient in the diagnostic "gray zone" in regard to acute chest pain who is discharged from the emergency department is contacted within 24 hours. Any patient who voluntarily recontacts or revisits the emergency department because of persistent or recurrent chest pain is strongly considered a candidate for admission. Such a patient is evaluated as if he had a "new" chief complaint to avoid assuming the diagnosis made on the first visit is still operative.

Chest Pain Centers/Clinical Decision Units

The cost per life saved to hospitalize a patient to rule out MI is about $1.5 million. By establishing an "observation" or clinical decision unit (CDU) and performing serial ECGs and cardiac enzymes, the patient with acute MI can be identified at 20% to 50% of the cost of inpatient admission. Critical to success is an active protocol to aggressively assess low- to moderate-risk patients. Patients are continuously monitored and serial enzymes and ECGs assessed to detect any change in status. Additionally, during the 12- to 14-hour observation period, testing such as stress ECG with or without thallium 201 or ^{99m}Tc-sestamibi imaging or stress echocardiography may be performed. Recent studies have demonstrated benefit of the CDU in patients with unstable angina. A decrease in resource use without increased patient risk was shown. Patient satisfaction surveys have demonstrated a preference for the CDU approach. The CDU may become the ancillary site in emergency medicine to help protect the 3% to 4% of patients with acute MI who currently are inappropriately discharged from the emergency department.

FINAL POINTS

- Acute chest pain is a complex complaint that requires a careful, detailed history.
- The physician examination focuses on signs of catastrophic illness, arteriosclerosis, and duplicating the chest discomfort.
- The initial differential diagnosis of acute chest pain may be based on the location and character of the pain.
- The six potentially catastrophic illnesses to be considered first are myocardial infarction, unstable angina, pneumothorax, dissection of the aorta, pulmonary embolism, and esophageal rupture.
- A single ECG is helpful for ruling in IHD if it shows positive results. "Normal" results do not rule it out.
- Cardiac enzyme concentrations as presently available are not absolute in "ruling out" IHD in most patients with acute chest pain evaluated in the emergency department. The accuracy and value of this testing continues to improve.
- Patients without a clear diagnosis are best reevaluated and the case discussed with another physician. If a clear decision cannot be reached, it is preferable to admit the patient for observation and further evaluation.
- Elderly or diabetic patients with IHD may present without chest pain. A high index of suspi-

cion is necessary in this age group, as delays in diagnosis and treatment are frequent.
- The emergency physician should always ask about drug use and consider cocaine-induced chest pain as a diagnosis.
- Women are currently underevaluated and undertreated after presenting with chest pain.

- Selected groups (e.g., postmenopausal women) have substantial risk.
- Clinical decision units have demonstrated benefit in allowing further time and testing for low risk, complex, or confusing patients.

CASE *Study*

The 73-year-old woman was at home when the lower chest discomfort and nausea began 12 hours earlier. The rescue squad was called by her family, and they brought the patient to the emergency department. The rescue squad reports the patient's pain was in the lower chest. It was described as a "burning indigestion," moderate in intensity and lasting about 12 hours. The patient complained of nausea, belching, and increasing pain during the past 4 hours. Vital signs are blood pressure, 180/90 mm Hg; pulse, 100 beats per minute; and respirations, 18 breaths per minute. The patient is approximately 5 feet tall and weighs 200 pounds. She is sweating moderately and slightly pale. She seems in distress but is tolerating the pain. The patient had taken Alka-Seltzer without experiencing relief. The squad placed oxygen via a nasal cannula at 2 L/min and started an intravenous line with dextrose/water 5% at a keep-open rate. A monitored rhythm showed sinus tachycardia. Transport time was 15 minutes. The patient has known hypertension, treated with a daily "water pill."

The patient is brought into the acute care area, and the physician is asked to see her. Her family is referred to registration. All points of the assessment and stabilization routine were accomplished, and her status remained unchanged. No nitroglycerin or aspirin was given. Repeat vital signs were blood pressure, 200/100 mm Hg; pulse, 100 beats per minute; and respirations, 18 breaths per minute. She was afebrile. Her color was slightly pale. The monitor showed a sinus tachycardia with an occasional premature ventricular beat.

Even when busy, it is useful to observe quickly the arrival of a chest pain patient. This is the best opportunity to meet the patient and further question the rescue personnel, who may leave otherwise. One must shift from the "audio" impression given by prior radio contact to the "video" reality of the patient's presence. It is surprising how many patients change abruptly,

seldom for the better, on arrival at the hospital. In this patient, there was little change from the vital signs taken in the field. Further intervention (e.g., nitroglycerin, aspirin) could wait until more data were gathered.

Although nothing "catastrophic" is apparent, the patient's age, weight, pain pattern, associated symptoms, and slightly increased blood pressure and pulse should raise suspicions about serious illness. Because the history is atypical for IHD, administration of nitroglycerin was not indicated in the field. Aspirin could be given, but Alka-Seltzer was taken. Ambulance transport and observation with cardiac monitoring was appropriate. At the close of radio contact it is useful to request the rescue squad to bring in the patient's medication. The rescue personnel are expected to allay the initial fears of the patient and family about coming to the hospital.

Note: From this point on the case is written to demonstrate errors leading to an unfortunate outcome. Evaluating patients with chest pain has a number of pitfalls. Many are included here.

The physician's history from the patient was not amplified in the chart. There was a brief nursing note repeating the history given by the paramedic. The physician wrote: "History as above" and went on to the physical examination. Information available from the daughter in the waiting room was not obtained.

This is pseudoefficiency. Time demands of emergency medicine may compromise one's assessment, but the basic principles of care, such as "A detailed history is the most important diagnostic tool in chest pain assessment" and "If it isn't recorded on the chart, it wasn't done," cannot be ignored. This may not be the situation literally, but in this case the history the physician actually obtained is lost forever. Shortcuts of this type tend to reflect shortcuts in the interview. Current documentation requirements for insurance purposes have complicated the lives of emergency physicians, but they preclude this type of error.

Additional history the physician may have learned was instead of 12 hours' lower chest and epigastric pain only, during the last 4 hours the patient's pain had changed from epigastric to substernal and was more a "fullness" and "burning" sensation than pain. There was no radiation of pain. She came to the hospital after trying Alka-Seltzer but experiencing no relief. She noted a little "sweatiness" earlier in the day and was mildly nauseated at the time. A lesser sensation of pressure was noted on two occasions during the last 2 days, each lasting 10 to 15 minutes before disappearing. The patient denied any previous pain history. She gave a family history of hypertension and stated two brothers and one uncle had died of "heart attacks." The daughter in the waiting room would have added her mother was rather stoic and distrustful of doctors. Two days earlier she had called her and complained of "pressure between her breasts" when going out into the cold air.

The patient looked her stated age of 73 years. She was obese and in mild distress from the discomfort. Vital signs were blood pressure, 170/100 mm Hg; pulse, 90 beats per minute; respirations, 18 breaths per minute; and afebrile temperature. The results of the physical examination were recorded as follows:

Thorax: WNL, some xiphoid tenderness

Lungs: clear

Heart: distant heart tones (pendulous breasts), no murmur

Abdomen: mild epigastric discomfort and tenderness

Extremities: pulses symmetric, no edema, no cyanosis

This record provides adequate information, although data on the head, cervical spine status, eye, and patient's response to bedside tests or maneuvers were not recorded. The xiphoid area almost always has some tenderness. From the chart it is difficult to tell the patient's pain tolerance.

The patient's condition was preliminarily categorized as central chest pain of nonischemic origin. An ECG and chest radiograph were ordered.

The major reason for not emphasizing cardiac ischemia as the cause of the patient's symptoms was an inadequate history, at least as recorded on the chart. In patients with acute chest pain, a cardiac etiology is the first diagnosis to rule out. A serious error in emergency medicine is forming an early diagnosis and not reconsidering it throughout the examination. An early diagnosis can give the physician a false sense of security and limit the search for more information.

An ECG was obtained and interpreted as having only nonspecific ST segment/T wave changes in the chest leads. An old ECG was available to the physician, but it was "in another building." No comparison of new and old ECGs was done. No other laboratory tests were performed.

Comparison of old and new ECG results does not greatly improve the predictive capability of the test for IHD. Interestingly, "new" ECG changes based on comparison of ECG test results lead to increased frequency of admission to the hospital. The impact of ECG comparison on critical care versus monitored bed selection is unknown.

This patient's ECG results showed subtle changes of an ischemic nature compared with the ECG taken 1 year earlier. Although not definitive, the opportunity for a raised level of suspicion was missed by not pushing for more responsiveness from the hospital record retrieval system.

With the history, physical examination, and laboratory test results assembled by the physician, the most likely origin of the pain was thought to be gastrointestinal. The highest probability in this category was esophagitis. Although the patient did not improve with one dose of antacid in the emergency department, she was readied for discharge.

No additional history or repeat physical examination was recorded. It must be assumed that the patient was relatively pain free or at least not actively complaining about it. Because of failure to gather complete data from all sources, the physician chose the wrong diagnosis. A careful history would have pointed to new-onset angina with a recent change in pattern. Therefore, this patient has unstable angina as a working diagnosis. Even at this late point in the care, the outcome can still be influenced in both the patient's and the physician's favor.

The patient was discharged home on antacid therapy. The following morning, just before the treating physician was leaving his night shift, she called the emergency department to speak

Continued on following page

to the physician. She described a slightly stronger pain in the epigastric area and a slight amount of sweating after going home. A second similar episode lasting 10 to 20 minutes awakened her just before her call. The physician stated the antacids take some time to work and suggested she avoid "hot" foods. The patient called back about 2 hours later, but the physician had left. She was found dead at her home approximately 4 hours later. An autopsy found a new inferior MI.

The most worrisome patients in emergency medicine are often the ones who are discharged home. This physician neglected a cardinal rule of emergency medical practice. "Listen to, rather than explain away, a patient who has returned. Do not form a rigid mindset about any diagnosis." Better patient education, a follow-up system in the emergency department, more responsiveness on the part of the treating physician, and arranged referral to the primary physician might have favorably influenced the outcome of this case. "Come on back, we'd like to see you again, particularly if things are not working out" must be the continual parting message in the emergency department. It is always smarter to rule out serious disease in the hospital than to have it ruled in at home.

Summary. The total documentation in this case read as follows:

History as above
Obese WF
Thorax: WNL, some xiphoid tenderness
Lungs: clear

Heart: distant heart tones (pendulous breasts), no murmur
Abdomen: mild epigastric tenderness
Extremities: no edema
Diagnosis: esophagitis
Treatment: antacids, D/C (discharge) to PMD (primary medical doctor)
ECG: WNL

The physician is vulnerable medicolegally because of poor documentation. Each element of the evaluation has a purpose in communication and if documented appropriately creates a high-quality record from the emergency department. The importance of a few sentences in documenting one's thoughts on a complex or confusing patient with acute chest pain who is being discharged from the emergency department is not to be underestimated.

Despite the untimely death of this patient, the hospital generated and forwarded a bill. The physician did not notify the risk management department of the hospital nor know that the bill had been sent. This action may cause a legal reaction. Total time in the emergency department was 2 hours and 45 minutes. Charges were:

Ambulance fee: $200.00
Hospital fee: Level III care: $250.00
Physician fee: Level III care: $155.00
ECG and interpretation: $90.00
Monitor: $30.00
IV: $15.00
Mylanta, first dose: $4.00
Total: $744.00

Bibliography

TEXTS/MONOGRAPHS

American College of Emergency Physicians: Revised Clinical Policy for Management of Adult Patients Presenting with a Chief Complaint of Chest Pain with No History of Trauma. Dallas, American College of Emergency Physicians, 1995.

Bahr RD, ed: Heart Attack: The Public Health Challenge for the New Millennium. Fourth National Congress of Chest Pain Centers in Emergency Medicine, 2001, Maryland Medicine (suppl).

Braunwald E (ed): Heart Disease, 5th ed. Philadelphia, WB Saunders, 1997.

Emergency Department: Rapid Identification and Treatment of Patients with Acute Myocardial Infarction. National Institutes of Health publication No. #93-3278. Bethesda, MD, U.S. Department of Health and Human Services, 1993.

Yusuf S: Evidence Based Cardiology. London, BMJ Books, 1998.

JOURNAL ARTICLES

Balk EM, Ioaunides JP, Salem P, et al: Accuracy of biomarkers to diagnose acute cardiac ischemia in the emergency department. Ann Emerg Med 2001; 37:478–494.

Brady WJ, Bosker G, Kleinschmidt K: Acute myocardial infarction and coronary syndromes: optimizing selection of reperfusion and revascularization therapies in the EP, Emerg Med Rep 2001; 22:235–250, 251–264.

Braunwald E, Autman EM, Beasely JW, et al: ACC/AHA guidelines for the management of patients with unstable angina and non–ST-segment elevation myocardial infarction. Circulation 2000; 102:1193–1209.

Diop D, Aghababian RV: Definition, classification, and pathophysiology of acute coronary ischemic syndromes. Emerg Med Clin North Am 2001; 19:259–268.

Gibler WB, Armstrong PW, Ohment EM, et al: Persistence of delays in prevention and treatment of patients with acute myocardial infarction: The GUSTO-I and GUSTO-III experience. Ann Emerg Med 2002; 39:123–130.

Goodacre S, Locker T, Morris F, et al: How useful are clinical features in the diagnosis of acute, undifferentiated chest pain? Acad Emerg Med 2002; 9:203–208.

Ioaunides JP, Salem D, Chew PW, Lau J: Accuracy of imaging technologies in the diagnosis of acute cardiac ischemia in the emergency department. Ann Emerg Med 2001; 37:471–477.

Jones ID, Slovis CM: Emergency department evaluation for the chest pain patient. Emerg Med Clin North Am 2001; 19:269–282.

Kleinschmidt K: Acute coronary syndrome (ACS). Emerg Med Rep 2000; 21(23):257–272; 21(24):273–284; 21(25):285–296.

Klompas M: Does this patient have an acute thoracic aortic dissection? JAMA 2002; 287:2262–2272.

Klones RA, et al: The effects of acute and chronic cocaine use on the heart. Circulation 1992; 85:2–10.

Lange RA, Hillis LD: Cardiovascular complications of cocaine use. N Engl J Med 2001; 345:351–358.

Lau J, Ioaunides JP, Balk EM, et al: Diagnosing acute cardiac ischemia in the emergency department. Ann Emerg Med 2001; 37:453–460.

Lee TH, Goldman L: Evaluation of the patient with acute chest pain. N Engl J Med 2000; 342:1187–1195.

Lee PY, Alexander KP, Hammill BG, et al: Representation of elderly persons and women in published randomized trials of acute coronary syndromes. JAMA 2001; 286:708–713.

Pope JH, Aufderheide TP, Ruthazer R, et al: Missed diagnosis of acute cardiac ischemia in the emergency department. N Engl J Med 2000; 342:1163–1170.

Pryor DB, Shaw L, McCants CB, et al: Value of the history and physical in identifying patients at increased risk for coronary artery disease. Ann Intern Med 1993; 118:81–90.

Ryan TJ, Autman EM, Brooks NH, et al: ACC/AHA guidelines for the management of patients with acute myocardial infarction: 1999 update. Available at *www.americanheart.org/scientific/statements*.

Savonitto S, Ardissino D, Grauger CB, et al: Prognostic value of the admission electrocardiogram in acute coronary syndromes. JAMA 1999; 281:707–713.

Schneider SM, Salluzzo R: Non-myocardial infarction chest pain. Emerg Med Rep 1995; 16(25): 247–254.

Sheifer SE, Manolio TA, Gersh B.T: Unrecognized myocardial infarction. Ann Intern Med 2001;135:801–811.

Storrow AB, Gibler WB: Chest pain centers. Ann Emerg Med 2000; 35:449–461.

Weber JE, Chudnofsky CR, Boczar M, et al: Cocaine-associated chest pain. Acad Emerg Med 2000; 7:873–877.

Yeghiazarians Y, Braunstein JB, Askari A, Stone PH: Unstable angina pectoris. N Engl J Med 2000; 342:101–114.

CHAPTER 9

Syncope

DOUGLAS WARD
TIMOTHY G. JANZ

CASE *Study*

A 25-year-old woman was brought to the emergency department by rescue squad after a syncopal episode at home. She had been ill for several days with left lower quadrant abdominal pain. The squad could not establish intravenous access while en route. Her blood pressure on arrival was 80/50 mm Hg, with a pulse of 120 beats per minute. The patient regained consciousness when the rescue squad evaluated her at home, but she had some confusion in recalling the event.

INTRODUCTION

Syncope is defined as a brief loss of consciousness characterized by loss of postural tone and collapse, with or without minor muscle twitching, with spontaneous recovery. After a brief period of unconsciousness, the patient has a complete recovery of function without a postictal phase. Unfortunately, neither patients nor health care providers consistently adhere to this strict definition. The variability of presentation and imprecise descriptions leave considerable room for confusion and misunderstanding in the diagnosis and discussion of "syncopal episodes" and has helped create the modified, but confusing term *near-syncope*. Presyncope or near-syncope is said to have occurred when symptoms abate before loss of consciousness.

Up to 3% of emergency department visits are for "syncope," and nearly 1% of all admissions are attributed to this complaint. The number of emergency department visits for presyncope is somewhat lower, owing to a maintained consciousness. The assessment and differential diagnosis change very little in evaluating presyncope or syncope, and generally these patients are treated the same.

Consciousness is maintained through activity of the reticular activating system in the brain stem. Loss of consciousness is caused by injury or disease in the reticular activating system or by bilateral cerebral hemispheric dysfunction.

Decreased blood flow to only one cerebral hemisphere during an embolic event, for example, will not cause a loss of consciousness. The etiology may be either a primary neurologic disease or secondary to toxins, inadequate nutrients, or inadequate cerebral blood flow. The primary nutrients for the brain are oxygen and glucose. Cerebral perfusion pressure is physiologically determined by the mean arterial pressure minus the intracranial pressure. Neurologic disease or injury can raise the intracranial pressure and compromise cerebral perfusion. Most commonly, patients with syncope experience a temporary decrease in mean arterial pressure. Arterial pressure is dependent on multiple factors as outlined in Figure 9–1, including cardiac output, peripheral vascular resistance, heart rate, stroke volume, myocardial contractility, preload, and afterload.

Circumstances affecting any of these hemodynamic parameters can decrease the arterial pressure and cerebral blood flow, causing syncope. If the heart rate is slowed from increased vagal tone or heart block, the cardiac output decreases and arterial pressure falls. Normally, the peripheral vascular resistance increases in an attempt to compensate for the bradycardia and raise the arterial pressure. Hypovolemia decreases the preload, stroke volume, and cardiac output. When a patient who is hypovolemic stands up, he or she may experience syncope because the cardiac

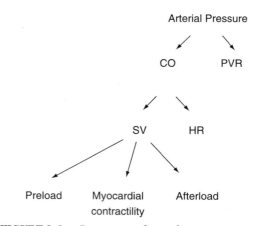

FIGURE 9–1 • Components of arterial pressure.

output is not adequate to support the cerebral perfusion pressure necessary to maintain consciousness. In attempting to compensate for hypovolemia, the heart rate and peripheral vascular resistance will generally increase.

Syncope may be caused by serious illness (e.g., cardiac dysrhythmias) or benign conditions (e.g., a simple faint). In approximately 40% of patients seen in the emergency department after a syncopal episode, a vasovagal or psychogenic cause is found. These patients have a benign clinical course even after several years of follow-up. Cardiac syncope occurs in approximately 13% of patients with transient loss of consciousness and heralds a poor long-term prognosis; 20% to 30% of patients with cardiac syncope will die within 1 year despite medical treatment. In other patients, almost one fifth have orthostatic hypotension and up to 40% of patients have no clear cause for the syncope. Patients who have cerebrovascular disease or drug related or metabolic causes of syncope have poorer long-term prognoses than the general population.

INITIAL APPROACH AND STABILIZATION

Rapid Assessment

The initial concern in the emergency department is to stabilize abnormal vital signs and anticipate a recurrence of the syncope.

1. The patient is asked to describe what happened and if this type of event has occurred previously. A brief medication history is taken.
2. The patency and protection of the airway and breathing are assessed.
3. Measurement of vital signs is repeated and the values compared with those reported by the rescue squad.
4. The physical examination is focused on whether the patient is alert, oriented, and aware of what happened. If the patient remains poorly responsive, it is more appropriate to classify the problem as altered mental status (see Chapter 31, Altered Mental Status) rather than syncope.
5. The patient is asked to move all extremities; signs of asymmetric motor strength potentially representing a gross neurologic deficit are sought.
6. The patient is questioned about any injury that may have occurred during the syncopal episode, and a brief physical examination is made of the affected area.

Early Intervention

1. The intravenous line, supplemental oxygen, and cardiac monitor are confirmed or started as necessary. Unstable vital signs may require aggressive volume resuscitation.
2. The cardiac monitor is continuously observed for any evidence of dysrhythmias.
3. If there is a persistent decreased level of consciousness, a clotted tube of blood (red top) is drawn, a bedside blood glucose level is measured, and consideration is given to administering the following medications: (a) 100 mg thiamine to treat Wernicke's encephalopathy; (b) 25 to 50 g of 50% dextrose to treat hypoglycemia; and (c) an initial 2 mg of naloxone to reverse the effects of having taken opiates or some of their derivatives.

CLINICAL ASSESSMENT

History

An accurate history of the event is crucial for determining the appropriate diagnosis. In one study, the etiology could be determined in 50% to 70% of syncopal patients enrolled. Almost 80% of the diagnoses were made based on the findings of the history and physical examination. It is often necessary to question family, friends, or bystanders, as well as the rescue personnel from the scene. Discussion with the patient's primary physician is often valuable. Syncope often manifests as a dynamic event in which the patient's status changes frequently.

Surrounding the Event

- Was there an *inciting event*? What events immediately preceded the syncopal episode? Physical or emotional stress such as a fight or extreme anger is common preceding syncope.
- Did the patient say anything immediately before the event? Was a *prodrome* experienced by the patient such as pallor, chest or abdominal pain, weakness, dizziness, confusion, diaphoresis, nausea, or anxiety? Each of these may point to a serious cause of the event.
- Was the event preceded by the patient suddenly *assuming* the *upright position*? Was there any *head turning* or *neck pressure*? The first question explores the possible role of postural hypotension, and the second investigates the possibility of a hypersensitive carotid sinus or vascular obstruction of one or more vessels supplying the brain.

- Did any *activity* such as urination, defecation, Valsalva maneuver, or hyperventilation occur before the syncopal episode? Were there any noxious stimuli?
- What occurred *during* the syncope? Tonic-clonic movements suggest seizure activity. A few myoclonic jerks are common in syncope.
- *Postsyncope* status is important. The patient should recover completely and rapidly. Confusion or postictal findings are suggestive of more serious causes.

Focused Review of Systems

- Is there any reason to suspect *dehydration* or *volume loss*? Dehydration could be caused by strenuous activity, diuretics, gastrointestinal losses, or poor fluid intake.
- Is there any history suggesting *chronic anemia* or *recent blood loss* (gastrointestinal tract bleeding or excessive menstrual loss)? Is there any possible occult blood loss from obscure but critical sites such as a leaking abdominal aneurysm or ruptured ectopic pregnancy?
- Was there any *chest pain, dyspnea,* or *palpitations*?
- Did the patient have any *seizure activity, weakness,* or other *neurologic symptoms*?
- Could the patient be *pregnant*?

- Was the *fall* the *cause* or the *result* of the loss of consciousness? Was there any *trauma* to the head, chest, abdomen, or extremities?

Past Medical History

- Has the patient ever *sustained* a *syncopal episode* before?
- Is there any history of *cardiac disease*? Is there any history of paroxysmal supraventricular tachycardia, heart blocks, ventricular dysrhythmias, valvular heart disease, cardiac medications, or prior placement of an external pacemaker?
- Does the patient have a history of *seizures, carotid artery disease, transient cerebral ischemia,* or *stroke*? Is there a history of an *abdominal aneurysm*?
- Is there a history of *bleeding problems* or *peptic ulcer disease*?
- Is the patient a *diabetic*? Insulin dependent? If so, what is the usual dose, when was it last given, and when was the last meal?
- Because pulmonary embolus can be a cause of syncope, careful inquiries should be made about past pulmonary embolus, venous thrombosis, and leg pain or swelling.
- A review of pertinent medications may be helpful (Table 9–1). Quinidine causes syncope in 0.5% of patients taking it, and it is an important cause of torsades des pointes, a life-threatening

---

TABLE 9–1. Pharmacologic Agents Associated with Syncope

Cardiovascular

β-Blockers
Vasodilators (α-blockers, calcium channel blockers, nitrates, hydralazine, angiotensin-converting-enzyme inhibitors, phenothiazines, sildenafil)
Diuretics
Central hypertensives (clonidine, methyldopa)
Other antihypertensives (guanethidine)
QT interval–prolonging agents (amiodarone, disopyramide, flecainide, procainamide, quinidine, sotalol, encainide)

Psychoactive

Anticonvulsants (carbamazepine, phenytoin)
Antiparkinsonian agents
Central nervous system depressants (barbiturates, benzodiazepines)
Monoamine oxidase inhibitors
Tricyclic antidepressants
Narcotic analgesics
Sedating and nonsedating antihistamines

Drugs with Other Mechanisms

Drugs of abuse (marijuana, cocaine, alcohol, heroin)
Digitalis
Insulin and oral hypoglycemics
Neuropathic drugs (vincristine)
Nonsteroidal anti-inflammatory drugs

ventricular dysrhythmia. In addition, digoxin, lithium, diuretics, nitroglycerin, propranolol, and other β blockers can contribute to orthostatic hypotension or syncope. Antihypertensives and antidepressants are the most common medication-related causes of syncope. Other intoxicants such as cocaine can cause cardiac dysrhythmias, and alcohol and narcotics produce an altered mental status. Marijuana use can also be an inciting factor, secondary to the Valsalva maneuver many users practice after inhaling the drug.

Physical Examination

The goal of the physical examination is to determine whether there are findings that confirm the origin of the patient's syncope and whether injuries resulted from the episode. Specific elements of this examination are listed in Table 9–2. By necessity, a complete examination of the cardiovascular and neurologic systems is completed.

CLINICAL REASONING

After the history and physical examination, the emergency physician formulates a preliminary differential diagnosis that can be developed by answering the following questions.

Does the Patient Have True Syncope?

Syncope is often confused with other conditions such as dizziness, weakness, vertigo, "faintness" or "lightheadedness," transient confusion, or inability to stand. Occasionally, stroke, coma, transient cerebral ischemia, or seizures are labeled syncope. Furthermore, some patients with incomplete loss of consciousness, altered mental status, or loss of postural tone are described as having "presyncope." The history of a transient loss of consciousness with sudden collapse and spontaneous recovery is important for a diagnosis of true syncope.

Did a Life-Threatening Event Cause the Syncope? Is It Ongoing?

The patient's vital signs and the cardiac monitor will generally indicate any immediate threats. Specific diseases to be considered first include the following:

1. *Cardiac dysrhythmia with hypotension.* Vital signs, chest pain, level of mentation, and the cardiac monitor may indicate a dysrhythmia that must be treated immediately.

2. *Myocardial ischemia.* Up to 10% of patients with myocardial infarction present with syncope.
3. *Acute blood loss.* The patient will often exhibit orthostatic hypotension and be pale and cold ("shocky"). The physical examination usually indicates the source of blood loss, such as abdominal pain or vaginal bleeding.
4. *Obstructive cardiomyopathy.* Critical aortic stenosis or hypertrophic cardiomyopathy may present as syncope during exercise.
5. *Hypoxia.* An acute pulmonary event such as a pulmonary embolus may cause syncope. Stress or exercise may also cause syncope if the patient has a limited physiologic ability to respond (e.g., if the patient has hypertrophic cardiomyopathy).
6. *Hypoglycemia.* The patient often has a history of diabetes mellitus and usually responds to an infusion of 50% dextrose.
7. *Cerebrovascular disease.* Stroke or subarachnoid hemorrhage may present as a history of syncope.

If There Is No Immediate Life-Threatening Process, What Organ Systems Are Likely To Be Involved?

The major systems to be assessed are the cardiovascular, neurologic, metabolic, and psychological systems (Table 9–3). Most of these patients have cardiovascular problems that cause decreased blood flow to the reticular activating system. Primary neurologic diseases are the next most common cause. Metabolic abnormalities or psychological problems are also significant causes of syncope. A specific cause of syncope is not determined even after a full hospital or outpatient evaluation in almost 20% of patients.

DIAGNOSTIC ADJUNCTS

Routine screening laboratory tests, radiographs, and electrocardiograms (ECGs) performed on all patients with temporary loss of consciousness or syncope yield few results and are not cost effective. A young person with a simple faint precipitated by a plausible situation who is now fully recovered may not benefit from any additional tests. Diagnostic adjuncts are considered in all older patients and in those younger patients in whom the cause is unclear.

Laboratory Studies

1. *Hematocrit-hemoglobin* is ordered for patients in whom anemia or active blood loss is

TABLE 9–2. Directed Physical Examination in Patients with Syncope

Area of Examination	Important Tests and Findings	Significance
Vital signs	Pulse—rate and regularity	Atrial or ventricular tachycardias (pulse > 100 beats per minute). Heart blocks can cause bradycardias and syncope. Irregular pulse may indicate premature contraction or heart blocks
	Blood pressure, orthostatic pressure, and pulse	Shock from any cause can decrease cerebral blood flow and cause syncope. Orthostatic pressure and pulse changes may indicate hypovolemic cause
	Respiratory rate	Tachypnea may indicate hypoxia or pulmonary embolus
	Temperature	Fever may indicate sepsis
General appearance	Responsiveness, skin color, diaphoresis	Signs of decreased organ perfusion
Head, eyes, ears, nose, throat	Point tenderness or ecchymosis	May indicate trauma from fall
	Funduscopic examination, papilledema	Increased intracranial pressure, diabetic retinopathy, retinal hemorrhages from central nervous system bleeding
	Breath, oral mucosa	Ketones from ingestion, ketoacidosis, or dehydration
Neck	Tenderness, carotid bruits	Cervical spine trauma, source of cerebral emboli
Lungs	Percussion, auscultation: consolidation, decreased breath sounds, rales, wheezing	Hypoxia from pulmonary embolus, infection, bronchospasm, or congestive heart failure
Cardiac system	Systolic ejection murmur, particularly changing with the Valsalva maneuver; gallop, rub, prosthetic valves	Aortic stenosis murmur decreases and the hypertrophic myopathy murmur increases with Valsalva maneuver; new murmur
Abdomen and rectum	Pulsatile masses, peritoneal signs, stool Hematest	Abdominal aneurysm, intra-abdominal catastrophe, gastrointestinal bleeding
Pelvis	Uterine bleeding, tenderness, adnexal mass	Ectopic pregnancy, pelvic infection
Extremities	Cyanosis, pallor, capillary refill, leg pain, swelling	Evidence of peripheral perfusion and deep vein thrombophlebitis
Neurologic	Cranial nerves, motor, sensation, reflexes, mental status	Focal neurologic signs may indicate intracranial process or primary neurologic disease

TABLE 9–3. Etiology of Syncope and Temporary Loss of Consciousness

Cardiovascular System

Vasovagal faint
Cardiopulmonary
Aortic dissection
Aortic stenosis, hypertrophic cardiomyopathy, atrial myxoma
Myocardial infarction
Dysrhythmias
  (rapid: paroxysmal supraventricular or ventricular tachycardia)
  (slow: sick sinus syndrome, atrioventricular blocks)
Pericardial tamponade, pericarditis
Faulty prosthetic valve
Pacemaker failure
Pulmonary embolus
Carotid sinus hypersensitivity
Orthostatic hypotension
Medications
Chronic illness
Autonomic neuropathy
Volume loss
Sudden massive occult blood loss
Leaking abdominal aneurysm
Gastrointestinal hemorrhage (acute or chronic)

Situational Syncope

Micturition, defecation, cough, Valsalva maneuver

Pregnancy

Anemia, hemodynamic predisposition to faint
Ruptured ectopic pregnancy (blood loss)

Neurologic System

Transient ischemic attack
Stroke (completed or stroke in evolution)
Subarachnoid hemorrhage
Seizures
Occult head trauma

Metabolic

Hypoglycemia
Hypoxia
Intoxication
  Alcohol, sedative hypnotics, opiates, carbon monoxide
Medications
  Cardiac, hypertensive drugs

Psychologic

Anxiety disorders
Conversion disorders
Panic disorder, breath-holding spells

Uncertain Etiology

Miscellaneous reflex
Cough, sneeze
Post micturition

suspected by the history and physical examination. Measurements may be repeated if blood loss continues.

2. *Blood type and crossmatch* are obtained for patients who are orthostatic or hypotensive or if massive blood loss is suspected, as in patients with ectopic pregnancy or leaking abdominal aneurysm.

3. *Electrolytes* are obtained in patients taking diuretics or when severe dehydration is suspected based on orthostatic measurements and clinical history.

4. *Serum glucose* value is checked in all patients with persistently altered mental status before administration of glucose.

5. *Arterial blood gases* are obtained in patients who have unexplained pleuritic chest pain, shortness of breath, or tachypnea associated with syncope.

6. A *pregnancy test* (urine or serum β-human chorionic gonadotropin) may be needed, because ectopic pregnancy must be considered in all women of childbearing age with syncope.

Electrocardiogram

All patients with unexplained syncope and possible cardiovascular disease receive a 12-lead ECG and cardiac monitoring. The ECG has been demonstrated to aid diagnosis more than any other single diagnostic adjunct. In one study, 74% of patients presenting with syncope had an abnormal ECG and 6% had diagnostic findings.

Radiologic Imaging

Computed tomography of the head is indicated for patients with focal neurologic signs, unexplained seizures, or persistently altered mental status post syncope. A careful clinical assessment is essential before ordering imaging studies unlikely to be of benefit.

Special Tests

Holter Monitor. A Holter monitor may provide useful information in patients who are discharged from the hospital but need to have additional ECG recordings made during their normal activity at home. The ECG monitor is attached to the patient and worn for 24 hours while the patient keeps a diary of all symptoms and activities. Subsequently, the ECG record is analyzed for dysrhythmias and correlated with symptoms.

An "event" monitor is similar to a Holter monitor, but the patient must activate the unit when symptomatic to begin recording the rhythm. The obvious drawback is in a patient without prodromal symptoms who can not begin the recording before losing consciousness. It can be useful, however, in patients with less frequent symptoms who require the unit for a longer period of time.

Electroencephalogram. Routine electroencephalographic testing for all syncopal patients is unnecessary. It is performed in patients in whom seizure is the most likely cause of syncope and in those difficult patients with no other likely cause of syncope in whom an occult seizure disorder is being ruled out. It is seldom performed in the emergency department.

EXPANDED DIFFERENTIAL DIAGNOSIS

The history, physical examination, and ancillary tests support a definitive diagnosis in most patients presenting with syncope. Table 9–4 reviews the common causes of syncope. These include vasovagal faint, cardiac dysrhythmias, orthostatic hypotension, seizures, situational syncope, primary neurologic diseases, and metabolic abnormalities.

Vasovagal Faint

The vasovagal faint is the most common cause of syncope in patients younger than age 40. Less frequently, fainting may occur in older patients and pregnant women. It occurs in approximately 20% of patients presenting to the emergency department with syncope. It typically is caused by diminished venous return associated with a reflex increase in sympathetic tone. This activity stimulates the parasympathetic nervous system and results in peripheral vasodilations and relative bradycardia. Accordingly, when such a patient has collapsed and is unconscious, the pulse rate is usually slow at 40 to 60 beats per minute and blood pressure is less than 100 mm Hg systolic.

Given the right set of circumstances, almost anyone can experience a fainting episode. Predisposing conditions associated with a vasovagal faint are hunger; exhaustion; alcohol; a stuffy, closed warm room; strong smells; or noxious sensory input. Noxious stimulation includes any unpleasant physical or psychological event. Additionally, medical conditions such as anemia, dehydration, certain medications (vasodilators), and electrolyte abnormalities may predispose patients to a vasovagal faint. "Weight lifter's blackout" is syncope caused by the Valsalva maneuver during an exercise.

Many patients who faint experience a prodrome lasting a few moments before actually collapsing. Observers may report that the patient had pallor and was sweating. The patient is aware of

TABLE 9–4. Common Causes of Syncope

Disease Entity	History	Physical	Ancillary Tests	Comments
Vasovagal faint	Past fainting history; predictable stimulus; sudden collapse with complete recovery	Young, healthy. Immediate recovery after event: low blood pressure, slow pulse, then normal examination results	Unremarkable	Young, healthy. Rapid return to normal
Orthostatic hypotension	Past illness, prolonged bed rest, dehydration, medications; sudden upright position associated with collapse	May be unremarkable except for postural changes in vital signs	Orthostatic changes in blood pressure and heart rate	Check for dehydration or sudden blood loss; review medications.
Cardiac dysrhythmias	Past medical history: cardiac history, sudden collapse, older patient, may be associated with chest pain	May be within normal limits or may have irregular heart rate	Monitor rhythm, electrocardiogram, rule out myocardial infarction. Outpatient Holter monitor helpful	Older patients with cardiac history have serious 1-yr mortality with syncope. Admit patient with pacemaker and syncope.
Situational syncope	May have had similar prior experience; sudden collapse. History of Valsalva or micturition, or cough	May be within normal limits	Not generally helpful. Results of carotid sinus massage may be dramatic.	Be careful with carotid massage.
Seizure	Usually positive past history; loss of bladder control, tongue biting, generalized convulsion	Postictal state is common post event; otherwise physical may be within normal limits	Electroencephalogram may be helpful.	In simple syncope, motor activity is usually not generalized and is not accompanied by tongue biting or loss of bladder control.
Metabolic abnormality	Usually *not* sudden collapse with complete recovery as in true syncope	Generalized weakness, associated confusion	Serum glucose	Most often related to glucose abnormality or exogenous toxins
Primary neurologic disease	Older patients, atherosclerosis or hypertensive vascular disease	Fixed or transient neurologic deficit. Blood pressure elevated	Computed tomography of head may be positive.	Simple true syncope is rarely associated with a neurologic deficit.

feeling uncomfortable and often complains of being warm and diaphoretic, lightheaded, or nauseated. The patient may be confused just before collapsing and may try to sit or lie down. This frequently results in an unprotected fall and possible injury. While lying on the ground unconscious, the patient may exhibit eye rolling, lip smacking, a few generalized muscle spasms, or tonic movement. Very rarely, urinary incontinence, tongue biting, or true tonic-clonic movements occur. The faint is rapidly resolved within 1 or 2 minutes as the cardiac output increases while the patient is lying in a horizontal position. There is no postictal state, and the patient becomes alert and responsive. The rate of the resolution may vary because of age, the continued presence of noxious stimuli, and possible injury from the fall.

Cardiac Syncope

Cardiac causes of syncope are responsible for approximately 20% of all syncope-related visits to the emergency department. This type of syncope frequently has a serious predisposing cause and a worse prognosis than vasovagal faint. Valvular heart disease such as aortic stenosis and hypertrophic cardiomyopathy may be associated with syncope. Exertional syncope may be a serious herald of a critical outflow obstruction and perhaps coronary artery hypoperfusion. The classic systolic murmur heard at the base of a hypertrophic dynamic heart may be the only finding.

As many as 10% of patients with acute myocardial infarction will have syncope. In some patients, syncope is related to ventricular dysrhythmias; and in others, it is related to sudden uncompensated changes in cardiac output. A careful history and the ECG record are necessary in making the diagnosis.

A number of cardiac conduction disorders can cause an abrupt fall in cardiac output and subsequent syncope. Many of these are associated with atherosclerotic coronary artery disease and acute ischemia or chronic degeneration of the conduction system. Conduction disorders are manifest as heart blocks at the sinoatrial node (sick sinus syndrome), atrioventricular node (second- or third-degree block), or bundle of His (fascicular block). Tachycardias such as ventricular tachycardia or supraventricular tachycardia can also decrease cardiac output and lead to syncope. Pacemaker failure unmasks the underlying cardiac disorder and must have a consistent approved.

The *sick sinus (brady-tachy) syndrome* is characterized by abnormal sinoatrial function causing episodes of bradycardia as well as tachycardia. The bradycardia can consist of sinus rhythm, usually less than 50 beats per minute, or sinus arrest

with junctional escape beats. Syncopal episodes occur most frequently during bradycardia. Sick sinus syndrome can be caused by degeneration of the sinus node, atherosclerotic heart disease, rheumatic heart disease, cardiomyopathy, or congenital abnormalities of the conduction system. Electrophysiologic studies can help to define the sick sinus syndrome if the diagnosis is uncertain.

Carotid sinus syndrome is caused by hypersensitivity of the carotid sinus stretch receptors. Approximately 80% of patients with this syndrome experience bradycardia only. Up to 10% suffer from hypotension without bradycardia, with the remainder having a mixed disorder. Both types can cause syncope and are often associated with neck malignancies as well as head turning and tight shirt collars. The elderly are the most common group experiencing syncope from carotid sinus hypersensitivity, but an estimated 10% of the population actually has the syndrome.

Atrioventricular blocks are seen in approximately 11% of patients with cardiac syncope. First-degree heart block, a prolongation of the PR interval, indicates disease in the atrioventricular conduction system but by itself should not be associated with syncope (Fig. 9–2).

In *second-degree heart block* some supraventricular impulses are conducted to the ventricles whereas others are not. In Mobitz type I block, the PR interval increases until a P wave is not conducted (Fig. 9–3). It is associated with myocardial infarction, digitalis toxicity, and increased vagal tone. Type I block generally has a benign prognosis and is not usually the cause of syncope. Mobitz type II block is characterized by a fixed PR interval with dropped beats in a regular or irregular pattern (Fig. 9–4). Type II block can cause significant hemodynamic compromise and syncope. Causes include myocardial infarction, myocarditis, and degenerative disease of the conduction system.

Third-degree heart block is marked by complete atrioventricular dissociation (Fig. 9–5). Causes include acute myocardial infarction, digitalis toxicity, congenital anomalies, and degenerative disease of the conduction system. Third-degree heart block can lead to significant hemodynamic compromise and syncope. Adams-Stokes attacks occur when the ventricular escape beats cannot maintain cerebral perfusion during complete heart block resulting in a syncopal episode.

Fascicular blocks are another important consideration in cardiac causes of syncope. The bundle of His bifurcates into right and left bundle branches. The left bundle further divides into anterior and posterior fascicles. Thus three fascicles transmit impulses to the ventricles. There is concern that patients with syncope who demonstrate bifascicu-

FIRST-DEGREE ATRIOVENTRICULAR BLOCK

Diagnostic Criteria	Causes
Rate: 60–100/min *Rhythm:* regular *P wave:* normal *P:QRS:* 1:1; PR interval is >0.20 sec	Coronary artery disease, digoxin, rheumatic fever, congenital conditions

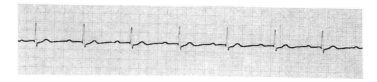

First-degree atrioventricular block

FIGURE 9–2 • First-degree atrioventricular block. (From Eisenberg MS, Cummins RO, Ho MT [eds]: Code Blue: Cardiac Arrest and Resuscitation. Philadelphia, WB Saunders, 1987.)

SECOND-DEGREE ATRIOVENTRICULAR BLOCK, MOBITZ TYPE I (WENCKEBACH)

Diagnostic Criteria	Causes
Rate: atrial rate is greater than ventricular rate *Rhythm:* atrial rhythm is regular; ventricular rhythm is irregular *P wave:* normal *P:QRS:* PR interval becomes progressively lengthened until a QRS is dropped; PP interval remains constant	Myocardial infarction, rheumatic fever, digitalis toxicity

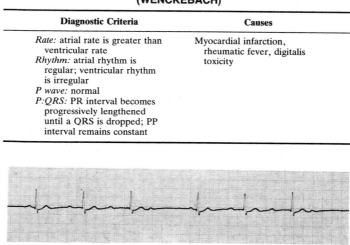

Second-degree atrioventricular block, Mobitz Type I (Wenckebach)

FIGURE 9–3 • Second-degree atrioventricular block, Mobitz type I (Wenckebach). (From Eisenberg MS, Cummins RO, Ho MT [eds]: Code Blue: Cardiac Arrest and Resuscitation. Philadelphia, WB Saunders, 1987.)

lar disease on an ECG may be predisposed to complete heart block. Patients with left bundle branch block or right bundle branch block with left anterior hemiblock have bifascicular blocks. These patients need continued cardiac monitoring and electrophysiologic studies to define their conduction disease and subsequent treatment.

A number of *cardiac medications* (see Table 9–1) can lead to serious toxicity and may cause conduction disturbances and syncope. Digoxin toxicity can cause sinus node stimulation with the atrioventricular node conduction delay resulting in paroxysmal supraventricular tachycardia with block. Quinidine can cause conduction delays marked by QT prolongation and eventually

bizarre ventricular dysrhythmias such as torsades. Calcium channel blockers and β blockers can cause conduction delays and bradydysrhythmias.

Orthostatic Hypotension

A fall in blood pressure after a quick change in position from lying to standing is a frequent cause of syncope or near-syncope. The causes of orthostatic hypotension include prolonged inactivity and bed rest, medications (vasodilators, antihypertensive drugs), central nervous system disorders (Parkinson's disease), and autonomic neuropathies (chronic alcoholism and diabetes). Other causes of orthostatic hypotension include acute blood loss

SECOND-DEGREE ATRIOVENTRICULAR BLOCK, MOBITZ TYPE II

Diagnostic Criteria	Causes
Rate: atrial rate is greater than ventricular rate *Rhythm:* atrial rate is regular; ventricular rate may be regular or irregular *P wave:* normal; PR interval is normal, and QRS usually shows bundle branch block *P:QRS:* ratio may be 2:1, 3:1, 4:1, or 3:2; ratio may vary over time; ratios of 2:1 are difficult to distinguish from Mobitz Type I; if in doubt, treat as Mobitz Type II	Myocardial infarction, digitalis toxicity

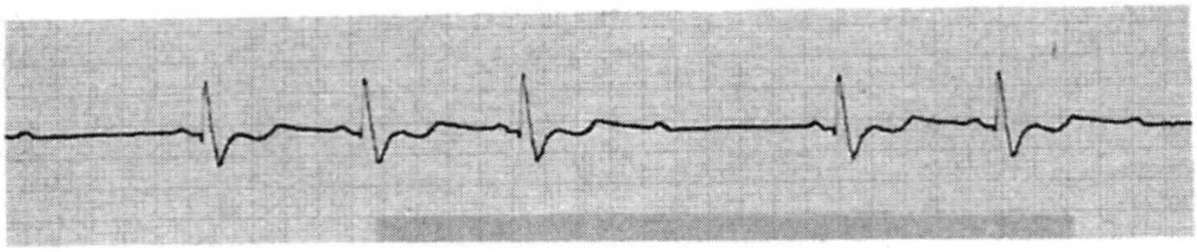

Second-degree atrioventricular block, Mobitz Type II

FIGURE 9–4 • Second-degree atrioventricular block, Mobitz type II. (From Eisenberg MS, Cummins RO, Ho MT [eds]: Code Blue: Cardiac Arrest and Resuscitation. Philadelphia, WB Saunders, 1987.)

THIRD-DEGREE ATRIOVENTRICULAR BLOCK, COMPLETE HEART BLOCK

Diagnostic Criteria	Causes
Rate: atrial rate is greater than ventricular rate *Rhythm:* atrial rate is 60–100/min; ventricular rate is 40–60/min if junctional escape beats occur; ventricular rate is 20–40/min if ventricular rate escape beats occur *P wave:* normal *P:QRS:* no relationship; atria and ventricles are independently contracting *QRS:* normal if junctional escape beats occur; >0.11 sec if ventricular escape beats occur	Coronary heart disease, myocardial infarction, myocarditis, drug toxicity (digitalis, procainamide, quinidine, verapamil)

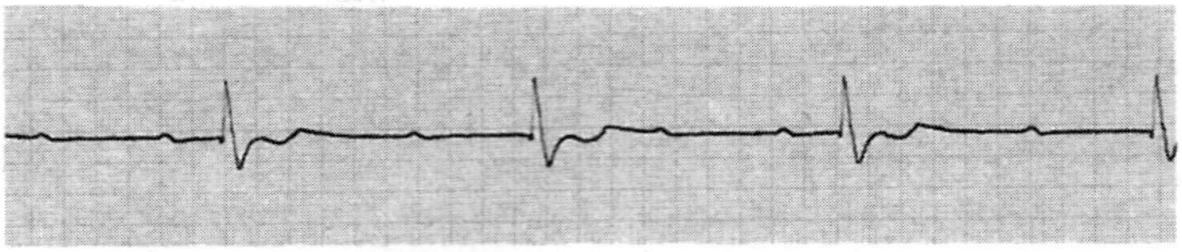

Third-degree atrioventricular block, complete heart block

FIGURE 9–5 • Third-degree atrioventricular block, complete heart block. (From Eisenberg MS, Cummins RO, Ho MT [eds]: Code Blue: Cardiac Arrest and Resuscitation. Philadelphia, WB Saunders, 1987.)

and dehydration due to diuretics, poor oral intake, excess sweating, or gastrointestinal loss.

Orthostatic vital signs are used to help detect positional hypotension. The blood pressure and heart rate are recorded while the patient is supine, then sitting or standing. A decrease in systolic pressure of 20 to 30 mm Hg or more and/or an increase in pulse rate by 20 to 30 beats per minute from supine to standing indicate a positive test. If any patient becomes symptomatic with dizziness or near-syncope during the test, the result is also considered positive. Symptoms are a more reliable indicator of this type of syncope than changes in pulse rate and blood pressure. Many sources use only this criterion as a positive test result.

Situational Syncope

Situational syncope may occur under specific circumstances. It has been described after micturition, defecation, cough, and the Valsalva maneuver. The inciting event produces vagal stimulation and bradycardia without immediate sympathetic stimulation, resulting in transient loss of consciousness.

Seizures can cause a temporary loss of consciousness. The patient is frequently seen in a postictal state, which gradually resolves. The evaluation and management of seizures in the emergency department are discussed in Chapter 33, Seizures.

Metabolic Abnormalities

Metabolic abnormalities such as hypoxia, hypoglycemia, and hyponatremia can be associated with syncope. Hypokalemia, hypomagnesemia, and hypocalcemia are also predisposing conditions that can result in cardiac arrhythmias with prolonged QT intervals. Generalized weakness and confusion often accompany these conditions.

Neurologic Diseases

Primary neurologic diseases such as stroke can produce syncope. These are often accompanied by focal neurologic deficits and are discussed further in Chapter 34, Stroke.

Psychiatric Diseases

Psychiatric disorders are an important category in the cause of syncopal episodes. One study found 35% of patients with syncope as a presenting complaint in the emergency department had a psychiatric disorder. Most common was major depression followed by generalized anxiety disorder and panic disorder. Vertigo and dizziness are often associated with a psychiatric cause, although many patients with cardiac diseases also complain of similar symptoms. These disorders are considered after more immediate life-threatening causes are excluded.

PRINCIPLES OF MANAGEMENT

Management of the patient with syncope is based on the following general principles:

1. Reversible causes of syncope are immediately addressed.
2. Recurrences or complications are anticipated.
3. Specific causes of syncope are addressed.

As discussed previously, airway and breathing are assessed and supplemental oxygen is provided. Circulation is maintained with intravenously administered isotonic crystalloid. An ECG monitor is placed, and dysrhythmias are promptly treated. Thiamine, glucose, and naloxone are given if the patient does not have a normal level of consciousness when initially seen.

Vasovagal Faint

Patients who clearly have had a simple vasovagal faint are observed for 1 to 2 hours, rechecking the vital signs including orthostatic measurements and observing the cardiac rhythm. No specific treatment is required other than reassurance and patient education. Effective prophylaxis is usually achieved with β blockers. These are prescribed by the primary physician in cases of recurrent vasovagal syncope.

Cardiac Dysrhythmias

Tachycardia. Patients with ventricular tachycardia or ventricular fibrillation require defibrillation, intravenous amiodarone or lidocaine, and additional medication as necessary to control their dysrhythmias. These patients may have an irritable cardiac focus, owing to acute ischemia, ventricular aneurysm, electrolyte imbalance, or digoxin toxicity.

Bradycardia. Patients with a bradycardic dysrhythmia usually have serious disease in the conduction system or acute or cardiac medication toxicity. If they are symptomatic, these patients may be treated with intravenous atropine. If atropine is unsuccessful in decreasing the symptoms, a transcutaneous or transvenous pacemaker is indicated. Dopamine, epinephrine, and isoproterenol have been used temporarily if a pacemaker cannot be promptly inserted.

Orthostatic Hypotension

Patients presenting with syncope caused by orthostatic hypotension are rehydrated with normal saline until the symptoms and orthostasis improve. A search for the source of volume depletion is mandatory. If blood loss is the cause of orthostasis, blood transfusion and surgical consultation must be considered, depending on the cause of the bleeding. Some patients with chronic illness and multiple medications will have orthostatic hypotension and syncope after rapidly rising from the horizontal position. These patients may only need reassurance and education.

Other Causes

Situational syncope requires no specific emergency department treatment. Patients are educated about the inciting events. Metabolic abnormalities are treated according to the laboratory test results. Patients with seizures and primary neurologic diseases are treated for specific entities in conjunction with neurologic consultants.

UNCERTAIN DIAGNOSIS

In a substantial number of patients the precise diagnosis or etiology is not clear in the emergency department. For this group of patients, hospitalization is considered under the following circumstances:

1. Elderly patients. Mortality for syncope increases for patients older than 70 years of age.
2. Patients with demonstrated or suspected heart disease.
3. Patients who have an abrupt onset of syncope without prodrome (consistent with a dysrhythmia).
4. Patients who fall and sustain a significant injury.

In approximately 40% of patients presenting with syncope, a clear etiology is not identified even after extensive inpatient evaluation. The reported 1-year mortality for syncope of unknown etiology is 6%, and from noncardiovascular causes it is 12%. Increasing age (>70) and comorbidity are important risk factors.

The importance of suspected cardiac disease cannot be overemphasized. When a cardiac cause is not ruled out, the patient must be treated as if this is the true cause of syncope. Admission for further evaluation is the prudent conclusion.

SPECIAL CONSIDERATIONS

Pediatric Patients

Syncope or near-syncope is relatively common in the pediatric population. Between 15% and 50% of children experience at least one episode. The most common causes of syncope in children are vasovagal episodes, orthostatic hypotension, and breath-holding spells. Cardiovascular disease is much less common than in adults; when present, it is frequently associated with congenital heart disease such as aortic or pulmonic stenosis, tetralogy of Fallot, or pulmonary hypertension.

Supraventricular tachycardia is the most common dysrhythmia of childhood. Standard therapies, including adenosine, have demonstrated effectiveness in the emergency department. It is sometimes difficult to distinguish true syncope from seizures. The clinical history, postictal state, and associated signs and symptoms such as incontinence and tongue biting may help the clinician to make the appropriate diagnosis. Children with syncope should be scheduled for follow-up visits to a pediatrician.

Elderly Patients

A substantial percentage of patients with true syncope in the geriatric age-group will be found to have a serious and potentially fatal cause for the disorder. These causes include acute myocardial infarction, bradydysrhythmias or tachydysrhythmias, cerebrovascular accident, or serious blood loss.

Geriatric patients presenting with apparent orthostatic syncope often require an extensive evaluation. This finding is noted in up to 20% of patients older than 65 years of age. These patients may be taking a number of medications capable of causing syncope, such as β blockers, calcium channel blockers, and diuretics. Drug-drug interactions are considered an important cause in this group. Assessment of these patients may be complicated by poor history (either given by the patient or taken by the physician), mild dehydration, autonomic nervous system dysfunction, and recent prolonged bed rest. Hypertension is a known risk factor.

Testing for orthostatic hypotension must be done carefully in this age group, because there is a significant risk for falls and syncope. Minimal cardioacceleration (<10 beats per minute) with hypotension suggests an impaired baroreceptor reflex or cardiac response. Symptoms are of utmost importance when testing for orthostatic hypotension and constitute a positive finding.

Geriatric patients should be carefully evaluated for serious causes and sequelae of syncope. They need to be observed, educated, and protected to avoid a secondary injury related to a syncopal episode.

DISPOSITION AND FOLLOW-UP

Admission

The disposition of patients with syncope depends on the presumed cause. Patients with the following causes are admitted to the hospital.

Cardiac Disorders. Patients with syncope due to cardiac causes have a 20% to 30% 1-year mortality. Therefore, admission to a cardiac-monitored bed is mandatory. These patients include those with ventricular tachycardia, second- or third-degree heart block, bifascicular conduction defects, or paroxysmal supraventricular tachycardia with hypotension. Some of these patients require sophisticated diagnostic testing procedures in the coronary catheterization or electrophysiology laboratory to precisely determine the dysrhythmia and its origins.

Patients with a pacemaker who present with syncope may need admission to the hospital even if their pacemaker appears to be functioning adequately. In many of these patients a malfunction of the pacemaker, of the battery, or at the electrode-cardiac muscle implant site may be beginning. Although they now appear stable, their syncopal episode may herald pacemaker malfunction. Cardiology consultation is necessary before discharge is considered.

Patients with newly diagnosed aortic stenosis causing syncope are admitted for monitoring, catheterization, and valvular intervention. Other patients with a known prosthetic valve who have a new or changed murmur or any evidence suggesting valvular malfunction require admission to the hospital with cardiothoracic consultation to consider prosthetic valve replacement.

Orthostatic Hypotension. Patients with syncope caused by acute blood loss need urgent volume and blood resuscitation, surgical consultation, and admission to the hospital.

Situational Syncope. The unusual patient who is found to have new onset of situational syncope, such as micturition, defecation, or cough syncope, may benefit from admission to rule out other serious diseases.

Drugs. Patients with syncope that is attributed to medications need a review of their medication dose and indications by their primary care physician. Most patients with medication-induced syncope are admitted and observed in the hospital.

Discharge

Most of the patients (80% to 90%) seen in the emergency department can be discharged after a careful assessment. Patients may be discharged under the following circumstances.

Vasovagal Faint. The young person with a simple, clear vasovagal faint can be discharged after a brief period of observation. The patient is educated to avoid inciting stimuli and to take appropriate precautions when the prodrome occurs.

Cardiac Etiology. An exception to the rule to admit all syncopal patients with cardiac causes is the young patient with previously known, predictable, and controllable paroxysmal supraventricular tachycardia. If the dysrhythmia is easily converted and the patient has not been hypotensive or experienced chest pain, discharge with close follow-up by a primary physician is appropriate.

Orthostatic Hypotension. Dehydrated patients are rehydrated and sent home. Specific treatment is given for the cause of the dehydration, such as diarrhea and vomiting. On discharge, the patient should be able to tolerate oral fluids.

Situational Syncope. If situational syncope has been previously diagnosed and other causes of syncope have been ruled out, the patient is discharged with suggestions for altering behavior to minimize future risk; follow-up arrangements are made with the primary physician.

Drugs. Patients found to be intoxicated by alcohol are observed until their mental status is normal. They are examined and, if no serious problems are found, discharged. Care is taken to ensure that no other drugs have been ingested. Other, more serious intoxications (i.e., tricyclic antidepressants or opiates) will require specific and supportive therapy.

FINAL POINTS

- Syncope is defined as a transient loss of consciousness characterized by unresponsiveness and loss of postural tone with rapid and spontaneous recovery.
- The most common cause of true syncope in young people is a simple vasovagal faint. An appropriate predisposition, inciting event, and stressful environment are usually present.
- In as many as 40% of patients a precise diagnosis of the cause of the syncopal episode is not made.
- In approximately 15% of patients with syncope there is a cardiac cause. The 1-year mortality for this group is 20% to 30%.
- Older patients with syncope are assumed to have serious causes until proved otherwise.
- Syncope may present as an injury. Patients are questioned closely about the cause of falls, and secondary problems are actively sought in patients after a syncopal episode.

CASE *Study*

The 25-year-old woman was studying for an examination while at home when her syncope occurred, according to her boyfriend, who was found in the waiting room. She had gone to get something to drink when her boyfriend heard a "thud" and went in to the kitchen to investigate. He found her lying on the floor confused and unable to tell him what had happened. Apparently she was a previously healthy marathon runner but had recently been complaining of left lower quadrant abdominal pain. Her boyfriend stated she normally had low blood pressure, given her marathon status. She was cool, somewhat diaphoretic, and appeared pale. She spoke several incoherent words.

At the bedside, the physician spoke with the paramedics while assessing the patient's ABCs. Oxygen was started, and the patient was placed on a monitor. Verbal orders were given to start another large-bore intravenous line and to begin an infusion of isotonic crystalloid wide-open while the other intravenous line is also opened to continue the bolus. She was also given thiamine, glucose, and naloxone without any change in her mental status. A complete blood cell count, electrolytes, glucose, urine pregnancy, and blood type with crossmatch were ordered. No abdominal tenderness could be elicited.

This case underscores the importance of data gathering and initial stabilization of a syncope presentation. The physician must use time wisely, and it is necessary to ask the paramedics to remain as well as to seek out other family members or friends who might be available to give a more complete history. Initial assessment can often be performed while speaking with the paramedics. Interviewing the boyfriend at the bedside was necessary given the patient's condition.

Airway, breathing, and circulation are always the first priority, and this also includes attempts at stabilization of blood pressure should it be necessary. Intubation might have been prudent in this patient unless the airway was deemed appropriate with some type of speech and a good gag reflex. Still, the decision to intubate this patient would be reasonable because one cannot be confident where this case might lead. Early aggressive stabilization, intravenous access, cardiac monitoring, and laboratory testing are important in anticipating and preventing further sequelae from this as yet unknown cause.

After approximately 2 L of normal saline, the patient's mental status improved and she stated she felt "normal" and would like to go home to continue studying. Further history gathering is attempted with no new data, other than the feeling of being "lightheaded" just before the incident. She remembered everything up to the syncopal episode but not the transport by the rescue squad.

The patient is asked to remain in the emergency department to await the laboratory results and possible further evaluation. She reiterated her desire to leave, and her boyfriend joined the conversation attempting to convince the physician nothing was wrong. A rather lengthy discussion followed, but the patient finally agreed to stay until her laboratory results were available.

Until the physician is truly confident nothing life-threatening is going to occur, the patient should not be allowed to leave the emergency department unless it is unavoidable. Leaving "against medical advice" does not necessarily protect the physician from litigation, and every attempt should be made to reason with the patient. All such conversations should be documented in the chart.

An abdominal ultrasound could be performed if the physician was skilled in this procedure. It may have given a positive result, enabling the consultant to be called a bit earlier. Waiting for the pregnancy test result before contacting the consultant is reasonable in this case. It is not, however, critical to wait for all laboratory results if the physician has enough data to make the diagnosis.

An arterial blood gas analysis might also have been appropriate given the patient's initial presentation. Her altered mental status could have been attributed to a toxicologic etiology, and a toxicologic screen would also be appropriate, recognizing the limits of the test.

An ECG should be ordered to help with the workup for syncope. Although it probably would not have been useful in this case, it often has value in establishing the diagnosis.

If her condition had remained stable after the initial bolus, and her clinical assessment warranted it, computed tomography might also demonstrate another cause, such as a stroke, intracranial hemorrhage, or mass lesion.

While waiting for the laboratory results, the patient became confused and then lethargic. Repeat vital signs demonstrated a blood pressure of 70/40 mm Hg, pulse of 140 beats per minute, and respirations of 24 breaths per minute. Her extremities were cold and clammy, and a grimace to palpation of the left lower quadrant was noted on repeat examination.

This patient initially displayed a somewhat confusing presentation. Her abdominal tenderness was not immediately present. A repeat examination when the patient regained consciousness was warranted instead of waiting for her condition to deteriorate.

Calling the laboratory is sometimes appropriate to help laboratory personnel "triage" the specimens sent for evaluation for maximum efficiency. In this case, it may have been a lifesaving maneuver.

Fluid resuscitation was again initiated. Given the patient's age, abdominal pain, and gender, an ectopic pregnancy was suspected. The laboratory was called to expedite the urine pregnancy test. The obstetric consultant was contacted immediately after confirming the patient was indeed pregnant. She was taken to the operating room where an ectopic pregnancy was found and removed. Eight hundred milliliters of blood were in her peritoneal cavity.

It became clear after the patient's condition deteriorated she would be admitted to the hospital and possibly be taken directly to the operating room. What if her condition had remained stable and her laboratory test results showed no abnormalities and a positive pregnancy test?

At this point an ectopic pregnancy must be ruled out with ultrasound. (See Chapter 39, Pelvic Pain in Women.)

What if the pregnancy test was negative?

As discussed earlier, an ECG could have helped here. The cardiac monitor was already placed on the patient, but this is not a good method to determine all cardiac anomalies. If her condition had remained stable after the fluid bolus and ectopic pregnancy potential evaluated by ultrasonography, she still required admission for further evaluation. The same process had caused at least two episodes of hypotension and confusion. Computed tomography might also help complete the evaluation while in the emergency department.

This case emphasizes the importance of a good history and physical examination when evaluating the syncopal patient. Young patients most often have syncopal episodes from a vasovagal episode. This should not prevent a complete evaluation.

Formulating a working differential diagnosis while in the emergency department is always important, especially when the patient's condition is a complicated one. When no obvious cause can be determined, a cardiac cause should be entertained. Without some reasonable explanation for syncope, patients should receive further evaluation, even if in an outpatient scenario.

Bibliography

JOURNAL ARTICLES

Ahluwalia M, Quest M: Supraventricular tachycardia (SVT); strategies for diagnosis, risk stratification, and management in the emergency department setting. Emerg Med Reports 2002; 23(4): 41–52.

Bartfield JM: Syncope. Crit Decisions Emerg Med 1998; 12:7–11.

Day SC, Cook EF, Funkenstein H, et al: Evaluation and outcome of emergency room patients with transient loss of consciousness. Am J Med 1982; 72:15–23.

Driscoll DJ, Jacobsen SJ, Porter CJ, et al: Syncope in children and adolescents. J Am Coll Cardiol 1997; 29:1039–1045.

Gaeta TJ, Fiorini M, Ender K, et al: Potential drug-drug interactions in elderly patients presenting with syncope. J Emerg Med 2002; 2:159–162.

Hayes OW: Evaluation of syncope in the emergency department. Emerg Med Clin North Am 1998; 16:601–615.

Klein GJ, Lerman BB, Tavel ME: Syncope: Common clinical problem of diagnosis and management. Chest 1994; 105:1246–1248.

Linzer M, Yang BS, Estes M, et al: Diagnosing syncope: I. Value of history, physical examination, and electrocardiography. Ann Intern Med 1997; 126:989–996.

Linzer M, Yang BS, Estes M, et al: Diagnosing syncope: II. Unexplained syncope. Ann Intern Med 1997; 127: 76–86.

Mangrum JM, DiMarco JP: The evaluation and management of bradycardia. N Engl J Med 2000; 342:703–708.

Martin TP, Hanusa BH, Kapoor WN: Risk stratification of patients with syncope. Ann Emerg Med 1997; 29: 459–466.

Meyer MD, Handler J: Evaluation of the patient with syncope: An evidence based approach. Emerg Med Clin North Am 1999; 17:189–201.

Pancioli AM, McNeil PM, Arnold J: The clinical challenge of syncope: A cost-conscious and outcome-driven approach to patient evaluation and disposition. Emerg Med Rep 1998; 19:191–202.

Prodinger RJ, Reisdorff EJ: Syncope in children. Emerg Med Clin North Am 1998; 16:617–626.

Sarasin FP, Louis-Simoner M, Carballo D, et al: Prospective evaluation of patients with syncope: a population-based study. Am J Med 2001; 111:177–184.

CHAPTER 10

Hypertension

ARTHUR B. SANDERS

CASE *Study*

A 55-year-old obese woman complains of dyspnea, malaise, and vague chest and back pain. Her symptoms began 20 minutes earlier and became progressively worse. Vital signs are blood pressure, 230/150 mm Hg; pulse, 128 beats per minute; and respiratory rate, 32 breaths per minute.

INTRODUCTION

Hypertension affects more than 20% of the adult population and about 3% of the pediatric population. Chronic hypertension is a major cause of morbidity and mortality in the United States. Over the course of years, untreated hypertension causes substantial long-term morbidity and mortality due to stroke, congestive heart failure, peripheral vascular disease, sudden death, and, to a lesser extent, myocardial infarction.

Hypertension is a physical finding that is usually not accompanied by symptoms. Thus, detection of patients with hypertension is problematic and elevated pressures deserve appropriate follow-up. In the emergency department, an elevated blood pressure reading is often unrelated to the patient's chief complaint. Approximately one third of patients with elevated blood pressure measured in the emergency department have significant hypertension; another third have borderline hypertension, and the remainder are normotensive on follow-up visits.

Hypertension is classified according to the degree of elevation of the systolic or diastolic blood pressure. Table 10–1 lists the values that define optimal, normal, high normal, and stage 1, 2, and 3 hypertension. Stages 1 and 2 hypertension are the most common. Diagnosis of hypertension in asymptomatic cases requires two blood pressure measurements taken days apart. Severe hypertension is diagnosed and managed from a single blood pressure reading with or without symptoms indicative of organ damage.

Rarely, elevated blood pressure causes rapidly progressive end-organ damage. This is a *hypertensive emergency* and usually does not occur until the diastolic blood pressure is at least 115 mm Hg or more. Commonly, diastolic pressures are considerably higher, exceeding levels of 130 mm Hg. Prompt diagnosis and treatment of hypertensive emergencies may save organ function and the patient's life. Preeclampsia and eclampsia, both hypertensive emergencies of pregnancy, can occur at lower blood pressures (see Special Considerations). In emergency medicine most clinical management efforts are devoted to the diagnosis and management of hypertensive emergencies.

TABLE 10–1. Classification of Blood Pressure in Adults Older Than 18 Years

Category	Blood Pressure (mm Hg)		
	Systolic		*Diastolic*
Optimal	<120	and	<80
Normal	<130	and	<85
High-normal	130–139	or	85–89
Hypertension, stage 1	140–159	or	90–99
Hypertension, stage 2	160–179	or	100–109
Hypertension, stage 3	≥180	or	≥110

From the Joint National Committee on Prevention, Detection, Evaluation and Treatment of High Blood Pressure, National Heart, Lung and Blood Institute. Arch Intern Med 1997; 157: 2413–2445. Copyright © 1997, American Medical Association.

In the past, patients with elevated blood pressures but no acute end-organ effects were termed *hypertensive urgencies* and treatment was recommended to lower the blood pressure before the patient left the emergency department. Recent medical literature has called this practice into question and addressed whether hypertensive urgencies really exist. Most of these patients probably have chronic hypertension, and the danger of urgent treatment in the emergency department generally outweigh the benefits.

Hypertension results from any disorder affecting the circulation that increases cardiac output or total peripheral resistance. These changes can result from normal and pathologic processes in the autonomic, cardiovascular, renal, and endocrine systems. Each of these systems is eventually evaluated in the assessment of the hypertensive patient.

The organ systems primarily involved in hypertensive emergencies are also insidiously damaged by mild and moderate hypertension. These are the central nervous, cardiovascular, and renal systems. In the central nervous system (CNS), excessive elevation of blood pressure produces cerebral hypoperfusion, dilation of arterioles, and loss of the integrity of the blood-brain barrier. These effects in turn result in increased intracranial pressure, cerebral edema, and, eventually, decreased blood flow. Patients with chronic, uncontrolled mild-to-moderate hypertension may reset their cerebral autoregulation mechanism. In these patients, adequate cerebral blood flow is not maintained when the arterial pressure is low. Therefore, overzealous treatment of the hypertensive patient may result in significant compromise of cerebral blood flow. In the cardiovascular system, acute significant elevations in the diastolic pressure cause increases in the cardiac afterload. This increase results in increased myocardial work and oxygen demand to maintain cardiac output. This cardiovascular stress can lead to angina, myocardial infarction, or heart failure. The kidney is subject to arteriolar vasoconstriction, arteriolitis, parenchymal damage, and hormonal changes that can result in decreased renal function.

INITIAL APPROACH AND STABILIZATION

Priority Diagnosis

The ability to diagnose and treat hypertensive emergencies before the patient arrives in the emergency department is limited. Prehospital management is directed toward the presenting symptom, such as chest pain, shortness of breath, or headache.

Patients classed as having hypertensive emergencies are seen immediately and are placed in the resuscitation area. These emergencies are suspected in patients with diastolic pressures greater than 115 mm Hg who have evidence of end-organ damage. The accompanying finding may be altered mental status, severe headache, new focal neurologic deficits (including visual problems), seizures, chest or back pain, dyspnea, tachypnea, or hematuria.

Rapid Assessment

The initial assessment is devoted to the patient's symptoms, hypertensive history, possible causes of the acute presentation, and specific organ physical examination findings.

1. Is there chest or abdominal pain? When did it start? Was the onset sudden or insidious? What is the character of the pain? Does anything make the pain better or worse?
2. Is there a severe headache, weakness, visual problems, or change in mentation?
3. Is there any trouble breathing?
4. Is the patient known to be hypertensive? Has he or she ever been given medications for high blood pressure?
5. What medications does the patient take? Is there any circumstantial evidence of drug abuse such as needle tracks or drug paraphernalia at the scene?
6. For females of childbearing age, is the woman pregnant? If she is, is there an antecedent history of obstetric problems?
7. *Cardiovascular system.* Does the patient have rales, distended neck veins, or peripheral edema?
8. *Neurologic system.* Does the patient's mental status appear to be appropriate? Are there any gross neurologic deficits?
9. *Funduscopic examination.* Does the patient have papilledema or retinal hemorrhage?

Early Intervention

Patients undergo diagnostic and therapeutic maneuvers simultaneously.

1. Blood pressure measurement is repeated in both arms. Pulses are compared in all extremities. Blood pressure testing is repeated every 3 to 5 minutes early in the course of care.
2. An oxygen supplement is maintained at 2 to 4 L/min by nasal cannula. Higher flow rates may be necessary.

3. Intravenous access is established or confirmed. Dextrose/water 5% is given at a keep-open rate.
4. A cardiac monitor is placed, followed by a 12-lead electrocardiogram (ECG).
5. Immediate laboratory studies including urinalysis, complete blood cell count, and determination of serum electrolytes, blood urea nitrogen, creatinine, and glucose levels are ordered.
6. Emergency management consists of administering parenteral antihypertensive medications in hypertensive emergencies. The medications are selected depending on the end organ affected (Table 10–2). They are reviewed in detail under "Principles of Management."

CLINICAL ASSESSMENT

Once early stabilization and monitoring are established, a more detailed history and physical examination allow the physician to assess the end-organ effects and search for primary causes of hypertension.

History

Symptoms. What are the *time course* and *character* of the symptoms? Hypertensive emergencies usually have a rapid onset and fast (minutes to hours) progression.

Neurologic Signs. Does the patient have *headache, seizures,* and *visual disturbances* or other *focal neurologic findings* that are found with hypertensive encephalopathy, intracranial hemorrhage, eclampsia or preeclampsia, or pheochromocytoma?

Chest Pain. Is *chest pain* present? Ischemic cardiac pain is typically dull and boring and is often described as a feeling that something heavy is sitting on the patient's chest. Pain from a dissecting aortic aneurysm often radiates to the back and is described as a "tearing" sensation.

Congestive Heart Failure. Is there *shortness of breath, dyspnea* on exertion, *orthopnea,* or *peripheral edema* that may be suggestive of congestive heart failure?

Hematuria. Is *hematuria* present? A history of hematuria is highly suggestive of accelerated renal hypertension; this condition may have few other signs or symptoms until other organ systems start to fail.

Pregnancy. Is the patient *pregnant*? If so, the diastolic blood pressure at which the patient may have a hypertensive emergency or urgency is lowered to 100 mm Hg.

Similar Episodes. Have *similar episodes* occurred in the *past?* Are there precipitating factors? Are there treatments that have been effective? Episodes of congestive heart failure, pulmonary edema, aortic aneurysm, coronary artery ischemia, and eclampsia or preeclampsia tend to recur.

Past Medical History. Is there a history of hypertension, cardiovascular disease, or renal disease? Does the patient have a history of endocrinopathy, especially diabetes, medullary carcinoma of the thyroid, or pheochromocytoma? Diabetics are at increased risk of underlying renal disease, ischemic heart disease, and peripheral arterial disease. Patients with medullary carcinoma of the thyroid are at increased risk of developing pheochromocytoma.

Drug History. The *medication* history, including illicit drugs, alcohol, and compliance with prescribed medications, is important. The use of "uppers," including cocaine or amphetamines, can increase blood pressure, sometimes dramatically. Young, healthy patients can develop myocardial infarction and stroke as a side effect of these medications. Similar problems occur when patients on a monoamine oxidase inhibitor (e.g., phenelzine [Nardil]), prescribed for depression, ingest food with tyramine or certain drugs (e.g., pseudoephedrine). Sudden cessation of antihypertensive medication, especially clonidine, may lead to rebound hypertension, a condition in which the blood pressure rises above the level it was before treatment was begun.

Physical Examination

Appearance. Level of consciousness, evidence of distress, diaphoresis, and skin color are assessed.

Blood Pressure. Blood pressure in these patients can be very labile. The evolving underlying disease and the drugs used for treatment can cause wide swings that require close monitoring. Blood pressure measurements are taken in both arms and repeated every 3 to 5 minutes early in the course of care.

Noninvasive blood pressure measurements can be notoriously inaccurate. The blood pressure cuff must be of the appropriate size. The bladder of the cuff should encircle at least two thirds of the arm, and the width of the cuff should be 40% of the circumference of the arm at the midpoint (or 20% wider than the diameter). Most cuffs are labeled so that the appropriate size can be verified for each patient. Palpation of an artery while the blood pressure cuff is being inflated or released is one of the least accurate ways of determining

TABLE 10-2. Intravenous Drugs for Hypertensive Emergencies

Drug	Class	Dose and Route	Onset	Duration	Comments
Nitroprusside	Vasodilator	0.25–10 µg/kg/min	<1 min	2–5 min	Potent; titratable with short duration of action impairs cerebral autoregulation. Suspected coronary ischemia; titratable
Nitroglycerin	Vasodilator	5–100 µg/min	2–5 min	3–10 min	
Labetalol	α and β blocker	1–2 mg/min; max 300 mg	5 min	3–8 hr	Contraindicated in asthma, chronic obstructive pulmonary disease, heart block
Magnesium sulfate	Vasodilator; nerve stabilizer	2–4 g over 5 min then 1–2 g/hr	Minutes	Hours	Eclampsia and preeclampsia
Hydralazine	Arteriolar dilator	10–20 mg	10–30 min	2–6 hr	Causes tachycardia and can precipitate angina; useful in eclampsia/preeclampsia
Fenoldopam	Selective dopamine DAI receptor agonist	0.1–1.5 µg/kg/min	15 min	15 min (50% effect lost)	Preserves renal function. Intermediate onset and duration. Infusion approved for less than 48 hours.

blood pressure. Auscultating for Korotkoff sounds is the standard means of measurement. After the pressure is increased 20 to 30 mm Hg above the point where a palpable medial pulse is lost, the systolic pressure is recorded when the heart beat is heard clearly and at every beat as the cuff pressure is lowered. The diastolic level is recorded when the heart beat sounds begin to muffle and when they disappear. Which of the two points is more accurate is still controversial. The point at which sound becomes absent is more commonly recorded.

Oscillometric devices, also called automatic noninvasive blood pressure monitors, are useful when repeated measurements are necessary. They most accurately measure mean pressure; systolic and diastolic readings are subject to greater error. These devices can be set to measure automatically every few minutes.

Compared with noninvasive methods, invasive blood pressure measurement with an arterial line is considerably more accurate and gives continual information. This monitoring method is feasible in some emergency departments and is the ideal method for monitoring unstable hypertensive patients. When this method cannot be used, the best alternative is to use an oscillometric device that automatically repeats measurements.

Eye. Papilledema, fundal hemorrhage, and vasospasm occur as acute, ongoing hypertensive damage. The term *malignant hypertension* is applied to a diastolic blood pressure of more than 130 to 140 mm Hg with funduscopic pathology. Although the term is used less now than formerly, it appropriately describes the high potential for morbidity and mortality that is associated with these two findings. Chronic changes of hypertension (arteriovenous nicking, silver wiring) or diabetes (arteriolar aneurysms, cotton-wool exudates) may suggest an undiagnosed or longstanding underlying problem.

Cardiovascular Examination. The heart is auscultated for murmurs, gallops, and extra sounds; the neck is inspected for jugular venous distention; pulmonary rales and peripheral edema are sought. Patients with congestive heart failure may have S_3 gallops, rales, jugular venous distention, and peripheral edema. Aortic dissections involving the aortic root may cause a diastolic murmur of aortic regurgitation. Continuous (lasting through systole and diastole) murmurs may be heard in patients with coarctation of the aorta. Peripheral edema is often seen in pregnant patients with preeclampsia.

Pulmonary Findings. The major findings are those of pulmonary edema secondary to congestive heart failure. Increased respiratory rate and effort combined with diffuse fine rales are highly suggestive findings.

Abdomen. The gravid uterus and elevated blood pressure are usually diagnostic of eclampsia/preeclampsia. If the uterus is gravid, fetal heart tones are sought, usually with bedside Doppler-assisted ultrasound. The abdomen and flanks are carefully auscultated for bruits. The presence of a bruit suggests the presence of an arterial aneurysm or stenosis; the absence of a bruit does not rule them out. A pulsatile abdominal mass is palpated in up to 60% to 70% of cases of aortic aneurysm. If found, an aneurysm is assumed to be present until proven otherwise.

Peripheral Pulses. If a dissecting aneurysm is suspected, peripheral pulses are compared and rechecked often. Other conditions can cause different blood pressures in arteries of different extremities, such as peripheral arteriosclerosis or coarctation of the aorta.

Neurologic Findings. The neurologic examination includes an estimate of the mental status and cranial nerve, motor, sensation, deep tendon reflex, and plantar (Babinski) responses. Altered mental status and focal deficits may be seen with hypertensive encephalopathy, intracranial hemorrhage, and eclampsia or preeclampsia.

CLINICAL REASONING

After gathering the data, the emergency physician considers the following questions.

Is a Hypertensive Emergency Present?

The answer to this question is defined by demonstrated ongoing end-organ damage manifested by progressive CNS (including the eye), cardiovascular, or renal dysfunction.

Central Nervous System. Hypertensive encephalopathy and cerebrovascular accidents due to severe hypertension may cause significant neurologic dysfunction and damage. Hypertensive encephalopathy involves the entire brain, although the damage is not uniform. At autopsy, petechial hemorrhages and multiple small infarctions are found, often accompanied by edema. Some areas are relatively spared, and other areas are more heavily damaged. Thus, neurologic manifestations vary from patient to patient. Typically, hypertensive encephalopathy evolves over hours to days. Patients complain of headache, nausea, and vomiting. They may have an altered mental status or focal neurologic findings, including blindness, cranial nerve dysfunction, aphasia, and hemiparesis. In addition to or separate from encephalopathy, patients with severe hypertension often develop intracerebral hemorrhage. Differentiation between hypertensive encepha-lopathy and intracranial hemorrhage is important because treatment of hypertensive encephalopathy is more aggressive than for hypertension associated with intracranial hemorrhage. Intracranial hemorrhages are usually seen on CT, and a hemorrhage too small to be seen on CT is unlikely to result in an elevated blood pressure.

Cardiovascular System. Patients with cardiovascular damage secondary to hypertensive crisis may manifest hypertensive pulmonary edema, aortic dissection, myocardial infarction, or unstable angina. Myocardial oxygen consumption is increased because of the greater afterload in patients who are hypertensive. This increase can lead to ischemia in patients with underlying cardiovascular disease. One third of patients with a myocardial infarction have diastolic pressures of over 100 mm Hg. This elevation usually lasts for only a few hours.

Pulmonary edema is often the initial manifestation of a hypertensive emergency. An acute ischemic cardiac event or other factors such as salt overload may be considered as precipitants. More often, there is no clear precipitating event. Pulmonary edema may be present in a subtle or dramatic manner. The patient may complain of orthopnea and dyspnea on exertion or may demonstrate fine rales, mild tachypnea, and anxiety. Severe pulmonary edema manifests as extreme dyspnea, cough, frothy sputum, profound diaphoresis, cyanosis, pallor, and an anxious appearance.

Aortic dissection classically presents (in 75% to 85% of cases) with a sudden onset of severe tearing chest pain. The pain radiates to the epigastrium, extremities, or, more typically, the back. These patients may have diminished blood pressure distal to the site of the dissection. This finding varies from patient to patient. The findings for a given patient often change as the dissection progresses. If the aneurysm involves a carotid artery or the coronary arteries, the event may present as a cerebrovascular accident or myocardial infarction. Proximal aortic dissection may lead to acute aortic insufficiency or dissection into the pericardium, which can cause acute cardiac tamponade. Up to 20% of patients have some degree of congestive heart failure. Although hypertension is the rule, patients may be normotensive or hypotensive. The finding of unequal blood pressures or pulses or ischemia in two sites is consistent with a dissecting aneurysm.

Renal System. Acute renal failure may present as a hypertensive emergency. The patient may complain of hematuria or peripheral edema. Laboratory testing is usually necessary to confirm this diagnosis.

Is the Hypertension Essential or Secondary to Another Disease Process?

This question may not be pertinent to most management decisions in the emergency department. It is important to maintain a broad differential outlook and consider definitive care beyond the emergency department. The great majority (90% to 95%) of patients have essential hypertension with no underlying cause. Of those 5% to 10% of patients with secondary hypertension, approximately half have diseases in which the hypertension is potentially curable. The most common causes of secondary hypertension are chronic renal disease, renal artery stenosis, primary aldosteronism, coarctation of the aorta, Cushing's syndrome, pheochromocytomas, and drug-induced hypertension.

Renal Artery Stenosis. Renal artery stenosis is the most common potentially curable cause of hypertension. It is seen in 1% to 5% of hypertensive patients. Compromised renal perfusion caused by the stenosis promotes the secretion of renin. Renin produces an increase in angiotensin II, a potent vasoconstrictor, which also increases sympathetic vasomotor activity. Renal artery stenosis occurs most commonly in two groups of patients, elderly men with atherosclerotic disease and young women with fibrous dysplasia of the renal artery. An abdominal bruit is present in 40% to 80% of patients with renal artery stenosis. Other clinical findings that have been associated with renovascular hypertension include severe hypertensive retinopathy (papilledema, flame hemorrhages, cotton-wool exudates), acute onset of severe hypertension, hypertension resistant to treatment, thin body habitus, and hypokalemia. Diagnostic studies include renal arteriography and renal vein renin sampling.

Aldosteronism. Mineralocorticoid excess or aldosteronism is an uncommon but potentially curable cause of hypertension. Patients with mineralocorticoid excess experience sodium retention, volume expansion, and increased cardiac output. The degree of hypertension is usually mild to moderate. Patients typically demonstrate hypokalemia and increased potassium excretion on laboratory evaluation. Aldosteronism may be caused primarily by an adrenal adenoma or hyperplasia or may be secondary to other diseases such as Cushing's syndrome, congenital adrenal hyperplasia, or exogenous mineralocorticoids such as heavy ingestion of licorice that contains glycyrrhizic acid. Patients have elevated levels of aldosterone that do not suppress normally with volume expansion.

Renal Disease. Chronic renal disease is the most common form of secondary hypertension. It occurs in more than 80% of patients with end-stage renal disease.

Pheochromocytoma. Pheochromocytoma is an uncommon cause of reversible hypertension. It represents a tumor of chromaffin cells, usually in the adrenal medulla, producing excess catecholamines, epinephrine, and norepinephrine that cause paroxysmal hypertension. Ten percent of pheochromocytomas are extra-adrenal. Patients usually complain of a pounding, severe headache, palpitations, and excessive perspiration. Episodes of hypertension may be paroxysmal with normotensive, symptom-free intervals in 50% of patients. Laboratory tests may show hyperglycemia. Pheochromocytomas are associated with specific diseases, including medullary thyroid carcinoma, hyperparathyroidism, neurofibromatosis, cerebellar hemangioblastoma, mucosal neuromas, and intestinal ganglioneuromatosis. About 10% of patients have a family history of pheochromocytoma. Biochemical tests such as those determining fasting levels of plasma catecholamines and urinary vanillylmandelic acid can help to make the diagnosis.

Drugs. Medications are an important cause of secondary hypertension. Drugs such as cocaine and amphetamines may produce severe hypertensive crisis. In addition, withdrawal from drugs such as alcohol or clonidine may precipitate severe hypertension. Finally, some drugs such as monoamine oxidase inhibitors may react with tyramine-containing foods such as red wine, aged cheese, beer, and pickled herring to produce a hypertensive emergency.

DIAGNOSTIC ADJUNCTS

Diagnostic tests help to confirm the presence of end-organ damage caused by severe hypertension and can help to differentiate primary from secondary causes of hypertension.

Laboratory Studies

Blood Urea Nitrogen, Creatinine, Electrolytes, Glucose, and Complete Blood Cell Count. These tests are indicated in all patients with significant hypertension. Blood urea nitrogen and creatinine values may rise steeply, indicating a significant loss of renal function. An elevated glucose concentration may disclose the existence of diabetes mellitus. Hypokalemia may indicate the presence of hyperaldosteronism or high-renin forms of hypertension. Microangiopathic hemolytic anemia is suspected if broken red cells are noted in the peripheral smear and the red cell count is decreased.

Urinalysis. Urinalysis is indicated in all patients with significant hypertension. In patients with ongoing renal damage, blood and protein leak into the urine and are usually discovered by testing with a urine dipstick. These tests are quite sensitive, although other causes besides hypertensive renal damage may result in protein or blood being found in the specimen. Test strips can also detect glucosuria, which may be caused by diabetes mellitus. On microscopic examination, red cell casts imply glomerulonephritis and white cell casts suggest pyelonephritis. Proteinuria with red cells or red cell casts often indicates the presence of acute renal dysfunction secondary to hypertension.

Drug Screen. Urine or serum drug analysis is indicated in any hypertensive patient in whom drug abuse is suspected. Drug screening can clarify whether the patient suffers from the toxic effects of cocaine or other "uppers." Screening tests detect the presence of cocaine and most amphetamines; they do not give quantitative information about the amount of substance ingested by the patient.

Electrocardiogram

A 12-lead ECG is indicated for all patients with severe hypertension. Patients with ischemic heart disease may have ECG evidence of ischemia. Most patients with an evolving myocardial infarction will develop ECG changes within hours after the onset of the infarction. Left ventricular hypertrophy is very suggestive of chronic hypertension. The ECG is abnormal in 80% of 90% of patients with aortic dissection.

Radiologic Imaging

Radiographs. Posteroanterior and lateral chest radiographs are ordered in patients with hypertensive emergencies. They are highly sensitive for findings of pulmonary edema. Early in the process of pulmonary edema, vascular markings become blurred and interstitial edema may be seen. These changes are subtle and can be missed. Normally, the dependent vessels are larger than the upper ones. As pulmonary edema progresses beyond the early stages, the upper vessels enlarge. This is called *cephalization* of flow. In the latter stages of pulmonary edema the lungs become diffusely hazy. Frequently, cardiomegaly or left ventricular hypertrophy is noted. When the disease has progressed to this advanced stage, the changes are easy to see and are universally present.

Chest radiographs of patients with aortic aneurysms typically show widening of the superior mediastinum with "blurring of the aortic knob." If the vascular intima is calcified, the aortic wall will appear abnormally thick. These diagnostic findings are present in 80% of cases. Coarctation of the aorta can appear on the chest radiograph as disproportionate widening of the arteries proximal to the site of the coarctation; there may also be a narrowing described as a "three sign" of the aorta at the site of the coarctation. In asymptomatic patients the left ventricle is often enlarged, suggesting a chronic problem.

Computed Tomography. CT of the head is necessary for the patient with neurologic findings. CT will detect an intracranial hemorrhage and possibly indicate another pathologic process such as a stroke.

Aortography, Computed Tomography of Chest. Aortography or a chest CT scan is indicated for the patient in whom a dissecting aortic aneurysm is suspected. Both tests reveal the dissection with a very high degree of accuracy, although a few false-negative tests have been reported. CT is usually performed more quickly than aortography, but aortography usually provides more accurate information about the location of intimal tears. This information is important for surgical management. Performance of both tests improves the diagnostic accuracy.

PRINCIPLES OF MANAGEMENT

General Management

The management of patients with hypertensive emergencies depends on the following principles:

1. Blood pressure is gradually lowered using intravenous medication as appropriate for the degree of crisis. The general goal is to lower the mean arterial pressure no more than 25% in less than 2 hours. Treatment is directed toward the 160/100 mm Hg range over 2 to 6 hours. Rapid decreases in the blood pressure may precipitate cerebral, coronary, or renal ischemia.
2. Complications of hypertensive crisis including myocardial infarction, CNS hemorrhage, pulmonary edema, and renal failure are treated.
3. The possibility of underlying secondary hypertension is addressed.

As with other conditions seen by emergency physicians, it is prudent to search for the most cat-astrophic illnesses first. There is no need to correct the blood pressure to "normal" levels, and it is often dangerous to do so.

Pharmacologic agents are necessary for the treatment of patients with hypertension. Patients with hypertensive emergencies are treated with intravenous medications under close hemodynamic supervision and with cardiac monitoring. Optimally, an arterial catheter continuously measures the systolic, diastolic, and mean blood pressures. Serial external measurements by blood pressure cuff usually suffice. The intravenous medication is titrated to the desired blood pressure and the clinical response. Three of the most common drugs used to control hypertensive emergencies listed in Table 10–2 are briefly discussed next.

Drugs for Hypertensive Emergencies

Nitroprusside is widely used for hypertensive emergencies and is often the initial medication of choice. It is an arterial and venous dilator that acts rapidly, thus decreasing both preload and afterload. It has minimal effect on cardiac output and myocardial blood flow. When nitroprusside is administered over a prolonged period of time, thiocyanate intoxication may occur. This is generally not a concern for the initial treatment in the emergency department.

Nitroglycerin is an arterial and venous dilator that also dilates the large coronary arteries. It has a greater effect on the capacitance (venous) vessels. Administered intravenously, it is effective in lowering the preload and afterload immediately. It is particularly useful for hypertensive emergencies with coronary insufficiency.

Labetalol is an α_1 and β blocker that has a direct vasodilatory effect. It reduces systolic arterial pressure and total peripheral vascular resistance without producing reflex tachycardia. Cerebral and renal blood flows are maintained despite reductions in blood pressure. It is safe for patients with severe renal insufficiency.

Fenoldopam is a newly approved dopamine-receptor agonist that has potential benefit in hypertensive emergencies. It has an intermediate time of onset and duration of action, is tolerated well, and may uniquely protect renal blood flow. It is approved for infusions of less than 48 hours, and has had limited exposure in emergency medicine practice.

Management of Specific End-Organ Hypertensive Emergencies

Hypertensive Encephalopathy. Ongoing neurologic damage necessitates prompt control of blood pressure, ideally within 1 hour. Normally, sodium nitroprusside is the drug of choice for these patients because it produces no inherent CNS side effects. Intravenous labetalol can also be used.

Other Intracranial Hypertensive Emergencies. Subdural and epidural hematomas are best treated with prompt surgery. Treatment of intra-parenchymal and subarachnoid hemorrhages is problematic. Unfortunately, most cerebrovascular hemorrhages caused by hypertension belong in these categories. In many patients, the CNS "baro-stat" is reset, and some elevation in the mean arterial pressure is necessary to maintain cerebral perfusion. Therefore, it is dangerous to lower the pressure too quickly. The blood pressure is initially reduced by only 15% to 20%. The patient is then reassessed, and, if stable, another 15% to 20% decrease is attempted. The goal is to lower the diastolic pressure into the 100- to 110-mm Hg range. Nitroprusside and labetalol are the drugs of choice. These patients may benefit from other treatments that reduce intracranial pressure, such as mannitol.

Hypertensive Pulmonary Edema. Nitrates are excellent drugs in this situation. They dilate both arteries and veins, reducing preload and afterload. Nitroglycerin also dilates the coronary arteries and is especially useful when patients have concomitant angina. Nitroprusside is relatively more effective in dilating the peripheral arteries and reducing afterload. Furosemide (Lasix) and bumetanide (Bumex) are also used to increase venous capacitance and diurese excess water. Morphine sulfate is given intravenously to reduce sympathetic overflow, dilate the veins, and reduce anxiety. The goal of blood pressure reduction is to maximize perfusion and minimize cardiac work. This is attained most precisely by titrating the antihypertensive drugs while following arterial pressure, pulmonary artery wedge pressure, and cardiac output.

Acute Aortic Dissection. The therapeutic goal is to quickly reduce the mean arterial blood pressure and the rate of rise of aortic pulse pressure during the cardiac cycle (dP/dt). Nitroprusside is administered with a β blocker such as propranolol or esmolol to decrease mean arterial pressure while reducing dP/dt. The β blocker is titrated to avoid sudden heart failure or bronchial spasm. Invasive arterial line monitoring is especially useful in these patients because it allows one to see the pressure wave and monitor dP/dt. Labetalol may be used by itself or in combination with nitroprusside. Trimethaphan is rarely used because of the unpleasant side effects of ganglionic blockade. Type A aneurysms, which involve the ascending aorta, require surgical inter-

vention. Uncomplicated type B (DeBakey type III) aneurysms, which involve only the descending aorta, may be treated medically. Early mortality occurs in up to 50% of these patients if they are not treated properly.

Hypertensive Renal Failure. Symptoms of this emergency may not become evident until the patient suffers severe renal failure. Prompt treatment may salvage some damaged but still viable renal tissue. Because almost all of these patients have elevated renin levels, angiotensin-converting enzyme inhibitors captopril and enalapril are useful. Unfortunately, it takes a few hours for these drugs to produce an antihypertensive effect. Initial parenteral treatment is usually begun with nitroprusside or labetalol.

Pharmacologically Induced Hypertension. In hypertension induced by circulating catecholamines (e.g., by monoamine oxidase inhibitors, sympathomimetic agents such as cocaine or amphetamines) or by pheochromocytoma, phentolamine (Regitine) may be used as a potent α blocker. If the initial response to these drugs is inadequate, nitroprusside is often effective. Pure β blockers may result in unopposed α-adrenergic stimulation and worsen the situation.

Withdrawal from Antihypertensives. Relatively sudden withdrawal from antihypertensive agents may lead to "rebound" hypertension above baseline hypertensive states. This rebound is not a problem with diuretics, but it is with agents that block sympathetic tone, especially clonidine (Catapres). It occurs in 1% to 5% of patients who abruptly stop taking the drug. The time course varies with the agent involved. With clonidine, the onset of rebound hypertension typically begins 18 to 20 hours after the last dose. This condition responds well to reinstitution of the drug. Patients with specific end-organ damage may be treated like patients with the other hypertensive emergencies described earlier.

Withdrawal from CNS Depressants. As patients withdraw from CNS depressants they enter a relatively sustained hyperadrenergic state characterized by tachycardia, tachypnea, hypertension, and fever. The time course of the withdrawal process varies with the involved drug. In general, the longer the half-life of the drug, the longer the withdrawal process. Ethanol withdrawal evolves over a period of about 4 days, and diazepam (Valium) withdrawal lasts over about 9 days. If untreated, withdrawal sometimes progresses to profound vasomotor instability, characterized by alternating hyperadrenergic and hypoadrenergic states such as delirium tremens. Delirium tremens has a significant mortality, so it is important to diagnose and treat these patients early. A wide variety of sedative-hypnotic medications have been used successfully to treat withdrawal. The benzodiazepines are the drugs of choice. Lorazepam (Ativan), chlordiazepoxide (Librium), and diazepam are frequently used because they have desirable pharmacokinetic properties and cause minimal respiratory depression. These agents can be used to treat most patients with depressant withdrawal. Narcotic withdrawal usually does not require any treatment; if treatment is necessary, clonidine or methadone is often used.

Hypertensive Urgencies: An Uncertain Diagnosis

The category of hypertensive urgency is clouded by controversy. The term has been used in the literature to describe a state in which the blood pressure is severely elevated (stage 3 and higher, see Table 10–1) but the patient does not have evidence of end-organ dysfunction. For several years, the strategy for these patients was to lower their blood pressure gradually over a few hours with oral agents such as sublingual nifedipine or oral clonidine. Recently, some authorities have questioned whether the term *hypertensive urgency* has any real meaning. The widespread treatment of patients with *hypertensive urgencies* (asymptomatic stage 3 blood pressure readings) with sublingual nifedipine has resulted in significant adverse effects in some patients, including stroke and acute myocardial infarction. The Joint National Committee on the Prevention, Detection, Evaluation, and Treatment of High Blood Pressure notes that "elevated blood pressure alone, in the absence of symptoms or new or progressive target organ damage, rarely requires emergency therapy" (Sixth Report, 1997). There is also evidence that when patients with asymptomatic blood pressure elevations are reassured and put in a quiet room, the blood pressures decrease gradually over time with no medication. There is no clear evidence that acutely lowering the blood pressure of asymptomatic patients over several hours improves their outcome. Nifedipine should not be used for acutely lowering the blood pressure because its effects cannot be well controlled. If an oral agent is needed for gradual reduction of the blood pressure, clonidine is a safer alternative.

In the majority of emergency department patients, asymptomatic hypertension is a chronic disease. If the blood pressure is in the range of stage 3 or higher, the patient will need chronic treatment with antihypertensives. If the patient is on antihypertensive medication, the treatment regimen needs to be reevaluated by the primary physician. Thus, the most important emergency department management principle for the patient with asymptomatic hypertension is ensuring follow-up for chronic care. A telephone consultation is made with the primary physician to decide on a management strategy and ensure prompt follow-up within a few days to a week. Most commonly, patients with newly diagnosed hypertension are started on a diuretic or β blocker as first-line treatment. However, treatment must be individualized based on the patient factors and comorbid diseases.

Moderate and Mild Hypertension

Patients with relatively mild high blood pressure (stages 1 and 2) and no ongoing end-organ damage need no emergency department intervention. They are referred for follow-up.

SPECIAL CONSIDERATIONS
Pregnancy

Pregnant patients are more sensitive to the effects of hypertension than are other adults. The American College of Obstetrics and Gynecology defines *hypertension of pregnancy* as (1) a diastolic pressure of greater than 90 mm Hg or greater than 15 mm Hg above baseline or (2) a systolic pressure of greater than 140 mm Hg or 30 mm Hg above baseline. These patients are at increased risk for complications, including fetal mortality, eclampsia, and preeclampsia. Preeclampsia may involve hypertension, edema, proteinuria, microangiopathic hemolytic anemia, thrombocytopenia, and abnormal results of liver enzyme tests. Eclampsia is preeclampsia accompanied by new-onset seizures. Eclampsia and preeclampsia occur only in the latter part of gestation, so in most cases the diagnosis of pregnancy is not in doubt. Pregnant patients are at increased risk for preeclampsia if

1. Previous episodes of preeclampsia have occurred.
2. Multiple gestations exist.
3. A hydatidiform mole is present.
4. There is a family history of preeclampsia.
5. The patient belongs to the lower socioeconomic classes. (This finding may relate to adequacy of prenatal care.)
6. The patient is a child or an older primigravid woman.

Patients with eclampsia or preeclampsia typically have hyperactive deep tendon reflexes. Reflex reactivity may be serially assessed as a means of monitoring therapy. The visual and optic funduscopic changes described in the earlier section on hypertensive encephalopathy place these patients at risk for cerebral hemorrhage. Magnesium sulfate is the drug of choice for treatment of the neurologic symptoms, and it may also help to lower the blood pressure. Hydralazine is the drug of choice for blood pressure control, especially antepartum, because it preserves uterine blood flow. Although these agents help to control the disease, delivery of the infant is the only cure for preeclampsia and eclampsia.

Pediatric Patients

The issue of asymptomatic hypertension in children has been the source of much discussion. There is evidence that many of these children, if left untreated for an extended period of time, will develop the complications of hypertension as adults. It is prudent to refer children with high blood pressure to specialists for further evaluation. To determine which children are hypertensive one must refer to tables or graphs of normal values for children. Children are considered hypertensive if they consistently have blood pressures above the 95th percentile for age.

Elderly Patients

Hypertension is common in patients 60 years and older. The treatment of hypertension in older adults has been demonstrated to decrease the risk of stroke, cardiovascular disease, and congestive heart failure and improve mortality. Older persons may have elevated systolic pressures or large pulse pressures (systolic minus diastolic pressure). This may indicate reduced vascular compliance and is correlated with cardiovascular disease, stroke, renal failure, and higher mortality. Interpreting blood pressure measurements in older persons is a complex task. Some have pseudohypertension owing to excessive vascular stiffness in major arteries. Others may be prone to "white coat" hypertension caused by the stress of the emergency department environment. Older persons more commonly have orthostatic changes in their blood pressure. Thus, multiple blood pressure readings in different environments may be important for diagnosis. However, treatment by a primary physician is essential for lowering the risk of complications from chronic hypertension in older persons.

DISPOSITION AND FOLLOW-UP

Disposition of the patient depends on accurate classification of the hypertension, assessment of end-organ damage, and response to treatment.

Admission

All patients with hypertensive emergencies are admitted. Essentially, all require close monitoring in the intensive care unit. Rarely, patients are sent to a "monitored bed" if the blood pressure has been controlled in the emergency department and there is no longer a need for intravenous agents. Repeated blood pressure measurements are still necessary.

Discharge

Patients with asymptomatic stage 3 hypertension are discharged from the emergency department with follow-up in a week or less by a primary physician. The plan for treatment is discussed with the physician. An agreement is necessary on outpatient medication and a follow-up appointment. If follow-up cannot be arranged, the patient should return to the emergency department in 24 hours for a reassessment.

Patients with stage 1 or 2 blood pressure readings are referred for follow-up to their primary physician. Many patients with isolated elevated blood pressure measurements are found to have chronic hypertension, and their long-term prognosis is greatly improved if they are correctly diagnosed and treated.

FINAL POINTS

- Most of the patients seen in the emergency department with elevated blood pressure have mild or moderate hypertension. They do not need immediate treatment and are referred for further care.
- Patients with severe hypertension are immediately evaluated for end-organ involvement, which defines a hypertensive emergency. The end-organ systems at special risk are the neurologic system (including the eyes), the cardiovascular system, and the renal system.
- The blood pressure cuff must be of the appropriate size and must be correctly applied. The blood pressure is measured in at least two extremities, and the pulses are palpated in all extremities.
- A careful physical examination is important to search for end-organ effects of severe hypertension.
- The treatment of a hypertensive emergency is a controlled decrease in blood pressure over time to specific pre-determined levels. This is optimally accomplished with intravenous medication and serial reassessments.

- Drugs, especially cocaine, are in wide use and may cause hypertensive emergencies. Abrupt cessation of antihypertensive medications can produce severe rebound hypertension.
- Pregnant women become hypertensive at relatively low blood pressures. Their blood pressure readings must be compared with baseline values for the same patient.
- Patients sent home with hypertension are given clear instructions for follow-up with a primary physician.

CASE Study

The patient is a 55-year-old woman with a blood pressure of 230/150 mm Hg and cardiopulmonary symptoms. The rescue squad stated the patient was in moderate respiratory distress. Rales were heard halfway up the lung fields. Her neck veins (external jugular) were distended, and she had 2+ pitting edema in the lower extremities. Medications found in the patient's home included furosemide (Lasix), clonidine (Catapres), glyburide (DiaBeta), and alprazolam (Xanax).

This patient has serious disease. Her potential diagnoses include myocardial infarction, pulmonary edema, dissecting aortic aneurysm, and clonidine or alprazolam withdrawal. Oxygen, nitroglycerin, furosemide, and morphine are ordered for treatment of hypertension, chest pain, and probable pulmonary edema. Because a dissecting aneurysm is a possibility, early chest CT is considered.

On further examination, the patient was markedly dyspneic; she gave only brief answers to questions. She was not accompanied by her family. She had developed dyspnea during the past 2 hours that had worsened in the past 30 minutes. Her vague, nonlocalized chest and back pain came on at the same time and persisted. She described previous hospitalizations for "heart trouble" but could not give any details. She denied a history of renal disease, hematuria, or flank pain. She confirmed taking the medication brought in by the rescue squad. She denied taking any other prescribed, over-the-counter, or recreational drugs. She stated that she complied with the prescribed medication regimens.

The patient was sitting forward, using accessory muscles of respiration, and breathing at a rate of 36 breaths per minute. She had rales extending throughout both lung fields. Seven centimeters of jugular venous distention were present. Heart sounds were difficult to hear over the rales. Results of the neurologic and abdominal examinations were unremarkable. Repeat blood pressure measurements were about 240/130 mm Hg in all extremities. The pulse rate was 130 beats per minute.

The woman was in acute distress. The blood pressure, rales, jugular venous distention, respiration distress, and history identified her as a patient with a hypertensive emergency, probably with hypertensive pulmonary edema, although an aortic dissection was a possibility.

The cardiac monitor showed a sinus rhythm with a heart rate of 130 beats per minute. Twelve-lead ECG was interpreted as a sinus tachycardia with borderline left ventricular hypertrophy. There were no ischemic changes. A portable chest radiograph was read as marked cardiomegaly and distended pulmonary vasculature with cephalization of flow. The aorta appeared normal. A Foley catheter was placed and drained 100 mL of clear yellow urine, which on dipstick testing proved negative for glucose, protein, and blood.

The laboratory findings reinforced the working diagnosis of hypertensive congestive heart failure with pulmonary edema. In this patient, as in others, more than one cause may be producing the situation—for instance, both clonidine withdrawal and hypertensive pulmonary edema could be operative. The chest radiograph findings and the normal peripheral pulses made an aortic aneurysm unlikely. The normal results of urinalysis made renovascular disease improbable. The normal neurologic findings decreased the possibility of an intracranial event. The patient was not of childbearing age. The relatively normal ECG findings suggested that ischemic heart disease was unlikely, but this could not be ruled out. The patient continued to require cardiac monitoring, cardiac enzymes, and serial ECGs during treatment and recovery.

The patient was given 12 mg of morphine over 40 to 60 minutes in 2- to 3-mg increments. Furosemide, 80 mg, was given intravenously and an intravenous nitroglycerin drip was started. The patient's blood pressure decreased to 180/90 mm Hg, and her anxiety diminished in concert with her improved ability to breathe.

Continued on following page

This patient was appropriately treated for hypertensive pulmonary edema. Lowering the blood pressure decreased the afterload and myocardial oxygen consumption. She needs continued intensive care monitoring of her arterial and pulmonary artery wedge pressures. Because the chest radiograph demonstrated a normal aorta and her chest pain symptoms resolved with limited improvement in blood pressure, it was reasonable to not order an emergency chest CT scan to rule out a thoracic aneurysm.

The patient's condition continued to stabilize in the emergency department. She was transferred to an intensive care unit, where she spent 2 days. She was discharged from the hospital after 5 days with a diagnosis of hypertensive congestive heart failure. She was well at 4-month follow-up.

Bibliography

TEXT

Kaplan NM: Kaplan's Clinical Hypertension, edn. 8. Philadelphia: Lippincott, Williams and Wilkins; 2002.

Mancia G: Manual of Hypertension. Edinburgh: Churchill Livingstone; 2002.

JOURNAL ARTICLES

Chaing WK, Jamshahi B: Asymptomatic hypertension in the ED. Am J Emerg Med 1998; 16:701–704.

Elliot WJ: Hypertensive emergencies. Crit Care Clin 2001; 17:435–451.

Grossman E, Messerli FH, Grodzicki T, Kowey P: Should a moratorium be placed on sublingual nifedipine capsules given for hypertensive emergencies and pseudoemergencies? JAMA 1996; 276:1328–1331.

Hyman DJ, Pavlik VN: Characterizations of patients with uncontrolled hypertension in the United States. N Engl J Med 2001; 345:479–486.

Murphy MB, Murray C, Shorten GD: Fenoldopam: a selective peripheral dopamine-receptor agonist for the treatment of severe hypertension. N Engl J Med 2001; 345:1548–1557.

Pitts SR, Adams RP: Emergency department hypertension and regression to the mean. Ann Emerg Med 1998; 31: 214–218.

Sixth Report of the Joint National Committee on Prevention, Detection, Evaluation and Treatment of High Blood Pressure. Arch Intern Med 1997; 157:2413–2445.

Thach AM, Schultz PJ: Nonemergent hypertension: New perspective for the emergency medicine physician. Emerg Med Clin North Am 1995; 13:1009–1035.

Zampaglione B, Pascale C, Marchisio M, Cavallo-Perin P: Hypertensive urgencies and emergencies: Prevalence and clinical presentation. Hypertension 1996; 27:144–147.

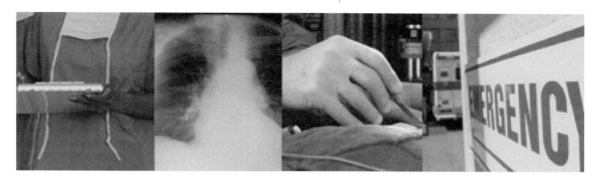

CUTANEOUS DISORDERS

CHAPTER 11

Rash

ALEXANDER T. TROTT

CASE *Study*

A 50-year-old ill-appearing man was brought to the hospital with fever and weakness. The illness began with the appearance of a rash on his legs. Several small, dark purple spots covered both of his ankles. Because he appeared ill, the triage nurse brought him to the acute care area of the emergency department.

INTRODUCTION

The emergency physician is confronted with a wide variety of skin disorders. In some settings complaints related to the skin make up 5% to 8% of all visits. Skin findings contribute to diagnosis and management decisions in another 5% of emergency department patients. Although rarely life threatening, skin lesions and rashes are a source of considerable discomfort and anxiety. Dermatologic diagnoses are often missed, treated incorrectly, and referred (or not) inappropriately. As the clinician who sees dermatologic problems when they first present, the emergency physician must have a clear understanding and organized approach to the patient presenting with "rash."

The skin is composed of three layers: the epidermis, the dermis, and the subcutaneous layer. In addition to these layers, the skin contains various adnexal structures such as hair follicles, nails, sebaceous glands, eccrine sweat glands and apocrine sweat glands, and cutaneous blood vessels and nerves (Fig. 11–1).

The epidermis is the outermost layer of skin. In this layer reside the melanocytes, which produce the skin pigment melanin. Melanin serves as the protective filter against ultraviolet radiation. The outermost layer of the epidermis, the stratum corneum, with its interlocking sheets of keratin and lipid is responsible for the barrier function of the skin. The dermal-epidermal junction is a complex region. It is the site of immunoglobulin and complement depositions and of blister formation in many vesiculobullous diseases. The dermis makes up the bulk of the skin. Major components of the dermis are the collagen and elastin fibers and the ground substance, which is responsible for the strength and elasticity of the skin. The subcutaneous layer consists mostly of fat cells intermingled with connective tissue. It provides a protective cushion against trauma.

The cutaneous blood supply consists of arterioles connected to capillary loops, which are associated with venules to form the vascular network in the dermis. These blood vessels regulate temperature by vasodilation and vasoconstriction. Cutaneous sensation is mediated by both myelinated and nonmyelinated sensory nerves terminating in the dermis. Itching is a unique cutaneous sensation that probably represents a type of weak pain. Scratching converts the intolerable sensation of itching to the more familiar sensation of pain and can relieve the pruritus.

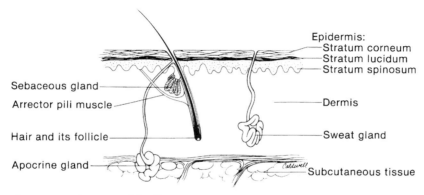

FIGURE 11–1 • Cross-sectional anatomy of the skin.

The skin serves as a strategic interface between the body and the external environment. It functions as a physical barrier, maintains temperature control, offers protection from ultraviolet light, and operates as a source of sensory input to the body.

To describe a cutaneous disorder appropriately, a common language must be used and understood by all clinicians. These descriptive terms are crucial in the development of a differential diagnosis.

A *lesion* is a general term for any single, small area of skin disease. *Rash* is a more extensive process that is generally made up of many lesions. See Tables 11–1 and 11–2 for further terms and definitions.

INITIAL APPROACH AND STABILIZATION

Most cutaneous disorders presenting in the emergency department are not life threatening, and the patient is not systemically ill. In these cases, it is appropriate to begin with a detailed dermatologic history and a physical examination. However, the clinician must recognize the patient with a serious cutaneous disorder or a cutaneous manifestation of a serious systemic illness.

PRIORITY DIAGNOSES

The most likely life-threatening disorders that can present with a rash include the following:

- Meningococcemia
- Urticaria angioedema with anaphylaxis
- Cellulitis with sepsis
- Erythema multiforme major
- Pemphigus vulgaris/bullous pemphigoid.

Initial Assessment

Each of the following symptoms should be explored, because they commonly accompany a potentially serious rash:

- *Hoarseness, voice change, or difficulty swallowing:* These features may be associated with upper airway edema secondary to anaphylaxis.
- *Shortness of breath:* This may be caused by anaphylaxis, allergic reactions, and urticaria.
- *Neck stiffness, headache:* Meningitis can be accompanied by a nonspecific maculopapular rash or petechiae.
- *Abdominal pain, nausea, vomiting:* Anaphylaxis and Rocky Mountain spotted fever are disorders that affect the gastrointestinal tract.

TABLE 11–1. Basic Terminology

Primary Skin Lesions: Initial, Basic Lesion

Macule:	An area of color change <2 cm in diameter. Is not palpable. Visible margins only. May be red, brown, yellow, or white.
Patch:	Macules >2 cm in diameter.
Papule:	A palpable mass <1.5 cm in diameter. May be red, brown, yellow, white, or skin-colored. May be flat topped, dome shaped, or pointed. May have a smooth surface or have surface changes, such as scale, crust, erosion, or ulceration.
Plaque:	A flat-topped, palpable lesion >1.5 cm in diameter. Papule that has enlarged in length and width but not depth.
Nodule:	A papule that has enlarged in length, width, and depth. More than 1.5 cm in diameter. May be solid, edematous, or cystic and may be dome shaped or have sloped shoulders.
Wheal:	An edematous papule containing nonloculated fluid.
Vesicle:	A fluid-filled papule <1 cm in diameter in which the fluid is loculated. Usually skin colored because they contain clear fluid.
Bulla:	A vesicle >1 cm in diameter.
Petechiae:	A circumscribed deposit of blood <0.5 cm in diameter.
Purpura:	A circumscribed deposit of blood >0.5 cm in diameter.

Secondary Skin Lesions

Scales:	They may develop during the evolutionary process of the cutaneous disorder or are created by scratching or infection. Shedding of excess keratin from surface epithelial cells. Reflects abnormal keratinization. Loose flakes of scale are white or gray and rough on palpation. Compacted scale is translucent and shiny and smooth on palpation.
Crust:	A collection of dried serum and cellular debris. Usually yellow or yellow-brown unless red blood cells are involved—then the crust is black.
Excoriation:	Linear or angular erosions due to scratching.
Lichenification:	An area of thickened epidermis that results from habitual rubbing. The normal skin markings are accentuated and may be accompanied by a mild amount of scaling.

TABLE 11–2. Other Descriptive Terms

Margination:	The shape of a lesion as viewed in cross section, representing the transition from normal to diseased skin. If that transition occurs abruptly (dome-shaped, square shoulders), the lesion is sharply marginated. If the transition zone is gradual (slope shoulders), it is poorly marginated. This term is helpful in distinguishing the papulosquamous diseases with their sharp margins from the eczematous diseases, which have poor margination.
Configuration:	The shape of a lesion as viewed from above.
Linear or angular:	Suggests that external factors are causative agents, as in contact dermatitis.
Annular:	A ring-shaped lesion. This shape implies outward extension with central clearing.
Discoid:	A lesion with outward extension without central clearing.
Nummular:	A coin-shaped lesion without central clearing.
Iris or target:	A ring-shaped lesion with a central bull's-eye.

- *Arthralgias:* Many disorders, such as gonococcemia and Lyme disease, are manifested by rash with joint symptoms.
- *Easy bruisability, mucosal bleeding:* Leukemia and drug toxicity that suppress bone marrow often present as these signs.

The physical examination is targeted to the following areas:

- *General appearance:* Most patients who are systemically ill look toxic.
- *Head and neck:* A patient with urticaria may have laryngeal edema or stridor indicating airway compromise. Mucosal involvement can occur in several serious skin disorders. Neck stiffness or pain with flexion is always a serious finding in acutely ill patients with a rash.
- *Chest:* Wheezing can accompany urticaria or a severe allergic response.
- *Abdomen:* Anaphylaxis can cause abdominal tenderness.
- A brief survey of the lesion(s) or rash is performed. Location, extent, pattern, and appearance are noted until a more thorough examination can be performed.

Early Intervention

- Patients with rash are sometimes not immediately recognized as seriously ill and are triaged to a basic examination room. Transfer to a higher-level care area within the emergency department may be necessary.
- Oxygen per nasal cannula can be beneficial, particularly in a patient with compromised respiration. Occasionally, more definitive airway management may be necessary.
- Intravenous access is established. An isotonic crystalloid solution is the fluid of choice when hypotension is present.
- Early use of intravenous corticosteroids is indicated in patients with anaphylaxis, severe urticaria, or allergic responses. They are considered in patients with suspected adrenal failure secondary to meningococcemia.
- Early administration of antibiotics is indicated in suspected meningococcemia or sepsis.

CLINICAL ASSESSMENT

History

1. *Date of onset:* This will help determine if the patient has an acute process such as contact dermatitis or a chronic problem such as psoriasis.
2. *Site of onset:* The site of onset of the rash is the most important first clue as to its cause. From onset, the patient is carefully questioned as to spread and sparing, if present.
3. *Periodicity:* Hand lesions that improve on weekends are probably caused by a work-related irritant dermatitis.
4. *Factors that worsen or improve the rash:* Pruritus associated with urticarial lesions will improve with cool compresses and worsen with a hot shower.
5. *Exposure history:* Scabies and flea bites can affect the entire household. Other close contacts may have similar lesions.
6. *Occupation, hobbies, and recreational activities:* Patients often try to relate their rash to some work-related factor such as use of chemicals. Hobbies involving pets can lead to dermatologic manifestations.
7. *Associated symptoms:* A painless penile lesion may be the chancre of primary syphilis, whereas painful penile lesions may represent chancroid. Patients with lesions of scabies or urticaria almost always describe intense pruritus.
8. *Prior treatments:* Many patients attempt to treat their condition before seeking medical advice. The treatment may alter the appearance of the rash.
9. *Medication use:* In the case of a possible drug eruption rash, this information is crucial. It is important to ask about over-the-counter medications, herbal remedies, and contraceptives.

10. *Allergies:* Explore potential allergies to external agents, foods, and medications.
11. *Past medical history:* The past medical history should include any previous cutaneous disorders. Disorders such as diabetes, cancer, sarcoid, and lupus erythematosus may have significant dermatologic manifestations.

Physical Examination

The physical examination is crucial in making the correct diagnosis, because dermatology is a visual specialty. Although the focus is on the skin and its related structures, the patient may have a potentially life-threatening dermatosis and other organ involvement.

1. Adequate exposure and lighting are needed. The entire skin needs to be examined to avoid missing important information.
2. A lesion can change over time or with scratching or rubbing and can confuse the examiner. A fresh lesion, if present, is most helpful in pinpointing the diagnosis.
3. The lesion or rash is palpated wearing gloves. If the rash is palpable, texture is noted. Moisture can be palpated that cannot be seen. Warmth in the surrounding area may be an important finding if present (e.g., cellulitis).
4. The size and configuration of the lesion or rash are noted.
5. Whether a colored lesion (red or blue) is blanchable is noted. The color disappears with direct pressure over the lesion.
6. It is noted whether the lesion or rash has sharp margins or is poorly marginated.
7. The distribution of the lesions or rash is described accurately.
8. A general physical examination is completed to find other associated findings that may contribute to the diagnosis.

CLINICAL REASONING

The descriptive approach to dermatology based on the Lynch algorithm allows placement of an unknown lesion or rash into a major diagnostic group. To begin the process of developing a differential diagnosis, the questions listed in Figure 11–2 are asked to describe the lesion or rash. This information is then used to make an accurate diagnosis based on the choices in the major diagnostic groups (Table 11–3).

DIAGNOSTIC ADJUNCTS

A few simple tests done in the emergency department can give immediate information that can aid in making the diagnosis of a cutaneous disorder.

Diascopy

A glass slide is firmly placed against a solid, red, nonscaling lesion. It is used to determine whether the lesion blanches with pressure (e.g., wheals of urticaria). A nonblanchable lesion implies extravasated blood such as occurs in the petechiae of meningococcemia.

Potassium Hydroxide (KOH) Preparation

This test is helpful in confirming or ruling out the presence of a fungal infection and in identifying the causative mite in suspected cases of scabies. To determine the presence of fungal disease, the lesions are scraped vigorously with the edge of a microscope slide or a No. 15 scalpel blade after moistening the skin slightly with tap water. The best areas to use for obtaining a specimen include the underside of the roof of a blister, moist macerated areas, the rim of a lesion, under the nail or paronychial fold, and the base of a plucked hair. The scrapings are placed on a glass slide, one to two drops of 10% potassium hydroxide (KOH) solution are added, and the slide is covered with a glass coverslip. The specimen is gently heated over an alcohol flame. Right after heating, the specimen is examined under the microscope at 10x and 40x objective power with low illumination. The presence or absence of hyphae or spores is determined. They may resemble grapes on a branch or spaghetti and meatballs, or long thin hyphae may be present with few spores.

For the diagnosis of scabies, a fresh lesion at the end of a burrow should be selected. The best areas are the wrist, between the fingers, and the shaft of the penis. With a No. 15 scalpel blade, the top of the lesion is removed. The base of the lesion is scraped and the specimen is placed on a glass slide. Two drops of 10% KOH solution are added, and a coverslip is put in place. The specimen is viewed under 10x magnification, searching for the mite, egg, or fecal deposits. No heating is necessary.

Tzanck Smear

The presence of multinucleated giant cells with intranuclear inclusions on a specially prepared smear is diagnostic of herpes simplex, herpes zoster, and varicella. To make a Tzanck smear, the top of the vesicle or bulla is removed with a scalpel blade. The base of the lesion is gently scraped and the material smeared on a microscope slide. After letting it air dry, the specimen is stained with Giemsa or routine Wright's stain. A coverslip and drop of immersion oil are added,

Text continued on page 196

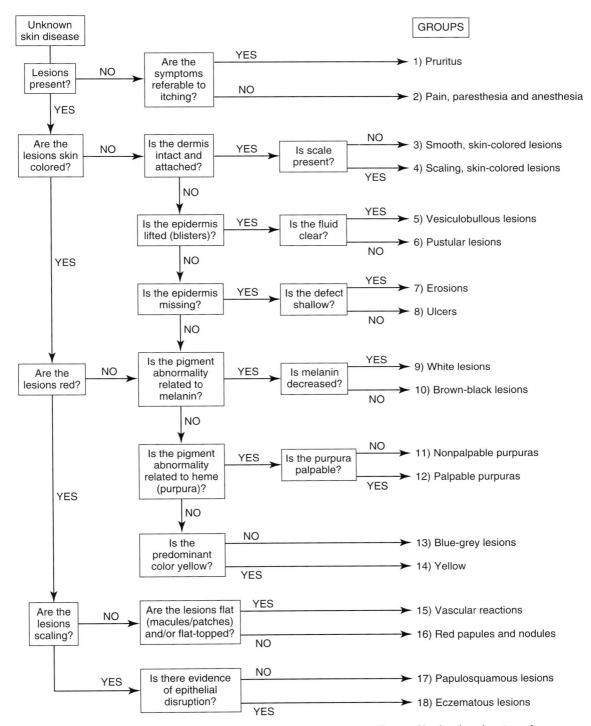

FIGURE 11–2 • A rapid method to place rashes into major diagnostic groups is illustrated by this algorithm. Basic descriptors for the consistency, color, and appearance of the rash allow for the initial group selection. (Modified from Lynch PJ: Problem oriented diagnosis. In Sams WM, Lynch PJ (eds): Principles and Practice of Dermatology, 2nd ed. New York, Churchill Livingstone, 1996; with permission.)

TABLE 11–3. Major Diagnostic Groups in Dermatology

Group 1: Pruritus

Pruritus due to inapparent skin conditions
    Xerosis (atopics, ichthyosis, excess bathing)
    Acquired immunodeficiency syndrome (AIDS)
    Pediculosis (pubic, head, and body lice)
    Scabies
Pruritus due to systemic disorders
    Lymphoma (especially Hodgkin's disease)
    Renal disease
    Hepatic disease (biliary cirrhosis, obstructive disease)
    Polycythemia vera
    Pregnancy
Pruritus of functional origin
    Anxiety (especially obsessive-compulsive persons)
    Depression (especially in the elderly)

Group 2: Pain

Pain in the absence of lesions
    Postherpetic neuralgia
    Trigeminal neuralgia
    Other neuralgias
    Reflex sympathetic dystrophy
    Formication (sensation of "crawling" under the skin) occurs in true infestation and in delusional states
    Peripheral neuropathy (especially diabetes)

Group 3: Smooth Skin-Colored Lesions

Papules, nodules
    Warts (flat warts, genital warts)
    Basal cell carcinoma (early)
    Molluscum contagiosum
    Lipomas
    Nevi (intradermal, neural)
    Scars (hypertrophic, keloid)
    Neurofibroma
    Squamous cell carcinoma (early)
    Skin tags (acrochordons)
    Closed comedones
    Pearly penile papules
    Rhinophyma
Cysts (synovial, mucinous, epidermoid, pilar, etc.)
Edema and pseudoedematous states (e.g., angioedema, lymphedema, scleredema, scleromyxedema, eosinophilic fasciitis, chronic genital edema, Melkersson-Rosenthal syndrome)
Flat and atrophic lesions (e.g., striae, lipoatrophy, lipodystrophy, pitted keratolysis)

Group 4: Scaling Skin-Colored Lesions

Papules and nodules
    Warts (verruca vulgaris, paronychial, and plantar)
    Actinic keratoses, some squamous cell carcinomas
    Corns and calluses
    Seborrheic keratoses (these are usually pigmented)
    Keratoacanthoma
Plaques and disseminated disease
    Xerosis (chapping)
    Ichthyosis (many types)
    Tinea manuum, pedis
    Postinflammatory desquamation and exfoliation

Group 5: Vesiculobullous Lesions

Vesicular
    Herpes simplex
    Varicella zoster (herpes zoster)
    Dyshidrosis (pompholyx)

TABLE 11–3. Major Diagnostic Groups in Dermatology *Continued*

    Vesicular tinea pedis
    Scabies
    Id reaction of the hand
    Vesicular insect bites
    Molluscum contagiosum (may simulate vesicles)
    Dermatitis herpetiformis
Bullous
    Contact dermatitis (especially poison ivy type)
    Frictional blisters
    Burns
    Bullous impetigo
    Pemphigoid (including cicatricial type)
    Pemphigus (more erosions than blisters)
    Epidermolysis bullosa (all types)
    Epidermolysis bullosa acquisita
    Erythema multiforme bullosum (Stevens-Johnson syndrome)
    Fixed drug eruption

Group 6: Pustular Lesions

Pustular diseases
    Folliculitis (bacterial and fungal)
    Acne vulgaris (acne conglobata, pyoderma faciale)
    Rosacea
    Candidiasis
    Stye
    Perioral dermatitis
    Erythema toxicum neonatorum
    Pustular psoriasis
    Chronic gonococcemia
    Acneiform lesions from medications (especially corticosteroids)
    Follicular retention diseases (hidradenitis suppurativa, folliculitis decalvans, dissecting cellulitis, acne keloidalis)

Group 7: Erosions

Erosions
    Unroofed vesiculobullous and pustular lesions
    Excoriations
    Impetigo
    Candidiasis (intertrigo, balanitis, vulvitis)
    Toxic epidermal necrolysis
    Staphylococcal scalded skin syndrome
Ulcers
    Traumatic (especially excoriations)
    Stasis ulcers
    Decubitus ulcers
    Hypertensive ulcers
    Arteriosclerotic ulcers
    Neuropathic ulcers
    Ulcerating tumors (e.g., basal cell cancer, squamous cell cancer)
    Gangrenous ulcers (multiple causes)
    Aphthous ulcers (of the mouth)
    Pyoderma gangrenosum, malignant pyoderma
    Genital infections (e.g., primary syphilis, chancroid, granuloma inguinale)
    Self-induced (factitial) ulcers

Group 9: White Lesions

White papules
    Milium and other epidermoid cysts
    Keratosis pilaris
    Acne vulgaris (early, before the keratotic plug liquefies)
    Molluscum contagiosum
    Sebaceous gland hyperplasia (may be yellow-white)
    Nits (on hairs)
    Hair casts
    White piedra (on hairs)
    Lichen nitidus

Continued on following page

TABLE 11–3. Major Diagnostic Groups in Dermatology *Continued*

Tophus
Calcinosis cutis
Scars
Patches and plaques
  Vitiligo
  Vitiligo-like lesions of scleroderma
  Postinflammatory hypopigmentation
  Pityriasis alba
  Tinea (pityriasis) versicolor
  Sarcoid
  Albinism
  Chemically induced hypomelanosis (e.g., hydroquinone, phenolic compounds)
  Atrophie blanche (depressed scar)
  Mucous membrane white lesions (e.g., lichen planus, secondary syphilis, lupus erythematosus, candidiasis, leukoplakia, white hair leukoplakia, biting, trauma)

Group 10: Brown-Black Lesions

Macules, papules, and nodules
  Nevus (junctional, compound, and intradermal)
  Nevus, dysplastic
  Lentigo (including lentiginosis syndromes)
  Freckles
  Seborrheic keratoses
  Dermatofibroma
  Skin tag (acrochordon)
  Open comedone (blackhead)
  Angiokeratoma (usually violaceous)
  Pigmented basal cell carcinoma
  Acanthosis nigricans (confluent, linear array of papules)
  Urticaria pigmentosa
Patches and plaques
  Café-au-lait patch
  Café-au-lait–like birthmark
  Congenital pigmented nevus
  Tinea (pityriasis) versicolor
  Postinflammatory hyperpigmentation
  Fixed drug eruption
Generalized hyperpigmentation
  Scleroderma
  Porphyria (cutanea tarda and variegate)
  Addison's disease
  Hemochromatosis
  Ichthyosis (several types)
  Wilson's disease
  Whipple's disease
  Medication-related pigmentation (e.g., phenothiazines, metals, cancer chemotherapeutic agents)

Group 11: Nonpalpable Purpuras

Primarily petechial
  Medication-related (especially thiazides)
  Benign pigmented purpuras (multiple types of capillaries)
  Dysproteinemias (especially cryoglobulinemia)
  Hydrostatic petechiae (as in lower-leg stasis)
  Black-dot toes and heels
  Bacteremia (e.g., staphylococcal, meningococcal, bacterial endocarditis)
  Histiocytosis X
  Intravascular coagulation defects (usually with ecchymoses)
Ecchymotic (with or without petechiae)
  Actinic (senile) purpura
  Steroid purpura
  Disseminated intravascular coagulation (multiple causes)
  Anticoagulant therapy (excess dose, idiosyncratic and immune reactions)
  Trauma
  Scurvy
  Amyloidosis (primary type)

TABLE 11–3. Major Diagnostic Groups in Dermatology *Continued*

Intravascular coagulation defects (e.g., platelets, erythrocytes, coagulation proteins)
Necrotizing fasciitis

Group 12: Palpable Purpuras

Venulitis, arteritis
  Henoch-Schönlein purpura
  Leukocytoclastic vasculitis (e.g., hypersensitivity angiitis, rheumatoid vasculitis, allergic vasculitis)
  Dysproteinemias (more often nonpalpable, see above)
Bacteremia (more often nonpalpable, see above)
Rocky Mountain spotted fever, typhus, and other rickettsial infections
Histiocytosis X (not a true vasculitis, lesions often not palpable)
Nonvasculitic (pseudopurpura)
  Angiokeratoma
  Cherry angioma
  Kaposi's sarcoma
  Pyogenic granuloma

Group 13: Blue-Grey Lesions

Papules and nodules (includes more violaceous lesions)
  Blue nevus
  Kaposi's sarcoma (especially the classic type)
  Acroangiodermatitis (arteriovenous fistula, pseudo-Kaposi's disease)
  Leukemia cutis (all types)
  Hemangiomas (especially cavernous and verrucous types)
  Angiosarcoma
  Pyogenic granuloma
Macules and patches
  Heliotrope eyelids of dermatomyositis
  Fixed drug eruption
  Medication-related (e.g., gold, silver, other metals, phenothiazines, antimalarials, minocycline)
  Lead, graphite, asphalt, and other foreign body tattoo
  Hemochromatosis

Group 14: Yellow Lesions

Papules, plaques, and nodules
  Xanthelasma
  Xanthomas (tendinous, tuberous)
  Sebaceous gland hyperplasia (usually yellow-white)
  Histiocytic lesions (various types)
  Tophus
  Amyloidosis (nodular, usually red-orange)
  Cysts (more often white or skin-colored)
Macules and patches, generalized
  Necrobiosis lipoidica diabeticorum
  Xanthomas (plantar, palmar)
  Amyloidosis (primary, macular)
  Pseudoxanthoma elasticum
  Keratoderma of the palms and soles
  Carotenemia
  Jaundice

Group 15: Vascular Reactions

Transient lesions (evolve and resolve in minutes to hours)
  Flushing syndromes (e.g., emotional, pheochromocytoma, carcinoid, mastocytosis, medications)
  Anaphylactic reactions
  Urticaria
  Contact urticaria
  Dermographism, other physical urticarias
  Erythema marginatum
Persistent erythema: livedo (reticular) patterns
  Livedo vasculitis
  Livedo reticularis
  Cholesterol emboli

Continued on following page

TABLE 11–3. Major Diagnostic Groups in Dermatology *Continued*

    Polyarteritis (and other large vessel vasculitis)
    Fifth disease (erythema infectiosum)
    Poikiloderma (e.g., Civatte-type, collagen vascular disease, cutaneous lymphoma)
Persistent erythema: gyrate, serpiginous, and annular patterns
    Erythema annulare centrifugum
    Erythema chronica migrans (Lyme disease)
    Subacute cutaneous lupus erythematosus
    Erythema multiforme
    Granuloma annulare (may mimic the vascular annular lesions)
    (See also papulosquamous diseases, because sometimes the scale on tinea cruris, tinea corporis, psoriasis, etc., is inapparent.)
Persistent erythema: telangiectatic patterns
    Essential telangiectasia
    Unilateral nevoid telangiectasia
    Telangiectasia of collagen vascular disease (CREST syndrome)
    Ataxia-telangiectasia (eyes, ears)
    Angioma serpiginosum
    Radiodermatitis
Persistent erythema: plaques
    Cellulitis
    Erysipelas
    Erysipeloid
    Erythema multiforme
    Hypocomplementemic vasculitis (urticarial vasculitis)
    Erythema nodosum
    Nodular vasculitis
    Panniculitis (multiple types)
    Sweet's syndrome
    Juvenile rheumatoid arthritis
    Pruritic urticarial papules and plaques of pregnancy (PUPP)
    Fixed drug eruption
    Relapsing polychondritis (ear)
    Bee stings, some other bites and stings
    Granuloma faciale
Persistent erythema: diffuse and morbilliform patterns
    Toxic epidermal necrolysis (early)
    Toxic shock syndrome
    Staphylococcal scalded skin syndrome
    Scarlet fever (streptococcal and staphylococcal)
    Viral exanthems (e.g., rubella, rubeola, roseola, erythema infectiosum)
    Kawasaki disease (mucocutaneous lymph node syndrome)
    Graft-versus-host disease
Persistent erythema: macular localized patterns
    Groin: intertrigo, erythrasma, tinea cruris, seborrheic dermatitis (moisture in these areas obscures the presence of scale)
    Hand: erythromelalgia, acrocyanosis, liver disease, hereditary redness of the palm, secondary to chemotherapy, etc.
    Face: lupus erythematosus, dermatomyositis, seborrheic dermatitis, photosensitivity reactions
    Various locations: pernio (chilblains)
    Tinea (pityriasis) versicolor
    Fixed drug eruption
    Basal cell carcinoma (superficial-type)
    Bowen's disease (usually some scale is present)

Group 16: Red Papules and Nodules

Papules
    Insect bites and stings
    Cherry angioma
    Pyogenic granuloma
    Pityriasis rosea (usually macular)
    Secondary syphilis
    Scabies, human and animal
    Mite infestation (bird, grain, *Cheyletiella*)
    Foreign-body granuloma
    Diaper granulomas
    Papular urticaria
    Coral and marine animal contact
    Eruptive xanthoma (pink color)
    Granuloma annulare (papules usually confluent in the form of rings)

TABLE 11–3. Major Diagnostic Groups in Dermatology *Continued*

Sarcoid
    Chondrodermatitis nodularis (ears)
    Stye and hordeolum (eyelid)
    Kaposi's sarcoma (epidemic type)
Nodules and plaques
    Furuncle, carbuncle
    Inflamed cyst
    Acne cyst (acne conglobata, pyoderma faciale)
    Hidradenitis suppurative, dissecting cellulitis
    Erythema nodosum
    Nodular vasculitis (erythema induratum)
    Panniculitis (erythema induratum)
    Polymorphous light eruption (face)
    Lupus erythematosus
    Bites, stings
    Sporotrichosis
    Mycobacterial infection (especially *M. marinum*)
    Lymphoma and leukemia cutis
    Hemangioma
        Sarcoma, angiosarcoma
    Kaposi's sarcoma (especially epidemic-type)
    Vasculitis, large vessel and granulomatous types (especially polyarteritis nodosum)
    Sweet's syndrome
    Granuloma annulare (subcutaneous-type)
    Rheumatoid nodules

Group 17: Papulosquamous Lesions

Papules predominate
    Pityriasis rosea
    Secondary syphilis
    Lichen planus (some plaque formation)
    Pityriasis lichenoides
    Psoriasis (gluttate type)
    Viral exanthems (rubella, rubeola)
Plaques predominate
    Psoriasis
    Tinea capitis, corporis, cruris, pedis
    Lupus erythematosus
    Parapsoriasis, small and large plaque
    Mycosis fungoides
    Pityriasis rubra pilaris
    Reiter's syndrome
    Bowen's disease (often solitary)
    Superficial basal cell carcinoma (often solitary)
    Lichen striatus (linear, usually arms, legs)
    Ichthyosis (multiple types)
    Photosensitivity eruptions
    Pellagra

Group 18: Eczematous Lesions

Prominent excoriation
    Atopic dermatitis
    Neurodermatitis
    Lichen simplex chronicus (variable excoriations)
    Stasis dermatitis
    Dyshidrotic eczema
    Dermatitis herpetiformis
    Exfoliative erythrodermatitis (especially with T-cell lymphoma)
    (The itch-scratch cycle with attendant excoriations can be superimposed on almost any other disease.)
Minimal excoriation
    Irritant contact dermatitis
    Allergic contact dermatitis
    Xerotic eczema (asteatotic eczema, winter itch)
    Perioral dermatitis
    Seborrheic dermatitis

Continued on following page

TABLE 11–3. Major Diagnostic Groups in Dermatology *Continued*

Photosensitivity syndromes
Tennis-shoe foot (juvenile palmar-plantar dermatitis)
Infectious eczematoid dermatitis
External otitis
Lichen striatus (linear, usually arms or legs)
Paget's disease (mammary and extramammary)
Impetigo
Acrodermatitis enteropathica and related nutritional diseases
Histiocytosis X (Langerhans cell histiocytosis)
Nummular eczema
Autoeczematization

---

and the specimen is examined under 10x and 40x objective power for the multinucleated giant cells.

Gram's Stain

Gram's stain is rarely helpful in making the diagnosis of a cutaneous lesion. Pustules, crusts, or exudates may have overlying skin colonization with bacteria, making interpretation of the Gram-stained specimen confusing. In the case of gonorrhea, a Gram-stained specimen of the cervical or penile discharge that exhibits gram-negative intracellular diplococci is diagnostic for the disease. The organisms are not recoverable from the skin lesions in patients with disseminated gonococcemia.

Wood's Lamp Examination

A Wood's lamp is a low-output ultraviolet lamp. Examination of certain skin lesions with a Wood's lamp will show a characteristic fluorescent pattern. In patients with tinea capitis caused by *Microsporum*, sharply marginated, bright blue-green patches are visible on the scalp when it is examined with the Wood's lamp. In patients with erythrasma, which is an erythematous patch affecting the intertriginous areas and caused by a bacterium, a red fluorescence of the skin is seen on examination with a Wood's lamp. This sign is extremely helpful because erythrasma looks very similar to the lesions of tinea cruris, which do not fluoresce. Hypopigmented lesions do not fluoresce but are more visible when examined under a Wood's lamp in a darkened room. This procedure may also lead to better identification of the skin lesions of tinea versicolor and vitiligo and the ash-leaf spots of tuberous sclerosis.

VDRL/RPR

A serologic test (Venereal Disease Research Laboratories [VDRL]/rapid protein reagin [RPR]) is performed in any case of suspected syphilis or in patients who have a rash, usually in a generalized,

maculopapular distribution, that cannot be explained. Syphilis can masquerade as other, more benign dermatoses, such as pityriasis rosea.

EXPANDED DIFFERENTIAL DIAGNOSIS

Using the major diagnostic groups as a guideline, several dermatologic manifestations of serious systemic illness and common dermatologic disorders can be described in more detail.

Potentially Life-Threatening Dermatoses

Vesiculobullous Diseases

Erythema Multiforme Major. Erythema multiforme major is a variant of erythema multiforme characterized by bullous lesions. *Stevens-Johnson syndrome* is erythema multiforme with extensive mucosal lesions as well as bullous cutaneous lesions. *Toxic epidermal necrolysis* is a variant of erythema multiforme characterized by extensive cutaneous bullae associated with epidermal sloughing. Causes of erythema multiforme and its variants include medications, especially sulfa, nonsteroidal anti-inflammatory drugs, and anticonvulsant drugs; bacterial (*Staphylococcus, Mycoplasma*); viral (herpetic); and fungal infections and autoimmune diseases. One half of the cases have no identified etiology.

Patients with Stevens-Johnson syndrome present with vesicles and ulcerations of the mucous membranes of the lips, buccal cavity, eyes, nostrils, and genitalia. Bullous lesions appear on the hands and feet and the trunk. These patients appear extremely toxic and have a high fever and malaise. They have difficulty with oral intake, and urinary retention may result from the painful mucosal lesions. Eye involvement can be severe, and blindness can result. Mortality is 5%.

The rash of toxic epidermal necrolysis begins on the face and is followed by widespread erythema and extensive formation of bullae. The bullae and large sheets of epidermis can be lifted off the dermis. Because of the subepidermal cleavage plane, extensive fluid loss can occur. The mucous membranes, including prolabial and ocular surfaces, are usually involved as in Stevens-Johnson syndrome and toxic epidermal necrolysis. These patients are extremely toxic with fever and malaise. They have signs of dehydration and vascular collapse owing to fluid losses. Mortality is 10% to 30%. Early dermatologic consultation is important in these cases. Management approaches may be complex, including fluids, corticosteroids, antibiotics, and other therapies. Death may occur from complicating sepsis and fluid and electrolyte disorders.

Pemphigus Vulgaris/Bullous Pemphigoid. Pemphigus vulgaris (PV) is an autoimmune, mucocutaneous disease characterized by intraepidermal blistering. It once carried a poor prognosis, but currently less than 10% of patients die. Bullous pemphigoid (BP) occurs primarily in the elderly, with an average age at presentation of 70 years. It has a better long-term prognosis than PV. Autoantibodies have been identified in PV.

PV can present as vesicles or bullae centered on the head, trunk, and mucous membranes. The clear bullae become turbid and rupture after 3 to 5 days. These denuded areas are painful and often become infected. Nikolsky's sign is positive in PV.

BP usually occurs in areas of skin folds. The blisters may be large and associated with pruritus and burning. Lesions may occur in the mouth and usually heal quickly.

Treatment in both diseases includes fluid resuscitation and electrolyte replacement. The eroded areas are treated as burns. High doses of systemic corticosteroids, as well as immunosuppressive therapy, may be initiated in consultation with a dermatologist.

Pustular Diseases

Gonococcemia. Disseminated gonococcemia occurs in 1% to 3% of patients with gonorrhea. It usually occurs 3 to 21 days after the initial infecting contact. The skin lesions are often few in number and tend to occur on the palms, fingers, and soles. The lesions are umbilicated pustules with a red halo. Occasionally, erythematous macules, tender hemorrhagic papules, or hemorrhagic necrotic bullae may be seen. A flu-like illness precedes the migratory polyarthralgias and the pustules by 1 to 3 weeks. Although gonococcemia is relatively benign, life-threatening complications of meningitis, endocarditis, myocarditis, pericarditis, or hepatitis can develop if the disease is left untreated.

Vascular Reactions

Meningococcemia. Meningococcemia is a rapidly progressive and potentially lethal infection caused by *Neisseria meningitidis*. It usually presents as a combined central nervous system and systemic infection, but it may present as either. Most victims are younger than 20 years of age, but anyone is at risk. It often follows a mild upper respiratory tract infection and is commonly reported in the winter and spring. The patient looks toxic, has a fever, and may complain of headache, nausea, and vomiting. Meningeal signs may or may not be present. Mental status changes, such as aggressive behavior, confusion, or stupor, may occur. Seventy-five percent of patients have skin lesions on presentation that consist of palpable petechiae with pale gray centers. They usually occur on the wrists, ankles, and flanks and in the axillae. The lesions may progress to purpura fulminans. Five to 10 percent of patients have a fulminant onset characterized by vasomotor collapse and shock. Mortality rates range from 5% to 30%, depending on the timing of diagnosis and treatment.

Rocky Mountain Spotted Fever (RMSF). This tick-borne rickettsial disease (*Rickettsia rickettsii*) occurs primarily (95%) in the spring and summer. Despite its name, it occurs most frequently in the mid- and southern Atlantic states. The incubation period from tick bite to illness is about 7 days. The classic triad of symptoms of RMSF is fever, rash, and a history of tick exposure; this triad occurs in only 67% of patients with the disease. RMSF begins with a prodrome of fever (94%), chills, severe frontal headache (88%), arthralgias, and myalgia (85%). The rash begins on day 2 to 4 of the illness as erythematous macules, which become palpable petechiae over the next 2 to 4 days, and finally hemorrhagic vesicles. The rash begins on the palms, wrists, soles, and ankles and spreads to involve the entire body. It may be more difficult to diagnose in darkly pigmented individuals. Abdominal pain, hepatomegaly, splenomegaly, conjunctivitis, lymphadenopathy, and meningismus are frequently seen. Mortality in untreated cases ranges from 20% in children to 70% in adults.

Urticaria/Angioedema with Anaphylaxis. Urticaria represents the skin manifestations of an allergic reaction. They occur at least once in approximately 20% of the population. Urticarial lesions are transient edematous papules or wheals that extend to form large flat plaques. Urticaria can involve any part of the body. Most lesions resolve in 1 to 3 hours. Itching is usually a prominent feature. Urticaria is triggered by a wide variety of agents. Possible causes include medications, infections, insect venom, autoimmune diseases, dysproteinemias, inhalants, malignancies, physical stimuli, and foods, dyes, and preservatives. The acute triggering events were identified in 5% to 60% of cases. The trigger ultimately results in the release of histamine and other allergic mediators.

Angioneurotic edema is a variant of urticaria with painless subcutaneous swelling of the face involving the eyelids, lips, and tongue. It may be hereditary or sporadic and may result in laryngeal edema and airway compromise. Angioedema also can occur in the hands, feet, and genitalia. There is usually mild pruritus, and skin lesions resolve over 24 hours.

IgE-mediated systemic involvement in addition to skin lesions represents anaphylaxis and is a true emergency (see Chapter 12, Anaphylaxis). The hallmarks of anaphylaxis include hoarseness, trouble in swallowing, stridor, wheezing, and respiratory arrest. Hypotension and vascular collapse may occur, owing to vasodilation and capillary permeability. Other findings include apprehension, a sense of impending doom, headache, increased lacrimation, rhinorrhea, abdominal pain, and pelvic pain from uterine contractions. Intravenous antihistamines (H_1 and H_2 blockers), corticosteroids, and subcutaneous epinephrine may be necessary.

Cellulitis. Cellulitis is a localized deep infection involving both the dermis and the subcutaneous tissue. It is usually caused by *Streptococcus pyogenes* or *Staphylococcus aureus* and is often precipitated by minor trauma or preexisting lymphatic stasis. Cellulitis occurs most frequently on the extremities and the face. The lesion is deeply indurated, erythematous, warm, edematous, tender, and poorly marginated. Regional adenopathy may be prominent. There may be systemic spread of the infection manifested by fever and malaise. Necrotizing fasciitis is the most extreme, deep form of cellulitis. It is frequently associated with *Streptococcus,* and can be a rapidly progressive, deadly disease. Early diagnosis can be very difficult, and rapid mobilization of consultants, including infectious disease and surgery, is essential. Aggressive resuscitation, antibiotics, and surgical debridement are the current therapies. Mortality may approach 80%.

Common Dermatoses

Vesiculobullous Diseases

Herpes Simplex. Herpes simplex is caused by *Herpesvirus hominis* types 1 and 2. It manifests as herpes labialis or herpes genitalis eruptions. Recurrent infections are quite common and are triggered by sunburn, coryza, fever, and stress for type 1 and trauma during intercourse, vaginitis, menses, and stress for type 2. There is a preeruptive syndrome that consists of burning and tingling of the skin before the appearance of lesions. Herpes labialis lesions present as a tight cluster of small vesicles on an erythematous base or arising from normal skin in the perioral area. The vesicles are fragile and rupture easily, leaving an irregularly shaped erosion. Herpes genitalis is similar to herpes labialis in appearance except that more vesicles are present, and they are less tightly clustered. Primary and recurrent lesions are painful. The diagnosis can be confirmed by Tzanck smear or viral culture.

Scabies. This infestation is caused by the mite *Sarcoptes scabiei.* The female mite burrows within the stratum corneum and deposits eggs within the epidermis. Transmission of the disease usually depends on direct person-to-person contact but can occur through contaminated clothing or bed linens. Once contracted, it is spread by scratching. The lesions of scabies are quite pruritic, especially after several weeks of infestation, when allergic sensitization occurs. Although scabies is a vesicular disease, few intact vesicles are seen because of the intense scratching, which leaves excoriated inflammatory papules. If present, the vesicles are oval or elongated, reflecting their development as a burrow for the mite. The lesions are distributed in the web spaces of the hands, around the elbows, on the anterior axillary folds, and over the buttocks. The breasts in women and the penis in men are often involved. Long-standing cases involve the trunk and extremities, but the face is spared (except in infants). The diagnosis is confirmed by demonstration of the mite, eggs, or feces in material obtained from unroofing the lesion.

Papulosquamous Diseases

Tinea. Tinea is a superficial fungal infection affecting the feet, the groin area, the body, or the scalp. The diagnosis can be made from KOH preparations and fungal cultures. Tinea pedis involves the feet and usually begins with fissures in the web space between the fourth and fifth toes that appear white and macerated. The infection can spread to involve the toenails, but it does not extend to the dorsal surface of the foot. It is worsened by occlusive footwear, which promotes a warm, moist environment that encourages growth of the dermatophyte.

Tinea cruris involves the groin area and begins as a sharply marginated red plaque in the inguinoscrotal crease. It advances to the inner thighs and may extend to the gluteal cleft and buttocks but tends to spare the penis and scrotum. It is more common in men and does not occur before puberty. Tinea corporis involves the neck, arms, legs, or trunk. Annular tinea corporis is the classic "ringworm" infection, which begins as an erythematous, sharply marginated, scaling plaque that enlarges and becomes clear in the center. The annular form rarely consists of more than one or two lesions. Other forms of tinea corporis present as multiple annular lesions with gyrate or serpiginous borders.

Tinea capitis involves the scalp and occurs in two forms. The noninflammatory form presents with patchy, scaling areas containing short stubby hairs. If the hairs are broken off at the surface of the scalp, a characteristic black dot appearance results. The inflammatory type consists of exudative, crusted patches, draining nodules, or large swellings with multiple pustules and draining sinuses; it can easily be confused with a bacterial infection. To make the diagnosis in either type, a plucked broken-off hair rather than scalp scrapings should be used for the KOH preparation or culture.

Tinea can be complicated by an "id" reaction, an idiopathic vesicular eruption of the palms and lateral borders of the fingers distant from the fungal infection site.

Pityriasis Rosea. This disorder most often affects healthy young people between the ages of 10 and 30 years. The cause is unknown. Most patients are asymptomatic, but some may complain of extreme pruritus. Because secondary syphilis can mimic the rash of pityriasis rosea, it is advisable to perform a VDRL/RPR test in most instances. In 50% of patients a large erythematous scaling plaque may be present that may be oval or annular and precedes the rash. This is known as the herald patch. This patch is followed by an eruption of 50 to 100 isolated, oval, erythematous, nonconfluent papules 1 cm in diameter. These oval lesions run parallel to the rib lines in the typical Christmas tree distribution. The lesions are found on the trunk, neck, and inner aspects of the arms and thighs. The face is always spared.

ECZEMATOUS DISEASES

Exfoliative Dermatitis. This can be an abrupt cutaneous reaction to medications, allergens, or malignancy. It is characterized by generalized erythema with flaking and tightness of the skin. The skin is generally not tender, but heat loss and volume shifts are complications. Consultation with a dermatologist is necessary because there are many approaches to treatment. Inpatient care may be necessary, and a potentially chronic course is common.

Contact Dermatitis. Contact dermatitis is an inflammatory response of the skin to an external agent. There are two major types: irritant contact dermatitis and allergic contact dermatitis.

Irritant contact dermatitis is more common than allergic contact dermatitis. Strong irritants will produce skin changes almost immediately after a single exposure. Examples of these are thermal burns and chemical burns due to strong acid or alkaline solutions. These are painful lesions. Weak irritants cause skin changes after repeated exposures to the irritant; these are caused by changes in the moisture content of the skin. The changes result in skin that is too dry or too wet. Examples of weak irritants are detergents, hot water, and solvents. Irritant dermatitis can involve any area of the skin, but the hands are most frequently affected. Exposure to strong irritants produces erythema, swelling, blister formation, ulceration, or skin necrosis. Low-grade irritants causing drying of the skin result in minimal redness with cracks and fissure and scale formation. When exposure to low-grade irritants results in maceration, the area is bright red with small amounts of weeping, and scale formation is not prominent.

Allergic contact dermatitis is the result of inflammatory changes that are caused by sensitization to chemical antigens. The inflammatory response does not occur on the first exposure to the antigen, and sensitization may not occur for months or years. The most common antigens responsible for allergic contact dermatitis are pentadecacatechols of poison ivy, nickel, formaldehyde, neomycin, benzocaine, parabens, ethylenediamine, chromates in cements and cutting oils, and uncured epoxy resins in fiberglass. Proof of causation can be made by patch testing. The affected area exhibits prominent erythema and edema. Weeping and crusting will be present in acute cases, whereas in chronic cases scale formation is more prominent. Vesicles are seen only in poison ivy dermatitis. Asymmetric or unilateral lesions may suggest an external causation. Linear configuration of lesions is a clue to causation by external agents. Pruritus is usually a prominent feature.

Drug Eruptions

Drug eruptions transcend classification because they can present in many different forms. Cutaneous vasculitis from a blood vessel is the common underlying lesion inflammation. The vasculitis may be confined to the skin or involve other organ systems. No drug is "safe," and drugs vary in their ability to produce a reaction. The same drug can produce a variety of reactions. Drug reactions often occur after a course of therapy has been completed. The most likely culprit is the drug most recently prescribed. However, a reaction can develop after a drug has been taken continuously for months or years. Symptomatic relief is necessary, and corticosteroids are used for serious or extensive involvement.

Exanthems. A morbilliform rash is the most common expression of a drug rash and accounts for 50% of all cases. This rash appears as discrete or confluent erythematous macules and papules distributed on the trunk, face, and extremities. Palms, soles, and mucous membranes are not usually involved. The penicillins, sulfonamides, phenytoin, and barbiturates are the most frequent causes of this type of drug eruption.

Urticaria. Typical urticarial lesions consist of edematous papules or wheals, and anaphylaxis accounts for 25% of drug rashes. Penicillin and its derivatives are the most common drugs associated with urticaria and anaphylaxis. Aspirin and nonsteroidal anti-inflammatory agents also cause this type of rash. Codeine causes urticaria by triggering the release of histamine by nonimmunologic mechanisms. Serum sickness is characterized by urticaria, fever, myalgias, arthritis, and lymphadenopathy. It usually begins 7 to 10 days after administration of the drug and is caused by circulating immune complexes. Penicillin, sulfonamides, phenytoin, and thiazides can produce this type of reaction.

Erythema Multiforme and Erythema Multiforme Bullosum. The penicillins, phenytoin, sulfonamides, thiazide diuretics, phenothiazines, chlorpropamide, pyrazolone, and allopurinol have been implicated in erythema multiforme. The rash may present as the typical minor form of erythema multiforme or may progress to the life-threatening bullous forms (toxic epidermal necrolysis, Stevens-Johnson syndrome).

Acneiform Dermatitis. Acneiform dermatitis has the appearance of acne vulgaris but without the formation of comedones and cysts. It has a sudden onset and is commonly caused by corticosteroids, phenytoin, or lithium.

Vasculitis or Palpable Purpura. Vasculitis results in a petechial rash or widespread palpable purpura that affects the legs most severely. Sulfonamides, thiazide diuretics, pyrazolone, thiouracil, phenytoin, penicillin, indomethacin, cimetidine, and quinidine are the most likely culprits.

Localized Reaction. Drug eruptions may also manifest as localized reactions. A fixed drug reaction presents as a recurrent, erythematous oral plaque in the same site with each exposure to the drug. It is associated with tetracycline, chlordiazepoxide, sulfonamides, and phenobarbital. The tender erythematous plaques or nodules of erythema nodosum may occur in response to oral contraceptive use or sulfonamide, penicillin, or salicylate therapy. These lesions are extremely painful and are most always located on the anterior legs.

Photosensitivity. Certain drugs may be responsible for photoeruptions. A phototoxic eruption resembles an exaggerated sunburn in light-exposed areas. Compounds that absorb ultraviolet energy, such as tetracycline and its derivatives, can cause this condition. A photoallergic reaction is the result of a cell-mediated immune response that is elicited by light exposure. It resembles an allergic contact dermatitis and is usually due to topical drugs.

PRINCIPLES OF MANAGEMENT

Management of a cutaneous lesion or rash includes general therapeutic techniques of skin care as well as specific therapy for the particular disease state.

General Therapy

Wet Dressing. Wet dressings are indicated for any scaly eruption of an acute nature such as eczema as well as for crusted, exudative lesions. They provide an antipruritic effect, cause evaporative heat loss, which reduces inflammation, and effectively débride crusts to prevent secondary infection and maceration from fluid entrapment. There are three types of wet dressings: compresses (wet cloths soaked in solution), soaks (immersion of the involved part in solution), and baths. Soaking solutions include normal saline, Burow's solution (1 tablet of Domeboro [aluminum sulfate and calcium acetate] diluted in a pint or quart of cold water), acetic acid (1/4 cup vinegar in 1 quart of cool water), and Aveeno (colloidal oatmeal added to a cool bath).

Topical Medications and Lubricants. Topical medications and lubricants are commonly used in the treatment of cutaneous disorders. They come in a variety of different vehicles, including powders, lotions (water-based suspension of powder), gels, creams (water-based emulsion of oil), ointments (oil based), and pastes. Powders work best for intertriginous areas because of their ability to absorb moisture and alleviate maceration. Lotions are mild lubricants. Calamine lotion also absorbs moisture and dries out exudative lesions. Gels spread easily and work well in hair-bearing areas. Creams are good lubricants for acute exudative processes and are associated with the best patient compliance. Ointments are the best lubricants and should be the first choice for a dry chronic disorder. They should not be used on acutely oozing lesions because they are nearly occlusive.

Antipruritics and Anesthetics

Topical. Anesthetics such as lidocaine (5% ointment) may be helpful in relieving pain and itching. Benzocaine (Americaine) preparations can cause allergic contact sensitization. Antihistamines, such as diphenhydramine (Benadryl) cream and diphenhydramine mixed with calamine lotion (Caladryl), are very popular over-the-counter remedies. They are prescribed cautiously because of the risk of allergic sensitization. Mixtures that contain menthol, phenol, and camphor can be mixed together and added to a standard lotion or cream. They produce a cooling sensation and are helpful in relieving itching.

For painful oral ulcerations and erosions it is useful to know how to prescribe "magic mouthwash." It consists of 4 oz of diphenhydramine elixir, 4 oz of Kaopectate, and 100 mL of viscous lidocaine. The patient is instructed to swish and swallow 1 teaspoon 30 minutes before each meal.

Systemic. Antihistamines are most helpful in cases of itching from urticaria. There are approximately 30 H_1 antagonists, and there is little difference between their antipruritic capabilities. Diphenhydramine is probably the most sedating and should be used only at night. H_2 blockers (cimetidine and ranitidine) may be helpful in patients with chronic urticaria used in conjunction with an H_1 antihistamine. Although not a true antihistamine, hydroxyzine (Atarax) has both antihistaminic and tranquilizing properties. It is often the drug of choice for the relief of itching. Subcutaneous epinephrine (1:1000) may be used in adults and children for severe acute urticaria or severe pruritus associated with these lesions. The benefits can be rapid and substantial, lasting up to 1 hour. Initial dosage is 0.3 to 0.5 mL for the average adult and 0.01 mL/kg in children (not to exceed 0.3 mL).

Specific Therapy

Corticosteroids

Topical. Corticosteroids of various potency have been incorporated into lotions, gels, creams, and ointments. They are extremely useful for treatment of the eczematous disease group, moderately useful for the papulosquamous disease group, and somewhat useful for the vesiculobullous disease group. The topical corticosteroids are divided into groups based on potency (Table 11–4). It is only necessary to learn one or two products from each group. The low-potency corticosteroids will work for almost all acute and subacute eczematous diseases. The intermediate-potency group is used for resistant eczematous diseases and for most papulosquamous diseases. The high-potency group is necessary for eczematous diseases of the palms and soles and for resistant papulosquamous diseases. Only low-potency, nonfluorinated preparations are used for the face and groin; otherwise the patient can develop steroid acne and cutaneous atrophy or groin striae. Corticosteroids are generally applied twice a day, although there are advocates for a single daily application. A good time is right after bathing.

TABLE 11–4. Topical Corticosteroids

Potency	Use
Low Potency	Acute and subacute eczematous disorders
Fluocinolone acetonide (Synalar 0.025%) Hydrocortisone 1%, 2.5% Hydrocortisone valerate 0.2% (Westcort) (OTC) Desonide 0.05% (Tridesilon) Triamcinolone acetonide 0.025% (Kenalog, Aristocort)	
Intermediate Potency	Resistant eczematous discomforts, papulosquamous disorders
Fluticasone propionate 0.05 (Cutivate) Triamcinolone acetonide 0.1% (Kenalog, Aristocort)	
High Potency	Eczematous disorders of palms and soles, resistant papulosquamous disorders
Desoximetasone 0.25% (Topicort) Triamcinolone acetonide 0.5% (Kenalog, Aristocort) Fluocinonide 0.05% (Lidex, Topsyn)	
Super High Potency (Class I)	Psoriasis, other severe or persistent skin disorders
Diflorasone diacetate (Psorcon 0.05%) Clobetasol propionate (Temovate 0.05%) Halobetasol propionate (Ultravate 0.05%)	

Systemic. Systemic corticosteroids are necessary when the severity or extensiveness of the cutaneous disorder precludes topical use. For example, an allergic contact dermatitis that involves the face or the trunk as well as the extremities is treated with systemic corticosteroids. Other dermatoses treated with systemic corticosteroids include erythema multiforme bullosum, urticaria, and several other disease states affecting a large total body surface area. Chronic eczema and psoriasis are not treated with systemic corticosteroids in spite of their effectiveness. Their effect on a chronic illness is only transient, and there is an increased risk of adverse effects with long-term use of corticosteroids. The most effective way to give systemic corticosteroids is by the short-burst method. Forty to 60 milligrams of prednisone is given daily for 7 to 10 days, then discontinued without tapering. There do not appear to be any problems with pituitary-adrenal suppression using this approach. A longer treatment period usually involves a tapering schedule.

Antifungal Agents

Topical. Both clotrimazole (Lotrimin) and miconazole (Monistat) are effective against yeasts and dermatophytes. They are effective for all candidal infections as well as in tinea corporis, tinea cruris, and tinea versicolor. They are applied twice a day for 2 to 4 weeks.

Systemic. Newer systemic antifungal agents are gaining favor for the treatment of a wide range of acute and chronic fungal dermatoses. Fluconazole in single or repeat weekly oral doses can treat conditions such as tinea corporis and local *Candida* infections. With their improved side effect profile and reduced toxicity, these newer agents have replaced griseofulvin for chronic and deep skin and nail mycoses.

Antibacterial Agents

Topical. Topical antibiotics are helpful in the treatment of mild impetigo. Mupirocin ointment (Bactroban) is effective against both staphylococcal and streptococcal organisms. Studies have shown it to be as efficacious as oral erythromycin in the treatment of impetigo. It is applied to the affected area three times a day for 5 days.

Systemic. Ninety percent of all skin infections are caused by *Staphylococcus aureus* or group A *Streptococcus*. Agents that cover for both organisms are recommended because it is difficult to be certain as to the cause. As well, infections can be mixed. First-generation cephalosporins (cephalexin, cefadroxil) are effective. Erythromycin provides coverage against both organisms and is useful for patients allergic to β-lactam drugs. Clindamycin and ciprofloxacin are second-line antibiotics for skin infections. Deep, life-threatening skin lesions are treated with broad-spectrum antibiotics. Ampicillin-sulbactam or ticarcillin with clavulanic acid are effective single agents for this setting. Combination antibiotics include a second- or third-generation cephalosporin with an aminoglycoside.

Scabicides

Lindane (Kwell cream, lotion, or shampoo) is the treatment of choice for scabies. It is also effective against head and pubic lice. It is safe in infants and children if used properly. Crotamiton (Eurax) 10% cream or lotion is somewhat less effective than lindane, but it is also less toxic and an antipruritic.

UNCERTAIN DIAGNOSIS

Uncertain diagnosis of dermatologic lesions is common in emergency medicine. Emergency physicians tend to be trained in "classic patterns of rash," and patients do not always cooperate. The lesion may be early or late in its natural course, topical therapies may mask typical findings, and other diseases may influence the visual appearance of a lesion. It is essential for the potentially serious causes of the skin lesion to be considered before accepting an uncertain diagnosis. A well-indexed, quality atlas of dermatologic photographs should be available for reference in the emergency department. In all cases of suspected serious processes, dermatologic consultation is necessary. Discharge from the emergency department with an uncertain diagnosis should be clearly explained to the patient and family and the serious concerns ruled out and well documented.

SPECIAL CONSIDERATIONS
Pediatric Patients

Emergency dermatologic treatment transcends all age groups. However, the age of the patient can help to key in to the appropriate diagnosis. The pediatric age group deserves special mention because there are several cutaneous disorders that are more likely to occur in this group as well as some that are not likely to occur. For example, allergic contact dermatitis is unusual in this age group because it takes several months or even years to become sensitized to most common allergens. The typical cutaneous disorders in children are often infectious in origin. Some pediatric age-specific cutaneous disorders are listed in Table 11–5.

DISPOSITION AND FOLLOW-UP

Several general principles are recommended to arrange appropriate follow-up for the patient.

Admission

Patients with cutaneous disorders who have lost the generalized protective barrier function of the skin are admitted. Examples of disorders in this category include toxic epidermal necrolysis and Stevens-Johnson syndrome. Also, patients with evidence of extensive systemic involvement, airway compromise, suspected sepsis, or an immunocompromised state require inpatient therapy. Gonococcemia, meningococcemia, Kawasaki syndrome, and anaphylaxis usually lead to the admission of the patient.

Emergency Department Observation

Emergency department observation with discharge within 12 to 24 hours or less is appropriate for disorders that resolve rapidly after emergency department therapy. These disorders include anaphylaxis (not requiring intubation and responding promptly to therapy), angioneurotic edema, and urticaria.

Discharge

Most cutaneous disorders take at least a week or longer to resolve. It is important to schedule follow-up appropriately to allow time for improvement or resolution. It is also important to let the patient know how long the condition will last to prevent unrealistic expectations and frustration if the condition is not cured immediately.

Close Follow-Up. Close follow-up implies physician contact in 24 to 48 hours by phone, a repeat emergency department visit, or an appointment with the referral physician. This is appropriate for cutaneous disorders with minimal systemic involvement. The patient must be able to tolerate the prescribed outpatient therapy. Examples of disorders in this group include cellulitis and the childhood exanthems.

Expedient Follow-Up with a Dermatologist. In certain situations the patient is referred to a dermatologist within a week or less. Examples include unknown or unclear cutaneous disorders, suspected melanoma, and known treatment failures.

Routine Dermatology Follow-Up. Certain cutaneous disorders are always referred to a dermatologist for follow-up. These include chronic dermatologic disorders such as psoriasis, acne, tinea pedis, tinea capitis, onychomycosis, chronic urticaria, and atopic dermatitis and disorders requiring specific dermatologic workups.

Appropriately Timed Follow-Up with a Primary Physician. Patients with minor cutaneous disorders that do not meet the criteria for the preceding categories are referred after a course of therapy to the patient's primary physician.

FINAL POINTS

- Although the majority of patients who present to the emergency department with rashes do not have serious complications of that rash or an underlying systemic disorder, the possibility has to be kept in mind.
- All patients require a systemic overview before focusing on the cutaneous complaint.
- By learning the appropriate terminology and descriptors and then performing a thorough dermatologic history and physical examination, the algorithm shown in Figure 11–2 will lead the clinician to a workable differential diagnosis.
- The emergency physician has a finite number of dermatologic therapies available. The benefits and risks of each are to be well understood before prescribing them to the patient.

Bibliography

JOURNAL ARTICLE

Nguyen T, Freednan J: Dermatological Emergencies: diagnosing and managing life-threatening rashes. Emerg Med Pract 2002;4:1–28.

TABLE 11–5. Pediatric Cutaneous Disorders

Disease	Cause	Skin Presentation	Associated Signs and Symptoms	Therapy
Scarlet fever	Group A β-hemolytic *Streptococcus*	Nearly confluent punctate papules, sandpaper texture. Begins on neck and chest and spreads to abdomen and extremities. Petechiae may be found in creases. Desquamation occurs	Fever, exudative pharyngitis and tonsillitis, strawberry tongue, cervical lymphadenopathy	Penicillin, erythromycin
Roseola (measles)	Paramyxovirus	Erythematous maculopapular rash begins on face and spreads to body and extremities. Desquamation occurs except on palms and soles. Koplik spots: white papules on red base on buccal mucosa opposite second molar	Fever, coryza, cough, conjunctivitis. Pneumonia, encephalitis, and hemorrhagic measles can occur.	Supportive/symptomatic
Rubella (German measles)	Togavirus	Erythematous maculopapular rash begins on face and spreads to trunk and extremities	Upper respiratory symptoms, fever, malaise, lymphadenopathy. Arthritis, encephalitis, hemorrhagic German measles are complications.	Supportive/symptomatic
Varicella (chickenpox)	Varicella virus	Vesicles (2–4 mm) on an erythematous base progress to pustules and crusts. Rash begins on trunk and face and spreads to extremities. Lesions are present in all stages simultaneously. Pruritus is present. Patient may have mucous membrane lesions and almost always has scalp lesions. Tzanck smear is positive	Fever, malaise. Varicella bullosum, pneumonia, encephalitis, disseminated intravascular coagulation, and secondary infection of lesions are complications.	Cool compresses, calamine lotion. Antibiotics for secondary infection
Erythema infectiosum (fifth disease)	Probably caused by parvovirus	Erythematous plaques on cheeks; "slapped cheeks" appearance 2–4 days later, a reticulated erythema appears on extensor surfaces of extremities and buttocks. No mucous membrane involvement	Headache, malaise, nausea, myalgias	Supportive/symptomatic
Roseola infantum	Response to several different viruses: echovirus, coxsackievirus, adenovirus	Discrete pink macules begin on trunk and may spread to extremities. Face is usually spared.	High fever, rash coincides with defervescence.	Supportive/symptomatic
Hand-foot-and-mouth disease	Coxsackievirus A16, B5	Maculopapular and vesicular lesions on palms and soles. Vesicles and ulcerations on tongue, buccal mucosa, soft palate, and gums	Pharyngitis, fever	Supportive/symptomatic
Exanthem	Coxsackievirus A9, B5	Pinkishred maculopapular rash. Occasionally petechiae are present. A9 virus causes generalized face and trunk lesions. B5 virus causes	Fever, adenopathy. Aseptic meningitis can occur.	Supportive/symptomatic

Impetigo	Nonbullous: *Streptococcus*	generalized lesions. No mucous membrane involvement. Nonbullous: erythematous papule or vesicle that spreads to form an erosion covered with honey-colored crust. Usually involves the face.	None	Nonbullous: penicillin, erythromycin
	Bullous: *Staphylococcus*	Bullous: erythematous macules that vesiculate and enlarge to produce bullae that contain purulent exudate. Rupture easily, usually involve face, trunk, or buttocks.		Bullous: oxacillin, dicloxacillin, erythromycin. Both: gentle washing with soap and water three times a day
Kawasaki syndrome (mucocutaneous lymph node syndrome)	Unknown	Erythematous rash; resembles urticaria involving trunk and extremities. Can be maculopapular as in measles. Vesiculopapular eruption may occur on knees and elbows. Oral cavity: edema and erythema of lips, strawberry tongue; no mouth ulcers.	Major criteria: fever, conjunctivitis, firm indurated edema of hands and feet that later desquamates. Lymphadenopathy present. Associated signs: urethritis, arthritis, aseptic meningitis, diarrhea, hepatitis, jaundice. Twenty percent of patients will have cardiac involvement: congestive heart failure, pericardial effusion, dysrhythmias, coronary artery aneurysms, valvular dysfunction.	Hospitalize. High-dose aspirin therapy: 80 mg/kg/day until fever subsides, then 10 mg/kg/day

CASE *Study*

A 50-year-old ill-appearing man was brought to the hospital with fever and weakness. The illness began with the appearance of a rash on his legs. Several small, dark purple spots covered both of his ankles. Because he appeared ill, the triage nurse brought him to the acute care area of the emergency department. The patient was pale and lying quietly on the stretcher. He complained of malaise and chills. He had a headache, felt sleepy, and said that the light bothered his eyes. He had never been seriously ill, and his past medical history was unremarkable. His temperature was 102°F (38.9°C), blood pressure was 100/70 mm Hg, and pulse was 120 beats per minute. His respiratory rate was 20 breaths per minute. He complained of neck discomfort on flexion. His chest was clear to auscultation, and there were no murmurs, rubs, or gallops on heart examination.

Even without recognizing the skin lesions, it is apparent that a serious process is ongoing. The patient is systemically ill. The patient may not volunteer information about "insignificant skin lesions"; therefore, it is imperative that the patient be fully undressed and the entire body examined.

As soon as it is recognized that the patient is potentially hemodynamically unstable, two intravenous lines are placed with isotonic crystalloid running. Oxygen by mask is started, and the patient is placed on a cardiac monitor. While these resuscitative steps are under way, the examination continues to ensure its completeness. This patient had several solid, reddish purple, nonscaling, flat-topped lesions around his ankles. They were 0.5 cm or less in diameter and slightly raised to palpation. They did not blanch to pressure.

Following the diagnostic algorithm, it is apparent that these lesions belonged in the non-red heme origin group. Because they did not blanch on pressure, the differential diagnosis lay with the purpuric lesions. These lesions most likely fall into the venulitis/vasculitis group. This type of vasculitis is caused by medications, infection, autoimmune disease, and certain malignancies. The lesions of neutrophilic or leukocytoclastic vasculitis consist entirely of petechiae and are associated with perivascular inflammation resulting in palpable lesions (palpable purpura). They may also be nonpalpable in a number of bacteremias. This description corresponds to the lesions found on this patient. Because the clinical presentation and findings are consistent with a severe infection, with involvement of the meninges, the rash is most likely due to meningococcemia.

A lumbar puncture was performed without delay. Because meningococcemia can cause acute adrenal failure, high-dose corticosteroids were administered, along with the saline infusions. The Gram stain of the cerebrospinal fluid revealed many polymorphonuclear leukocytes and small gram-negative diplococci consistent with *Neisseria meningitidis*. The third-generation cephalosporin ceftriaxone, 2 g, was administered, and the patient was transferred to the intensive care unit.

Bibliography

TEXTS

Fitzpatrick BT, et al (eds): Color Atlas and Synopsis of Clinical Dermatology, 3rd ed. New York, McGraw-Hill, 1997.

Sams WM, Lynch PJ (eds): Principles and Practice of Dermatology, 2nd ed. New York, Churchill Livingstone, 1996.

JOURNAL ARTICLES

Brady WJ: Selected dermatologic emergencies: Recognition, differential diagnosis, and initial therapeutic considerations for the emergency physician. Emerg Med Rep 1998; 19(pt 1):132–143; 19(pt 2):144–153.

Cohen DJ, MacKay M: Emergency room dermatology: Common acute disorders. Comp Ther 1994; 20:410–413.

Fader RM, Johnson TM: Medical issues and emergencies in the dermatology office. J Am Acad Dermatol 1997; 36:1–16.

Howard RM, Frieden IJ: Dermatophyte infections in children. Pediatr Infect Dis 1999; 14:73–107.

Kaplan AP: Chronic urticaria and angioedema. N Engl J Med 2002; 346:175–179.

Lesher JL Jr: Oral therapy of common superficial fungal infections of the skin. J Am Acad Dermatol 1999; 40:s31–s34.

Raimer SS: New and emerging therapies in pediatric dermatology. Dermatol Clin 2000; 18:73–78.

Shivaram V, Christoph RA, Hayden GF: Skin disorders encountered in a pediatric emergency department. Pediatr Emerg Care 1993; 9:202–204.

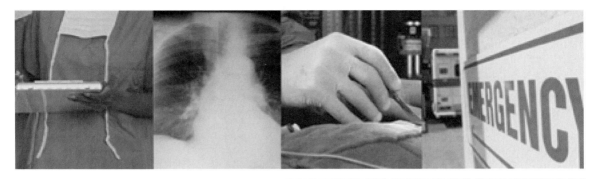

IMMUNOLOGIC DISORDERS

CHAPTER 12

Anaphylaxis

RHODESSA CAPULONG

CASE *Study*

A 28-year-old woman was brought to the emergency department with a chief complaint of diffuse itching, chest tightness, and a sensation of being unable to swallow. According to her friends, the patient's symptoms started after dinner at a local seafood restaurant.

INTRODUCTION

Hypersensitivity reactions present with symptoms ranging from mild (urticaria, pruritus) to severe (hypotension, airway compromise). Anaphylaxis is an acute, often life-threatening, immunoglobulin E (IgE) antibody-antigen–mediated hypersensitivity reaction. The signs and symptoms of anaphylaxis include airway obstruction, cardiovascular collapse, and death. A variety of substances are known to trigger anaphylaxis (Table 12–1). In general, the more rapid the onset, the more severe the reaction to the inciting agent. All age groups are susceptible to anaphylaxis, but the elderly generally tend to have more severe episodes. Males and females are equally affected. Early

TABLE 12–1. Common Causes of Anaphylaxis

Drugs

  Penicillins
  Aspirin
  Sulfa-containing medications
  Nonsteroidal anti-inflammatory agents

Foods and Additives

  Shellfish
  Nuts
  Milk products
  Eggs
  Monosodium glutamate
  Nitrates and nitrites

Other

  Hymenoptera stings
  Radiographic contrast material

recognition and aggressive management of anaphylaxis in the emergency department is essential.

There are 400 to 800 deaths per year in the United States caused by anaphylaxis. Fatalities are most commonly caused by parenterally administered penicillin (100 to 500), Hymenoptera stings (50 to 200), radiographic contrast media, and food reactions. Anaphylaxis does not recur in 100% of repeat exposures, but it is most frequently recurrent after Hymenoptera stings (40% to 60%).

An anaphylactoid reaction has similar signs and symptoms as a true anaphylactic reaction. It is not antigen-antibody mediated, but it is a mast cell degranulation by direct substance stimulation or other mechanisms yet unknown. Reactions to radiopaque contrast media, nonsteroidal anti-inflammatory agents (NSAIDs), and aspirin account for most anaphylactoid-induced fatalities.

An anaphylactic reaction results from the massive release of numerous chemical mediators from mast cells, basophils, and platelets. The cascade begins with an initial exposure to an antigen causing the production of antigen-specific IgE antibodies by B lymphocytes. These antigen-specific antibodies either freely circulate or attach themselves to the surface of mast cells, basophils, and platelets. Reexposure to the antigen leads to antibody-antigen complex formation on the cell surface. This complex triggers the release of preformed granules containing chemical mediators, including histamine and leukotrienes. These mediators cause vasodilation and increased vascular permeability, leading to hypotension, urticaria, and angioedema of the upper airways and gastrointestinal tract. Bronchoconstriction may be caused by leukotriene release. In addition to the IgE antibody-antigen–mediated release of chemical mediators, other pathways also contribute to the process of anaphylaxis on the cellular level. These include activation of the complement system, a non–immune-mediated reaction, and an alternate complement pathway.

The following medications modulate mediator release from mast cells or alter the end-organ response to these mediators (Fig. 12–1).

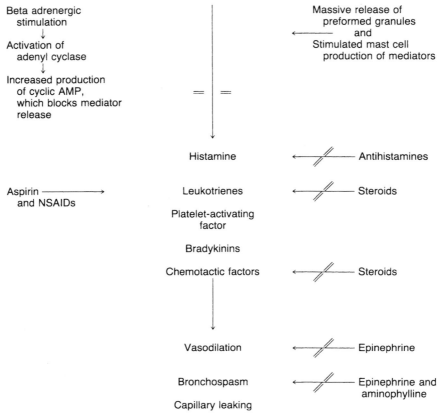

FIGURE 12–1 • Mechanism of anaphylactic reactions. AMP, adenosine monophosphate; NSAIDs, nonsteroidal anti-inflammatory drugs.

1. β-Adrenergic drugs promote the synthesis of cyclic adenosine monophosphate (AMP) inside mast cells. Increased intracellular cyclic AMP inhibits degranulation of mast cells, slowing the reaction and dilating bronchial smooth muscle.
2. Antihistamines competitively block histamine at its tissue receptor sites (H$_1$ and H$_2$).
3. The anti-inflammatory action of steroids appears to have a delayed benefit in decreasing angioedema and relieving bronchospasm. Corticosteroids may interfere with leukotriene release and stabilize mast cell membranes.
4. Aspirin and NSAIDs block the cyclo-oxygenase enzyme, shunting prostaglandin synthesis to leukotriene production.

INITIAL APPROACH AND STABILIZATION
Priority Diagnoses

True anaphylaxis or extreme hypersensitivity reaction involves airway or breathing com-promise and hemodynamic instability/hypotension. As with any threat to life, the question of anaphylaxis must be aggressively explored and answered.

Rapid Assessment

1. Did the patient complain of itching, localized or generalized edema, voice change, difficulty in breathing, lightheadedness, or fainting?
2. Did symptoms begin after exposure to medications or other possible allergens such as bites or stings?
3. Does the patient have a history of previous allergic reactions?
4. Vital signs are obtained immediately.
5. Is there evidence of a rash, wheals, or urticaria?
6. Is there facial, lip, or tongue swelling?
7. Does the patient exhibit stridor or wheezing?
8. Is there tachycardia or hypotension?

Early Intervention

- Laryngeal edema and upper airway obstruction can progress rapidly. If there is evidence of airway compromise, early intubation to establish airway control is essential. One must also be prepared for a cricothyroidotomy should endotracheal intubation be unsuccessful because of massive angioedema of the oropharynx and upper airway.
- High-flow supplemental oxygen is given via non-rebreather mask, and large-bore intravenous line access is established for fluid and medication administration.
- The patient is placed on a cardiac monitor, and oxygen saturation is monitored by continuous pulse oximetry.
- Crystalloid administration is essential for volume expansion. Otherwise healthy adults should receive at least a 1- to 2-L bolus of crystalloid. Children may be given 20 mL/kg boluses up to 60 mL/kg. In the elderly or those with heart disease, frequent monitoring for fluid overload is mandatory. In cases of refractory hypotension despite fluid administration, initiation of vasopressors, such as epinephrine or dopamine infusions, is indicated.
- Antihistamines are given to block the action of histamine at the target cell level. The dosage of diphenhydramine is 25 to 50 mg intravenously or intramuscularly in adults and 1 to 2 mg/kg in children. Alternatively, an H_2 blocker such as cimetidine 300 mg IV can be used in adults who are hypotensive or for whom sedation is best avoided.
- Epinephrine is the mainstay of therapy for acute anaphylactic reactions. Its β-adrenergic effects inhibit the release of chemical mediators from mast cells by increasing cyclic AMP, and bronchial smooth muscle relaxation is promoted. α-Adrenergic effects result in vasoconstriction, reversing hypotension and decreasing tissue edema. The dose and route of administration are dependent on the severity of the anaphylactic reaction and on the age, size, and cardiovascular status of the patient. In mild-to-moderate cases, epinephrine can be given subcutaneously or intramuscularly. The dosage is 0.3 to 0.5 mL of 1:1000 solution subcutaneously or intramuscularly in an adult and 0.01 mL/kg in a child. This dose may be repeated at 10- to 15-minute intervals, as needed based on clinical response. For patients with airway obstruction or with hemodynamic instability, epinephrine, 0.3 to 0.5 mg of 1:10,000 dilution, is administered intravenously. Should intravenous access be difficult, direct injection into the sublingual plexus or femoral vein or endotracheally is an alternative.

CLINICAL ASSESSMENT

Once the patient's condition has stabilized, the focus can be placed on further historical data gathering and completing a more detailed physical examination.

History

Patients suffering from an anaphylactic reaction are often unable to provide historical information. Reliance on family members, friends, and emergency services personnel is important for complete data gathering. Key historical features to be obtained are as follows.

Onset. What were the *initial symptoms*, and how did they *progress*? Symptoms may develop immediately after exposure and are usually present within 30 minutes. Exposure to antigens by the oral route may result in a delay of symptom onset of 2 to 3 hours. The severity of the reaction is proportionate to the rapidity of onset; an eruption occurring over a few minutes tends to be more severe (greater systemic involvement) than a reaction that develops over hours or days.

Route. Was their *exposure* to possible *antigens* by an invasive route? The more direct the access to the systemic circulation, the greater the likelihood of severe reaction. Intravenous exposure is the most dangerous, followed by intramuscular, subcutaneous, intradermal, mucous membrane, and skin exposures.

Timing and Dosage. Have there been frequent *recurrent exposures* to the possible antigen? Recurrent exposures increase the risk of sensitization.

Antigen Potency. What are the *possible offending agents*? A review of the patient's step-by-step actions during the previous 4 hours will usually identify potential agents. Antibiotics are a common etiologic factor, with penicillin being the most common cause of life-threatening anaphylaxis. Stings of insects of the order Hymenoptera are the second most common cause. Foods, especially nuts and shellfish, as well as common analgesics such as aspirin and the NSAIDs, are also common offenders and are specifically inquired about.

Duration. *How long* have the *symptoms persisted*? There is wide clinical variability, but symptoms generally do not last for more than 3 to 4 hours. Angioedema, however, is very slow to resolve and may last for 6 hours or more.

Physical Examination

In general, patients with anaphylaxis have symptoms related to the skin or respiratory tract, but objective findings may be very subtle (Table 12–2)

TABLE 12–2. Symptoms and Signs of Anaphylaxis

Reaction	Symptoms	Signs
Urticaria	Itching	Raised wheals diffusely wandering, evanescent
Angioedema	Nonpruritic tingling	Swelling of lips, eyes, hands; without heat or erythema
Laryngeal edema	Hoarseness	Inspiratory stridor, intercostal and supraclavicular retractions, cyanosis
	Dysphagia	
	Lump in throat	
	Airway obstruction	
	Sudden death	
Bronchospasm	Cough, dyspnea, chest tightness	Wheezing, tachypnea, retractions
Vasodilation	Dizziness	Hypotension (mild to severe), tachycardia, oliguria
	Syncope	
	Confusion	
Rhinitis	Nasal congestion, itching	Rhinorrhea
Conjunctivitis	Tearing	Lid edema and injection
	Itching	
Gastroenteritis	Cramping	Normal examination or increased bowel sound activity
	Diarrhea	
	Vomiting	

1. *Vital signs:* Tachycardia, tachypnea, and hypotension are common findings. In general, fever is not part of the clinical picture of anaphylaxis. When fever is present, an infectious etiology or a drug reaction is considered.
2. *General appearance:* Does the patient look sick, apprehensive, pale, cyanotic? Does the voice sound hoarse? Are there supraclavicular retractions?
3. *HEENT:* Is there edema of the lips, uvula, tongue, or posterior pharynx?
4. *Lungs:* Auscultation for inspiratory stridor, wheezing, and air exchange is performed and retractions are noted. Bronchospasm is relatively rare with anaphylaxis unless there is an underlying history of asthma.
5. *Heart:* In anaphylaxis, myocardial ischemia and dysrhythmias can occur, especially in the elderly or those with underlying cardiovascular disease. Cardiac auscultation for rate and rhythm is important. Cardiac involvement in the setting of anaphylaxis is typically secondary to hypoxia, hypotension, or epinephrine administration.
6. *Abdomen:* The abdominal examination is generally normal, although patients may complain of abdominal cramping.
7. *Skin:* Over 90% of patients with anaphylaxis present with urticaria or angioedema. Urticaria is edema of the upper dermis. It characteristically appears as widely distributed erythematous wheals, and the patient complains of pruritus. In contrast, angioedema is edema of the deep dermis. It is painless, nonpruritic, and generally localized to the face, lips, and hands.

CLINICAL REASONING

After data gathering and observing the initial response to any treatment, two important questions can usually be answered when confronted by a patient in shock or with acute upper respiratory distress.

Could This Be Anaphylaxis and, If Not, What Other Problem Is Present?

The diagnosis of anaphylaxis is obvious when antigen exposure is rapidly followed by urticaria, angioedema, bronchospasm, upper airway edema, and hypotension. When there is a delay in the development of symptoms so that cause and effect are not clear or expression of the syndrome is only partial, other entities are considered (Table 12–3).

If the Problem Is Anaphylaxis, What Is the Precipitating Agent?

The agents most likely to be responsible for anaphylaxis are identified in Table 12–1.

DIAGNOSTIC ADJUNCTS

There are no tests that diagnose anaphylaxis; however, when the diagnosis is uncertain, there are radiographic, laboratory, and bedside tests that can help rule out other causes of shock, detect complications resulting from anaphylaxis, or follow treatment progress.

Laboratory Studies

• *Complete blood cell count:* The CBC may be helpful in assessing the patient for systemic

TABLE 12–3. Differential Diagnosis of Anaphylaxis

Anaphylactoid reactions
Acute, severe urticaria
Acute, severe bronchospasm
Hereditary angioedema
Upper airway infections
Scombroid fish poisoning
Chinese restaurant syndrome
Systemic mastocytosis
Carcinoid syndrome
Munchausen's syndrome

infection, hematologic abnormalities, or neoplastic processes.

- *Serum electrolytes and renal function tests:* These are useful guides for patients who are undergoing massive fluid resuscitation secondary to shock.
- *Arterial blood gas analysis:* This is used to assess the patient's oxygenation, ventilatory, and acid-base status.

Radiologic Imaging

- *Chest radiograph:* In the setting of severe anaphylaxis, the chest film is useful after endotracheal intubation, for visualization of tube position and assessment of lung expansion.
- *Lateral soft tissue of the neck:* Other causes of upper airway obstruction (e.g., retropharyngeal tissue swelling, foreign body) should be assessed, as necessary.

Electrocardiogram

In elderly patients and in those with underlying cardiovascular disease, the stress of airway obstruction or profound hypotension may result in myocardial ischemia, conduction abnormalities, or dysrhythmia.

PRINCIPLES OF MANAGEMENT

The therapeutic approach to the patient with anaphylaxis includes general supportive care, removal of the inciting antigen, and inhibition of the process at the biochemical level.

General Supportive Care. All patients with suspected anaphylaxis should be given oxygen, have an intravenous line established, and have cardiac monitoring instituted. Airway control and aggressive fluid resuscitation should be initiated immediately when there is evidence of airway compromise or hypotension.

Cessation of Antigen. Removal of the suspected trigger of the anaphylactic reaction is essential. In the case of Hymenoptera stings, an effort should be made to remove the stinger. A constrictive band may be applied proximal to the sting to slow the spread of the venom. If the reaction is due to medication, further delivery should be stopped immediately and future administration of the drug prevented.

Specific Medications in Anaphylaxis

As illustrated in Figure 12–1, the biochemical cascade involved in anaphylaxis may be altered at several levels. Table 12–4 lists the medications commonly used in treatment. These medications are discussed in the paragraphs that follow.

Epinephrine is the drug of choice in anaphylaxis. Its α-adrenergic effects result in increased peripheral resistance and reversal of peripheral vasodilation and vascular permeability, lessening hypotension. The β-adrenergic effects dilate bronchiolar smooth muscle, increase the chronotropic and inotropic state of the heart, and increase the production of cyclic AMP. The clinical results are bronchodilation, enhanced cardiac activity, and inhibition of further chemical mediator release.

Antihistamines competitively block the action of histamines at the target cell level. H_1 and H_2 antagonists are often used together because of their synergistic effect. Diphenhydramine and hydroxyzine are examples of H_1 blockers, whereas ranitidine and cimetidine are H_2 antihistamines. Most studies have evaluated the combined effectiveness of cimetidine (H_2) and diphenhydramine (H_1).

Corticosteroids inhibit the degranulation of chemical mediators from mast cells and are believed to block the effects of leukotrienes.

β-Adrenergic agents administered by inhalation are useful for patients who have a component of bronchospasm.

Methylxanthines, such as aminophylline and theophylline, in the past, have been recommended for patients with severe, persistent bronchospasm despite epinephrine and inhaled β-agonist therapy. However, recent literature does not recommend the use of methylxanthines in the treatment of anaphylactic reactions.

Glucagon is a pharmacologic adjunct to consider in patients who chronically use β-adrenergic blocking agents. These patients may have exaggerated anaphylactic reactions resistant to standard epinephrine therapy. It is thought that glucagon, like epinephrine, increases the intracellular synthesis of cyclic AMP, thereby leading to positive chronotropic and inotropic effects on the heart, smooth muscle relaxation, and prevention of further chemical mediator release. Side effects include nausea, vomiting, hyperglycemia, and dizziness. Glucagon may be helpful for the rare patient in whom epinephrine administration is contraindicated.

TABLE 12–4. Common Medications Used in the Treatment of Anaphylaxis

Drug	Adult Dose	Pediatric Dose
Catecholamines		
Epinephrine	0.3–0.5 mg (1:1,000 SC/1:10,000 IV)	0.01 mg/kg SC/IV
Corticosteroids		
Methylprednisolone	125 mg IV	1–2 mg/kg IV
Hydrocortisone	500 mg IV	4–8 mg/kg/dose IV
Prednisone	60 mg PO	1 mg/kg PO
Antihistamines		
H$_1$		
Diphenhydramine	50 mg IV	1–2 mg/kg slow IVP
Hydroxyzine	50 mg/IV	1–2 mg/kg slow IVP
H$_2$		
Ranitidine	50 mg IV	
Cimetidine	300 mg IV	
β-Adrenergic Agents		
Albuterol sulfate*	5 mg/dose by inhalation PRN	1.25–2.5 mg/dose by inhalation PRN
Other		
Glucagon	1 mg IV	

Note: albuterol nebulization solution: 5 mg/mL or 2.5 mg in 3 mL of normal saline

UNCERTAIN DIAGNOSIS

When a patient presents with a history of antigen exposure (e.g., bee sting) followed by clinical manifestations consistent with an anaphylactic reaction (e.g., urticaria, laryngeal edema, or hypotension), the diagnosis is not difficult. More diagnostic challenge occurs when the patient presents with only a portion of the clinical syndrome or is in extremis with airway obstruction or cardiovascular collapse and no clear history of events. While standard measures for securing the airway, providing ventilation, and shock resuscitation are proceeding, the differential diagnosis must be considered (see Table 12–3). Anaphylactic reactions are an important part of the differential diagnosis of shock status and acute airway compromise. It must not be overlooked, even when there is no clear history of a precipitating event.

SPECIAL CONSIDERATIONS

Elderly and Cardiac Patients

In the elderly and patients with underlying cardiovascular disease, administration of epinephrine should be done with caution, especially if the reaction is mild. However, in extremis with airway compromise and profound hypotension, epinephrine and aggressive administration of crystalloid should not be withheld.

Although full doses of subcutaneous epinephrine are shown to be safe in the treatment of elderly asthmatics, an initial test dose of 0.15 mL (1/1000) subcutaneously is prudent in cardiac patients with mild to moderate reactions. They are monitored carefully for 15 minutes after the dose is given. If no chest pain or dysrhythmias develop, another test dose or a full dose may be administered. Intravenous epinephrine is avoided in this patient group unless severe reactions and shock are present.

β-Adrenergic Blocker–Aggravated Anaphylaxis

Patients who experience anaphylactic reactions and are on β-blocker therapy may be resistant to standard treatment. They may suffer from profound elevation in blood pressure after epinephrine administration because the alpha effects of the epinephrine are unopposed. Glucagon may be given in these cases. Prophylactic glucagon administration should be considered in any patient suffering from anaphylaxis who is on β-blocker therapy.

DISPOSITION AND FOLLOW-UP

Disposition depends on the severity of the reaction and the degree of resolution that occurs with emergency department treatment and observation.

Admission

- Any patient who has had life-threatening manifestations such as shock or upper airway obstruction, even if resolved with acute therapy
- Patients with a slow or incomplete response to therapy (unless urticaria or very minimal angioedema of skin or uvula remains)
- Patients with any worsening of symptoms during emergency department evaluation and treatment
- Elderly, debilitated, or cardiac patients

Admission to Critical Care Unit

- Patient with hypotension not responding to fluid resuscitation and (subcutaneous or intramuscular) epinephrine
- Patient with potential upper airway obstruction, with persistent symptoms or signs of upper airway angioedema
- Any patient requiring intravenous epinephrine
- Patients on β-blocker therapy, complicating anaphylaxis and therapy

Discharge

A patient with complete and rapid resolution of symptoms after minimal therapy (e.g., one or two doses of subcutaneous epinephrine) and observation in the emergency department for 3 to 4 hours can be discharged. A companion should observe the patient at home, overnight, for symptom recurrence.

Treatment at home includes the following:

1. Prednisone, 40 mg, given initially and once per day for 5 to 7 days. In a small percentage of patients, a secondary exacerbation of symptoms occurs within 12 hours of the initial onset despite earlier complete resolution. Corticosteroids appear to be effective in preventing this late recurrence.
2. Diphenhydramine, 25 mg, every 4 to 6 hours for rash or itching over 2 to 3 days. Another H_1 or H_2 antagonist may be considered.
3. Avoid any potential exposure to antigen.
4. Arrange for physician follow-up in 24 hours.

Long-Term Care

Counseling on avoidance of the known or strongly suspected trigger is needed for prevention of a repeat attack. Patients who are identified as being predisposed to moderate-to-severe anaphylactic reactions should be taught to immediately self-administer an oral antihistamine and to self-inject epinephrine after a known exposure. Patients should be encouraged to wear a medic alert identification bracelet. Patients who have suffered from insect venom anaphylaxis should consider venom immunotherapy for desensitization. Patients with a known radiocontrast allergy should avoid future studies that use that contrast medium. If studies and procedures are absolutely required, pretreatment with diphenhydramine and corticosteroids is mandatory.

FINAL POINTS

- Anaphylaxis is an acute, potentially life-threatening condition in which airway compromise and cardiovascular collapse are the most common causes of morbidity and mortality.
- Anaphylaxis is the result of the systemic reaction (of multiple organs) to an antigen by IgE antibody release of chemical mediators in previously sensitized individuals.
- Immediate stabilization of the airway is essential when patients with anaphylaxis present with symptoms and signs of upper airway obstruction secondary to angioedema.
- Hypotension is treated with aggressive fluid resuscitation.
- Epinephrine is the mainstay of therapy for anaphylaxis.
- Consider admitting all patients but those with the mildest anaphylactic reactions.

CASE *Study*

A 28-year-old woman is brought to the emergency department with a chief complaint of diffuse itching, tightness in the chest, and sensation of being unable to swallow. According to her friends, these symptoms started after the patient had dinner at a seafood restaurant.

The patient appeared in mild to moderate respiratory distress. She was unable to give further history, but her friends stated that she had had a similar episode in the past after eating shrimp.

Previous history of similar event aids the clinician in determining the etiology of the illness. When an accurate history is unavailable, stabilization and treatment should be initiated while simultaneously searching for the cause of the signs and symptoms.

The physical examination was as follows:

Vital signs: temperature, 98.7°F; pulse, 124 beats per minute; respiratory rate, 28 breaths per minute; blood pressure, 80/62 mm Hg

General appearance: anxious and pale

HEENT: mild upper lip and left-sided tongue swelling; uvula midline; no inspiratory stridor; her voice was slightly hoarse

Lungs: clear to auscultation

Heart: tachycardic without murmurs, gallops, or rubs

Abdomen: soft, nontender

Skin: multiple raised erythematous wheals on arms, legs, and trunk

The patient was placed on oxygen, an intravenous line was established, and cardiac monitoring was initiated. A 2-L fluid bolus of normal saline was given and her repeat blood pressure was 124/80 mm Hg. Epinephrine, 0.3 mg, was given subcutaneously every 15 minutes for three doses. There was improvement of angioedema of the lip and tongue. In addition, she received methylprednisolone, 125 mg, and diphenhydramine, 50 mg, intravenously.

If there is any evidence of airway compromise or hemodynamic instability, aggressive management should be initiated immediately. Stabilization of the airway and cardiovascular system is paramount in conjunction with administration of epinephrine, antihistamines, and corticosteroids to treat and prevent progression of the anaphylactic reaction.

The patient's condition continued to improve with complete resolution of symptoms after 6 hours of observation in the emergency department. She gave further history that she had had a similar episode after taking penicillin for "strep throat" as a child. After discussion with her primary physician, the patient was discharged with a prescription for oral antihistamines and a 7-day course of oral corticosteroids with strict instructions to return to the emergency department if symptoms recurred. She was educated in the importance of avoiding consumption of shrimp and possibly other seafood in the future.

Extended observation of patients with anaphylaxis is essential to monitor progression of symptoms or recurrence after an initial clinical improvement. Referral and early follow-up is mandatory. Patient education on the avoidance of the causative agents and recommending keeping auto-injectable epinephrine close at hand is warranted depending on the severity of the attack.

Bibliography

TEXT

McGrath KG: Anaphylaxis. In Patterson R, Grammer LC, Greenberger PA (eds): Allergic Diseases: Diagnosis and Management, 5th ed. Philadelphia, Lippincott-Raven, 1998.

JOURNAL ARTICLES

Atkinson TP, Kaliner MA: Anaphylaxis. Med Clin North Am 1992; 76:841.

Bochner BS, Lichtenstein LM: Anaphylaxis. N Engl J Med 1991; 324:1785–1790.

Ewan PW: Anaphylaxis. BMJ 1998; 316:1442–1445.

Freeman TM: Anaphylaxis: Diagnosis and treatment. Prim Care 1998; 25:809–817.

Howarth PH: Assessment of antihistamine efficacy and potency. Clin Exp Allergy 1999; 29(Suppl 3):87–97.

Javeed N, Javeed H, Javeed S, et al: Refractory anaphylactoid shock potentiated by beta-blockers. Cathet Cardiovasc Diagn 1996; 39:383–384, 1996.

Joint Task Force on Practice Parameters, American Academy of Allergy, Asthma, and Immunology, American College of Allergy, Asthma, and Immunology, and the Joint Council of Allergy, Asthma, and Immunology: The diagnosis and management of anaphylaxis. J Allergy Clin Immunol 1998; 101(6 pt 2):S465–S528.

Kay AB: Allergy and allergic diseases (part 2). N Engl J Med 2001; 344:109–113.

O'Brien J, Howell JM: Allergic emergencies and anaphylaxis: How to avoid getting stung. Emerg Med Pract 2000; 2:1–20.

Robinson SM: Treatment of acute anaphylaxis: Investigations help confirm diagnosis. BMJ 1995; 311:1435.

Salkind AR, Cuddy PG, Foxworth JW: Is this patient allergic to penicillin? JAMA 2001; 285:2498–2505.

Sampson HA: Peanut allergy. N Engl J Med 2002; 346:1294–1299.

CHAPTER 13

Approach to HIV in the Emergency Department

DENIS J. FITZGERALD

ALEXANDER T. TROTT

JENNIFER M. BOCOCK

CASE *Study*

The rescue squad brings a 33-year-old man to the emergency department. He appears ill, complains of weakness, and states that he is HIV positive.

INTRODUCTION

Acquired immunodeficiency syndrome (AIDS) was first recognized as a separate disease approximately 20 years ago. In 1981, unusual opportunistic infection patterns were found among a population of previously healthy homosexual men. Retrospective analyses of blood samples from the original patients have shown the presence of antibodies to human immunodeficiency virus type 1 (HIV). The presence of antibodies to HIV has been demonstrated in virtually all patients who have developed AIDS. In every region or country where AIDS has developed, positivity for the HIV virus also has been documented, clearing linking the virus and the development of AIDS.

In the emergency department a dual approach is taken when caring for HIV-infected patients. The primary duty is treating patients with potential HIV infection with compassion and a comprehensive focus. This focus includes a high index of suspicion for occult HIV infection in young patients presenting with high-risk behavior history or with atypical infections and the aggressive pursuit of the infectious complications unique to this immunocompromised state. Second, all health care providers must meticulously follow universal precautions while caring for these patients to prevent the spread of this potentially fatal disease. Understanding the protocols for prophylaxis in individuals with accidental parenteral exposure is a necessity.

HIV infection was initially considered inevitably fatal. Intense study of the causative agent, disease development, and complications for 2 decades has improved longevity and health quality for persons infected with this virus. Discoveries in diagnosis, opportunistic infection prophylaxis and treatment, and antiretroviral therapies have contributed to these health care advances. The developments in antiretroviral therapy, particularly over the past 10 years, have dramatically altered the course of the viral infection and slowed the progression of the disease. These new antiretroviral agents can have severe side effects that also bring the HIV-infected patient to the emergency department. The complexity of current treatment regimens requires early communication with the primary health care provider to best coordinate patient care.

Pathophysiology

HIV is a retrovirus, a member of the lentivirus family. Genetic information is carried by single-stranded RNA. HIV has an affinity for lymphocytes with the CD4 cell surface molecule, found primarily on the surface of helper T cells. These cells are critical to the normal cell-mediated immune response. Once infected, a person has a flu-like illness, accompanied by a rapid viral replication phase. After a few weeks, a long asymptomatic latency period (up to 10 years) develops. The patient is contagious throughout the latency period, despite a lack of symptoms or signs of illness. The route of infection involves an exchange of body fluids, as can occur with unprotected sexual intercourse (vaginal or seminal fluids), parenteral transmission (blood product transfusion or intravenous drug abuse), or perinatal or postnatal transmission (amniotic fluid or breast milk). The course of the illness renders the infected individual progressively more immunocompromised as helper T cell numbers diminish. Patients contract a variety of infections, many of which are opportunistic. These infectants are normally prevented from manifesting as clinical disease by an intact cellular immune system response. Emergence of opportunistic infections commonly marks the transition between asymptomatic HIV infection and the diagnosis of AIDS. Patients with HIV infection, without an opportunistic infection, may also be diagnosed with AIDS, based on laboratory tests evaluating immune status. The point in the disease process when AIDS is diagnosed represents an overwhelmed immune system with limited ability to regenerate.

Epidemiology

In December 2000, the World Health Organization (WHO) estimated 22 million people had died of HIV infection and AIDS and another 36.1 million had either HIV infection or AIDS at that time. Approximately 75% of all HIV-infected and AIDS patients live in underdeveloped countries. AIDS has become the second leading global cause of death from infectious disease. In May 2001, the Centers for Disease Control and Prevention (CDC) estimated that approximately 900,000 persons are HIV positive in the United States, and many of them are unaware they are infected with the virus.

An estimated 40,000 people are newly infected annually in this country, a decrease from the originally estimated 150,000 annual cases in the late 1980s. Approximately 450,000 people have died of AIDS. In the United States, AIDS is the fifth leading cause of death in the 22- to 44-year age group, and in the African-American population it is the first and second leading causes of death among men and women, respectively.

High-risk behavior for contracting HIV has been studied and shown to include unprotected sexual activity between homosexual men, unprotected sexual activity between heterosexual men and women, intravenous drug abuse with shared, nonsterile equipment, and nonoccupational nonsexual exposures (needlesticks, tattooing, piercing, body fluid contact with mucous membranes or abraded skin).

Approximately 95% of patients who have received a transfusion of one unit of HIV-infected whole-blood product will seroconvert. The risk of infection from exposure to HIV-positive blood by intravenous needle is 0.67%, and by percutaneous needlestick exposure it is 0.3% to 0.4%. Mucous membrane exposures have been demonstrated to have a transmission risk of 0.09% per exposure. The risk of virus transmission with repetitive sexual encounters varies from 0.1% to 3% (penile-rectal) to 0.1% to 0.2% (receptive vaginal intercourse).

Almost 50% of the health care workers diagnosed with documented HIV infection after an occupational exposure have developed AIDS, with no other known risk factors. Occupational exposures include the exposure to patients' blood and/or body fluids in health care, laboratory, and public-safety settings. Factors influencing the risk of transmission may include the volume of blood or body fluids involved in the exposure (visible blood contamination or hollow-bore needle), the viral load (copies per milliliter) of the source patient, terminal illness status of the source patient, increased depth of exposure site/wound, and the immune status of the person exposed.

Patients can present to the emergency department with known disease, disease complications, suspected occult disease with high-risk behavior, or occupational exposures. The emergency physician must be educated in the most appropriate care choices for all of these patient situations, from prophylactic management to those critically ill who require care for end-stage AIDS.

INITIAL APPROACH AND STABILIZATION

HIV-infected patients presenting to the emergency department may have subclinical, blunted, subtle, or florid life-threatening illness. There are many life-threatening conditions affecting multiple organ systems that may be attributed to the primary disease process or to opportunistic infections secondary to immune compromise. A high degree of suspicion must be maintained for severe illness. The basic rule in the treatment of HIV-positive patients is "They are often much sicker than they appear."

Priority Diagnoses

HIV-infected and AIDS patients may present with severe medical complaints both related to and unrelated to their viral infection. Conditions that interfere with airway and respiratory status, cause hemodynamic instability, or present as altered mental status that may be secondary to infections or mass lesions are among the priority diagnoses in the emergency department.

Rapid Assessment and Early Intervention

A primary survey of airway, breathing, and circulation is followed by a systematic assessment of the patient. Universal precautions are strictly maintained by all members of the health care team. The primary assessment is followed by the management of medical issues compromising the patient's condition, with an additional awareness of possible HIV-related complications:

1. The airway is managed with standard protocols (see Chapter 2, Airway Management), with particular attention to the potential for airway compromise secondary to altered mental status or intracerebral disease. When intubation is necessary for patients with advanced AIDS, oropharyngeal infection with *Candida* can complicate the procedure and should be anticipated.

2. Respiratory compromise occurs from a variety of causes, primarily infectious in nature. *Pneumocystis carinii* pneumonia (PCP) produces hypoxemia and respiratory distress in the AIDS patient, with minimal physical examination findings. Pulse oximetry provides a rapid measurement of respiratory status and oxygenation, but it may be compromised by poor distal perfusion. Supplemental oxygen is provided to all patients with respiratory complaints.

3. Circulatory status is thoroughly assessed, and patients with compromise require continuous cardiac monitoring. Sepsis in HIV infection can produce signs and symptoms of shock in young patients, with no change in body temperature. Orthostatic vital signs may be evaluated in patients with suspected hypovolemia (bleeding, dehydration). Two large-bore intravenous lines with rapid normal saline infusion are indicated in any patient with hypotension, tachycardia, poor perfusion, and other signs of shock. If cardiac or pulmonary disease is suspected, careful reassessment for signs of pulmonary edema or fluid overload is needed after therapeutic interventions. If hemodynamic status does not improve, pressor infusion may be necessary.

4. Altered mental status may be the only presenting problem in HIV-infected patients and can occur from both infectious and noninfectious causes. Common causes, such as hypoglycemia and hypoxia, must not be forgotten while evaluating these patients. Signs of elevated intracranial pressure (altered level of consciousness, abnormal breathing pattern, pupil abnormalities, seizure) require aggressive measures to alleviate the insult. Intubation may be necessary to ensure airway control in the presence of severe mental status decline.

CLINICAL ASSESSMENT

Obtaining a clear and sequential history is potentially challenging in the patient with HIV infection and those who have progressed to AIDS. Developing a coherent story about a complex disease requires patience. An accompanying relative, significant other, or care provider may offer crucial information and helpful insights, especially if the patient has an altered mental status. The primary physician managing the patient's disease is often helpful, particularly those who specialize in patient care for the HIV-infected person.

History

Presenting Complaint. The chief complaint is the first data point received and may often be linked to an HIV-related complaint. It is often necessary to separate the acute complaints from the recurrent chronic conditions. HIV-infected patients have both common and uncommon causes for any given complaint, and their presenting complaints may *not* be directly related to their underlying HIV infection.

History of Present Illness. The origin of the presenting complaints from an HIV patient can be broad, with four main sources to explore: (1) symptoms arising from a new complication of HIV infection, (2) new or changing symptoms from established HIV-related conditions, (3) symptoms of adverse drug reactions or side effects (not uncommon), and (4) symptoms unrelated to the underlying HIV infection. Of the major presenting complaints of HIV-infected patients, respiratory and neurologic complaints are the most common. Infectious symptoms, such as fever, chills, cough, or headaches, are also common. Altered mental status is a particularly worrisome complaint. Cardiac complications also have been reported.

Review of Symptoms. A review of symptoms in the HIV-infected patient is likely to be positive for many secondary complaints. Careful questioning will help distinguish between pertinent acute symptoms and those that are chronic. Fever, chills, and night sweats may be chronic or part of the current presentation. Changes in appetite, weight loss, vomiting, and diarrhea may be chronic (drug effect) or acute (bacterial, fungal, or parasitic gastrointestinal infection).

Past Medical History. The past medical history can be extensive in patients with established AIDS. It is important to obtain detailed information regarding past and current conditions. The most recent CD4 count is important in understanding the stage of the disease, and therefore the potential for an opportunistic infection.

Medications/Allergies. A detailed history of current medications (prescribed and taken) is important. Regimens are often complex, compliance can be difficult, and adverse drug reactions are frequently seen in the HIV-infected patient. The current medication list is also needed to prevent medication interaction during the acute course in the emergency department.

Questions to Ask if HIV Infection Is Suspected but not Diagnosed

In patients with suspected disease who present with otherwise unexplained fever, myalgia, adenopathy, lethargy, rash, pharyngitis (seroconversion phase symptoms), or stigmata of immune compromise or opportunistic disease, questions regarding high-risk behavior or exposures should be asked.

- Has the patient been tested for HIV previously? Up to 30% of HIV patients may not spontaneously reveal their status when seeking medical care. Also, unrecognized HIV infection is common, especially in women and the elderly.
- What are the patient's sexual activity behaviors? Has there been unprotected intercourse (penile-anal, penile-vaginal, oral-genital) or more than one sexual partner?
- Is the patient an intravenous drug abuser with contaminated or shared needles?
- Has there been contact with blood/body fluids from nonsexual, nonoccupational exposure (e.g., piercing, tattooing)?
- Does the patient have a hematologic disease that requires multiple blood or blood product transfusions?

Physical Examination

General. A general assessment of the patient's overall appearance can help rapidly categorize the patient's condition as potentially unstable. Altered mental status is of particular concern. Pallor, tachypnea, and diaphoresis are also signs of serious illness that require prompt attention. Patients who appear malnourished, dehydrated, cachectic, and chronically ill also require careful evaluation.

Vital Signs. Vital signs are an important index of systemic illness, despite an overall nontoxic appearance. Fever is particularly notable in the immunocompromised patient when present, but the lack of a febrile response does not rule out severe systemic illness. Septic HIV-infected patients may not mount a high temperature because the immune system is too seriously compromised. The degree of fever is not indicative of disease severity or etiology. Fever is a nonspecific warning signal and can be the result of any number of viral, bacterial, fungal, or protozoan infec-

tions. It also can complicate a number of drug reactions, including neuroleptic malignant syndrome.

Blood pressure measurements are monitored closely in patients who appear ill. Systemic disease, shock, hypovolemia, and drug reaction/response are a few of many potential diagnoses causing hemodynamic instability.

Patients are assessed for the presence of tachypnea, which may herald pulmonary disease, even in the presence of normal auscultatory findings. Tachypnea or an abnormal oxygen saturation are both indications for a chest radiograph.

Tachycardia may represent systemic response to fever, pain, hypoxia, or hypovolemia, or it may be of cardiac etiology.

Skin. Skin examination is especially important because it may reveal nutritional deficiencies, malignancies. Kaposi's sarcoma, adverse drug reactions, "track marks," injury, and infection. Certain skin infections or skin changes, in an otherwise healthy young adult (e.g., new-onset seborrheic dermatitis, multiple violaceous plaques, or herpes zoster), require that the emergency physician inquire about risk factors and prior testing for HIV.

HEENT. Funduscopic examination may detect cotton-wool hemorrhagic spots typical for cytomegalovirus retinitis. If untreated, this viral infection can lead to blindness. Evaluation of the fundus for evidence of papilledema is also important (elevated intracranial pressure). Oral lesions may include oral candidiasis, hairy leukoplakia, or Kaposi's sarcoma. These should be actively sought. The ears and pharynx should be evaluated for infection.

Neck. Meningitis and other intracranial infections occur commonly in HIV-infected patients, and it is important to assess for evidence of meningismus and lymphadenopathy.

Heart. New murmurs can be indicative of bacterial endocarditis. Prior intravenous drug use is a common vector for HIV infection. Cardiac rub may indicate myocarditis or pericarditis. Tachycardia should be noted, and evidence of ectopic or dropped beats should be further evaluated using an electrocardiogram. The patient should remain on a cardiac monitor.

Lung. Evidence of tachypnea, pleuritic pain, wheezes, rales, rhonchi, or rubs should be noted. Pulmonary infections in the HIV-infected patient are often diagnosed in the emergency department and may be the first presentation of a severe immune compromise.

Abdomen. Intra-abdominal processes, including infection, must be considered in any HIV-infected patient presenting with acute abdominal complaints and particularly those with peritoneal signs. Diarrhea afflicts more than 50% of patients with AIDS, and a stool sample for culture and parasite evaluation is recommended in patients with this complaint.

Genitourinary. The close association between HIV and a sexually transmitted disease mandates a thorough genitourinary examination. Infection with *Neisseria gonorrhoeae, Chlamydia,* and herpesvirus are common in these patients. The genitalia are inspected for any lesions, and a serologic test for syphilis is recommended. A pelvic examination is performed in females, and complete genital assessment is performed in males. Recognition of coexistent pregnancy is particularly important for the protection and health of the fetus, as well as the mother.

Neurologic. Altered mental status, other neurologic symptoms, and respiratory complaints are the majority of chief complaints of emergency department patients with HIV infection. A thorough neurologic evaluation, including the mental status, is mandatory. Neurologic disease may include (1) focal neurologic deficits from mass lesions; (2) altered mental status secondary to encephalitis, meningitis, or dementia; and (3) peripheral neuropathies. All patients with new (or changing) neurologic signs and symptoms require computed tomography (CT) of the head. In the absence of a mass lesion or findings of elevated cerebrospinal fluid pressure on a CT scan, a lumbar puncture will usually be the next step in the diagnostic evaluation.

CLINICAL REASONING

From the start of the visit to the final disposition, the emergency physician must address the key questions that will ultimately guide patient care.

How Ill Is this Patient?

This question is the crux of the patient's case. As mentioned previously, patients with HIV infection can be much sicker than they initially appear. The immunocompromised state may prevent the development of clear signs of serious disease. Attention should be directed to subtle signs (fatigue, erythema, pallor) and minor behavior changes, as well as to the emergent issues.

Does the Condition Require Surgical Intervention?

Most of the findings in the patient with HIV infection do not require surgical intervention; however, these patients can have the same common surgical diseases found in noninfected patients, such as appendicitis and cholecystitis. A change in mental status may be secondary to a subdural hematoma, atypical brain abscess, encephalitis, or AIDS-related dementia.

What Is the Acute Change in the Patient, and What Is the Chronic Disease State?

It can be a challenge to determine the acute condition among the chronic medical issues that patients might have. Key symptoms of acute disease are fever, new shortness of breath, decreases in level of consciousness, or altered behavior patterns.

What Is the HIV Infection Pattern, and What Findings Suggest Progression to AIDS?

Seroconversion occurs 3 to 6 weeks after exposure to and infection with HIV. At the time of seroconversion, the patient can experience an acute syndrome that resembles mononucleosis. Fever, malaise, arthralgia, and myalgia occur with the appearance of lymphadenopathy. Weight loss and a nonspecific rash may also occur. This syndrome subsides in 1 to 2 weeks and is followed by a long asymptomatic period. An astute clinician, when confronted by this symptom-complex in a young adult, may ask about any risk factors for HIV infection.

After primary HIV infection, the average adult develops the first AIDS-defining illness in 7 to 9 years. In children, the asymptomatic period is shorter, usually 2 years. A positive test for HIV, a CD4 count of less than $200/mm^3$, and one of the following opportunistic infections indicate that the patient status has progressed to AIDS.

- Esophageal candidiasis
- Pulmonary tuberculosis
- Cryptococcosis
- Cryptosporidiosis
- Cytomegalovirus retinitis
- Herpes simplex virus
- Kaposi's sarcoma
- Brain lymphoma
- *Mycobacterium avium* complex
- *Pneumocystis carinii* pneumonia
- Progressive multifocal leukoencephalopathy
- Brain toxoplasmosis
- HIV encephalopathy
- HIV wasting syndrome
- Disseminated histoplasmosis
- Isosporiasis

- Disseminated *Mycobacterium tuberculosis* disease
- Recurrent *Salmonella* septicemia
- Invasive cervical cancer.

Is the Emergency Department and Hospital Capable of Providing the Breadth of Care Required by the Patient?

Patients with HIV-associated illness are commonly cared for in large medical centers with clinical programs able to support their needs. Most patients with HIV infection have readily identifiable caregivers within the health care system. Early contact with the primary caregivers is important, because complex treatment regimens can be reviewed and current CD4 counts and viral loads may be discussed. If the patient needs admission, transfer to the patient's primary health care facility may be arranged at the patient's (or physician's) request, when the initial medical evaluation is completed and the patient is stabilized for safe travel.

Are Appropriate Support Systems in Place for Outpatient Management?

Because of the complexity of HIV-associated diseases and their management, patients require well-coordinated support. Family members, social workers, case managers, and home infusion therapists all play a role in the care of these patients, in addition to physicians and nurses. Before discharge from the emergency department, the treatment and follow-up plan should include appointments with these health care providers.

DIAGNOSTIC ADJUNCTS

Laboratory Studies

Liberal use of laboratory testing is essential in the assessment of the HIV-infected patient. An aggressive search for a large number of potential diagnoses must be maintained. The tests described in the paragraphs that follow are performed routinely in HIV-infected patients with all but minor complaints and provide a broad overview of current clinical status.

Complete Blood Cell Count. Anemia, secondary to blood loss, hemolysis, or chronic disease, is not uncommon. The white blood cell (WBC) count, while not specific, provides a measure of the patient's response to disease. Sepsis, drug effect, and advanced disease diminish the WBC count, which is a poor prognostic sign. A CD4 count may be difficult to obtain in a timely manner. Therefore, an absolute lymphocyte count (ALC) may be calculated using total WBC count × lymphocyte percentage. Patients with ALCs less than 1000 cells/mm^3 are at higher risk for infection, and this level is almost always proportional to a CD4 count of less than or equal to 200/mm^3. If the ALC is greater than 2000/mm^3, less susceptibility is suggested.

Electrolytes and Renal Function. Nausea and vomiting are common side effects of the new antiretroviral drugs. HIV-related diarrhea can be prolonged and severe. Both vomiting and diarrhea lead to electrolyte imbalance with renal insufficiency and azotemia.

Urinalysis. In addition to testing for infection, the urinalysis can provide simple but useful information, such as specific gravity. A high specific gravity indicates urinary concentration, occurring with dehydration and volume loss.

Oxygen Saturation. Respiratory compromise in patients with HIV can be subtle. A careful observation of respiratory rate and effort, as well as determination of oxygen saturation with pulse oximetry, is carried out.

Liver Function/Amylase. Infectious hepatitis, acute and chronic, is often found in patients with HIV. Elevation of liver enzymes can be a side effect of antiretroviral agents, and elevation of amylase (e.g., pancreas injury secondary to medications) may also occur.

Cardiac Enzymes/Electrocardiogram. Chest pain can be the result of coronary artery disease, but pericarditis, pericardial effusion, and endocarditis are also considered. Risk factors for coronary artery disease, when present in patients with pain, support the decision to pursue enzyme and electrocardiographic testing.

Cerebrospinal Fluid. Bacterial meningitis may not be a clear-cut diagnosis in patients infected with HIV. Other causes of fever, headache, and altered mental status, such as brain abscess or viral infection, can also raise intracranial pressure. For these presentations, antibiotics should be administered before CT and lumbar puncture. They will not jeopardize the cerebrospinal fluid Gram stain or culture result. Blood, urine, sputum (if obtainable), and other indicated cultures are collected before giving the antibiotic, if possible. After the CT, if no intracranial mass is visualized, a lumbar puncture is carried out immediately. Because a myriad of infectious causes are possible, all suspected sites should be cultured. In addition to routine bacteriologic samples, mycobacterial, viral, and fungal cultures are obtained, as clinically indicated. The microbiologic complexity of these cases is best managed by laboratories that routinely handle specimens from HIV-infected patients.

Blood Cultures. These should be obtained in higher-risk patients such as intravenous drug users, toxic-appearing patients, those with indwelling devices, and patients with low CD4 counts or neutropenia.

Radiologic Imaging

Chest Radiograph. Most patients with fever, shortness of breath, or other systemic complaint require a chest film, even with normal auscultatory findings. Extensive *Pneumocystis carinii* pneumonia (PCP) can present with minimal symptoms and few findings on physical examination. Lobar infections, mediastinal adenopathy, and other findings may be revealed.

Computed Tomography. CT is a mainstay in the evaluation of patients with complaints related to HIV infection. Altered mental status, fever and headache, and headache alone (>3 days, different in quality) are indications for CT of the head. CT is performed with and without contrast medium enhancement to best define the potential findings. A CD4 count of less than or equal to 200/mm^3 is an important risk factor for a positive CT in HIV-positive patients presenting with uncomplicated headache.

Scans of the brain may detect elevated intracranial pressure (narrow ventricles, swollen or effaced brain) from many causes, including tumor, mass, abscess, hemorrhage, and encephalopathy. Evidence of midline shift, ventricular dilatation, and cerebral degeneration may be seen on unenhanced scans, whereas tumor, abscess, and vascular changes may be seen with the addition of contrast medium. In cases with strongly suspected central nervous system disease, and a normal CT, magnetic resonance imaging (MRI) is then performed. It is important that CT not delay administration of antibiotics in patients with suspected meningitis.

Computed tomography of the abdomen has become increasingly effective in diagnosing causes of abdominal pain, including intra-abdominal abscesses, masses, adenopathy, or other more typical pathologic processes, seen in nonimmunocompromised patients.

Electrocardiogram

An ECG is part of the evaluation of the suspected AIDS patient. Cardiac complications include dysrhythmias, myocarditis, pericarditis, and infective endocarditis.

Specific HIV-related Testing

CD4 Counts. Although not rapidly measurable in the acute care setting, the total CD4 T-cell count is one of the most important measures of patient stage of illness and potential condition when dealing with HIV-positive patients (Table 13–1). CD4 counts correlate roughly with the stage of disease and likelihood of certain infections. Normal CD4 range (± 2 SD) is 500 to 1400 cells/mm^3. The absolute CD4 count is the result of three other test variables: the total WBC count, the percent of lymphocytes, and the percent of the lymphocytes with CD4 receptor sites. Also contributing to the CD4 count are physiologic changes from season, time of day, other acute illnesses, acute corticosteroid therapy, or laboratory test variability. A count of 500 to 1000 cells/mm^3 is seen in early disease, at the time of seroconversion and acute HIV. Counts of less than 200 cells/mm^3 are associated with advanced disease and severe opportunistic infections such as *P. carinii* pneumonia and cytomegalovirus infections.

Viral Load. In recent years, the direct measurement of HIV genomic RNA has allowed for actual viral activity or "load" to be quantified. Viral load measurements correlate with stage and severity of disease more closely than CD4 counts. They are used to assess the effect of antiretroviral agents, acute HIV infection, and disease prognosis. On admission to the emergency department, the emergency physician should review the patient's medical records to determine the most recent cell counts and viral load. Of recent interest are possible gender differences in the viral loads of asymptomatic patients, with lower numbers in the female population. Further evaluation of these data is necessary to avoid a delay in medical therapy. Any gender difference in viral load count vanishes when the patients progress to symptomatic disease.

HIV Testing. Testing for HIV is not routinely done in the emergency department. It may be ordered for patients with a strong clinical suspicion of undiagnosed disease, for a health care worker with a significant occupational exposure, or occasionally during a sexual assault assessment. Appropriate pretest counseling and paperwork must be completed before phlebotomy and appropriate outpatient follow-up for results, posttest counseling, and treatment (if necessary) should be arranged.

Standard testing protocols are used by laboratories when analyzing specimens for HIV antibodies. This involves a highly sensitive enzyme-linked immunosorbent assay (ELISA) as the first step. If this test is negative, no further testing is done on

TABLE 13–1. Correlation of Complications with CD4 Cell Counts

CD4 Cell Count	Infectious Complications	Noninfectious complications
> 500/mm^3	Acute retroviral syndrome Candidal vaginitis	Persistent generalized lymphadenopathy Guillain-Barré syndrome Myopathy Aseptic meningitis
200–500/mm^3	Pneumococcal and other bacterial pneumonia Pulmonary tuberculosis Herpes zoster Oropharyngeal candidiasis (thrush) Cryptosporidiosis, self-limited Kaposi's sarcoma Oral hairy leukoplakia	Cervical intraepithelial neoplasia Cervical cancer B-cell lymphoma Anemia Mononeuronal multiplex Idiopathic thrombocytopenic purpura Hodgkin's lymphoma Lymphocytic interstitial pneumonitis
< 200/mm^3	*Pneumocystis carinii* pneumonia Disseminated histoplasmosis and coccidioidomycosis Miliary/extrapulmonary tuberculosis Progressive multifocal leukoencephalopathy	Wasting Peripheral neuropathy HIV-associated dementia Cardiomyopathy Vacuolar myelopathy Progressive polyradiculopathy Non-Hodgkin's lymphoma
< 100/mm^3	Disseminated herpes simplex Toxoplasmosis Cryptococcosis Cryptosporidiosis, chronic Microsporidiosis Candidal esophagitis	
< 50/mm^3	Disseminated cytomegalovirus Disseminated *Mycobacterium avium* complex	Central nervous system lymphoma

the specimen. If the ELISA is positive, a confirmatory Western blot assay is then done, evaluating for the presence of antibodies to three major viral proteins (a core protein and two envelope proteins). A positive result indicates antibodies to two of these major proteins. Sensitivity and specificity of current testing standards is greater than 99%. Rapid HIV testing (home kits, urine analysis, saliva analysis) is currently available but is not in widespread use.

PRINCIPLES OF MANAGEMENT

General Principles

A general management principle involved in the care of HIV-infected patients is "Anticipate the worst possible outcome and protect them against the consequences." Appropriately aggressive care to uncover and eliminate life-threatening problems is crucial, because HIV-infected patients are subject to the same problems as the noninfected population, in addition to HIV-related diseases.

Specific Principles

The three general categories of HIV-related problems that require specific management guidelines

are infectious, noninfectious, and adverse drug reactions.

Infectious Etiology. Patients with infectious complaints, including fever, are thoroughly evaluated. Hypotensive patients are presumed septic and resuscitated aggressively. Stable patients receive a thorough workup, as indicated by clinical scenario, including complete blood cell count, bacterial cultures (blood, urine, sputum, wound), urinalysis, chest radiograph, CT of head, and lumbar puncture. Antibiotics should be given as early as possible in the emergency department and are initially chosen for broad-spectrum activity, until sensitivity test results are completed (Table 13–2).

Noninfectious Etiology. The most significant noninfectious problem for the HIV-infected patient is malignancy, primarily lymphoma. Patients with focal neurologic abnormalities should always have CT of the head to rule out the presence of lymphoma or other focal processes (Table 13–3).

Adverse Drug Reactions. HIV patients are prone to adverse drug reactions from the multiple medications they are taking. These medications may include antiretroviral agents, prophylactic antibiotics, and antibiotics for current infections. The reactions are variable, with dermatologic,

TABLE 13–2. Common Infectious Complications of HIV Infection

Organism	Common Manifestations
Streptococcus pneumoniae	Community-acquired pneumonia
Haemophilus influenzae	Community-acquired pneumonia
Mycobacterium tuberculosis	Pulmonary tuberculosis
Candida species	Oropharyngeal and vaginal candidiasis
Herpes simplex virus	Orogenital herpes
Varicella zoster virus	Dermatomal zoster (shingles)
Epstein-Barr virus	Oral hairy leukoplakia
Cryptosporidium parvum	Self-limited diarrhea
Pneumocystis carinii	Pneumonia
Cryptosporidium parvum	Chronic diarrhea
Toxoplasma gondii	Encephalitis
Microsporidia	Diarrhea
Candida species	Esophagitis
Cryptococcus neoformans	Meningitis
Mycobacterium tuberculosis	Disseminated or extrapulmonary tuberculosis
Herpes simplex virus	Disseminated or aggressive herpes
Varicella zoster virus	Disseminated herpes zoster
Epstein-Barr virus	Primary central nervous system lymphoma
Mycobacterium avium complex	Disseminated *Mycobacterium avium* complex
Cytomegalovirus	Retinitis, gastrointestinal disease, encephalitis

TABLE 13–3. Noninfectious Complications of HIV Infection

Pulmonary	Kaposi's sarcoma Interstitial pneumonitis Primary pulmonary hypertension
Gastrointestinal	Esophagitis—60% to 75% *Candida albicans* Esophageal Kaposi's sarcoma Esophageal lymphoma Hepatic lymphoma Acalculous cholecystitis Drug-induced cholecystitis Drug-induced pancreatitis Pancreatic lymphoma or Kaposi's sarcoma Large and small bowel lymphoma or Kaposi's sarcoma
Hematologic	Bone marrow suppression Anemia Leukopenia Immune-mediated thrombocytopenia
Oncologic	Systemic lymphoma Primary central nervous system lymphoma Anogenital neoplasm
Neurologic	Aseptic meningitis Encephalopathy Headache Neuropathy (early and late onset) AIDS dementia Myopathy Seizures Transient ischemic attacks and strokes
Renal	HIV-associated nephropathy Renal tubular acidosis (hyporeninemic hypoaldosteronism) Adrenal insufficiency and necrosis
Ophthalmic	Microangiopathic retinopathy Ophthalmic lymphoma or Kaposi's sarcoma
Dermatologic	Acute HIV dermatitis Drug reactions Nutritional deficiency (acrodermatitis enteropathica, pellagra, scurvy) Kaposi's sarcoma Squamous cell carcinoma T-cell lymphoma B-cell lymphoma Nail changes, hair loss, psoriasis, seborrhea, pruritus Reiter's syndrome

nephrotoxic, hepatotoxic, and anaphylactoid occurrences. Early recognition is critical, as is discontinuation of the medication and symptom-specific therapy as indicated (Table 13–4).

SPECIAL CONSIDERATIONS

Pediatric Patients

HIV infection of the pediatric population occurs through three routes: (1) mother to child, (2) transfusion of infected blood, and (3) sexual abuse by an HIV-positive assailant. HIV infection is difficult to detect in the pediatric population for several reasons. The persistence of maternal IgG anti-HIV antibodies confounds standard tests (transplacental transfer) and may lead to positive tests for several months. Typically, by 9 months, 15% to 30% of these children are found to have actual infection, although maternal antibodies have been shown to remain for up to 18 months. Age-related changes in CD4 counts complicate use of this laboratory assay as an index of immunocompetence. Children may present with clinical presentations that are different from adults and often are unable to provide historical elements that guide the workup. There are several classifications for pediatric HIV patients, based on immunologic suppression, CD4 counts, and clinical presentation standards determined by the CDC.

Fever without a source in the pediatric HIV population is a special challenge, particularly in patients younger than 3 years of age. As in the infected adults, the WBC count may not be reliable for these children. A thorough evaluation and very low threshold for admission are needed when caring for these patients because of an increased risk for sepsis. HIV infection is maintained in the long list of differential diagnoses for these patients.

Antiretroviral therapy is recommended in children with clinical symptoms associated with HIV infection, immune suppression, and any younger than 12 months old. In children older than 1 year, with a normal immune status and who are HIV positive, there are two schools of thought: (1) those who treat regardless of the age or symptoms and (2) those who defer until situations of clinical risk of disease progression (increasing viral load, declining CD4 count, or clinical symptoms) occur. When therapy is initiated, typically a combination of a highly active protease inhibitor and two nucleoside analogue reverse transcriptase inhibitors are recommended. There are other recommended regimens and those specifically for extreme clinical situations, all of which should be initiated and monitored by a pediatric infectious disease specialist.

Hospital Staff HIV Exposure

Occupational exposure to HIV is a concern for all health care providers. When universal precautions are followed appropriately, the risk of exposure becomes minimal, but, unfortunately, accidents do occur. In the emergency department, the potential for mishaps is increased by the urgency of care needed by patients who may be at high risk for HIV seropositivity. The cumulative risk of HIV infection over an emergency department career of 30 years may be as high as 1.4%. The overall risk of infection after a single parenteral exposure to HIV-infected blood is estimated to be 0.3%. At the time of exposure, the exposed health care providers are tested for a baseline HIV status. Testing is done in a confidential manner, with accompanying pretest and posttest counseling. Because of the phase of infection to seroconversion, antibody testing should be repeated at 6 weeks, 12 weeks, 6 months, and 1 year. Emergency physicians need to be familiar with elevated risk associated with different types of parenteral exposures and must be aware of the indications for chemoprophylaxis (Tables 13–5 and 13–6). Currently, a three-drug regimen is recommended for significant blood exposures from a known positive source. Zidovudine (ZDV), lamivudine (3TC), and indinavir (IDV) are all prescribed for 4 weeks. Other combinations of these or similar drugs, at different doses, are given for less risky exposures. These prophylaxis schedules are accompanied by high rates of side effects that cause many patients to stop before completion of the regimen.

DISPOSITION AND FOLLOW-UP

Admission

Admission is straightforward for most cases of HIV patients presenting with a new complaint or a complication of an existing problem. The following guidelines are for less sick patients who need to be admitted:

- *Fever of unknown source:* Some patients with AIDS have persistent fevers that have sources. These patients are often managed in the outpatient setting.
- *New-onset neurologic event:* The CT in the emergency department may be unremarkable and an MRI is indicated.
- *Hypoxia:* Suggested *Pneumocystis* pneumonia and other pulmonary processes may be complicating factors.
- *Systemic changes:* Severe weakness, weight loss, uncontrolled diarrhea, fevers, and anorexia may be noted.

Text continued on page 231

TABLE 13-4. Adverse Reactions to Drugs for HIV Infections

Class/Agent	Common (>5%)	Uncommon (1–5%)	Rare (<1%)
Antiretroviral Agents			
Zidovudine (AZT)	Anemia, leukopenia, headache, nausea, other gastrointestinal intolerance, and malaise	Myalgia, insomnia, and nail pigmentation	Myopathy, rash, seizures, steatosis, cardiomyopathy (children), and mania
Didanosine	Diarrhea, pancreatitis, and peripheral neuropathy	Nausea, vomiting, rash, neutropenia, hyperuricemia, and hepatitis	Cardiomyopathy and steatosis
Zalcitabine (ddC)	Peripheral neuropathy and flu-like syndrome	Pancreatitis, aphthous ulcers, rash, and hepatitis	Thrombocytopenia and leukopenia
Stavudine (D4T)		Peripheral neuropathy, anemia, and leukopenia	Pancreatitis and rash
Nonnucleoside Reverse Transcriptase Inhibitors (NNRTIs)			
Nevirapine (Viramune; NVP)	Rash (including cases of Stevens-Johnson syndrome), fever, nausea	Headache, hepatitis, and increased liver function tests	
Delavirdine (Rescriptor; DLV)	Rash (including cases of Stevens-Johnson syndrome), nausea, diarrhea	Headache, fatigue, and increased liver function tests	
Efavirenz (Sustiva; EFV)	Rash (including cases of Stevens-Johnson syndrome), insomnia, somnolence	Dizziness, trouble concentrating, and abnormal dreaming	
Protease inhibitors (PIs)			
Indinavir (Crixivan; IDV)	Nausea, abdominal pain	Nephrolithiasis and indirect hyperbilirubinemia	
Nelfinavir (Viracept; NFV)	Diarrhea, nausea, abdominal pain	Weakness and rash	
Ritonavir (Norvir; RTV)	Weakness, diarrhea, nausea, circumoral paresthesia	Taste alteration and increased cholesterol and triglycerides	
Saquinavir (Fortovase; SQV)	Diarrhea, abdominal pain, nausea	Hyperglycemia and increased liver function test results	
Amprenavir (Agenerase; AMP)	Nausea, diarrhea, rash, circumoral paresthesia	Taste alteration and depression	
Lopinavir/ritonavir (Kaletra)	Diarrhea, fatigue, headache, nausea	Increased cholesterol and triglycerides	
Anti–*Pneumocystis*-*Toxoplasma* Drugs			
Trimethoprim-sulfamethoxazole (Bactrim, Septra)	Fever, rash, pruritus, leukopenia, nausea and vomiting (dose related)	Hepatitis, hyponatremia (IV form), and photosensitivity	Renal failure, hyperkalemia, hemolytic anemia, neuropathy, depression, Stevens-Johnson syndrome, and pancytopenia
Dapsone	Anemia (hemolytic) and rash	Methemoglobinemia, nephrotic syndrome, headache, insomnia, irritability, and nausea	Optic atrophy, peripheral neuropathy, aplastic anemia, fever, jaundice, and adenopathy
Pentamidine	Renal insufficiency, hypoglycemia and hyperglycemia, and sterile abscess (intramuscular injection), bronchospasm (aerosol)	Anemia, leukopenia, thrombocytopenia, hepatitis, and gastrointestinal intolerance	Pancreatitis, seizures, dysrhythmias, rash, and hypotension (use slow IV infusion)

Continued on following page

227

TABLE 13–4. Adverse Reactions to Drugs for HIV Infections Continued

Class/Agent	Common (>5%)	Uncommon (1–5%)	Rare (<1%)
Atovaquone	Headache, diarrhea, nausea, vomiting, rash, and fever	Hyponatremia and pruritus	
Trimetrexate (requires folinic acid)	Anemia, leukopenia, and thrombocytopenia	Nausea, vomiting, renal insufficiency, and hepatitis	Mucositis and rash
Pyrimethamine (requires folinic acid)		Anemia, leukopenia, and thrombocytopenia, and gastrointestinal intolerance	Ataxia, tremor, seizures, headache, fatigue, depression and insomnia
Clindamycin	Diarrhea (*Clostridium difficile* toxin associated) rash, nausea, and vomiting		Severe colitis
Primaquine		Hemolytic anemia and gastrointestinal intolerance	Headache, rash, pruritus, and methemoglobinemia
Antifungal Agents			
Amphotericin B	Fever and chills with infusion (may be treated with acetaminophen, hydrocortisone), renal insufficiency, hypokalemia, anemia, nausea, vomiting, headache, and phlebitis	Taste perversion and hypomagnesemia	Rash, pruritus, peripheral neuropathy, blurred vision, convulsion, gastrointestinal bleeding, arrhythmias, diabetes insipidus, hearing loss, pulmonary edema, hepatitis, and liver failure, eosinophilia, leukopenia, and thrombocytopenia
Ketoconazole	Nausea	Elevated transaminase levels, impotence, gynecomastia, menstrual irregularities, headache, dizziness, pruritus, rash, asthenia, nausea, vomiting, headache, abdominal pain, and diarrhea	Fulminant hepatitis, anaphylaxis, lethargy, fever, cytopenias, and hypothyroidism
Fluconazole		Elevated transaminase levels, nausea	Thrombocytopenia, Stevens-Johnson syndrome, and fulminant hepatitis
Itraconazole	Gastrointestinal intolerance	Elevated transaminase levels	Fulminant hepatitis
Antiviral Agents			
Foscarnet	Electrolyte abnormalities, renal impairment	Twitching and tremors, penile ulcers	Headache, nausea
Ganciclovir	Anemia, leukopenia, neutropenia	Elevated transaminases	Psychosis, nausea
Acyclovir	Nausea, vomiting (PO), irritation at injection site (IV)	Transient renal impairment, headache	Central nervous system: agitation, disorientation, encephalopathy

Modified from Kelen GD (ed): HIV interface with emergency medicine. Emerg Med Clin North Am 1995; 13: 134–135; with permission.

TABLE 13–5. Recommended HIV Postexposure Prophylaxis (PEP) for Percutaneous Injuries

Exposure Type	Infection Status of Source				
	HIV-Positive Class 1*	HIV-Positive Class 2*	Of Unknown HIV Status†	Unknown Source‡	HIV-Negative
Less severe§	Recommended basic 2-drug PEP	Recommended expanded 3-drug PEP	Generally, no PEP warranted; however, consider basic 2-drug PEP‖ for source with HIV risk factors¶	Generally, no PEP warranted; however, consider basic 2-drug PEP‖ in settings where exposure to HIV-infected persons is likely	No PEP warranted
More severe**	Recommend expanded 3-drug PEP	Recommend expanded 3-drug PEP	Generally, no PEP warranted; however, consider basic 2-drug PEP‖ for source with HIV risk factors¶	Generally, no PEP warranted; however consider basic 2-drug PEP‖ in settings where exposure to HIV-infected persons is more likely	No PEP warranted

*HIV-Positive, Class 1—asymptomatic HIV infection or known low viral load (e.g., <1500 RNA copies/mL). HIV-Positive, Class 2—symptomatic HIV infection, AIDS, acute seroconversion, or known high viral load. If drug resistance is a concern, obtain expert consultation. Initiation of PEP should not be delayed pending expert consultation, and, because expert consultation alone cannot substitute for face-to-face counseling, resources should be available to provide immediate evaluation and follow-up care for all exposures.

†Source of unknown HIV status (e.g., deceased person with no samples available for HIV testing).

‡Unknown source (e.g., a needle from a sharps disposal container).

§Less severe (e.g., solid needle and superficial injury).

‖The designation "consider PEP" indicates that PEP is optional and should be based on an individualized decision between the exposed person and the treating clinician.

¶If PEP is offered and taken and the source is later determined to be HIV negative, PEP should be discontinued.

**More severe (e.g., large-bore hollow needle, deep puncture, visible blood on device, or needle used in patient's artery or vein)

From MMWR, June 2001.

TABLE 13–6. Basic and Expanded HIV Postexposure Prophylaxis (PEP) Regimens

Drug	Dosage	Advantages	Disadvantages
Basic Regimen			
Zidovudine (ZDV; AZT) + lamivudine (3TC) (available as Combivir)	ZDV: 600 mg PO daily, divided into a two-dose or three-dose per day format 3TC: 150 mg PO twice daily May be given as a single Combivir tablet, PO twice daily	Serious toxicity in PEP use in rare Side effects are predictable and manageable with antiemetics and antimotility drugs Probably safe regimen for PEP in pregnant workers May be given as a single tablet	Side effects may result in poor compliance Source virus may be resistant
Alternate Basic Regimens			
Lamivudine (3TC) + stavudine (d4T)	d4T: 40 mg PO twice daily (if < 60 kg, 30 mg PO twice daily)	Well-tolerated, twice-daily doses, improving compliance Rare serious toxicity	Source virus may be resistant
Didanosine (ddI) + stavudine (d4T)	ddI: 400 mg PO daily on empty stomach (if <60 kg, 125 mg PO daily) d4T: 40 mg PO twice daily (if < 60 kg, 30 mg PO twice daily)	Likely to be effective versus source virus on 3TC and ZDV	ddI is unpalatable and difficult to take May interfere with other drug absorption Side effects are common Serious pancreatic, hepatic, and neurologic toxicities occur
Expanded Regimen (basic regimen plus one of the following drugs)			
Indinavir (IDV)	IDV: 800 mg PO every 8 hours on an empty stomach	Potent HIV inhibition	Serious nephrotoxicity Hyperbilirubinemia may occur Acid milieux for absorption (empty stomach) Multiple drug interactions, cannot take with ddI
Nelfinavir (NFV)	NFV: 750 mg PO three times daily, with meals or snack, *or* NFV: 1250 mg PO twice daily, with meals or snack	Potent HIV inhibitor	Multiple drug interactions
Efavirenz (EFV)	EFV: 600 mg PO daily, at bedtime	Improved compliance with twice-daily dosing May be active earlier than other agents as no phosphorylation is required for drug activation Improved compliance with once-daily dosing	May accelerate clearance of concomitant medications Early-onset drug rash can progress to Stevens-Johnson syndrome Seroconversion rash and early drug rash may be difficult to differentiate Nervous system toxicity and psychiatric symptoms are common and may be severe May be teratogenic in pregnancy
Abacavir (ABC) (available as Trizivir, a combination of ZDV, 3TC, and ABC)	ABC: 300 mg PO twice daily	Potent HIV inhibitor Well tolerated	Serious or life-threatening drug interactions may occur Severe hypersensitivity reactions in first 6 weeks

- *Hematologic derangement:* Leukopenia, anemia, and/or thrombocytopenia may occur.
- *Social reasons*: Poor intake, inability to manage medications, poor support, and poor compliance are factors to consider.

Observation

Patients qualify for observation when the reasonable expectation of their clinical course is the resolution of the acute problem and symptoms in the next 24-hour period. An example of an observation scenario is nausea and vomiting responsive to antiemetics and fluid administration.

DISCHARGE AND FOLLOW-UP

A patient with HIV-related acute complaints can be discharged when the issues have been thoroughly addressed. Vital signs (including orthostatic) have to be within a normal range, and oxygenation is appropriate. Mental status should be normal or unchanged from baseline. The patient and the caregivers must have a clear understanding and acceptance of the clinical treatment and the follow-up plan. Finally, the patient's primary physician is contacted, and a timely follow-up visit is scheduled.

FINAL POINTS

- HIV is the cause of an epidemic and infection often is fatal because of the incapacitating effects on the immune system, particularly the CD4 lymphocytes.
- Initial stabilization focuses on the "ABCs" with an awareness that HIV-infected patients are often sicker than they appear.
- Maintaining blood and body fluid precautions is essential in managing any patient, particularly those infected with HIV. Any critical patient who requires an invasive procedure creates a risk for the health care provider.
- History taking is often a process of determining what is a new-onset disorder versus a deterioration or change in an HIV-related illness.
- The most recent CD4 count and viral load is important for immune suppression information and infectivity.
- The onset of *Pneumocystis* pneumonia may be subtle, with hypoxia more severe than the clinical presentation would predict.
- Antiretroviral-related complications and medication side effects are very common and may be severe.
- Social support is as important as medical treatment in patients with an acute disorder related to their HIV infection.
- Antiretroviral therapy has become very effective, the prognosis for these patients has significantly improved, and the disease now behaves more like a chronic condition versus an inevitably fatal one.

CASE*Study*

The rescue squad brings a 33-year old man to the emegency department. He appears ill, complains of weakness, and states that he is HIV positive. The medics report they were called by the patient's roommate because the patient "was weak" and could not get out of bed. Vital signs at the scene were blood pressure, 100/50 mm Hg; pulse, 100 beats per minute; and respiratory rate, 24 breaths per minute. The patient was given oxygen by nasal cannula at 2 L/min with an open intravenous line of normal saline, at 100 mL/hr.

Generalized weakness is a common complaint of patients with AIDS. In this case, the weakness may be the result of an underlying infectious condition. The respiratory rate is of particular concern. The patient needs prompt attention from the emergency physician. Patients with AIDS are often sicker than they appear at the start of the visit.

As the initial evaluation and stabilization occurs, pulse oximetry on room air was measured at 92%. Attempts at obtaining orthostatic vital signs were discontinued when the patient became weak and dizzy when sitting. The pulse increased rapidly to 140 beats per minute. Oral temperature was 101.5°F (38.6°C). His mental status was normal. Chest examination revealed no rales, rhonchi, or rubs. A second intravenous line was placed, and oxygen by mask delivered at 100%. A liter of saline was delivered wide open followed by an infusion of 250 mL/hr. A rectal examination was negative for occult blood. A blood sample was drawn and sent for complete blood cell count, electrolytes and glucose determination, renal function, and blood cultures. A chest radiograph and arterial blood gas evaluation was ordered. Because of the hemodynamic instability of this patient, he was moved to a critical care bed in the emergency department.

Continued on following page

These steps complete the initial stabilization. The emergency team remains focused on the potential instability of the patient. The life-threatening problems (hypoxia and volume depletion) are addressed effectively. The basic screening tests are ordered. At this point, a more complete evaluation can take place.

A more complete history reveals that the patient has been HIV positive for 7 years. He was compliant with his antiretroviral therapy until recently, when he lost his job. His partner reveals that he has become increasingly depressed and was less compliant with his medications. Before this acute episode, the patient had had no AIDS-defining illness. Close questioning revealed weight loss for at least 1 month and bowel habit change, with the onset of persistent diarrhea. A thorough physical examination reveals evidence of weight loss and an erythematous rash with scaling plaques on the malar eminences, ears, and genitalia. Auscultation of the chest remains clear. His last CD4 count (4 months previously) was 400/mm³. A repeat count was ordered, with a viral load determination.

The patient's condition has deteriorated rapidly since his job loss. Maintaining a complicated antiretroviral regimen is a challenge for any motivated, stable HIV-infected patient. Many circumstances disrupt the regimen and lead to opportunistic infections and other complicating conditions. Weight loss, diarrhea, and the seborrheic dermatitis rash are consistent with advancing disease. His CD4 count while he was still "healthy" is of concern, at the level less than 500 cells/mm³.

The chest radiograph reveals diffuse, bilateral infiltrates consistent *with Pneumocystis carinii* pneumonia. His hematocrit was 34% with a WBC count of 3800 cells/mm³. The arterial pH was 7.48, the P_{CO_2} was 18 mm Hg, and the P_{O_2} was 55 mm Hg on room air. An antibiotic (trimethoprim-sulfamethoxazole) and a first dose of prednisone was given. Intravenous fluids were continued, and multivitamins were added to the solution. The patient's primary health care provider was contacted and agrees to the hospital admission. After discussing the treatment plan with the patient, his partner, and his family, the patient was transferred to a monitored bed for ongoing care.

The patient has developed a clear AIDS-defining illness, Pneumocystis carinii *pneumonia. Because of his hypoxia (P_{O_2} < 70 mm Hg), corticosteroids are given in addition to antibiotics. His weight loss and poor nutritional status should be addressed, and treatment is started with vitamins. In addition to informing the family and discussing treatment plans, the emergency physician may take the partner aside to discuss his HIV status and recommend testing if needed, completing the "total" care of this patient.*

Bibliography

TEXTS

Bartlett JG, Gallant JE: 2000–2001 Medical Management of HIV Infection. Baltimore, John Hopkins University, 2000.

Pizzo PA, Wilfert CM (eds): Pediatric AIDS: The Challenge of HIV Infection in Infants, Children, and Adolescents, 2nd ed. Baltimore, Williams & Wilkins, 1994.

JOURNAL ARTICLES

Armstrong WS, Katz JT, Kazanjian PH: Human immunodeficiency virus–associated fever of unknown origin: A study of 70 patients in the United States and review. Clin Infect Dis 1999; 28:341–345.

Barbaro G, Fisher SD, Giancaspro G, Lipshultz SE: HIV-associated cardiovascular complications: a new challenge for emergency physicians. Am J Emerg Med 2001; 19:566–574.

Carpenter CC, Cooper DA, Fischl MA, et al: Antiretroviral therapy in adults: Updated recommendations of the International AIDS Society—USA Panel. JAMA 2000; 283:381–390.

Centers for Disease Control and Prevention: Health-care workers with documented and possibly occupationally acquired AIDS/HIV infection, by occupation, reported through March 1993, United States. HIV/AIDS Surveillance Reports 1993; May 19.

D'Souza MP, Cairns JS, Plaeger SF: Current evidence and future directions for targeting HIV entry: Therapeutic and prophylactic strategies. JAMA 2000; 284:215–222.

Kelen GD (ed): HIV interface with emergency medicine. Emerg Med Clin North Am 1995; 13:134–135.

Kovacs JA, Masur H: Prophylaxis against opportunistic infections in patients with human immunodeficiency virus infection. N Engl J Med 2000; 342:1416–1429.

Levine AM: Evaluation and management of HIV-infected women. Ann Intern Med 2002; 136:228–242.

Moran GJ: Pharmacologic management of HIV/STD exposure. Emerg Med Clin North Am 2000; 18:829–842, viii.

Moran GJ, House HR: HIV-related illnesses: The challenge of ED management. Emerg Med Pract 2002; 4:1–28.

Park DR, Sherbin VL, Goodman MS, et al: The Harborview CAP Study Group. The etiology of community-acquired pneumonia at an urban public hospital: Influence of human immunodeficiency virus infection and initial severity of illness. J Infect Dis 2001; 184:268–277.

Rothman RE, Keyl PM, McArthur JC, et al: A decision guideline for emergency department utilization of noncontrast head computed tomography in HIV-infected patients. Acad Emerg Med 1999; 6:1010–1019.

Sepkowitz KA: Effect of prophylaxis on the clinical manifestations of AIDS-related opportunistic infections. Clin Infect Dis 1998; 26:806–810.

Shapiro NI, Karras DJ, Leech SH, et al: Absolute lymphocyte count as a predictor of CD4 count. Ann Emerg Med 1998; 32(3 pt 1):323–328.

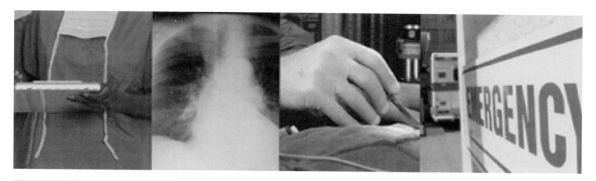

INFECTIOUS DISORDERS

CHAPTER 14

Febrile Adults

WESLEY EILBERT

CASE *Study*

A 36-year-old man presented to the emergency department complaining of fever and having "the flu" over the past 2 days. Triage vital signs were temperature, 101.8°F (38.7°C); pulse, 108 beats per minute; blood pressure, 112/70 mm Hg; and respirations, 20 breaths per minute.

INTRODUCTION

Fever can be defined as an elevation of the body temperature caused by a change in the hypothalamic set-point. In contrast, *hyperthermia* is caused by overwhelming or malfunction of the body's usual cooling mechanisms, in which heat production exceeds heat loss. Whereas fever rarely causes temperature elevations in excess of 105.8°F (41°C), hyperthermia may lead to temperatures well above this level. Most fevers are caused by infection, but other causes do exist (Table 14–1). Causes of hyperthermia include heatstroke,

TABLE 14–1. Noninfectious Causes of Elevated Temperature

Allergic reactions
Central nervous system
    Hypothalamic injury
    Subarachnoid hemorrhage
Connective tissue diseases
    Rheumatoid arthritis
    Systemic lupus erythematosus
    Vasculitides
Drug reactions
    Most commonly cocaine
Factitious fever
Familial fever
Heat illness
Hyperthyroidism/thyroid storm
Immunization reactions
Inflammatory disorders
    Sarcoid
    Crohn's disease
Malignant hyperthermia
Neoplasms
    Most commonly leukemia or lymphoma
Tissue injury or infarction

hyperthyroidism, and malignant hyperthermia due to medication. Fever of infectious origin is the primary focus of this chapter.

The baseline body temperature in humans varies among individuals, with the majority falling in the range of 96.8°F to 99.9°F (36°C to 37.8°C). A circadian rhythm is typically present with variations of up to 3.6°F (2°C) throughout the day. Temperatures are usually lowest around 4 AM and peak between 6 PM and 10 PM. This diurnal pattern persists in febrile individuals. Given the wide variations of normal it is difficult to assign a set temperature as a definition of fever. A reasonable guideline may be oral temperatures exceeding 99.6°F (37.5°C) in the morning hours and 100.4°F (38.0°C) in the evening.

The process by which the body produces fever is illustrated in Figure 14–1. Fever appears to have a beneficial effect on immune function by increasing the phagocytic and bactericidal activity of neutrophils and the cytotoxic effects of lymphocytes. Fever also lowers serum iron levels, making it more difficult for bacteria to reproduce. The febrile response places a significant metabolic burden on the body, increasing the basal metabolic rate 7% for each 1°F (0.55°C) increase in temperature. It also shifts the oxyhemoglobin dissociation curve to the right, resulting in lower serum oxygen saturation.

Fever with or without an associated symptom is found in about 6% of adult visits to the emergency department. Febrile illnesses are a major source of morbidity and mortality especially in the very young, the elderly, and the immunocompromised. An organized and thorough approach is necessary to differentiate a benign febrile illness from a potentially fatal or catastrophic one.

INITIAL APPROACH AND STABILIZATION

Priority Diagnoses

Any febrile patient with a significant abnormality of other vital signs warrants immediate assessment. Likewise, any patient with a fever and altered mental status should be evaluated without delay. Although any febrile illness has the potential for significant morbidity, the following priority

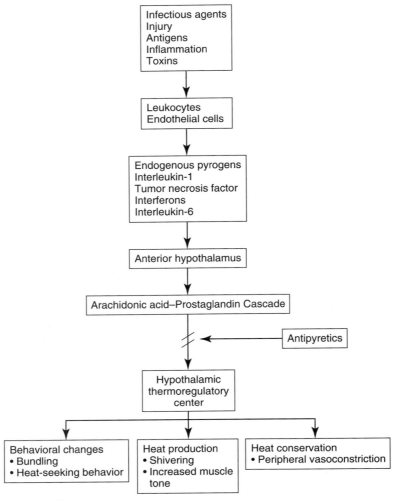

FIGURE 14–1 • Production of fever.

diagnoses require immediate identification given their rapidly fatal potential.

- Sepsis or septic shock
- Bacterial meningitis
- Infections causing potential airway compromise (epiglottitis and deep space infections of the lower face and neck)
- Pneumonia
- Acute bacterial peritonitis
- Suspected necrotizing fasciitis

Rapid Assessment

1. Is there any evidence of *current* or *impending airway compromise*? An immediate history of difficulty swallowing, hoarseness, or a distressing "lump" in the throat or physical findings of drooling, stridor, obvious edema, or the inability of the patient to tolerate certain neck postures should alert the physician to consider

immediate airway control. Distortion of the usual anatomy may necessitate using alternative airway techniques such as fiberoptic intubation, intubation under controlled conditions in the operating room (time permitting), or cricothyrotomy.

2. Is there evidence of *inadequate ventilation or impending respiratory failure*? Whereas fever itself may cause a mild increase in the respiratory rate, any patient with tachypnea out of proportion to the height of the fever or auscultatory findings consistent with pneumonia should be evaluated with pulse oximetry and placed on supplemental oxygen. Arterial blood gas analysis should be performed. Intubation and mechanical ventilation is considered if the infectious process is causing inadequate ventilation or uncorrectable hypoxia.

3. Is there *hypotension or tachycardia out of proportion* to the height of the fever? (The pulse

can be expected to rise 10 beats per minute for every 1°F (0.55°C) rise in body temperature.) Evidence of hypoperfusion or hypotension with fever implies sepsis and should be treated initially with aggressive fluid resuscitation.

4. Is there any change in the *patient's mental status*? Altered mental status with fever should be presumed to be caused by meningitis until proven otherwise. Septic patients are often noted to have an altered sensorium.

5. Is a *characteristic rash* present? Although several different illnesses may present as fever and rash, the petechial rash of meningococcemia should not be missed. This rash may initially have a maculopapular appearance before progressing to petechiae and eventually purpura. It may be present anywhere on the skin or mucous membranes but is most common on the trunk and extremities.

6. Is there *evidence of peritonitis*, such as a rigid abdomen, absence of bowel sounds, or severe abdominal pain with any movement?

7. Are there any *clinical findings* consistent with *rapidly expanding deep cellulitis*, especially in diabetics or other immunosuppressed individuals?

Early Intervention

In suspected sepsis or septic shock, or any priority diagnosis, the following interventions are instituted:

1. Two large-bore intravenous lines with isotonic crystalloid running.
2. Aggressive volume resuscitation with 1 to 2 L being administered over the first 30 to 60 minutes, unless contraindicated.
3. Cardiac and pulse oximetry monitoring.
4. Frequent repeat monitoring of vital signs.
5. Early administration of appropriate antibiotics (within 1 hour of initial assessment). Empirical dosing based on suspicion of the infecting agent is common (Table 14–2).
6. Early administration of antipyretics, unless contraindicated.
7. Early consultation with the appropriate consultant, for example, a surgeon should be consulted for necrotizing fasciitis, as extensive debridement is an integral component of therapy.

CLINICAL ASSESSMENT

History

A thorough history is often the most important step in determining the cause of a patient's fever. A significant percentage of patients complaining of subjective fever are found to be afebrile on examination.

Characteristics of the Fever

Duration. Some infectious diseases may cause fevers lasting 2 weeks or more. However, a fever persisting for over 3 weeks without a source requires extensive workup beyond what is possible in the emergency department.

Pattern. Although classic fever patterns are described for several illnesses, their value in this age of frequently used antipyretics is quite limited.

Concomitant Symptoms

Pain. Many febrile illnesses, classically those of viral etiology, can cause diffuse myalgia. Most localized inflammatory processes cause pain at the site, and this complaint should help focus the history and physical examination.

Headache. Although fever alone may cause a headache, meningitis should be considered in any febrile patient with this complaint.

Sore Throat. Pharyngitis is a very common cause of fever with a sore throat. However, other potentially life-threatening illnesses, such as epiglottitis, may present these complaints.

Chest Pain. Fever with chest pain, especially if pleuritic, should prompt a careful evaluation for pneumonia.

Abdominal Pain. Any complaint of abdominal pain with fever should be treated as a potential surgical emergency until proven otherwise.

Chills and Rigors. Chills, a sensation of cold despite an elevated body temperature, are common with all febrile illnesses and therefore of little diagnostic value. Rigors, profound chills with shivering and teeth chattering, are reportedly more common with bacterial or protozoal diseases. However, this distinction is of questionable clinical value.

Nausea, Vomiting, and Anorexia. Although the presence of any of these features suggests an intra-abdominal source of the fever, they are neither sensitive nor specific in this regard.

Past Medical History

Several preexisting conditions may compromise a patient's host defenses and predispose the patient to serious illness (Table 14–3). Any patient with an indwelling foreign body, such as an intravenous catheter, urinary catheter, prosthetic joint, or heart valve is at increased risk to develop infections related to these devices.

TABLE 14–2. Empirical Antibiotic Choices for Community-Acquired Adult Infection

Setting	Common Organism	Primary Antibiotic	Alternate Antibiotic
Urinary tract	E. coli or Enterococcus	Fluoroquinolone,[†] trimethoprim/sulfamethoxazole, or third-generation* cephalosporin	Broad-spectrum penicillin[§] or imipenem or meropenem
Biliary tract	Enterobacter, Enterococcus	Anti-pseudomonal penicillin,[‡] imipenem or meropenem, broad-spectrum penicillin,[§] ampicillin + gentamicin	Third-generation* cephalosporin + clindamycin or metronidazole
Peritonitis, secondary	Gram-negative aerobes and anaerobes: Enterobacteriaceae, enterococci, Bacteroides	Cefoxitin, cefotetan, broad-spectrum penicillin,[§] imipenem or meropenem	Third-generation* cephalosporin or cefepime or aztreonam or fluoroquinolone + clindamycin or metronidazole
Pneumonia			
Previously healthy	Streptococcus pneumoniae, Haemophilus influenzae, Mycoplasma, Chlamydia	Azithromycin or enhanced spectrum[†] fluoroquinolone or third-generation* cephalosporin + erythromycin	Third-generation* cephalosporin + azithromycin
COPD, DM, ETOH	As above + anaerobes and Klebsiella	Imipenem or meropenem or broad-spectrum penicillin,[§] cefepime	Enhanced-spectrum fluoroquinolone[†]
Neutropenic	As above + fungi	As above + amphotericin B	Fluconazole for fungal coverage
AIDS	Pneumocystis carinii, Mycobacterium tuberculosis	Trimethoprim/sulfamethoxazole	Clindamycin + primaquine
Viral	Influenza virus A or B, other viruses	Zanamivir or oseltamivir	Influenza virus A only: amantadine or rimantadine
Bacterial meningitis			
Previously healthy	S. pneumoniae, meningococcus	Ceftriaxone or cefotaxime	Meropenem
Elderly, DM, ETOH abuse	As above + Listeria and gram-negative bacilli	As above + ampicillin	
AIDS	Above + Cryptococcus	As above + amphotericin B	Fluconazole for Cryptococcus coverage
Decubitus ulcer	Mixed aerobes and anaerobes	Imipenem or meropenem or broad-spectrum penicillin[§]	Enhanced-spectrum fluoroquinolone[†] + clindamycin or metronidazole
Unknown Source			
Previously healthy	Staphylococcus, Streptococcus, gram-negative bacilli, anaerobes	Ticarcillin/clavulanate or piperacillin/tazobactam or imipenem or meropenem	Cefepime or third-generation* cephalosporin + metronidazole or clindamycin
Neutropenic	Above + Pseudomonas + fungi	Imipenem or cefepime or ceftazidime	

*Third-generation cephalosporins include cefotaxime, ceftriaxone, ceftazidime, ceftizoxime, and cefoperazone.
[†]Enhanced-spectrum fluoroquinolones include levofloxacin, gatifloxacin, and moxifloxacin.
[‡]Anti-pseudomonal penicillins include mezlocillin, piperacillin, and ticarcillin.
[§]Broad-spectrum penicillins include ticarcillin/clavulanate, piperacillin/tazobactam, and ampicillin/sulbactam.
COPD, chronic obstructive pulmonary disease; DM, diabetes mellitus; ETOH, ethanol.

TABLE 14–3. Preexisting Conditions That Predispose to Serious Febrile Illness

Active malignancy or recent chemotherapy
Chronic corticosteroid use
Chronic debilitating illness
Chronic renal failure
Congenital or acquired immunodeficiency syndromes
Diabetes mellitus
Extremes of age
Organ transplant recipients
Sickle cell anemia
Splenectomy

Other key points in the past medical history include recent immunizations and any noninfectious medical illness that may produce a fever (see Table 14–1). Chronic conditions that limit the patient's ability to meet the increased metabolic demands of fever, such as chronic obstructive pulmonary disease or decompensated congestive heart failure, should be identified.

Human Immunodeficiency Virus (HIV) Risk Factors

Given the obvious clinical importance of this illness (see Chapter 13, Approach to HIV in the Emergency Department), a thorough history from any febrile patient in the emergency department should include the following:

• Sexual preference and practices
• Prior blood product transfusions
• Intravenous drug use
• Occupational history

Social History

Tobacco and alcohol use should be determined. Intravenous drug use is a risk factor not only for HIV infection but also for several other blood-borne infections and endocarditis. A sexual history, occupational history, and recent travel history should be sought. Finally, any recent household or other contacts with ill individuals should be identified.

Family History

A few febrile illnesses affect only certain ethnic groups, such as Mediterranean fever. Other noninfectious causes of fever, such as connective tissue disease, may have a familial pattern.

Medications and Allergies

The patient's current medications, prescription and nonprescription, should be reviewed. Use of antipyretics and antibiotics (prescription and self-prescribed) are important to determine. Despite a commonly held belief to the contrary, the response of the fever to antipyretics does not help to distinguish bacterial from nonbacterial infections.

Review of Systems

This part of the history can be more focused if the source of the fever is obvious and should be expanded when the cause of the fever is unknown.

Physical Examination

Examination of the febrile patient in the emergency department is directed primarily by the concomitant symptoms. Patients without a likely source of their fever require a more extensive physical examination.

Body Temperature Measurement

Standard "glass" thermometers have been used for years to measure body temperature and still are considered the clinical "gold standard." Digital electronic thermometers allow a more rapid temperature assessment and are reasonably accurate. Liquid crystal thermometers are plastic strips containing compounds that alter their molecular structure and change color in response to varying temperature. Although easy to use and read, they are imprecise. Infrared detectors used to measure tympanic membrane temperatures have become popular in recent years. These thermometers offer the theoretical advantage of measuring a true core temperature as reflected by the tympanic membrane. The accuracy of these thermometers may be compromised however by the effects of ambient temperature and otitis media.

A true *core temperature*, as measured in the esophagus, pulmonary artery, or bladder, is usually not obtainable in the emergency department. A *rectal temperature* gives a reasonably accurate measurement of the core temperature but may not be practical for all patients. *Oral temperatures* are convenient and easily tolerated by patients. Oral temperatures vary by up to 2.9°F (1.6°C) depending on where the probe is positioned in the mouth. Ideally, the temperature should be measured under the tongue. Oral temperatures are usually 1.3°F (0.7°C) lower than rectal temperatures and can be significantly influenced by respiratory rate, heart rate, recent smoking, and recent ingestion of hot or cold liquids. *Axillary temperatures* are reportedly 1.3°F (0.7°C) lower than oral temperatures but are notoriously inaccurate and not appropriate for most patients.

Although certain infectious processes can cause fevers of characteristic magnitude (e.g., the "low grade" fever of appendicitis), fever height by itself is of limited diagnostic value. Furthermore, fever magnitude has not proved helpful in predicting the presence of bacteremia in adult patients. Patients at extremes of age or who are immunocompromised may not mount a fever in response to infection.

Other important components of the physical examination are listed in Table 14–4.

CLINICAL REASONING

The approach to the febrile adult patient in the emergency department is outlined in Figure 14–2. It can be summarized by answering the following four questions.

Is There Evidence of an Acute Life-Threatening Illness?

Characteristics of the acute life-threatening febrile illnesses are listed in Table 14–5. If a catastrophic illness is suspected, stabilization and empirical therapy take precedence over establishing the definitive diagnosis.

Are Concomitant Symptoms or Signs Present That Indicate a Possible Source of the Fever?

Most febrile illnesses will have symptoms or clinical findings suggestive of a particular illness or related set of illnesses.

Does the Patient Have Risk Factors for Specific Illnesses or Is the Patient Elderly or Immunocompromised?

Without an obvious other source, diagnostic efforts should be directed toward those illnesses for which the patient is at risk. Immunocompromised patients and the elderly often have atypical presentations of common illnesses and therefore require more extensive evaluation when the source of the fever is unknown.

Is Further Laboratory or Other Ancillary Testing Indicated?

In the absence of a source of the fever, certain diagnostic investigations may be used to screen for common infections.

DIAGNOSTIC ADJUNCTS

Laboratory Testing

Complete Blood Cell Count (CBC). Despite its well-known limitations, the CBC is frequently used to screen for serious bacterial illness. It may be more appropriately viewed as a confirmatory examination. White blood cell (WBC) counts above the normal range, especially those greater than 15,000/mm^3, have been found to be predictive of serious illness in adults. Likewise, a higher than normal percentage of immature band forms, greater than 10%, has been found to be a predictor of serious illness. However, both the total WBC and band count may be elevated by noninfectious processes and therefore have limited specificity (Table 14–6). The sensitivity of these findings is also of limited value, especially in the elderly and immunocompromised. A serious bacterial infection cannot be excluded on the basis of a normal CBC.

A low WBC count may be associated with some viral illnesses, or secondary to a depletion of the bone marrow storage pool of polymorphonuclear leukocytes (PMNs), signifying an overwhelming bacterial infection. For this reason, neutropenia in the setting of septic shock is a particularly ominous sign.

Certain morphologic changes have been identified in PMNs that may be predictive of significant bacterial disease. The presence of toxic granules, Döhle bodies, and cytoplasmic vacuoles has been found to be relatively sensitive yet rather nonspecific in detecting bacterial infections.

C-Reactive Protein (CRP). CRP is an acute-phase reactant that typically elevates in the presence of bacterial infection. It has demonstrated some use in predicting the presence of serious bacterial illness in some patient populations. Although sensitive for bacterial illness, CRP is relatively nonspecific.

Blood Cultures. Blood cultures remain the gold standard for identifying bacteremia. They are often routinely ordered on febrile patients in the emergency department. Only 5% to 7% of all blood cultures sent from the emergency department yield positive results, and a significantly smaller percentage will result in a change in management. This high cost-to-benefit ratio has lead to the development of several clinical models to identify those patients whose care might be significantly influenced by blood culture results. Patients with the following disorders or features should have blood drawn for culture when presenting to the emergency department with fever:

TABLE 14–4. Important Components of the Physical Examination in Febrile Adults

Area of Examination	Important Components	Comments
General appearance	Apparent state of health State of awareness Signs of distress Posture and gait	Often a good indicator of current immunologic status. May be altered in sepsis or central nervous system infection. Often present in life-threatening illness. Frequently altered to compensate for pain.
Skin	Inspection	Many rashes are characteristic of the underlying illness. Petechiae and purpura may signify the presence of sepsis or disseminated intravascular coagulation. May be flushed in early sepsis or pale in late sepsis. Examine nails for cyanosis (often present with hypoxia and hypotension) and splinter hemorrhages, which may be present with bacterial endocarditis. Inspect the sacral area and heals for decubitus ulcers or any evidence of infection, and note any areas of localized erythema indicating cellulitis.
	Palpation	Note areas of localized warmth. Crepitus may represent early necrotizing fasciitis or gas-producing organisms. Cool, moist ("clammy") skin may be present with septic shock. The presence of diffuse lymphadenopathy may be a marker of previously undiagnosed HIV infection.
HEENT		
Ears	Inspection	Note appearance and mobility of the tympanic membrane.
Sinuses	Transillumination Percussion	Inability to transilluminate suggests mucosal thickening or fluid in the sinus. Overlying tenderness suggests sinusitis.
Pharynx	Inspection	Note any erythema, exudates, or uvular displacement, which may be caused by peritonsillar abscess.
Mouth	Inspection Percussion	The presence of oral candidiasis may be a marker of previously undiagnosed HIV infection. Tenderness to percussion over teeth characteristically present with dental abscesses.
Neck	Inspection Auscultation	Note any swelling. Stridor is a concerning sign of airway impingement that may be present with epiglottitis, retropharyngeal abscess, and Ludwig's angina.
	Palpation	Note any enlarged lymph nodes. Pain or resistance to neck flexion/extension is frequently present with meningitis.
Chest		
Heart	Auscultation	Note any unusual murmurs or rubs.
Lungs	Inspection Auscultation Percussion	Note any retractions or accessory muscle use. Check the symmetry and quality of breath sounds. Dullness may indicate pneumonia or effusion.
Breast	Palpation	In postpartum women, warmth or tenderness may be a sign of mastitis.
Abdomen	Inspection	A guarded posture (i.e., to avoid any jarring of the peritoneum) is suggestive of peritonitis. Pain with coughing or bed shaking is a relatively sensitive indicator of peritonitis.
	Auscultation Percussion Palpation	Decreased or absent bowel sounds usually noted with peritonitis. Note any costovertebral angle tenderness, seen with pyelonephritis Check for rigidity, localized tenderness and rebound tenderness.
Genital		
Female	Inspection Palpation	Note any lesions or unusual discharge. Cervical motion tenderness and adnexal tenderness are signs of pelvic inflammatory disease. The presence of an adnexal mass may be noted with a tubo-ovarian abscess.
Male	Inspection Palpation	Check for urethral discharge and penile lesions suggestive of sexually transmitted disease. Epididymal and testicular tenderness and swelling are indicative of epididymitis and orchitis, respectively.
Rectal	Inspection Palpation	Note any perianal redness or swelling suggestive of a perirectal abscess. Check for masses, tenderness, or fluctuance of the prostate.
Musculoskeletal	Inspection Palpation	Note any swelling/erythema around joints or Osler's nodes or Janeway lesions in infective endocarditis. Check for increased warmth or effusions in joints suggestive of septic arthritis.

HIV, human immunodeficiency virus.

241

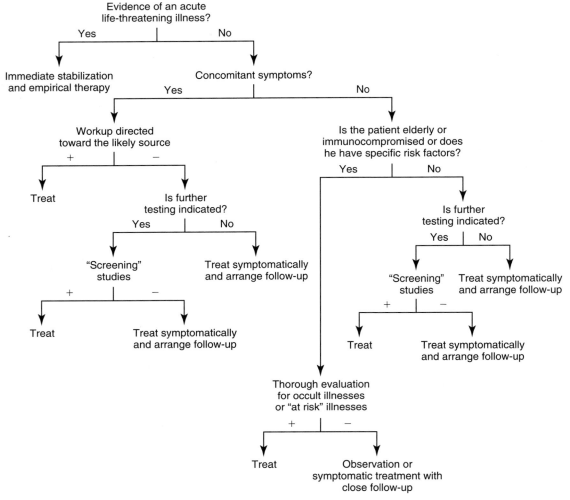

FIGURE 14–2 • Approach to the febrile adult in the emergency department.

- Chronic debilitating illness
- Extremes of age
- History of intravenous drug abuse
- Immunocompromised
- Identifiable focus of serious infection (e.g., pneumonia)
- Indwelling catheter (urinary or venous) or prosthetic device
- Residence in an institution
- Intensive care unit admissions
- Presumed catastrophic illness
- Splenectomy

Two sets of blood cultures, each including an aerobic and anaerobic specimen, are recommended in most cases. Each set should be drawn from a separate venipuncture site. If an indwelling venous catheter is present, one set of cultures should be drawn from it and the other drawn peripherally. At least 10 to 15 mL of blood should be collected for each culture. If endocarditis is suspected, multiple sets of samples are drawn over time. Blood cultures should ideally be obtained before the administration of antibiotics.

Urinalysis. Urinalysis is frequently ordered as a screening examination for urinary tract infection (UTI) in febrile patients. Approximately 75% of UTIs will cause a positive nitrite or leukocyte esterase result as measured by dipstick. The majority of UTIs will also cause at least 5 to 10 WBC per high-powered field on microscopic examination. The presence of bacteria seen on microscopic examination is the most sensitive indicator of UTI if the urine was collected in a sterile fashion (i.e., midstream collection in men and sterile catheterization or suprapubic aspiration in women).

TABLE 14–5. Characteristics of the Acute Life-Threatening Febrile Illnesses

Illness	Risk Factors	Supporting History	Concomitant Symptoms	Prevalence in the Emergency Dept.	Physical Examination	Diagnostic Aids	Additional Comments
Sepsis	Immunosuppression, chronic debilitating illness, diabetes, active malignancy or recent chemotherapy, lymphoproliferative disease, advanced age (>75 years), intravenous drug use, splenectomy, the presence of a chronic indwelling catheter or prosthetic heart valve.	Frequently, symptoms of the initial source of infection are present. Intra-abdominal processes are the most common source of sepsis in adults. Other common causes include meningitis, pneumonia, gynecologic infections, pyelonephritis, and cellulitis.	Chills, malaise, and symptoms of inadequate perfusion, most commonly mental status change. Symptoms may be blunted or absent in the elderly or immunocompromised.	Common	Some patients may be euthermic or even hypothermic. Tachycardia, wide pulse pressure, and tachypnea are typically present. Mental status change (usually obtundation) is frequently noted. Warm, flushed skin is often noted early in sepsis, with cold pale skin predominating in its later stages. Hypotension is an especially ominous sign. Physical findings of the initial focus of infection are usually present.	No single reliable laboratory test can definitively diagnose sepsis. Complete blood cell count. The WBC count is often, though not always, elevated with a left shift. Leukopenia may occur. Thrombocytopenia may occur. Blood cultures. At least two sets from different sites should be obtained. Baseline tests. Liver function tests, PT/PTT, renal function tests, electrolytes, chest radiograph, and ABG analysis. Other more specific testing for the source of infection should be guided by the history and physical examination.	Adult respiratory distress syndrome, acute tubular necrosis, liver dysfunction, and disseminated intravascular coagulopathy all may occur in the setting of sepsis.
Bacterial meningitis	Advanced age (>60 years), male gender, low socioeconomic status, crowded living conditions, splenectomy, sickle cell disease, alcoholism, diabetes, immunosuppression, recent intracranial surgery, contiguous infection (e.g, sinusitis), household contact with meningitis, intravenous drug use, ventriculoperitoneal shunt, active malignancy.	Often a 1- to 3-day history of fever and generalized malaise precedes the illness. There may be symptoms of a contiguous source of infection—most commonly sinusitis or otitis media. Altered mental status.	The classic triad of fever, headache, and stiff neck is present in the majority of cases. Seizures occur approximately 25% of the time. Nausea and photophobia are frequently present.	Infrequent	The majority of patients will have some evidence of meningeal irritation (i.e. pain with passive neck flexion or Brudzinski or Kernig's sign). Some evidence of cerebral dysfunction is often present, marked by confusion or a declining level of consciousness. Twenty-five percent of cases will have a focal neurologic deficit. Certain pathogens may cause a characteristic rash.	Lumbar puncture and CSF analysis is the primary mode of diagnosis. Head CT to rule out intracranial mass should be performed first if there is evidence of increased intracranial pressure or a focal neurologic deficit. Pertinent CSF studies include cell count, protein, glucose, Gram stain, culture, and antigen detection	Empirical antibiotics should not be delayed before performing the lumbar puncture if the likelihood of meningitis is high.

Continued on following page

TABLE 14-5. Characteristics of the Acute Life-Threatening Febrile Illnesses *Continued*

Illness	Risk Factors	Supporting History	Concomitant Symptoms	Prevalence in the Emergency Dept.	Physical Examination	Diagnostic Aids	Additional Comments
						studies. It should be noted that normal initial studies do not exclude the possibility of meningitis.	

Infections with Potential Airway Compromise

Illness	Risk Factors	Supporting History	Concomitant Symptoms	Prevalence in the Emergency Dept.	Physical Examination	Diagnostic Aids	Additional Comments
Epiglottitis	Classically described in the pediatric age group. Now increasingly recognized in adults, usually ages 20 to 40.	A 1- to 3-day history of a benign upper respiratory tract infection, followed by a severe sore throat.	Dysphagia, pharyngeal pain out of proportion to physical findings. Respiratory difficulty usually not present until late in the illness.	Rare	Dysphonia and a muffled voice are common. Laryngeal tenderness to palpation may be present. Stridor and drooling are signs of impending airway obstruction.	Lateral soft tissue neck radiographs may be helpful. Indirect or direct laryngoscopy needed for definitive diagnosis.	Frequently misdiagnosed as streptococcal pharyngitis. Laryngoscopy in the emergency department should only be performed on stable patients.
Ludwig's angina	Diabetes, alcoholism, immunodeficient states. However, most patients are healthy adults age 20 to 60 years.	Recent dental disease, usually of the lower molars, is typically present. Other proximate causes include recent mandibular fracture and lacerations to the floor of the mouth.	Dysphagia, neck pain with restricted neck movement, muffled voice, sore throat, and pain in the floor of the mouth.	Rare	Bilateral submandibular swelling and elevation of the tongue are the main findings. A firm consistency of the floor of the mouth and induration of the anterior portion of the neck may be present. The presence of stridor indicates impending loss of airway.	Though diagnosis is based primarily on clinical grounds, soft tissue radiographs of the neck may be used to confirm the diagnosis. CT and MRI are useful but are contraindicated if the patient cannot tolerate a supine posture.	Although rare, mediastinal involvement can occur and is life-threatening.
Retropharyngeal and parapharyngeal abscesses	Retropharyngeal abscesses are primarily an illness of childhood. Both illnesses occur more commonly in immunocompromised patients and diabetics.	A history of preceding dental or pharyngeal infection is common. Local trauma from dental procedures and upper airway manipulations (e.g., intubation) are frequent causes.	Patients with retropharyngeal abscesses typically complain of sore throat, voice change, and feeling a "lump" in their throat. Parapharyngeal abscesses often cause pain in the neck, odynophagia, and occasionally torticollis.	Rare	Edema and erythema of the posterior pharynx and cervical lymphadenopathy are typically present with retropharyngeal abscesses. Parapharyngeal abscesses classically present with medial displacement of the tonsillar pillar or a tender swelling at the angle of the mandible.	Lateral soft tissue radiographs are 88% sensitive in diagnosing retropharyngeal abscesses but of limited value with parapharyngeal abscesses. CT and MRI, if tolerable, are quite useful in diagnosing both illnesses.	Both infections may spread to cause mediastinal involvement or neurovascular complications in the head and neck.

Other Infections

	Risk Factors	Symptoms	Frequency	Physical Findings	Diagnostic Studies	Comments
Necrotizing fasciitis	Patients at increased risk: diabetes, peripheral vascular disease, malnutrition, obesity, IV drug use. Can occur in previously healthy without warning.	Pain out of proportion to local findings is common. Usually acute onset with rapid progression.	Rare. Earliest stages can be missed.	Cellulitis (90%), edema (90%), fever (70%), cutaneous gangrene (50%), altered mental status (40%), skin discoloration/crepitus (30%), shock (25%).	Usually with elevated white blood count. Anemia is common. CT and MRI are imaging studies of choice to differentiate from cellulitis.	Delay in treatment increases mortality. Can be 40%–80% death rate. Full and adequate débridement is essential.
Pneumonia	Alcoholism, diabetes, smoking, chronic debilitating illnesses, seizure disorder, splenectomy, advanced age, and any illness causing a depressed mental status or gag reflex.	A history of a preceding upper respiratory tract infection may be present.	Cough is present in most cases. Other classic symptoms include shaking chills, cough productive of purulent sputum, and pleuritic chest pain. The atypical pneumonia agents may cause more flu-like symptoms such as headache, sore throat, and a nonproductive cough.	Common	Tachypnea and tachycardia are often present. Decreased breath sounds, bronchial breath sounds, egophony, and crackles may be noted. Scattered rales and rhonchi with pharyngeal erythema and cervical adenopathy may be the main findings with pneumonias caused by the atypical pneumonia agents.	Chest radiograph is the most helpful diagnostic test but may occasionally be normal in the presence of pneumonia. Sputum analysis, if properly performed, may be of benefit. Assessment of respiratory function, usually by pulse oximetry or ABG analysis, should be done. Blood cultures should be sent on all hospitalized patients.	The etiologic agent of the pneumonia can be predicted by its radiographic appearance, but sputum Gram stains, and sputum and blood cultures are important.
Acute bacterial peritonitis	Immunosuppression, advanced age, and chronic debilitating illness.	A preceding history of the original illness causing the peritonitis is typically present. The most common causes of peritonitis are appendicitis and perforations caused by diverticuli, peptic ulcer disease, gangrenous cholecystitis, and small bowel obstruction.	Abdominal pain initially localized then becoming diffuse is invariably present. Nausea and anorexia are common.	Common	Abdominal tenderness and signs of peritoneal irritation (i.e., pain with any agitation of the peritoneal contents) are typically present. These symptoms may be localized initially, then become diffuse as the inflammation spreads. Bowel sounds are usually diminished or absent.	The WBC count is usually, though not always, elevated. Abdominal radiographs may show free air. Typically an ileus pattern is present.	Immunosuppressed patients and patients on chronic corticosteriods may have fewer symptoms and physical findings.

ABG, arterial blood gas; CSF, cerebrospinal fluid; CT, computed tomography; MRI, magnetic resonance imaging; PT, prothrombin time; PTT, partial thromboplastin time; WBC, white blood cell.

TABLE 14–6. Noninfectious Processes That Can Cause an Elevation of White Blood Cell and Band Counts

Asthma
Diabetic ketoacidosis
Cushing's syndrome
Hemorrhage
Hemolysis
Inflammation
Malignancy
Medications (most commonly epinephrine, lithium, and
 corticosteroids)
Myeloproliferative disorders
Physical or emotional stress
Pregnancy
Splenectomy
Seizures

Urine Culture. The urine culture is the definitive study used to diagnose urinary tract infection. Most uncomplicated UTIs in previously healthy women may be treated without culture if evidence of UTI is present on the urinalysis. Other groups in which a urine culture is usually indicated are listed in Table 14–7. Proper collection of the urine specimen is vital to avoid contamination. A midstream clean-catch specimen is acceptable in most men. Sterile catheterization is the collection method of choice in women, because clean-catch specimens are notoriously contaminated in this group. Urine taken from chronic indwelling catheters is inadequate because these devices have bacterial colonization over time.

Radiologic Imaging

Chest Radiographs. Standard anteroposterior and lateral films are used by many emergency physicians as a screening assessment in patients who have no other obvious source for fever. The posteroanterior and lateral chest films are probably most useful in elderly, immunocompromised, and chronically debilitated patients. They are of little value in young, otherwise healthy, febrile patients who do not have concomitant respiratory complaints.

Other Imaging. Occult infection sites (e.g., sinusitis, paraspinous abscess, deep cellulitis, pelvic abscess) may require more sophisticated imaging techniques, including ultrasonography, computed tomography, or magnetic resonance imaging.

EXPANDED DIFFERENTIAL DIAGNOSIS

Once it has been determined that an acute life-threatening febrile illness is not present, the evaluation of the febrile patient can proceed as directed by concomitant symptoms and specific risk factors. Table 14–8 lists some of the common, non–life-threatening infectious causes of fever in patients seen in the emergency department.

PRINCIPLES OF MANAGEMENT

General Principles

Addressing the underlying cause should be the first priority in the treatment of the febrile patient. Treatment of the fever itself is somewhat controversial, because there is substantial evidence that fever benefits the host's defense response during illness. Nevertheless, antipyretic therapy has become routine mainly for reasons related to patient comfort. Three main antipyretic agents are routinely used to suppress fever: acetaminophen, aspirin, and nonsteroidal anti-inflammatory drugs. There appears to be

TABLE 14–7. Patient Populations with Fever in Whom Urine Culture Is Indicated

Children
Adult men
Immunosuppressed patients
"Treatment failures" (recently completed course of antibiotics with persistent urinary symptoms)
Patients with symptoms in excess of 4 to 6 days
Elderly patients at risk for developing bacteremia
Toxic-appearing patients with signs and symptoms suggestive of pyelonephritis or bacteremia
Pregnant women
Patients with known chronic or recurrent renal infection
Patients with known anatomic urologic abnormalities
Patients in whom urinary tract obstruction is suspected (e.g., stones, benign prostatic hypertrophy)
Patients with serious medical diseases, to include diabetes mellitus, sickle cell anemia, cancer, or other debilitating diseases
Patients with alcoholism, drug dependence
Recently hospitalized patients
Patients recently taking antibiotics
Patients recently instrumented (e.g., cystoscopy, catheterization)
Chronic indwelling catheter

TABLE 14–8. Common Non-Life-Threatening Causes of Fever in the Emergency Department

Cause	Risk Factors	Supporting History	Concomitant Symptoms	Physical Examination	Diagnostic Aids	Additional Comments
Pharyngitis	Most commonly seen in adolescents and young adults.	Those of viral etiology are often preceded by nasal congestion and cough.	Pharyngeal pain aggravated by swallowing is the most common symptom. Headache, malaise, and myalgias are common.	Enlarged erythematous tonsils are typically present. Tonsillar exudates and cervical lymphadenopathy occur classically with streptococcal pharyngitis. Generalized lymphadenopathy and splenomegaly are often present with mononucleosis.	CBC of limited value, but may show predominantly lymphocytes with greater than 10% atypical lymphocytes and mild thrombocytosis with mononucleosis. Rapid strep tests are usually 60%–95% sensitive and 70%–100% specific. Throat culture is approximately 90% sensitive for streptococcal infection. Monospot testing approximately 80% sensitive and 90% specific for infectious mononucleosis.	The main goal in the emergency department is to identify and treat streptococcal pharyngitis. Left untreated, suppurative (peritonsillar abscess) and nonsuppurative (rheumatic fever) complications can occur.
Infectious enteritis	May be related to certain foods—often fried rice, eggs or raw seafood, or drinking of untreated water. Viral infections often occur in community outbreaks, usually in the winter or spring, and are common in infants and children.	Fever often low grade in viral infections and can be quite high with some bacterial causes.	Diarrhea is usually the predominant complaint. Vomiting and abdominal cramping are often present.	Variable degrees of abdominal tenderness are often present. Rectal examination may reveal heme-positive stool or frank blood. Signs of dehydration may be present.	Often not needed in mild cases. CBC may show a left shift, and fecal leukocytes are often present with bacterial infections. Blood cultures should be sent on all toxic-appearing patients. Stool cultures usually of high yield if fecal leukocytes are present.	Viral infections usually produce mild symptoms and require supportive care only.
Influenza	Occurs almost exclusively in the winter, often in epidemics. Infection rates are highest in young children and adolescents.	Onset of symptoms is usually quite abrupt.	Myalgias, headache, rhinorrhea, sore throat, and arthralgias. Respiratory symptoms, most commonly a nonproductive cough, predominate.	Often unremarkable in uncomplicated cases. Abnormal breath sounds (rhonchi, wheezes, or rales) may occasionally be heard.	Often of little value in the emergency department. Chest radiograph may show infiltrates in cases of viral pneumonia. Rapid assay ~ 75% sensitive	While usually a benign illness in otherwise healthy individuals, influenza may cause significant mortality in the elderly, immunocompromised, and chronically debilitated.

Continued on following page

247

TABLE 14–8. Common Non-Life-Threatening Causes of Fever in the Emergency Department *Continued*

Cause	Risk Factors	Supporting History	Concomitant Symptoms	Physical Examination	Diagnostic Aids	Additional Comments
Urinary tract infection (UTI)	Female gender, especially if sexually active. Pregnancy. Indwelling bladder catheter or recent instrumentation. Diabetes. Congenital bladder abnormalities. Any obstruction of urinary outflow—most commonly prostatic enlargement. Neurogenic bladder dysfunction.	Fever often low grade if infection confined to the bladder and higher in pyelonephritis.	Dysuria, frequency, suprapubic pain, and cloudy or bloody urine are typically present with cystitis. Shaking chills, nausea, vomiting, and flank pain are more common with pyelonephritis.	Mild suprapubic tenderness is typically present with cystitis. Patients with pyelonephritis often have a more toxic appearance and costovertebral angle tenderness to percussion.	The majority of UTIs will be detected on routine urinalysis. Urine culture is used for definitive diagnosis. CBC is usually of little value in uncomplicated cystitis, but it may show an elevated WBC count in pyelonephritis. Blood cultures should be sent on all toxic-appearing patients.	Clinical and laboratory findings are often unreliable in differentiating cystitis from pyelonephritis.
Pelvic inflammatory disease (PID)	Frequent sexual activity with multiple partners, adolescence, the presence of an intrauterine device, prior history of PID, any recent invasive gynecologic procedure (e.g., dilatation and curettage, endometrial biopsy, hysterosalpingography).	The onset of symptoms typically occurs 3 to 5 days after menses.	Symptoms often begin with a vaginal discharge and dysuria, then progress to a dull pelvic pain. Abnormal vaginal bleeding may be present. Advanced cases may have diffuse abdominal pain consistent with peritonitis.	Cervical motion tenderness is the hallmark finding. A purulent cervicitis is frequently noted on speculum examination. Fundal and adnexal tenderness, as well as adnexal swelling, may be noted on bimanual examination. In advanced cases signs of peritonitis may be present.	In the emergency department, PID is primarily a clinical diagnosis. CBC reveals an elevated WBC count in approximately 60% of cases. Cervical cultures for gonorrhea and chlamydia should be obtained.	Less than 65% of patients with the presumptive diagnosis of PID are found at laparoscopy to have the disease.

CBC, complete blood cell count; WBC, white blood cell.

little difference in the efficacy of these drugs in treating fever.

Rarely do infectious causes of fever result in a temperature greater than 105°F (41°C). However, during cases of extreme pyrexia, physical methods of cooling may be used in conjunction with antipyretic agents to lower the body temperature (see Chapter 17, Heat Illness). Air-circulating fans and sponging with tepid water is perhaps the most practical method. Cooling blankets are rarely necessary, and the patient must be closely monitored to avoid iatrogenic hypothermia.

Dehydration from increased metabolic rate and insensible losses is common with fever, especially in elderly and debilitated patients. Aggressive volume repletion with isotonic crystalloid is frequently necessary in these cases.

Specific Principles and Antibiotic Recommendations

Sepsis

Removal of the source of infection should be the first priority. Drainage of abscesses or débridement of necrotic tissue is performed as soon as possible. Likewise, indwelling venous catheters or obstructed urinary catheters are promptly removed.

Empirical antibiotic therapy is directed toward the initial source of infection. If the source of infection is unknown, the choice of empirical antibiotics should be directed by the patient's specific risk factors (see Table 14–2). Patients at risk for sepsis due to gram-positive organisms include those with indwelling venous catheters and intravenous drug users. Appropriate empirical antibiotics in these patients include nafcillin or vancomycin combined with an anti-pseudomonal aminoglycoside such as gentamicin or tobramycin. In healthy, nonimmunocompromised adults with no clear source of infection and no specific risk factors, treatment is aimed at gram-negative bacteria with broad-spectrum coverage. Monodrug therapy with imipenem or meropenem or two-drug therapy with a third-generation cephalosporin or ticarcillin/clavulanate combined with an anti-pseudomonal aminoglycoside can be used.

Bacterial Meningitis

Rapid administration of parenteral antibiotics capable of crossing the blood-brain barrier is of utmost importance in patients with bacterial meningitis. Timing of the first dosage (<1 hr) is an important role of the emergency physician. Young (<50 years), otherwise healthy adults can be treated empirically with cefotaxime or ceftriaxone. Patients older than 50 and known alcoholics should receive cefotaxime or ceftriaxone combined with ampicillin. Immunocompromised patients are at particular risk for meningitis caused by Listeria and gram-negative bacilli and should be treated with ampicillin and ceftazidime. Because of the increasing problem of cephalosporin-resistant Streptococcus pneumoniae, many authorities recommend the addition of vancomycin in the empirical treatment of all adult meningitis. Finally, those patients with a ventriculoperitoneal shunt who are suspected of having meningitis should receive vancomycin plus rifampin.

Epiglottitis

Close observation with emergency airway equipment at the bedside is required given the risk of sudden obstruction in patients with epiglottitis. Empirical antibiotic therapy should be started. In otherwise healthy adults, cefuroxime, ceftriaxone, and cefotaxime are considered drugs of choice. The use of corticosteroids to reduce airway edema is advocated by some authorities.

Ludwig's Angina

As with all infections causing potential airway compromise, vigilant observation is necessary in patients with Ludwig's angina. High-dose penicillin with metronidazole, or cefoxitin alone, is the therapy of choice. Other options include clindamycin, ticarcillin/clavulanate, and ampicillin/sulbactam. Surgical débridement is indicated if there is crepitus or the presence of purulent collections.

Retropharyngeal and Parapharyngeal Abscesses

Airway management is the main priority. The majority of patients will require incision and drainage by a specialist. Antibiotics are given in the emergency department and are the same as for Ludwig's angina.

Community-Acquired Pneumonia

Community-acquired pneumonia is now commonly treated with oral antibiotics on an outpatient basis in otherwise healthy adults without evidence of respiratory compromise. Empirical treatment options include second- or third-generation cephalosporins, doxycycline, and macrolides, with the latter two providing coverage for "atypical" agents seen with increasing prevalence in young and middle-aged adults. Patients who are elderly, have underlying comorbidity, have nosocomial transmission, or are suspected of being septic should be admitted for intravenous antibiotics (see Table 14–9 for admission criteria). These patients may benefit from broader coverage with an enhanced-spectrum fluoroquinolone, such as levofloxacin, or an aminoglycoside combined with either a third-generation cephalosporin or one of the β-lactamase resistant β-lactams. Supplemental oxygen is provided for all hypoxic patients. Intubation may be necessary in cases of severe hypoxia or inadequate ventilation.

Acute Bacterial Peritonitis

Emergent surgical consultation is indicated, with operative intervention almost always required for patients with acute bacterial peritonitis. Antibiotic options include cefoxitin, cefotetan, ticarcillin/clavulanate, and ampicillin/sulbactam.

Urinary Tract Infection

Although most urinary tract infections (UTIs) are treated on an outpatient basis, they also account for approximately 1 million hospitalizations per year and are the most common cause of nosocomial infections and gram-negative sepsis. Because of structural or functional changes in the genitourinary system, elderly patients and pregnant women are particularly prone to develop UTIs and subsequent complications. Most patients are cognizant of signs and symptoms associated with UTI, such as suprapubic pain, dysuria, frequency, or gross hematuria. However, elderly patients or those with indwelling catheters may only manifest

a change in mental status as a sign of urosepsis; thus, in such patients, a urologic workup is imperative in the evaluation of fever without another source. Diagnosis is made by urinalysis, which is both sensitive and specific when the sample is properly collected. In fact, the presence of both nitrites (a by-product of bacteria metabolism) and leukocyte esterase (evidence of leukocyte degradation) are nearly 100% predictive of UTI, whereas the diagnosis of UTI is highly unlikely if both of these indicators are absent. The severity of infection correlates with the number of leukocytes found on urine microscopy, with more than 10 WBC per high-power field indicating simple lower tract infection and 50 to 100 WBC per high-power field usually present with pyelonephritis. The presence of WBCs in the urine is nonspecific and may also be secondary to peritonitis, such as that caused by pelvic inflammatory disease or acute appendicitis. Definitive diagnosis is made by urine culture, which should be ordered on any patient who is hospitalized or believed to be at risk for a complicated UTI (e.g., prostatitis or pyelonephritis). Blood cultures are of limited value in the evaluation of urosepsis, because they almost invariably confirm the same organism(s) determined by urine culture.

Treatment is based on the severity of infection and underlying risk factors. Patients who are ambulatory and otherwise healthy are usually treated on an outpatient basis with oral antibiotics that concentrate in the urine. Coverage is primarily aimed at gram-negative pathogens, most commonly acquired from fecal contamination (*Escherichia coli* is implicated in 90% of cases). Trimethoprim/sulfamethoxazole is inexpensive and 80% to 90% effective in treating uncomplicated UTIs; however, resistance has emerged in some communities. Other choices include nitrofurantoin and cephalosporins, both of which may

---

TABLE 14–9. Admission Criteria for Community-Acquired Pneumonia

Age > 65 years
Comorbid conditions:
    Alcoholism, asplenia, cancer, congestive heart failure, chronic lung disease (includes asthma, cystic fibrosis, chronic obstructive pulmonary disease), chronic liver disease, chronic renal failure, diabetes, immunocompromised (e.g., leukemia, AIDS, chronic corticosteroids), malnutrition, sickle cell disease.
History:
    Intubation or hospital admission within the past 1 year, suspected aspiration
Physical findings
    Respiratory rate > 30 breaths per minute, acute mental status changes, evidence of shock
Laboratory findings:
    WBC count < 4,000/mm^3 or > 30,000/mm^3
    Po$_2$ < 60 mm Hg or /saturation < 90% on room air
    Metabolic acidosis
    Hemoglobin < 9 g/dL, hematocrit < 30%, creatinine > 1.4 mg/dL
    Chest radiograph showing multilobar involvement, cavitation, or effusion

be used during pregnancy. The fluoroquinolones, although significantly more expensive, are more than 95% effective against urinary pathogens, including *Pseudomonas* and other more antibiotic-resistant organisms. Uncomplicated infections may be effectively treated with a 3- to 5-day course of therapy, whereas ascending infections or pyelonephritis may require 10 to 14 days of therapy for effective cure. Hospitalization for intravenous antibiotics should be considered for patients with pyelonephritis during pregnancy, those with concurrent kidney stones or structural abnormalities, or those at increased risk of sepsis, including elderly or chronically debilitated patients with upper tract infections. Intravenous antibiotic options include the fluoroquinolones, anti-pseudomonal penicillins (ticarcillin/clavulanate, ampicillin/sulbactam, piperacillin/tazobactam), imipenem, or meropenem. Addition of an aminoglycoside may be considered in the treatment of sepsis.

UNCERTAIN DIAGNOSIS

Healthy febrile adults who are younger than 60 years old and have no evidence of serious illness, risk factors for particular illnesses, or abnormality on screening examinations represent a diagnostic dilemma for the emergency physician. The first step in these situations is to review the history and physical findings, repeating certain aspects if necessary. Key parts of the history may be revealed during the second encounter, such as any sick contacts, foreign travel, tick bites, or a history of intravenous drug abuse that was initially denied. Other noninfectious causes of fever should be considered (see Table 14–1). Occult infections, especially tuberculosis, tumors, and connective tissue diseases are the three most common causes of fever that is initially of unknown etiology. Finally, it may be helpful to ask the assistance of a colleague in reevaluating the patient or to obtain consultation from a primary physician who has personal knowledge of the patient's past medical history.

SPECIAL CONSIDERATIONS

Nursing Home Patients

Both advanced age and residence in a long-term care facility increase the susceptibility of an individual to infection. When compared with younger patients from the community, the presence of fever in an elderly nursing home resident is much more likely to signify a serious bacterial infection. Furthermore, the elderly in general do not mount as significant a febrile response as do their younger counterparts and 20% to 30% of the elderly patients with a serious infection will be afebrile. Some elderly patients may only manifest a decline in mental status as a sign of sepsis. For these reasons, the presence of fever, even a "low grade" fever, in an elderly nursing home resident warrants a thorough evaluation in the emergency department.

The three most common sources of infection in nursing home patients are the respiratory tract, the urinary tract, and the skin and soft tissue. The urinary tract is the most common cause of bacteremia in nursing home residents, being responsible for over 50% of cases in most studies. Patients with a history of stroke may be prone to aspiration pneumonia resulting from dysphagia. The bacteria causing infections in nursing home residents are frequently resistant to commonly used antibiotics and require more extensive antimicrobial coverage. Specifically, the high prevalence of methicillin-resistant *Staphylococcus aureus* and pseudomonal infections warrants the liberal use of vancomycin and extended-spectrum penicillins or cephalosporins in combination with aminoglycosides as empirical therapy. Given this high prevalence of resistant organisms and the increased frequency of comorbid conditions, the emergency physician should have a low threshold for admitting elderly febrile patients from long-term care facilities.

Chemotherapy Patients

Neutropenia caused by recent chemotherapy predisposes patients to serious bacterial illness. Chemotherapy-induced neutropenia usually reaches its nadir between 10 and 14 days after treatment, with a return to normal usually by day 28. An absolute neutrophil count (ANC) less than 500/mm^3 renders patients at high risk for bacterial infection. *Note: The total ANC count can be calculated using the following equation: (Percent of PMNs and bands on the peripheral smear) × (WBC count).* Compounding this problem is the fact that as the absolute neutrophil count falls below 1000/mm^3, the signs and symptoms commonly associated with infection and inflammation become less prominent. Fever without signs of a localized infection is the most common clinical presentation in neutropenic patients. After consultation with their primary physician, reverse isolation should also be strongly considered.

The risk of developing a fever during a course of chemotherapy is between 40% and 70%. Bacteremias represent approximately 20% of these febrile episodes. A diligent search for the source of the fever is necessary. In those febrile patients with an ANC less than $500/mm^3$ or less than $1000/mm^3$ with a further decline anticipated, and in whom no source of the fever can be found, empirical antibiotic therapy is indicated. Either ticarcillin, piperacillin, or imipenem in combination with gentamicin is a reasonable option, as is ceftazidime or cefoperazone combined with gentamicin, aztreonam, or ciprofloxacin. In those patients with a possible indwelling venous catheter–related infection, vancomycin combined with ceftazidime is a reasonable choice. Although most febrile neutropenic patients require inpatient treatment, outpatient therapy may be an option in some low-risk groups.

Transplant Patients

Fever is one of the most common complications experienced by transplant recipients and represents a diagnostic challenge for the emergency physician. Noninfectious causes of fever in these patients include graft rejection in solid organ recipients, graft-versus-host disease in bone marrow transplant recipients, and drug fever. Infection is a major cause of morbidity and mortality and may be masked by the immunosuppressant medications taken by these patients.

Infections occurring in the first month after transplantation are frequently related to the procedure itself, such as wound infections and catheter-related infections. After the first month, the transplant recipient is unusually susceptible to viral, fungal, and protozoal infections. Infection with cytomegalovirus is the most common life-threatening infection. Transplant-specific infections are common and include urinary tract infections in renal transplant patients, mediastinitis after heart transplantation, lung infections in lung transplant recipients, and cholangitis and peritonitis after liver transplantation.

Treatment of the febrile transplant patient should include consultation with a transplant surgeon to ensure optimal care.

Intravenous Drug Users

The presence of fever in an intravenous drug user should raise suspicion for certain characteristic illnesses. Pneumonias, skin and soft tissue infections, and, of greatest concern, bacterial endocarditis all commonly occur in these persons. Forty-two percent of all febrile intravenous drug users were found to be bacteremic in one study. Additionally, many intravenous drug users are HIV positive.

Fever without an identifiable source is of special concern. Many of the classic findings of bacterial endocarditis, such as murmurs and petechial and splinter hemorrhages, occur infrequently or too late in the course of the illness to be of diagnostic value. For this reason, many authorities advocate routine admission of these patients, obtaining several blood cultures, liberal use of echocardiography to detect valve pathology, and the empirical administration of antibiotics. Drugs of choice include nafcillin or vancomycin combined with gentamicin, or ceftizoxime, cefotaxime, or ceftriaxone given alone.

HIV-Positive Patients

Fever is one of the most common presenting complaints in HIV-positive patients (see Chapter 13, Approach to HIV in the Emergency Department). The initial approach to the febrile HIV-positive patient should be guided by the stage of the patient's disease, if known. Patients with CD4 cell counts between $200/mm^3$ and $500/mm^3$ are relatively immunocompetent yet still predisposed to certain febrile illnesses. Pneumococcal pneumonias, pulmonary tuberculosis, *Salmonella* infections, and varicella-zoster commonly occur in this group. Those febrile individuals with CD4 cell counts less than $200/mm^3$ are at high risk for *Pneumocystis carinii* pneumonia, disseminated herpes simplex, toxoplasmosis, extrapulmonary tuberculosis, cryptococcosis, and disseminated fungal infections. Other noninfectious causes of fever to be considered in all HIV-positive patients are malignancies and drug fevers.

Diagnostic evaluation can be guided primarily by clinical findings in those patients with CD4 counts greater than $200/mm^3$. In those patients with more advanced disease, a more extensive diagnostic evaluation is often necessary. However, the emergency physician should resist the temptation to focus exclusively on opportunistic and exotic pathogens in these patients.

Patients with Sickle Cell Disease

Adult patients with sickle cell disease have increased susceptibility to infection owing to their chronic disease state and functional asplenism. Although symptoms such as dyspnea, abdominal pain, or arthralgias may be attributable to vaso-occlusive phenomenon, the presence of fever should prompt a thorough evaluation to rule out pneumonia, peritonitis, or septic arthritis. The management of these patients is discussed separately in Chapter 19, Sickle Cell Disease.

The Foreign Traveler

Patients who have returned from foreign travel within the previous month warrant special consideration. Although the majority of cases will be caused by a self-limited viral illness, patients may have had exposure to pathogens not endemic to the United States. Among these, the most common diseases are malaria, hepatitis A, typhoid, and dengue fever. The current Centers for Disease Control and Prevention (CDC) guidelines are useful in determining which areas of the globe harbor risk for which pathogens. Emphasis should be placed on ruling out those pathogens that may be potentially fatal if untreated (e.g., malaria and typhoid). Table 14–10 lists the areas of special concern during the history and physical examination that are applicable to patients who have traveled abroad. The following laboratory tests may be helpful: CBC (may show leukopenia or thrombocytopenia), liver enzymes, peripheral blood smear, blood cultures, and stool culture and analysis for ova and parasites. Although culture results may not be conclusive for 48 to 72 hours, hospitalization for supportive care and empirical antibiotic coverage should be considered for patients with high or persistent fever, petechial rash, or other signs of sepsis. Infectious disease consultation is requested early in the course of care.

Pediatric Patients

Fever in pediatric patients is covered in Chapter 26, Febrile Infants.

DISPOSITION AND FOLLOW-UP

Febrile Patients Requiring Admission

Any patient with evidence of a catastrophic illness requires admission to the hospital. Patients with a presumptive diagnosis of sepsis, an infection causing potential airway compromise, bacterial meningitis, acute bacterial peritonitis, or pneumonia with hypoxia fall into this category. Patients with less serious illnesses but with significant potential for deterioration should also be admitted. A kidney transplant recipient with an early pneumonia would be an example. Admission is necessary for any patient requiring services only available in the hospital, such as surgical débridement. Finally, those patients who are unable to comply with outpatient therapy will need to be admitted. An example of this is a patient with pyelonephritis and intractable vomiting.

Admission to the Intensive Care Unit

Any patient who required intubation or other type of invasive airway control in the emergency department will need to be admitted to an intensive care unit (ICU). Patients requiring close observation and nursing care, such as those with Ludwig's angina, should also be admitted to the ICU. Other indicators of the need for ICU care are reflected in the patient's vital signs and mental status. Patients with significant tachypnea, tachycardia, or hypotension that does not correct with intravenous administration of fluids and antipyretics are considered as lacking physical stability and

---

TABLE 14–10. Special Considerations in History and Physical Examination of Patients Returning from Foreign Travel

---

History

Specific countries visited (also rural vs. city)
Prior vaccinations
Use of H_2 blockers (increases risk of enteric pathogens)
Whether prophylactic antibiotics were taken with proper compliance
Diet that included food that was not boiled or fully cooked
Ingestion of unpeeled fruit or vegetables
Use of local water sources (i.e., nonbottled)
Insect bites and use of insecticides
Sexual activity with foreign natives
Onset and timing of febrile episodes
Whether any other travelers became ill

Physical Examination Findings

Scleral icterus
Lymphadenopathy
Hepatosplenomegaly
Rashes or petechiae

should not be managed on the general medical floor.

Febrile Patients Who May Require Admission

Some patients with febrile illnesses that could otherwise be treated at home will require admission because of comorbid factors or less than desirable social situations. Elderly patients, those with impaired immune function, diabetics, and patients with chronic debilitating illnesses may need to be admitted for certain infectious diseases that could otherwise be treated at home in young, healthy individuals. Similarly, unreliable patients, those without access to appropriate follow-up, and patients without adequate social support systems should be considered for admission. One last consideration is the magnitude of the fever when viewed in light of the patient's age. One study found that of patients 60 years and older presenting to the emergency department with a temperature greater than 101°F (39°C), 92.5% had a serious illness requiring admission. Although directed toward community-acquired pneumonia, Table 14–9 contains several risk factors that can be applied to other febrile illnesses.

Febrile Patients Not Requiring Admission

Those patients without an indication for admission as just discussed may be treated as an outpatient with appropriate follow-up. In general, patients with infections that have the potential to worsen despite antibiotics (e.g., pneumonia, cellulitis, pyelonephritis) should be reevaluated in 1 to 2 days. Patients with other less-concerning illnesses, such as influenza, can be reexamined in 4 to 5 days. Follow-up should ideally be arranged with the patient's primary or referral physician. It is not unreasonable, however, to reevaluate the patient in the emergency department if no other alternatives exist.

FINAL POINTS

- Fever can be defined as an elevation of the body temperature caused by a change in the hypothalamic set-point and varies depending on the individual and the time of day.
- Tachycardia, hypotension, and tachypnea are "red flags" for life-threatening febrile illnesses.
- Temperature measurement is significantly influenced by the type of thermometer used as well as body location and technique.
- If a catastrophic illness is suspected, stabilization and empirical therapy take precedence over establishing the definitive diagnosis.
- Evaluation of the febrile patient should be directed by concomitant symptoms or signs and the patient's risk factors for specific illnesses.
- The complete blood cell count, urinalysis, and chest radiographs can be used as screening studies in febrile patients without an obvious source of infection on physical examination.
- Foremost in the treatment of the febrile patient is to address the underlying cause, rather than the fever itself.
- Removal of the source of infection should be the first priority in the management of sepsis.
- Nursing home residents, chemotherapy patients, transplant recipients, foreign travelers, intravenous drug users, and patients who have HIV infection or sickle cell disease require special consideration when presenting to the emergency department with a fever.
- Comorbid conditions and social situation need to be taken into account when considering possible admission for a febrile illness.

CASE *Study*

A 36-year old man presented to the emergency department complaining of fever and having "the flu" over the past 2 days. Triage vital signs were temperature, 101.8°F (38.7°C); pulse, 108 beats per minute; blood pressure 112/70 mm Hg; and respirations, 20 breaths per minute. The patient had been in his usual state of health before developing a fever with a dry cough and generalized body aches 2 days before coming to the emergency department. He had no vomiting, diarrhea, rash, chest pain, or shortness of breath. He specifically requests "some antibiotics to help me get over this." Past medical history is remarkable for a groin abscess requiring outpatient incision and drainage 2 years ago. Social history is remarkable for one pack of cigarettes a day for the past 20 years. He denies alcohol or illegal drug use. Family history is unknown because he had not kept in contact with his parents or siblings over the past 10 years.

At this point there is no evidence of an acute life-threatening illness. Other than a mild tachycardia, which is expected given the fever, the vital signs are stable.

The patient is noted to be a thin, unkempt white man in no distress. Several old "needle tracks" are noted on his arms. Head and neck examination is essentially unremarkable. Chest examination reveals clear and equal breath sounds. There is a normal S_1 and S_2 with no murmurs. The abdomen is noted to be soft and nontender with normal bowel sounds and no masses. A brief dermatologic examination reveals no rashes.

The emergency physician informs the patient that he is concerned about a potential lung problem and needs to "check a blood test and a chest film." A CBC, pulse oximetry, and radiographs are ordered.

This otherwise healthy patient with flu-like symptoms, relatively stable vital signs, and an unremarkable physical examination could be diagnosed as having a "viral upper respiratory infection" (especially if it was midwinter) and discharged with symptomatic therapy and appropriate follow-up. However, experienced emergency physicians develop a "sixth sense" about patients. This "sixth sense" is often derived from the patient's general appearance, demeanor, cultural background, profession, and even their location of residence. In this case, the total cost of the "screening studies" will be approximately $300.

The nurse notes that it was difficult to obtain blood from the patient because several of his veins were sclerosed. The physician confronts the patient about potential drug use, and he admits to previous intravenous drug abuse. He states he hasn't "shot up" for over 1 year. He had tested HIV negative 2 years ago at an outside clinic. While the patient is in radiology, the registration clerk informs the physician the patient's significant other is in the waiting room and "wants to know how her boyfriend is doing."

In speaking with the significant other it is discovered the patient recently resumed intravenous drug use and has been "using" every day for the past month.

Information gleaned by the nursing and ancillary staff is often extremely valuable and should not be ignored or discounted. Also, it is essential to maintain communication with the patient's family or friends both for additional history and good patient relations.

The CBC revealed a mild normocytic anemia with a hemoglobin of 10.3 g/dL and a mildly elevated WBC of 13,200/mm^3. A manual differential showed 70% PMNs, 17% bands, 10% lymphocytes, and 3% monocytes. The oxygen saturation was 98%, and the chest film showed no acute pathologic process.

Given the extra history of recent intravenous drug use and the finding of an elevated WBC with a high percentage of band forms, the emergency physician is highly suspicious of bacterial endocarditis. Other possibilities include an HIV-related illness (especially Pneumocystis carinii pneumonia or tuberculosis) or a viral upper respiratory tract infection. Blood cultures are ordered and the patient's permission for HIV testing is obtained.

The patient is admitted to the medical service. Nafcillin and gentamicin are given parenterally after discussion with the consultant. Echocardiography performed the next day revealed vegetations on the tricuspid valve. *Staphylococcus aureus* was growing in three of the four blood cultures on the third hospital day. The patient was found to be HIV negative and was discharged after 14 days of intravenous antibiotic therapy.

This case demonstrates the importance of obtaining a thorough history and performing an appropriately focused physical examination on febrile adults in the emergency department.

Bibliography

TEXTS

Brillman JC, Quenzer RW (eds): Infectious Disease in Emergency Medicine, 2nd ed. Philadelphia, Lippincott-Raven, 1998.

JOURNAL ARTICLES

American Thoracic Society: Guidelines for the initial management of adults with community-acquired pneumonia. Am Rev Respir Dis 1993; 148:1418–1426.

Butler KH: Urinary tract infection: I and II. Emerg Med Rep 2001; 22:58–68, 69–80.

Chapnick EK, Abter EJ: Necrotizing soft-tissue infections. Infect Dis Clin North Am 1996; 10:835–855.

The choice of antibacterial drugs. Med Lett Drugs Ther 2001; 43(1111–1112):69–78.

Donowitz GR: Fever in the compromised host. Infect Dis Clin North Am 1996; 10:129–148.

Fine MJ: Prediction rule to identify low-risk patients with community-acquired pneumonia. N Engl J Med 1997; 336:243–250.

Fischer SA, Trenholme GM, Levin S: Fever in the solid organ transplant patient. Infect Dis Clin North Am 1996; 10:167–183.

Gallagher EJ, Brooks F, Gennis P: Identification of serious illness in febrile adults. Am J Emerg Med 1994; 12:129–133.

Gupta K, Hooton TM, Stamm WE: Incurring antimicrobial resistance and the management of uncomplicated community-acquired urinary tract infections. Ann Intern Med 2001; 135:41–50.

Henker R: Evidence-based practice: Fever-related interventions. Am J Crit Care 1999; 8:481–486.

Hughes WT, Armstrong D, Bodey GP, et al: 1997 Guidelines for the use of antimicrobial agents in neutropenic patients with unexplained fever. Clin Infect Dis 1997; 25:551–573.

Klein NC, Cunha BA: Treatment of fever. Infect Dis Clin North Am 1996; 10;211–216.

Leinicke T, Navitsky R, Cameron S, Brillman J: Fever in the elderly: How to surmount the unique diagnostic and therapeutic challenges. Emerg Med Pract 1999; 1:1–24.

Mylonakis E, Calderwood SB: Infective endocarditis in adults. N Engl J Med 2001; 345:1318–1330.

Shah SM, Searls L: The febrile adult: I and II. Emerg Med Rep 1998; 19:173–182, 183–190.

Sullivan M, Feinberg J, Barlett JG: Fever in patients with HIV infection. Infect Dis Clin North Am 1996; 10: 149–166.

Thanassi M, Thanassi WT: Fever in returning travelers: Evaluation, differential diagnosis, and treatment. Emerg Med Rep 1998; 19:22.

Weisse AB, Heller DR, Schimenti RJ, et al: The febrile parenteral drug user: A prospective study in 121 patients. Am J Med 1993; 94:274–280.

Yoshikawa TT, Norman DC: Approach to fever and infection in the nursing home. J Am Geriatr Soc 1996; 44:74–82.

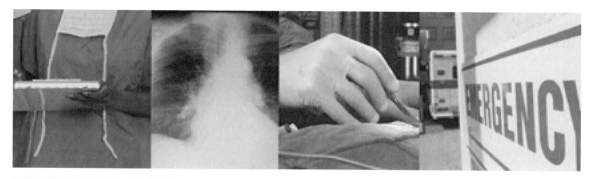

TOXICOLOGY/ENVIRONMENTAL DISORDERS

CHAPTER 15

The Poisoned Patient

ROBERT WILSON

LESLIE WOLF

CASE *Study*

A 45-year-old man was unresponsive when his son found him at home.

CASE *Study*

A 15-year-old girl was brought to the emergency department by her parents after she took 10 "sleeping pills" after an argument with them. She was alert and asymptomatic. The parents want to take the patient home because she has no symptoms. On physical examination, her only significant finding is a heart rate of 120 beats per minute.

CASE *Study*

A 65-year-old man with chronic obstructive pulmonary disease (COPD) and congestive heart failure presented with nausea, palpitations, and the "jitters."

INTRODUCTION

The American Association of Poison Control Centers (AAPCC) annually reports over 2 million cases of poisonings. Many persons who die at home or present directly to the emergency department do not involve a poison control center, resulting in the total number of poisonings each year being underreported. According to some authors, poisoning is the third leading cause of death in the United States.

The peak ages for pediatric poisoning are 10 months and between 2 and 4 years. Many pediatric exposures occur in children with a prior history of poisoning, and they tend to repeat with the same type of substance. The most common agents in children are household products and pharmaceuticals, and in adults the most common substances are analgesics, psychotropics, and hypnotic agents. Although children younger than 6 are involved in over half of the poisonings, they only represent approximately 4% of fatalities. Fatalities are more common after adult, intentional exposure. The most common fatal exposures in children occur from gases/fumes/vapors (including carbon monoxide), toxic alcohols, analgesics, iron, antidepressants, cleaning substances (from aspiration), and cardiovascular toxins. Fatalities in adults are most commonly caused by carbon monoxide, antidepressants, drugs of abuse, cardiovascular toxins, analgesics, and theophylline. Carbon monoxide continues to be the most common cause of poisoning death in children and adults.

Although pediatric accidental ingestion represents the most common exposure, other groups are at risk for poisoning. Child abuse must be considered in exposures in children younger than 1 year of age, and overdose in children older than age 5 years often represents suicidal intent. Patients with depression or other psychiatric conditions are also at high risk for poisoning. Chemical exposures are common in the workplace, yet toxicity often is undetected. Because of the common presence of "polypharmacy," diminishing eyesight, and potentially impaired mental capacity, the elderly population is at particular risk for accidental overdose, chronic drug toxicity, and drug interactions.

Many persons with exposures and poisonings, as well as substance abuse problems, present first to the emergency department, giving the clinician a unique opportunity for intervention. Although the understanding of the evaluation and stabilization of the poisoned patient is a critical skill in emergency medicine, education and exposure prevention in our patient population is essential.

INITIAL APPROACH AND STABILIZATION

Rapid Assessment

Because a reliable history may not be available, the rescue squad can be invaluable in obtaining information from family members, friends, or other witnesses at the scene. Whenever possible, the scene is surveyed for prescription bottles, syringes, open containers of chemicals, and other potentially valuable diagnostic clues. When possible, the following information is obtained:

1. Type, amount, and timing of ingestion or exposure
2. Symptoms since exposure
3. Circumstances leading to the exposure (accidental or intentional)
4. Home treatment rendered (e.g., syrup of ipecac)
5. Past medical or psychiatric history
6. Allergies
7. Medications (routine or others found in the home, medications of family members)
8. Occupation of patient and family members
9. Alternative therapy use (e.g., herbs)

A brief physical examination is also conducted to establish the need for immediate management. The examination includes assessment of (1) patency and protection of the airway; (2) gross adequacy of ventilation; (3) vital signs; (4) mental status; and (5) pupillary size and reactivity.

Early Intervention

Airway. When ventilation is compromised or airway protective mechanisms are impaired, airway management should begin immediately (see Chapter 2, Airway Management). Assisted ventilation is instituted whenever ventilation is of insufficient rate or depth.

Oxygen. Supplemental oxygen is administered at an initial rate of 2 to 4 L/min. If exposure to a toxic gas is suspected or if pulmonary effects can occur after a specific exposure, high flow oxygen (10 to 12 L/min) is given by mask.

Intravenous Access. If a significant ingestion is suspected, intravenous access is established.

Cardiac Monitor. Cardiac monitoring is useful to observe the effects of cardiotoxic drugs or in any hemodynamically unstable patient.

Decontamination. Prompt decontamination of the skin or eyes with copious irrigation may significantly reduce exposure to agents absorbed by these routes.

Elimination. Syrup of ipecac–induced emesis, although advocated for prehospital use by some, is generally reserved for use with ingestions of highly toxic substances when transport times are prolonged. Its efficacy is maximized if given within 15 minutes of ingestion. Syrup of ipecac is contraindicated in patients with altered mental status, in children younger than 6 months old, after caustic or hydrocarbon ingestion, and in patients at risk for seizure or rapid clinical deterioration. If activated charcoal or other oral antidotes are indicated, syrup of ipecac will delay administration of these agents. Although ipecac may have selected usefulness in the home, it is seldom used in the emergency department.

Treatment of Altered Mental Status

Hypoglycemia Screening. A 25% to 50% dextrose solution (25 to 50 g) is administered intravenously to reverse the effects of hypoglycemia. If available, a rapid quantitative glucose determination using a glucose oxidase reagent strip is obtained before empirical treatment. Intravenous glucose is recommended in patients with altered mental status who have a serum glucose value less than 80 mg/dL. Also, thiamine, 100 mg intravenously or intramuscularly, should be given, if available.

Empirical Treatment for Narcotic Overdose. Naloxone (Narcan) may be given to reverse the effects of opioid toxicity. The initial goal of naloxone administration is reversal of respiratory depression. Initial doses of 2 mg are generally preferred unless opioid dependence is suspected. In this situation, smaller doses (0.2 mg) are used and are titrated to the clinical response, while attempting to avoid acute withdrawal. If clinical assessment suggests opioid toxicity and there is no response to the initial naloxone dose, repeat doses up to a total of 10 mg may be necessary. Because the half-life of naloxone is only 1 hour, careful monitoring after dosing is necessary, because repeat dosage may be required.

CLINICAL ASSESSMENT

History

Although the history is important in the poisoned patient, it may be difficult to obtain or unreliable. The potential of a toxic exposure is considered in patients with unusual presentations, in children with an acute onset of illness, in patients who become symptomatic in the workplace, in patients who present with altered mental status, in drug and alcohol abusers, in health care personnel, and in patients with psychiatric illness. Aggressive evaluation of fire victims for inhalation of toxic gases should be done in concert with the treatment of thermal injuries. Intoxication is also considered in any trauma patient. It is important to obtain historical information from all potential sources, such as emergency services personnel, family, coworkers, friends, and police.

1. If the situation is that of a possible but still unverified toxic ingestion and the patient is

unable to provide a history (as in Case 1), the following information may be valuable:

a. *Situational history. Where* was the patient *found* and *what* were the *circumstances?* Were there pills or drug paraphernalia in the area?

b. *Occupational history.* Is the patient *exposed* to *toxic substances?*

c. *Past medical history.* Preexisting medical problems may influence therapeutic options, and chronic or terminal illnesses may predispose patients to depression and suicidal ideation. What *medications* has the patient been prescribed in the past?

d. Is there a previous *history* of *mental illness?*

e. Is there a history of *substance abuse?*

f. Are there other *family members' medications* available in the home?

g. Is there a detailed *psychiatric history* from the patient's chart or from other individuals?

h. Were any *empty pill bottles* found at home or on the person?

i. Was there a *suicide note?*

2. When the exposure is known and the patient is alert and able to provide a reasonable history (as in Case 2), the following questions may elicit useful information:

a. What *medications* or *compounds* were *ingested?* The ingestion of multiple drugs is common, although specific questioning is often necessary to obtain the details.

b. *How much* of each agent was *ingested?* This information is confirmed whenever possible by checking the prescription bottle. The pharmacist may be called to confirm the number of pills and contents in a prescription.

c. *When* and *how* did the *exposure take place?* Timing of exposure is extremely important, particularly when considering gastric decontamination. Asymptomatic patients should be observed for 4 to 6 hours in the emergency department after most reported ingestions.

d. Were there any *symptoms after* the exposure?

e. Was the exposure *accidental* or *intentional?*

f. Was any *treatment* given *at the scene?* Dilution with water or milk, home remedies, and attempts to induce vomiting are common.

3. Occasionally an alert patient will present with symptoms of an unsuspected toxic exposure (as in Case 3). The following information may aid with the diagnosis:

a. The *chronology* of the presenting complaint(s)

b. *Medications*, including any recent dose changes or health store products

c. Any *special diets* or *dietary supplements*

d. Detailed *situational* and *occupational history*

Physical Examination

The physical examination may be normal immediately after a toxic ingestion. However, as toxicity develops, the patient may manifest signs that serve as clues to the nature of the agent. A thorough examination is necessary and may identify subtle findings. These findings may be useful in evaluating ingestions of both known and unidentified toxins. Importantly, the clinical picture may corroborate or contradict the preliminary history. It also may reveal clues implicating a previously unsuspected intoxicant. Furthermore, the physical examination can help determine the extent of the poisoning, reveal the presence of a toxic syndrome, establish the baseline for underlying disease, and expose underlying trauma. Abnormal physical signs are routinely sought with a detailed examination.

Vital Signs. Abnormalities of pulse, respiratory rate, blood pressure, and temperature are helpful in the identification of the agent or agents involved and are used to guide therapeutic intervention (Table 15–1).

Cardiopulmonary System. The lungs are auscultated to assess the adequacy of air movement. Wheezes, rhonchi, or rales may indicate the presence of pneumonitis resulting from inhalation of toxic gases, aspiration of gastric contents, or exposure to direct pulmonary toxins. Pulmonary edema may result from ingestion of cardiotoxic drugs or agents that produce noncardiogenic pulmonary edema (e.g., heroin, salicylates)

Neurologic System. Many toxic agents produce alterations in mental status, and some produce pupillary changes that are helpful in differentiating a specific class of agent involved. Focal findings on the motor, sensory, or reflex examination may suggest causes other than intoxication. However, hypoglycemia as a result of poisoning can produce focal findings.

Mental Status. Altered mental status may suggest the involvement of particular intoxicants. Delirium, often accompanied by severe agitation, is suggestive of sympathomimetic or phencyclidine (PCP) overdose, anticholinergic toxicity, or withdrawal from opioids, alcohol, or sedative-hypnotics. Depressed mental status occurs with narcotics, sedative-hypnotic agents, carbon monoxide, and many other toxins.

TABLE 15–1. Vital Sign Abnormalities Associated with Intoxication

Abnormality	Mechanism	Class of Compound
Hypoventilation	CNS depression	Opioids, sedative-hypnotics, alcohols
Hyperventilation	CNS stimulation	Sympathomimetics, theophylline, salicylates, phencyclidine
		Drug withdrawal, toxin-based metabolic acidosis
	Tissue hypoxia	Carbon monoxide, cyanide, methemoglobinemia, methane (asphyxia), opioids (noncardiogenic pulmonary edema)
	Metabolic acidosis	See Table 15–4
Bradycardia	Parasympathetic	Organophosphates, carbamates
	CNS depression	Opioids, sedative-hypnotic agents, ethanol
	Cardiotoxicity	Digoxin, calcium channel blockers, β blockers, clonidine
Tachycardia	CNS stimulation	Sympathomimetics, drug withdrawal
	Direct cardiac effect	Theophylline, sympathomimetics (cocaine)
	Cholinergic blockade	Cyclic antidepressants, antihistamines, belladonna alkaloids
Hypotension	Cardiotoxicity	Cyclic antidepressants (sodium channel blockade), β blockers, calcium channel blockers
	Loss of vasomotor tone	Cyclic antidepressants, antihypertensive agents, calcium channel blockers, theophylline, clonidine
	CNS depression	Opioids
	Volume depletion	Iron, other heavy metals, diuretics, lithium (diabetes insipidus), organophosphates (diarrhea)
Hypertension	α-Adrenergic stimulation	Sympathomimetics, drug withdrawal, thyroid supplements, nicotine
	Cholinergic blockade	Anticholinergic agents
Hypothermia	CNS depression	Barbiturates, opioids, oral hypoglycemics, insulin
	Loss of thermoregulation	Phenothiazines, ethanol, carbon monoxide
Hyperthermia	CNS stimulation	Sympathomimetics, phencyclidine, salicylates, drug withdrawal (ethanol, others), nicotine
	Cholinergic inhibition	Cyclic antidepressants, other anticholingic agents
		Phenothiazines
	Loss of thermoregulation	Belladonna alkaloids, antihistamines, cyclic antidepressants
	Vasodilatation	Ethanol

CNS, central nervous system.

Pupillary Changes. Abnormalities can be very specific for certain classes of intoxicants (Table 15–2). Although careful inspection is often necessary, the pupillary changes associated with poisons typically are symmetric, and reactivity to light is retained. This is an important differentiating point between toxicologic and structural causes of altered mental status. Structural causes (e.g., brain edema, hematoma) often cause pupillary asymmetry and inhibit light reactivity.

Skin. Skin color, moisture, and the presence of lesions or needle tracks are noted. The skin examination further aids in determining the class of agent involved. Large blisters or bullae may be present in areas subjected to pressure after exposure to carbon monoxide, barbiturates, glutethimide, or other sedative-hypnotic agents. Needle tracks from intravenous drug abuse are typically associated with heroin or cocaine use.

ENT Examination. The oral mucosa is evaluated for evidence of burns from caustic ingestions, and any specific odor of the breath should be noted (Table 15–3). Dry mucous membranes are seen with anticholinergic toxicity. Ulcerated lesions of the nasal mucosa may be observed in chronic cocaine abusers.

CLINICAL REASONING

Has This Patient Experienced a Toxic Ingestion?

Most commonly, this question is asked after a patient presents with an altered level of consciousness. Other causes of mental status change are outlined in Chapter 31, Altered Mental Status. The variability of presentations of toxic ingestions makes it prudent to consider poisoning in any patient who presents with any mental status abnormality of unclear origin. An obvious ingestion involving an identified intoxicant usually presents no diagnostic dilemma. In most such cases, the physician needs to establish whether toxicity has occurred or the likelihood that it will.

Is There a Diagnostic Pattern of Clinical Findings, That Is, a Toxidrome?

Therapeutic decision making for the poisoned patient must often precede specific identification of the agent by history or laboratory results. In these situations, decisions are based on an understanding of human physiology and the response to

TABLE 15–2. Toxic Pupillary Abnormalities

Abnormality	Mechanism	Compound
Miosis	Central nervous system depression	Opioids Chloral hydrate
	Cholinergic stimulation	Organophosphates, carbamates Pilocarpine
	α-Adrenergic block	Labetalol, clonidine Phenothiazines
Mydriasis	Cholinergic inhibition	Cyclic antidepressants, antihistamines, belladonna alkaloids
	α-Adrenergic stimulation	Sympathomimetics, drug withdrawal

a toxic insult. Fortunately, many drugs or toxins betray their presence by leaving physiologic fingerprints. These occur in the form of syndromes or groups of signs, termed *toxidromes*, that result from the pharmacologic action of the agent(s) involved. Most toxidromes represent agonist or antagonist effects on the autonomic nervous system. Drugs that serve as agonists at opiate receptors also produce a discernible pattern of response. Withdrawal from ethanol or other sedative-hypnotic agents has also been classified as a separate toxidrome, although historical information is required to differentiate it from the sympathetic toxidrome. A toxidrome may not be part of the patient's initial presentation. Delayed toxidromes may occur by enteric-coated agents, slowed gastrointestinal motility, drug concretions, slow production of toxic metabolites, or prolonged duration of action of the intoxicant.

Opioid Toxidrome

Opioids are central nervous system (CNS) depressants and are capable of causing global depression of vital functions. The classic triad for opioid intoxication is

TABLE 15–3. Odors Associated with Toxic Agents

Fruity	Ethanol, ketoacidosis
	Isopropanol
Mothballs	Camphor
	Naphthalene
	Paradichlorobenzene
Bitter almonds	Cyanide
Silver polish	Cyanide
Rotten eggs	Hydrogen sulfide
Garlic	Arsenic, organophosphates, thallium, selenium, DMSO
Wintergreen	Methylsalicylate
Peanuts	Vacor (rodenticide)
Vinyl upholstery	Ethchlorvynol
Pears	Chloral hydrate
Shoe polish	Nitrobenzene
Cleaning solution	Tetrachloride

- Coma
- Respiratory depression
- Pinpoint pupils

Hypotension and bradycardia may also be present. Hypothermia, decreased bowel sounds, and decreased reflexes often occur with this toxidrome. Noncardiogenic pulmonary edema can also occur, usually after injection of heroin.

Agents associated with the opioid toxidrome include

- Codeine
- Diphenoxylate (Lomotil)
- Heroin
- Propoxyphene
- Pentazocine
- Morphine
- Meperidine
- Fentanyl
- Hydrocodone

Cholinergic Toxidrome

There are two kinds of cholinergic toxidromes, the muscarinic and nicotinic. Features of the clinical presentation of the muscarinic toxidrome can be remembered by the mnemonic **DUMB BELS**.

    Diarrhea
    Urination
    Miosis
    Bradycardia
    Bronchorrhea
    Emesis
    Lacrimation
    Salivation

Agents that produce the muscarinic toxidrome include

- Organophosphate insecticides
- Pilocarpine
- Carbamate insecticides
- Carbachol
- Betel nuts

Features of the nicotinic toxidrome are more muscle related and include

- Tachycardia
- Hypertension
- Muscle fasciculations
- Weakness or paralysis

Agents that produce the nicotinic toxidrome include

- Organophosphate/carbamate insecticides
- Indian tobacco
- Nicotine (e.g., gum, patches)
- Black widow spider venom

Anticholinergic Toxidrome

A mnemonic for the clinical presentation of the anticholinergic toxidrome is *"Red as a beet, dry as a bone, mad as a hatter, blind as a bat, hot as Hades."* The features include

- Flushed skin
- Dry skin and mucous membranes
- Mydriasis
- Delirium
- Hyperthermia
- Hypertension
- Tachycardia
- Urinary retention
- Absent bowel sounds

Several common agents produce the anticholinergic toxidrome:

- Antihistamines (including most over-the-counter sleep aids)
- Antimotility agents
- Phenothiazines
- Tricyclic antidepressants
- Scopolamine
- Jimsonweed
- Belladonna alkaloids

Sympathomimetic Toxidrome

Compounds such as cocaine and amphetamines are not only CNS stimulants but also have a significant effect on the sympathetic portion of the autonomic nervous system. Therefore, the toxidrome seen with overdoses of these compounds cause a systemic hyperdynamic state. Drug withdrawal from ethanol and other substances of abuse can manifest a similar hyperadrenergic state. This syndrome is characterized by

- Hypertension
- Tachycardia
- Hyperpyrexia

- Mydriasis
- Anxiety or delirium

Toxicity due to phencyclidine (PCP), although it is not a sympathomimetic agent, may present in a similar manner. Seizures, hypotension, and dysrhythmias may occur in severe cases.

Sedative-Hypnotic Toxidrome

Compounds such as barbiturates and benzodiazepines cause depressed mental status. Barbiturates can cause severe respiratory depression. Unlike with opioids, pupillary changes with these drugs are unpredictable, although a slowing in reaction to light is common. The barbiturates may cause vesicles or bullae to develop at pressure points. Persistence of the pupillary light reflex in the presence of deep coma is characteristic of a barbiturate overdose. Characteristic signs are

- Confusion or coma
- Respiratory depression
- Hypotension
- Hypothermia
- Variable pupillary changes
- Vesicles or bullae ("barb burns")
- Seizures

Salicylate Toxidrome

Salicylates are common components of both prescription and nonprescription preparations. Toxicity may result from intentional or accidental overdose and is common in all age groups. Characteristic signs are

- Fever
- Tachypnea
- Vomiting and dehydration
- Altered mental status (rarely coma)
- Tinnitus
- Seizure

Other Symptom Complexes Associated with Poisoning

AGENTS ASSOCIATED WITH SEIZURES

A list of agents that can produce seizures can be recalled using the mnemonic **OTIS CAMPBELL.** Agents that cause hypotension or hypoxia may result in secondary seizure activity. Drug withdrawal can also present with seizures.

O: Opioids (meperidine, propoxyphene), organophosphates, oral hypoglycemic agents
T: Theophylline, tricyclic antidepressants
I: Isoniazid, insulin

S: Salicylates, sympathomimetic agents, serotonin agonists

C: Camphor, cocaine, cyanide, carbon monoxide, caffeine

A: Amphetamines, anticholinergic agents, antihistamines

M: Methylxanthines, mushrooms (*Gyromitra*)

P: PCP, phenothiazines, plants (e.g., Jimsonweed, belladonna alkaloids, water hemlock)

B: Belladonna alkaloids, β blockers (propranolol)

E: Ethanol withdrawal, ergotamine

L: Lindane, lidocaine

L: Lithium, lead, LSD

AGENTS THAT BLOCK SODIUM CHANNELS

The presence of a wide QRS complex can occur after poisoning by agents that cause blockade of fast sodium channels. Other findings include ventricular dysrhythmias (especially torsades de pointes), hypotension, atrioventricular block, asystole, and bradycardia.

- Propranolol, sotalol
- Orphenadrine (Norflex)
- Local anesthetic agents, including cocaine
- Propoxyphene
- Antihistamines
- Cyclic antidepressants
- Type IA and IC antiarrhythmic agents
- Phenothiazines

DIAGNOSTIC ADJUNCTS

Laboratory Studies

Serum Electrolytes. The value of these measurements in evaluating the poisoned patient is in the determination of the "anion gap."

$$\text{Anion gap} = Na^+ - (HCO_3^- + Cl^-)$$

The normal anion gap of 8 to 12 mEq/L is caused by the presence of unmeasured anions such as sulfates, phosphates, and negatively charged proteins. Poisoning with some agents can produce an increase in the anion gap, as more unmeasured anions are formed. This finding is usually associated with a metabolic acidosis (Table 15–4).

Arterial Blood Gas. Arterial blood gas analysis is necessary for evaluating respiratory status and acid-base abnormalities, especially in patients presenting with altered mental status or seizure.

Serum Glucose. Hypoglycemia or hyperglycemia may result from toxic exposures, and the serum glucose concentration may have prognostic, diagnostic, and therapeutic significance.

TABLE 15–4. Causes of a High Anion-Gap Metabolic Acidosis (MUDPILES)

Methanol
Uremia
Diabetic ketoacidosis*
Paraldehyde, phenformin, metformin
Iron,[†] isoniazid[†]
Lactic acid, carbon monoxide,[†] cyanide[†]
Ethylene glycol, ethanol[†]
Salicylate

*Ethanol and starvation can also lead to ketoacidosis.
[†]These agents also produce lactic acidosis.

Fingerstick glucose measurement should be performed in any patient presenting with altered mental status.

Serum Osmolality. Serum osmolality is useful when an osmotically active agent, including methanol, ethylene glycol, isopropanol, mannitol, glycerol, or ethanol is suspected. These compounds result in an increase in the osmolal gap, the difference between the calculated and measured osmolality. The calculated osmolality is determined by the equation:

$$\text{Osmolality} = 2[Na] + \frac{[\text{glucose}]}{18} + \frac{[BUN]}{3} + \frac{[\text{ethanol}]}{4}$$

This result is compared to the measured osmolality, determined by freezing point depression. The normal range is 285 to 295 mOsm/L. A difference greater than 10 mOsm/L reflects the presence of one or more of the aforementioned compounds.

Toxicology Screens. These "screens" are a diverse group of *qualitative* assays used to identify the presence of a predetermined array of compounds in the urine, blood, or gastric fluid. However, the toxicology screen results are rarely useful in emergency department management decisions. Stat results are often unavailable, and screens are frequently inaccurate, demonstrating significant limitations in both sensitivity and specificity. They are also relatively expensive. A standard toxicology screen may be of use when there are occupational, medicolegal, or forensic issues.

One method commonly used in the emergency department is the enzyme-mediated immunoassay (EMIT). This assay is simple and fast, with turnaround times of 2 to 4 hours, and has intermediate accuracy and specificity. The EMIT screen for common drugs of abuse (Table 15–5) is performed on a urine sample. When interpreting screen results the physician must remember that a "negative" result may occur when drugs are present in undetectable quantities or with the presence of agents not detected by the assay. Ideally,

TABLE 15–5. Drugs Screened by the Enzyme-Mediated Immunoassay for Toxins (EMIT)

Amphetamines	Marijuana
Barbiturates	Opiates
Benzodiazepines	Phencyclidine
Cocaine	Tricyclic antidepressants
Ethanol	

this screen is obtained when the result will affect management.

Quantitative Toxicology Studies. Quantitative blood levels can be obtained for a variety of compounds (Table 15–6). Acetaminophen levels are performed on all intentional overdoses because it is often a co-ingestant or present in overdosages of combination drugs. If ingestion of acetaminophen is known or suspected, a properly interpreted drug blood level can provide both diagnostic and prognostic information. Furthermore, treatment of acetaminophen poisoning is based on the serum level and the timing of ingestion, regardless of symptoms. The most useful information is obtained when the blood sample is taken at or near peak concentration. Unfortunately, individual variations in absorptive capacity and unreliable information about the actual time of ingestion often make it impossible to know when this peak occurs. Early blood levels may be useful for prognoses before peak concentration is reached. Serial quantitative levels are often required to determine whether drug concentration is rising or falling.

Complete Blood Cell Count and Differential. The presence of leukocytosis in the differential cell count may suggest a stress demargination or infection, but ingestions of iron, theophylline, lithium, and hydrocarbons may produce an absolute leukocytosis.

Blood Urea Nitrogen and Creatinine. In the poisoned patient, these tests are useful to identify the presence of a preexisting renal dysfunction that could influence management of toxins with renal excretion and for providing a useful baseline when the poison involved is nephrotoxic.

TABLE 15–6. Clinically Useful Quantitative Blood Levels

Acetaminophen	Lithium
Carbamazepine	Methanol
Carbon monoxide (carboxyhemoglobin)	Methemoglobin
Digoxin	Phenobarbital
Ethanol	Phenytoin
Ethylene glycol	Procainamide
Heavy metal	Quinidine
Iron	Salicylate
Isopropanol	Theophylline
Lidocaine	Valproic acid

Radiologic Imaging

Imaging studies can play three separate roles in the poisoned patient. They can (1) assist in the diagnosis, (2) help guide management, and (3) reveal complications from the exposure.

Chest Radiography. The chest radiograph is useful in patients exposed to agents with a direct pulmonary effect, including hydrocarbons, toxic gases, intravenous injection of mercury, or paraquat. It may also be useful in the baseline assessment of patients who ingest potentially toxic quantities of drugs associated with noncardiogenic pulmonary edema (e.g., salicylates, methaqualone, heroin).

Abdominal Radiography. A plain abdominal film may reveal radiopaque agents in the gastrointestinal tract. Compounds visualized include chloral hydrate, enterically coated tablets, carbon tetrachloride, ferrous sulfate, and other heavy metals. The radiograph is also useful for evaluation of "body packers," individuals who swallow large amounts of illicit drugs encased in balloons or condoms for purposes of smuggling. A popular acronym for radiographically opaque toxins is CHIPES (Table 15–7).

Plain films of the abdomen can also be used to follow the efficacy of gastrointestinal decontamination. Films obtained after gastric lavage with persistent pill fragments mandate continued lavage and/or whole-bowel irrigation or invasive removal by gastrotomy or endoscopy.

Electrocardiogram

An electrocardiogram (ECG) is obtained to exclude conduction delays or dysrhythmias. Agents that block fast sodium channels result in QRS widening and torsades de pointes. Tricyclic antidepressants can also produce tachydysrhythmias and rightward axis deviation of the frontal plane. Anticholinergic or sympathomimetic agents can cause sinus tachycardia, supraventricular tachycardia, ventricular tachycardia, or ventricular fibrillation. β Blockers or calcium channel blockers produce bradycardias or conduction delays. Although the most common electrocardio-

TABLE 15–7. Radiographically Opaque Toxins

C	Chloral hydrate, calcium carbonate, crack vials
H	Heavy metals, health foods (bone meal)
I	Irons, iodides
P	Psychotropics, potassium (enteric coated), phosphates, and packages (illicit drugs)
E	Enteric-coated preparations
S	Slow-release preparations, solvents (CCl_4, $CHCl_3$)

graphic change seen with digitalis toxicity is ventricular ectopy, digitalis overdose can result in severe atrioventricular block and other dysrhythmias. The most common cause of paroxysmal atrial tachycardia with block is digitalis toxicity.

PRINCIPLES OF MANAGEMENT

Although the gathering of clinical and laboratory data is essential for accurate identification of both the toxic compound and the degree of toxicity, medical management often cannot be delayed until a definitive diagnosis is made. Diagnosis and management are therefore dynamic and interrelated processes. Because of the vast array of potentially toxic compounds and the diversity with which ingestions of these are managed, assistance in management is routinely sought from standard references. The most comprehensive and practically useful reference is the regional poison control center.

Certain principles of management have general applicability in the poisoned patient:

1. Emergency stabilization
2. Decontamination
3. Minimization of absorption
4. Maximization of elimination
5. Use of antagonist agents

Emergency Stabilization (also see "Initial Approach and Stabilization")

As always, initial stabilization requires attention to the ABCs. Early airway control with intubation should be considered, especially in patients with altered mental status and those requiring gastric lavage.

Treatment of Hypotension

A cardiac monitor is placed to assess dysrhythmia as a cause of hypotension, and the first intervention is an intravenous fluid bolus. Pressor agents should be tailored to the pharmacology of the toxic agent, when known. With agents that cause fast sodium channel blockade, hypotension can result from the negative inotropic effect, even if the QRS interval is not prolonged. These cases often respond well to sodium bicarbonate therapy (see Acute Metabolic Acidosis and Metabolic Alkalosis, Chapter 21).

Treatment of Altered Mental Status

Standard empirical treatment with glucose, thiamine, oxygen, and naloxone is considered (as previously mentioned). Although flumazenil, a benzodiazepine receptor antagonist, is available, it has no place in the emergency department management of the *unknown* overdose.

Treatment of Seizure

Initial treatment should include oxygen and glucose. Benzodiazepines are administered for continued seizure activity. If ineffective, barbiturates are given. Routine administration of phenytoin is not recommended because toxin-induced seizures rarely respond and phenytoin can produce unwanted cardiac effects. If seizures continue despite these measures, pyridoxine should be administered for reversal of toxicity from isoniazid and *Gyromitra esculenta* (false morel mushroom). Sustained seizure activity may require neuromuscular paralysis with continuous electroencephalographic monitoring.

Decontamination

Decontamination includes clothing removal and copious irrigation of the eyes and skin as well as the gastrointestinal tract.

Minimize Absorption

Limiting the absorption of a compound can be accomplished several ways. With inhaled agents, limiting pulmonary absorption can occur with access to fresh air and oxygen administration. When the agent is dermally absorbed, as with organophosphate pesticides, the skin should be decontaminated using a series of detergent washings. Gastrointestinal decontamination includes gastric emptying, activated charcoal administration, and catharsis.

Gastric Emptying. Gastric emptying is achieved by one of two methods: *induced emesis* or *gastric lavage*. Historically, emesis has been achieved in a variety of ways, including forced ingestion of salt water (an extremely dangerous practice), pharyngeal stimulation, and drug induction. The most reliable method is the use of the drugs apomorphine or syrup of ipecac, which results in emesis in over 90% of cases. Although apomorphine is no longer used because of its side effects, syrup of ipecac is still widely available. Although syrup of ipecac can be purchased without a prescription, it should be used judiciously. Contraindications to its use are summarized in Table 15–8. Optimally, this compound is administered as early as possible after the ingestion. Because it is efficacious only in the first 15 minutes after ingestion, its use has been abandoned in the emergency department. Its greatest clinical

TABLE 15–8. Contraindications to Syrup of Ipecac Usage

Age <6 months
Third trimester of pregnancy
Actual or potential loss of airway reflexes due to coma, seizure, cardiovascular collapse
Rapidly acting central nervous system depressant (e.g., cyclic antidepressants, isoniazid, propoxyphene, propranolol)
Suspected caustic ingestions
Certain hydrocarbon ingestions with high aspiration risk and little systemic toxicity
Hemorrhagic diathesis
Need to administer an oral antidote

use is in the management of pediatric ingestions in the home for witnessed acute ingestions. After telephone contact with the poison center, parents or guardians are instructed to give 15 mL of syrup of ipecac by mouth. Even then, ipecac-induced emesis results in only partial emptying of stomach contents, ranging from 20% to 75% depending on the time since ingestion and volume of ipecac administered. Vomiting secondary to ipecac administration can persist for up to 2 hours.

The alternative to induced emesis is gastric lavage. The procedure involves passage of a large-bore orogastric tube (36 to 40 French in an adult) into the stomach and flushing the stomach of its contents with normal saline. Multiple 200- to 300-mL aliquots of fluid are sequentially instilled into the tube, allowed to mix with the gastric contents, and then drained by gravity. Recommendations for the volume of fluid that constitutes an optimal lavage vary. The most practical guideline is to continue lavage until the fluid is clear of any débris.

Gastric lavage is associated with potential adverse effects. Hemorrhage, laryngospasm, esophageal tears, gastric perforation, pyriform sinus trauma, and aspiration can all occur. The most imminent danger is that of aspiration. Before lavage, the physician must assess the ability of the patient to protect the airway. If airway protection is tenuous or if the patient ingested a drug likely to produce rapid deterioration (e.g., a tricyclic antidepressant), the patient must be intubated before placement of the orogastric tube. Even if the patient is able to protect the airway or is intubated, there is still a small risk of aspiration. This risk can be minimized by placing the patient in the Trendelenburg and left lateral decubitus positions during lavage.

Like syrup of ipecac–induced emesis, gastric lavage cannot be relied on to completely empty the stomach of its contents. It is particularly inefficacious when pill fragments are large or are slow-release tablets. Gastric lavage is preferred over ipecac-induced emesis in the emergency department.

There is a declining emphasis on gastric emptying because improvement in outcome is rarely demonstrated, and a trend toward a more selective approach to the use of this intervention is occurring. Emptying is no longer indicated for the management of ingestions of minimally toxic or nontoxic potential. It is also unlikely to be beneficial for the removal of rapidly absorbed drugs such as ethanol and acetaminophen or if spontaneous emesis has already occurred. Furthermore, gastric emptying is contraindicated when the risks of intervention are outweighed by the potential benefits, such as in patients with caustic ingestions, ingestions of sharp objects, and pills too large to fit through a lavage tube or in any patient unable to protect the airway. Finally, gastric lavage must be performed within 1 hour of the ingestion or its effectiveness is significantly diminished.

Activated Charcoal. Activated charcoal has rapidly gained favor as the most effective modality for reducing the gastrointestinal absorption of toxic compounds. It has a gritty texture and is unpalatable; therefore, patients are frequently reluctant to drink charcoal and it often causes vomiting. Despite these shortcomings, activated charcoal has become a highly regarded therapeutic modality.

Activated charcoal is produced by heating wood pulp, washing it, and then activating it with steam or acid. It provides a large surface area for direct adsorption of agents in the gastrointestinal tract. It can also produce "gut dialysis" by pulling substances from the blood into the gastrointestinal tract (e.g., chronic theophylline toxicity) and is useful for eliminating agents with enterohepatic recirculation. Although this is difficult to estimate in practice, a 10:1 ratio of activated charcoal to ingested compound is recommended. The volume of diluent necessary to facilitate administration of activated charcoal limits the maximum tolerated dose to 1 to 2 g/kg.

Studies have demonstrated the superiority of activated charcoal in comparison with syrup of ipecac–induced emesis in limiting the absorption of certain compounds. Although there are no absolute contraindications to its use and it is nontoxic, activated charcoal is withheld in patients who have ingested caustic substances to avoid obscuring endoscopic examination, and in patients who have ingested pure petroleum distillates to avoid emesis. Furthermore, activated charcoal does not bind well to lithium, metals, caustic agents, or alcohols. It may still be recommended in these poisonings, when there is a risk of co-ingestion. As with gastric lavage, activated charcoal should be given within 1 hour of ingestion for maximal effectiveness.

Cathartics. Cathartics, such as sorbitol, can counteract the constipating effect of activated charcoal and decrease the intestinal transit time of the drug-charcoal complex, potentially reducing the amount of drug that desorbs from charcoal during its intestinal passage. Sorbitol also improves the palatable nature of the charcoal slurry. The vigorous catharsis that often follows the use of sorbitol is associated with stomach cramps and can result in fluid and electrolyte abnormalities, especially in small children. If a cathartic is used in combination with activated charcoal, it should be limited to a single dose. In addition, studies have not proved effectiveness of cathartics and their routine use is not recommended.

Whole-bowel irrigation is accomplished by using large volumes of a balanced polyethylene glycol lavage solution such as Golytely. Because these solutions are isotonic, their use does not result in fluid or electrolyte imbalance. Theoretically, whole-bowel irrigation should not routinely be used in conjunction with activated charcoal, because it can displace or occupy toxin-binding sites on the activated charcoal and thereby increase bioavailability of the toxin. It may be particularly beneficial in removing packets found in "body packers" and large quantities of compounds not well adsorbed by activated charcoal, such as iron or lithium. Whole-bowel irrigation also can be considered with massive overdoses of sustained-release products or with substances that cause concretion or bezoar formation.

Maximize Elimination

Although gastric emptying, activated charcoal, and whole-bowel irrigation are useful for limiting the absorption of many compounds, by the time these interventions are made a significant amount of compound may already be absorbed. Elimination of selected toxins can be enhanced by hemodialysis, hemoperfusion, enhanced renal elimination, or multidose activated charcoal therapy.

Hemodialysis. Hemodialysis involves the circulation of blood through a semipermeable membrane. Dialysis is more effective for compounds that are water soluble, are poorly protein bound, and have a low molecular weight (Table 15–9).

Hemoperfusion. Hemoperfusion is similar to hemodialysis, but the blood passes through a column filled with adsorbent material, which is usually some form of activated charcoal. Because hemoperfusion does not involve passive diffusion of molecules, some poorly dialyzable, lipid-soluble, protein-bound compounds can be elimi-

TABLE 15–9. Intoxicants for Which Dialysis Is Especially Useful

Methanol	Salicylate
Ethylene glycol	Lithium
Ethanol	Procainamide
Isopropanol	

nated in significant quantities by this process. Hemoperfusion is recognized as the most valuable modality for eliminating theophylline. It is also useful for eliminating carbamazepine, ethchlorvynol, and barbiturates.

Enhanced Elimination. The rate of elimination of some drugs can be enhanced by alkalinization of the urine. Salicylates, chlorpropamide, and phenobarbital are weak acids and, in an alkaline solution, are more ionized, resulting in decreased absorption in the renal tubule. This "ion trapping" results in increased excretion of these substances. The goal of urinary alkalinization is a urine pH of 7.5 to 8.0 and can be accomplished by administration of 1 mEq/kg bolus of sodium bicarbonate followed by an infusion of approximately 7.5% $NaHCO_3$ at 1.5 to 2 times maintenance. This may be approximated by diluting 3 ampules of $NaHCO_3$ (50 mEq each) in 1 L of dextrose 5% in water. Serum pH should remain less than 7.55. Although elimination of weak bases such as amphetamines and phencyclidine is enhanced by acidification of the urine, the cardiovascular and neurologic dangers associated with this practice far outweigh the advantages.

Physiologic Antagonists (Antidotes)

Antagonist agents are a diverse group of compounds that block, reverse, slow, or lessen the adverse effects of various intoxicants through a variety of mechanisms. With some exceptions, the actions of antagonists are generally quite specific against certain classes of toxic compounds. Therefore, the physician must know the type of toxic compound involved before choosing an individual antagonist agent. Notable exceptions to this rule include oxygen and naloxone (Narcan), both of which can be used safely early in the course of management. Antidotes are listed in Table 15–10.

EXPANDED DIFFERENTIAL DIAGNOSIS

Some agents are either commonly encountered or cause significant morbidity if not recognized and properly treated, and each is discussed in this section. Ethanol is discussed at greater length in Chapter 16, Alcohol Intoxication.

TABLE 15–10. Toxins and Specific Antidotes

Toxin	Antidote	Dosage and Comments
Acetaminophen	N-Acetylcysteine	Initial dose 140 mg/kg PO followed by 17 doses of 70 mg/kg every 4 hr
Anticholinergic agents	Physostigime	1–2 mg IV. Use only for severe toxicity.
Venom	Antivenin	Rattlesnakes, copperhead (rarely needed), water mocassin
	Crotalid	Eastern coral snake
	Coral snake	Black widow spider
	Latrodectus	
Benzodiazepines	Flumazenil	0.2 mg IV over 30 sec. If there is no response after 30 sec, give 0.3 mg, then 0.5 mg over 30 sec at 1-min intervals up to a total dose of 3 mg. Note contraindications in text. May be useful in iatrogenic benzodiazepine toxicity. Contraindications to flumazenil use include seizure disorder, benzodiazepine dependence, or concomitant tricyclic antidepressant ingestion.
β Blockers	Glucagon	Starting dose 5–10 mg IV titrate to response (normalization of vital signs). Maintenance dose of 2–10 mg/hr may be used.
Calcium channel blockers	Calcium chloride	1 g IV over 5 min
	Glucagon	See β Blockers
Carbon monoxide	100% and hyperbaric O₂	Hyperbaric oxygen (3 ATA) for 90 minutes; can repeat; usefulness remains controversial.
Coumadin	Vitamin K₁	25–50 mg IV slowly at 1 mg/min. Takes 4–6 hr for effect.
	Fresh frozen plasma	Reserved for active bleeding
Cyanide	Sodium nitrite	10 mL of a 3% sodium nitrite
	Sodium thiosulfate	50 mL of 25% sodium thiosulfate IV
	Hydroxycobalamin	Adjust doses for children. Not approved in United States
Digitalis glycosides	Digoxin-specific antibodies	One vial binds 0.6 mg digoxin.
Phenothiazines (extrapyramidal reactions)	Diphenhydramine	5–100 mg
	Cogentin	1–2 mg IM
Heparin	Protamine sulfate	1 mg per 100 units heparin, 50 mg maximum dose
Iron	Deferoxamine	15 mg/kg/hr IV infusion; max 6 g/day
Isoniazid *Gyromitra esculenta* (false morel)	Pyridoxine	Gram-per-gram equivalent. If amount ingested is unknown, start with 5 g IV.
Lead, mercury, arsenic	Dimercaprol, BAL	Consult toxicologist for specific recommendations
Methanol, ethylene glycol	Ethanol	Loading dose: 10 mL of 10% solution. Maintenance: 1–2 mL/kg/hr 10% EtOH to maintain serum at 100 mg/dL.
	4-Methyl-pyrazole	Consult toxicologist for specific recommendations.
Nitrites	Methylene blue	1–2 mg/kg/IV as a 1% solution, given slowly over 5 min. A second dose can be given after 1 hr.
Opiates	Naloxone	0.2 mg–10 mg
	Nalmefene	0.5 mg/70 kg IV
Organophosphates	Atropine	2 mg IV over 5 min. Repeat until bronchorrhea resolved
	Pralodoxine	2–4 mg IV
Carbamates	Atropine	See organophosphates.
Tricyclic antidepressants and other fast sodium channel blockers	Sodium bicarbonate	1–2 mmol/kg IV for QRS complex widening, ventricular dysrhythmias, hypotension

Acetaminophen

Acetaminophen is remarkably safe at therapeutic dosages but can cause fatal hepatic necrosis after overdose. Hepatic metabolism to nontoxic glucuronide and sulfate conjugates accounts for 90% to 95% of the disposition of acetaminophen. A small fraction (1% to 2%) is excreted unchanged in the urine. The remaining drug is converted to a highly reactive, potentially destructive intermediate through the cytochrome P450 mixed function oxidase system. Normally, this intermediate is quickly conjugated with glutathione to nontoxic metabolites. After acetaminophen overdose, however, the rate of glutathione use exceeds the rate of regeneration, glutathione stores become depleted, and the unconjugated toxic intermediate reacts with and destroys hepatocytes. The same reaction can occur in the kidneys, and abnormal results on renal function tests occur in about 10% of patients with hepatotoxicity and, rarely, in patients without liver injury. The true "toxic" dosage of acetaminophen is variable, but ingestions of 7.5 g in an adult and 150 mg/kg in a child are considered potentially toxic.

Within a few hours of overdose, nonspecific signs and symptoms such as nausea, vomiting, pallor, and diaphoresis may occur, but even severely poisoned patients may remain asymptomatic. During the initial 18 to 24 hours (stage 1) there is no laboratory evidence of hepatic or renal injury. If hepatotoxicity develops, aminotransferase levels begin to rise after 18 to 24 hours (stage 2). Accompanying symptoms (nausea, vomiting, right upper quadrant pain), signs (hepatic enlargement and tenderness, jaundice), and laboratory abnormalities (hyperbilirubinemia, increased prothrombin time) occur. Peak hepatotoxicity (stage 3) usually occurs 72 to 96 hours after overdose. Although massive necrosis of the liver can occur, recovery is the rule. Recovery (stage 4) usually occurs over a few days; and if patients survive, recovery is complete, without evidence of chronic hepatotoxicity.

The most important feature of acetaminophen poisoning is that although the signs and symptoms of hepatotoxicity are delayed for 18 to 36 hours, antidotal therapy is most effective if started within 8 to 10 hours. Because drug histories are unreliable, the plasma acetaminophen concentration is the only reliable method of predicting potential toxicity. It should be measured in all cases of suspected acetaminophen overdose, polydrug overdose, and overdose of drugs of abuse often combined with acetaminophen (e.g., codeine, propoxyphene). The Rumack-Matthew nomogram (Fig. 15–1) is used to predict the severity of toxicity and the need for antidotal therapy. Proper use requires that the blood sample be drawn at least 4 hours after ingestion. Patients with acetaminophen concentrations above the line shown in the treatment nomogram are treated with N-acetylcysteine (NAC).

NAC serves primarily as a glutathione precursor, but it also is a glutathione substitute, and it increases the supply of substrate for the nontoxic sulfate conjugation pathway. Oral NAC (intravenous NAC is not yet FDA approved in the United States but is currently the preferred therapy in Europe) is an extremely effective antidote if started within 8 hours of overdose; and although its efficacy starts to decline thereafter, the current standard of care is to treat patients as late as 24 hours after overdose. The decision to treat with NAC can await determination of acetaminophen levels if this information is available within 8 hours of ingestion. If it is not available, it is best to initiate NAC treatment while awaiting laboratory results and then to discontinue or continue it accordingly.

Aspirin

The therapeutic index of aspirin (acetylsalicylic acid) is low, and toxicity often occurs after repeated dosing with normal or slightly above normal amounts as well as after single acute overdose. Aspirin has effects on several organ systems. It stimulates the central respiratory system directly, uncouples oxidative phosphorylation, inhibits the Krebs cycle and amino acid metabolism, and interferes with normal hemostasis. As a result, the possible signs and symptoms of poisoning are varied and numerous. Tinnitus, nausea, vomiting, and hyperpnea (with or without tachypnea) are common. Although lethargy and confusion may occur in moderately severe cases, hyperpyrexia or profound CNS abnormalities (seizure, coma) imply life-threatening toxicity. Noncardiogenic and cardiogenic pulmonary edema may also occur in severe cases.

Alkalemia (pH of greater than 7.45) is the most common acid-base disorder caused by mild or early salicylism. It is caused initially by pure respiratory alkalosis and later by mixed respiratory alkalosis with a lesser metabolic acidosis. In severe cases, especially in children, metabolic acidosis eventually predominates, leading to acidemia (pH of less than 7.35). In addition to primary salicylate-induced acid-base disorders, fever, hyperpnea, and vomiting frequently lead to secondary dehydration and electrolyte abnormalities, which may complicate management. The accumulation of "unmeasured" anions (ketoacids, salicylate,

PLASMA ACETAMINOPHEN LEVELS VS. TIME

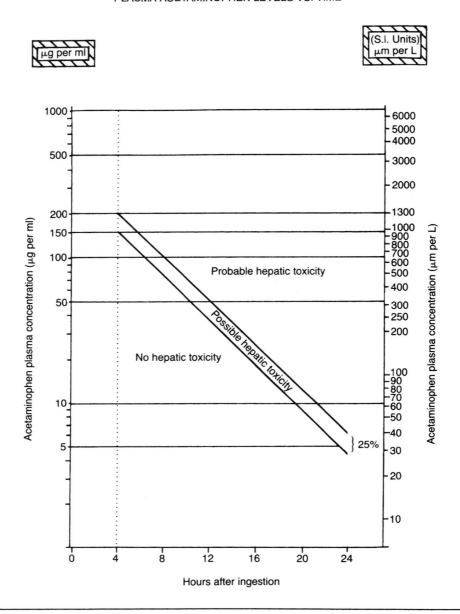

CAUTIONS FOR USE OF THIS CHART:

1) The time coordinates refer to time of ingestion.
2) Serum levels drawn before 4 hours may not represent peak levels.
3) The graph should be used only in relation to a single acute ingestion.
4) The lower solid line 25% below the standard nomogram is included to allow for possible errors in acetaminophen plasma assays and estimated time from ingestion of an overdose.

FIGURE 15–1 • Rumack-Matthew nomogram for acetaminophen poisoning. (With permission from Micromedex, Inc. Adapted from Pediatrics 55[6], June 1975, with permission from the authors and the publisher. Copyright Micromedex, Inc. 1974–1985. All rights reserved.)

lactate) causes an increase in the anion gap, and salicylate toxicity should be considered in the presence of an increased anion-gap metabolic acidosis. Evaluation of the urine may be helpful in making the diagnosis. Urine ketones are often present, owing to the interference of salicylate with normal glucose and amino acid metabolism. Urine ferric chloride testing provides an extremely sensitive but nonspecific test. This reagent, when mixed with salicylate-containing urine, turns purple.

Hepatic salicylate metabolism is limited, and enzyme saturation occurs even at therapeutic doses. As a result, after an acute overdose or after drug accumulation from repeated doses (chronic toxicity), other routes of elimination are important. Salicylate exists in both ionized and nonionized forms. Both are readily filtered into the urine, but only the nonionized form is reabsorbed. Because the ratio of ionized to nonionized drug increases 10-fold for each pH unit increase, alkalinization of the urine increases the proportion of ionized salicylate and prevents drug reabsorption (ion trapping). The pK_a of salicylate is 3.5; therefore, increasing urine pH to 7 or higher by administering sodium bicarbonate significantly enhances urinary elimination of the drug. Alkalemia will also minimize CNS salicylate concentrations. The potential for complications from treatment with sodium bicarbonate include hypernatremia, hypokalemia, fluid overload, and congestive heart failure. The risk of these complications can be decreased by the use of an isotonic solution of sodium bicarbonate made by adding 3 ampules of sodium bicarbonate to 1 L D_5W with a goal of urine pH of 8.0.

When alkalinization is not possible or ineffective or when more rapid drug removal is indicated, hemodialysis is required. Indications for dialysis include renal failure, pulmonary edema, seizures, any significant alteration in mental status, severe acid-base or electrolyte disturbance, coagulopathy, lack of response to sodium bicarbonate therapy, or, in the absence of these, a salicylate level of above 100 mg/dL in acute overdose or 65 mg/dL in chronic overdose.

Serious errors occur when treatment decisions are based solely on serum levels, rather than clinical presentation. Levels are useful in confirming diagnosis, and serial levels predict drug absorption/excretion. Treatment should primarily be based on signs and symptoms. Because patients with chronic toxicity often present more insidiously, the diagnosis can be delayed and the seriousness underestimated. Patients with chronic salicylate toxicity are at higher risk for serious complications and should be treated more aggressively. Salicylate toxicity should always be considered in elderly patients with altered mental status and in patients with unusual presenting signs and symptoms accompanied by characteristic acid-base abnormalities.

Tricyclic Antidepressants

Overdose of tricyclic antidepressants (TCAs) is a common toxicologic cause of morbidity and mortality, despite advances in diagnosis and treatment. Fortunately, many newer agents differ in toxicity from earlier products and result in fewer serious effects. TCAs produce toxicity by three primary pathophysiologic effects. They have significant anticholinergic effects, produce α blockade, and produce membrane-depressant (quinidine-like) effects.

The first clue to the diagnosis of TCA overdose is the finding of anticholinergic signs. The onset of toxicity usually occurs early (1 to 3 hours after overdose), and the progression from asymptomatic or minor toxicity to major toxicity is often very abrupt. Sinus tachycardia is present in more than 80% of cases and alone is not considered a sign of major toxicity. However, persistent sinus tachycardia greater than 120 beats per minute may indicate continued absorption. Other conduction defects and serious rhythm disturbances are caused by quinidine-like effects. Inhibition of fast inward sodium channels (action potential phase 0) prevents normal rapid depolarization of myocardial cells, slowing conduction and promoting ectopy. On the ECG, abnormal depolarization may appear only as subtle changes in QRS morphology and vector analysis, or there may be obvious QRS or QT prolongation with major rightward axis deviation, leading to ventricular tachycardia or torsades de pointes. Sinus tachycardia with aberrant conduction is common and is often mistaken for ventricular tachycardia. The QRS duration is the best predictor of subsequent risk for seizures or ventricular dysrhythmias. A QRS interval of greater than 0.10 second within 6 hours of overdose appears to be associated with increased risk for subsequent seizures. A QRS interval greater than 0.16 second is associated with ventricular dysrhythmias.

Because decompensation is rapid and seizures can occur, syrup of ipecac is contraindicated. Gastric lavage is recommended for TCA overdose up to 1 hour after ingestion. Airway protection with endotracheal intubation may be necessary before lavage. Activated charcoal with sorbitol should also be administered. Because significant enterohepatic recirculation occurs, administration of multiple doses of activated charcoal enhances the rate of drug elimination. However, clinical improvement has not been established. Treatment of conduction defects and tachydysrhythmias begins with alkalinization of the serum to pH 7.45 to 7.55. Unlike salicylate poisoning, in which alkalinization is undertaken primarily to raise the urine pH and enhance elimination, alkalinization of the serum after cyclic antidepressant overdose is done to diminish the toxic effects of the overdose. The mechanism is still controversial, but serum alkalinization rapidly improves conduction. Both sodium bicarbonate and hyperventilation have been used, but experimentally the use of bicarbonate appears to be faster and somewhat more effective. Many toxicologists recommend alkalinization whenever the QRS interval is increased and in patients with hypotension or ventricular dysrhythmias. If alkalinization fails, lidocaine may be used to treat ventricular dysrhythmias. Class Ia agents and Ic agents and phenytoin should be avoided. Magnesium can also shorten the QT interval and suppress torsades de pointes and ventricular ectopy when given intravenously.

Neurologic manifestations include coma and seizures and are treated with airway protection, ventilatory support, and administration of benzodiazepines. Seizures should be rapidly controlled to prevent acidosis and worsening cardiotoxicity. If benzodiazepines are ineffective, phenobarbital should be administered. Phenytoin is not recommended because of its limited efficacy and dysrhythmic effects. Failure of seizures to respond to phenobarbital is an indication for neuromuscular blockade and general anesthesia with continuous electroencephalographic monitoring.

Hypotension is caused by both decreased inotropy (quinidine-like effect) and peripheral α-adrenergic blockade. Decreased inotropy is best treated with alkalinization, but in many cases additional treatment is necessary. A fluid challenge (500 to 2000 mL of isotonic crystalloid solution) may correct hypotension, but vasopressor therapy is often required. Dopamine may be ineffective secondary to the antidepressant-induced blockade of catecholamine uptake, but direct-acting α-adrenergic agents such as norepinephrine or Neo-Synephrine are effective. Despite its ability to reverse anticholinergic signs and symptoms transiently, *physostigmine is contraindicated* and has been associated with increased mortality in the treatment of TCA toxicity.

Serotonin Syndrome

Serotonin syndrome was first recognized in the early 1950s and 1960s associated with monoamine oxidase inhibitors. It is characterized by altered mental status, autonomic dysfunction, and neuromuscular abnormalities. Selective serotonin reuptake inhibitors (SSRIs) are replacing TCAs as drugs of choice for the treatment of depression. Although much less toxic after overdose, serotonin syndrome is more common and can be life-threatening.

With a known ingestion of a serotoninergic agent, even without intentional overdose, serotonin syndrome is considered to be present if three of the following criteria are met: (1) mental status changes; (2) agitation; (3) myoclonus; (4) hyperreflexia; (5) diaphoresis; (6) shivering; (7) tremor; (8) diarrhea; (9) incoordination; (10) fever; (11) restlessness, especially of the feet; and (12) extreme fear. Other possible causes of a similar symptom profile have to be excluded, such as infection, metabolic disorders, substance abuse, or withdrawal. Neuroleptic malignant syndrome (NMS) can also be mistaken for serotonin syndrome. Distinguishing features of NMS include a history of neuroleptic agent usage, lead pipe rigidity rather than myoclonus or hyperreflexia, and an absence of mydriasis (pupillary dilatation present in serotonin syndrome). In the emergency department, care must be exercised in medication administration to patients who are taking SSRIs. Agents that should be avoided include dextromethorphan and meperidine.

Fortunately, serotonin syndrome can typically be treated with discontinuation of the offending medication and conservative measures, which include external cooling, sedatives, paralytics, anticonvulsants, antihypertensives, and mechanical ventilation. In more severe cases, more specific serotonin antagonists can be used. Propranolol and nonspecific 5-hydroxytryptamine (serotonin) antagonists, to include methysergide and cyproheptadine, have been shown to be effective, especially against myoclonus. Benzodiazepines have been shown to relieve muscular hyperactivity and sympathetic symptoms. Dantrolene, which inhibits influx of calcium into muscle cells, is recommended for the treatment of hyperthermia associated with hyperrigidity. Cyproheptadine is probably the most commonly used antidote for serotonin syndrome. It is especially effective against myoclonus and is given at a dosage of 4 mg/hr.

Bupropion/Lithium

Bupropion is an antidepressant that acts as a dopamine agonist and reuptake inhibitor. It also has anxiolytic properties. It has gained popularity as an antidepressant agent because of its lack of anticholinergic side effects and cardiotoxic effects. It is also commonly prescribed as an adjunctive treatment for smoking cessation. The most significant adverse effect is seizure. Other symptoms associated with overdose include sinus tachycardia, tremor, and decreased level of consciousness. Sinus tachycardia has not been associated with other dysrhythmias or QRS widening. Seizures are readily treated with benzodiazepines in conjunction with decontamination procedures.

Lithium carbonate is an inorganic salt that is prescribed for the treatment of recurrent manic-depression. It has been proposed for treatment of several other psychiatric disorders. Toxicity from lithium is often unintentional. It has a narrow therapeutic window with a therapeutic serum range of 0.6 to 1.2 mEq/L. Levels above 1.5 mEq/L often result in toxicity and those above 2.0 mEq/L usually produce some toxicity. Seventy-five to 90 percent of patients on long-term therapy experience signs or symptoms of toxicity. Factors that predispose patients to toxicity include a high serum concentration, a long duration of lithium exposure, and individual tolerance to lithium. Any process that limits excretion can also produce toxicity. Dehydration, dietary restriction of sodium, anorexia, vomiting or diarrhea, and strenuous activity have all been implicated. Interaction with other medications that hinder lithium excretion, including diuretics or nonsteroidal anti-inflammatory medications, also can produce toxicity.

Toxic manifestations range from mild and nonspecific to severe. Neurologically, the patient can exhibit decreased memory, impaired concentration, fine tremor, fatigue or weakness, hyperreflexia, or extrapyramidal symptoms. These will progress to a coarse tremor, dysarthria, tinnitus, ataxia, or myoclonus. In severe cases, seizures, stupor, fasciculations, rigidity, paralysis, and coma can occur. With acute toxicity, nausea, vomiting, and diarrhea are usually present. In chronic toxicity, cerebrovascular deterioration, cerebellar dysfunction, and T-wave abnormalities can develop. The ECG initially may show T-wave changes with interventricular conduction defects. These can progress to ventricular dysrhythmias and cardiovascular collapse. Serum lithium levels cannot be used alone to gauge the seriousness of toxicity. Chronic use of lithium has resulted in mild to moderate symptoms with levels of 1.5 to 2.5 mEq/L and serious symptoms with 2.5 to 3.5 mEq/L; levels above 3.5 mEq/L are considered life-threatening. The increased risk from chronic toxicity is caused by the increased distribution of lithium throughout the intracellular and extracellular compartments after chronic use.

Acute overdoses can be associated with very high serum levels yet produce minimal or no symptoms.

Treatment of lithium toxicity after acute overdose should begin with gastric lavage. Activated charcoal does not bind lithium and, therefore, is not recommended in isolated overdose. Whole-bowel irrigation has been reported to decrease absorption by 67% when performed within 1 hour of ingestion. Polyethylene glycol electrolyte solution is administered at 2 L/hr until rectal effluent is clear. Dehydrated patients should receive intravenous fluids, but forced diuresis is ineffective and not recommended. Hemodialysis is the treatment of choice for severe lithium toxicity. Indications for hemodialysis include moderate to severe lithium intoxication that fails to improve after conservative therapy. Specific indications for dialysis include patients with severe neurologic dysfunction, including seizures, patients with hemodynamically unstable dysrhythmias, patients who cannot tolerate intravenous fluids (e.g., those with congestive heart failure), and patients with chronic intoxications with serum levels from 2.5 to 4.0 if symptomatic or greater than 4.0 regardless of symptoms. In most cases, neurologic symptoms resolve after treatment. However, long-term neurologic sequelae such as ataxia, persistent tremor, and dysarthria can occur.

Carbon Monoxide

Carbon monoxide (CO) poisoning is a leading cause of death due to poisoning in the United States, resulting in over 5000 deaths per year. Complex combustion of any organic fuel generates CO; thus, in addition to suicidal exposures, accidental home exposures (gas water heaters, furnaces, space heaters, fireplaces, barbecues, automobile exhaust) and occupational exposures (gasoline-powered tools and machinery) are common. The diagnosis is often difficult because the exposure is not recognized and the symptoms are nonspecific. A history of several members in a household with similar "flu-like" symptoms and presentation of these symptoms at the onset of cold weather should raise clinical suspicion of CO poisoning.

CO combines with hemoglobin to form carboxyhemoglobin (COHb) and causes toxicity in many ways: decreased oxygen-carrying capacity (COHb cannot transport oxygen), decreased oxygen delivery (the oxyhemoglobin dissociation curve shifts to the left in the presence of CO), and, possibly, decreased oxygen utilization, especially by myoglobin in the heart, which has an affinity for CO 40 times greater than oxygen. CO also acts to stimulate guanosine monophosphate activity, resulting in smooth muscle relaxation and hypotension. In animal studies, delayed neurologic sequelae from CO poisoning have been associated with episodes of hypotension. CO also produces lipid peroxidation in the brain, which is probably responsible for delayed neurologic effects.

There are no methods available to determine levels of tissue CO; thus, blood COHb levels are used to assess exposure. The clinical role of COHb measurement is to determine if a CO exposure has occurred. Measurements greater than 10% are considered abnormal. Smokers may normally have levels up to 15%. The correlation between COHb levels and severity of toxicity is very poor. Therefore, clinical symptoms in association with an elevated COHb level are the primary determinants of treatment. Early symptoms include headache, fatigue, dyspnea, and exertional angina. Moderate symptoms include dizziness, ataxia, and cardiac dysrhythmias. More prolonged severe exposures are associated with syncope or loss of consciousness, seizures, altered mental status, coma, marked acidosis, and even death.

Treatment consists of supportive care and oxygen administration. The higher the concentration of oxygen delivered, the more rapidly CO is eliminated from both blood and tissue. Although there is great variation, the half-life of COHb is 4 to 6 hours when breathing room air, 40 to 90 minutes after breathing normobaric 100% oxygen, and 20 minutes with hyperbaric oxygen (HBO) at 3 ATA. All symptomatic patients should receive 100% oxygen, initially.

Indications for HBO are controversial but generally include evidence of significant tissue anoxia, as manifested by loss of consciousness, chest pain, ischemic electrocardiographic changes, acidosis, hypotension, or any cognitive or neurologic abnormality, including abnormal bedside neuropsychiatric testing. In the absence of these signs and symptoms, each HBO center establishes a COHb level above which HBO is offered. These levels vary from 25% to 40%. Because the fetus tolerates CO very poorly, pregnant victims should receive HBO if they have COHb levels greater than or equal to 15% or if they are symptomatic. High-risk or difficult to assess groups such as infants, the elderly, and patients with abnormal baseline cardiovascular function also should receive HBO at lower COHb levels.

Supportive care can be complex, because of the multisystemic nature of postanoxic injury. Myocardial infarction, dysrhythmias, shock, pulmonary edema, anoxic encephalopathy, rhab-domyolysis, and renal failure have all been described after CO poisoning. In addition, delayed and permanent neuropsychiatric and neurologic abnormalities occur. The most serious errors in management result from failure to consider the diagnosis, neglecting HBO therapy in the presence of low COHb levels in patients with ongoing organ dysfunction (i.e., ongoing tissue toxicity), failure to consider that other victims (family members, neighbors, coworkers) must be assessed, and failure to identify and eliminate the source of CO.

Caustic Agents

Although caustic agents can cause significant morbidity, particularly after intentional ingestion, management of these patients is controversial. Alkaline agents produce liquefaction necrosis, resulting in acute and chronic gastrointestinal effects after ingestion. The esophagus is most commonly affected, and patients with acute injury may develop esophageal strictures and esophageal carcinoma years after initial exposure. Acidic agents (except hydrofluoric acid) produce coagulation necrosis and more commonly affect the stomach. Significant ingestions usually produce gastrointestinal symptoms. Patients may develop dysphagia, oropharyngeal lesions, vomiting, or abdominal pain.

The first priority in management of caustic ingestion is airway management. Upper airway edema can occur, particularly after large ingestions. If any airway signs or symptoms occur, intubation should be performed early. Preparation for early surgical airway management should also occur, because severe edema can result in difficult airway placement and rapid decompensation.

Spontaneous vomiting is common after caustic ingestions, but induction of emesis or gastric lavage is contraindicated because increased gastrointestinal injury may occur. Activated charcoal is also contraindicated because it does not effectively adsorb caustic agents, can increase the risk of emesis, and obscures endoscopic visualization. The use of corticosteroids to decrease stricture formation after alkali ingestion is controversial, although efficacy has not been adequately demonstrated.

Accidental ingestion or questionable ingestion of caustic agents in children is particularly difficult to manage, because predictive signs and symptoms of significant gastrointestinal injury have not been established. If there are no signs or symptoms of toxicity after a possible alkaline ingestion, administration of oral fluids should be attempted. If the patient remains asymptomatic, discharge is usually appropriate. However, if the patient has symptoms or evidence of oropharyngeal injury, flexible endoscopy is recommended. Endoscopy is recommended after all acid ingestions or in any patient with a history of intentional ingestion, regardless of symptoms.

Hydrocarbons

Hydrocarbons are a diverse group of organic compounds that include petroleum distillates (aromatic or aliphatic) and turpentine. They are also often mixed with other toxic agents, such as insecticides or heavy metals. Effects from exposure can be pulmonary, neurologic, or cardiovascular. Chemical pneumonitis from aspiration is a common toxic effect that depends on the physical characteristics of the agent. High viscosity, high volatility, and low surface tension all increase the risk of aspiration.

Patients, particularly after accidental exposure, can be asymptomatic on presentation to the emergency department. Symptoms can include oral pain, vomiting, abdominal pain, dyspnea, coughing, headache, and altered mental status. Gastric decontamination, including charcoal administration, is contraindicated in the majority of hydrocarbon exposures because aspiration risk is increased.

Patients who remain asymptomatic after 6 hours of observation can be discharged. Chest radiographs and oxygenation status should be evaluated in symptomatic patients. Airway and ventilatory management may be required in the emergency department, although severe toxicity is often delayed. No benefit has been demonstrated from the use of corticosteroids or antibiotics in the management of hydrocarbon pneumonitis.

Abuse of aromatic hydrocarbons (e.g., toluene, xylene) has become more common in adolescents as a method to induce euphoria. Paint products are placed on a rag and "sniffed" or placed in a bag and "huffed." Tragically, this practice has resulted in death, referred to as "sudden sniffing death." Death is believed to occur because aromatic hydrocarbons sensitize the myocardium to catecholamines, resulting in fatal cardiac dysrhythmias. Because of this effect, administration of catecholamine agents is contraindicated after aromatic hydrocarbon exposure. Chronic abuse can lead to irreversible neurologic sequelae. Most patients who present after aromatic hydrocarbon exposure are asymptomatic, and no treatment is required. However, parents should be educated to prevent further abuse.

Theophylline

Theophylline poisoning generally occurs in one of three settings: (1) acute intentional overdose, (2) acute on chronic overdose, and (3) chronic overdose. Any interference with the hepatic metabolism of theophylline can cause toxicity. Alcoholic liver disease, liver congestion due to right-sided heart failure, medications (e.g., erythromycin, propranolol, or cimetidine), and some infections slow metabolism and can result in theophylline toxicity.

Gastrointestinal symptoms (nausea, vomiting, diarrhea) are common regardless of the severity of toxicity. Cardiovascular effects may include sinus tachycardia, premature atrial contractions, supraventricular tachycardias, atrial flutter or fibrillation, ventricular ectopy, ventricular tachycardia, ventricular fibrillation, and refractory hypotension. However, sustained supraventricular and ventricular tachyarrhythmias are uncommon. CNS effects include tremor, anxiety, agitation, and seizures. Laboratory abnormalities are also common and include hypokalemia, lactic acidosis, leukocytosis, hyperglycemia, hypomagnesemia, and hypophosphatemia.

Serum theophylline levels are useful but must be interpreted cautiously. Chronic overdoses result in serious toxicity at much lower drug levels than acute overdoses. In all cases, the degree of symptomatology is the most important factor in determining therapy, but many authors consider a drug level of 40 to 60 μg/mL in a patient with a chronic overdose roughly equivalent in significance to a level of 70 to 100 μg/mL after an acute overdose. Because morbidity and mortality are significant above these levels, they are used as indications for hemoperfusion. A common, and potentially lethal, mistake is failure to consider the pharmacokinetics of theophylline when interpreting serum levels. Most currently prescribed theophylline preparations are sustained-release formulations, which achieve peak levels as late as 8 to 12 hours after ingestion in therapeutic doses and even later after overdoses. If theophylline levels are obtained earlier, the severity of the overdose may be underestimated unless serial levels are obtained to illustrate the rate of rise and the efficacy of initial attempts to limit absorption. As a result, levels much lower than the commonly used "critical values" may still indicate a need for hemoperfusion.

Syrup of ipecac is contraindicated because of the risk of seizures and because it may interfere with the administration of activated charcoal. Orogastric lavage is indicated in ingestions that have occurred within 1 hour. Activated charcoal is a critical part of treatment because it is highly effective in both limiting gastrointestinal absorption and enhancing elimination of theophylline. Large initial doses of activated charcoal (1 to 2 g/kg up to 100 g) should be used, and repeated doses (0.5 to 1.0 g/kg every 4 hours) are given until toxicity has resolved and drug levels have declined. Antiemetics are often required, but phenothiazines are contraindicated, owing to their ability to decrease the seizure threshold. Slow nasogastric instillation may facilitate retention of charcoal. Hypokalemia is a common complication but should be corrected conservatively. It occurs secondary to an intracellular shift of potassium; therefore, replacement of potassium too vigorously can cause hyperkalemia as theophylline toxicity resolves. Seizure control is often difficult. Rapid-acting intravenous agents such as benzodiazepines are used initially, followed by phenobarbital. Phenytoin is not recommended. Refractory seizures are treated by induction of general anesthesia with barbiturates and continuous electroencephalographic monitoring.

Fluid administration is the first-line treatment of hypotension, but in severe cases vasopressors, although often ineffective, may be administered. In such cases, when hypotension is associated with evidence of shock (increasing acidosis, worsening mental status, or inadequate urine output), β blocker therapy should be initiated while hemoperfusion is being arranged. Life-threatening hypotension is probably caused more by β_2-adrenergic–mediated vasodilatation than to decreased cardiac output from β_1-adrenergic–mediated tachycardia. Esmolol has been useful experimentally and clinically in treating victims of severe theophylline toxicity, but caution must be exercised with its use in asthmatics, secondary to the risk of β blocker–induced bronchospasm.

Extracorporeal theophylline removal using hemodialysis or charcoal hemoperfusion is effective in enhancing drug elimination. Because theophylline is highly protein bound, hemoperfusion is more effective than hemodialysis and is the preferred method of removal of theophylline. Indications for extracorporeal removal include seizures, hemodynamically significant dysrhythmias, hypotension, or extremely high theophylline levels (greater than 80 mg/L in acute ingestions or greater than 40 to 50 mg/L for chronic ingestions). Patients with rapidly rising drug levels, those unable to take multiple dose charcoal, or those with worsening symptoms despite supportive care and multidose charcoal are also candidates for hemoperfusion.

Cocaine, Amphetamines, and Phencyclidine

Amphetamine and cocaine intoxication both produce the classic sympathomimetic toxidrome, but other causes must be entertained, including pheochromocytoma, sepsis, and thyrotoxicosis. The findings may be difficult to distinguish from phencyclidine (PCP) intoxication or alcohol/sedative-hypnotic withdrawal. The most appropriate initial treatment for these clinical entities is benzodiazepines. They act to calm the patient while concurrently increasing the seizure threshold and reducing catecholamine output.

PCP is not a sympathomimetic agent, and thus cardiovascular and pupillary findings are much less consistent. Tachycardia and hypertension are common but are not always present. Although pupillary findings vary, miosis is common with PCP. Bidirectional nystagmus and rotary nystagmus are the most consistent physical examination findings after PCP intoxication, but they may be absent. Two final distinguishing features are the waxing and waning mental status of PCP-overdosed patients and their surprising strength and pain tolerance when resisting physical restraint methods. PCP-poisoned patients may alternate rapidly and unpredictably between violent agitation and deep coma. As in drug-induced agitation from other causes, rhabdomyolysis, hyperthermia, and intracranial hemorrhage can occur from PCP intoxication.

Amphetamines are predominantly synthetic agents, which vary in their stimulant effect on the central and peripheral nervous system. CNS actions are caused by the increased release and decreased reuptake of dopamine and serotonin. They cause increased peripheral effects by stimulating release of norepinephrine at the postganglionic synapses. This leads to both α- and β-adrenergic effects.

Cocaine is an alkaloid compound derived from the leaves of the *Erythroxylon coca* plant. It may be smoked in its free-base or alkaline form as "crack" or snorted in its hydrochloride form. Intravenous injection is also common. Acute overdose will present as the sympathomimetic toxidrome with hypertension, tachycardia, hyperpyrexia, mydriasis, diaphoresis, and anxiety or delirium. Other symptoms can include repetitive activities such as grinding teeth (bruxism) or tactile hallucinations ("formications"), preoccupation with one's thought processes, or acute psychosis.

Cocaine use often produces chest pain and is a common reason for cocaine users to present to the emergency department. In a study of hospitalized patients with cocaine-related chest pain, 31% had acute myocardial infarction whereas 13% had myocardial ischemia. Although cocaine acutely produces vasospasm, thrombosis can occur several days after use, and chronic use is associated with an increased risk of atherosclerotic heart disease. Like myocardial infarction from other causes, cocaine-induced infarction often presents as atypical chest pain and a nondiagnostic ECG. Therefore, patients who present with chest pain associated with cocaine use should have myocardial infarction ruled out, despite other risk factors. Chest pain can also be caused from barotrauma after crack inhalation, causing pneumothorax, pneumomediastinum, and pneumopericardium. Therefore, a chest radiograph is indicated in all patients with cocaine-associated chest pain.

Treatment of ischemic chest pain from cocaine use is similar to that from other causes. Initial management of cardiovascular complications is with intravenous administration of benzodiazepines. Patients should receive oxygen, nitrates, and aspirin. However, because they can produce unopposed α-adrenergic effects and coronary artery spasm, β blocker use is contraindicated in patients with cocaine toxicity. Calcium channel blockers and phentolamine appear to be safe. Thrombolytic agents are also used less frequently in patients with cocaine-induced myocardial infarction because there is an increased risk of bleeding from concomitant hypertension. Patients with cocaine-induced infarction have fewer complications and lower mortality. Lidocaine should be avoided, because it may increase cocaine toxicity during early treatment. Hypertension is common after cocaine use and can often be controlled with benzodiazepine use alone. If hypertension persists, nitroprusside and/or calcium channel blockers and phentolamine may be effective.

Seizures can occur after exposure to any sympathomimetic agent. Twenty-six percent of all new-onset seizures in adult patients are caused by cocaine use. Cocaine-induced seizures are usually generalized, single, brief, and without neurologic sequelae. Other CNS manifestations can include subarachnoid hemorrhage, migraine-like headaches, altered level of consciousness, tremors, dizziness, and, rarely, focal neurologic deficits. Computed tomography and lumbar puncture should be considered in any patient with neurologic symptoms or signs. First-line treatment of seizures should be intravenous benzodiazepines. If recurrent or prolonged seizures occur after benzodiazepine treatment, phenobarbital or general anesthesia should be considered.

Hyperthermia can be severe and should be aggressively treated with external cooling.

Sedation and intravenous hydration may also help, but patients with refractory hyperthermia may require neuromuscular paralysis. Because of the hyperactive state, hyperthermia, seizures, and muscle ischemia, patients are also at risk for rhabdomyolysis and acute renal failure. Creatine phosphokinase levels should be determined and a urinalysis done, especially if the patient complains of myalgia, muscle tenderness, weakness, or dark urine. Standard treatment, including alkalinization of urine and intravenous fluid administration, should be instituted.

Psychiatric manifestations of acute cocaine, amphetamine, or PCP use are initially treated with benzodiazepines. The chronic cocaine or amphetamine abuse state may present as weight loss, restlessness, or insomnia. Although there is no physiologic withdrawal, the psychologic withdrawal syndrome from cocaine or amphetamine abuse typically presents as severe psychological dysphoria or depression. Depression may have suicidal implications as well as severe fatigue, anxiety, increased appetite, and psychomotor retardation. All patients should be referred for substance abuse counseling and further psychiatric care, as there is a high risk of postwithdrawal depression.

Opiates

Opiate toxicity can result from use of single agents or combined exposures such as intravenous heroin and cocaine ("speedball") or pentazocine and tripelennamine ("T's and blues"). The numerous opioid products available for street use are far exceeded by available prescription formulations (analgesics, cough suppressants). The result is that opioid toxicity is common, comes in many forms, and should always be considered in the differential diagnosis of altered mental status. Because opioids are often combined with antipyretic agents (acetaminophen or salicylate), toxicity from these agents must also be considered. Opioids characteristically cause sedation, respiratory depression, and miosis. Bradycardia is also common. The opioid antagonist naloxone (Narcan) will rapidly reverse these effects and will precipitate acute withdrawal in opioid-dependent patients. Unlike sedative-hypnotic withdrawal, adult opioid withdrawal is not life-threatening.

In patients with respiratory depression and decreased mental status, naloxone, 2.0 mg, should be administered intravenously. The pediatric dose is the same. A lower dose regimen (0.1 to 0.4 mg) can be given to the known opioid-dependent patient with decreased mental status without significant respiratory depression. If this treatment is only partially effective, repeat doses can be given. Some agents (e.g., propoxyphene, fentanyl) may require large doses of naloxone for reversal, and lack of response to naloxone administration should only be concluded after a total of 10 mg has proved to be ineffective. Because the half-life of naloxone is shorter than that of most opioids, repeat administration may be required and no patient should be discharged before 1 hour after naloxone administration. Any recurrence of symptoms, exposure to a long-acting opioid, or continued exposure from concretion of pills or heroin bags within the gastrointestinal tract requires continued intravenous infusion of naloxone. The starting dosage is two thirds the initial dose needed to reverse respiratory depression per hour.

SPECIAL CONSIDERATIONS

Pediatric Patients

In patients younger than the age of 6 months, poisoning is a result of inadvertent administration of an incorrect agent or dose, intentional administration by a parent or sibling, or passive exposure. In any child younger than age 1 who presents with poisoning, child abuse/neglect must be considered. Poisonings in children have certain characteristics: exposures are usually unintentional, a small amount is ingested, nontoxic ingestions are common, morbidity and mortality are relatively low, and presentation to a health care facility occurs quickly.

Adequate history may be difficult to obtain in pediatric ingestions, but information is gathered about the number of pills or volume of liquid missing and about exposures outside the home (with alternative caregivers). Because children generally ingest small amounts of minimally toxic agents, gastric decontamination is often unnecessary. If gastric emptying is required, the use of smaller tubes in children may limit the removal of large tablets. Syrup of ipecac may be useful if administered in the home immediately after ingestion; however, it is recommended that its use be directed by the poison control center.

In children older than age 5, suicidal intent must be considered. The leading lethal agents in children are carbon monoxide, iron, and hydrocarbons. Agents that can cause fatal toxicity in a toddler after ingestion of one swallow or one tablet include camphor, chloroquine, imipramine, desipramine, quinine, methyl salicylate, theophylline, thioridazine, chlorpromazine, imidazolines, benzocaine, diphenoxylate, acetonitrile, and selenious acid. In adolescents, hydrocarbons, antidepressants, and analgesic agents lead the list of fatal agents. Adolescents commonly experience toxicity from misadventures in drug experimentation. Parents must be cautioned about storing agents in tempting containers (e.g., placing pesticides in a soda bottle). They should also be reminded to store substances out of the reach of children and to use child-resistant containers.

Elderly Patients

Although the elderly represent a minority of the poisoning victims, their mortality is the highest. This increase in mortality is the result of several factors: underlying disease, polypharmacy, unrecognized toxicity with delay in diagnosis, unexpected side effects due to alterations in pharmacodynamics, atypical symptoms and signs of toxicity, delayed manifestations of toxicity, availability of highly toxic agents, increased risk of chronic toxicity, and an increased rate of suicide as age progresses. Impaired vision and hearing and dementia also increase the risk of toxicity and/or overdose in the elderly. Because drug dependence may not be considered in older patients, withdrawal may occur, particularly in hospitalized patients.

As age increases, several pharmacokinetic characteristics change. Renal function decreases (50% decrease in glomerular filtration rate between ages 30 and 80), hepatic blood flow declines, hepatic enzyme activity may fall, body fat content increases, and protein synthesis declines. All these changes combine to alter drug metabolism, distribution, and excretion in often unpredictable ways.

Gastric decontamination indications are the same in the elderly as in younger patients. Because of diminished renal function and an increased risk of heart failure, intravenous fluids and bicarbonate must be judiciously used in the elderly, and extracorporeal drug removal may be indicated earlier. The same safeguards to prevent pediatric poisoning often apply to the elderly population.

Substance Abuse Patients

Substance abuse or drug abuse is difficult to define. In addition to the direct toxicity of various agents, those who use agents multiple times have the added risks of dependence, prostitution, criminal activities, violence, and homelessness. For obvious reasons the epidemiology of substance abuse is difficult to accurately determine.

The presence of contaminants in "street drugs" and their associated toxicity must always be considered. Common adulterants include local anesthetics, quinine, talc, phencyclidine, LSD, sugars, and sodium bicarbonate. Some are added with malicious intent (strychnine, thallium), and clandestine laboratories may accidentally produce toxic agents because of erroneous synthesis.

Medical complications must always be considered in the differential diagnosis, requiring a detailed history and physical examination in substance abusers. This population often self-administers antibiotics before seeking medical care, making diagnosis more difficult. Intravenous drug users represent a group at particular risk for medical problems, including complications of human immunodeficiency virus infection, hepatitis, endocarditis, skin and soft tissue infections, thrombophlebitis, abscesses, mycotic aneurysm, osteomyelitis, CNS infections, and sexually transmitted diseases.

Although the relationship may be difficult to establish, the emergency department is usually the first and only contact that the substance abuser has with the health care system. This circumstance offers the unique opportunity to intervene socially as well as medically.

UNCERTAIN DIAGNOSIS

If overdose or intoxication is suspected, the most important clue to the class of agent is the presence of a toxidrome. The presence of specific symptom complexes, such as sodium channel blockade or seizure, are added clues. Although the laboratory rarely aids in diagnosis, the presence of an elevated anion-gap acidosis or an osmolal gap can provide valuable information. Altered mental status protocol should be followed regardless of the history or physical findings, because patients may present with multiple medical problems.

Although the patient who presents with a reliable history of overdose of a specific agent or agents may be straightforward, many toxicology cases must be addressed in the manner of a jigsaw puzzle. Patients are often brought to the emergency department by prehospital care providers, family, friends, or even law officers with a presumed history of overdose or intoxication. Just as it is dangerous to not rule out other medical problems in this group, including associated trauma and metabolic disease, one must also always consider toxicology problems in patients who present with presumed medical or traumatic injuries.

DISPOSITION AND FOLLOW-UP

Appropriate patient disposition depends on many variables. Consideration must be given to both the medical aspects and the psychosocial circumstances before a final decision is made.

Medical Considerations

Medical considerations are based on the nature of the ingested compound and its manifested or potential toxicity. In the absence of other reasons for admission, patients with nontoxic ingestions (Table 15–11) are usually discharged after simple reassurance. It is imperative to confirm ingredients of products before discharge. Similarly, those who have been exposed to compounds with minimal toxicity can usually be discharged after initial emergency department treatment and a suitable observation period. In patients with a questionable history or those who become asymptomatic, medical clearance can usually be accomplished after a 6-hour observation period.

Patients who manifest persistent, significant clinical evidence of toxicity are usually admitted to the hospital. Those patients who are found to have drug levels in the toxic range may also require admission, even in the absence of symptoms or clinical findings. Although admitted patients tend to require intensive care and monitoring, this is not always necessary. The need for intensive care is generally based on the presence of, or risk for, cardiopulmonary or CNS complications that may affect vital functions.

Psychosocial Considerations

The psychosocial elements associated with each case are also taken into account. Toxic ingestions are either intentional or accidental. Intentional ingestions are usually suicide attempts but may also be gestures. Accidental ingestions or intoxications, on the other hand, are usually caused by either excessive intake of chronically ingested medications, reckless substance abuse, or a child's oral curiosity.

Any *intentional ingestion* that is believed to be the consequence of a suicide attempt requires psychiatric consultation. The patient who is a danger to himself or herself may be hospitalized even without patient consent, if necessary. Unfortunately, this issue is not always straightforward. An intentional ingestion is sometimes the result of a suicide *gesture* rather than a suicide *attempt*. The distinction is often difficult to determine. When in doubt, the patient is presumed to be suicidal until determined otherwise by a psychiatric evaluation.

Accidental ingestions present other dispositional concerns. For example, the patient who becomes intoxicated after unwittingly ingesting an

TABLE 15–11. Substances That Are Nontoxic When Ingested in Small Amounts

Abrasives	Ink (black, blue)
Adhesives	Iodophil disinfectant
Antibiotics	Laxatives
Baby-product cosmetics	Lipstick
Ballpoint inks	Lubricants
Bath oil	Lubricating oils
Bathtub floating toys	Magic Markers
Bleach (household)	Make-up
Body conditioners	Matches
Bubble-bath soaps	Mineral oil
Calamine lotion	Newspaper
Candles	Paint (indoor, latex)
Caps (toy pistols)	Pencil (graphite, coloring)
Chalk	Perfumes
Cigarettes or cigars	Petroleum jelly (Vaseline)
Clay (modeling)	Phenolphthalein laxatives
Colognes	Play-Doh
Contraceptive pills	Porous-tip marking pens
Corticosteroids	Putty (less than 2 oz)
Cosmetics	Rouge
Crayons (marked by AP, CP on label)	Rubber cement
Dehumidifying packets	Shampoo (liquid)
Detergents (phosphate)	Saving creams, lotions
Deodorants	Soap
Deodorizers	Spackles
Eye make-up	Suntan cream, lotions
Fabric softeners	Sweetening agents (saccharin, cyclamates)
Fertilizer (unless insecticides or herbicides added)	Teething rings
Fishbowl additives	Thermometers (mercury)
Glues and pastes	Toilet water
Grease	Toothpaste (with or without fluoride)
Hair tonics	Vitamins (with or without fluoride)
Hand lotions	Warfarin (most rat poisons)
Hydrogen peroxide (3%)	Water colors
Indelible markers	Zinc oxide

Adapted from McPherson MC, Greensheer J: Controversies in the prevention and treatment of poisonings. Pediatr Ann 1977; 6:60.

excessive quantity of a therapeutic drug must be educated about the proper use of the drug before discharge. Although such patients are usually admitted for further treatment and observation until sufficient drug metabolism has taken place, some can be safely treated as outpatients. Arrangements are made for timely medical reevaluation and rechecking of blood levels.

The *substance abuser* represents a very special category of patient who frequently requires extensive counseling or rehabilitation to prevent the chronic recurrence of drug toxicity. Although these patients rarely intend to hurt themselves, they are often as self-destructive as suicidal patients. Every effort is made to arrange rehabilitative care for these patients before discharge. An emergency department visit provides an excellent opportunity for treatment of the substance abuser.

Children who accidentally ingest toxic compounds are also at risk for recurrence. An effort is routinely made to counsel parents about home safety. At the same time, the family situation is assessed to determine whether the ingestion could be a sign of abandonment, abuse, or an unsafe family situation. Children who are 5 years old or older must be considered suicide risks when ingestion occurs.

FINAL POINTS

Although the incidence of poisoning is high, resultant morbidity and mortality can be limited by early diagnosis and appropriate treatment. However, the pitfalls associated with the management of toxic ingestions are many. The following caveats can markedly reduce the risk of error:

- A poisoning has occurred but may not be apparent. Be suspicious, particularly in high-risk groups!
- Historical information is almost always more important than diagnostic testing for identifying

the specific intoxicant(s). Considerable detective work and use of all available individuals and resources are often necessary to get the information needed.

- When interpreting physical findings, toxidromes—combinations of symptoms and signs that suggest a particular class of intoxicant—are a useful means of identifying the offending agent.
- Laboratory studies have value and limitations. Potentially spurious results from poorly chosen tests can cloud the diagnostic picture and provide a false sense of security.
- Blood levels of the various intoxicants are interpreted in light of the timing of the specimen.

Multiple levels may be required to make proper conclusions.

- Preventive and supportive therapy of the poisoned patient should be aggressive. An innocuous clinical presentation can change dramatically over a short period of time.
- When toxicity is in doubt, admission to a setting in which careful monitoring can take place is the indicated course.
- Psychosocial problems and needs may far outweigh the medical concerns. The ingestion or overdose may be a "cry for help."

CASE*Study*

A 45-year-old man was unresponsive when his son found him at home. The patient was spontaneously breathing with a weak gag reflex. The presence of several empty pill bottles strongly suggested drug overdose. The rescue squad responding to the call established an intravenous line and initiated cardiac monitoring and oxygen therapy. There was no response to administration of 50% dextrose, thiamine, or naloxone. On arrival in the emergency department, the airway was reassessed.

Even if a patient does appear to be ventilating properly, lack of a gag reflex in an unresponsive patient represents an unprotected airway and requires endotracheal intubation. Manual ventilation may be necessary immediately in an apneic or bradypneic patient, as well as later if the ventilatory pattern deteriorates. Blood pressure, pulse, and cardiac rhythm are also reassessed. If there is a partial response or if the dose given is inadequate, the medications for altered mental status may be readministered.

This patient was brought, unresponsive, to the emergency department by paramedics, who stated that he took an overdose of an unknown substance. The patient could provide no history.

In many cases in which paramedics are involved, evidence in the form of pills or prescription bottles is brought to the hospital with the patient. If this has not been done, a relative or police officer may be sent to the home to retrieve such evidence. A commitment to an aggressive and extensive search for information while the patient is being stabilized will usually yield results.

This patient was found unresponsive at home with empty pill bottles nearby. One bottle had contained thirty 1-mg tablets of lorazepam, the other, fifty 325-mg tablets of acetaminophen. Laboratory results were obtained as follows: blood glucose, 90 mg/dL; blood urea nitrogen, 14 mg/dL; sodium, 140 mEq/L; potassium, 4.0 mEq/L; chloride, 100 mEq/L; bicarbonate, 10 mEq/L; pH, 7.26; and serum osmolality, 350 mOsm/kg. Acetaminophen level was unavailable. Computed tomography of the head was negative.

One must be careful to avoid missing other causes of altered mental status; therefore, computed tomography of the head was performed, despite the presumptive history of overdose. The patient had acidosis. Without arterial blood gas measurements it could not be clearly determined if there was a respiratory component. However, the anion gap ($Na^+ - [Cl^- + HCO_3^-]$) was abnormally elevated at 30 mEq/L and the serum bicarbonate value was low. Therefore, the acidosis was partly metabolic. Because neither lorazepam nor acetaminophen causes metabolic acidosis, another problem existed. The osmolal gap gave a clue in that it was elevated at 50 mOsm/L. Two compounds that can cause a high anion-gap metabolic acidosis, as well as increasing the osmolal gap, are methanol and ethylene glycol. It was reasonable to presume that the patient had ingested one of these compounds. Specific blood level measurements were ordered, and treatment was started for presumptive methanol or ethylene glycol intoxication (see Chapter 16, Alcohol Intoxication). The methanol level subsequently proved to be 30 mg/dL.

CASE *Study*

A 15-year-old girl was brought to the emergency department by her parents after she took 10 "sleeping pills" after an argument with them. She was alert and asymptomatic. The parents want to take the patient home because she has no symptoms. On physical examination, her only significant finding is a heart rate of 120 beats per minute.

This patient had no symptoms and the only abnormal sign was tachycardia. One must not ignore abnormal vital signs. However, even if this patient's examination was completely normal, the possibility for deterioration must be entertained. In this case, the patient developed rapid mental status depression and hypotension. It was subsequently determined that the "sleeping pills" were amitriptyline, 75-mg tablets, a tricyclic antidepressant. Overdoses of this medication can result in

rapid and profound alterations in mental status, seizures, and cardiovascular collapse, even with a normal initial examination. This patient was managed aggressively with an intravenous line and cardiac monitoring. Rapid sequence intubation was performed before gastric lavage to protect the airway. The patient also received a bolus injection of sodium bicarbonate, which resulted in an improved blood pressure.

The case also demonstrates the potential adverse outcome if patients are discharged too early. All patients with intentional ingestions must be observed for at least 6 hours from the time of ingestion to determine if toxicity will occur. Although this can put the physician in an awkward position, the parents must receive a detailed explanation.

CASE *Study*

This 65-year-old patient with a past history of COPD and congestive heart failure presented with symptoms of nausea, palpitations, and tremor.

Any chronically medicated patient, especially an elderly patient, who presents with nonspecific symptoms should be suspected of drug toxicity. In many cases the patient will be able to list the medications he or she is taking. In other cases, however, the names of the medications are unknown and must be inferred from the nature of the illness. Corroborating information is then obtained either by reviewing the patient's medical record or, once again, by having someone retrieve pill bottles from the home.

This patient was observed to have frequent premature ventricular contractions, and a theophylline level of 40 µg/mL was noted. His serum potassium level was normal.

The theophylline level of this patient was in the toxic range. Because theophylline is cardiotoxic,

we must assume that the frequent premature ventricular contractions were a consequence of the excessive serum concentration of this compound. Such a patient is at risk for more serious ventricular dysrhythmias. Because the half-life of theophylline is prolonged in patients with congestive heart failure and with increasing age, we would anticipate metabolism to take place more slowly.

Although the patient demonstrates theophylline toxicity, no indications for charcoal hemoperfusion are present. Because of the patient's underlying disease, age, and the presence of chronic theophylline toxicity, he was admitted to the intensive care unit for monitoring. The patient received oral activated charcoal in the emergency department. On admission, the patient received multiple doses of activated charcoal every 4 hours and serial theophylline levels were monitored for clearance of the drug.

Bibliography

TEXTS

Ellenhorn MJ, Schonwald S, Ordog G, Wasserberger J (eds): Ellenhorn's Medical Toxicology: Diagnosis and Treatment of Human Poisoning, 2nd ed. Baltimore, Williams & Wilkins, 1997.

Ford MD, Delaney KD, Ling LJ, Erickson T (eds): Clinical Toxicology. Philadelphia, WB Saunders, 2001.

Goldfrank LR, Flomenbaum NE, Lewin NA, et al (eds): Goldfrank's Toxicologic Emergencies, 6th ed. Stamford, CT, Appleton & Lange, 1998.

Haddad LM, Shannon MW, Winchester JF (eds): Clinical Management of Poisoning and Drug Overdose, 3rd ed. Philadelphia, WB Saunders, 1998.

JOURNAL ARTICLES

Acute reactions to drugs of abuse. Med Lett Drugs Ther 2002; 44:21–24.

Barceloux D, McGuigan M, Hartigan-Go K: Position Statement: Cathartics. American College of Clinical Toxicology; European Association of Poison Centres and Clinical Toxicologists. J Toxicol Clin Toxicol 1997; 35:743–752.

Bond GR: The role of activated charcoal and gastric emptying in gastrointestinal decontamination: A state-of-the-art review. Ann Emerg Med 2002; 39:273–286.

Bosse G, Matuynas NJ: Delayed toxidromes. J Emerg Med 1999; 17:679–690.

Erickson TB, AKS SE, Gussow L, et al: Toxicology update: A rational approach to managing the poisoned patient. Emerg Med Pract 2001; 3:1–28.

Ernst A, Zibrak JD: Carbon monoxide poisoning. N Engl J Med 1998; 339:1603–1608.

Ford MD, Olshaker JS (eds): Concepts and controversies in toxicology. Emerg Med Clin North Am 1994; 12(2).

Giorgi DF, Jagoda A: Poisoning and overdose. Mt Sinai J Med 1997; 64:283–291.

Groleau G: Lithium toxicity. Emerg Med Clin North Am 1994; 12:511–532.

Larsen LC, Fuller SH: Management of acetaminophen toxicity. Am Fam Physician 1996; 53:185–190.

Liebelt EL, Shannon MW: Small doses, big problems: A selected review of highly toxic common medications. Pediatr Emerg Care 1993; 9:292–296.

Litovitz TL, Klein-Schwartz W, White S, et al: 1999 Annual Report of the American Association of Poison Control Centers Toxic Exposure Surveillance System. Am J Emerg Med 2000; 18:517–574.

Martin TG: Serotonin syndrome. Ann Emerg Med 1996; 28:520–526.

Minton NA, Henry JA: Treatment of theophylline overdose. Am J Emerg Med 1996; 14:606–609.

Perrone JM, Hoffman RS, Goldfrank CR: Special considerations in gastrointestinal decontamination. Emerg Med Clin North Am 1994; 12:285–300.

Proudfoot AT: Paracetamol (acetaminophen) poisoning. Lancet 1995; 346:547–552.

Prybyskm KM, Melville KA, Hanna JR: Polypharmacy in the elderly: Clinical challenges in emergency practice (I, II). Emerg Med Rep 2002; 23(11,12):145–152, 153–162.

Shannon M: Ingestion of toxic substances by children. N Engl J Med 2000; 342:186–191.

Storrow AB: Bupropion overdose and seizure. Am J Emerg Med 1994; 12:183–184.

CHAPTER 16

Alcohol Intoxication

NATALIE M. CULLEN

CASE *Study*

A 43-year-old man was found lying in the gutter with the heavy odor of ethanol on his breath and clothes. He was arousable only with a painful stimulus. His hair was matted, his clothes were torn and wet, and he was without shoes. There was dried blood around his right eyebrow. The police had previously found him in a similar condition.

INTRODUCTION

Epidemiology

The use and abuse of ethanol is of enormous social and medical importance. Alcoholism, as defined by the National Council on Alcoholism of the American Medical Association, is "a chronic progressive and potentially fatal disease." It is characterized by tolerance and physical dependency or pathologic organ changes or both. These features are the direct or indirect consequence of the alcohol ingested. There are an estimated 18 million alcoholics in the United States and certainly millions more who present intoxicated in the emergency department. Fifty percent of motor vehicle accidents involve ethanol abuse, and 25% to 40% of trauma patients incur the trauma while under the influence of alcohol. Driving under the influence of alcohol (DUI) is considered illegal when the serum ethanol level is greater than or equal to 80 to 100 mg/dL. This can be tested by serum level or estimated by breath alcohol testing. The prevalence of alcohol dependence or abuse in emergency department patients is estimated to be as high as 40% in some populations.

Ethanol consumption ranges from acute intoxication to chronic use with "tolerance" but insidious pathologic effects. Chronic consumers may be difficult to identify. Contrary to the image of the "derelict drinker," alcoholics may be well dressed, successful, and avid deniers of their disease.

Pathophysiology

Evaluating and managing the acutely intoxicated patient is a complicated clinical pursuit. The uncooperative, often belligerent intoxicated patient frequently poses obstacles to the simplest aspects of evaluation and care. Ethanol is associated with pathologic changes in almost every system of the body (Table 16–1). The impairment of judgment and motor coordination significantly increases the risk of serious injury, and depression of the level of consciousness masks many of the usual responses to pain and underlying diseases. The effects of the drug can be complicated by environmental conditions (e.g., hypothermia, trauma).

The toxic alcohols include ethanol, ethylene glycol, methanol, and isopropyl alcohol. In this chapter ethanol is emphasized and the other alcohols are briefly addressed under "Special Considerations." Alcohols are rapidly absorbed and widely distributed throughout the body. They have properties similar to those of general anesthetics, acting primarily at the cellular membrane level. They are principally metabolized in the liver by the enzyme alcohol dehydrogenase to form a variety of metabolites. Ethanol is converted into acetaldehyde, which is rapidly cleared by acetaldehyde dehydrogenase. Alcohol dehydrogenase is the rate-limiting step of metabolism and has a fixed rate of activity (zero-order kinetics). Therefore, the metabolism of ethanol for any individual will be constant regardless of the initial blood level. The average rate of metabolism is 20 to 30 mg/dL/hr. There are wide individual variations secondary to induction of the liver's microenzyme system with chronic abuse, ethnic differences, and genetic predispositions.

The metabolism of ethanol affects many other metabolic pathways. Of prime concern is the inhibition of gluconeogenesis, which results in hypoglycemia, a common finding in intoxicated patients, especially those at the extremes of age. Hypoglycemia is further exacerbated by the depleted glycogen stores in the liver secondary to chronic malnutrition.

TABLE 16–1. Systemic Effects of Chronic Alcoholism

Nervous System	Cardiac Effects
Cerebellar degeneration	Cardiomyopathy
Brain cell degeneration	**Musculoskeletal System**
Peripheral neuropathy	
Seizures	Skeletal myopathies
Gastrointestinal Tract	**Hematologic System**
Esophagitis	Anemia
Gastritis	Thrombocytopenia
Esophageal varices	Impaired leukocyte function
Ulcer disease	Hemolytic syndromes
Impaired intestinal absorption	
Liver	**Metabolic Effects**
Fatty liver	Hypoglycemia
Alcoholic hepatitis	Hypokalemia
Cirrhosis	Hypomagnesemia
	Hypocalcemia
Pancreas	Hypophosphatemia
	Hyperuricemia
Pancreatitis	Hyperlipidemia

INITIAL APPROACH AND STABILIZATION

Priority Diagnoses

The initial approach to the intoxicated patient first addresses the status of the airway, breathing, circulation, and the cervical spine. Ethanol consumption is often associated with respiratory depression and a decreased gag reflex. Significant trauma and environmental exposure are frequently associated findings. *Therefore, the initial approach to the intoxicated patient with altered consciousness is based on the presumption that the patient has underlying significant trauma or medical illness.* Because active resistance to treatment may occur, physical intervention and restraint may be necessary.

Rapid Assessment/Early Intervention

1. Airway patency and protection are established. A nasopharyngeal airway is often helpful if the gag reflex is intact. Suctioning equipment is placed at the bedside. If the gag reflex is not intact, the patient can no longer adequately protect the airway and intubation may be necessary.
2. Adequate oxygenation and ventilation is supplied as necessary.
3. The cervical spine is evaluated and immobilized in anticipation of discovery of an injury. Immobilization is maintained and a cross-table lateral plain view of the neck is obtained in any uncooperative patient or those in whom there is a possibility of trauma. Nonradiologic clearance of the cervical spine is inappropriate in the intoxicated patient.
4. If not previously done, intravenous access is established. An isotonic crystalloid solution is infused at a rate appropriate to the need for volume replacement.
5. Naloxone, 2 mg, given intravenously may help to identify and reverse concomitant narcotic abuse in patients with decreased conscious. In patients with decreased consciousness, it may improve the depressed mental status secondary to ethanol ingestion. Naloxone is primarily indicated for respiratory depression. Caution should be used in administering naloxone because it may cause an otherwise controllable patient to become agitated and difficult to treat.
6. Thiamine, 100 mg, is administered intravenously. Thiamine stores are often diminished in alcoholic patients. Thiamine is an important coenzyme in glucose metabolism. If it is absent, the administration of glucose may precipitate Wernicke's encephalopathy. This encephalopathy is recognizable by the triad of ocular abnormalities (primarily horizontal nystagmus or a bilateral sixth nerve palsy, ataxia, and global confusion). It has a time-dependent reversibility, and a residual deficit can be found in up to 40% of patients. Thiamine is given to *all* patients with altered mental status who are suspected to be consuming a poor diet, regardless of whether they are alcoholic.

The thiamine is administered before glucose administration or, if glucose was given in the field, on arrival in the emergency department.

7. Initial serum blood levels are measured with glucose test strips. Dextrose, 25 to 50 g, is administered to treat hypoglycemia as necessary or if it is suspected. A 75- to 125-mg/dL increase in serum glucose per ampule can be anticipated. The serum glucose value is remeasured if dextrose is given.

8. An accurate body temperature is obtained. The intoxicated patient rarely cooperates to allow an accurate oral temperature to be recorded. An accurate temperature is valuable in determining the likelihood of hypothermia, which may be associated with infection, co-ingestion, or hypothermia, which is often associated with environmental exposure. Rectal or tympanic membrane measurements are more dependable.

9. The patient is undressed to allow for a full examination. This important step is often ignored, leading to missed injuries and illnesses.

10. Other responses are determined by the patient's clinical condition.

CLINICAL ASSESSMENT

Providing good medical care for an intoxicated, often belligerent, patient is difficult. Patients may place both themselves and the medical personnel at risk for injury. Patience, thoroughness, and a clear sense of purpose are essential in evaluating and treating an intoxicated patient.

History

The patient may not provide any history. Any information obtained from the patient is potentially unreliable. It is essential to listen to the patient's story, but the information must be corroborated by alternative sources. The patient's belongings are searched for phone numbers or addresses, and prior hospital records are requested. Additional information is obtained from family, friends, or bystanders. The emergency medical services squad may provide invaluable information about the situation as well. If available, the following information is sought:

1. *When* was the patient *last seen*? What is the patient's *usual mental status*? Acute changes in mental status are often due to intoxicants, hypoglycemia, head trauma, or a combination of the three. Each is explored if the history supports evidence of an abrupt alteration in content or level of consciousness.

2. *How much* and what *type of alcohol* has been *ingested* (gross approximation)? What are the patient's *usual drinking patterns*? Preferences? Volumes? Most patients are notoriously inaccurate in describing the volume of ethanol they ingest. The purpose of this questioning is to determine whether variations from the patient's usual drinking habits have occurred and to gain insight into the severity of the patient's alcoholism and the possibility of nonethanol intoxicants.

3. Is the patient a potential *polydrug abuser*? Although most alcoholics stay with ethanol, it often is a "chaser" in polydrug abusers.

4. Does the patient have *known complications* of chronic alcoholism? Table 16–1 provides a helpful list of potential sites of organ damage.

5. Has the patient had *withdrawal symptoms* from ethanol? If so, what type of symptoms have occurred (see "Special Considerations")?

6. Could *trauma* be a *causal* or *contributing* factor in the patient's condition?

7. What is the *past medical history*? Have there been any medical, surgical, or psychiatric illnesses? Have there been recent hospitalizations, particularly for detoxification? What efforts have been attempted to treat alcoholism? What medications (e.g., disulfiram [Antabuse]) does the patient take? Are there known allergies?

8. The potential for alcohol addiction may be evaluated by asking the patient the CAGE questions (C = Do you feel the need to *cut* down?, A = Are you *annoyed* by criticism of your use of alcohol?, G = Do you have *guilty* feelings about things done while drinking?, E = Do you need an *"eye* opener" in the morning to get going?). A "yes" to any question suggests a significant alcohol problem.

Physical Examination

A careful physical examination is particularly important in the intoxicated patient, because the history is often inaccurate. The intoxicated state can mask a variety of findings, particularly related to pain awareness. Serial examinations are necessary to ensure the patient "sobers up" and to discover new unmasked findings. Special attention is paid to findings that support the common complications of alcohol intoxication, including head trauma, cervical spine trauma, trauma to the extremities, aspiration pneumonia, pancreatitis, gastrointestinal bleeding, hypoglycemia, and alterations in thermal regulation. Chapters 31,

Altered Mental Status, and 15, The Poisoned Patient, offer additional information.

General Appearance. The general appearance of the patient is noted, including cautious sampling of the breath odor for ethanol or fruity ketosis. The presence of "alcohol on the breath" is noteworthy, but it does not correlate with blood levels of alcohol, nor does it explain an altered mental status. Signs of chronic alcoholism are sought, including muscle wasting, spider angiomas, palmar erythema, and jaundice (see Table 16–1). Evidence of medical illness such as pallor, abdominal tenderness, or abnormal breath sounds is sought. A general inspection for evidence of trauma is also performed at this time, noting lacerations, bruises, or deformities. Evidence of trauma is sought by examining the patient and the immediate surroundings. The patient found at the bottom of a flight of stairs or down on the sidewalk must be treated as if trauma was incurred even if there is no external evidence of injury on physical examination.

Vital Signs. Vital signs may be "unobtainable," owing to poor hygiene, multiple layers of thick dirty clothes, or belligerence. These are not adequate reasons for avoiding these essential measurements. To the degree possible, vital signs (including temperature) are obtained on all patients, especially intoxicated patients. Blood pressure measurements are taken supine and positional in a search for dehydration or blood loss. Accurate temperature measurements may reveal (1) hypothermia caused by exposure and (2) underlying disease or fever caused by ingestants or infection. Increased respiratory rate may be consistent with volume depletion, sepsis, or acidosis.

Head. The skull and facial bones are inspected and palpated for signs of trauma.

Eyes, Ears, Nose, and Throat. The tympanic membranes are visualized and pupillary and funduscopic examinations are performed. Evidence of horizontal nystagmus and bilateral sixth nerve palsy is sought when examining the eyes as evidence of Wernicke's syndrome. The oral cavity and nose are examined for signs of trauma, and the neck is palpated for the position of the trachea. The patient is evaluated for neck stiffness (after radiographic clearance). Clinical clearance of C-spine injury is impossible with a patient with altered mental status. Any patient with neck pain or mechanism of injury that could result in neck injury should have a radiologic assessment.

Thorax. The thorax is inspected for evidence of trauma and palpated anteriorly and posteriorly for crepitus or deformity. The lungs and heart are auscultated with attention to the presence of rales or consolidation. These may represent aspiration or underlying infection.

Abdomen. An enlarged abdominal girth may mask or be caused by ascites. Liver and spleen are specifically examined for both size and tenderness. A palpable spleen tip connotes splenomegaly and potential portal hypertension.

Rectum. The rectum is examined for tone, and stool testing is done for gross or occult blood.

Extremities. The extremities are inspected and palpated for bony crepitus, deformity, and pulses.

Neurologic Examination. The level and content of consciousness are evaluated, as are the response to stimulation and the presence of spontaneous movements. An active search for focal neurologic deficiencies is essential. Eye movements and pupillary findings are assessed. Cranial nerves are evaluated if the patient is cooperative. Deep tendon reflexes are tested, including plantar responses, and cerebellar function with gait testing is observed if the patient is able and allowed to walk.

CLINICAL REASONING

Acute intoxication can be associated with many serious conditions. The first decision priorities center around the following questions.

Does the Patient have an Altered Mental Status? If so, What are the Possible Causes Other than Ethanol?

This is one of the most important questions to ask in this situation. The major sources of altered mental status associated with alcoholism are listed in Table 16–2. (See also Chapter 31, Altered Mental Status.)

Rapidly reversible conditions are considered and treated first in all intoxicated patients. These include hypoxia, hypotension, hypoglycemia, hypothermia, and substance abuse. If acute trauma has occurred, epidural hematoma, subarachnoid hemorrhage, cerebral contusion or concussion, or subdural hematoma is considered. Subdural hematoma is seen in alcoholics secondary to both repeated trauma and cerebral atrophy leading to spontaneous rupture of the communicating veins. Seizure disorders are commonly associated with alcoholism, and many patients present in a postictal state. Phenytoin toxicity, with signs of ataxia and dysarthria, often mimics acute intoxication but does not usually produce coma. Other considerations include other toxic alcohol ingestions, especially in suicidal patients

TABLE 16–2. Differential Diagnosis of Impaired Level of Consciousness in the Alcohol-Intoxicated Patient

Metabolic

Hypoglycemia, diabetic ketoacidosis, uremia, hyponatremia, hypercalcemia, hepatic encephalopathy

Respiratory

Hypoxia

Environmental

Hypothermia

Toxicologic

Narcotics, benzodiazepines, sedative-hypnotics, ethanol, methanol, ethylene glycol, isopropyl alcohol, carbon monoxide

Infectious

Meningitis/encephalitis, sepsis

Trauma

Hypotension, epidural hematoma, subarachnoid hemorrhage, concussion, or contusion

Central Nervous System Disorders

Cerebrovascular accident, tumor, seizure or postictal state, subdural hematoma

and chronic alcoholics. The degree of assessment needed to find these causes may vary from nothing beyond data gathering to the full use of laboratory studies and radiologic imaging. The methods of assessment used depend on the patient's symptoms and their course during treatment. How far to go with an individual patient is based on experience in emergency medical practice. When in doubt, the physician should err on the side of added assessment.

What Role does Ethanol Play in the Patient's Presentation?

Although the blood ethanol level does not need to be measured in all cases of alcohol intoxication, it is necessary in patients with depressed mental status, known polydrug ingestion, and in those who are not improving in the emergency department (see "Diagnostic Adjuncts"). The possibility that other alcohols (methanol, ethylene glycol, and isopropyl alcohol) are contributing to and complicating the patient's condition must be considered (see "Special Considerations"). It is rare for polyalcohol ingestion to occur, but desperate circumstances can prompt this admixture.

Are Any Potential Complications of Acute or Chronic Alcoholism Present?

The patient cannot be considered a chronic alcohol abuser without searching for the pathophysiologic effects of the abuse. Table 16–1 serves as a guide for examination and also offers a checklist of possible problems that could affect a satisfactory outcome. The most common disorders associated with chronic alcohol abuse in patients seen in the emergency department are gastrointestinal hemorrhage, seizures, hepatic dysfunction, pancreatitis, anemia, thrombocytopenia, and hypokalemia. Evidence of each of these problems is actively sought in the alcohol-intoxicated patient.

DIAGNOSTIC ADJUNCTS

Because the history and the physical findings are often confusing or nondiagnostic, the intoxicated patient with altered mental status usually requires laboratory and radiologic evaluation.

Laboratory Studies

The laboratory workup of a patient with an altered mental status and alcohol on the breath has essential and optional components:

Essential Tests

1. Blood ethanol level (some controversy)
2. Serum electrolytes (including anion-gap determination)
3. Blood urea nitrogen/creatinine
4. Blood glucose
5. Arterial blood gases
6. Complete blood cell count
7. Urinalysis

Optional Tests

1. Toxicology screen
2. Liver function test
3. Amylase/lipase concentration
4. Hemostatic studies
5. Serum osmolality

Blood Ethanol Level. Intoxicated patients without significant depression of level of consciousness presenting for care of an isolated injury or problem do not need a measured ethanol level. This test has specific value in evaluating the remainder of intoxicated patients. The value has a rough correlate with the expected level of consciousness (Table 16–3). If the level does not correlate (e.g., when it is zero), an intensive search to explain the patient's condition is necessary. A blood ethanol level less than 250 mg/dL in a chronic alcohol consumer does not adequately explain a significantly depressed mental status (e.g., responsive to deep pain only). Interestingly, blood ethanol levels correlate poorly with the expected degree of intoxication because of the broad response of the population to acute and chronic ethanol use. Measurements of ethanol levels are available rapidly but have the disadvantage of measuring the serum ethanol concentration only. Methanol, ethylene glycol, and isopropyl alcohol levels have to be specifically requested.

Serum Electrolytes. Electrolyte disturbances are common in patients suffering from complications of chronic alcohol abuse. Hyponatremia may be responsible for significant alterations in mental status. An increased anion-gap metabolic acidosis is also a common finding. A common cause of an anion-gap metabolic acidosis in an alcoholic patient is alcoholic ketoacidosis. This is a result of chronic ethanol abuse and poor nutritional habits associated with protracted vomiting. Other causes of anion-gap metabolic acidosis are listed in Table 16–4 using the mnemonic MUD PILES. Calculation of the anion gap in an intoxicated patient can be very useful (see Acid-Base Disorders, Chapter 21).

Blood Urea Nitrogen/Creatinine Concentrations. These tests are useful in evaluating hydration and renal status. Renal failure is another cause of altered mental status. Increases in blood urea nitrogen may occur with blood loss or dehydration. Increases in creatinine secondary to renal failure may occur with toxins such as ethylene glycol.

TABLE 16–3. Serum Ethanol Levels and Corresponding Clinical Findings

0–100 mg/dL
    Altered judgment
    Decreased inhibitions
    Decreased coordination
100 mg/dL
    Legal limit for driving in most states
100–200 mg/dL
    Slurred speech
    Ataxia
    Poor balance
200–300 mg/dL
    Lethargy
    Altered equilibrium
300–400 mg/dL
    Coma, respiratory depression

Note: Chronic ethanol consumption produces tolerance, which results in much higher ethanol levels producing the same clinical findings.

Common Drinks	Absolute Ethanol Content
1 oz 100 proof whiskey	15 mL
One 6-oz glass wine (12% ethanol)	22 mL
One 12-oz beer (5% ethanol)	18 mL

For a 70-kg person, 15 mL of absolute ethanol will increase the blood alcohol level 25 mg/dL.

TABLE 16–4. Anion-Gap Metabolic Acidosis

M-Methanol
U-Uremia
D-Diabetic ketoacidosis
P-Paraldehyde
I-Isoniazid
L-Lactic acidosis
E-Ethylene glycol
S-Salicylates

Blood Glucose Concentration. Frequently, hypoglycemia, although initially assessed by reagent strip determination or by empirical treatment with dextrose, is documented or ruled out more definitively by the laboratory determination. Both hyperglycemia as well as hypoglycemia can be responsible for altered mental status as well as focal neurologic deficits.

Arterial Blood Gases. Blood gas determinations are extremely helpful in evaluating adequacy of oxygenation (aspiration pneumonia), ventilation (depressed mental status), and acid-base status (ingestion of toxic alcohols).

Complete Blood Cell Count. A complete blood cell count including a platelet estimate is useful if there are signs of bleeding or infection. Bone marrow suppression by chronic ethanol abuse can lead to anemia and thrombocytopenia as well.

Urinalysis. Urinalysis may provide evidence of dehydration, infection, toxin-related crystals, myoglobin, or bleeding.

Serum Amylase Concentration. Amylase determination is most useful in patients complaining of abdominal pain who may have acute pancreatitis from alcohol abuse. Lipase, although less sensitive, is more specific for pancreatitis than amylase.

Liver Function Tests. Patients who have evidence of hepatic dysfunction on physical examination are screened for adequacy of hepatic function. This is a late finding of hepatic injury.

Hemostatic Studies. Patients with hepatic dysfunction will have a prolonged prothrombin time. This test result appears early in the course of hepatic dysfunction and can be used as a screening test.

Toxicology Studies. Determinations of specific drug levels are ordered as indicated by the history and results of the physical examination. A general screening test is of very limited utility. Rarely does this test offer any additional guidance in the care of the intoxicated patient.

Serum Osmolality. The serum osmolality is measured by assessing the freezing point depression of a liquid. The measured value (normal = 285 – 295 mOsm/kg) is most useful when it is compared with the calculated value.

$$\text{Calculated osmolality} = 2\,[\text{Na}^+ \text{ level}] + \frac{\text{glucose}}{18} + \frac{\text{BUN}}{3} + \frac{\text{ethanol}}{4}$$

If the difference between the measured and calculated values is greater than 10 mOsm/kg, unmeasured osmotically active molecules are present in the specimen. The alcohols—ethanol, methanol, isopropanol, and ethylene glycol—are the most commonly encountered osmotically active agents.

Radiologic Imaging

Radiologic evaluation is often difficult, because of the poor cooperation of the patient. Initial films may be performed in the emergency department. Only the cooperative and stable patient is allowed to leave the emergency department for more complete imaging studies. Important radiologic studies to be considered include studies of the cervical spine, chest, pelvic area, and extremities and computed tomography of the brain.

1. *Cervical spine* evaluation is frequently necessary in an intoxicated patient. If there is any history of head trauma or evidence of head trauma on examination, the neck is immobilized and a portable, lateral neck film is obtained in the emergency department. There is an 80% sensitivity with this study. A complete cervical spine series (minimum of three views) is obtained when the patient's condition permits it. This must be correlated with clinical findings. If the patient has a normal C-spine series and still complains of pain, a CT or MRI may be necessary to rule out serious injury.
2. A *chest radiograph* may reveal an occult pneumonia or evidence of trauma. If there is any evidence of chest trauma, fever, or abnormal findings on lung examination, a chest radiograph is obtained.
3. *Computed tomography of the head* should be performed when there is evidence of head trauma or skull fracture, major mechanisms of injury and/or altered mental status, focal findings on neurologic examination, new-onset or persistent seizures, inappropriate level of responsiveness when the alcohol level is known, or if there is no improvement in, or worsening of, the neurologic findings with time.

Electrocardiogram

A 12-lead electrocardiogram is useful for detecting concomitant cardiac disease. In alcoholic patients this can range from the ischemic heart disease problems to dysrhythmogenic alcoholic cardiomyopathy.

PRINCIPLES OF MANAGEMENT

The goals of management are to protect patients from hurting themselves or others, to treat potentially life-threatening conditions without delay, to reexamine and monitor to verify findings caused by ethanol, to discover unmasked findings as patients' ethanol levels decrease, and to ensure appropriate disposition and follow-up. These goals are realized through several management principles.

Observation and Frequent Measurements of Vital Signs and Neurologic Assessment

Close observation with frequent neurologic assessment of the intoxicated patient is essential. Vital signs and mental status checks are initially performed every half hour, and a more complete assessment is made every hour until the patient becomes easily arousable. Examinations can then be made every 2 hours to follow the improvement in neurologic function. The mental status examination is the primary tool in the serial assessment of the intoxicated patient, not the absolute blood ethanol level.

Aggressive Evaluation of Nonimproving or Deteriorating Mental Status

At any point during the observation, a deterioration of neurologic function should prompt an intensive search for the cause. If the patient has shown progressive improvement, a thorough examination is performed. New symptoms or complaints may be uncovered as the patient becomes more aware and further studies are often needed at this point. The sober patient can more reliably report symptoms and is essentially considered a "new" patient requiring a complete assessment.

Continued Observation

This is done until the patient is able to function and care for himself.

Intravenous Hydration and Nutrition

Maintenance fluids with multivitamins will allow maintenance of venous access and supply some nutrition for these chronically malnourished patients. Dextrose is included in the intravenous fluids given. A repeat serum glucose determination may be obtained if the patient's condition does not improve during the observation period. Nevertheless, neither intravenous fluids, multivitamins, nor dextrose hastens the metabolism of ethanol.

Restraint by Physical or Chemical Means When Needed (to Protect the Patient or Others)

At times, restraints are needed to protect the patient and the staff. Physical restraints are most commonly used when the patient cannot be controlled without adding new medications. These may complicate the assessment of a patient whose consciousness is already depressed. Adequate personnel, usually at least four people, are necessary to apply the leather restraints to an agitated patient. Care is taken to check any patient in physical restraints frequently to ensure distal circulation of the extremities and proper placement of the restraints. As the patient becomes more cooperative, restraints can be removed first from two opposite extremities (e.g., left arm and right leg). When the patient is fully cooperative, they are completely removed. Careful documentation of the reason for the restraints is recorded on the chart. There have been recorded deaths associated with excessive force during the restraining process; therefore, careful serial examinations must be done by the physician while the patient remains restrained. Other complications of physical restraints include rhabdomyolysis and hyperthermia. Family members or friends, if present, are also informed about the reason for the restraints.

The chemical restraint of choice in the agitated intoxicated patient is one of the benzodiazepines. Dosages can be easily titrated to the individual patient needs. Lorazepam can be given intramuscularly or intravenously starting with 0.5- to 2-mg increments. Haloperidol has been used in the past as well. Although haloperidol causes minimal sedation with excellent behavior control, it may decrease the seizure threshold, placing the chronic alcoholic at increased risk for seizures. Chemical restraints are often very effective used in conjunction with physical restraints to protect the severely agitated patient.

Monitoring of Physical/Chemical Dependency

Withdrawal from ethanol poses a life threat to the patient. Signs of withdrawal include tachycardia, hypertension, agitation, and diaphoresis. Symptoms include feelings of anxiety, tactile hallucinations, and agitation.

UNCERTAIN DIAGNOSIS

Alcohol intoxication can mask other serious conditions, and serious pathologic processes may masquerade as acute alcohol intoxication. Clinical judgment and experience have a major role in decisions about the extent of workup directed to the acutely intoxicated patient. If there is any doubt about the role of alcohol in the patient's presentation, the earlier the alcohol (ethanol) level is tested, the better. Even with a level in the range consistent with the patient's clinical status, a through assessment for other potentially life-threatening causes is necessary.

SPECIAL CONSIDERATIONS
Pediatric Patients

Whether the patient is a toddler who drank mouthwash (up to 20% ethanol, 40 proof) or a child who experimented in the liquor cabinet, hypoglycemia is much more common in this age group, since children have lower glycogen reserves than adults. In one study of intoxicated pediatric patients, hypoglycemia was found in 24%. Fluids with 5% dextrose are given, after initial bolus therapy with 25% dextrose, and the serum glucose level is monitored frequently.

Because these patients have not been previously exposed to ethanol, much smaller amounts and lower serum levels produce significant and even fatal effects. Respiratory depression is common, and support of respiratory function is often needed until ethanol is metabolized. "Experimenting" adolescents are considered in this high-risk group as well.

Legal Requests for Ethanol Levels

Serum ethanol determinations may be requested by law enforcement agencies or by employers for nonmedical purposes. Care is necessary to guarantee that patients' rights are not violated. Individual emergency departments usually have specific protocols to direct this type of evaluation. Although currently used laboratory techniques for ethanol determination do not measure concentrations of other alcohols, skin preparation is done with nonalcoholic preparations to avoid any question about contamination of specimens that are drawn for legal or employment purposes.

Patients Who have Ingested Other Alcohols: Methanol, Ethylene Glycol, Isopropanol

Although methanol and ethylene glycol differ in toxicity, there are many chemical similarities between them, and the treatment of patients intoxicated with either is essentially identical. Neither agent is itself dangerous, although ethylene glycol and, to a lesser extent, methanol can cause ethanol-like intoxication. Serious toxicity is caused by the metabolites formed after metabolism by alcohol dehydrogenase. These by-products include various organic acids that increase the anion gap; therefore, methanol and ethylene glycol intoxications are always considered in the differential diagnosis of increased anion-gap metabolic acidosis. Because laboratory determinations of methanol and ethylene glycol serum levels are not readily available, indirect measures such as the anion and osmolal gaps are useful. Before they are metabolized, these agents do not increase the anion gap or cause acidosis, but they do cause an increased osmolal gap. After metabolism is complete, the opposite is true. Methanol metabolites (e.g., formic acid) can cause sometimes irreversible visual impairment, complete blindness, and central nervous system damage. Ethylene glycol by-products can cause coma, cardiopulmonary complications, and renal failure. Oxalic acid production from ethylene glycol leads to formation of calcium oxalate crystals in the urine.

Treatment of both methanol and ethylene glycol intoxication includes attempts to block metabolism of the parent compounds to their toxic by-products, increasing the rate of metabolism of toxic metabolites, and removing both the parent compound and its metabolite using hemodialysis. Alcohol dehydrogenase has a much higher affinity for ethanol than for methanol or ethylene glycol; thus, metabolism of these agents can be prevented by administration of ethanol either intravenously or orally. Another newly approved alcohol dehydrogenase blocker is fomepizole (4-methyl pyrazole). Fomepizole (approved by the U.S. Food and Drug Administration in 1998 for the treatment of ethylene glycol) competitively inhibits alcohol dehydrogenase more effectively and reliably than ethanol. Ethanol and fomepizole therapy does not alter the toxicity of previously formed metabolites. Once alcohol dehydrogenase is blocked, there is no other effective route of elimination of the parent compound. As a result, hemodialysis is almost always required for patients with serious intoxications. In addition, recent studies have suggested the use of folic acid or leucovorin (given parenterally) at the first sign of methanol intoxication enhances the elimination of the toxic metabolite formate. Additional therapy for ethylene glycol should include thiamine and pyridoxine. Thiamine may shunt glycolic acid to α-hydroxy-β-ketoadipic acid, decreasing the production of the toxin oxalic acid. Pyridoxine (in the presence of magnesium) may shunt the metabolism from the toxic metabolite glycolic acid to glycine, which is harmless.

Isopropanol, unlike the other alcohols, is metabolized to acetone. Serum acetone levels in such patients will be very high, but there is little or no acidosis. Isopropanol is a strong gastric irritant, and gastritis with bleeding often develops. Otherwise, the presentation of patients with isopropanol intoxication is similar to that of persons with ethanol intoxication, but the condition resolves much more slowly. By doubling the serum isopropanol level, the emergency physician can approximate the equivalent serum ethanol level.

Patients with Ethanol Withdrawal

Alcoholic patients may present to the emergency department with acute intoxication or with onset of symptoms caused by the sudden reduction or cessation of ethanol intake. Ethanol withdrawal is traditionally divided into four stages:

> *Stage 1: Minor withdrawal:* insomnia, irritability, tremor, anorexia, nausea, tachycardia, hypertension, and hyperthermia (mild)
> *Stage 2: Hallucinosis:* visual hallucinations (auditory, tactile, and olfactory hallucinations are less common)
> *Stage 3: Seizures:* generalized, often multiple
> *Stage 4: Major withdrawal:* global confusion, sympathetic hyperactivity with agitation and diaphoresis

Ethanol withdrawal is best viewed as a continuum of symptoms rather than as a series of distinct stages. The vital signs often give an early clue about impending minor withdrawal syndromes. Tachycardia and mild hypertension are almost always present as early findings and, when not due to other medical or traumatic conditions, are predictors of the development of ethanol withdrawal. The onset of major withdrawal symptoms is signified by disorientation to person, place, and time. Some degree of confusion occurs in 5% to 10% of ethanol withdrawal cases, but the profound global confusion traditionally described as delirium tremens occurs in only 1% to 2% of cases. Hallucinations and seizures may occur after minor or major withdrawal syndromes. They are superimposed on other symptoms, rather than being distinct stages of withdrawal.

The pathophysiology of ethanol withdrawal has been extensively studied. Although many factors are involved in the full expression of these syndromes, the effect of ethanol on the inhibitory neurotransmitter γ-aminobutyric acid (GABA) and the subsequent removal of this effect are believed to be the most important mechanisms. There are chloride-dependent receptor sites for GABA in the central nervous system (CNS), and alcohol has been shown to increase the flow of chloride into these receptor sites, producing depression of the CNS. With chronic ethanol use, this effect is reduced or eliminated, and there is a reduction in the influx of chloride, a decrease in the inhibitory effect of GABA, and a resultant sympathetic hyperactivity mediated by norepinephrine. Other contributing factors to the ethanol withdrawal syndromes are metabolic effects (hypomagnesemia, hypokalemia, zinc deficiency), prostaglandin deficiency, and endocrine effects (cortisol excess).

Management of the ethanol withdrawal syndromes is primarily based on preventing the progression of symptoms to the major withdrawal stage by supplying an alternative CNS depressant that can be gradually withdrawn. Additionally, patients may require treatment for tremor, hallucinations, seizures, hyperthermia, dehydration, and malnutrition.

The benzodiazepines are the drugs of choice as temporary replacements for the withdrawn ethanol. They have similar effects in the CNS. Although their primary clinical usefulness lies in their ability to reduce agitation and tremor, they also have significant anticonvulsant activity. Diazepam, lorazepam, or chlordiazepoxide, either orally or intravenously, provide good control and can be titrated to the desired effect.

In major withdrawal reactions, the sympathetic hyperactivity may be so great that the benzodiazepines are not sufficient to control the tremor, tachycardia, and hypertension that occur. β-Adrenergic blocking agents such as propranolol and α-adrenergic blocking agents such as clonidine have been used for further control of sympathetic hyperactivity.

Alcoholic hallucinosis often requires no specific intervention. However, in severe cases or when the patient is significantly upset by the hallucinations, treatment is indicated. Haloperidol, administered intramuscularly, may control hallucinations in ethanol withdrawal. Phenothiazines are effective but may potentiate seizure activity; therefore, benzodiazepines are probably a safer choice.

Alcohol withdrawal seizures may occur singly or in multiples (two to four) and do not usually require specific anticonvulsant therapy. Status epilepticus, a rare occurrence, is treated as outlined in Chapter 33, Seizures. If the patient has not had alcohol withdrawal seizures before, a full laboratory and radiologic evaluation to rule out other causes of seizures is indicated.

Associated hyperpyrexia, a temperature over 104°F (40°C), is aggressively treated with a cooling blanket or sponging with tepid water and administering acetaminophen. Aspirin is contraindicated, because of its inhibitory effect on platelet aggregation. Any anticoagulant effect is potentially harmful because the alcoholic patient is already at risk for hemorrhagic complications.

Marked dehydration, associated with electrolyte disturbances and malnutrition, is common in patients with major withdrawal syndromes. Isotonic crystalloid (typically 4 to 8 L) is used to correct fluid losses. Serum electrolyte levels are measured and corrected as indicated. *Hypokalemia* and *hypomagnesemia* are especially common. Depletion of glycogen stores secondary to chronic malnutrition makes *hypoglycemia* a concern. Bedside screening with glucose oxidase reagent strips or empirical treatment with dextrose is indicated. *Thiamine* is essential to prevent the development of Wernicke's encephalopathy, and its administration precedes or is concurrent with the use of dextrose. *Magnesium* and *multivitamin supplements* are also recommended.

The disposition of the patient with ethanol withdrawal will vary depending on the severity of the syndrome. Patients with major withdrawal symptoms and those with status epilepticus require management in an intensive care unit. Ethanol withdrawal patients frequently have significant medical conditions secondary to chronic ethanol abuse that will dictate the type of disposition needed. Common examples are gastrointestinal bleeding, hepatic failure, and cardiomyopathy. If there is no evidence of coexisting medical or traumatic illness and the patient has symptoms consistent with a minor withdrawal syndrome, outpatient management is appropriate, with follow-up scheduled in a detoxification program.

DISPOSITION AND FOLLOW-UP

Admission

Admission to the hospital for alcohol intoxication is usually prompted by concomitant disease processes or trauma. Intoxicated patients with pneumonia, hepatitis, pancreatitis, or trauma often warrant admission because patient reliability is poor, self-care inadequate, and follow-up practically nonexistent. Direct admission to a detoxification unit may be possible, but this requires thorough knowledge of the unit and its capabilities. In general, if medical problems are present, a medical admission is the safest course. Transfer to an appropriate detoxification unit can be made 1 or 2 days later once the patient's condition has stabilized.

Intensive Care Unit Admission

Intensive care unit admission is usually reserved for patients with severe overdose requiring intubation, major withdrawal symptoms, injuries resulting from major motor vehicle accidents, ingestions of methanol or ethylene glycol, or concomitant medical problems such as sepsis, hemorrhage, and myocardial infarction.

Referral

Alcohol abuse needs to be addressed openly and nonjudgmentally by the examining physician. Referral for counseling through a detoxification program or a primary physician is an extremely important and often ignored part of discharge planning. CAGE questions must be evaluated in an attempt to determine alcohol dependency/addiction.

Discharge

Most acutely intoxicated patients can be safely discharged after appropriate observation in the emergency department. If supportive family or friends are willing and capable of observing the patient at home, earlier discharge from the emergency department may be possible. If no support system is available, the patient is observed in the emergency department until he (or she) is able to care for himself (or herself). Patients must be capable of eating and walking with a steady gait, and oriented to their surroundings before discharge is considered. This may require extended observation.

FINAL POINTS

- It is inappropriate to record only that a patient was "drunk" or "intoxicated." Recording "alcohol on the breath" and describing the behavior that occurred during the emergency department visit is reasonable. The documentation is descriptive and not judgmental.
- Other information includes history of the event, known complications of ethanol abuse, and pertinent past medical history.
- Physical examination findings, including stigmata of chronic abuse, are reported.

- If restraints were used, the indications for the restraints (e.g., protecting the patient or the staff) need to be recorded.
- Serial observation (especially mental status) is the key to successful management of these patients, and a record of the results of these examinations must be maintained.
- Laboratory findings, including the ethanol level, are reported.

- Of utmost importance is the discharge examination. The now sober patient is essentially a new patient. The patient's mental status, response to his or her environment, ability to walk, and ability to care for himself or herself should be documented.
- Plans for disposition and referral must be clearly understood by the patient and supporting individuals.

CASE*Study*

The 43-year-old man with odor of ethanol found lying in a gutter was a frequent emergency department visitor. The rescue squad reported the patient was arousable with painful stimuli but then fell back asleep. Dried blood was noted over his right eyebrow.

The paramedics followed standing orders for similar cases that included airway inspection, cervical spine immobilization, administration of oxygen, and measurement of vital signs. The patient's vital signs, taken in the field, were blood pressure, 160/90 mm Hg; pulse, 96 beats per minute; and respirations, 18 breaths per minute. The patient was transported quickly to the emergency department. His injury potential was considered to be high.

In the emergency department the patient was somnolent and snoring. He swore profusely when aroused, spit occasionally, and then fell back to sleep. Lying on a backboard with a rigid cervical collar in place, he had an aroma of alcohol, rotten socks, and urine. Repeat vital signs taken in the emergency department were blood pressure, 140/80 mm Hg; pulse, 90 beats per minute; respirations, 16 breaths per minute; and temperature, 96.5°F (39.8°C) orally. An intravenous line was established, supplemental oxygen was continued by nasal cannula, and naloxone, 2 mg, thiamine, 100 mg, and 1 ampule of 50% dextrose were given. A cross-table lateral neck radiograph was read as negative. The cervical collar was left in place until a complete cervical spine series could be done. A repeated temperature taken rectally was 99°F (37.2°C). The patient was completely undressed and placed in a gown. On being asked his name, he replied "None of your business." When asked, "Have you ever been to the hospital before?" he replied, "Just leave me alone and get out of here!" The staff was not pleased at having the patient in the emergency department.

Initial examination revealed normal vital signs and some semi-oriented hostile responsiveness,

which is better than no responsiveness. Close immediate attention is mandatory for accurate assessment of such patients. Many of these patients are not easy to manage in a caring manner. Just as in the prehospital setting, a clear sense of purpose and priorities is essential.

The patient fell into a light sleep. He was unable to give any history. Old medical records documented the existence of multiple previous visits for acute intoxication, no allergies, no medications, and a history of withdrawal seizures. On physical examination a 2-cm laceration was found over the right eyebrow, and equal breath sounds were present bilaterally with ecchymosis and crepitus of the right lower ribs in the midaxillary line. The patient was spontaneously swallowing and thought to be protecting his airway. The abdomen was soft; there was no guarding, and no grimace was noted on rebound. Bowel sounds were decreased. The spleen was not palpable, and the liver was palpated 2 cm below the right costal margin. Total liver span was 12 cm. No focal deficiencies were found on neurologic testing, including symmetrical reflexes and spontaneous movement of all four extremities. The results of rectal examination and stool hemoglobin testing were normal.

Initial examination of this patient did not reveal any immediate life-threatening conditions. He appeared to be intoxicated with no focal neurologic deficits and perhaps to have a broken rib on the right side and a laceration over his right eye.

It is dangerous to allow this first impression to produce a false sense of security. The apparent intoxicated state is a great masquerader. Many of the items listed in the differential diagnosis have been ruled out by the initial examination. Those remaining include drug ingestion other than ethanol, intracranial processes, and a seizure with a resultant postictal state. Phenytoin toxicity would be unlikely with this patient's depressed

Continued on following page

level of consciousness and lack of nystagmus. Laboratory assessment is necessary, and an expanded differential diagnosis needs to be developed. The patient is monitored with serial examinations.

The abdominal and neurologic examination results are most difficult to interpret because alcohol intoxication can hide significant pathology. Serial examinations, preferably by the same examiner, are essential for accurate evaluation of the intoxicated patient.

This patient's alcohol level was found to be 420 mg/dL; the sodium level was 136 mEq/L, with potassium, 4.0 mEq/L; chloride, 100 mEq/L; CO_2, 24 mEq/L; and glucose, 66 mg/dL. The urinalysis showed no evidence of blood.

The anion gap, Na − (Cl + CO_2), was 12 mEq/L, with a normal range of 8 to 16 mEq/L. There was no evidence of an anion-gap metabolic acidosis based on this calculation.

Does the alcohol level correspond to this patient's level of responsiveness (see Table 16–3)? It is important to note that chronic alcohol abusers become increasingly tolerant of the effects of alcohol. Although this patient is somnolent with an alcohol level of 420 mg/dL, an expected finding based on his previous history of ethanol consumption, a novice drinker may well be somnolent with an ethanol level in the 200- to 300-mg/dL range.

The patient was escorted to the radiology area. A complete cervical spine series was done that showed no abnormalities. A chest radiograph was performed because of the findings of crepitus and ecchymosis of the right chest wall. An isolated seventh rib fracture with no hemothorax or pneumothorax was noted. On his return from the radiology department to the emergency department, the laceration over his right eye was repaired. A repeat examination revealed no new findings, and there was a slight improvement in his willingness to cooperate and in his level of responsiveness.

A cross-table lateral cervical spine film will rule out significant fractures of the cervical spine in only 85% to 90% of cases. It is imperative that a complete cervical spine series be obtained when the patient's condition permits. The ability to complete other medical care (e.g., suturing) varies greatly with the patient's willingness to cooperate. Some areas, such as wounds, may be cleansed and covered.

The patient had normal vital signs, no evidence of respiratory compromise, no focal findings on neurologic examination, normal laboratory values, no acidosis, and an elevated serum ethanol level. Although pure ethanol intoxication was the most likely diagnosis, intracranial lesions are not yet ruled out and other ingestions could also be involved. Serial examinations made over a period of time should further refine this differential diagnosis. This patient was certainly intoxicated. If his blood alcohol level had been 30 mg/dL, the index of suspicion for a concomitant drug ingestion or a significant intracranial process would be raised. Computed tomography of the head would be needed, and more aggressive monitoring would be indicated. However, because the ethanol level was high and the patient had shown slight improvement on neurologic examination, and because the only other findings were a laceration above the eye and an isolated rib fracture, serial examinations were adequate to follow this patient as his alcohol level fell. Intracranial hemorrhage and drug ingestion were not entirely ruled out at this time, but they are less likely diagnoses than pure ethanol intoxication with minor trauma. Again, care must be taken to continue close monitoring and periodic reassessment. At a metabolic rate of 30 mg/dL/hr, this patient will need an estimated 14 hours to be alcohol free. Because he was a chronic abuser, he should be easily arousable and completely awake several hours before then.

The patient was awake and alert 8 hours after his arrival in the emergency department. He walked to the bathroom on his own and ate a full meal without difficulty. He stated that he was ready to go home. It appeared that the patient had returned to his normal level of functioning and could safely look after himself. Discharge was appropriate after counseling and referral for treatment of alcoholism. He may be unlikely to follow through, but good practice requires that he be provided with the opportunity to obtain help.

Intoxicated patients are commonly seen in the emergency department; they often have little insight into their own illness or injury and may be openly hostile and belligerent. A consistent approach to these patients is imperative to avoid overlooking a pathologic process. The following approach is suggested:

- The patient is completely undressed and fully examined.
- Injury to the cervical spine must be ruled out if trauma was possible.

- Reversible conditions are identified and treated, such as hypotension, hypothermia, hypoglycemia, hypoxia, and other substance abuse.
- Deterioration or lack of improvement on serial examination needs aggressive evaluation.
- Observation, serial examinations, and a complete discharge examination are performed.
- Appropriate referral for treatment of alcoholism is an important part of care.
- Consider early toxicologic consultation and administration of antidotes when appropriate.

Bibliography

TEXTS

Ellenhorn M, Darceloux D: Alcohols and glycols. In: Ellenhorn's Medical Toxicology: Diagnosis and Treatment of Human Poisoning, 2nd ed. Philadelphia, Lippincott Williams & Wilkins, 1997, pp 1127–1165.

Ford MD, Delaney KA, Ling LJ, Erickson T: Clinical toxicology. Philadelphia: WB Saunders, 2001.

Graham AW, Schultz TK, eds: Principles of Addiction Medicine, 2nd ed. Chevy Chase, Md: American Society for Addiction Medicine, 1998.

JOURNAL ARTICLES

Brent J, McMartin K, Phillips S, et al: Fomepizole for the treatment of ethylene glycol poisoning. Methylpyrazole for Toxic Alcohols Study Group. N Engl J Med 1999; 340:832–838.

Burns MJ, Graudins A, Aaron CK, et al: Treatment of methanol poisoning with intravenous 4-methylpyrazole. Ann Emerg Med 1997; 30:829–832.

Church AS, Witting MD: Laboratory testing in ethanol, methanol, ethylene glycol and isopropanol toxicities [review]. J Emerg Med 1997; 15:687–692.

Cydulka RK, Eversman G: The alcoholic patient: Recognition, assessment and management of urgent and life-threatening emergencies: I and II. Emerg Med Rep 1995; 16:149–170.

Davis DP, Bramwell KJ, Hamilton RS, Williams SR: Ethylene glycol poisoning: A case report of a record high level and a review [review]. J Emerg Med 1997; 15:653–667.

D'Onfrio G, Rathlev NK, Ulrich AS, et al: Lorazepam for the prevention of recurrent seizures related to alcohol. N Engl J Med 1999; 340:915–919.

Ewing JA: Detecting alcoholism: The CAGE questionnaire: A critical review. JAMA 1984; 252:1905–1907.

Fiellin D, Reid MC, O'Connor PG: Outpatient management of patients with alcohol problems. Ann Intern Med 2000; 133:815–827.

Garbutt JC, West SL, Carey TS, et al: Pharmacological treatment of alcohol dependence: A review of the evidence. JAMA 1999; 218:1318–1325.

Glaser DS: Utility of serum osmol gap in the diagnosis of methanol or ethylene glycol ingestion. Ann Emerg Med 1996; 27:343–346.

Jacobsen D, McMartin KE: Antidotes for methanol and ethylene glycol poisoning [review]. J Toxicol Clin Toxicol 1997; 35:127–143.

Rathlev NK, Ulrich A, Fish SS, D'Onofrio G: Clinical characteristics as predictors of recurrent alcohol-related seizures. Acad Emerg Med 2000; 7:886–891.

Shannon M: Toxicology Reviews: Fomepizole—a new antidote. Pediatr Emerg Care 1998; 14:170–172.

Sturmann K, Ryan MT: Alcohol-related emergencies: A new look at an old problem. Emerg Med Pract 2001; 3:1–24.

Sullivan-Mee M, Solis K: Methanol-induced vision loss. J Am Optom Assoc 1998; 69:57–65.

Swift RM: Drug therapy for alcohol dependence. N Engl J Med 1999; 340:1482–1490.

Wiese JG, Shlipak MG, Browner WG: The alcohol hangover. Ann Intern Med 2000; 132:897–902.

CHAPTER 17

Heat Illness

JOHN A. GUISTO

CASE *Study*

A 37-year-old male construction worker complained of nausea and dizziness, then fainted. The patient was working on the roof of a house in the afternoon of a humid August day.

INTRODUCTION

References to heat illness date as far back as 24 BC, when an entire Roman army succumbed to an illness that "attacked the head, and caused it to become parched," killing most of those affected. Exposure to excessive heat results in an average of 240 deaths per year in the United States alone, even during years with no "heat wave." In years when a heat wave has occurred, deaths have reached into the thousands. In Chicago, during the heat wave of July 1995, at least 700 deaths were attributed to heat-related illness. Populations at risk include the very young, and elderly and debilitated persons, as well as young and otherwise healthy individuals who exercise strenuously in adverse conditions. Heat illness is the second leading cause of death in athletes (head and spine injuries are number one). One percent of marathon runners suffer heat illness.

Physiology

Humans are homeotherms and attempt to maintain a core temperature of about 98.6°F (37°C) regardless of environmental conditions. Heat is gained from the environment and internal production. It is offset by heat loss through four main mechanisms: radiation, convection, conduction, and evaporation. The environmental heat load is influenced by the ambient temperature, relative humidity, and degree of exposure to sunlight. For example, direct sunlight can result in a heat gain of 150 kcal/hr. Internal heat production from basal metabolism generates about 70 kcal/hr. A 70-kg man would experience a 1°C rise in temperature per hour if there were no mechanism to dissipate this heat. Exercise can produce tremendous amounts of heat, even exceeding 1000 kcal/hr. Without heat dissipation, the temperature of a vigorously exercising man would increase 5°C to 15°C/hr.

The body accomplishes heat dissipation with behavioral and physiologic changes aimed at alteration of one or more of the heat loss mechanisms:

1. *Radiation.* The physical transfer of heat between the body and the surrounding environment by electromagnetic waves is called radiation. This mechanism accounts for approximately 65% of heat transfer under normal climate conditions. To facilitate this mechanism, peripheral blood flow can increase by a factor of 20 in response to heat stress. Clothing alteration may also produce a significant effect on heat loss or gain but may interfere with evaporation as a cooling method.
2. *Convection.* The energy transfer between a surface and a gas or liquid is called convection. This is affected by the temperature gradient, motion at the interface, and the ability of the involved substances to accept and store heat energy. Wind currents that disturb the insulating layer of warmth that surrounds the body can be responsible for 12% to 15% of heat loss. This mechanism can be altered by vasomotor response, as well as behavioral responses such as changing clothing and moving in or out of a particular environment.
3. *Conduction.* Direct transfer of heat energy between two surfaces is conduction, and it accounts for a small proportion of heat loss under normal circumstances. It can also be affected by vasomotor changes. Behaviors such as immersion in cool water can enhance heat loss through this mechanism by a factor of 32, as compared with air. Interposition of insulation changes this mechanism significantly.
4. *Evaporation.* This is the most important mode of cooling under extreme heat stress, although under temperate conditions evaporation accounts for only 25% of heat loss. Just under 600 kcal of heat energy is lost for every liter of sweat that evaporates from the body. A conditioned athlete can produce up to 3 L of sweat

per hour. Relative humidity of greater than 85% causes evaporation to be ineffective, and clothing use may interfere with this process.

Heat illness is not a single entity but a *spectrum* of physiologic disorders that occur as the body attempts to maintain a normal temperature in the presence of heat stress. These disorders range from usually self-limited heat cramps to life-threatening heatstroke.

INITIAL APPROACH AND STABILIZATION

Priority Diagnoses

Heatstroke symptoms are the first consideration in suspected heat illness. Patients with serious disturbances in heat regulation can have signs and symptoms of central nervous system pathology: headache, syncope or near-syncope, disorientation, or coma.

Rapid Assessment

1. What is the exact nature of the problem for which the patient summoned help?
2. What was the ambient temperature and relative humidity in the immediate environment?
3. What level of physical activity was the patient involved in?
4. How much liquid and what type of liquid was consumed immediately before and during this episode?
5. Is there any airway, breathing, or circulatory compromise? What are the vital signs?
6. What is the patient's skin color and temperature? Temperature is usually not determined until initial evaluation and stabilization have been completed; however, when patients are known to have developed problems while in hot environments or during vigorous exercise, or when the patient's skin feels very warm, temperature needs to be measured early. Only a core or rectal temperature will be accurate in these circumstances. Many standard hospital thermometers only register up to 107.6°F (42°C). It may be necessary to use a thermometer capable of registering a higher temperature.
7. Is there evidence of sweating? Lack of sweating in heat illness suggests impairment of heat-regulating mechanisms, which may lead to, or be seen in, heatstroke.

Early Intervention

1. Cardiopulmonary evaluation is followed by stabilization as needed (the ABCs).

2. If heat illness is suspected, cooling measures are quickly initiated. A markedly elevated temperature requires immediate reduction to minimize the ill effects of hyperthermia. These include moving the patient to the coolest environment available, removing all excess clothing, moistening the skin with water (i.e., cool moist or wet sheets), and fanning the patient to expedite evaporative heat loss. In severe cases, a cooling blanket or placement of ice packs in the groin and axillae can be helpful. More aggressive cooling measures, such as cold water immersion or body compartment lavage, are seldom needed and are generally impractical or invasive.
3. Fluids are replaced in alert patients by giving them cold liquids by mouth; in those with a depressed level of consciousness an intravenous line is used to administer an isotonic crystalloid at room temperature. Infusion of fluid should be based on the patient's response. Urine output and signs of fluid overload (e.g., pulmonary edema, new S_3 sounds, or distended neck veins) are monitored.

CLINICAL ASSESSMENT

The history and supporting physical findings form the basis for the diagnosis of heat illness.

History

1. What are the *symptoms* and over what *time frame* did they develop? Alert patients who are suspected of having heat illness usually come to the emergency department with symptoms of muscular cramping, weakness, nausea, vomiting, headache, or syncope.
2. What was the *ambient temperature* and *relative humidity* in the environment at the time? Vigorous activity in a hot environment is the most common predisposing situation, but very young, elderly, or debilitated patients can suffer adverse effects from heat with no activity at all, since they may have inadequate means for dissipating body heat.
3. What *types of fluids* have been *ingested* and *how much* has been ingested? Replacement of fluid losses with hypotonic solutions such as water can lead to heat cramps or, if excessive, to serious reductions in the serum sodium concentration. Curiously, conditioned athletes are more prone to develop these problems because of their ability to sweat larger volumes.
4. What *risk factors for the development of heat illness* are present (Table 17–1)?

TABLE 17–1. Risk Factors for Development of Heat Illness

External Heat Load

Ambient temperature
Humidity
Environmental situation (e.g., full sun exposure)

Internal Heat Load

Work or exercise

Preexisting Illness

Cardiovascular compromise
   Cardiac disease
   Dehydration/hypovolemia
Spinal cord injury associated with impaired sweating
Impaired mentation
Skin or sweat follicle abnormality
   Burns
   Cystic fibrosis
   Ectodermal dysplasia (congenital absence of sweat glands)
   Scleroderma
Increased motor activity
   Parkinsonism
   Pheochromocytoma
   Hyperthyroidism
Obesity

Drugs

Drugs that inhibit sweating
   Anticholinergics, antihistamines, phenothiazines, cyclic
     antidepressants
Drugs that increase metabolic activity
   Amphetamines, phencyclidine, LSD, cocaine
Diuretics (due to potential for dehydration)
Alcohol

Miscellaneous

Previous history of heat stroke
Lack of acclimatization
Fatigue
Lack of sleep
Infection
Constrictive clothing
Extremes of age

---

5. What *baseline medical problems* are present that may influence current care or suggest causes other than heat illness for the patient's disorder?
   a. *All debilitated patients* are at increased risk for heat illness because of inability to dissipate endogenous heat loads. Patients who also have abnormal mental status may not be able to communicate the feeling of thirst and have an increased risk of heat illness.
   b. Patients with *previous episodes* of *serious heat illness* are prone to develop recurrences. There is evidence that heat stress on the day before the development of symptoms may increase susceptibility to heat illness.
   c. Patients taking *diuretics* (baseline fluid depletion) and *phenothiazines* or *tricyclic antidepressants* (anticholinergic sweat inhibition) are at increased risk of heat illness.
   d. Patients with a history of *drug abuse* (e.g., cocaine, amphetamines, or alcohol) may develop hyperthermia due to these drugs.

In patients who have a depressed level of consciousness, an accurate history is difficult, if not impossible, to obtain. Family, friends, and paramedics are usually able to supply a good deal of information about the events that led to the patient's present condition and the past medical history.

Physical Examination

Analysis of vital signs and physical findings is necessary to confirm the suspicion of heat illness and assess its impact on the patient.

Vital Signs

Blood Pressure. Changes in blood pressure range from orthostatic changes that respond promptly to fluid therapy to frank hypotension, which is caused by pump failure (cardiac microinfarcts and petechial hemorrhages), volume depletion, or peripheral vasodilation.

Respiratory Rate. Respirations are frequently increased as an accessory mechanism for dissipating heat, and musculoskeletal cramps can result from hypocapnia.

Pulse. Tachycardia usually is compensatory for hypovolemia and hypotension.

Temperature. It is important to obtain and monitor the core temperature in significant heat illness. This will often require use of a temperature probe bladder catheter or a rectal probe in patients who are not fully alert.

Cutaneous Signs. Skin temperature, presence or absence of sweating, rashes, and tissue turgor are important signs to be noted. Muscular fasciculations and spasms may also occur.

Cardiovascular System. A murmur, thrill, or lift on examination, an abnormal pulse rate and rhythm, and orthostatic changes may suggest a cardiovascular cause for syncope rather than primary heat illness. A hyperdynamic cardiovascular state suggests a compensatory response to increase heat dissipation.

Neurologic System. Focal deficits, neck stiffness, or Trousseau's or Chvostek's signs suggest alternative causes for the patient's condition. Mental status changes are consistent with primary heat illness, and neurologic abnormalities are the sine qua non of heatstroke.

Endocrine System. In the presence of hyperventilation, the odor of acetone on the breath may suggest diabetic ketoacidosis. Hyperthyroidism is suggested by a goiter, skin and eye findings, as well as a hyperdynamic cardiovascular status.

CLINICAL REASONING

In addressing the patient with possible heat illness, the physician asks the following questions.

Is this Primarily a Heat-Related Illness?

Primary heat illness is suspected when the presenting signs and symptoms and the situation in which they developed are consistent with that diagnosis. In some instances, those factors, along with the rapid resolution of symptoms on removal to a cool environment, may be sufficient to justify the diagnosis. In general, other conditions must be ruled out before the diagnosis of heat illness is confirmed (see Febrile Adults, Chapter 14).

If So, Which Form of Heat-Related Illness—Heat Cramps, Heat Exhaustion, Heat Syncope, or Heatstroke?

Although there are various types of heat illness, heat cramps, heat exhaustion, heat syncope, and heatstroke are the major forms encountered by emergency physicians (Table 17–2).

Heat Cramps. Heat cramps typically occur in the setting of heavy workload in a heat-stressed environment. Cramping of muscles working the hardest is typical. Dilutional hyponatremia is the cause, usually resulting from hypotonic (water only) fluid replacement. Conditioned athletes are often affected. Other causes of cramping such as hyperventilation, hypocalcemia, or hypokalemia can be suspected on the basis of the history, particularly anxiety or use of diuretics (Table 17–3).

Heat Exhaustion. A variety of symptoms, including dizziness, nausea, vomiting, malaise, fever, weakness, and occasionally syncope may occur with heat exhaustion. A combination of these symptoms in a heat-stressed patient with profuse sweating typically suggests heat exhaustion. There are no mental status changes. This is the most common form of heat illness, and it has a low morbidity and mortality. Heat exhaustion is, however, a step along the continuum of heat illnesses, leading to heatstroke.

Depletion of total body stores of water or salt may be the cause of symptoms. This develops over a period of days. Salt depletion occurs when sweat losses are replaced only by hypotonic solutions, and symptoms are thought to be due to hyponatremia (Table 17–4). Water depletion occurs when patients are unable to satisfy their thirst, causing dehydration and hypernatremia. This situation often occurs in nursing home patients. The temperature may be normal or elevated in the salt-depletion type of illness; with water-depletion, the temperature is usually elevated and risk of progression to heatstroke is great.

Heat Syncope. Heat stress may lead to the combination of intravascular volume depletion with peripheral vasodilation and loss of vasomotor

TABLE 17–2. Differentiation of Types of Primary Heat Illness

Condition	History	Temperature	Mentation	Skin Signs
Heat edema	Extremity swelling with exertion	Normal	Normal	Edema
Heat syncope	Brief syncope Prolonged heat exposure Mild dehydration	Normal	Normal	Sweating or none
Heat cramps	Muscle cramps	Normal	Normal	Sweating, muscle spasms
Heat exhaustion	Weakness Headache Syncope	102.2°–106°F (39°–41.1°C)	Normal	Profuse sweating
Heat stroke	Coma Seizures Confusion	106°–108°F (41.1°–42.2°C)	Impaired	Dry or sweating*

*Sweating is absent in classic heat stroke, but it may be present or absent in exertional heat stroke.

TABLE 17–3. Differential Diagnosis of Heat Cramps

Potential Diagnosis	Pertinent History	Pertinent Findings on Physical Examination	Pertinent Laboratory Findings
Hyperventilation	Stress/Anxiety	Rapid respiratory rate	Decreasing P_{CO_2}, increasing pH
Hypocalcemia	Neck surgery	Trousseau's sign Chvostek's sign Carpopedal spasm	
Hypokalemia	Malabsorption symptoms	Trousseau's sign Chvostek's sign Tetany Convulsions Skeletal abnormalities	Hypocalcemia Soft tissue calcification on radiograph
Heat cramps	Gastrointestinal losses Diuretic use Inadequate diet	Weakness Decreased or absent reflexes	Hypokalemia
	Conditioned athlete Exercise Sweat loss Water as main fluid replacement Previous similar illness	Muscle spasms/tetany Sweating Normal temperature	Hyponatremia

tone. The resulting syncope from postural hypotension is referred to as heat syncope. Simple heat syncope is nearly always treated with removal from the heat stress and rehydration. The difficulty with this syndrome is distinguishing it from other more serious problems (see Table 17–4).

Heatstroke. Heatstroke is the most severe form of heat illness, carrying a mortality of 10% to 20% with current therapy. Presentation will include high fever and neurologic deterioration. This may be altered mental status, focal deficits, seizure, or coma. Heatstroke occurs when the body's heat loss mechanisms are overwhelmed (Table 17–5). The classic symptom triad in heatstroke is hyperpyrexia, central nervous system dysfunction, and anhidrosis, although sweating may be present in some patients.

Classic heatstroke commonly occurs in older persons and develops over a period of days.

Dehydration leads to confusion, agitation, and lethargy. Patients may actually stop sweating and present with hot, dry skin.

Exertional heatstroke occurs in young, active, healthy individuals who overwhelm their body's capability to dissipate heat. It can develop during 1 hour or less. Signs of dehydration may or may not be present. Sweating is frequently present in this subgroup.

What Potential Complications of Heat Illness May Exist?

Complications of heatstroke are common, and there are several prognostic factors that indicate, when present, high mortality. They become more significant if treatment delay occurs (Table 17–6). Hepatic failure and disseminated intravascular coagulation are two of the most common compli-

TABLE 17–4. Differential Diagnosis of Heat Exhaustion—Symptom Complex: Weakness, Headache, Mild Disorientation, Syncope, or Near-Syncope

Potential Diagnosis	Pertinent History	Pertinent Findings on Physical Examination	Pertinent Laboratory Data
Head trauma	Injury, anticoagulant therapy	External trauma Focal neurologic deficit	Brain CT: hemorrhage
Subarachnoid hemorrhage	Sudden onset of severe headache during straining or exercise, family history, history of aneurysm	Variable level of consciousness, neck stiffness (Kernig's or Brudzinski's sign), retinal hemorrhages	Brain CT: hemorrhage Lumbar puncture (if CT negative): increased RBCs, xanthochromia
Aortic outflow tract stenosis (HCM or congenital valve disease)	Murmur known, exertional syncope	Murmur, precordial thrill or lift	ECG Cardiac echocardiography Cardiac catheterization
Dysrhythmia	Sudden onset of lightheadedness, palpitations, previous history	Abnormal heart rate, rhythm, and peripheral pulses; symptoms present during dysrhythmia	Cardiac monitor, ECG
Vascular dilatation	Postural symptoms, allergy (e.g., bee sting), drugs	Orthostatic changes, hives, wheezing	
Hypovolemia	Postural symptoms, fluid loss (e.g., sweat, blood, or gastrointestinal loss)	Orthostatic changes, decreased tissue turgor, sweating, rectal blood	Hemoglobin/hematocrit: decreased BUN/creatinine: elevated
Diabetic ketoacidosis	Polyuria, polydipsia, polyphagia, family history	Fruity odor of breath, decreased tissue turgor, hyperventilation, orthostatic changes	Serum and urine ketones: elevated Arterial blood gases: metabolic acidosis
Poison/adverse medication	Exposure: skin, ingestion, and inhalation	Odor, toxidrome (e.g., anticholinergic syndrome)	Drug level Drug screen Arterial blood gases: acid/base abnormality Carboxyhemoglobin
Encephalitis/meningitis	Fever, prodromal illness, severe headache, chills	Temperature, neck stiffness (Kernig's and Brudzinski's signs)	Lumbar puncture: elevated WBCs, positive Gram's stain, cultures
Heat exhaustion	Hot environment, exercise, sweat loss	Temperature, sweating, orthostatic changes	Serum sodium: hyponatremia BUN/creatinine: elevated Asparate aminotransferase: slightly elevated

BUN, blood urea nitrogen; CT, computed tomography; ECG, electrocardiogram; HCM, hypertrophic cardiomyopathy; RBCs, red blood cells; WBCs, white blood cells.

TABLE 17–5. Differential Diagnosis of Heat Stroke—Symptom Complex: Altered Mental Status/CNS Symptoms, Hyperthermia

Potential Diagnosis	Pertinent History	Pertinent Findings on Physical Examination	Pertinent Laboratory Data
Encephalitis/meningitis	Fever, prodromal illness, severe headache, chills	Temperature, neck stiffness (Kernig's and Brudzinski's signs)	Lumbar puncture: elevated WBCs, positive Gram's stain, cultures
Malaria	Exposure, travel history, previous history	Fever pattern, confusion	Peripheral blood smear
Typhoid fever, typhus	Exposure, travel history	Fever pattern	Titers: Weil-Felix reaction, complement fixation
Sepsis	Fever, age extreme, immunocompromised	Fever, confusion, coma, focal infection	Chest radiograph WBCs: elevated; cultures: blood, urine, cerebrospinal fluid
Hypothalamic hemorrhage	Hypertension, anticoagulant therapy	Coma and fever, focal neurologic findings	Brain CT: hemorrhage
Thyroid storm	Preexisting hyperthyroidism (e.g., Graves' disease); risk factors include stress or surgery, trauma, infection, failure to take antithyroid medication	Goiter, tachycardia, seizures, hypotension	Thyroid function studies: T_3 and T_4
Malignant hyperthermia/neuroleptic syndrome	Inhalation anesthetic, major antipsychotic medication, succinylcholine	Muscle fasciculations	Arterial blood gases: acidosis Electrolytes: hyperkalemia, hypermagnesemia AST: elevated WBC: elevated
Heat stroke	Risk factors (see Table 17–1), exposure to heat load, exercise	Hot, flushed skin, confusion, agitation, seizures, tachycardia, hypotension, vomiting, diarrhea, muscle tenderness	Electrolytes: hyperkalemia or hypokalemia, hyponatremia, hypocalcemia, hypophosphatemia Arterial blood gases: metabolic acidosis Urine: myoglobin; clotting factors: decreased; blood glucose: variable

AST, aspartate aminotransferase; CNS, central nervous system; CT, computed tomography; WBCs, white blood cells.

TABLE 17–6. Heat Stroke—Poor Prognostic Factors

Temperature greater than 106°F (41.1°C)
Aspartate aminotransferase greater than 1000 IU
Coma
Rhabdomyolysis
Renal failure
Hypotension

---

cations. Rhabdomyolysis and renal failure are much more common (25%) in exertional heatstroke than in classic heatstroke (5%). Although neurologic findings are the hallmark of heatstroke, very rarely do patients have residual neurologic abnormality.

What Else could be Causing the Patient's Problem? What is the Differential Diagnosis for Each of the Heat-Related Illness Syndromes?

The approach is to determine the type of primary heat illness being considered and then work through the differential diagnosis for that specific illness (see Tables 17–3, 17–4, and 17–5).

DIAGNOSTIC ADJUNCTS

There is no single ancillary test that is specific for heat illness. Patients with heat cramps or syncope and mild heat exhaustion that rapidly resolves usually require no ancillary tests. Patients with more severe conditions (e.g., severe heat exhaustion or heatstroke) require extensive evaluation to rule out other problems and to detect complications (Table 17–7).

Laboratory Studies

Complete Blood Cell Count with Differential. The white blood cell count is usually elevated but is less than 30,000/mm^3. A high percentage of immature neutrophils (bands) may be seen, but this is more common with underlying infection. Hemoglobin and hematocrit levels may be increased owing to depleted intravascular volume. When syncope events occur, anemia and occult bleeding are evident in the differential and may be detected with this test.

Electrolytes. Abnormalities of sodium and potassium may be detected. These levels may vary with patient's fluid status, renal status, and degree of rhabdomyolysis.

Blood Urea Nitrogen/Creatinine. Blood urea nitrogen and creatinine levels may be elevated, secondary to impaired renal function or dehydration.

Urinalysis. The urinalysis is used to monitor the hydration status and to detect the presence of rhabdomyolysis (the urine sample is positive for hemoglobin but negative for red blood cells).

Liver Enzymes. The liver is perhaps the organ most sensitive to heat stress. Elevation of transaminase levels can occur in heat exhaustion and is common in heatstroke. Levels peak 24 to 48 hours after injury. The severity of illness correlates well with the magnitude, as well as duration, of aspartate aminotransferase elevation. Aspartate aminotransferase levels in excess of 1000 IU predict severe illness with complications, especially renal failure.

Serum Glucose. Depending on the body's metabolic response to excessive heat load, the serum glucose may be high or low. It is helpful in the diagnostic workup of altered mental status and gives information about the general metabolic status of the patient.

Arterial Blood Gases. The PaO_2 is useful to assess the systemic maintenance of oxygen at times of high demand. It may also provide a reason for an altered mental status. The pH and $PaCO_2$ are necessary for calculating the degree of acid-base abnormality. Lactic acidosis is commonly associated with severe heat-related illnesses, as well as diseases that mimic heat illness.

TABLE 17–7. *Possible* **Laboratory Findings in Heat Stroke**

CBC	WBC elevated (20,000–30,000/mm^3)
Electrolytes	Hypokalemia, hyponatremia, hypophosphatemia, hypocalcemia, occasionally hyperkalemia from muscle breakdown
Arterial blood gases	Metabolic acidosis
Liver function	Elevated aspartate aminotransferase, lactic dehydrogenase, creatine phosphokinase
Glucose	Normal or low
Clotting	Picture of DIC may occur (deceased platelets, prolonged PT and PTT and increased fibrin split products)
ECG	Supraventricular tachycardia, nonspecific ST segment/T wave change

CBC, complete blood cell count; DIC, disseminated intravascular coagulation; ECG, electrocardiogram; PT, prothrombin time; PTT, partial thromboplastin time; WBC, white blood cell.

Coagulation Profile. This test is reserved for patients with severe heat illness. It includes a platelet count, prothrombin time, and activated partial thromboplastin time. Both severe heat illness and sepsis can trigger disseminated intravascular coagulation.

Cultures. Heatstroke presents less frequently than sepsis. Cultures of blood and urine are part of the evaluation of these patients.

Radiologic Imaging

A chest radiograph is included in the diagnostic evaluation. Infection is included in the differential diagnosis of moderate to severe heat illness.

Computed tomography is necessary in any patient with acute mental status changes not rapidly responding to therapeutic intervention. Subarachnoid and intracranial hemorrhage may cause associated central temperature elevation.

Electrocardiogram

A 12-lead electrocardiogram should be considered in any patient with moderate to severe heat illness, on any patient with syncope, or for those with a history of cardiovascular disease. Increased metabolic demands, electrolyte abnormalities, and cardiovascular stress can predispose to myocardial ischemia and dysrhythmias.

PRINCIPLES OF MANAGEMENT

Management principles for heat illnesses include

1. Elimination of excess heat
2. Correction of fluid losses and electrolyte imbalances
3. Treatment of complications

Elimination of Excess Heat

The initial intervention is the removal of the patient from the heat-stress environment. *Elimination of excess heat* may then be accomplished through radiation, conduction, convection, or evaporation.

Placing patients in a cool environment hastens heat loss through radiation; clothing removal enhances radiation and increases *convection* heat loss as air currents contact the skin. Fanning the patient further enhances *convection* and *evaporative* heat loss. Dissipation of heat by *conduction* is accomplished by covering the patient in cold wet sheets or placing ice packs in contact with the body. Immersion is frequently impractical, because it is logistically difficult and inhibits

access to the patient. Ice or cold water immersion also causes vasoconstriction, which theoretically retards heat loss.

Evaporation is the most clinically effective mechanism. Spraying the skin with a mist and then fanning the patient is easily accomplished and highly effective. Room temperature water should be used to avoid triggering vasoconstriction and shivering, to quickly evaporate, and to increase efficiency of the method.

Other cooling methods include ice water lavage of body cavities (i.e., stomach, bladder, or peritoneum) and cardiopulmonary bypass. These measures are rarely employed because simpler and less invasive techniques are very effective. Antipyretics are NOT effective in patients with heat illness, and acetaminophen is contraindicated because of the risk of liver injury.

The rapid cooling of the patient lowers mortality. Active cooling should stop when the patient's temperature has reached 102.2°F (39°C), to avoid iatrogenic hypothermia.

Correction of Fluid Loss and Electrolyte Imbalance

In patients with heat cramps or mild heat exhaustion, *fluid losses and electrolyte imbalances* can be corrected by having the patient drink oral fluids such as Gatorade or Pedialyte. Patients with syncope, severe heat exhaustion, or heatstroke require intravenous fluid replacement with isotonic crystalloid. In water-depletion–type illnesses, the fluid is switched to a hypotonic solution when the volume deficit has been replaced. The water deficit can be approximated as shown below:

$$\text{Normal total body water (TBW) (in liters)} = (0.6) \times (\text{wt in kg})$$

$$\begin{matrix} \text{Water} \\ \text{deficit} \\ \text{(in liters)} \end{matrix} = \text{TBW} - \left[\frac{\text{TBW} \times (\text{normal Na}^+ \ 140)}{(\text{actual measured Na}^+)} \right]$$

Example: 60-kg man with measured Na^+ of 160 mEq/dL

$$\text{Normal TBW} = (0.6) \times (60) = 36\text{L}$$

$$\begin{matrix} \text{Free water} \\ \text{deficit} \\ \text{(in liters)} \end{matrix} = 36 - \left[\frac{36 \times 140}{160} \right] = 4.5 \text{ L}$$

One half of the calculated amount of a free water deficit is given over 24 hours. The replacement fluid is hypotonic (i.e., D_5W). In addition, maintenance requirements and ongoing losses are corrected with an isotonic fluid.

In patients with salt-depletion type illness, normal saline is administered at a rate of 250 to 500 mL/hr. Monitoring is done with urine output measurements or, in severe cases, with central venous or pulmonary artery pressure measurements. Salt tablets are no longer recommended because an appropriate dose is not known and gastrointestinal upset occurs. Hypernatremia and fluid losses from vomiting or diarrhea can worsen clinical status.

Treatment of Heatstroke Complications

Shivering. During the cooling process, patients may begin to shiver, creating more heat. Chlorpromazine, 12.5 to 50 mg, given intravenously can be used for shiver suppression.

Hypotension. Hypotension may be induced by volume depletion, vasodilation, or cardiac failure secondary to heat damage. Fluid replacement must be cautious in such cases to avoid overloading the patient's pump function. Central venous monitoring is helpful in determining the cause of hypotension and can guide fluid therapy. In elderly patients with preexisting heart disease, a pulmonary capillary wedge pressure monitor may be more useful. Perfusion should be monitored closely with serial assessment of blood pressure, heart rate, skin temperature, and urine output. Dobutamine may be effective in the patient with cardiogenic hypotension.

Rhabdomyolysis. Rhabdomyolysis more frequently occurs in the exertional form of heatstroke (vs. the classic form). The cause is direct heat damage to muscle. If myoglobin is present in the urine, mannitol (0.25 g/kg) is given intravenously for osmotic diuresis. A urine output of 70 to 75 mL/hr is recommended. Alkalinization of the urine with administration of sodium bicarbonate helps prevent precipitation of myoglobin in the renal tubules.

Renal Failure. Renal failure occurs in 25% of exertional heatstroke victims and in 5% of those with classic heatstroke. The cause is multifactorial—dehydration with hypotension, poor renal perfusion, direct heat damage to the kidneys, and myoglobin blocking the renal tubules. The renal failure is usually reversible and requires only temporary dialysis therapy.

Future Directions in Treatment

Recent research has indicated possibilities for prevention of serious heat illness. For example, when under heat stress there is increased gastrointestinal permeability, release of gram-negative endotoxins, and cytokine activation. Binding agents or antibodies to lipopolysaccharides may prove helpful in altering this cascade.

Additionally, the hypothalamic-pituitary-adrenal axis is activated during heat stress and immune system suppression occurs. Possible attenuation of this response with hypnosis, biofeedback, and stress conditioning may maintain immune competency.

Hyperkalemia during heatstroke may be a significant contributor to the pathophysiologic progression. Agents to control efflux of potassium or increase cellular uptake may be beneficial in slowing the disease course.

Finally, heavy exertion in hot environments may increase cell death apoptosis, a process by which cells break down into chromatin vesicles and are phagocytosed by surrounding cells, is indicated. This is postulated as an explanation for the higher risk of heatstroke the day after heavy heat stress. Interleukin-6 and endogenous "heat shock proteins" may be protective. Agents to increase levels of these substances may be an arena for successful treatment research.

UNCERTAIN DIAGNOSIS

The primary origin of the uncertain diagnosis is acceptance of the patient's presentation (as being environmentally based) without exploration of other differential diagnoses. Delayed response to treatment should reinforce the need for an expanded differential diagnosis.

SPECIAL CONSIDERATIONS

Hyperthermia in the Agitated, Intoxicated Patient

Temperature measurement is very important in patients who are agitated or intoxicated. Any preexisting physical or mental impairment that results in failure to take protective measures in response to heat (such as meeting the thirst need or moving to a cooler environment) predisposes the individual to heat illness.

Agitation can be the result or the cause of heat illness. Agitation may be *caused* by a wide variety of conditions, such as primary metabolic disorders, serotonin syndrome, primary neurologic disorders, sepsis, or drug use (e.g., phencyclidine [PCP], cocaine, or amphetamines). Alternatively, agitation *causes* heat illness by virtue of the tremendous internal heat load resulting from increased muscular activity. It is difficult to reduce core temperature until the increased internal heat load is under control. Goals of therapy should include treating the primary disorder, in addition to cooling the patient.

Pediatric Patients

Smaller children have an increased surface area to body mass ratio and can rapidly take on heat from a thermal stress environment. They may be unable to utilize behavioral compensation methods, such as leaving the stressful environment, obtaining fluid replacement, or removing clothing, because of developmental stage or ability level.

Two settings in which children are at high risk for heat problems include the febrile infant wrapped in excessive blankets and the small child left unattended in the car with closed windows. Parent education is essential to eliminate these causes of preventable heat illness.

Elderly Patients

Heat illness as the sole cause of fever in the elderly is a diagnosis of exclusion. When environmental conditions are conducive to heat illness, a high index of suspicion is appropriate. Fever in the elderly is common, and sepsis frequently occurs in those who are debilitated with chronic illnesses or compromised immune status. Common sources of sepsis in elderly persons are pneumonia, urinary tract infection, and skin infections.

Elderly patients are at high risk for heat illness, based on several factors (see Table 17–1):

1. Inability to take appropriate behavioral measures (drink fluids, move to a cooler environment) to protect against a hot environment because of physical or mental impairment
2. Poor physical conditioning
3. Inability to mount an adequate physiologic response to heat loads, with impaired sweating and cardiovascular response
4. Medication use (e.g., diuretics, β blockers) that may predispose to heat illness

DISPOSITION AND FOLLOW-UP

The disposition for patients with heat illness varies from discharge home to intensive care unit admission, depending on the type and severity of the illness.

1. *Heat cramps* are self-limited and are not associated with serious sequelae. After cramp resolution, these patients are discharged home with instructions for oral fluid/electrolyte replacement and advice on preventive measures.
2. *Heat exhaustion* is a relatively benign condition that generally responds well to treatment in the emergency department. Patients may be discharged after treatment and 4 to 6 hours observation, with instructions about fluid therapy and prevention. Heat exhaustion patients who have any elevation in aspartate aminotransferase should refrain from any exercise and heat exposure for 48 to 72 hours, because they are at high risk for recurrent heat illness. Admission is considered when the patient has ongoing symptoms such as vomiting or orthostatic hypotension, or if other serious diagnoses have not been ruled out.
3. *Heat syncope* patients are usually treated with fluid repletion in the emergency department and discharged home when they are no longer symptomatic and are able to continue oral hydration. As with all patients with heat illness, counseling about prevention is mandatory at the time of discharge from the hospital.
4. *Heatstroke* victims require admission to a critical care unit. All patients with unexplained coma need critical care and aggressive monitoring of the airway, neurologic status, cardiac rhythm, and vital signs. Factors indicating a poor prognosis in these patients are listed in Table 17–6.

Prevention

Before discharge, all victims of heat illness should be advised on *prevention*:

1. All heat illness is theoretically preventable by avoidance of the heat stress. Encourage patients to avoid situations for which they are not properly prepared, especially if not absolutely necessary. Parents of small children and caretakers of debilitated persons should be instructed on avoiding risky situations for their dependents.
2. Thirst poorly indicates the degree of dehydration present. Patients need to drink fluids before exercise or heat stress and to hydrate during the stress, regardless of their thirst. An oral regimen for an active healthy adult is 8 to 12 ounces every half-hour.
3. The more knowledgeable patient can be instructed on parameters such as urine output, urine color, or body weight as indications of dehydration.
4. Acclimatization is the process by which the body adapts to extremes of heat. With acclimatization, sweating becomes more efficient (less salt lost and higher peak volumes) and starts at lower temperatures. Plasma volume increases, and vasodilation starts at lower body temperatures. Patients should be

advised that acclimatization to a hot environment is a process that takes 1 to 2 weeks. During this time it is advisable to take frequent breaks, to cool down, and to correct fluid losses aggressively. Gradual increase of exercise time and wearing light-colored, lightweight clothing also helps.

FINAL POINTS

- The common forms of heat illness are heat cramps, heat exhaustion, heat syncope, and heatstroke.

- Heat cramps are caused by sodium depletion, are benign, and are self-limited.
- Heat exhaustion and heat syncope usually respond rapidly to a cool environment and correction of fluid losses with water and electrolytes as needed.
- Heatstroke is a serious illness with significant mortality requiring aggressive therapy to reduce complications, morbidity, and mortality.
- Heat illness is preventable. Public education efforts on prevention continue to be necessary.

CASE*Study*

A 37-year-old male construction worker complained of nausea and dizziness, then fainted. The patient was working on the roof of a house in the afternoon of a humid August day. This patient fainted during significant heat stress. ABCs of resuscitation were instituted immediately, and the patient responded easily. History includes water intake of approximately 1 L in the Past 6 hours, with high ambient temperature and humidity. The patient had a rapid heart rate and a low blood pressure, and his skin was very warm and moist.

The paramedics were instructed to do the following:

1. Start an intravenous line and give a 500-mL bolus of normal saline.
2. Place the patient on a cardiac monitor.
3. Start oxygen by nasal cannula at 3 L/min.
4. Cool the patient by undressing him, misting him with water, and fanning.
5. Transport the patient to the emergency department for further evaluation and treatment.

The setting and skin signs raise the possibility of heat illness. The rescue squad appropriately institutes cooling measures.

The patient has mild residual nausea, dizziness, and cramping. He was engaged in similar work the day before and has had a previous episode similar to this.

The patient was tachycardic to 130 beats per minute and had orthostatic changes in blood pressure and pulse rate. His core temperature was 102.2°F (39°C). His skin was flushed and moist, and his mucous membranes were dry.

In such cases, simply removing the patient from the hot environment is a primary component of the treatment. In addition, the history of poor fluid intake, cramps, and syncopal episode suggest dehydration and possible electrolyte depletion. Intravenous and oral rehydration is appropriate in this case.

With a history of a syncopal episode, an electrocardiogram, complete blood cell count, electrolyte profile, and serum glucose measurement were ordered. All values were normal. The laboratory tests add significantly to the cost of the patient's care; however, it is arguable that the history and physical examination warrant these tests before discharge. The waiting time needed for laboratory results can be viewed as a "cost," but the need for treatment and observation negates this concern.

This patient was treated with removal to a cool environment, intravenous fluids, and an antiemetic to control his nausea. The original temperature of 102.2°F (39°C) came down to 99°F (37.2°C) over the next 2 hours, and the patient began producing urine. Once nausea was controlled, the patient started oral rehydration. History, physical examination, and laboratory evaluation uncovered no additional abnormalities. His diagnosis was heat exhaustion with syncope. This patient was discharged home with instructions for prevention of future heat illness.

Bibliography

TEXT

Hubbard RW, Gaffin SL, Squire DL: Heat-related illnesses. In Auerbach PS, (ed): Management of Wilderness and Environmental Emergencies, 4th ed. St. Louis, Mosby–Year Book, 2001.

JOURNAL ARTICLES

Bouchama A: Heatstroke: A new look at an ancient disease [editorial]. Intensive Care Med 1995; 21:623–625.

Centers for Disease Control and Prevention: Prevention and management of heat-related illness among the spectators and staff during the Olympic games—Atlanta, July 6–23, 1996. JAMA 1996; 276:593–595.

Centers for Disease Control and Prevention: Heat-related deaths—Los Angeles County, California, 1999–2000, and United States, 1979–1998. MMWR Morb Mortal Wkly Rep 2001; 50:623–626.

Gaffin SL, Hubbard RW: Experimental approaches to therapy and prophylaxis for heat stress and heatstroke. Wilderness Environ Med 1996; 4:312–334.

Khosla R, Guntupalli KK: Heat-related illnesses. Crit Care Clin 1999; 15:251–263.

Semenza JC, Rubin CH, Falter KH, et al: Heat-related deaths during the July 1995 heat wave in Chicago. N Engl J Med 1996; 335:84–90.

Stewart C: The spectrum of heat illness in children. Pediatr Emerg Med Rep 1999; 4:41–52.

CHAPTER 18

Hypothermia

E. BRADSHAW BUNNEY

CASE *Study*

A 63-year-old man was found collapsed in an alley after a cold night in December. Concerned neighbors called the rescue squad. The patient does not respond to verbal stimulation and groans to painful stimulation. His pulse rate is 50 beats per minute, blood pressure is 90/60 mm Hg, and respiratory rate is 10 breaths per minute and shallow.

INTRODUCTION

Definitions

Hypothermia is defined as a core temperature of less than 35°C (95°F). It is either accidental (primary) or secondary to other disease processes. Development of complications depends on many factors, the most important of which is the degree of hypothermia. Additional factors that affect morbidity and mortality are age, concomitant injury, preexisting or predisposing illness, localized hypothermia, immersion in water, and intoxication.

Well-publicized accounts of survival after accidental hypothermia due to mountaineering accidents and submersion in cold water have brought the subject of hypothermia to the attention of the general population. Far more common, however, are cases of hypothermia that develop subtly in urban settings. Severe cold and prolonged exposure are not necessary for a person to develop hypothermia. It is possible to develop hypothermia on a 60°F day if the victim is inappropriately dressed and has significant risk factors. Six percent to 10% of cases of mild-to-moderate hypothermia occur in warm seasons and may go unrecognized.

Hypothermia is usually classified as mild, moderate, or severe.

- *Mild hypothermia (34°C to 36°C [93.2°F to 96.8°F]).* The only manifestations of mild hypothermia may be slowing of mental processes producing slurred speech, mild incoordination, and inappropriate judgment or behavior. The shivering reflex is preserved in this temperature range.
- *Moderate hypothermia (30°C to 34°C [86°F to 93.2°F]).* There is a progressive decrease in the level of consciousness in this temperature range. Oxygen consumption and carbon dioxide production both drop. Coma is likely at temperatures of less than 30°C. The victim appears cyanotic and will develop tissue edema. Shivering is replaced by muscle rigidity. Respiratory activity and pulses may be difficult to detect. The gag/cough reflexes become depressed, and the risk of aspiration increases.
- *Severe hypothermia (Less than 30°C [86°F]).* The victim is usually comatose with dilated and unresponsive pupils. It may be impossible to detect any vital signs, and the distinction between death and profound hypothermia may be difficult to make. Respiratory arrest and ventricular fibrillation often occur in older patients at temperatures less than 28°C.

Epidemiology

Within the United States the annual death rate from hypothermia is approximately 2 to 4 per million persons. The very young and the very old are the most susceptible. Infants cool much faster because they have a greater ratio of body surface area to body mass and inadequate subcutaneous tissue. The elderly have a slower metabolic rate and more difficulty maintaining body temperature in cool weather. Over half of the cases of hypothermia in the urban setting are associated with central nervous system disease or alcohol or drug intoxication.

Pathophysiology

There are four mechanisms of heat loss that threaten thermostability:

1. *Radiation.* Radiation accounts for 55% to 65% of heat loss and is modified by insulation (clothing, subcutaneous fat layer) and skin blood flow.
2. *Conduction.* Conduction is normally not a major source of heat loss, but conductive heat

loss increases 5 times in wet clothing and 25 to 30 times in cold water.

3. *Convection.* Wind currents and body motion markedly increase heat loss. The wind chill effect significantly increases the likelihood of hypothermia developing at a given temperature.

4. *Evaporation.* Evaporation and losses through respiration account for 20% to 30% of the heat loss in dry, windy conditions. Sweating also accounts for evaporative heat loss.

Factors that have been found to predispose individuals to the development of hypothermia include

- Endocrine or metabolic derangement (hypoglycemia, hypopituitarism, hypothyroidism, and hypoadrenalism)
- Infection (meningitis, sepsis)
- Intoxication (alcohol, opiates, barbiturates, benzodiazepines, phenothiazines, cyclic antidepressants)
- Intracranial pathology (cerebrovascular accident, traumatic, congenital, tumors, Wernicke's encephalopathy)
- Submersion injury
- Environmental exposure
- Dermatologic (burns and exfoliative dermatoses)
- Iatrogenic (cold intravenous fluids, exposure during treatment)
- Acute debilitating conditions (diabetic ketoacidosis, trauma)

The mortality from hypothermia is directly related to the associated underlying disorder and is highest in submersion injury.

When the core body temperature begins to drop, the preoptic anterior hypothalamus senses blood cooling and immediately initiates sympathetic neurogenic signals that cause an increase in muscle tone and metabolic rate. This is most evident in the shivering reflex, which is an attempt by the body to increase heat production by involuntary muscle contraction. Heat production can be increased to about four times the normal rate in this way. The sympathetic nervous system also causes cutaneous vasoconstriction, thereby shunting blood toward the vital organs and defending against further heat loss. As the body cools, metabolic rate is reduced, resulting in a decrease in carbon dioxide production and slowing of the heart rate (Fig. 18–1).

Hypothermia affects the entire body, and the major signs and symptoms result from involvement of the cardiovascular, central nervous, respiratory, renal, and gastrointestinal systems. Apnea and asystole can occur very quickly.

Cardiovascular Effects. After an initial tachycardia, the heart rate decreases as the temperature falls. The "normal" heart rate is reduced by half at a body temperature of 28°C (82.4°F). The mean arterial pressure decreases progressively, and cardiac output drops to 45% of normal at 25°C (77°F).

Atrial dysrhythmias commonly appear at temperatures below 32.2°C (90°F) and generally do not need to be treated because they resolve upon warming. In contrast, ventricular ectopy is initially suppressed by the cold until the body reaches a temperature of 30°C to 28°C (86°F to 82.4°F). At these temperatures, electrical conduction through the myocardial muscle fibers is faster than through the His-Purkinje system, greatly increasing the risk of ventricular fibrillation, which can lead to asystole.

On the electrocardiogram or rhythm strip a J wave (Osborne wave or hypothermic hump) may be present at the junction of the QRS complex and ST segment. Although the J wave is *not* pathognomonic, it is frequently associated with the diagnosis of significant hypothermia (Fig. 18–2). Other common electrocardiographic findings include T-wave inversion and prolonged PR, QRS, and QT intervals.

Core temperature *afterdrop* is a term referring to the continued drop in temperature after rewarming is started. Afterdrop results when cold, acidotic, hyperkalemic blood returns to the core after heat is applied directly to the extremities and vasoconstriction is reversed.

Central Nervous System Effects. Neuronal activity decreases as the temperature falls. Enzyme systems become less functional, and there is a linear decrease in cerebral metabolism. Cerebral perfusion is maintained until vascular autoregulation becomes ineffective at 25°C (77°F). At 20°C (68°F), the electroencephalogram becomes flat. Associated with these changes is a decrease in cerebral oxygen requirement, which may provide a "brain protective" effect against anoxia and ischemia.

Common neurologic findings include dysarthria, hyporeflexia, ataxia, and coma. Psychiatric symptoms range from a peculiar "flat" affect to impaired judgment, as may be evidenced by paradoxical undressing.

Respiratory Effects. Cold initially stimulates the respiratory drive. Later, as metabolism slows, there is progressive depression of the respiratory minute volume. Bronchorrhea, brought on by the inhalation of cold air, can be severe, simulating pulmonary edema.

Renal Effects. The kidneys respond rapidly to hypothermic fluid sequestration. Although

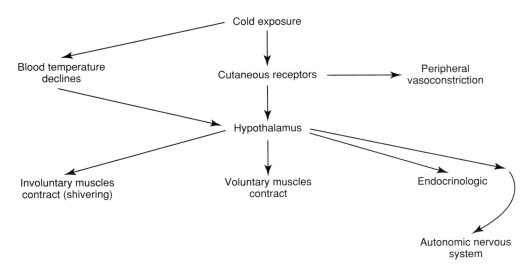

FIGURE 18–1 • Physiologic responses in hypothermia.

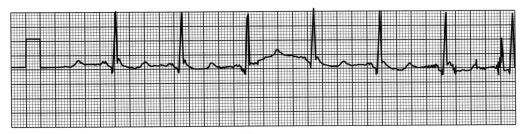

FIGURE 18–2 • Example of a J wave noted in a 73-year-old woman.

renal blood flow drops progressively, there is a large diuresis of dilute glomerular filtrate resulting from an initial central hypervolemia caused by vasoconstriction in the extremities. Ethanol can double the amount of volume loss. Cold water immersion may increase this diuresis by three and one-half times. Because of the decreased renal blood flow and myoglobinemia, acute tubular necrosis can result.

Gastrointestinal Effects. Hypothermia decreases gastrointestinal motility. Gastric dilatation, ileus, constipation, and poor rectal tone commonly result. Although the precise cause is unknown, inflammatory changes in the pancreas and hyperamylasemia are often found in the hypothermic patient. The decreased hepatic function can result in toxic levels of drugs usually metabolized by the liver (e.g., lidocaine).

INITIAL APPROACH AND STABILIZATION

Priority Diagnoses

The priority diagnoses to consider initially in the hypothermic patient include

- Hypoxemia
- Hypoglycemia
- Opiate overdose or alcohol intoxication
- Other medication or illicit drug overdose
- Drowning or near-drowning
- Shock (traumatic, septic, cardiovascular, neurologic)
- Cerebrovascular accident or other neurologic disorders
- Cardiac dysrhythmias

Most patients with significant hypothermia are brought in by ambulance, usually with a chief complaint of "altered mental status." Most ambulances are not equipped with thermometers, so the temperature of the patient may not be known on arrival. It is important to talk to the paramedics to find out where the patient was found (inside or outside, wet or dry). The paramedics may be able to provide past medical history obtained from bystanders or family or to report findings at the scene, such as pills, liquor bottles, or drug paraphernalia. When first approaching the patient with "altered mental status" it is important to maintain a broad differential diagnosis.

Rapid Assessment and Early Intervention

Priorities in the initial stabilization of the patient with hypothermia are the same as with all critically ill patients. The patient is handled gently to avoid precipitating ventricular fibrillation.

Airway. Is the patient awake and talking to you? If so, the airway is open for now. If the patient is severely obtunded, endotracheal intubation is necessary to maintain an open airway and to reduce the risk of aspiration of stomach contents. For further information, refer to Chapter 2, Airway Management.

Breathing. What is the patient's respiratory rate? Is the patient taking symmetric and deep breaths, or are respirations shallow and slow? If the patient is unable to ventilate properly, endotracheal intubation is indicated. A pulse oximetry reading should be obtained and the patient should be placed on warmed humidified oxygen (42°C to 46°C[107.6°F to 114.8°F]).

Circulation. Does the patient have peripheral pulses? If the patient does not have a radial pulse, does the patient have a carotid or femoral pulse? In severe cases of hypothermia even these pulses can be absent. The patient should be placed on a cardiac monitor, the rhythm assessed, and heart tones listened for with a stethoscope. Only life-threatening dysrhythmias (ventricular fibrillation, asystole) should be acutely treated because the rest correct with rewarming. An intravenous line should be placed. In the presence of hypothermia, cardiopulmonary resuscitation (CPR) is not started if there is any sign of perfusion. Iatrogenic ventricular fibrillation *may* result if external chest compressions are inadvertently applied in a patient who is *not* in cardiac arrest. Warmed intravenous fluids should be administered to patients with temperatures less than 34°C (93.2°F).

Disability (Neurologic Status). The patient's level of consciousness needs to be determined. AVPU is a quick way to categorize a patient's level of consciousness:

A = Alert
V = Responds to Verbal stimulation
P = Responds to Painful stimulation
U = Unresponsive to all stimulation

A glucose check should be done to rule out hypoglycemia as a cause of the altered mental status. Naloxone should be administered if an opiate overdose is suggested. Thiamine should be administered to all symptomatic adults, especially if Wernicke-Korsakoff syndrome is suggested. If the potential for traumatic injury exists, cervical spine immobilization, until clearance, is essential.

Exposure. The patient should be completely undressed, rapidly assessed for traumatic injuries and peripheral perfusion, and then covered in warm blankets. Patients with life-threatening dysrhythmias need rapid, immediate rewarming using all techniques available (see later under "Principles of Management").

While the assessment of the ABCs is proceeding, the rest of the vital signs should be obtained. This should include measuring blood pressure, pulse rate, respiratory rate, and temperature. If the initial temperature is low, a thermometer that can accurately read the core temperature is needed. This is usually done as a rectal probe, because standard thermometers read no lower than 34.4°C (93.9°F).

Patients may become hypothermic after they collapse for other reasons. A rapid physical assessment may reveal signs of other problems such as gastrointestinal hemorrhage, myocardial infarction, head trauma, or intoxication.

CLINICAL ASSESSMENT

History

The hypothermic patient is often unable to give an adequate history because of unconsciousness, confusion, or intoxication. Other sources of information are used as necessary.

1. What were the *circumstances surrounding the exposure? Where* did it occur? What was the *ambient temperature*? Was *submersion in water* involved? Was the patient's *skin or clothing wet* for other reasons?
2. *How long was the patient exposed* to these conditions?
3. Has the patient or others noted *mental status changes* or *incoordination*?
4. Has there been any *trauma*? The origin of the exposure must be explained. Trauma is a common antecedent.
5. Was the patient *acutely ill before the onset* of the current problem? Is the patient taking *any prescribed medications*?
6. Does the patient have any *chronic medical problems*? Is there a history of *alcohol or drug abuse*?

Factors that may predispose patients to the development of hypothermia are listed in Table 18–1.

Physical Examination

The key pathophysiologic findings in patients with hypothermia and the temperature level at which they occur are depicted in Table 18–2.

TABLE 18–1. Common Factors That Predispose to Hypothermia

Decreased Heat Production	Increased Heat Loss
Insufficient fuel	Environmental exposure
Hypoglycemia	Lack of acclimation, immersion, drowning
Starvation	Dermatologic abnormalities
Major exertion	Burns
Endocrinologic failure	Erythrodermas
Thyroid	Iatrogenic
Adrenal	Cold fluid infusions
Pituitary	Neonatal resuscitations or deliveries
Neuromuscular	Prolonged extrications
Age extremes	
Inactivity	**Miscellaneous**
Impaired Thermoregulation	Sepsis
	Multisystem organ failure
Centrally	Hypovolemia
Pharmacologic (e.g., anticholinergics)	Gastrointestinal hemorrhage
Toxicologic (e.g., opiates)	Myocardial infarction
Traumatic	
Peripherally	
Spinal cord injury	
Diabetes	

TABLE 18–2. Pathophysiologic Changes during Hypothermia

Centigrade	Fahrenheit	Findings
37.6	99.6	Normal rectal temperature
37	98.6	Normal oral temperature
35	95.0	Maximal shivering; increased metabolic rate
33	91.4	Apathy, ataxia, amnesia, dysarthria
31	87.8	Progressive decrease in level of consciousness, pulse, blood pressure, respiratory rate. Shivering stops
29	85.2	Dysrhythmias may occur, insulin not effective, pupils dilated; poikilothermia
27	80.6	Reflexes absent, no response to pain, comatose
25	77	Cerebral blood flow one-third normal, cardiac output one-half normal, significant hypotension
23	73.4	No corneal reflex, ventricular fibrillation risk is maximal
19	66.2	Asystole, flat electroencephalogram
16	60.8	Lowest temperature survived from accidental hypothermia
9	48.2	Lowest temperature survived from therapeutic hypothermia

Vital Signs. The core temperature defines the severity of hypothermia. Pulse, blood pressure, and respiratory rate are correspondingly depressed. The pulse rate decreases by 50% at a body temperature of 82.9°F (28.3°C). A Doppler-aided stethoscope is often required to detect blood flow. Tachycardia in the setting of significant hypothermia suggests concomitant problems such as sepsis, hypoglycemia, hypovolemia, or drug ingestion.

General Appearance. Initially, the patient will shiver, a reaction that is maximal at a temperature of 95°F (35°C). Shivering ceases by the time the temperature has fallen to 87.8°F (31°C). The skin is typically cold, firm, pale, or mottled.

Localized cutaneous damage from frostbite may be present.

Neurologic Examination. Early signs of hypothermia may be vague and include disorientation, moodiness, apathy, poor judgment, slurred speech, and ataxia. By the time the body temperature falls to 80.6°F (27°C), the patient is usually comatose, unresponsive to pain, and without reflexes. The Glasgow Coma Scale (see Chapter 31, Altered Mental Status) can serve as a means of tracking the patient's mental status. Focal neurologic deficits may occur secondary to hypothermia alone.

Complete Physical Examination. Because the effects of hypothermia involve multiple systems, cardiovascular, pulmonary, abdominal, rectal, and extremity examinations may demonstrate significant findings. Signs of trauma or concomitant or predisposing medical illness are also often noted. The abdominal examination is particularly unreliable in hypothermic patients because of cold-induced ileus and spasm of the rectus muscles. This examination is repeated as the patient's body temperature increases.

CLINICAL REASONING

In caring for the hypothermic patient, several key questions need to be addressed.

How Severe Is the Hypothermia?

The patient who is only mildly hypothermic (temperature above 93°F [34°C]) is not likely to develop complications and may be warmed slowly by passive external rewarming measures. With a body temperature below this level, dysrhythmias may occur, and rewarming should be more aggressive using active external and core rewarming techniques.

Is the Patient's Hemodynamic Status Appropriate for the Level of Temperature Depression?

Unexpectedly elevated or disproportionately depressed vital signs raise the question of concomitant disorders, such as trauma, hypovolemia, or endocrine disorders.

Is the Hypothermia Due to Primary Exposure, or Is It Secondary to Another Medical Problem?

Primary hypothermia, even when relatively severe, has a good prognosis when it is aggressively and appropriately treated. Secondary hypothermia is likely to be more difficult to treat and likely to respond more slowly. Treatment must include therapy for the underlying problem, as well as rewarming therapy. Extensive diagnostic testing is often necessary to confirm the underlying problem. The differential diagnosis is outlined in Table 18–3.

DIAGNOSTIC ADJUNCTS

The extent of ancillary testing depends on the degree of hypothermia, associated conditions, and response to rewarming. Mild accidental cases of hypothermia usually require no diagnostic tests.

TABLE 18–3. Causes of Hypothermia

Environmental Factors

    Exposure
    Near-drowning

Infections

    Meningitis
    Encephalitis
    Sepsis
    Pneumonia

Metabolic/Endocrine Factors

    Hypoglycemia
    Diabetic ketoacidosis
    Hypopituitarism
    Myxedema
    Addison's disease
    Uremia
    Malnutrition

Toxicologic Factors

    Alcohol
    Anesthetic agents
    Barbiturates
    Carbon monoxide
    Cyclic antidepressants
    Narcotics
    Phenothiazines

Neurologic Disorders

    Degenerative diseases
    Head trauma
    Spinal cord trauma
    Subarachnoid hemorrhage
    Cerebrovascular accidents
    Intracranial neoplasm

Vascular Factors

    Shock
    Pulmonary embolism
    Gastrointestinal hemorrhage

Dermatologic Factors

    Burns
    Erythrodermas
    Exfoliative dermatoses

Iatrogenic Factors

    Cold fluid infusion
    Exposure during treatment or delivery
    Prolonged extrication

On the other hand, secondary hypothermia and patients with a core temperature below 89.6°F (32°C) require extensive evaluation.

Laboratory Studies

Arterial Blood Gases. Oxygenation is impaired during hypothermia. There is decreased tissue perfusion, and the oxyhemoglobin dissociation curve is shifted to the left, leading to further impairment of oxygen release at the tissue level (Fig. 18–3). Some authorities have recommended correcting blood gas results for the body temperature. Correction actually leads to a false elevation of the PO_2. Therapeutic decisions are best based on the measured (uncorrected) PO_2 value.

The buffering capacity of cold blood is markedly reduced. As an example, a PCO_2 change of 10 mm Hg at 82.4°F (28°C) reduces the pH by approximately 0.16, whereas at normal body temperature the pH would change by only 0.08.

Complete Blood Cell Count. The hemoglobin may be decreased secondary to chronic blood loss or illnesses such as malnutrition, leukemia, or uremia. The hematocrit increases 2% for each 1°C drop in temperature. In severe cases, the increased hematocrit may interfere with the diagnosis of acute blood loss or chronic anemia.

The white blood cell count is reduced by sequestration and bone marrow depression during hypothermia. Even in the presence of serious infections, leukocytosis may not be seen.

Serum Electrolytes. Temperature has no consistent effect on sodium, chloride, or potassium concentrations. Serial measurements are needed during the rewarming process to assess the need for intervention. The serum potassium level is followed closely because hypokalemia is the most common finding. It is frequently caused by inappropriate antidiuretic hormone secretion or hypopituitarism. If hyperkalemia is identified, the patient is evaluated for evidence of renal failure or rhabdomyolysis.

Renal Function. Blood urea nitrogen and serum creatinine may be abnormal because of preexisting renal disease or dehydration. These tests are poor indicators of fluid status in hypothermic patients, but they may be useful in establishing baseline renal function because acute tubular necrosis is not uncommon after rewarming, especially in patients suffering from chronic hypothermia.

Serum Glucose Concentrations. Acute cold exposure elevates the serum glucose level because of catecholamine-induced breakdown of glycogen. An additional cause is the inactivity of insulin below 28°C to 30°C (82.4°F to 86°F). Persistently elevated glucose levels suggest pancreatitis or diabetic ketoacidosis.

Hypoglycemia usually results from glycogen depletion in the elderly, malnourished, or alcoholic patient.

Hemostasis Profile. Hemostatic studies including prothrombin time, partial thromboplastin time, platelet count, and fibrinogen level are performed in all patients with moderate-to-severe hypothermia. Cold induces thrombocytopenia, and clotting times are very prolonged in patients with core temperatures below 68°F (20°C). With rewarming, the coagulation profile usually returns to normal. Persistent changes suggest development of disseminated intravascular coagulation.

Serum Amylase and Lipase. Pancreatitis may be preexisting or may develop secondary to hypothermia. Because the abdominal examination is unreliable in the hypothermic patient, serum amylase or lipase elevation may be the only clue to the presence of pancreatitis. Hyperamylasemia has been shown to correlate with poor outcome in the hypothermic patient.

Toxicologic Studies. A full toxicologic screen is considered when there is a history suggestive of ingestion. Ethanol intoxication is one of the most common predisposing factors in hypothermia.

Urinalysis. The specific gravity is low (less than 1.010), because of cold-induced diuresis. There are no other consistent findings, but occult trauma or urinary tract infection is suggested by the finding of red blood cells or white blood cells and bacteria, respectively.

Cultures. Cultures of urine, sputum, and blood are indicated in all moderate-to-severe cases of hypothermia. Cultures from other body sites may also be indicated as suggested by the history and physical examination. Sepsis is a common cause of hypothermia and may also develop as a complication of accidental hypothermia.

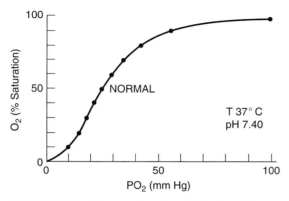

FIGURE 18–3 • The normal oxyhemoglobin dissociation curve at 37°C (98.6°F). Hypothermia shifts the curve to the left, as with alkalosis, and impairs oxygen release.

Radiologic Imaging

Plain Films. *Cervical spine films* are considered if trauma is suspected. Consider the possibility of a diving accident in all hypothermic submersion cases. A *chest radiograph* is necessary because pulmonary edema may develop during rewarming. Aspiration is relatively common in people with depressed mental status. Pneumonia and pneumothorax may be difficult to diagnose on physical examination in hypoventilating patients, making the chest radiograph even more important. An *abdominal series* may demonstrate pancreatic calcifications, pneumoperitoneum, ileus, or gastric dilatation.

Computed Tomography. Cranial computed tomography is considered if the mental status does not improve during rewarming or if there is evidence of head trauma.

Electrocardiogram

A 12-lead electrocardiogram is ordered in any patient with a temperature below 89.6°F (32°C). Atrial and ventricular arrhythmias are common in such patients, as is silent myocardial ischemia. A J or Osborne wave (see Fig. 18–2) may be present if the core temperature is below 89.6°F (32°C).

PRINCIPLES OF MANAGEMENT

Management principles for hypothermia include

- Prevention of further heat loss
- Initiation of life support techniques
- Rewarming the patient

Prevention of Heat Loss

All cold, wet clothing is cut off without manipulating the patient, a core temperature is obtained, and then the patient is covered with dry blankets. Respiratory heat loss is prevented by the administration of heated humidified oxygen.

Advanced Life Support

The recommendations for advanced life support in hypothermic patients continue to evolve. It has been suggested that endotracheal intubation can precipitate ventricular fibrillation in the hypothermic patient. Although the cold myocardium is susceptible to fibrillation, hypoxia, acidosis, and electrolyte disturbances are more common causes of ventricular fibrillation than mechanical stimulation. Because airway protection is critical, preoxygenation followed by careful intubation is still recommended in cases of severe hypothermia.

CPR is begun whenever asystole or ventricular fibrillation is seen on the cardiac monitor. The cold myocardium is resistant to defibrillation as well as to pharmacologic agents. After initial defibrillation with 200 J, 300 J, and then 360 J, CPR is resumed, and the patient is rewarmed to at least 86°F (30°C) before defibrillation is repeated. Many patients spontaneously convert to an organized cardiac rhythm at a core temperature of between 32°C and 35°C (89.6°F and 95°F).

The lower the temperature, the greater the protein binding of drugs. Therefore, most drugs will not be effective at normal doses. If large doses are used, toxicity can develop after rewarming. Generally, pharmacologic attempts to alter the pulse or blood pressure with vasopressors and cardiac medications are to be avoided. Sodium bicarbonate is rarely indicated. Lidocaine and procainamide are largely ineffective at cold temperatures, but bretylium has demonstrated some beneficial actions at low temperatures. Magnesium sulfate has also been shown to induce spontaneous defibrillation in patients with ventricular fibrillation.

Rewarming Techniques

The critical initial decision in rewarming the patient is determining the need for active versus passive rewarming. Patients with core temperatures of above 93°F (34°C) are candidates for passive external rewarming, whereas those with temperatures below 93°F require active rewarming.

Passive External Rewarming. Previously healthy patients who are only mildly hypothermic usually reheat themselves safely in a warm environment if they are covered in dry insulating materials. This technique is termed *passive external rewarming*. It is simple and noninvasive and can produce rewarming at a rate of 0.5°C to 1.0°C/hr.

Candidates for passive external rewarming must be able to generate sufficient endogenous heat. A variety of associated conditions can render patients unable to spontaneously rewarm (Table 18–4).

Active External Rewarming. There are a variety of active external rewarming techniques (Table 18–5). Direct application of heat to the extremities can be dangerous. This is particularly true in elderly and chronically hypothermic patients, in whom acute peripheral dilatation can result in rewarming shock. Core temperature afterdrop develops as the cold peripheral blood is shunted centrally. Active external rewarming of the trunk only is less likely to produce rewarming shock.

TABLE 18–4. Conditions Requiring Active Rewarming

Cardiovascular instability	Spinal cord injury
Core temperature below 90°F	Vasodilatation—pharmacologic, toxicologic
Extremes of age	Central nervous system disorders—cerebrovascular accident, trauma,
Fuel depletion—glycogen, fat, blood sugar	degenerative disease
Endocrinologic insufficiency	Failure to rewarm passively

TABLE 18–5. External Rewarming Options

Passive

Elimination of ongoing heat loss
Dry blankets in warm environment

Active

Hot packs
Electric blankets
Immersion

Use of active external rewarming is generally limited to young, previously healthy, acutely hypothermic patients. The most common forms of active external rewarming are warmed blankets and warmed forced air blankets. These allow for continuous monitoring of the patient and easy access in the event of an emergency. Rewarming baths and heating pads have been used in the past and are still available. Baths make monitoring and resuscitation difficult and defibrillation impossible. Heating pads are used with great care because cold, vasoconstricted skin is highly susceptible to thermal injury.

Active Core Rewarming. The techniques for active core rewarming are listed in Table 18–6. *Heated humidified oxygen* (40°C to 45°C) will transfer more heat when administered through an endotracheal tube than through a mask. Either way, further respiratory heat loss is prevented. As an additional advantage, supplemental oxygen is supplied. This technique is useful alone in mild

TABLE 18–6. Core Rewarming Options

Heated humidified oxygen
    Tube
    Mask
Heated intravenous fluids
Irrigation
    Bladder
    Stomach
    Colon
    Mediastinum
Peritoneal dialysis
Extracorporeal
    Hemodialysis
    Cardiopulmonary bypass
Diathermy

cases of hypothermia and is combined with other techniques in severe cases.

Intravenous fluids are *heated* to 40°C to 42°C. The heat transferred by this means becomes significant only when large volumes of fluid are required. Most patients with a body temperature of 32°C (89.6°F) will benefit from a 250- to 500-mL fluid challenge of heated 5% dextrose in isotonic crystalloid.

Heat transferred by means of *irrigation* of the stomach, bladder, and colon is limited. Mediastinal and thoracostomy tube irrigation are very invasive options. Peritoneal lavage with heated fluid is probably the preferred method of irrigation for rewarming. Delivery of heat by means of a 40°C to 45°C dialysate is expedited when two catheters and suction are used. Rewarming by means of peritoneal lavage is indicated in severe cases of hypothermia and in hypothermic patients with cardiac arrest prior to the availability of extracorporeal rewarming.

Extracorporeal rewarming is the most rapid method of rewarming. However, even in those facilities possessing the equipment and personnel for this technique, time is required to mobilize the resources. One technique that can be performed rapidly is partial cardiopulmonary bypass via the femoral vein and artery, if the equipment is available. Ideal candidates are patients with hypothermic cardiac arrest and patients with completely frozen extremities.

UNCERTAIN DIAGNOSIS

Once considered, uncertainty about the potential of hypothermia in a patient is easily assessed with a suitable core temperature measurement. Far more common is not thinking of potential hypothermia in patients at risk (see Tables 18–1 and 18–3) and trusting standard measuring devices that may not have the ability to measure low temperatures.

SPECIAL CONSIDERATIONS
Victims of Cold Water Drowning

Victims of drowning in water that is at or below 60°F (16°C) are far more likely to respond to resuscitative efforts than victims who have drowned in warm water. The protective effect of hypothermia is even more pronounced in children, one of whom reportedly recovered without neurologic sequelae after 66 minutes of immersion in icy water. Both the brain and the heart are protected by the cold. The mammalian diving reflex, often very effective in children, results in bradycardia and shunting of blood to the central circulation, both of which provide further protection.

In victims of cold water drowning, rewarming takes place in concert with other resuscitative maneuvers. Prolonged resuscitation efforts are indicated until the body temperature can be brought to near normal. Return of effective cardiac rhythm and recovery without neurologic sequelae may occur even after prolonged cardiac arrest.

Pediatric Patients

The most common form of hypothermia in children is neonatal hypothermia. The newborn, if unprotected, has very high conductive and convective heat losses because of a large body surface area compared to weight. Large evaporative heat losses also occur if the newborn's skin is not promptly dried of its covering of amniotic fluid. When childbirth occurs in emergency situations, attention to heat conservation is essential to prevent hypothermia. Radiant warmers are ideal for this purpose because they prevent heat loss without restricting access to the neonate.

Beyond the neonatal period, sepsis is the most common cause of hypothermia in infants. The finding of a low body temperature should prompt a thorough evaluation for a source of infection and early initiation of broad-spectrum antibiotics.

In older children, hypothermia is rare. Causes of hypothermia are similar to those seen in adults, the most common nonaccidental cause being malnutrition.

Patients with Local Hypothermia and Frostbite

Localized injury to the skin and underlying structures is commonly referred to as frostbite. Exposure to cold produces intense vasoconstriction in the cutaneous vessels, leading to impaired tissue perfusion. Persistent ischemia results in necrosis. Ice may form in the tissue as well, disrupting cell membranes and leading to further tissue destruction.

Localized hypothermia is described pathophysiologically in terms similar to those used for burns. Mild, first-degree frostbite is limited to the superficial epidermis. Erythema and mild edema occur and resolve without sequelae. Second-degree frostbite results in deeper epidermal involvement and presents as large, clear bullae. Third-degree injury is that due to full-thickness skin injury. In very severe cases, muscle, bone, and tendon injury may also occur.

The treatment of localized hypothermia is rapid rewarming. Thawing in circulating lukewarm water (40°C to 42°C) is the preferred technique. Reperfusion can be very painful, but complete thawing is essential to minimize tissue loss. Narcotic analgesics may be required during rewarming. Rewarmed body parts are highly susceptible to refreezing, leading to even greater tissue loss. If reexposure is anticipated, it is better not to thaw the tissue. In mild cases, topical ointments and nonsteroidal anti-inflammatory agents are adequate treatment. Topical aloe vera cream (Dermaide) is applied, and ibuprofen is given. The need for tetanus and streptococcal prophylaxis is also considered.

After localized hypothermia has occurred, it is very difficult to determine the viability of the involved tissue. Débridement is best delayed, sometimes for weeks, to preserve as much tissue as possible. Most patients are admitted for continued treatment and pain control.

DISPOSITION AND FOLLOW-UP

Admission

Patients presenting with moderate or severe hypothermia (core temperature of less than 89.6°F [32°C]) require admission to a monitored bed in the presence of

- Cardiovascular instability
- Significant predisposing factors (see Table 18–1)
- Metabolic or toxicologic abnormalities, such as renal insufficiency, electrolyte abnormalities, persistent hypoglycemia, or significant drug ingestion
- Delayed rate of rewarming. This is influenced by the rapidity of the patient's cooling. Those with gradual induction (usually the secondary causes) are rewarmed more slowly, at a rate of 1°C to 1.5°C per hour, because of dehydration and fluid sequestration problems.

Immediate transfer to a tertiary care facility is indicated only when the need for extracorporeal rewarming is anticipated. Examples are impending cardiac arrest in profoundly hypothermic patients and patients with completely frozen extremities.

Most with more severe secondary hypothermia will need to be admitted for further workup and care.

Discharge

Patients with mild primary accidental hypothermia (core temperature of 95°F to 89.6°F [35°C to 32°C]) can be safely rewarmed in the emergency department and discharged to a warm environment if they have no significant underlying disease. Caution is necessary to ensure that the patient is not discharged to return to the same environment that caused the hypothermia. Admission may be necessary while a safe disposition is worked out for the patient.

FINAL POINTS

- Endotracheal intubation is not contraindicated in patients with hypothermia. When indicated, intubation is preceded by preoxygenation and performed gently.
- Cold hearts fibrillate easily. Hypothermic patients are handled as gently as possible, but indicated procedures *are not* withheld.

- Pulses may be very difficult to palpate. An ultrasonic stethoscope is often required to detect blood flow. Chest compressions are started only after the cardiac monitor has documented asystole or ventricular fibrillation.
- Defibrillation of a cold heart is rarely successful in patients with a core temperature below 86°F (30°C). Defibrillation is indicated when ventricular fibrillation is recognized and is performed to a maximum of three times but *is not* repeated until the temperature is above 86°F (30°C).
- Most patients with a body temperature of 93°F (34°C) will benefit from a 250- to 500-mL fluid challenge of heated 5% dextrose in isotonic crystalloid.
- Passive external rewarming is ideal for most healthy patients with mild hypothermia.
- Active rewarming is necessary when the core temperature is below 93°F (34°C) and whenever thermogenesis is insufficient.
- Active external rewarming of the extremities may result in core temperature afterdrop.
- With hypothermia, protein binding of drugs increases and target organs become unresponsive. Pharmacologic therapy is frequently ineffective until rewarming is achieved.

CASE*Study*

A 63-year-old man was found collapsed in an alley after a cold night in December. Concerned neighbors called the rescue squad. The patient did not respond to verbal stimulation and groaned to painful stimulation. His pulse rate was 50 beats per minute, blood pressure 90/60 mm Hg, and respiratory rate 10 breaths per minute and shallow with breathing.

The patient arrived in the emergency department and was placed on a stretcher by the paramedics. He was recognizable to the staff as one of the "regulars," a homeless alcoholic. Because this ambulance run was the fourth in 15 minutes the stretcher was left in the hall as the staff took care of the more "critical" ambulance runs. A medical assistant who was sent to get a nitroglycerin drip for a patient with chest pain noticed that the man on the stretcher was blue and said to a nurse "he doesn't look good." The nurse stated "he always looks like that" and "hurry with that nitro." A few minutes later, another nurse passed the patient in the hall and found him blue and not breathing. At this point the patient became a priority.

Two cardinal rules about emergency medicine were broken in the care of this patient. First, every patient who comes in should be immediately screened for acuity of illness and stability. This patient had abnormal vital signs in the field and was not likely to have corrected them by the time he arrived. The second rule is that whenever another staff member, no matter what his or her "rank," states someone does not look good, this is cause for immediate evaluation. One of the biggest areas for mistakes to occur in the emergency department is becoming complacent with the "regulars."

The patient was found to be apneic and was intubated immediately. His pulse was not palpable in the radial area but was found to be 40 beats per minute in the carotid area. No blood pressure was obtainable. As the staff cut the clothes off his legs and arms, they noticed his skin to be cyanotic, mottled, and cold. A core temperature revealed a temperature of 85°F (29.4°C). The rest of his physical examination revealed the following:

HEENT: Abrasion/contusion to the left temporal area, otherwise normal
Heart: Bradycardic, no murmurs or rubs
Lungs: Decreased breath sounds on the left, no wheezes, rales, or rhonchi
Abdomen: No bowel sounds, no tenderness or masses
Neurologic: Glasgow Coma Scale score = 3

Continued on following page

Extremities: Cold, mottled, cyanotic, no deformities

The Glasgow Coma Scale comprises three categories: eye opening 1–4, verbal response 1–5, and motor response 1–6. The total score range is from 15, which is normal, to 3. This patient had no eye opening, no motor response, and no verbal response, giving him a total score of only 3, the lowest possible score.

The endotracheal tube was withdrawn 2 cm because the cause of the decreased breath sounds on the left was believed to be a right mainstem intubation. The breath sounds did not improve. As the staff pulled the clothes out from under the patient, blood was noticed on the patient's shirt. The patient was log rolled, and a single stab wound was seen on his left back. A chest tube was placed in the left chest, which produced 200 mL of blood and a rush of air. The breath sounds were now equal and clear.

Another cardinal rule is to talk to the paramedics, particularly when the patient cannot give a history. No one talked to the paramedics for this patient because he was a "regular" and everyone assumed they knew the story. The paramedics would have said they noticed a small amount of bleeding but could not figure out where it was from.

The tests that were performed and the results were as follows:

Cardiac monitor: Sinus bradycardia
Electrocardiogram: Sinus bradycardia
Chest radiograph: Chest tube in place on the left, lungs normal
C-spine radiograph: Normal
Complete blood cell count: Leukocytes, 10,200/mm^3; hemoglobin, 9.2 g/dL; hematocrit, 27.5%; platelets, 100,000/mm^3
Blood chemistries: Sodium, 139 mEq/L; potassium, 4.0 mEq/L; chloride, 100 mEq/L;bicarbonate, 19 mEq/L; blood

urea nitrogen, 22 mg/dL, creatinine, 1.0 mg/dL
Ethanol: 356 mg/dL
Toxicology screen: Negative
Computed tomography of the head: Atrophy, otherwise normal

To rewarm the patient the following measures were implemented:

- A warm forced air blanket was applied.
- Warmed humidified O_2 was administered through the endotracheal tube.
- Warmed crystalloid solutions were administered intravenously.
- Warmed crystalloid was irrigated through the chest tube.
- Because the stab wound was below the scapula, and therefore an intra-abdominal injury was suspected, a peritoneal lavage was performed. The return showed no evidence of blood, so warmed crystalloid was irrigated through the peritoneal catheter.

The patient was rewarmed over the next 8 hours and admitted to the intensive care unit. He was extubated the next day, and the chest tube was removed 2 days later. The patient was discharged to a shelter on the sixth hospital day.

Two other pearls for the emergency physician are demonstrated by this case. First, even if you have not had time to fully assess the patient, consider the chief complaint and the level of stability of each patient so that you can begin to form triage priorities and the order in which you will fully assess your patients. Second, patients can have more than one problem. This patient had four: hypothermia, stab wound to the chest, alcohol intoxication, and a forehead contusion. Do not narrow your differential diagnosis list until you have adequately ruled out critical life-threatening diagnoses.

Bibliography

TEXT

Danzl DF, Pozos RS, Hamlet MP: Hypothermia. In Auerbach P (ed): Wilderness Medicine: Management of Wilderness and Environmental Emergencies, 4th ed. St. Louis, CV Mosby, 2001.

JOURNAL ARTICLES

Antretter H, Dapunt OE, Bonatti J: Management of profound hypothermia. Br J Hosp Med 1995; 54:215–220.

Giesbrecht GG, Schroeder M, Bristow GK: Treatment of mild immersion hypothermia by forced-air warming. Aviat Space Environ Med 1994; 65:803–808.

Kloeck W, Cummins RO, Chamberlain D, et al: ILCOR Advisory statement: Special resuscitation situations. Circulation 1997; 95:2196–2210.

Larach MG: Accidental hypothermia. Lancet 1995; 345:493–498.

Steele MT, Nelson MJ, Sessler DL, et al: Forced air speeds rewarming in accidental hypothermia. Ann Emerg Med 1996; 27:476–484.

Weinberg AD: Hypothermia. Ann Emerg Med 1993; 22:370–377.

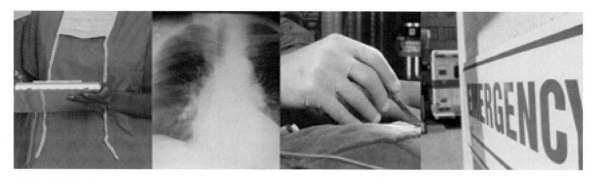

HEMATOLOGIC DISORDERS

CHAPTER 19

Sickle Cell Disease

PATRICIA LEE

CASE*Study*

A 27-year-old black man presents complaining of his "usual sickle pain" in the chest, abdomen, and back. It was unresponsive to home analgesics—acetaminophen with codeine. Initial examination reveals an anxious patient in obvious pain. His vital signs are blood pressure, 110/74 mm Hg; heart rate, 112 beats per minute; respiratory rate, 28 breaths per minute, and temperature, 101.5°F. The patient is requesting parenteral narcotics for pain control.

INTRODUCTION

Sickle cell disease (SCD) is the most commonly encountered genetic disease seen in patients presenting to the emergency department. It accounts for approximately 75,000 hospitalizations per year in the United States with an estimated average cost of $6,500 per hospitalization. SCD represents a challenging complex of manifestations, which range from mild discomfort to life-threatening catastrophe. To prevent serious morbidity and mortality, it is important to recognize and properly treat the manifestations and complications of sickle cell anemia.

Pathophysiology

Normal adult hemoglobin A (HbA) consists of four heme groups and four polypeptide chains: two α and, most commonly, two β chains. Sickle cell anemia is the result of the presence of a hemoglobin variant, hemoglobin S (HbS), which occurs when a single amino acid valine substitutes for glutamine at the sixth position of the β-hemoglobin chain. The gene of HbS is inherited as an autosomal recessive trait and is found in 8% to 10% of African Americans (sickle trait). The red cells of patients with sickle trait (HbAS) have an HbS concentration of 30% to 50%. In patients with sickle cell anemia (HbSS), 70% to 98% of hemoglobin is of the S type. Sickle cell trait is primarily asymptomatic, but hematuria and sickle complications can occur under severe dehydration, temperature or pressure change, or body stress.

Disease develops in persons who are homozygous for HbS or in heterozygous HbS patients possessing another abnormal hemoglobin, such as hemoglobin C (HbSC) or hemoglobin S β-thalassemia (HbS-βthal). In hemoglobin C there is a substitution of lysine for glutamic acid in the sixth amino acid position of the β-globin chain. β-Thalassemias are the result of a mutation that diminishes or eliminates the production of the β-globin subunit of hemoglobin. Sickle cell anemia, hemoglobin C, and hemoglobin S β-thalassemia comprise the majority of sickle cell syndromes. In persons who are homozygous for SCD, almost all hemoglobin is HbS with small amounts of hemoglobin F (HbF) and hemoglobin A_2. In the heterozygous state, only half of the hemoglobin is HbS.

Hemoglobin F has a protective role in SCD; higher HbF levels are associated with less sickling and a milder disease. In children, HbF is produced and falls to adult levels by the age of 4 to 5 months of age, accounting for the lack of symptoms in this age group.

When oxygenated, HbS shows near-normal solubility. When deoxygenated, HbS tetramers polymerize, forming long parallel rods within the red blood cell. These sickle-shaped cells cannot modify their shape while traveling though the capillary beds. They become trapped in the microcirculation, resulting in an increased blood viscosity and sludging. Sludging reduces blood flow and leads to local tissue hypoxia and acidosis, local blockage of circulation, and tissue ischemia. In addition, the "hard" sickle cells can physically damage the endothelium. The endothelium may vasoconstrict and release specific factors that promote more sludging and occlusion. Blockage can occur in virtually any organ in the body, leading to the painful "sickle crisis."

Sickling is enhanced when the oxygen-dissociation curve shifts rightward, as occurs with acidosis or increased 2,3-diphosphoglycerate or under conditions of vascular stasis, dehydration, high concentrations of HbS, and low oxygen tension. Sickling can be reversed to a degree with reoxygenation, but repetitive sickling and unsickling ultimately damages the red blood cell membrane. The spleen and liver remove the damaged cells, creating anemia. Sickled red blood cells are rapidly hemolyzed and may survive only 10 to 20 days, as compared with the normal red blood cell life span of 120 days.

The spleen and kidney have extensive capillary beds and often undergo multiple infarctions during a single sickle cell crisis. The end result is that most patients are functionally asplenic early in life and are highly susceptible to infection. Most patients are unable to concentrate urine because of a damaged renal countercurrent exchange system.

Epidemiology

It is estimated that 70,000 Americans of different ethnic backgrounds have SCD, including persons with eastern Mediterranean, Indian, or Saudi Arabian ancestry. About 0.2%, or 1 in 400, African Americans have sickle cell anemia (HbSS disease). After the first decade, two distinct groups of patients emerge. The first group, consisting of 10% to 15% of patients with SCD, continues to have frequent crises requiring hospital admission. The second (and larger) group rarely requires admission. After the first decade, the mortality rate decreases markedly and is spread evenly over the next four decades. As the result of treatment advances, children with SCD have about an 85% probability of reaching 20 years of age. The median age of death is 42 years for men and 48 years for women (SS disease). Eighteen percent of deaths are caused by organ failure (renal disease, congestive heart failure, or complications of chronic stroke). The majority of deaths result from complications of infectious disease.

Risk factors associated with poor outcomes in SCD are low levels of fetal hemoglobin and an elevated baseline white blood cell count. Improved health care programs for patients with SCD have reduced the incidence of hospital visits from 17.9 visits per year per patient in 1982 to 3.5 visits per year per patient in 1998.

Current Research

Research is ongoing to find new treatments for acute vaso-occlusive episodes using drugs to reduce sickling and sludging and treatments for preventing end-organ ischemia and infarction. Artificial blood is under development and could provide small molecules of hemoglobin that would allow oxygen to be transported through partially obstructed microvasculature. The future for patients with SCD is optimistic. The benefits of genetic engineering offer a cure for this devastating chronic disease. Recently, two parents with sickle cell trait achieved an unaffected pregnancy using preimplantation genetic diagnosis.

INITIAL APPROACH AND STABILIZATION

The initial approach to a patient with sickle cell anemia focuses on rapid assessment of vital signs, consideration of disease manifestations, and management of complications. Early treatment proceeds concomitantly with evaluation.

Priority Diagnoses

All sickle cell patients are considered at risk for the major crises associated with this disease:

- Infection
- Sequestration
- Aplastic anemia
- Vaso-occlusion of cerebral or myocardial vessels

Patients are aggressively managed if any of the following high-risk factors exist:

- Fever greater than 101°F (38.3°C)
- Severe abdominal pain
- Acute pulmonary symptoms
- Neurologic symptoms
- Pain associated with extremity weakness or loss of function
- Acute joint swelling
- Recurrent vomiting
- Pain not relieved by conservative measures
- Priapism

Rapid Assessment/Early Intervention

Every patient with sickle cell anemia, regardless of presenting complaint, requires rapid evaluation of vital signs and level of consciousness. Patients with altered mental status, hypotension, or fever are seen immediately by an experienced physician. Signs of the potentially life-threatening illnesses are actively sought during the assessment.

Initial management includes the following steps:

1. If the patient has tachycardia or hypotension, an intravenous line is established for venous access and possible hydration. If the patient is normotensive and able to tolerate liquids, oral hydration may be provided.
2. A pain assessment is made and adequate analgesia is provided. Analgesia is provided in quantities sufficient to resolve the patient's

complaint of pain. Studies have failed to support the finding of overwhelming addiction in patients with SCD and, in fact, have repeatedly found that these patients are usually undertreated.

3. Controversy exists about the use of oxygen in sickle cell crisis because experts state that chronic use will decrease erythropoiesis. However, any sickle cell patient in respiratory distress or with documented hypoxia is given oxygen.

4. Early antibiotic therapy directed at potential pathogens should be initiated for febrile or septic-appearing patients.

5. Cardiac monitoring is maintained.

Patients with stable vital signs and no neurologic symptoms usually do not require immediate treatment. They may be triaged for urgent evaluation.

CLINICAL ASSESSMENT

Patients with SCD are usually well aware of their diagnosis. The goals of the clinical assessment are to determine the usual nature of their disease, identify the types of crises, identify precipitating causes, screen for complications of SCD, and diagnose causes of pain unrelated to SCD.

History of Present Illness

Pain. Pain is the most common complaint. It is often, but not always, the result of vaso-occlusive crisis and ongoing ischemia. The history should include questions designed to determine whether the crisis is *similar to prior painful crises*, whether any identifying *precipitating cause* exists, and whether any *occult complications* of SCD exist.

The pain is qualified by asking if the pain is different in location, quality, or intensity from that of previous crises. The patient is asked what *alleviates* or *exacerbates* the *pain*, what has been *done to treat* the pain, and what *associated symptoms* exist.

The majority of patients with painful crises complain, in decreasing order of frequency, of pain in the lumbosacral spine, the thigh and hip, the knee, the abdomen, the shoulder, and the chest. The pain is frequently described as gnawing or throbbing. Pain that differs from previous patterns needs to be considered as a separate but often related process (e.g., cholecystitis, pulmonary infarction, osteomyelitis, or myocardial infarction).

Fever. Fever is a cause for serious concern in patients with SCD because of their decreased ability to fight certain infections. This immune defect, the result of a functional asplenia, primarily affects the ability to destroy encapsulated organisms such as *Streptococcus pneumoniae, Haemophilus influenzae,* and *Neisseria meningitidis.* Overwhelming sepsis remains a leading cause of death. Questions should be designed to determine the *potential focus of the infection,* such as acute chest syndrome, sinusitis, sepsis, or urinary tract infection.

Neurologic Symptoms. The occurrence of *new-onset focal neurologic deficits* or *altered mental status* is a devastating complication of SCD. As many as 6% to 13% of patients younger than the age of 10 may present with a cerebral infarction.

Other Symptoms. *Generalized weakness, fatigability,* and *nonspecific complaints* may relate to profound anemia or severe hemolysis.

Precipitating Factors. *Common precipitants* are infection, dehydration, increased anemia, acidosis from any cause, emotional stress, extreme temperature exposure, or ingestion of substances such as alcohol or other recreational drugs. A history of 3 or more pain crises per year is a marker of severe disease and early mortality. Less than 10% of patients with SCD have three or more pain crises per year.

Past Medical History

Previous SCD Crises. Many patients are very familiar with the manifestations of their disease and can clearly identify whether the present crisis is similar to those previously. Many patients are also aware of past complications, hospitalizations, treatment plans, and baseline hemoglobin. In adults, frequently no precipitating factor can be identified. In children, viral illness is believed to be the most frequent trigger.

Known Complications. Chronic organ damage is one of the devastating sequelae of SCD. A review of high yield areas for complicating problems is essential in developing the clinical assessment. Table 19–1 outlines an organ system approach to common complications.

Surgical History. Determination of previous surgical procedures can be of great benefit in evaluating a painful abdomen (e.g., previous cholecystectomy or appendectomy).

Medications. Assessing to what degree the patient benefited from previous medications is important to help devise the current treatment plan. Knowledge of previous home, emergency department, and hospitalization medications is useful in understanding the nature of the patient's disease, individual pain tolerance, and likelihood of effectiveness of emergency department treatment.

TABLE 19–1. Organ Systems Approach to the Physical Examination and Complications of Sickle Cell Disease

System	Specific Component	Physical Finding	Known Complications
Vital signs	Temperature	Fever in children may indicate infectious disease. In adults low-grade fever often accompanies vaso-occlusive crisis. Elevations greater than 101°F should be considered secondary to infection	Relative immunosuppression, especially against encapsulated bacteria
	Blood pressure	Hypotension could result from splenic sequestration or septic shock	Relative immunosuppression, as above
	Heart rate	Tachycardia may indicate fever, sepsis, impending shock	Relative immunosuppression, as above
	Respiratory rate	Tachypnea may indicate pulmonary disease or acute anemia	Relative immunosuppression or aplastic crisis; pulmonary embolism, infarct, or infection
Head, eyes, ears, nose, and throat	Ears, throat	Signs of otitis media, upper respiratory infection	Common source of encapsulated bacteria
	Eyes	Decreased visual acuity, funduscopic examination that is "blurry" or shows retinal damage	Retinal hemorrhages are common
		Pale conjunctiva	Suggests severe anemia
	Neck	Meningeal signs	Meningitis is 600 times more common in children with sickle cell disease
Cardiac		S_3 gallop, rub, or ischemic murmurs	Congestive heart failure, myocardial infarction
Pulmonary		Rales, pleural rub, decreased breath sounds with dull percussion from effusion, signs of consolidation	Intrapulmonary shunting, embolism, infarct, infection
Gastrointestinal		Guarding and rebound are common in abdominal crisis. Presence of bowel sounds is best physical finding consistent with crisis rather than with acute surgical abdomen. Enlarged spleen in children may indicate splenic sequestration	Hepatitis, liver infarcts. Bilirubin gallstones are common. Mesenteric infarcts. Splenic sequestration. Abdomen is common site of painful "crisis" without obvious site of injury.
Genitourinary	Kidney	Costovertebral angle tenderness	Hyposthenuria, hematuria, papillary necrosis, urinary tract infections
	Genitalia	Complete examination warranted particularly in abdominal crisis or priapism	Impotence, priapism, decreased fertility
Skeletal	Hands and feet	Painful swelling of dorsa of hands and feet	Hand and foot syndrome
	Joints and long bones	Painful swollen joints, point tenderness on a long bone	Osteomyelitis, infarction, septic necrosis of hips
Central nervous system		Focal defect or altered mental status	Meningitis and cerebrovascular accident type is more frequent in sickle cell disease
Skin		Pretibial or malleolar ulcers, signs of cutaneous infection	Stasis ulcers

Family History. Family history may be useful in establishing the initial diagnosis of sickle cell anemia.

Physical Examination

Because SCD affects the total body, a rapid, but complete and systematic examination should be performed to identify potential complications and manifestations of SCD. The physical examination should focus on hematologic, infectious, neurologic, chest, abdominal, and musculoskeletal findings, with special attention directed at the bony skeleton, lungs, heart, skin, and sinuses (see Table 19–1).

CLINICAL REASONING

The following questions are addressed.

Is the Patient Having an Acute Crisis? If so, Can It Be Categorized into the Major Types?

Unless the patient has no previous record of sickle cell anemia or the suspicion for drug-seeking behavior is very high, the physician should assume that the "crisis" is real and focus on identification of the type and initiation of appropriate workup and management.

The following questions are designed to assist the physician in determining the predominant crisis type:

1. *Is pain the major problem? If so, where is it located?* Pain is the overwhelming symptom of vaso-occlusive crisis. As a general rule, a patient's vaso-occlusive crisis pain is similar to that of previous crises.
2. *Is fever present?* Sepsis is a life-threatening complication of SCD. Fever may occur with sepsis or other infectious manifestations.
3. *Are there any neurologic complaints or focal deficits?* Neurologic crisis is the only vaso-occlusive crisis that is painless.
4. *Are the patient's vital signs normal?* Hypotension may occur with splenic sequestration. Shock may occur as a result of dehydration or sepsis.

Figure 19–1 is designed to assist in working through the differential diagnosis for the patient with SCD.

Most patients with SCD have multiple crises that may be categorized as hematologic, infectious, or vaso-occlusive. *Hematologic crises* usually involve decreased red cell mass, owing to increased cell destruction or occasionally acute decreased production. *Infectious crises* result from infections with encapsulated bacteria, such as *S. pneumoniae, H. influenzae, N. meningitidis,* and *Salmonella.* When repetitive episodes of vascular obstruction lead mostly to pain, they are called painful or vaso-occlusive crises. More severe episodes of vascular occlusion can lead to tissue infarction. *Vaso-occlusive crises* result in ischemia to a variety of organs, usually those with high blood flow, such as lung, brain, and spleen. One crisis type may coexist with another either as a cause or effect (e.g., aplastic crisis with infection, vaso-occlusive crisis at more than one location).

Hematologic Crisis

The spleen and liver remove sickled red blood cells after they become trapped in the reticuloendothelial system. The result is a chronic hemolytic anemia and a compensatory reticulocytosis. Eventually the spleen becomes irreparably damaged by recurrent vaso-occlusion and ischemia. By puberty, most patients' spleens are scarred down to a small nonfunctional fibrous mass.

Hyperhemolytic crisis is characterized by an increased rate of red blood cell destruction, as evidenced by decreasing hemoglobin levels and increased reticulocyte count and indirect bilirubin and lactate dehydrogenase levels. This crisis may occur during a sickle cell pain crisis. The etiology is variable and may include infectious causes, such as *Mycoplasma,* delayed hemolytic transfusion reactions, and coexistent glucose-6-phosphate dehydrogenase (G6PD) deficiency with oxidant stress.

Splenic sequestration crisis occurs usually in children younger than 6 years old. Cases have been reported in young adults. Sickled cells obstruct the splenic outflow, causing massive sequestration and removal of large amounts of red blood cells from circulation. Because as much as 30% of their blood volume may be sequestered, these patients may present in profound hypovolemic shock and may require aggressive fluid and transfusion therapy. The cause of this massive sequestration is unknown, but many authorities suspect viral illness as the precipitating factor. Treatment is aggressive transfusion or red cell exchange transfusion.

Hepatic sequestration crisis may also occur; however, it is seen later in life. The patient has a rapidly enlarging liver and falling hematocrit.

Aplastic anemia may occur in any age group, although it typically is seen in patients 6 months to young adulthood. Normally, the bone marrow of patients with SCD operates at the upper limits of

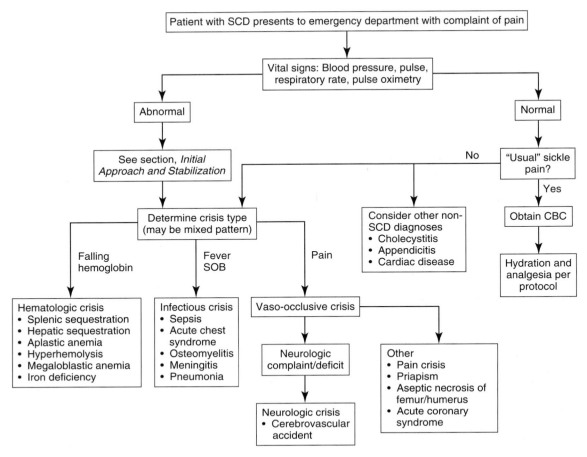

FIGURE 19–1 • Algorithm for sickle cell disease (SCD) differential diagnosis.

erythropoiesis. Aplastic anemia occurs when the patient's bone marrow is suppressed or undersupplied and fails to adequately compensate for the ongoing destruction of sickled cells. An aplastic crisis is manifested by a significant drop in the baseline hemoglobin combined with a low reticulocyte count. Viral infection with parvovirus B19 (the causative agent of "fifth disease" or erythema infectiosum) is a common cause of aplastic crisis, but other organisms, such as pneumococci, *Salmonella*, streptococci, and Epstein-Barr virus, also have been implicated. Folate deficiency and bone marrow toxins, such as phenylbutazone, are other common causes. Commonly, a prodrome of symptoms precedes the onset of aplastic anemia (e.g., fever, headache, abdominal pain, and upper respiratory tract symptoms). Aplastic crisis usually terminates spontaneously after 5 to 10 days.

Megaloblastic anemia may occur as a result of folate deficiency caused by lack of supplementation or poor dietary intake. Folic acid becomes rapidly depleted in patients with SCD, because of enhanced erythropoietic activity. Folate supplementation is important to replenish stores and lower high homocysteine levels, which have been linked to cardiovascular and cerebrovascular disease.

Iron deficiency anemia may be encountered in patients with SCD because of increased erythropoiesis and demands for iron metabolism. SCD is typically associated with a normocytic, normochromic anemia. Iron deficiency is characterized by hypochromic microcytic red cell morphology, and iron supplementation should be provided when it occurs.

Infectious Crisis

Infectious crises are the most frequent complication resulting in hospitalization and death (in all ages). Patients with SCD are immunocompromised secondary to functional asplenia, a defective complement system, and inadequate opsonins. They are susceptible to infections with encapsulated organisms, and septic shock may be associated with functional asplenia.

Overwhelming sepsis is the leading cause of death in sickle cell patients younger than 5 years of age. Encapsulated organisms, such as *S. pneumoniae, H. influenzae,* and *N. meningitidis* are common pathogens. *S. pneumoniae* is the predominant pathogen for children younger than 5 years of age. Other frequently encountered organisms are *Mycoplasma pneumoniae, Escherichia coli, Staphylococcus aureus*, and *Salmonella*.

The source of infection is frequently otitis media or a pulmonary source, but it may often be occult. Meningitis, pneumonia, and osteomyelitis are not uncommon. *Salmonella* osteomyelitis should be suspected in patients with fever and bone pain.

Acute chest syndrome is a complex of pulmonary symptoms that includes a pulmonary infiltrate. Thirty percent of adults initially present with extremity pain crisis. In children, primary infection is believed to be the cause; in adults, infarction generally precedes the syndrome. This clinical illness tends to be severe, prolonged, and difficult to treat; SCD patients with acute chest syndrome may suddenly experience deterioration of their condition. Hypoxia associated with the acute chest syndrome may promote even more sickling and other manifestations of the disease.

Vaso-occlusive Crisis

Vaso-occlusion, also called a sickle pain crisis, is the most common crisis seen in patients with SCD. Pain crises account for more than 90% of SCD hospital admissions. Vaso-occlusion may occur in any organ, and patients may present with resultant disease in any organ system. The most common complaints of pain are abdominal, bone and joint, priapism, hand and foot, pulmonary, and renal. Pain frequently occurs at more than one site (e.g., abdomen and bone). It can be difficult to sort out vaso-occlusive pain from a more serious underlying pathologic process, such as appendicitis. The frequency of pain crises varies with each individual and depends on the patient's hemoglobin phenotype, physical condition, concurrent illness, and psychological or social factors.

1. Vaso-occlusive pain is a self-limited and reversible pain that may last minutes to weeks.
2. There are no laboratory findings pathognomonic for pain crisis. The hemoglobin level is generally at baseline, and the white blood cell count is mildly elevated. If the white blood cell count is markedly elevated above baseline, an infectious cause should be sought.

3. *Neurologic crisis* is a subset of vaso-occlusive crisis. Any patient with SCD who presents with a neurologic deficit is a true emergency. Immediate consultation is recommended, with a plan for emergency exchange transfusion.

Has the Patient Had, or Is the Patient Having, a Significant Complication Related to the SCD?

The initial challenge when seeing a patient with sickle cell anemia is to identify which major manifestation is present and then evaluate for associated life-threatening complications (see Table 19–1). The following mnemonic **HBSS PAIN CRISIS** also is useful in remembering the *common complications* seen in patients with SCD:

Hemolysis, hand-foot syndrome
Bone marrow hyperplasia/infarction
Stroke: thrombotic or hemorrhagic, subarachnoid hemorrhage
Skin ulcers (usually leg)
Pain crisis, priapism, psychosocial problems
Anemia, aplastic crisis, avascular necrosis
Infections: central nervous system, pulmonary, genitourinary, bone, joints
Nocturia: urinary frequency from hyposthenuria
Cholelithiasis, cardiomegaly, congestive heart failure, acute chest syndrome
Retinopathy, renal failure, renal concentrating defects
Infarction: bone, spleen, central nervous system, muscle, bowel, renal
Sequestration crisis in spleen or liver
Increased fetal demise
Sepsis

DIAGNOSTIC ADJUNCTS

Laboratory Studies

Ideally, a record of each patient's baseline laboratory values should be maintained and available for reference and comparison with current studies.

Complete Blood Cell Count (CBC). A CBC is mandatory to evaluate a patient's SCD. SCD erythrocytes typically are normocytic and normochromic. The mean corpuscular hemoglobin concentration is approximately 90 μm^3/cell (normal range: 86 to 98 μm^3/cell).

Hemoglobin/Hematocrit. The hemoglobin in SCD is usually low, between 7 and 8 g/dL (normal range, 14 to 18 g/dL in males, 12 to 16 g/dL in females) (Table 19–2). The measured hemoglobin/hematocrit should be compared with the patient's baseline values if known. A decrease of

TABLE 19–2. Mean Values and Ranges for Patients with Sickle Cell Anemia

	Mean	Range
Hemoglobin (g/dL)	7.5	5.5–9.5
Hematocrit (%)	22	17–29
Reticulocyte count (%)	12	5–30
White blood cell count (permm^3)	13,000	12,000–15,000

more than 2 g/dL in hemoglobin or 4% to 9% in hematocrit indicates aplastic crisis, splenic sequestration, hemolysis, or ongoing blood loss.

White Blood Cell Count. The white blood cell count is generally elevated in patients with SCD because of increased bone marrow activity secondary to the chronic anemic state. A white blood cell count greater than 20,000/mm^3, particularly if accompanied by a left shift, should raise the suspicion of a bacterial infection. It is important to know that significant infection may exist in spite of a normal band count.

Platelet Count. The platelet count is generally high, representing chronic increased marrow activity and "auto-splenectomy," because platelets are not stored in the nonfunctional spleen.

Peripheral Smear. A blood smear should reveal sickled cells. Howell-Jolly bodies are frequently seen with loss of normal splenic function. The presence of many nucleated red blood cells represents bone marrow stress and may indicate impending aplastic crisis, splenic sequestration, hemolysis, or ongoing blood loss.

Reticulocyte Count. The reticulocyte count is typically elevated. A reticulocyte count should be obtained whenever the patient's hemoglobin level has decreased from baseline (by 2 g/dL); for new patients, a reticulocyte count should be ordered with the initial CBC. In SCD the typical absolute reticulocyte count is three to four times the upper limit of normal. A reticulocyte count less than 3% or lower than the patient's usual value may suggest an aplastic crisis. A reticulocyte count of greater than 12%, particularly if accompanied by numerous nucleated red blood cells, may indicate rapid hemolysis and require admission for transfusion.

Electrolytes. As a general rule, electrolyte assays are not required; however, patients with SCD may have renal complications.

Urinalysis. A urinalysis is appropriate for any sickle cell patient presenting with fever or dysuria. Infection is suspected when pyuria is found. Hematuria or the presence of tissue in the urine suggests nephritis or papillary necrosis. Most patients with SCD have hyposthenuria or inability to concentrate the urine. Urine specific gravity is generally 1.010 to 1.012; and if it is more than 1.025, the patient may have sickle cell trait or drug-seeking behavior may be suspected.

Arterial Blood Gas (ABG) Analysis. It is appropriate to order arterial blood gas analysis when evaluating sickle cell patients who present with respiratory distress or a lower than normal pulse oximetry. Frequently, clinicians are surprised by the degree of hypoxemia, and an ABG analysis is appropriate for any sickle cell patient presenting with fever and pulmonary symptoms. Patients who are hypoxic with acute chest syndrome are at high risk for deterioration of their condition. Hypoxic patients with rapidly progressing pneumonia require intensive care and may require early endotracheal intubation.

Blood Cultures. Any sickle cell patient with unexplained fever should have at least two blood cultures obtained, from different sites or at different times.

Sputum Gram's Stain and Culture. Any sickle cell patient with pneumonia and productive cough ideally should have a sputum Gram's stain performed to assist in antibiotic selection. Sputum culture should be performed to identify a causative organism and guide therapy.

Radiologic Imaging

Chest Radiographs. Sickle cell patients with pulmonary signs or symptoms or unexplained fever should have a chest radiograph. Pneumonia occurs in patients with SCD at a rate four times that of those without the disease.

Bone Radiographs. Patients with sickle cell anemia commonly have bone changes, especially avascular necrosis. Bone films should be obtained when the patient presents with bone or joint pain that is well localized and different from that of previous pain crises. Osteomyelitis should be considered in patients with fever and well-defined bone pain; however, pain with early osteomyelitis and infarction may be poorly differentiated on the radiograph.

Bone Scan. A bone scan is the preferred method to evaluate for early osteomyelitis (the first 2 to 3 weeks of onset).

Abdominal Ultrasonography. Gallbladder disease is a frequent complication of SCD, owing to the increased hemolysis, with production of heme-pigmented gallstones. Ultrasonography is a useful noninvasive procedure for identification of stones within the gallbladder, gallbladder wall thickening, pericolic fluid, or other signs of cholecystitis.

Head Computed Tomography. Nonenhanced computed tomography of the brain should be immediately performed on any patient with SCD who presents with neurologic deficits.

EXPANDED DIFFERENTIAL DIAGNOSIS

Once the crisis has been determined to be of the hematologic, infectious, or vaso-occlusive type, it may be necessary to refine the differential diagnosis to include subsets of disease. Vaso-occlusive crisis is the most common. The primary symptom of pain may represent the "simple vaso-occlusive crisis," or it may reflect an underlying pathologic process in a specific organ system, such as cholecystitis. See Table 19–3 for a list of subsets of vaso-occlusive crisis. Hematologic and infectious crises are less common. A discussion of variations is found earlier under "Clinical Reasoning." A discussion of issues relevant to the pediatric patient is presented under "Special Considerations." The clinician must always maintain a healthy suspicion that the patient may have a medical illness that is a complication of SCD or that two crisis types present simultaneously.

PRINCIPLES OF MANAGEMENT

General Management

Analgesia and hydration are the predominant interventions for patients presenting with vaso-occlusive crisis. Additional management is directed at the specific crisis type.

Analgesia

Analgesia remains the mainstay of supportive therapy for patients with SCD. Approximately two thirds of all patients with SCD rarely seek hospital-based treatment and manage their pain crises at home. Inability to control pain at home is generally what brings the sickle cell patient to the emergency department. Pain crises generally occur over hours but may last weeks. Inadequate or ineffective pain control has led to many confrontations and suspicions on the part of both the emergency physician and the patient. Appropriate management of this disease should include adequate pain control. Emergency physicians should recognize that withholding adequate pain medication may have moral, ethical, sociologic, or even racial overtones and that the sickle cell patient in pain is under stress and may have diminished coping skills.

Many protocols and regimens have been developed to treat the pain of SCD. Pain therapy should use medications that are safe and rapid in onset of action (Table 19–4). Ideally, these medications should be given on a fixed time schedule and at an appropriate dosing interval for maximal response. This approach will allow for a steady-state serum drug level that will improve the control of pain, minimize complications, and decrease anxiety. Titration dose methods or patient-controlled analgesia (PCA) devices are the preferred treatment methods. The oral route of administration is the safest and should be encouraged. Side effects of narcotic analgesics include itching from histamine release, respiratory depression, nausea, vomiting, hypotension, constipation, increased bladder tone, urinary retention, and decreased seizure threshold. These agents should be used in a well-supervised manner. Analogue or "0 to 10" pain scales should be used to assess pain levels and response to therapy.

The most important element of pain management for sickle cell patients is consistency and the knowledge that a protocol is being followed. The use of a protocol is encouraged because it decreases the wide variety of analgesics prescribed by physicians, including placebo dosing, and improves overall patient satisfaction that medication will be dispensed reliably and in a timely manner. A sample protocol for pain management is outlined in Figure 19–2.

Hydration

Dehydration increases sickling, and rehydration remains a mainstay of therapy. Most sickle cell patients are volume depleted by 1 to 2 L at presentation. Ideally, the patient should be rehydrated orally. Years of venipunctures for blood collection and intravenous catheters may result in scarred veins, preventing easy venous access. Patients who cannot or will not drink 8 to 12 ounces of fluid an hour are given fluid intravenously. Usually one and one-half the patient's daily requirement is given at a rate of 250 mL/hr. Because of hyposthenuria, the use of dextrose 5% in 0.45 normal saline is recommended, although normal saline is used with good success. Theoretically, the lower hypotonic solution reduces sickling by lowering the serum osmolality, thereby moving water back into the red blood cell and reducing the intracellular concentration of HbS. Because these patients are at risk for congestive heart failure, a conservative, closely monitored volume replacement regimen is recommended.

Oxygen

Surprisingly, increasing the PaO_2 by using supplemental oxygen has not been shown to be effective

TABLE 19–3. Subsets of Vaso-occlusive Crises

Subset	Frequency	Supporting History	Physical Examination	Diagnostic Tests	Differential Diagnosis	Comment
Abdominal	Common	Relatively acute onset; diffuse, poorly localized visceral pain Repetitive pattern from crisis to crisis Occasionally more typical of cholecystitis, hepatitis	Signs of peritoneal irritation are uncommon Occasionally localized to organ involved, particularly gallbladder	Interpretation of complete blood cell count difficult. No other characteristic test, although gallbladder ultrasound useful	Mesenteric infarction, cholecystitis, appendicitis, pancreatitis, hepatitis, pelvic inflammatory disease	30% of patients have pigmented gallstones by age 10; 70% by age 30. Less than 10% are symptomatic. Acute hepatic crises with sinusoidal sickling may imitate acute cholecystitis.
Bone and joint	Most common presenting complaint in emergency department—up to 50% of adults	Patient usually >2 years old. Rapid onset of deep aching pain; once it peaks, it tends to remain at that level. Repetitive pattern from crisis to crisis. Frequency varies by individual.	Occasionally local tenderness. More often, deep bone pain without physical findings	Radiographs are seldom diagnostic unless there are chronic changes of osteomyelitis. Bone scan may be useful early in course.	Osteomyelitis, septic arthritis, rheumatic fever, gout	The slow sinusoidal circulation of the bone marrow is a common site for sickling.
Cerebrovascular	Common—occurs in up to 26% of patients with symptomatic disease	Acute onset of any neurologic symptom: aphasia, headache, hemiparesis, cranial nerve palsy, altered mental status, seizure Cerebrovascular accident more common in children and young adults. Mean age at onset is 10 years. Intracranial hemorrhage more common in older group	Consistent with type of process and location of injury	Computed tomography necessary in emergency department. If normal, follow with lumbar puncture to assess possible subarachnoid hemorrhage. Angiography may be necessary. Contrast material can cause sickling.	Subarachnoid hemorrhage, intracerebral hemorrhage	Represents 16% of all causes of death in children with sickle cell disease. Tendency to recur Central nervous system damage (nonfocal) in 5 to 9 times as many patients, primarily cognitive impairment.
Hand and foot syndrome	Most common initial presentation of sickle cell disease in infancy, rare thereafter	Usually occurs in children <3 years old. One to four extremities may be affected.	Painful nonpitting edema of dorsa of hands and feet	Radiologic changes of periosteal elevation and/or bone necrosis may not appear for 1 week or longer.	Osteomyelitis, septic arthritis, rheumatic fever	Etiology is microinfarction of carpal and tarsal bones.
Priapism	Rare as complaint in emergency department, although reported to occur in up to 30% of men	Painful prolonged nonsexual penile erection persisting more than several hours. Seventy-five percent of cases occur between 12	Painful erection may be partial	None	None in sickle cell disease, although can be seen in leukemia and hyperviscosity syndromes	A more common form is "stuttering priapism"—painful reversible erection. This may precede more severe form.

System	Incidence	Symptoms	Signs	Laboratory	Differential Diagnosis	Comments
	and 6 AM. Increases in frequency and severity with advancing age. Some degree of impotence in 25% of cases					Normal sexual function may remain in 40% to 60% of men.
Pulmonary	Common—occurs in up to 50% of patients, more common in pediatric and more severe in adults	Acute-onset pleuritic chest pain, cough and dyspnea. Often preceded by other vaso-occlusive crises	Fever associated more often with infectious cause. Often tachypnea. Occasionally pleural rub, signs of consolidation	Chest film usually normal at onset of symptoms. Infiltrate appears at 2–3 days. Multilobe involvement suggestive of pneumonia. Arterial blood gases are compared with patient's baseline, not "normal range." Lung scan interpretation is confusing. Angiography rarely necessary, and contrast material may induce more sickling	Rib infarction, embolism, pneumonia, ischemic heart disease	Accounts for 15% of admissions of sickle cell patients. Underlying pathology is pulmonary infarction secondary to vascular occlusion. Can be complicated by pneumonia
Renal	Common	Often asymptomatic. May have acute back pain or ureteral colic due to papillary necrosis	Costovertebral angle tenderness	Concentrating defect on specific gravity, hematuria, tissue in urine. Intravenous pyelogram may show irregular renal papillae.	Glomerulonephritis, nephrotic syndrome, urinary tract cancer	Loss of concentrating function occurs early. Increases obligatory urine losses. Hematuria from sickling occurs in vasa recta.

Reid CD, Charache S, Lubin B, et al: Management and Therapy of Sickle Cell Disease. NIH publication No. 95–2(17). Bethesda, MD, US Department of Health and Human Services, National Institutes of Health, 1995.

TABLE 19–4. Recommended Dose and Interval of Analgesics Necessary to Obtain Adequate Pain Control in Sickle Cell Disease

	Dose/Rate	Comments
Severe/Moderate Pain		
Morphine	*Parenteral*: 0.1–0.15 mg/kg/dose every 3–4 hours. Recommended maximum single dose 10 mg. *PO*: 0.3–0.6 mg/kg/dose every 4 hours	Drug of choice for pain, lower doses in the elderly and infants and in patients with liver failure or impaired ventilation.
Meperidine (Demerol)	*Parenteral*: 0.75–1.5 mg/kg/dose every 2–4 hours. Recommended maximum dose 100 mg. *PO*: 1.5 mg/kg/dose every 4 hours	Increased incidence of seizures. Avoid in patients with renal or neurologic disease or who receive monoamine oxidase inhibitors.
Hydromorphone	*Parenteral*: 0.01–0.02 mg/kg/dose every 3–4 hours *PO*: 0.04–0.06 mg/kg/dose every 4 hours	
Oxycodone	*PO*: 0.15 mg/kg/dose every 4 hours.	
Ketorolac	*Intramuscular*: Adults: 30 or 60 mg initial dose, followed by 15 to 30 mg every 6–8 hours. Children: 1 mg/kg load, followed by 0.5 mg/kg every 6 hours.	Equal efficacy to 6 mg MS, helps narcotic-sparing effect, not to exceed 5 days. Maximum 150 mg first day, 120 mg maximum subsequent days. May cause gastrointestinal irritation.
Butorphanol	*Parenteral*: Adults: 2 mg every 3–4 hours	Agonist-antagonist. Can precipitate withdrawal if given to patients who are being treated with agonists.
Mild Pain		
Codeine	*PO*: 0.5–1 mg/kg/dose every 4 hours. Maximum dose 60 mg.	Mild-to-moderate pain not relieved by aspirin or acetaminophen; can cause nausea and vomiting
Aspirin	*PO*: Adults: 0.3–0.6 mg/dose every 4–6 hours. Children: 10 mg/kg/dose every 4 hours.	Often given with a narcotic to enhance analgesia. Can cause gastric irritation. Avoid in febrile children.
Acetaminophen	*PO*: Adults: 0.3–0.6 g every 4 hours. Children: 10 mg/kg/dose.	Often given with a narcotic to enhance analgesia.
Ibuprofen	*PO*: Adults: 300–400 mg/dose every 4 hours. Children: 5–10 mg/kg/dose every 6–8 hours.	Can cause gastric irritation.
Naproxen	*PO*: Adults 500 mg/dose initially, then 250 every 8–12 hours. Children: 10 mg/kg/day (5 mg/kg every 12 hours).	Long duration of action. Can cause gastric irritation.
Indomethacin	*PO*: Adults: 25 mg/dose every 8 hours. Children: 1–3 mg/kg/day given 3–4 times.	Contraindicated in psychiatric, neurologic, renal diseases. High incidence of gastric irritation. Useful in gout.

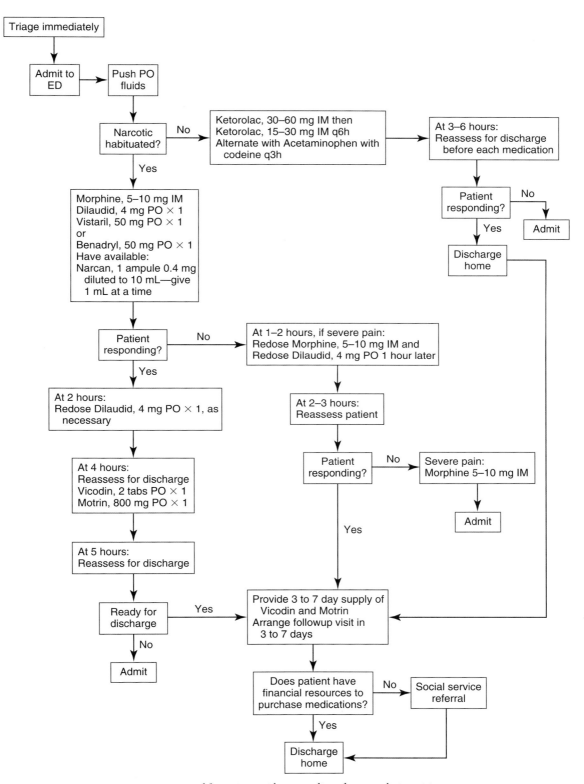

FIGURE 19–2 • Pain management protocol for patients with uncomplicated vaso-occlusive crisis.

in treating nonhypoxic patients. Pulse oximetry should be monitored but becomes less reliable as the severity of anemia increases. Any patient who is in respiratory distress or is hypoxic should be provided with oxygen supplementation to maintain the pulse oximetry above 92%. Long-term administration of oxygen may lead to suppression of erythropoiesis with exacerbation of anemia and should be discouraged. Hyperbaric oxygen therapy has been used with uncertain results for intracerebral sickling.

Transfusion

Transfusion should be reserved for specific indications in the treatment of patients with SCD. This may be done as a simple transfusion, exchange transfusion, or chronic transfusion. The goal of simple transfusion is to raise the hemoglobin to between 9 and 10 g/dL or return to the patient's baseline hemoglobin. Simple transfusion is indicated in the following situations:

- Severe anemia with profound symptomatology: high cardiac output, dyspnea, postural hypotension, angina, or cerebral dysfunction
- Aplastic anemia
- Splenic or hepatic sequestration
- Fatigue and dyspnea with hemoglobin less than 5.0 g/dL and associated erythroid hypoplasia or aplasia
- Hypoxia with PaO_2 greater than 60 mm Hg

Exchange transfusion removes sickled cells and replaces them with red cells containing HbA. The goal of exchange transfusion is the reduction of HbS to less than 30%. On occasion, such as with intrahepatic cholestasis, total blood exchange may be required. (Whole blood is removed and replaced with packed red blood cells and fresh frozen plasma.) Acute exchange transfusions are considered in the following instances:

- Severe hypoxia with PaO_2 less than 60 mm Hg
- Acute or suspected stroke and transient ischemic attack
- Hepatic failure
- Multiple organ system failure
- Fat embolization syndrome
- Acute chest syndrome unresponsive to other therapy
- Priapism unresponsive to therapy
- Intrahepatic cholestasis
- Surgery on the posterior segment of the eye. (Transfusion is not required for laser surgery.)
- Preparation for general surgery. (Recommended preoperative hemoglobin is 10 g/dL.)

Long-term chronic transfusion therapy has been found to prevent stroke, reduce pain crises, and reduce episodes of acute chest syndrome, sepsis, and hospitalization. A chronic transfusion program includes transfusion every 3 to 4 weeks to maintain HbA above 50% to 70%.

Transfusion has associated risks of disease transmission, red cell alloimmunization and transfusion reaction, iron overload, and vascular access problems as well as the suppression of erythropoiesis; thus, it should only be undertaken after consultation with the hematologist.

Bicarbonate

In documented severely acidotic patients, mild alkalinization may help to reduce sickling and improve patient condition. Two ampules of sodium bicarbonate to 1 L of 0.45 normal saline is given at a rate of 5 to 7 mL/kg/hr for the first 4 hours and then at a rate of 4 mL/kg/hr for the next 20 hours.

Rheology-Altering Agents

One goal of SCD therapy has been finding a means to improve the microvascular flow of sickled cells. Different substances have been used in the acute vaso-occlusive setting. One recent study using poloxamer 188, a nonionic surfactant, demonstrated a modest decrease in the duration of the painful crises. Other experimental strategies include fluorocarbon emulsions, antiadhesive integrin antibodies, and others. The search continues.

Specific Management Principles (See also Table 19–3.)

Painful Vaso-Occlusive Crises. Painful vaso-occlusive crises frequently arise simultaneously in the bones, joints, and abdomen. The first consideration must be given to ruling out a more serious underlying pathologic process and then treating the patient with hydration and analgesia as outlined earlier.

Susceptibility to Infection. Because patients with SCD are functionally hyposplenic, they have complement system abnormalities. Common sites of infection are the lungs, blood, bone, meninges, and urinary tract. The most common pathogens are *S. pneumoniae, H. influenzae, E. coli, S. aureus,* and *Salmonella.* Any patient with SCD who has a fever should be evaluated for the presence of sepsis; and if parenteral antibiotics are initiated, the patient should be hospitalized until all cultures are negative.

Acute Chest Syndrome. Acute pulmonary disease is the most common cause of death and the second most common cause of hospital admission. At presentation, pulmonary infarction and pneumonia may be difficult to differentiate.

Initial therapy begins with a search for infection, treatment with antibiotics, incentive spirometry, analgesia, hydration, and possible bronchoalveolar lavage to identify the pathogen. When positive, the chest radiograph may reveal one or more lobes involved, as well as a pleural effusion. Use of a broad-spectrum antibiotic directed against community-acquired organisms such as *S. pneumoniae, H. pneumoniae,* and *M. pneumoniae* is recommended. Because routine use of pneumococcal vaccine has reduced the incidence of pneumococcal pneumonia, gram-negative bacteria have emerged as a common infectious organism in adults. Suitable antibiotic choices might include a broad-spectrum cephalosporin or levofloxacin plus a macrolide. Sputum culture results can be used to further refine antibiotic selection. Although the disease is frequently self-limited, exchange transfusion may be necessary for rapidly progressive disease, respiratory insufficiency, or multiple-lobe involvement.

Aplastic Crisis. Aplastic crisis is the result of a rapid reduction in erythropoiesis. Treatment is generally supportive. Hematologic consultation should be obtained and the patient placed in respiratory isolation. A careful search for the underlying cause must be undertaken. Folate is given, because folate deficiency is a correctable cause of aplastic anemia. Transfusion is generally required to correct severe anemia; however, transfusion may inhibit recovery of erythropoiesis, and consultation with a hematologist is generally recommended. A bone marrow biopsy should be performed before beginning exchange transfusion for aplastic anemia. If the bone marrow shows elements of a recovering bone marrow, transfusion is avoided.

Neurologic Crisis. Stroke is a devastating complication of SCD that affects from 6% to 12% of patients. Neurologic crisis must be recognized and treated quickly. In children younger than the age of 10 years, cerebral infarction is most common. Hemorrhagic stroke is more commonly seen in the older patient. Once surgically correctable lesions are ruled out, hematology should be immediately consulted and exchange transfusion performed. The goal of exchange transfusion is to decrease the HbS to below 30%. Because strokes and transient ischemic attacks are associated with a 50% or greater recurrence rate, transfusion therapy is maintained for a minimum of 5 years.

To reduce problems with alloimmunization, transfusion-transmitted disease, and chronic iron overload, bone marrow transplantation is considered for young children with strokes. Transcranial Doppler ultrasonography may be used to identify children with SCD who are at high risk for stroke.

Priapism. Initial management should include bladder emptying, prostate massage, hydration with hypotonic intravenous fluids, and analgesia. Heat application may be useful in those patients without infarction-mediated priapism. Blood flow measurements should be obtained using technetium scintigraphy, infusion cavernosometry, color Doppler cavernosometry, or magnetic resonance imaging. If after 12 to 24 hours, the condition has not corrected, exchange transfusion is performed. Pharmacologic agents, such as α or β agonists, have been used with mixed success. Aspiration of the corpus cavernosum is a first-line surgical procedure that does not actually change the course of the disease but does decrease cavernous edema and reduce pain. Surgical drainage of the penis, such as a cavernosaphenous shunt or glans-cavernosum shunt, is recommended if detumescence does not occur within 24 hours of exchange transfusion.

Osteomyelitis. Osteomyelitis due to *Salmonella* may present as a result of deficient serum opsonins and should be suspected in any child presenting with fever and bone pain. Early consultation and prolonged antibiotic therapy are necessary.

Musculoskeletal Disorders. Infection of the bone and bone marrow is a frequent consequence of sickling. Treatment is with pain control, rest, local heat, and avoidance of weight bearing.

The differential diagnosis of joint effusions in patients with SCD includes synovial infarction or infarction of the long end of the bone (seen especially in the knee). Gout, septic arthritis, osteoarthritis, and rheumatic and collagen vascular disease must be ruled out using joint aspiration.

Hepatobiliary Disease. Gallstones occur in 75% of patients with SCD. The frequency of cholecystitis is variable. If cholecystectomy is required, it is best to schedule the procedure after the pain crisis has resolved. Whenever possible, the procedure should be performed laparoscopically.

Renal Disease. Sickling alters the blood flow to the kidney. The combination of hypoxia, hypertonicity, and acidosis leads to stasis and ischemia, resulting in interstitial nephritis, tubular dysfunction, and papillary necrosis. Water loss caused by hyposthenuria (an inability to concentrate the urine) is almost universally evident by 3 years of age. Hyposthenuria enhances dehydration, leading to increased sickling, which destroys the vasa recta causing hematuria and papillary necrosis. Gross hematuria occurs commonly and, on occasion, unilateral clot formation in the renal pelvis may cause renal colic. For severe cases, treatment is exchange transfusion and ε-aminocaproic acid. Patients with sickle trait or SCD may also have renal tubular acidosis, hyperkalemia, and proteinuria. Renal papillary necrosis is common in patients with SCD. It may be asymptomatic or present with hematuria or proteinuria. Twenty percent of patients older than age 40 years have renal failure contributing to their morbidity. Anemia secondary to renal failure may respond to treatment with erythropoietin, raising the hemoglobin level. Hypertension is a major risk factor for developing end-stage renal disease. Angiotensin-converting enzyme inhibitors, such as enalapril, have been effective in achieving blood pressure control and lowering urinary protein excretion.

Ocular Problems. Patients with SCD may present with nonproliferative or proliferative retinopathy, vascular occlusions, retinal hemorrhages, vitreous hemorrhage, hyphema, and neovascularization. Partial exchange transfusion is recommended for all patients with SCD preoperatively before eye surgery to prevent complications such as postoperative hyphema and ischemic necrosis of the anterior segment of the eye. Consultation with the ophthalmologist is recommended for any patient presenting with visual abnormalities. These patients are encouraged to have annual eye examinations.

Systemic Fat Embolization Syndrome. This is a rare but often fatal complication of SCD that occurs from widespread embolization of liquefied necrotic bone marrow that travels into the pulmonary vessels and then to the systemic circulation. It may occur during a severe vaso-occlusive crisis. The patient may present with bone pain, fever, chest pain, dyspnea, confusion, agitation, and coma and possibly renal failure, disseminated intravascular coagulopathy, and multiple organ system failure. Confirmation of the diagnosis is obtained by finding intracellular lipid in bronchial secretions, necrosis on bone marrow aspirates, refractile bodies on funduscopic examination, head and neck petechiae, or fat globules in the urine. Treatment is with early exchange transfusion.

Cardiac Disease. The cardiovascular system tolerates the anemia of SCD reasonably well for many years. Eventually, the chronic volume overload results in cardiac enlargement, with both dilation and hypertrophy occurring. Congestive heart failure may result. Symptoms of easy fatigability, dyspnea, and palpitations may lead physicians to a clinical misdiagnosis of heart failure. Without documented evidence of failure, treatment should be with transfusion and not with diuretics. Vaso-occlusion of coronary arteries may result in myocardial ischemia, which if not corrected can lead to infarction.

Long-Term Management

Sickle cell disease is a chronic illness. The goal of treatment is to prolong life and improve the patient's quality of life. Although emergency physicians manage the life-threatening events and complications of SCD patients, they should be knowledgeable about ongoing therapies designed to improve the patient's quality of life and decrease the frequency of hospital visits.

Patients with SCD are given folate daily to replenish the folate required for increased erythropoiesis. Iron preparations are avoided unless serum ferritin, iron, and total iron-binding capacity confirm a state of iron deficiency. As iron is recycled by the reticuloendothelium for reuse in erythropoiesis, iron overload may become problematic in later life. This is especially true for patients treated with repeated blood transfusions or aggressive iron supplementation.

In patients with chronic pain, NSAIDs with renal-sparing properties or long-acting narcotics, such as sustained-release oral morphine or oxycodone, or methadone may be used on a continuous basis. Transcutaneous nerve stimulation units, relaxation techniques, and occupational and physical therapy may be helpful in maintaining quality of life.

Hydroxyurea, a cytotoxic chemotherapeutic agent, augments the production of HbF in patients with SCD. HbF interferes with polymerization of HbS and with sickling. Recently, the advent of daily administration of oral hydroxyurea (Hydrea) has proven to be the first effective pharmacologic intervention, reducing pain events, hospital admissions, and the need for blood transfusions by 50%. A good clinical response is indicated by a rise in the patient's HbF, and total hemoglobin increases by more than 1 g/dL. The patients are closely monitored with CBCs for evidence of bone marrow suppression, as monocyte, neutrophil, and reticulocyte counts decrease, with lessening of endothelial damage and occlusion. Studies are showing early promise of improvement in pediatric populations, but long-term evaluation of benefits and side effects is ongoing.

Transfusions are recommended for patients with SCD who require surgery. The transfusions should be given to raise the hemoglobin level to 10 g/dL preoperatively. Chronic transfusions may be necessary to prevent recurrent strokes. Transfusion to hemoglobin levels above 10 g/dL may cause hyperviscosity, increasing sludging and complications.

Bone marrow transplantation has been used successfully to convert a small number of patients from HbSS to normal AA or AS. This experimental therapy is currently limited to patients who have had many complications from SCD and are at high risk for long-term complications and death. Transplantation is also done in children who have a sibling with an identical human leukocyte antigen match. This procedure has resulted in the *first* cures. Recently, unrelated stem cell transplantation has been undertaken with promising preliminary results.

UNCERTAIN DIAGNOSIS

It is nearly universal in the United States for infants to undergo sickle cell screening, and a "surprise" diagnosis of SCD is highly unlikely. When evaluating patients from other areas of the world, the physician should be suspicious when evaluating complaints that potentially could be from sickle cell anemia.

Making the Diagnosis

- A *sickle cell preparation* is a microscopic examination of the patient's blood looking for irreversibly sickled cells after the addition of sodium metabisulfite. The "sickle cell prep" can identify the presence of sickled cells, but it cannot identify the type of hemoglobinopathy.
- A microscopic *examination of the peripheral smear* may reveal sickled cells that can be used to validate the diagnosis.
- *Hemoglobin electrophoresis* confirms the type and relative percentage of hemoglobin. This is time consuming and is not available on an emergent basis.

Manipulative or drug-seeking behavior can be suspected if the patient's complaints do not fall into one of the just-listed categories and the laboratory tests fail to confirm sickle cell anemia. If the patient is known to have SCD, it is best to aggressively treat the patient, even if concerns exist regarding the possibility of drug-seeking behavior. Hematologic consultation or confirmatory testing for sickle cell anemia should be considered for new patients with unconfirmed disease.

SPECIAL CONSIDERATIONS

Pediatric Patients

Because of the limited life span of patients with SCD, many complications of SCD present in children and young adults (Table 19–5).

Life-threatening bacterial infection must be suspected in any child younger than 5 years of age who presents with a fever. Overwhelming sepsis is the leading cause of death in children with SCD younger than the age of 5. Because of an abnormal complement system and defective opsonins, all patients with SCD are susceptible to infection with encapsulated organisms, especially *S. pneumoniae*, whereas the advent of vaccination for *H. influenzae* has greatly reduced the incidence. Any child with SCD with a fever (102°F [38.9°C] or greater) should immediately be treated with broad-spectrum antibiotics with coverage against *S. pneumoniae* and *H. influenzae*. The child should be examined for causes of the fever, including otitis media, pneumonia, and urinary tract infection. The physician should have a low threshold for performing a lumbar puncture, particularly in the very young child. A workup should include blood and urine cultures and chest radiography. An appropriate empirical antibiotic is a broad-spectrum cephalosporin, such as ceftriaxone or cefuroxime, given as 50 mg/kg/dose.

Local practice varies on indications for admission for the febrile child. Consensus exists for the following parameters:

TABLE 19–5. Age Distribution of Sickle Cell Crisis Type

Types of Sickle Crisis	Age
Vaso-occlusive (pain) crisis	All ages
Acute chest syndrome	All ages
Sickle-stroke syndrome	All ages; usually children < 10 years
Splenic sequestration	1–6 years
Hepatic sequestration	Young adult–later life
Hand-foot syndrome (dactylitis)	6 months–6 years
Aplastic crisis	6 months to young adults
Overwhelming sepsis	All ages; usually children < 5 years

- Temperature greater than 104°F (38.9°C)
- Seriously ill appearance, hypotension
- Poor perfusion
- Dehydration
- Pulmonary infiltrate
- Corrected WBC count greater than 30,000/mm^3 or less than 5,000/mm^3
- Platelet count less than 100,000/mm^3
- Hemoglobin value less than 5 g/dL
- History of *S. pneumoniae* sepsis

Pediatric patients suitable for discharge must be considered at low risk for sepsis. They must have a good support system of family/physician follow-up with immediate ability to return to medical care should their condition worsen.

If septicemia is confirmed by positive blood culture, the child is hospitalized for a minimum of 5 to 7 days for antibiotic therapy.

Acute splenic sequestration is second only to sepsis as the leading cause of death in children with SCD. It generally occurs in children between the ages of 4 months and 3 years, but it may occur at any age to patients with HbSC or HbS-βthal disease. Twenty percent of children may present with splenic sequestration as their initial manifestation of SCD.

Patients with SCD have a 30% probability of having an acute splenic sequestration crisis by 5 years of age, with a potential mortality of 15% per event. Emergency care should be immediately initiated because these children may die rapidly. To maintain the cardiovascular system, the intravascular volume is repleted with a 20-mL/kg bolus of normal saline over 15 to 30 minutes. An ABG analysis, CBC, reticulocyte count, and type and screen should be performed. Hemoglobin and glucose should be rapidly performed. The child should be placed on supplemental oxygen and monitored. Transfusion of red blood cells may be lifesaving but is not always necessary, because the hematocrit may rise approximately 3 g/dL (or more) after the child receives intravenous fluids because the pooled splenic cells are mobilized. The child should be admitted to an intensive care unit. Children with repetitive sequestration crises may require chronic transfusion therapy or splenectomy.

Stroke in SCD occurs most commonly in children younger than the age of 10 years. Approximately 11% of patients with SCD have an acute thrombotic or hemorrhagic stroke by age 20. Seventy-five percent of all strokes in children are ischemic and present as cerebral infarction, whereas 25% of strokes are the result of subarachnoid or intracerebral hemorrhage. The incidence of hemorrhagic stroke seems to increase with age. Mortality is less than 5%, and motor recovery is common; however, intellectual impairment frequently results. Exchange transfusion is the primary treatment modality to prevent further sickling (decreasing the amount of HbS to less than 30%). Anticonvulsants are used to control seizures. The risk of recurrent stroke is 67% to 90%, and recurrence usually occurs within 3 years (without transfusion). Children are maintained on a chronic transfusion program, receiving transfusion every 3 to 4 weeks for a minimum of 5 years and possibly to continue indefinitely. Recurrent stroke in this group is approximately 10%.

Acute chest syndrome occurs with a frequency of 24.5 cases per 100 patient-years in children with SCD, with most cases occurring during the winter. The most common pathogens are *S. pneumoniae* and *H. influenzae*. In one study, bacteremia was present in 78% of children with acute chest syndrome associated with pneumococcus. Symptoms are fever and cough. A fall in hemoglobin of 1 to 2 g/dL is accompanied by a relative thrombocytopenia and leukocytosis. Radiography typically reveals upper or middle lobe pulmonary infiltrates.

Hand-foot syndrome or dactylitis occurs in children 6 months to 6 years of age and is frequently the initial presentation of disease. Although self-limiting and without permanent sequelae, dactylitis may provide the first clue that a child has SCD if not detected in a newborn screening program. Dactylitis is an acute non-pitting swelling of hands and feet that is accompanied by pain and low-grade fever. It may affect one to four extremities, and it is the result of bony infarcts of the metacarpals, phalanges, or metatarsals. Irritability or refusal to walk may be another early sign of SCD. With the protective effect of HbF, it rarely occurs before 6 months of age and, interestingly, rarely occurs after 6 years of age. Dactylitis may be confused with osteomyelitis, but in the absence of fever, elevated WBCs, elevated erythrocyte sedimentation rate, or signs of toxicity, osteomyelitis can be ruled out. Radiographs taken several days after the episode may show periosteal elevation. It is managed with hydration and adequate pain medication, titrated to crying. Infants with dactylitis should be hospitalized for pain control and hydration. Antibiotics should be given if the patient is febrile, until infection is ruled out.

Prophylactic penicillin has been very effective at reducing life-threatening complications, particularly infection with *S. pneumoniae*. Most states screen all newborns for SCD, and when they are identified they are placed on a prophylactic penicillin program. Prophylactic penicillin is begun at age 2 to 3 months and continues until the child is 6 years old. Prophylaxis in older children has not been shown to be necessary when pneumococcal vaccination is completed.

Routine vaccinations should be given on schedule. Pneumococcal vaccine at ages 2 and 6 and every 10 years is the standard of care. Beginning at 2 years of age, *H. influenzae* vaccine is given. Some clinicians recommend influenza vaccine be administered.

DISPOSITION AND FOLLOW-UP

Patient disposition is based on the presence of preexisting complications and the likelihood of clinical serious deterioration.

ICU admission is needed for patients with:

- Unstable vital signs or signs of toxicity
- Splenic sequestration, neurologic crisis, or infectious crisis
- Acute chest syndrome involving multiple lobes, respiratory distress, and hypoxia
- Treatment by exchange transfusion

Admission to an unmonitored medical bed is recommended for stable patients with:

- Aplastic crisis
- Vaso-occlusive crisis and persistent unrelenting pain
- Three or more emergency department visits for the same painful crisis
- Unexplained fever
- Cholecystitis
- Mesenteric sickling and bowel ischemia
- Swollen painful joints
- Renal papillary necrosis with severe renal colic or hematuria
- Hyphema and retinal detachment
- Acute abdomen
- Persistent priapism
- Acute dactylitis
- Treatment by simple transfusion

If a patient with vaso-occlusive crisis is discharged home, certain instructions should be given to include:

- Maintenance of adequate oral hydration.
- Prescription for analgesia for 3 to 5 days. Selection of analgesia is according to established protocol.
- Instructions to return if temperature is over 101°F (38.3°C) or there is increased pain, vomiting, or worsening of symptoms.

Follow-up should be arranged for reevaluation within 24 hours for children and 24 to 48 hours for adults. A long-term relationship with a primary or consulting physician is strongly encouraged.

FINAL POINTS

- Signs and symptoms of serious complications of SCD may be nonspecific. A complete history and physical examination are mandatory.
- The major crisis types are
  Hematologic
  Hyperhemolytic
  Aplastic anemia
  Splenic sequestration
  Infectious
  Vaso-occlusive–with neurologic changes as a subset
- The four true emergencies in SCD are
  - Sepsis
  - Splenic sequestration
  - Neurologic crisis
  - Aplastic crisis
- Patients with SCD are immunocompromised. Fever is a cause for serious concern. Overwhelming sepsis is a leading cause of death; a cause is sought and antibiotic therapy initiated immediately.
- Children are at greatest risk for the major complications of SCD.
- A CBC is mandatory for laboratory evaluation; a reticulocyte count is needed if the patient's hemoglobin has decreased from baseline by more than 2 g/dL.
- Transfusion is used to treat life-threatening vaso-occlusive or hematologic crisis.
- Analgesia, rest, and hydration are the mainstays of treatment for vaso-occlusive crisis.
- Pain is treated aggressively. Drug tolerance does not equal drug addiction. A pain protocol is used to ensure adequate analgesia and improve both patient and physician satisfaction.
- The warning signs that more serious disease may exist are
  - Pain that is unusual in quality, character, or location
  - WBC count over 20,000/mm^3
  - Fever
  - Hypoxia
  - Neurologic deficits
  - Abnormal vital signs
- Admission is warranted for any patient with ongoing or impending signs or symptoms of complications of sickle cell, unstable vital signs, or persistent pain.

CASE *Study*

A 27-year-old black man presented with a complaint of his "usual back pain" in the chest, abdomen, and back that did not respond to treatment at home with acetaminophen with codeine. Initial examination revealed an anxious patient in obvious pain. His vital signs were blood pressure, 110/74 mm Hg; heart rate, 112 beats per minute; respiratory rate, 28 breaths per minute, and temperature, 101.5°F. The patient requests parenteral narcotics for pain control.

This was the 12th visit for this patient to the emergency department in the past 10 months. He was considered by staff to be highly manipulative and was suspected of being a drug abuser. The nurses all "knew" this patient and believed that he did not appear ill despite his abnormal vital signs and complaints. He was triaged as a "green" to a routine bed for evaluation, and his chart was placed at the bottom of the stack.

Although the patient does not look ill, his elevated temperature and tachypnea indicate a potentially serious problem. By triaging the patient to a routine bed instead of requesting immediate physician evaluation, a common error has been committed. Patients who frequently visit the emergency department are often labeled as "abusers" and are treated casually. This ill-advised approach eventually leads to critical errors.

Forty-five minutes after the patient's arrival, a physician evaluated the patient. He was complaining of fatigue, dyspnea, cough, pleuritic chest pain, as well as pain to his back and abdomen. He was demanding narcotics for pain control. He was in moderate respiratory distress. Repeat vitals signs were blood pressure, 112/70 mm Hg; pulse rate, 120 beats per minute; respiratory rate, 30 breaths per minute; temperature, 101.5°F (38.6°C); and oxygen saturation by pulse oximetry, 89%. Pertinent physical findings included pale conjunctivae, inspiratory crackles in the left lung fields, a soft abdomen without organomegaly, and normal results on neurologic examination.

The patient complained of chest, back, and abdominal pain. Vaso-occlusive disease may be present, but the physical findings of fever, tachypnea, tachycardia, low pulse oximetry, and inspiratory crackles support a diagnosis of acute chest syndrome. The complaints of fatigue

fatigue and dyspnea are nonspecific and could be secondary to pulmonary disease. They also raise the possibility of acute hematologic crisis due to aplastic anemia. Confirmation of these suspicions awaits laboratory results. The patient was given analgesics according to the emergency department protocol: 5 mg of morphine initially intravenously, with 50 mg of hydroxyzine intravenously and 4 mg of hydromorphone orally for pain. Intravenous hydration was begun with dextrose 5% in 0.45 normal saline at 250 mL/hr. Blood was drawn for ABG analysis, CBC, and reticulocyte count. Sputum was collected for Gram's stain and culture. Chest radiography was ordered.

The results of the patient's laboratory studies were as follows: Arterial blood gas analysis showed a pH of 7.33, $PaCO_2$ of 32 mm Hg, and PaO_2 of 54 mm Hg. Hemoglobin was 5.4 g/dL (usual baseline 8.8 g/dL), reticulocyte count was 3.5% (baseline 8%), and WBC, 21,000/mm^3 with numerous sickled cells, 65% segmented neutrophils, 15% bands, and 15% nucleated red blood cells. The chest radiograph demonstrated bilateral lower lobe infiltrates. Sputum Gram's stain revealed multiple WBCs and gram-positive diplococci.

The patient's low hemoglobin and low reticulocyte count confirmed the initial impression of aplastic crisis. The radiographic findings and sputum Gram's stain supported the possibility of pneumococcal pneumonia. Blood, urine, and sputum cultures were collected.

The patient was immediately started on antibiotic therapy with ceftriaxone and azithromycin. He was admitted to the intensive care unit with a preliminary diagnosis of aplastic crisis and acute chest syndrome. Antibiotics were continued, and folate was added for the aplastic crisis. A bone marrow biopsy was performed and revealed active erythropoiesis. No transfusion was given.

This patient's disposition to the intensive care unit was appropriate because he had aplastic anemia with a coexisting pneumonia and hypoxia. Most experts agree that transfusion during aplastic crisis is best guided by bone marrow biopsy. If the biopsy reveals the return of active erythropoiesis, no transfusions are necessary and, in fact, may even be harmful by slowing the erythropoietic recovery.

The patient responded to treatment and was discharged on day 10 with hemoglobin of 7.4 g/dL and resolving chest radiography findings.

This case could have easily ended in disaster. The physician who finally evaluated this patient was thorough and discovered two coexisting and *potentially life-threatening disease processes. This case illustrates some important pitfalls in the care of the SCD patient. At every visit to the emergency department, the patient with SCD deserves a complete evaluation, during which the physician is always searching for more than one potential problem.*

Bibliography

TEXT

Reid CD, Charache S, Lubin B, et al: Management and Therapy of Sickle Cell Disease. National Institutes of Health publication No. 95–2117. Bethesda, MD, US Department of Health and Human Services, 1995.

JOURNAL ARTICLES/INTERNET

Adams R, McKie V, Hsu L: Prevention of a first stroke by transfusions in children with sickle cell anemia and abnormal results on transcranial Doppler ultrasonography. N Engl J Med 1998; 339:5–11.

Ballas SK: Complications of sickle cell anemia in adults: Guidelines for effective management. Cleve Clin J Med 1999; 66:48–58.

Charache S, Terrin M, Moore R, et al: Effect of hydroxyurea on the frequency of painful crises in sickle cell anemia. N Engl J Med 1995; 332:1317–1322.

Orringer EP, Casella JF, Ataga KI, et al: Purified poloxamer 188 for the treatment of acute vaso-occlusive crisis of sickle cell disease. JAMA 2001; 286:2099–2106.

Platt A, Eckman J: Sickle cell information—clinician summary, 1997. The Georgia Comprehensive Sickle Cell Center at Grady Health System, Atlanta, Georgia. Available at www.emory.edu/peds/sickle.

Steinberg M. Management of sickle cell disease. N Engl J Med 1999; 340:1021–1030.

Stephens CR: Sickle cell disease: A review of state-of-the art emergency management and outcome-effective therapy. Emerg Med Rep 1999; 20:183–192.

Vichinsky EP, Neumayr LD, Earles AN, et al: Causes and outcomes of the acute chest syndrome in sickle cell disease. National Acute Chest Syndrome Study Group. N Engl J Med 2000; 342:1855–1865.

Walters MC, Patience M, Leisenring W, et al: Bone marrow transplantation for sickle cell disease. N Engl J Med 1996; 335:369–376.

Wayne AS, Kevy SV, Nathan DG: Transfusion management of sickle cell disease. Blood 1993; 81:1109–1123.

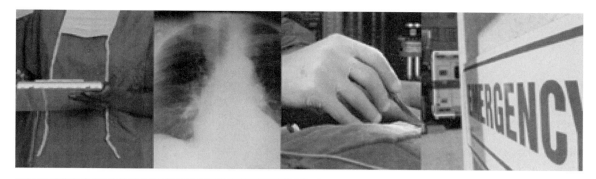

HORMONAL AND METABOLIC DISORDERS

CHAPTER 20

Diabetes

GARY R. STRANGE
CARL M. FERRARO

CASE *Study*

A rescue squad was called to the home of a 37-year-old diabetic woman. Her husband stated that she had been vomiting and became increasingly sleepy over the past 10 to 12 hours.

INTRODUCTION

Diabetes mellitus is a common disease affecting approximately 1% of the population. Over 11 million Americans are diabetic. The underlying metabolic defect is a deficiency of insulin, either absolute or relative. In type 1 diabetes, often referred to as insulin-dependent diabetes, there is an absolute deficiency of insulin. Type 1 diabetes usually begins during childhood, and patients with this type of diabetes are prone to develop ketosis. It is believed that type 1 diabetes results from autoimmune destruction of the insulin-producing pancreatic islet cells, thereby leading to a decreased synthesis of insulin. Type 2 diabetes, known as non–insulin-dependent or maturity-onset diabetes, is characterized by a relative lack of insulin and a resistance to ketosis. However, the occurrence of diabetic ketoacidosis (DKA) in type 2 diabetes, especially in obese black patients, is not as rare as once thought. The actual level of circulating insulin may be normal or low, and defective insulin receptors lead to a relative ineffectiveness of the circulating insulin. Although there is no known cure for diabetes, medications are available that can control the blood glucose level in an effort to prevent the neural, renal, and vascular complications of the disease.

Metabolic complications from diabetes are common and frequently present as an altered level of consciousness. Approximately 10% of all hospital admissions for diabetes are for altered mentation. Hypoglycemic states, DKA, and hyperosmolar hyperglycemic states (HHS) are the common causes. The incidence of DKA is five to eight episodes per 1000 diabetics annually.

Hypoglycemia is an extremely common problem and is considered in *all* patients who present in a coma. For many diabetics, hypoglycemia is a frequent event. The blood glucose concentration can fall because of an excess of insulin, a lack of substrate (glucose or glycogen), an overabundance of an oral hypoglycemic agent, or the action of other drugs. Ethanol predisposes to the development of hypoglycemia because of its inhibitory effect on glycogen storage and gluconeogenesis. Early signs and symptoms accompanying hypoglycemia result from sympathetic catecholamine release. They consist of tachycardia, diaphoresis, and anxiety. More subtle symptoms, such as hyperactivity, sleeplessness, or psychotic behavior, may be present in up to 25% of cases. Seizures occur in 10% of episodes. If the patient is taking a β-adrenergic blocking agent, coma may develop without premonitory symptoms.

DKA is characterized by hyperglycemia, ketonemia, and acidemia. It usually evolves over several days. The incidence of this condition may be increasing, and a 1% to 2% mortality rate has persisted since the 1970s. DKA results from hormonal imbalance, involving both insulin lack and an excess of counterregulatory hormones, which include glucagon, growth hormone, catecholamines, and cortisol. A complex interrelated metabolic cascade triggered by an insulin deficit occurs, leading to hyperglycemia, ketoacidosis, dehydration, and, if unchecked, to shock and ultimately death (Fig. 20–1).

HHS occurs in the setting of a relative insulin lack in which hyperglycemia may exist without concomitant ketosis. It may take days to weeks to become clinically evident. The extreme hyperosmolality accompanying this condition results in neurologic deficits more commonly than occurs in DKA. Mortality may be as high as 15% and is often caused by myocardial infarction or cerebrovascular accidents.

The initial diagnosis and management of the diabetic with an altered mental status in the emergency department is critical in determining the

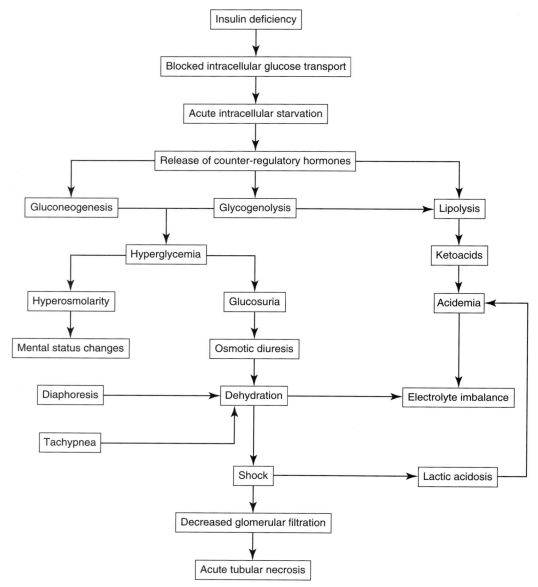

FIGURE 20–1 • Metabolic Cascade for diabetic ketoacidosis.

outcome. An early diagnosis with appropriate therapy can be lifesaving, whereas failure to differentiate the cause and initiate proper therapy may lead to significant morbidity or death.

INITIAL APPROACH AND STABILIZATION

Priority Diagnoses

This chapter will emphasize the primary diagnoses of importance to the emergency physician:

- Hypoglycemia
- Diabetic ketoacidosis
- Hyperosmolar hyperglycemic states
- Complications of diabetes

Rapid Assessment

The patient with a significantly altered level of consciousness will obviously require immediate evaluation by the emergency physician. Ambulatory diabetic patients who present with nonspecific complaints such as dizziness, fever, or vomiting may also have major metabolic disturbances that require prompt intervention. Triage personnel should be aware of the need to rapidly assess diabetic patients.

The following are indicated during the initial assessment:

1. The patency of the airway, the ability of the patient to protect the airway, and the adequacy of respirations are evaluated first. Airway and ventilatory support are rarely needed for patients with complications of diabetes, but prompt identification of the need for intervention is essential.
2. Hypotension requires immediate administration of isotonic crystalloid. Existing intravenous lines are checked for patency, and new lines are placed as needed.
3. Blood specimens are obtained and prepared for the laboratory. A glucose oxidase reagent strip is checked. Even if the glucose level was determined in the field, a recheck is indicated.
4. A cardiac monitor is placed, and the heart rhythm is assessed. The height and configuration of the T wave are specifically noted. This observation will be useful in guiding initial electrolyte replacement if the patient proves to have DKA and hyperkalemia.
5. Arterial blood gas measurements and venous blood determinations are ordered for patients who have not responded to any preceding interventions by an improvement in the level of consciousness. Measurement of serum electrolytes, blood urea nitrogen, creatinine, glucose, ketones, and osmolality and a complete blood cell count are important and are ordered immediately.
6. A urine sample is obtained, glucose and acetone concentrations are determined by dipstick, and a urinalysis is requested. For patients with significantly depressed mental status, mini-catheterization is usually necessary. This procedure carries a slight risk of infection in diabetics, but this risk is offset by the urgent need for information regarding the presence of glucosuria or ketonuria. The patient with DKA and HHS will continue to produce large amounts of urine even in the presence of moderate hypotension. Glucosuria and the subsequent osmotic diuresis will maintain urine production until shock leads to decreased glomerular filtration. In unstable, unconscious patients, an indwelling catheter is useful for monitoring urinary output.
7. The initial level of consciousness is assessed and recorded in terms that are descriptive and understandable by subsequent care providers. The Glasgow Coma Scale, as described in Chapter 31, Altered Mental Status, is a widely accepted system of objectively grading the level of consciousness.
8. A flow sheet is initiated for serial recording of vital signs, urine output, fluid intake, mental status, and biochemical parameters.

Early Intervention

1. Supplemental oxygen is provided for all patients with significant alteration in mental status.
2. Dextrose 50%, 1 to 2 ampules (25 to 50 g), may be administered intravenously. If the glucose oxidase reagent strip indicates hyperglycemia, dextrose may be held. However, administration of dextrose even to a patient with DKA is not likely to cause significant harm. On the other hand, withholding dextrose in a setting of hypoglycemia can cause substantial cerebral damage.
3. Naloxone, 2 mg, may be administered empirically to avoid missing an occult opioid intoxication.

The results of certain diagnostic tests are generally available during the initial assessment phase and will guide the initial therapy of the patient. A high blood or urine glucose level with ketonuria is sufficient data to prompt suspicion of DKA.

Reagent Strip Blood Glucose Determination. Commercially available reagent strips are based on the glucose oxidase reaction. The color change produced with varying levels of blood glucose can be discerned by the naked eye, but more accuracy can be obtained by observing it with a light meter. Because reagent strips are sensitive to light, heat, and moisture, care must be exercised to ensure they are properly stored and not left open to the environment.

Accuracy of reagent strips is better in the hypoglycemic range than in the hyperglycemic range. This is not a problem because strips are used primarily for hypoglycemic concerns and only to obtain a rough estimate of the blood glucose level. Laboratory determination of the exact blood glucose always follows the bedside estimate.

Urine Glucose and Acetone Concentrations. Urine glucose and acetone levels are determined using Clinitest and Acetest tablets or Chemstrips bG. Glycosuria results when the kidney is presented with a large glucose load. The level of glucose in the urine cannot be directly correlated with the serum glucose concentration, but the presence of glycosuria is supportive evidence for hyperglycemia as measured by the reagent strip. Similarly, ketonuria is supportive evidence for the presence of ketonemia, and, in the diabetic, it suggests DKA. The urine ketone dip test is a better screening test for DKA than the anion gap or serum bicarbonate level.

Arterial Blood Gas (ABG) Analysis. ABG test results, including the arterial pH, are usually available rapidly. A pH below 7.30 is suggestive of DKA. The Pco_2 is usually decreased and represents respiratory compensation (see Chapter 21, Acute Metabolic Acidosis and Metabolic Alkalosis).

Electrocardiogram (ECG). In the presence of DKA, the serum potassium value will usually be normal to high, but it falls precipitously when treatment is started. To avoid hypokalemia, potassium supplementation is started as early as possible. The T wave of the ECG is a fair gauge of the serum potassium level; and, if the T waves are normal or small, early potassium supplementation is considered. In the presence of tall, peaked T waves, which are consistent with hyperkalemia, potassium is held until the level is known.

The ECG also may be helpful in recognizing acute injury patterns that may be a precipitating factor in the development of DKA or the result of the metabolic stress. The ECG may reveal a silent myocardial infarction, which occurs more frequently in diabetics. An ECG should be ordered in diabetic patients presenting with nonspecific complaints such as dizziness, shortness of breath, or weakness.

CLINICAL ASSESSMENT

History

Information is obtained from all available sources with emphasis on a few key points:

1. Is the patient a *known diabetic?* Knowing that a patient is diabetic is helpful. However, complications of diabetes may occur as the initial presentation of the disease and must be considered even when the patient is not a known diabetic.
2. Has the patient experienced problems from *hypoglycemia* or *hyperglycemia previously?* How *frequently* has this occurred?
3. What *type of*, and *how much, insulin* does the patient usually take, or what type and dose of *oral hypoglycemic agent* is used? Has the patient *altered the dose recently?* Hypoglycemia is not uncommon when a patient's dose of insulin or oral agent is increased. Also, when a patient takes the regular dose but fails to eat, hypoglycemia may follow. On the other hand, a reduction in doses of medication or increases in dietary intake may result in hyperglycemia.
4. Has the patient's *food intake* been less than usual?
5. Is the patient taking a *β-adrenergic blocking agent?* The β-adrenergic blocking agents mask the signs of sympathetic release that are the warning signs for the development of hypoglycemia. Patients taking these agents may

therefore slip into coma without premonitory signs or symptoms.

6. Does the patient *take* or *have access to drugs* that may cause alterations in level of consciousness? Diabetics frequently take other medications that can result in alterations of level of consciousness. Sedative-hypnotics and cyclic antidepressants are commonly used agents that may be responsible for a diabetic's change in mental status.
7. Has the patient been *more active* than usual? Exercise increases glucose requirements.
8. What are the *events leading* to the patient's presentation? Can specific *precipitants* be identified? These include infection (no. 1 cause), alcohol abuse, pancreatitis, cerebrovascular accident, acute myocardial infarction, corticosteroids, thiazides, noncompliance, and lack of access to fluids. The classic triad of polyuria, polyphagia, and polydipsia strongly suggests hyperglycemia but is present in fewer than half of cases of DKA.
9. What is the patient's *usual mental status?* Over what *time course* did *changes develop?* Hypoglycemia may cause subtle forms of mental status change, such as personality changes or lassitude. True coma may follow. Coma is common in hyperosmolar coma but occurs in only 10% of patients with DKA and does not correlate with the degree of metabolic disturbance. The altered level of consciousness from hypoglycemia usually occurs abruptly, whereas hyperglycemic coma has a gradual onset.
10. Has the patient had any *gastrointestinal complaints?* Patients may complain of anorexia, nausea, vomiting, abdominal pain, or hunger with either high or low blood glucose levels. For patients with DKA, abdominal pain secondary to the metabolic acidosis may be severe, leading the physician to suspect intra-abdominal problems such as pancreatitis or appendicitis. Gastroenteritis is a common misdiagnosis in early DKA.
11. Has the patient been exposed to *specific stresses?* Any stress may lead to an alteration in insulin or glucose metabolism. Recent infections of the respiratory, genitourinary, or gastrointestinal tracts are frequently implicated. Recent trauma or surgery may also be a cause.
12. Does the patient have *known complications of diabetes?* These include neuropathy, retinopathy, nephropathy, and vascular disease.
13. Does the patient have potential *suicidal ideation?* Insulin overdose or non-compliance may be used by diabetics in an attempt to end their lives.

Physical Examination

The physical examination can provide useful clues to the etiology and severity of altered mental status in a diabetic and can be used to assess for end-organ damage from vascular changes.

General Appearance. Does the patient appear to be in shock? Is the skin pale or diaphoretic? Is the skin dry or lacking in turgor? In hypoglycemia, sympathetic hormone release may result in pallor and diaphoresis. DKA and HHS are both associated with significant dehydration, which can progress to hypovolemic shock.

Vital Signs. Pulse and respiratory rates, blood pressure, and temperature levels are assessed. Tachycardia is a manifestation of stress and is present in all forms of diabetes-related coma. Tachypnea is present in patients with DKA as a compensatory mechanism for the metabolic acidosis. Rapid, deep, sighing respirations, termed *Kussmaul respirations*, are very suggestive of the presence of DKA, and the fruity odor of ketones may be noted. Hyperventilation also can be caused by respiratory infection and by toxic ingestions (e.g., salicylates). Hypoventilation may be present with severe hypoglycemia.

Blood pressure is often elevated and associated with physiologic stress. As the dehydration of DKA and HHS progresses, however, hypotension and shock may ensue.

Elevated temperature is uncommon in the setting of DKA, even in the presence of serious infection. Infection is a common predisposing factor for HHS, and an associated elevated temperature will require a thorough search for a focus of infection. Hypoglycemia is not commonly associated with temperature changes.

Level of Consciousness. Is the patient alert? Does he or she respond to verbal or painful stimuli? Are responses appropriate? The Glasgow Coma Scale (see Chapter 31, Altered Mental Status) is an excellent means of quantitating and following the patient's mental status.

Head, Eyes, Ears, Nose, Throat. Are there signs of head trauma? Head injury may be responsible for the change in mental status, and external signs may be subtle. Falls caused by "dizziness" from metabolic disturbances may lead to combined metabolic and traumatic abnormalities.

Is any evidence of infection found? Infection is a common predisposing condition for the development of DKA. Some rare ear, nose, and throat infections occur almost exclusively in poorly controlled diabetics. Malignant otitis externa is a rapidly progressive, life-threatening condition that requires early diagnosis and aggressive therapy. Does the patient have a stiff or rigid neck?

Meningitis must be considered in any patient with an altered level of consciousness.

Do the fundi show diabetic changes? The retinal vessels are an externally visible reflection of the degree of end-organ damage caused by diabetes. The most common changes seen are increased width and tortuosity of vessels, microaneurysms, hemorrhages, and exudates. Diabetic retinopathy may be graded based on these observations and correlate with the severity of end-organ damage throughout the body.

Cardiovascular Signs. Is there adequate perfusion? Both DKA and HHS are associated with severe dehydration that can progress to shock. Is there evidence of a primary cardiac problem? DKA may result from the stress of acute myocardial infarction in a diabetic, and either hypoglycemia or hyperglycemia can result in myocardial infarction. Signs of congestive heart failure are sometimes seen in HHS patients; such patients require close monitoring during fluid replacement.

Pulmonary Signs. Is there adequate air exchange? Is there evidence of consolidation or infiltration? Pulmonary infection may be a predisposing condition for the development of DKA or HHS. Hypoglycemia may be associated with aspiration.

Abdomen. Is the abdomen distended? Distention from ileus or obstruction may be present. Are bowel sounds present? Electrolyte disturbances, especially hypokalemia, may result in diminished bowel sounds. Are peritoneal signs present? Patients with DKA may have abdominal pain, but careful examination should reveal an absence of peritoneal signs, such as guarding and rebound. Is there rectal tenderness or blood? Gastrointestinal bleeding can occur in conjunction with hyperglycemic states, such as mesenteric ischemia from dehydration and systemic hypotension.

Extremities. Is capillary refill adequate? Is skin turgor good? Poor peripheral perfusion and turgor are indicators of severe dehydration.

Neurologic Signs. Are there focal deficits or lateralizing signs indicating an intracranial event? Cerebrovascular accidents occur with increased frequency in diabetic patients and may be solely responsible for a change in mental status. Hypoglycemia may masquerade as a focal cerebrovascular accident.

CLINICAL REASONING

After completion of the history and physical examination, two questions are addressed.

Is a Cause of Altered Level of Consciousness Unrelated to Diabetes Suggested?

Common causes of coma that may occur in any patient, including diabetics, are head trauma, drug ingestion, meningitis, and cerebrovascular accidents. The diagnosis and initial management of these problems are discussed in Chapter 31, Altered Mental Status.

Is the Altered Mental Status Due to a Metabolic Derangement Caused by Diabetes? If So, What Specific Metabolic Derangement Is Present?

Altered level of consciousness from diabetes is differentiated as depicted in Figure 20–2.

Early in the approach to the patient, the glucose concentration is measured at the bedside by reagent strip testing. If the blood glucose level is low, hypoglycemia is diagnosed. If it is high, a hyperglycemic problem exists. The next step is to determine the acid-base status of the patient by assessing arterial blood gas values. A normal blood pH in the presence of significant hyperglycemia indicates HHS. A low blood pH indicates metabolic acidemia. The nitroprusside test is then used to assess the presence of serum ketones. If ketones are present in a dilution of 1:2 or greater, DKA is diagnosed. A commonly used working definition appropriate for most patients with DKA follows:

- Blood glucose level in excess of 300 mg/dL
- Ketonemia with serum ketones present in a dilution of 1:2 or greater
- Acidemia with a blood pH of less than 7.30 or a serum bicarbonate concentration of less than 15 mEq/L

DIAGNOSTIC ADJUNCTS

Laboratory Studies

Laboratory tests that are useful in evaluating diabetes-related coma are numerous. They can be grouped into two categories: those for which results are immediately available and those for which results are often delayed for 60 minutes or more. All tests are ordered immediately, but results become available at different times.

Tests for which results are available immediately and are therefore used to guide initial therapy include the following:

- Reagent strip blood glucose concentration
- Urine glucose and acetone levels
- Arterial blood gases
- Electrocardiogram

The use of these tests was discussed earlier under "Early Intervention." From these test results, an assessment of the degree of hypoxemia, acidemia, and hyperosmolality is obtained. Initial therapy is started on the basis of these test results while awaiting the following test results, which may modify the treatment course.

Complete Blood Cell Count and Differential. Even in the absence of infection, the white blood cell count is usually 15,000 to 20,000/mm^3 in patients with DKA. The white blood cell count correlates more closely with the severity of DKA than does the presence of sepsis. A left shift of the differential cell count is suggestive of an infectious process. The hemoglobin and hematocrit values are elevated if there is significant dehydration.

Serum Electrolytes. Sodium deficit in DKA is approximately 6 mEq/kg. In addition, the measured sodium level may be spuriously lowered by hyperglycemia. To obtain an approximate actual

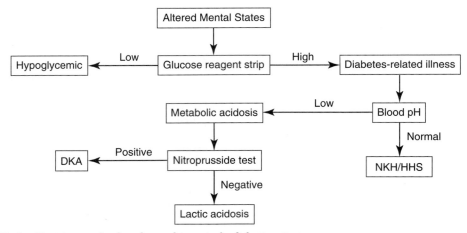

FIGURE 20–2 • Decision tree for altered mental status in the diabetic patient.

value, 1.6 mEq/L is added to the measured value for every 100 mg/dL of blood glucose over 100 mg/dL. Therefore, a highly elevated glucose concentration with a normal sodium level actually represents hypernatremia.

The potassium deficit averages 5 mEq/kg in patients with DKA. The initial level is usually normal to high, secondary to the extracellular shift that occurs as a compensatory mechanism for acidosis. With fluid and insulin administration, the level falls precipitously. To anticipate the amount of change, one should estimate that for every 0.1 change in pH, there is a 0.6 mEq/L change in potassium in the opposite direction.

Chloride loss in patients with DKA averages 4 mEq/kg. Replacement is easily accomplished with isotonic saline. In fact, overreplacement is common, leading to hyperchloremic acidosis.

Renal Function Tests. Blood urea nitrogen is elevated above the usual 10:1 ratio with creatinine because of dehydration. The serum creatinine level may be spuriously elevated from interference in testing by ketonemia.

Blood Glucose and Ketone Levels. Blood glucose determination is essential to confirm the results of urine and blood reagent strip estimates. Serum acetone and acetoacetate are measured by means of the nitroprusside reaction, which causes a color change when acetoacetate is present in the specimen. Acetoacetate usually exists in a 1:3 ratio with β-hydroxybutyrate. The equilibrium is shifted toward β-hydroxybutyrate in the presence of severe acidosis. Because β-hydroxybutyrate is not measured by the nitroprusside reaction, measured ketones may be spuriously low or absent in patients with severe DKA and may actually "appear or increase" as treatment takes effect. Recently, a quantitative test for β-hydroxybutyrate has become available that may offer a superior method for measurement of ketone bodies.

Serum Osmolality. Serum osmolality is measured and followed during therapy for patients with DKA and HHS to prevent a rapid decrease, which may be responsible for the development of cerebral edema. If measurements are unavailable, serum osmolality may be calculated as follows:

$$\text{Serum osmolality} = 2(\text{Na}) + \text{glucose}/18 + \text{BUN}/3 + \text{ETOH}/4$$

The normal range is 285 to 295 mOsm/L. Significant hyperosmolality exists at levels greater than 320 mOsm/L.

Urinalysis. Urinalysis may reveal glycosuria and ketonuria. Proteinuria and hyaline casts may also be present because of dehydration. White blood cells and bacteria may be present, indicating urinary infection, which is common in diabetics and may be a predisposing factor in the development of DKA.

Other Tests. Serum magnesium and phosphorus levels may be followed in patients with DKA. Changes in these electrolytes parallel those for potassium. Serum calcium levels are followed if phosphate is administered because hypocalcemia can be induced. Cultures of urine, blood, and cerebrospinal fluid may be indicated based on historical, physical examination, or laboratory evidence of infection.

Radiologic Imaging

Chest radiographs are used in the search for a common source of infection in patients with DKA or HHS. If the patient has been unconscious, the possibility of aspiration is assessed. Computed tomography of the head is considered if the altered mental status is possibly caused by a central nervous system disorder.

PRINCIPLES OF MANAGEMENT

There are several aspects of management to be considered for each diabetic state. Although the following principles may not apply in every situation, each is included when formulating a plan for the emergency department care of the diabetic with hypoglycemia, DKA, or HHS:

- Restoration of circulating volume
- Normalization of blood glucose level
- Clearance of ketones
- Correction of acidemia or acidosis
- Correction to, and maintenance of, normal serum electrolyte concentrations
- Gradual restoration of the equilibrium of the serum osmolality
- Close clinical and laboratory monitoring

Hypoglycemia

Patients who are hypoglycemic are usually not hemodynamically unstable and have an adequate intravascular volume. In the awake patient who is not at risk for aspiration, orally administered glucose is sufficient to reverse hypoglycemia. The initial dose should be followed by a meal containing some protein to ensure that continued glucose metabolism will occur.

If the patient is unable to ingest oral glucose, administration of intravenous dextrose is necessary. Twenty-five to 50 g in a 50% solution is a routine adult dose. This amount of dextrose should elevate the blood glucose level 75 to 125 mg/dL from the initial levels. If intravenous access cannot be obtained, intramuscular injection of glucagon can stimulate gluconeogenesis, provided the patient's liver glycogen stores are not depleted.

In hypoglycemia there are no significant ketones to clear and rarely are there electrolyte abnormalities. The patient's clinical response must be monitored to ensure resolution of lethargy or coma and maintenance of an alert state. A repeat blood glucose measurement is obtained to verify adequate glucose levels.

Diabetic Ketoacidosis

Restoration of Circulating Volume. Fluid administration is the most important component of therapy. Intravenous fluids not only restore circulating volume but also help to lower the blood glucose level and clear free fatty acids. The adult patient in diabetic ketoacidosis has an average fluid deficit of 6 L. If the patient is hemodynamically unstable, 15 to 20 mg/kg/hr of isotonic crystalloid is given while monitoring the patient's response. In the patient whose blood pressure does not respond adequately or whose clinical condition worsens after fluid administration, invasive hemodynamic monitoring may be indicated. In the stable patient in diabetic ketoacidosis, fluid is given as 1 L of normal saline during the first 30 minutes. The second liter is given over 1 to 2 hours. At this point, fluids are often changed to 0.5 normal saline and are given at a rate that ensures adequate urine output, typically 300 to 500 mL/hr.

Normalization of Blood Glucose Concentration. The administration of normal saline alone may account for a 15% to 20% decrease in blood glucose in 1 to 2 hours. The goal of therapy is to reduce blood glucose by about 100 mg/dL/hr. Insulin administration is not necessary during the first hour of fluid therapy and may lower blood glucose too rapidly, predisposing the patient to cerebral edema and hypoglycemia. The recommended method of insulin administration and the amount given vary. A loading dose of 0.1 unit/kg may be given by intravenous push during the first hour of fluid administration, but is not required. A continuous infusion of 0.1 unit/kg/hr is initiated after the first hour of fluid infusion. When a blood glucose level of 250 to 300 mg/dL is attained, the insulin infusion is reduced to 0.05 mg/dL/hr and dextrose is added to the fluids. The insulin infusion is continued until acidosis and ketonemia are resolved. Much lower doses, such as 1 unit/hr, have been used in an attempt to correct the metabolic abnormalities in a more gradual fashion and appear to be effective and associated with no complications. Correction of the serum glucose level

to a normal range is usually completed after the patient leaves the emergency department.

Clearance of Ketones. Fluid administration aids in the clearance of free fatty acids, the precursors of ketone bodies. The administration of insulin is important to halt intracellular starvation and leads to a decrease in the counterregulatory hormones and cessation of lipolysis and ketogenesis. Fluids and insulin are usually sufficient to effect clearance of ketones.

Correction of Acidemia. Bicarbonate therapy for acidemia may be associated with the development of cerebral edema, alkalosis, and paradoxical cerebrospinal fluid acidosis. Its use is not recommended in most patients. Even with severely acidotic patients with pH in the range of 6.9 to 7.1, there are no data to support its use. When used (usually in patients with pH less than 6.9), bicarbonate is given slowly as an infusion (1 to 2 mEq/kg over 2 hours). Bicarbonate may have a significant lowering effect on potassium. (See Chapter 21, Acute Metabolic Acidosis and Metabolic Alkalosis.)

Maintenance of Normal Serum Electrolytes. Administration of potassium should proceed in the patient who has urinary output and in whom there is no electrocardiographic evidence of hyperkalemia (peaked T waves). Potassium, 20 to 40 mEq, may be added to the second liter of fluid. One regimen is to give potassium, half as potassium chloride and half as K_3PO_4, since phosphate depletion also occurs in these patients. Except for patients with extreme hypokalemia, it is administered at a rate not to exceed 10 mEq/hr. In extreme situations, potassium may be given at rates of 80 to 100 mEq/hr, using central venous access and continuous cardiac monitoring. Further potassium therapy is guided by serum levels obtained hourly.

Replacement of magnesium in the patient who is hypomagnesemic may be accomplished by adding 4 g of magnesium to each liter of fluid after the initial rapid infusions are completed.

Close Clinical and Laboratory Monitoring. Hourly laboratory values are obtained in a patient with significantly severe diabetic ketoacidosis until improvement is noted. Parameters monitored hourly include

- Glucose
- Electrolytes
- Arterial blood gases (venous pH may be adequate after improvement begins)
- Vital signs
- Mental status
- Urine output

A flow sheet will aid in organizing the data and allow for easy recognition of trends. Vital signs are obtained frequently, and the patient's mental status is closely monitored, as is his or her handling of the fluid load. *If the patient's clinical status does not improve as the biochemical abnormalities are corrected, a search for additional problems (e.g., sepsis, meningitis, ingestion, or head trauma) is mandated.*

Most complications of DKA (and HHS) are treatment related. Hypoglycemia, hypokalemia, and rebound hyperglycemia can be prevented by serial monitoring of the patient's condition and laboratory boluses. Cerebral edema, especially in pediatric patients, is the most serious problem. It occurs in about 1% of pediatric DKA and can be prevented by careful fluid administration following prescribed guidelines.

Hyperosmolar Hyperglycemic States

Restoration of Circulating Volume. Normal saline is administered until hemodynamic stability is achieved. Fluids are then changed to 0.5 normal saline. Because of large fluid shifts and the frequency of associated disease, hemodynamic monitoring is frequently required.

Normalization of Blood Glucose Level. Again, the goal of therapy is to lower blood glucose by 100 mg/dL/hr. For patients with HHS, fluid administration can lower the blood glucose level by 25% to 30% during the first hour. Because there is a relative insulin lack, patients with HHS may be sensitive to insulin administration; therefore, an insulin dose of 0.02 to 0.05 unit/kg/hr given by infusion is used initially. This is especially important when the blood glucose concentration is more than 1000 mg/dL.

Clearance of Ketones and Correction of Acidemia or Acidosis. These patients have no or minimal ketosis.

Maintenance of Serum Electrolytes. As in patients with DKA, dehydration and fluid shifts will result in electrolyte imbalances. Potassium is administered as soon as urine flow is established and true hyperkalemia is ruled out. Major total body deficits of phosphate and magnesium are also frequently present.

Close Clinical and Laboratory Monitoring. A flow sheet is used to follow key parameters hourly:

- Glucose
- Electrolytes
- Osmolality
- Mental status
- Vital signs
- Urine output

The high association between HHS and other serious illnesses may make additional specific management necessary and may require modification of the treatment regimen outlined.

SPECIAL CONSIDERATIONS

Pediatric Patients

Metabolic complications of diabetes mellitus are not uncommon in children. Hypoglycemia is extremely common in critically ill children. Screening or empirical treatment with dextrose is indicated in all neonates and infants who present with critical illness or altered mental status. The lack of significant glycogen reserves leads to hypoglycemia in the presence of a wide variety of stresses.

Ninety-seven percent of children with diabetes have type 1 disease and are therefore prone to ketosis. An episode of diabetic ketoacidosis is the initial presentation of this disease in approximately 10% of cases. The diagnosis of DKA in children is achieved in essentially the same fashion as for adults, but the management varies considerably. Rapid shifts in osmolality lead to the complication of cerebral edema more frequently in children than in adults, and many children will die when cerebral edema develops. Therefore, every effort is made during treatment to bring the serum glucose level down gradually in an effort to prevent this dreaded complication.

Fluid resuscitation is begun with normal saline given at a rate of 20 mL/kg over the first hour (more rapidly if there are signs of shock). It is prudent to reduce the rate of fluid infusion to less than 10 mL/kg for the next 3 hours. Hydrating at a rate greater than 50 mL/kg in the first 4 hours has been shown to be associated with an increased risk of cerebral edema and brain herniation. Insulin is administered as a continuous infusion at a rate of 0.1 unit/kg/hour. No loading dose is recommended to provide a more gradual, linear decline in the serum glucose level.

Elderly Patients

Maturity-onset (type 2) diabetes mellitus is extremely common in the elderly population. These patients are frequently adequately treated with proper diet and an oral hypoglycemic agent. DKA is rare in this population, but HHS is not uncommon.

Elderly diabetic patients are likely to have a host of vascular complications of this disease. Proper evaluation and management require a high index of suspicion of peripheral vascular disease, renal failure, coronary artery disease, and cerebrovascular accidents.

DISPOSITION AND FOLLOW-UP

Hypoglycemia

Patients Requiring Admission. The patient who fails to respond to initial therapy, who has inadequate oral intake, or who relapses into a hypoglycemic state is admitted. The patient who has taken a long-acting hypoglycemic agent (long-acting insulin or one of the oral agents) is admitted.

Patients Requiring ICU Admission. Patients with profound hypoglycemia unresponsive to therapy, usually in the setting of a massive overdose with a hypoglycemic agent, require intensive care.

Patients Who Can Be Discharged. After the patient's blood glucose level is normalized, the hypoglycemic patient must be fully awake and alert before discharge is considered. If the cause of the patient's reaction is not clear, admitting the patient to investigate possible causes is recommended.

Hyperglycemia (DKA and HHS)

Patients Requiring Admission. If a patient cannot tolerate oral fluids (i.e., has continuous vomiting) or has moderate to severe diabetic ketoacidosis or HHS, admission is arranged. If the patient cannot monitor blood glucose closely at home or cannot administer the appropriate insulin dose, in-hospital therapy and education are advised.

Patients Requiring ICU Admission. Although all patients admitted for DKA or HHS are considered for ICU admission, some situations that generally make intensive care advisable are as follows:

- Age younger than 2 or older than 60 years

- pH less than 7.0
- Serious concurrent illness

If a separate metabolic unit is not available in the hospital, all patients with moderate to severe DKA or HHS should be monitored in the ICU for the first 24 hours.

Patients Who Can Be Discharged. Criteria for resolution of DKA include

- Glucose less than 200 mg/dL
- Bicarbonate of 18 mEq/L or greater
- pH greater than 7.3

An alert patient with mild symptoms, mild ketoacidosis without vomiting, reasonable intelligence, and accessibility to the hospital may be treated as an outpatient. If vomiting persists despite initial therapy, the patient is admitted. Essentially all HHS patients are admitted.

FINAL POINTS

- Patients with derangements in glucose metabolism most frequently present to the emergency department with a depressed level of consciousness.
- Rapid determination of blood glucose level is essential in the initial approach to all patients with an altered level of consciousness.
- Dextrose may be used empirically if blood glucose test strips are unavailable, because it will do no harm even in the hyperglycemic patient.
- In hypoglycemic patients, an adequate blood glucose level must be ensured before disposition is decided on. Long-acting agents may result in recurrent episodes of hypoglycemia.
- In hyperglycemic states, adequate fluid and insulin administration with careful monitoring of acid-base status and electrolytes are the *mainstays* of therapy.
- The dehydrated patient who is still voiding has DKA until proved otherwise.
- A discrepancy between the laboratory findings and clinical status should lead the emergency physician to consider other causes for the patient's condition.

CASE*Study*

The rescue squad is called to the home of a 37-year-old diabetic woman, whose husband states that the woman had been vomiting and had become increasingly sleepy over the past 10 to 12 hours. When the rescue squad arrives, the patient is responsive to verbal stimulation but gives no coherent answers to questions. The husband states that his wife has not been feeling well for a week or more. Yesterday she complained of abdominal pain and began to vomit. These complaints continued through today. She is a lifelong diabetic and takes daily

NPH insulin in a dose of 25 units each morning. She takes no other medications and has no known medical complications from the diabetes.

The patient's vital signs revealed a pulse rate of 120 beats per minute, a respiratory rate of 36 breaths per minute, and a blood pressure of 100/60 mm Hg. Respirations were deep, and there appeared to be adequate ventilation. The glucose reagent strip revealed a glucose level of 180 to 240 mg/dL. The paramedics were instructed to give the patient oxygen and to start an intravenous line of normal saline at a rate of 500 mL/hr.

Glucose reagent strips are very useful for estimating the blood glucose concentration but cannot be relied on conclusively. In the field, where these strips are more likely to be exposed to excess heat and moisture, the possibility of an error is significant. Administration of 50 mL of 50% dextrose will result in an increase of 75 to 125 mg/dL in the serum glucose level. Even in the hyperglycemic patient, this is unlikely to cause additional problems. Therefore, some physicians will elect to administer dextrose empirically to all patients with a significantly altered level of consciousness. In this case, the rescue squad has decided against supplemental dextrose because the history and physical findings are also consistent with a diagnosis of hyperglycemia as the origin of this patient's problem.

The patient is rapidly transported to the emergency department, where she is evaluated immediately. She remains responsive to verbal stimulation but is incoherent. Repeat vital signs reveal pulse rate, 128 beats per minute; respirations, 36 breaths per minute; and blood pressure, 90/50 mm Hg. Her temperature is 98.6° F (37°C) Oxygen was continued at 10 L/min by mask. The falling blood pressure is of great concern, and an additional large-bore intravenous line is initiated. Both lines are allowed to run wide open. Blood is obtained for laboratory studies, and the blood glucose level is rechecked at the bedside. The reagent strip gives a reading of greater than 240 mg/dL.

Because the reagent strip reading was elevated, the physician decided against dextrose administration. Although administration of dextrose will not cause significant harm metabolically, there are potential problems with it, owing to the hypertonicity of the solution. If 50% dextrose is administered into the subcutaneous tissue by error, a large area of skin may slough. An intravenous line should be specifically checked for patency before

50% dextrose is administered through it. The rest of the treatment and rapid focus on the complications of diabetes are appropriate.

The initial information supplied by the patient's husband is all that is readily obtainable. He has been married for only a short time and has no knowledge of previous similar episodes. Physical examination reveals a woman with no external evidence of trauma who is responsive to verbal stimulation with incoherent mumbling. Her skin is pale and dry. The oral mucosa is dry and cracked, and there is a strong fruity odor on the breath. Cardiac and lung examinations reveal no abnormalities. The abdomen is soft and nontender. There are no focal neurologic findings.

The history and physical examination failed to suggest causes of coma unrelated to diabetes, and the bedside glucose screening test reveals a modest elevation of the blood glucose level. The findings of hyperventilation, dehydration, and fruity odor of the breath are very suggestive of DKA. Arterial blood gas measurements will confirm the suspicion of acidosis, and a rapid check of the urine for glucose and acetone provides further support for this preliminary diagnosis.

Additional test results immediately available at the bedside reveal a urine glucose of 4+, urine ketones of 2+, arterial pH of 7.10, and a normal electrocardiogram with no T-wave abnormalities.

During the next 30 minutes to 1 hour, additional test results become available. They show a blood glucose level of 540 mg/dL, serum ketones present in a 1:8 dilution, and serum electrolytes as follows: sodium, 140 mEq/L; potassium, 4.0 mEq/L; and chloride, 100 mEq/L. The blood urea nitrogen value was 30 mg/dL, and the creatinine level was 1.8 mg/dL.

Treatment should proceed based on the immediately available test results. Even when laboratory results are rapidly available the delay is too great to allow initial therapy to be postponed pending their arrival.

Interpreting the laboratory test results provides the following information:

For every 100 mg/dL above 100 mg/dL of glucose, the serum sodium level falls 1.6 mEq/L, because of osmotic dilution. At a glucose level of 500 mg/dL, the serum sodium concentration should be falsely decreased. The true value is $140 + (1.6 \times 4) = 146.4$ mEq/L.

Continued on following page

Serum osmolarity can be calculated as follows:
2(Na) + glucose/18 + blood urea nitrogen/3 = osmolarity.
2(140) + 540/18 + 30/3 = 329 mOsm/L.

This is significant hyperosmolarity.

It may be useful to estimate what the potassium level would be if the pH were normal. To correct the pH to 7.4, the present 7.1 value needs to have 0.3 added to it. Because potassium moves 0.6 mEq/L in the opposite direction for each 0.1 change in the pH, the serum potassium would decrease by 3 × 0.6 = 1.8 mEq/L. Therefore, the present serum potassium of 4.0 mEq/L would fall to 2.2 mEq/L if the pH were corrected without supplemental potassium. This is a dangerously low level and can be avoided by the addition of a potassium supplement.

Because of the patient's fall in blood pressure, 2 L of normal saline is administered during the first 30 minutes in the emergency department. Blood pressure promptly rises to 110/60 mm Hg. Normal saline is continued, with the third liter given over the next hour. The patient has a normal ECG (normal T waves) and is producing copious urine. Potassium chloride, 20 mEq, and K_3PO_4, 20 mEq, are added to the third liter of normal saline.

Insulin is started through a second intravenous line after the first liter of fluid has been given. This 50-kg woman is started on an infusion at 5 units/hr. After 1 hour of insulin therapy and 1.5 hours of fluid therapy, the blood glucose level is 400 mEq/dL, the pH is 7.12, the potassium concentration is 3.5 mEq/L, and the bicarbonate value is 14 mg/L.

Slow resolution of the metabolic derangement is preferable. A general guide for the desired change in blood glucose concentration is a decrease of 10% per hour of therapy. Rapid falls predispose the patient to development of hypoglycemia, electrolyte disturbances, and cerebral edema. The potassium level in this patient, which was initially normal, became low-normal with therapy in spite of potassium supplementation. This change was anticipated by earlier calculations. Early potassium replacement is essential to prevent hypokalemia because the level will fall with therapy.

Although this patient's metabolic disturbance was not too great, her initial cardiovascular instability and her mental status made admission to the ICU advisable. The clinical findings, including mental status, did not correlate with the degree of metabolic disturbance found. Disposition decisions should take both of these aspects into consideration.

Bibliography

TEXTS

Quan M: Clinical Cornerstone: Diabetes. Hillsborough, NJ, Excerpta Medica, 2001
Wilson JD, Foster DW, Kronenberg HM, Larsen PR (eds): Williams Textbook of Endocrinology, 9th ed. Philadelphia, WB Saunders, 1998.

JOURNAL ARTICLES

American Diabetes Association: Hospital admission guidelines for diabetes mellitus. Diabetes Care 2000; 23(Suppl 1):S83.
Bonadio W: Pediatric diabetic ketoacidosis: Pathophysiology and potential for outpatient management of selected children. Pediatr Emerg Care 1992; 8:287–290.
Brink SJ: Diabetic ketoacidosis: Prevention, treatment and complications in children and adolescents. Diabetes Nutr Metab 1999; 12(2):122–135.
Cryer PE, Fisher JN, Shamoon H: Hypoglycemia. Diabetes Care 1994; 17:734–755.

Keller RL, Rivers CS, Wolfson AB: Update in diabetic ketoacidosis: Strategies for effective management. Emerg Med Rep 1991; 12:89.
Kitabchi AE, Wall BM: Management of diabetic ketoacidosis. Am Fam Physician 1999; 60:455–464.
Laffel L: Ketone bodies: A review of physiology, pathophysiology and application of monitoring to diabetes. Diabetes Metab Res Rev 1999; 15:412–426.
Mahoney CP, Vicek BW, DelAguila M: Risk factors for developing brain herniation during diabetic ketoacidosis. Pediatr Neurol 1999; 21:721–727.
Matz R: Management of the hyperosmolar hyperglycemic syndrome. Am Fam Physician 1999; 60:1468–1476.
Schwab TM, Hendey GW, Soliz TC: Screening for ketonemia in patients with diabetes. Ann Emerg Med 1999; 34:342–346.
Viallon A, Zeni F, Lafond P, et al: Does bicarbonate therapy improve the management of severe diabetic ketoacidosis? Crit Care Med 1999; 27:2690–2693.
Wagner A, Risse A, Brill HL, et al: Therapy of severe diabetic ketoacidosis: Zero-mortality under very-low-dose insulin application. Diabetes Care 1999; 22:674–677.

CHAPTER 21

Acute Metabolic Acidosis and Metabolic Alkalosis

GLENN C. HAMILTON

CASE *Study*

A 35-year-old man was escorted to the emergency department by the police for medical clearance before incarceration for public intoxication. The patient stated that he had no medical problems and had been drinking alcohol. He complained of vague abdominal pain.

The patient appeared intoxicated. He had slurred speech and a wide-based gait. Vital signs were blood pressure, 120/70 mm Hg; pulse, 112 beats per minute; respirations, 22 breaths per minute; and oral temperature, 37.0°C (98.6°F). Physical examination was unremarkable except for mild, nonspecific abdominal pain. The patient was discharged to police custody. He returned to the emergency department 12 hours later poorly responsive and hypotensive.

INTRODUCTION

Disturbances in acid-base equilibrium are common findings in the practice of emergency medicine. In every seriously ill patient, the presence and influence of an acid-base imbalance must be considered. The problem-solving approach in these disorders is usually different from that used in "symptom-oriented" presentations. Initial decision priorities and the preliminary differential diagnosis are established after laboratory test results are received. The information presented in this chapter is arranged to reflect this difference. After a review of basic pathophysiology, an approach to deciphering the laboratory values is given. This is followed by the differential diagnosis of metabolic acidosis and alkalosis.

Normal blood pH ranges from 7.36 to 7.44. The suffix "-emia" refers to blood pH; *acidemia* indicates a pH of less than 7.36, and *alkalemia* signifies a pH of greater than 7.44. Acidemia has a number of physiologic impacts in the body. Low pH can cause decreased myocardial contractility,

cardiac dysrhythmias, decreased central nervous system function, or hypotension from vasodilation and a decreased receptor responsiveness to catecholamines. Alkalemia may induce hypokalemia, tetany, cerebral vasoconstriction, and a shift in the oxygen-hemoglobin dissociation curve, causing less oxygen to be released to the tissues.

There are two basic types of acid-base disturbances: metabolic and respiratory. Respiratory disorders primarily alter the PCO_2, whereas metabolic disorders are characterized by changes in the plasma bicarbonate (HCO_3^-) concentration. Should a disease process occur that alters the blood pH, a compensatory response is initiated in the body. If the primary process alters the HCO_3^-, the initial compensatory response alters the PCO_2, and the reverse also occurs. The compensatory process is a normal physiologic response triggered by the primary acid-base disturbance. It is a physiologic attempt to move the plasma pH closer toward normal. If the source of the primary disorder is removed or resolved, compensation is often followed by "correction." This is the definitive process of returning the acid-base balance to normal.

Acidosis and *alkalosis* refer to primary processes that, if unopposed, result in a decrease and an increase in pH, respectively. Acidosis occurs secondary to the addition of acid or loss of HCO_3^-. Alkalosis results from the addition of HCO_3^- or loss of acid. A simple acid-base disorder is a single primary disturbance accompanied by its appropriate compensatory process. A mixed disorder implies the coexistence of two or more primary processes. The remainder of this chapter is devoted to a discussion of simple metabolic processes and their causes.

Physiology

Diagnosis and management of these disorders require an understanding of normal acid-base physiology, which involves generating hydrogen (H^+) and HCO_3^-, handling and eliminating these ions, and responding to excess ion loads from endogenous and exogenous sources.

Oxidative metabolism of carbohydrates and fats results in the generation of CO_2 ("volatile" acid) and water. Every day approximately 15,000 mmol of CO_2 is generated. Most of the CO_2 is transported from the tissues to the lungs in the form of plasma HCO_3^- and hemoglobin-bound carbamino groups. In the lungs, the transport forms are converted back into CO_2 and eliminated by normal ventilation. Approximately 200 mL/min of CO_2 is removed from the tissues at rest. During physical exertion up to 2000 mL/min is expired.

Dietary proteins and incompletely oxidized carbohydrates and fats are metabolized to "fixed" or "nonvolatile" acids. The metabolism of protein results in approximately 1 mEq of fixed acid for each gram of protein ingested, or about 60 to 80 mEq/day in the average American diet. This fixed acid is usually in the form of sulfuric or phosphoric acid. These new acids are chemically buffered by HCO_3^- to maintain pH within the narrow range necessary for the optimal performance of the body's numerous enzyme systems. To sustain acid-base equilibrium, the kidney compensates by secreting the fixed acid load and regenerating the HCO_3^- previously consumed by the buffering process. Disruption of this finely integrated balance between production, buffering, and compensation results in a metabolic acid-base disturbance.

In acid-base physiology, the bicarbonate/carbonic acid buffer system is quantitatively the most important of the body's buffers. The system operates through the chemical equation:

CO_2 (excreted via lung) + H_2O ↔ H_2CO_3 (carbonic acid) ↔ HCO_3^- (maintained via kidney) + H^+

This buffer system is unique because it is open ended, because the lung constantly excretes CO_2, and is self-regulating, and because the kidney excretes, reabsorbs, and regenerates HCO_3^-.

Renal reabsorption of HCO_3^- in the proximal tubule normally averages 80% to 90% of the filtered load. The fraction of reabsorbable HCO_3^- is relatively constant over a wide range of glomerular filtration rates and HCO_3^- concentrations. The reabsorption of HCO_3^- by the proximal tubule may be altered by extracellular volume, CO_2 tension, serum calcium, potassium level, and parathyroid hormone. For example, the existence of significant extracellular volume contraction or hypokalemia causes an increase in proximal tubular HCO_3^- reabsorption and may result in a metabolic alkalosis.

Within the distal nephron, that is, the distal convoluted tubule and collecting ducts, HCO_3^- is also reabsorbed to the extent that no HCO_3^- escapes into the urine during systemic acidosis. As shown in Figure 21–1, distal H^+ secretion not only mediates reabsorption of remaining HCO_3^- but the decreased tubule fluid pH also causes the existing cellular NH_3 and nonbicarbonate buffers to be trapped in the luminal fluid as NH_4 and titratable acid. The excretion of H^+ in these forms combined with regenerated HCO_3^- keeps the body in pH balance. Facilitation of HCO_3^- excretion occurs in response to extracellular volume expansion. However, other factors, including primary hyperaldosteronism, hypokalemia, and increased non-reabsorbable anion delivery, may independently enhance distal H^+ secretion, thus reducing or preventing the amount of HCO_3^- lost from the body.

Pathophysiology

Metabolic Acidosis

Metabolic acidosis is an acid-base disturbance created by a primary reduction in HCO_3^- concentration with a consequent fall in pH. It may be caused by one of three mechanisms: (1) increased production or addition of acids, (2) decreased renal excretion of acids, or (3) loss of alkali through the kidneys or gastrointestinal tract. This decrease in HCO_3^- is first limited by buffers such as hemoglobin and phosphate. Respiratory compensation follows as the central chemoreceptors respond to the fall in pH by stimulating the respiratory center, causing alveolar hyperventilation. This lowers the P_{CO_2} in an attempt to return the pH closer to normal. Therefore, a respiratory hyperventilation ($\downarrow P_{CO_2}$) is the normal compensatory response to an induced decrease in the HCO_3^- and pH level.

Metabolic Alkalosis

The hallmark of metabolic alkalosis is the primary elevation of the plasma HCO_3^- concentration, with a subsequent increase in pH. The compensatory response is alveolar hypoventilation. This process is limited by an upper limit of P_{CO_2} at 55 to 60 mm Hg. The development of metabolic alkalosis requires two physiologically distinct processes. Initially, there is loss of acid or addition of alkali to generate the metabolic alkalosis. Under normal circumstances, the efficiency with which HCO_3^- can be excreted by the kidneys is so great that it is difficult to induce more than a mild alkalosis even when 24 mEq/kg/day of $NaHCO_3$ is ingested. Thus, to maintain a metabolic alkalosis, enhanced renal reabsorption (or regeneration) of HCO_3^- must be present. Factors causing this

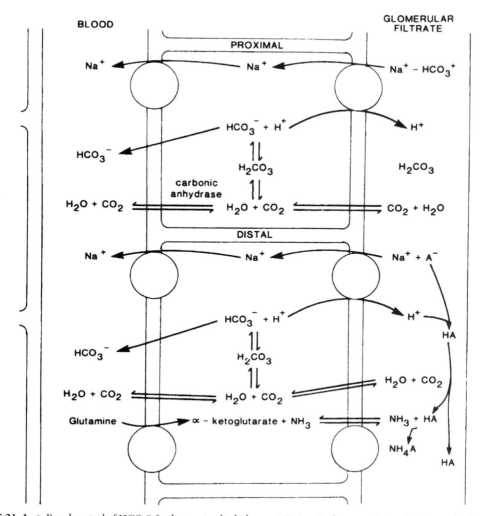

FIGURE 21–1. • Renal control of HCO_3^-. In the proximal tubule, most H^+ is actively secreted into the glomerular filtrate by a Na^+/H^+ exchange. It reacts with the filtered HCO_3^- to form carbonic acid (H_2CO_3). Carbonic anhydrase in the brush border of the luminal cell membrane rapidly catalyzes its breakdown to H_2O and CO_2 and a hydrogen ion gradient is not established. Water and CO_2 diffuse into the cell, where H_2O is split to H^+ and OH^-. The OH^- combines with CO_2 to form HCO_3^- in another carbonic anhydrase–facilitated reaction. This HCO_3^- then moves with Na^+ into the blood, and the H^+ moves into the lumen to react with another filtered HCO_3^-.

The distal tubule has carbonic anhydrase only within the cell. This allows a hydrogen gradient to become established. In the distal tubule, the rest of the HCO_3^- is reclaimed, and the tubular fluid is acidified. This added H^+ to the lumen results in a newly generated HCO_3^- moving into the blood. This balances the new "fixed" acid created in protein metabolism. The H^+ binds with ammonia, sulfate, or phosphate and is excreted. This process is influenced by urinary Na^+, intracellular K^+, aldosterone, and the HCO_3^- load reaching the distal nephron. (From Jehle D, Harchelroad FP: Bicarbonate. Emerg Med Clin North Am 1986; 4:150.)

include volume depletion, chloride deficiency, mineralocorticoid excess, and hypokalemia. The physiologic interplay of these factors in vomiting, a common cause of metabolic alkalosis, is diagrammed in Figure 21–2.

INITIAL APPROACH AND STABILIZATION

Priority Diagnoses

Suspicion of a metabolic disorder depends on recognizing the clinical settings in which it may occur. The patients at greatest risk for metabolic acidosis are those with altered mental status, diabetes mellitus, alcoholism, toxic ingestion, and renal or gastrointestinal disturbances.

Rapid Assessment

Patients with a metabolic acidosis often present with nonspecific symptoms. The clinical effects of metabolic acidosis are often overshadowed by the signs and symptoms of the underlying disorder.

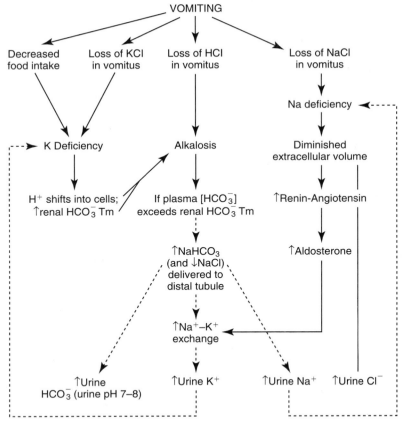

FIGURE 21–2. • Pathophysiology of metabolic alkalosis secondary to vomiting. (From Seldin DW, Rector FA: Symposium on acid-base homeostasis: The generation and maintenance of metabolic alkalosis. Kidney Int 1972; 1:306, with permission from Kidney International.)

Frequently, the only clue to the presence of a metabolic acidosis is an abnormality in the vital signs. Any patient with hyperventilation, altered mental status, and hemodynamic instability may be suspected of having a potentially significant decreased pH.

Metabolic alkalosis may occur in patients with prolonged vomiting, significant dehydration, or diuretic use. There are no specific signs or symptoms of metabolic alkalosis; thus, laboratory studies play an essential role in its assessment.

Early Intervention

Initial intervention is directed toward stabilizing the patient's vital signs. Most patients with a suspected acid-base disorder will require the following:

- Intravenous access
- Volume repletion, if clinically necessary
- Oxygen supplementation
- Cardiac monitoring for potential dysrhythmias

Early ordering of several laboratory tests is necessary to fully unravel an acid-base disorder. These tests include arterial blood gas (ABG) analysis, electrolyte levels, renal profile, and serum glucose concentration. Other tests such as osmolarity and specific toxicology screens are ordered only as necessary.

CASE *Study*

On reexamination, the patient was now poorly responsive with vomitus around his mouth. Vital signs were blood pressure, 100/50 mm Hg; pulse, 120 beats per minute; respirations, 40 breaths per minute; and temperature, 36.0°C (96.8°F). Initial stabilization included endotracheal intubation, ventilation with 100% oxygen, and intravenous access. After checking for normal breath sounds, 1 L of isotonic crystalloid was given over 15 minutes. The glucose oxidase test strip measured 120 mg/dL, and intravenous glucose was not given. Naloxone, 2 mg, and thiamine, 100 mg, were administered intravenously. After the initial resuscitation, the patient's blood pressure was 80 mm Hg (palpation) and pulse was 120 beats per minute. The skin was mottled and cold. He made no spontaneous noise and withdrew symmetrically from painful stimuli without posturing. His pupils were 8 mm bilaterally and were sluggishly reactive. Papilledema was noted on funduscopic examination. There was no evidence of trauma. A cardiac monitor, nasogastric tube, and indwelling urinary catheter were placed. Samples were sent for laboratory studies.

The only information available is that the patient had been "medically cleared" 12 hours earlier. He gave a history of alcohol intake and vague abdominal pain. He was tachycardic and tachypneic during the prior evaluation and became increasingly lethargic over the intervening hours. The medics reported that the patient was in a cell alone. There were no signs of trauma, and the possibility of drug ingestion in this setting was considered as slight.

Because of the altered mental status and unstable vital signs, metabolic acidosis may have a role, either as a cause or a complication. The primary goal is to stabilize the patient.

CLINICAL ASSESSMENT

There may be historical points or findings on physical examination suggestive of acid-base metabolic disorders. This information is often gathered after the laboratory results have identified the problem.

History

The history is directed to uncover high-risk settings in which a metabolic disorder is known to occur.

Metabolic Acidosis

1. Are there clinical *manifestations* that are *suggestive* of *diabetes mellitus,* including polyuria, polydipsia, and polyphagia?
2. Are there *gastrointestinal complaints,* especially abdominal pain or vomiting? These are frequently seen in diabetic, alcoholic, and starvation ketoacidosis.
3. Is there a history of *depression, suicidal ideation,* or *drug/alcohol abuse?* These may suggest a possible ingested poison.

4. Is there a history of *renal insufficiency?* Oliguria and pruritus are late manifestations.

Metabolic Alkalosis

1. Are there symptoms consistent with *volume depletion?* These include thirst, dry mouth, dizziness or syncope (often orthostatic), and decreased urine output.
2. Is there persistent or prolonged *vomiting* or *diarrhea?* This is one of the most common histories in patients with metabolic alkalosis.
3. Is the patient taking *diuretics?* This medication, particularly thiazide or loop diuretics, is most often associated with an elevated level of HCO_3^-.
4. Does the patient complain of *physical weakness* or *muscle cramps?* These symptoms can be noted in patients with changes in potassium, magnesium, or calcium concentrations.

Physical Examination

The major goal of the physical examination is to identify further the presence and etiology of the metabolic process. The vital signs and general appearance may indicate the body's response to a metabolic acidosis. Specific signs are few (Table 21–1). Findings in metabolic alkalosis are limited to those of dehydration or secondary complications, such as muscle weakness from hypokalemia or muscle irritability from hypocalcemia.

CASE *Study*

The physical examination findings that hint at an underlying metabolic acidosis are limited: alteration in vital signs (especially increased respiratory rate), depressed mental status, and peripheral skin changes consistent with a hyperadrenergic state. Papilledema may be an early indication of increased intracranial pressure. In the setting of metabolic acidosis, it also suggests a specific ingested toxin. Confirmatory laboratory testing is necessary to make the diagnosis of a metabolic acidosis.

DIAGNOSTIC ADJUNCTS

Laboratory Studies

Laboratory testing assists and usually reveals the diagnosis in acid-base disorders. In any patient suspected of metabolic acidosis or alkalosis, the following studies are ordered:

TABLE 21–1. Physical Examination Findings in Metabolic Acidosis (Nonspecific)

Examination Area	Components	Comments
Vital signs	Heart rate	Tachycardia common secondary to acidosis-induced epinephrine release
	Blood pressure	Decrease in myocardial contractility is balanced by positive inotropic effect of acidosis-induced epinephrine release. If pH < 7.20, there is progressive loss of catecholamine responsiveness and myoinhibitory effects dominate.
	Respiratory rate and depth	Tachypnea is compensatory respiratory response to metabolic acidosis. Hyperventilation (Kussmaul respiration) may be pronounced in acute metabolic acidosis, pH < 7.20. In chronic metabolic acidosis, the increased ventilatory rate may not be clinically apparent. However, tachypnea is not a specific sign of metabolic acidosis.
General appearance	Temperature	Fever points to an infectious process contributing to the acidosis.
	Skin	Evidence of poor perfusion and/or hydration; alcoholic liver disease or inadequate diet (palmar erythema, ecchymosis, or perifollicular hemorrhage); renal disease or infection. Signs of diabetes (e.g., necrobiosis)
Eyes	Tearing; funduscopic examination	Hydration. Papilledema or erythema may be present with toxic ingestions (e.g., methanol). Vascular changes may suggest diabetes (e.g., cotton-wool spots, hemorrhage, neovascularization).
Mouth	Breath	Smell for ketosis, wintergreen (methyl salicylate), cyanide
Lungs	Percussion and auscultation for signs of pneumonia	Infectious process may cause sepsis and metabolic acidosis.
Cardiac	Auscultation	Murmurs may suggest a hyperdynamic state, valvular heart disease, or endocarditis. S_3 gallop is present with congestive heart failure.
Abdomen	Inspection, auscultation, percussion, palpation	Presence of diffuse pain common in diabetic ketoacidosis and toxic ingestion. Appropriately localized pain may give evidence of pancreatic or small bowel fistula.
Neurologic	Altered sensorium	Common in all types of severe acidosis. May reflect toxic ingestion or coexistent hyperosmolar state

Sodium (Na⁺). This may give information on the origin of a change in volume status. Hyponatremia also may cause an altered mental status.

Potassium (K⁺). The serum level is influenced by cellular shifts in both acidemia and alkalemia. It is an important ion to monitor in all cases, because it can be significantly depleted in both metabolic acidosis and alkalosis. Potassium depletion can cause dysrhythmias and neuromuscular paresis.

Chloride (Cl⁻). In most cases, chloride moves in the direction opposite that of HCO_3^-. It is useful as part of the anion gap equation.

Bicarbonate (HCO₃⁻). Elevations and decreases of this ion are important in identifying metabolic disorders. Isolated values may be confusing because of mixed acid-base disturbances.

Glucose. The glucose concentration is important because of the high incidence of metabolic problems associated with diabetes and hyperosmolar states.

Blood Urea Nitrogen (BUN) and Creatinine (Cr). It is important to assess renal function. An elevated BUN to Cr ratio (>10:1) may indicate dehydration.

Arterial Blood Gas Analysis. This test is essential to determine the pH, Po_2, and Pco_2. Each has an influence on acid-base balance. There may be other useful information in the ABG values. The reported HCO_3^- level may be correlated with the serum level. It is usually a calculated value extrapolated from the pH and Pco_2. The measured percent hemoglobin saturation may indicate a variance from the expected hemoglobin saturation at the measured Po_2. This can occur if the hemoglobin is dysfunctional (e.g., carbon monoxide poisoning, methemoglobinemia).

Urinalysis. The specific gravity helps gauge dehydration and kidney function. Dipstick testing is valuable for measuring the urinary pH, presence of ketones, and urinary glucose. The microscopic evaluation may be diagnostic in urinary infections or certain ingestions (e.g., calcium oxalate crystals in ethylene glycol poisoning).

Other Tests. Other tests are selected on the basis of the foregoing values and the clinical setting:

1. *Venous pH.* This test can be used to measure pH and HCO_3^-, if oxygenation is not a major concern. The blood is drawn without a tourniquet from an unexercised arm. These limitations may preclude its availability if central access is not established.
2. *Urinary electrolytes (Na⁺, K⁺, Cl⁻).* Testing for urinary chloride levels is particularly useful in distinguishing "saline-responsive" from "saline-resistant" alkalosis.
3. *Serum and urine osmolality.* These tests may be valuable in hyperosmolar states and specific ingestions (e.g., alcohols).
4. *Calcium (Ca²⁺), potassium (K⁺), magnesium (Mg²⁺).* Serum levels for these electrolytes should be evaluated in rhabdomyolysis, chronic alcoholism, starvation, or metastatic carcinoma.
5. *Measures of specific endogenous or exogenous acids or toxins*, when suspected: lactic acid, salicylic acid, serum ketones, alcohols (ethanol, methanol, ethylene glycol, isopropanol), and serum iron.

Radiologic Imaging

There is no specific role for imaging in acid-base disorders. The abdominal plain film may be useful in identifying an ingested substance (e.g., iron tablets) or a gastrointestinal problem causing or complicating the acid-base imbalance (e.g., bowel obstruction, dead bowel).

Electrocardiogram

Cardiac monitoring is often useful. The ion changes accompanying acid-base disorders can have significant dysrhythmogenic effects. The 12-lead electrocardiogram is usually reserved for (1) clarification of the dysrhythmia, (2) monitoring changes due to elevated or decreased potassium, and (3) assisting in the diagnosis of ischemic heart disease in patients with nausea, vomiting, or epigastric pain.

CLINICAL REASONING

Once the laboratory values are available, and assuming they are accurate, several questions are asked in all metabolic acid-base disorders. These steps identify the process as acidosis or alkalosis, assess whether it is a simple or mixed acid-base disorder, and begin to differentiate between causes.

What Is the PH?

The pH measures the blood as acidemic or alkalemic. This identifies and specifies the primary process, because compensatory mechanisms do not overcorrect. That is, if the pH is acidemic (<7.35), the lung response (ΔPco_2) to a primary metabolic (ΔHCO_3^-) process will not bring the pH to normal.

What Is the Measured HCO_3^-?

The measured HCO_3^- is taken from the electrolytes. HCO_3^- is the major ion altered in a primary metabolic process, and the Pco_2 will change as part of compensation or another primary process. In metabolic acid-base disorders it will usually be abnormal. A low HCO_3^- (< 22 mEq/L) is consistent with metabolic acidosis. An elevated HCO_3^- (> 28 mEq/L) indicates a metabolic alkalosis.

What Is the Physiologic Compensation?

In metabolic acid-base disorders the compensatory response is respiratory.

If the primary process is metabolic acidosis (HCO_3^-), the normal compensatory response (hyperventilation) will lower the Pco_2 to equal

$$1.5 \times (\text{measured } HCO_3^-) + 8 \pm 2.$$

This equation calculates the expected range for an appropriate respiratory compensation. If the observed Pco_2 is not within this range, then an additional respiratory disorder coexists. The lower limit of compensation for the Pco_2 is 8 to 10 mm Hg.

If the primary process is metabolic alkalosis, the response (hypoventilation) will raise the Pco_2 to equal

$$(\text{measured } HCO_3^-) + 15 \pm 2.$$

If not in this range, a problem with respiration again coexists. The compensatory hypoventilation does not exceed a Pco_2 of 55 mm Hg, except in the person with chronic pulmonary disease.

What Is the Anion Gap?

The principle of electrical neutrality dictates the total milliequivalents per liter of cations that must equal the total milliequivalent per liter of anions. Serum Na^+ accounts for 90% of cations. Serum HCO_3^- and Cl^- represent 85% of all anions.

The anion gap estimates the amount of unmeasured anions that may be contributing to the acid-base disorder. It is most useful in determining the cause of metabolic acidosis. Only metabolic acidosis that results in the addition of acid (endogenous or exogenous) will create an anion gap. Metabolic acidosis caused by the loss of HCO_3^- results in a normal anion gap acidosis because the Cl^- rises as the HCO_3^- decreases. The gap originates as HCO_3^- is consumed to buffer organic acids and anions in the blood. Its usual calculation is

$$Na^+ - (HCO_3^- + Cl^-).$$

The anion gap has a range of 10 to 14 mEq/L. The normal gap does not misrepresent electrical neutrality, because the 12 mEq/L is made up of anions, such as albumin (the major contributor), phosphate, and sulfates. The gap may be influenced by plasma proteins, magnesium, calcium, or lithium.

Is a Primary Metabolic Acidosis Leading to Acidemia?

If this is the case, the differential diagnosis is categorized as an "increased" anion gap or "normal" anion gap.

Most acidoses are "increased" anion gap in origin, meaning endogenous or exogenous acid has been added (see Tables 21-2, 21-3 and 21-4). The clinician's task is to identify and treat, as necessary, the added acid(s). Most normal gap acidoses result from HCO_3^- being lost from the kidney or gastrointestinal tract. Electrical neutrality is maintained by the adjustment of Cl^-, and the calculated gap remains normal.

Is a Primary Metabolic Alkalosis Leading to Alkalemia?

If this situation exists, the differential is categorized as "saline-responsive" or "saline-resistant."

Most disorders are saline-responsive and may be differentiated by the patient having volume depletion and a urinary chloride of less than 10 mEq/L (see Table 21-5).

What Is the Potassium Level in Relation to the Abnormal PH?

Metabolic disorders may lead to cardiac dysrhythmias. One source of these abnormal rhythms is hyperkalemia or hypokalemia. Because of intracellular shift in exchange with H^+, K^+ moves in the opposite direction to the pH. That is, as the pH decreases, the serum potassium increases, and vice versa. It is helpful to calculate a "corrected" serum potassium level to determine approximately what the potassium level will be at a normal pH. This may be estimated by the formula: For each 0.1 change in the pH, the potassium level changes 0.6 mEq/L in the opposite direction.

What Is the Calculated Serum Osmolality?

If the sodium, glucose, and blood urea nitrogen levels are all elevated, or if one level is particularly high, it is advisable to calculate the estimated osmolarity with the formula:

$$\text{Calculated osmolality} = 2\ (Na^+) + \text{glucose}/18 + \text{BUN}/3 + \text{ETOH}/4.$$

If the result is elevated beyond the normal range of 285 to 295 mOsm/L, a serum osmolality is ordered to check its accuracy and to calculate the osmolal gap:

Measured mOsm/L – calculated mOsm/L.

An osmolal gap of greater than 15 to 20 mOsm/L is significant and represents low-molecular-weight osmotically active substances circulating in the blood. In patients with metabolic acidosis, methanol and ethylene glycol are possible causes. Metabolic acidosis and a widened osmolal gap require a search for these toxins.

CASE *Study*

Laboratory test results have returned to the emergency department. ABG analysis (taken soon after intubation) shows a pH of 6.95, P_{CO_2} of 14 mm Hg, and P_{O_2} of 50 mm Hg. Electrolyte concentrations were as follows: sodium, 136 mEq/L; potassium, 6.0 mEq/L; chloride, 100 mEq/L; and bicarbonate, 3 mEq/L. Glucose was 120 mg/dL, and BUN was 21 mg/dL.

Following the steps for analyzing the laboratory data:

1. A pH of 6.95 is an obvious acidemia.
2. The HCO_3^- is 3 mEq/L. This represents a severe metabolic acidosis, consistent with the pH.
3. The physiologic respiratory compensation range is

   $P_{CO_2} = 1.5 \times 3 \text{ (measured } HCO_3^-) + 8 \pm 2 = 10.5$ to 14.5 mm Hg.

   The measured P_{CO_2} of 14 mm Hg falls in the range; therefore, this is a simple, but severe, metabolic acidosis.
4. The anion gap is

   136 mEq/L – (100 mEq/L + 3 mEq/L) = 33 mEq/L.

This is an increased anion gap and places the origin of the acidosis as an added endogenous or exogenous acid. The BUN of 21 mg/dL makes renal failure unlikely, but the full urinalysis is not available.

This is an "elevated anion gap" simple metabolic acidosis. The patient's low pH with almost maximal respiratory compensation places him at great risk. Early replacement of HCO_3^- is necessary, and hyperventilation is maintained. To answer the other two important questions:

1. The potassium level is 6.0 mEq/L with a pH of 6.95. Increasing the pH 0.4 (4×0.1) to 7.35 would decrease the potassium 2.4 (4×0.6) mEq/L to 3.6 mEq/L. The elevated potassium level is consistent with the severity of acidemia. A slightly low normal potassium level is anticipated as the pH is corrected.
2. The calculated osmolality is

   2(136 mEq/L Na^+) + 120 mg/dL glucose/18 + 21 mg/dL BUN/3 = 285.7 mOsm/L.

This is within the normal range. By itself this gives no indication of the actual osmolal status.

The patient was treated initially with 2 mEq/kg of $NaHCO_3$ by intravenous bolus. The clinician initiated the search for the "added" acid by ordering the following tests: serum ketones, osmolality, serum lactate, toxicology screen, and urinalysis.

TABLE 21–2. Differential Diagnosis of Metabolic Acidosis

Normal Anion Gap (Hyperchloremic)	Increased Anion Gap (Added Acid)
Gastrointestinal loss of HCO_3^-	Ketoacidosis
Diarrhea	Diabetic
Small bowel or pancreatic fistula	Alcoholic
Ureterosigmoidostomy	Starvation
Ileal loop (obstructed or too long)	Renal failure (acute and chronic)
Anion exchange resins	Lactic acidosis
Ingestion of $CaCl_2$, $MgCl_2$	Exogenous toxins
Renal loss of HCO_3^-	Ethylene glycol
Renal tubular acidosis	Ibuprofen
Carbonic anhydrase inhibitors	Iron
Tubulointerstitial renal disease	Isoniazid
Hypoaldosteronism—deficiency or drug inhibition	Methanol
Hyperparathyroidism	Paraldehyde
Addition of hydrochloric acid	Salicylates/NSAIDs
Ammonium chloride, arginine HCl	Miscellaneous
Hyperalimentation	Nonketotic hyperosmolar coma
	Inborn errors of metabolism

EXPANDED DIFFERENTIAL DIAGNOSIS

Metabolic Acidosis

The differential diagnosis of metabolic acidosis is classified according to the amount of unmeasured anions (Table 21–2). The normal gap (hyperchloremic) acidoses may be divided further into three pathogenic categories: (1) gastrointestinal loss of HCO_3^-, (2) renal loss of HCO_3^-, and (3) addition of hydrochloric acid equivalents. This group tends to be less severe, with HCO_3^- levels rarely less than 12 mEq/L.

Diarrhea is the most common cause of normal anion gap acidosis and is always included in the differential diagnosis. The HCO_3^- concentration in diarrhea exceeds that of plasma, and potassium depletion is a frequent accompaniment. Small bowel or pancreatic drainage has an increased HCO_3^- concentration. Also, draining fistulas lead to a steady loss of HCO_3^- and eventual metabolic acidosis (normal anion gap).

The kidney is a less common source of HCO_3^- loss. In renal tubular acidosis (RTA) there is defective handling of H^+ or HCO_3^-. In proximal RTA, the defect is in proximal reabsorption of HCO_3^- and other filtered substances, such as glucose and uric acid. In distal RTA, the problem is in secreting adequate H^+ to maintain acid balance. Both are commonly associated with significant hypokalemia. An exception is hypoaldosteronism (RTA type IV), which results in a hyperkalemic distal RTA. Carbonic anhydrase inhibitors (acetazolamide) inhibit the hydrolysis of luminal carbonic acid to H_2O and CO_2. This impairs HCO_3^- reabsorption, resulting in a normal anion gap metabolic acidosis.

Elevated anion gap acidoses (addition of endogenous or exogenous acid) may be separated into five categories: (1) ketoacidosis, (2) lactic acidosis, (3) renal insufficiency, (4) exogenous toxins, and (5) miscellaneous. These acidoses are often seen in the emergency department. Table 21–3 outlines the pathogenesis and clinical manifestations of these common disorders.

Ketoacidosis

The production of ketones (β-hydroxybutyrate, acetoacetate, and acetone) is the hallmark of diabetic, alcoholic, and starvation ketoacidosis. Ketoacids rapidly dissociate into hydrogen ions and ketones (unmeasured anions), resulting in an anion gap acidosis. The diagnosis of ketoacidosis is based on finding a metabolic acidosis and serum ketones. The severity of the ketoacidosis cannot be followed by serum ketone measurements

TABLE 21–3. Common Anion Gap Metabolic Acidoses: Anions Involved and Diagnosis

Disorder	Anion	Diagnosis
Ketoacidosis		
Diabetic	Acetoacetate (AcAc)	Usually elevated glucose (but can be less than 350 mg/dL in 10%–15% of cases)
	β-hydroxybutyrate (βHB)	Decreased pH, ketones—βHB to AcAc ratio up to 8:1
Alcoholic	Predominantly βHB, smaller amount AcAc	Alcoholism, binge drinking, starvation, decreased pH, ketones—βHB to AcAc ratio up to 14:1
Starvation	AcAc, βHB	Decreased intake, $HCO_3^- \geq 18$ unless underlying problem
Lactic Acidosis	Lactic acid	Clinical setting with or without hypoxia (see Table 21–4)
Renal Failure	Sulfates, phosphates, other organic acids	Usually creatine > 4 mg/dL; acidosis may be more severe in acute renal failure owing to increased catabolic rate
Toxins		
Salicylate	Salicylate, lactate, ketones	Mixed acid-base, salicylate level
Methanol	Formate	Intoxicated, visual and gastrointestinal symptoms, optic nerve swelling and erythema, osmolal gap
Ethylene glycol	Glycolate	Intoxicated
	Glyoxalate	Osmolal gap (serious disease can occur without gap)
	Oxalate	Calcium oxalate crystals in urine
Paraldehyde	Unknown	Characteristic breath, sedation
Miscellaneous		
Hyperosmolar coma	AcAc, βHB, acetone	Increased glucose, absent or small amount of ketones

because β-hydroxybutyrate is not usually measured by the laboratory or bedside test. In addition, the usual 3:1 ratio of β-hydroxybutyrate to acetoacetate increases in conditions causing hypoxia or tissue ischemia. Paradoxically, when the patient begins to improve clinically and these conditions are reversed, an increase in measured ketones may be noted despite clinical improvement. This is from the conversion of β-hydroxybutyrate to measurable acetoacetate.

Diabetes mellitus is the most common cause of clinically significant ketoacidosis. It usually occurs in type 1 (juvenile-onset) diabetics who have little if any endogenous insulin. The lack of insulin causes an overproduction and undermetabolism of glucose and ketoacids. A history of chronic excessive alcohol intake, abdominal pain, and protracted vomiting is elicited from most patients with alcoholic ketoacidosis. Ethanol inhibits gluconeogenesis and promotes lipolysis. This process, in association with decreased caloric intake and a secondary lowering of the insulin level, promotes accelerated ketogenesis. Alcoholic ketoacidosis can be associated with lactic acidosis and metabolic alkalosis, from vomiting and volume depletion, to create a complex mixed acid-base disorder. Almost one half of these patients present as alkalemic. Prolonged starvation in the nonalcoholic patient results in a mild ketoacidosis. The plasma HCO_3^- is usually maintained above 18 mEq/L in these patients.

Lactic Acidosis

The most common form of elevated anion gap metabolic acidosis is lactic acidosis. Lactate is a metabolic end product of anaerobic glycolysis. It is in equilibrium with pyruvate. The major determinants of lactate concentration are the oxygenated state of the cell and the pyruvate concentration. A presumptive diagnosis of lactic acidosis is made when serum lactate concentrations of greater than 4 mmol are found in association with acidemia. Causes of lactic acidosis can be divided into those with overt systemic tissue hypoxia (type A) and those with clinically local or inapparent tissue hypoxia (type B). These are listed in Table 21–4.

Renal Insufficiency

Early in renal failure, there is a hyperchloremic metabolic acidosis secondary to impaired ammonia excretion and a variable deficiency in HCO_3^- reabsorption. As failure advances, there is impaired phosphate, sulfate, and organic anion excretion, leading to an increased anion gap. Generally, the anion gap does not begin to rise until the glomerular filtration rate drops to below 20 mL/min and the creatinine value is greater than 4 mg/dL. The HCO_3^- level is usually lowered into the 16 to 20 mEq/L range.

Exogenous Toxins

Ingested toxins are often causes of metabolic acidosis (see Chapter 15, The Poisoned Patient). Salicylate intoxication may occur secondary to attempted overdose or as a side effect of therapy for rheumatologic disorders. Levels above 30 mg/dL are toxic but correlate poorly with symptoms. In children, metabolic acidosis develops early and is the major acid-base disorder. In contrast, adults exhibit a mixed acid-base disturbance, with respiratory alkalosis predominating. Early symptoms include nausea, vertigo, and tinnitus.

Methanol is found in windshield wiper solution, fuel line de-icer, paint thinners, and an assortment of industrial solvents. It is occasionally substituted for ethanol in illicit alcohol production. It is metabolized by alcohol dehydrogenase to its toxic metabolites formaldehyde and formic acid. Clinical manifestations include abdominal pain, nausea, vomiting, and visual disturbances ranging from blurred vision to blindness. The appearance of symptoms may have a latent period of 12 to 72 hours because of the time lag in metabolism.

TABLE 21–4. Causes of Lactic Acidosis

Type A: Overt or Systemic Tissue Hypoxia	Type B: Local or Inapparent Tissue Hypoxia
Shock states	Ischemic bowel
Congestive heart failure	Diabetes mellitus
Hypoxia	Uremia
Anemia	Hepatic failure
Carbon monoxide poisoning	Seizures
	Leukemia
	Hereditary metabolic defects
	Drugs*

*Ethanol, fructose, strychnine, isoniazid, iron, cyanide, nitroprusside.

Simultaneous ingestion of ethanol will delay the onset of toxicity, because both methanol and ethanol are metabolized by alcohol dehydrogenase.

Ingestion of ethylene glycol, present in antifreeze and lacquer, is associated with central nervous system dysfunction, cardiovascular collapse, respiratory failure, severe metabolic acidosis, and renal failure. Toxicity is from its metabolites, glycolic and glyoxylic acids. As in methanol poisoning, the initial degradation by alcohol dehydrogenase can be slowed by ethanol. A clue to the diagnosis of ethylene glycol poisoning is the presence of monohydrate and dihydrate calcium oxalate crystals in the urine of 50% to 75% of patients. Methanol and ethylene glycol are among the rare causes of an anion gap above 50 mEq/L.

Metabolic Alkalosis

It is useful to divide the causes of metabolic alkalosis into two major subgroups: saline responsive and saline resistant (Table 21–5), based on history, volume status, and response to therapy. Urine chloride concentrations are required only occasionally in the diagnostic evaluation.

Saline-Responsive Metabolic Alkalosis

A saline-responsive metabolic alkalosis is maintained by volume and chloride deficits. Intravascular volume depletion is such a powerful stimulant that the kidneys sacrifice acid-base homeostasis to maintain plasma volume. Reduction of extracellular volume results in avid renal sodium conservation. Sodium is transported with HCO_3^- because of the relative unavailability of chloride, accelerating the rate of HCO_3^- reabsorption, thereby sustaining the alkalosis. In saline-responsive conditions, the urinary chloride concentration remains less than 10 mEq/L, unless diuretic action is still present. Sodium chloride replacement corrects the metabolic alkalosis.

Gastrointestinal disturbances can produce metabolic alkalosis either by loss of gastric contents or by diarrhea that is unusually rich in chloride. Vomiting or nasogastric suction can result in significant hydrogen, chloride, and volume losses. The loss of H^+ is not offset by HCO_3^- elimination, because of volume depletion. Chloride diarrhea is a rare congenital syndrome arising from a defect in intestinal chloride reabsorption, resulting in volume depletion and significant chloride losses. Occasionally, villous adenoma will result in a diarrhea with elevated chloride concentrations and secondary metabolic alkalosis, although diarrhea-induced metabolic acidosis is more common in this disease. All diuretics, except those that specifically block HCO_3^- reabsorption (acetazolamide) or acid excretion (spironolactone and triamterene), can result in a metabolic alkalosis. This is due to renal NaCl loss, enhanced acid excretion secondary to increased delivery of sodium to the distal tubule, and volume depletion. Cystic fibrosis can produce significant volume and chloride losses in the patient's sweat. Posthypercapnic alkalosis occurs as a consequence of delayed renal adjustment to the abrupt respiratory correction of chronic hypercapnia. Administration of the nonreabsorbable anions carbenicillin and penicillin to volume-depleted patients can produce an alkalosis secondary to enhanced distal renal acidification. In addition, hypercalcemia without hyperthyroidism increases renal HCO_3^- reabsorption. The mechanism underlying the elevation of HCO_3^- seen during carbohydrate feeding after starvation has been uncertain, although metabo-

---

TABLE 21–5. Classification of Metabolic Alkalosis

Saline-Responsive ($^uCl^-$ < 10 mEq/L)	Saline-Resistant ($^uCl^-$ < 10 mEq/L)
Gastrointestinal disorders	Mineralocorticoid excess
Vomiting	Hyperaldosteronism (primary or secondary)
Nasogastric suctioning	Cushing's syndrome
Chloride diarrhea	Licorice ingestion
Villous adenoma	Bartter's syndrome
Diuretic therapy	Severe hypokalemia
Cystic fibrosis	
Post hypercapnia	
Alkali administration	
Nonreabsorbable anion	
Refeeding alkalosis*	
Hypercalcemic/hypoparathyroid*	

*Classified as saline resistant by some workers despite extracellular volume contraction.

lism of ketones to HCO_3^- and extracellular volume contraction play an important role.

Excessive HCO_3^- administration can result in a metabolic alkalosis, if there is volume depletion with diminished renal reabsorption of HCO_3^-, or renal failure. It may occur from oral antacid therapy or parenteral administration of the citrate anticoagulant in transfused blood. Milk-alkali syndrome occurs in patients ingesting large amounts of calcium-containing antacids. In time, mild renal failure develops, limiting HCO_3^- excretion and promoting the maintenance of the metabolic alkalosis. In these disorders, removal of the HCO_3^- load is usually curative.

Saline-Resistant Metabolic Alkalosis

Maintenance of metabolic alkalosis in the saline-resistant disorders is caused by mineralocorticoid-induced stimulation of distal tubular acid secretion and the regeneration of HCO_3^-. A similar process can occur with severe hypokalemia (less than 2 mEq/L). Increased ammoniagenesis and chloruresis result in regeneration of HCO_3^-. Patients with saline-resistant disorders are neither volume nor chloride deficient; consequently, urinary chloride concentrations remain greater than 10 to 20 mEq/L, and therapy with sodium chloride is ineffective. Significant potassium depletion occurs in both the saline-responsive and saline-resistant disorders.

Primary hyperaldosteronism, Cushing's syndrome, and licorice ingestion produce metabolic alkalosis, hypokalemia, and hypertension secondary to excessive mineralocorticoid activity. The glycyrrhizic acid in licorice has a mineralocorticoid action. Bartter's syndrome is a rare condition found in children, characterized by increased renin and aldosterone production secondary to hyperplasia of the juxtaglomerular apparatus. The increased secretion of aldosterone results in a metabolic alkalosis, yet hypertension is usually absent. Profound hypokalemia can produce a metabolic alkalosis with increased urinary chloride concentrations, without evidence of increased mineralocorticoid effect.

CASE_Study_

The patient remained poorly responsive. Blood pressure was 90 mm Hg (palpation), and pulse was 115 beats per minute. The additional laboratory data were BUN, 9 mg/dL; creatinine, 0.8 mg/dL; glucose, 100 mg/dL; serum osmols, 340 mOsm/L; ethyl alcohol, 0 mg/dL; and ketones, none detectable. Urinalysis was unremarkable. Lactate level and complete toxicology screen were pending. An electrocardiogram showed a sinus tachycardia without acute ischemic changes.

The extremely high measured serum osmolality cannot be overlooked and must be compared with a calculated osmolality. In this case, the calculated osmolality is 286 mOsm/L. The osmolal gap is 340 − 286 = 54 mOsm/L. The osmolar gap is greater than 20 mOsm. Therefore, some substance is creating an anion gap metabolic acidosis, as well as a significant osmolal gap. The two most common causes of these findings are methanol and ethylene glycol.

PRINCIPLES OF MANAGEMENT

Treatment of acidosis and alkalosis is directed toward the underlying causative disorder and correction of the patient's acid-base disturbance. General principles of management include replacement of electrolyte and water deficits. This often may be sufficient for correction or improvement of the acid-base disturbance.

Metabolic Acidosis

If the acidemia is causing serious organ dysfunction, the patient's acidosis warrants correction. Therapy with $NaHCO_3$ is reserved for severe organic acidoses or those not easily reversed. Lactic or toxic acidemia generally requires treatment when the pH drops below 7.10 or the HCO_3^- falls below 8 mEq/L. In contrast, patients with ketoacidosis may not require $NaHCO_3$ therapy unless the metabolic acidosis is extremely severe with pH less than 7.0 or HCO_3^- less than 5 mEq/L, assuming there is no compromise of cardiac function. As the ketosis is reversed, the patients metabolize ketones to endogenous alkali, rapidly correcting their acid-base disorder. Chronic metabolic acidosis (e.g., in renal failure) is usually treated with supplemental $NaHCO_3$ when the HCO_3^- drops below 17 mEq/L to prevent skeletal demineralization.

The goal of therapy in acidemia is to raise arterial pH above 7.2. Unfortunately, there is no perfect formula for estimating HCO_3^- doses. One commonly used formula is

$NaHCO_3$ dose in mEq = (desired $[HCO_3^-]$ − observed $[HCO_3^-]$) × 50% of body weight in kg

The desired HCO_3^- is usually in the 12 to 15 mEq/L range. This target avoids alkalemia during correction, from organic anions being metabolized into HCO_3^- and persistent compensatory hyperventilation. One half of this dose is given initially, and further replacement is based on repeat laboratory testing. The formula is a rough guideline and tends to underestimate HCO_3^- replacement in severe acidosis (i.e., pH < 7.1, HCO_3^- < 5 mEq/L). In this case, 80% of body weight is used to estimate the HCO_3^- space in the calculation.

Bolus therapy is recommended only for those with severe acidosis or when there is hemodynamic compromise. Hypernatremia, hyperosmolality, volume overload, hypokalemia, and post-treatment alkalosis can complicate treatment of metabolic acidosis with $NaHCO_3$. A 50-mL ampule of $NaHCO_3$ has 50 mEq of sodium and the equivalent of 2000 mOsm/L. Usually 1 or 2 ampules are used as an initiating dose in acute situations, and then laboratory values are rechecked before additional treatment.

Patients with less life-threatening acidosis may be treated with an intravenous $NaHCO_3$ infusion. Two to three ampules of $NaHCO_3$ can be added to 1 L of D_5W. This results in a sodium concentration of 100 to 150 mEq/L. Normal saline has 150 mEq/L. Symptoms of hypocalcemia may occur secondary to a reduction in the ionized calcium fraction, although the total serum calcium level will remain unchanged. Paradoxical cerebrospinal fluid acidosis after $NaHCO_3$ administration exists but does not influence therapeutic decisions.

Specific therapy is directed to the underlying pathologic process. For example:

1. Diabetic ketoacidosis is treated with insulin, volume repletion, and electrolyte replacement, especially potassium (see Chapter 20, Diabetes).
2. Alcoholic ketoacidosis is treated with volume, glucose, and phosphate repletion (see Chapter 16, Alcohol Intoxication).
3. Methanol or ethylene glycol poisoning is treated with ethyl alcohol to block conversion to toxic metabolites. (Specific treatment guidelines are given in Chapter 15, The Poisoned Patient.)
4. Severe persistent lactic acidosis may require hemodialysis against an HCO_3^- dialysate.

Metabolic Alkalosis

Therapy for metabolic alkalosis is directed at the primary problem and the subsequent process maintaining the disorder.

1. The saline-responsive disorders are treated with saline (0.9 NS) volume replacement.

2. The saline-resistant disorders, with excessive mineralocorticoid activity, can be treated with aldosterone antagonists spironolactone or triamterene.
3. Potassium depletion is almost universally present in both forms. Supplements are administered as the chloride salt.
4. Persistent gastric acid losses can be diminished by the use of H_2 antagonists.
5. In patients in renal failure with neuromuscular irritability or cardiotoxicity, a pH of greater than 7.55 is treated with dialysis with a low HCO_3^- bath or acid administration. Parenteral hydrochloric acid may be administered through a central vein as a 0.1 to 0.2 mol solution, infusing up to 20 mEq/hr. Ammonium chloride administration may result in ammonium toxicity, and arginine chloride can cause significant hyperkalemia. These acidifying agents are used infrequently.
6. In life-threatening situations caused by severe alkalemia (pH > 7.6), the P_{CO_2} may be allowed to rise if ventilatory control is established and oxygenation is adequate. This may be accomplished by volume repletion, sedation, and, if necessary, by paralysis and mechanical ventilation.

CASE *Study*

The nurse at last was able to contact a member of the patient's family by phone. The family had been looking for him and were concerned for his welfare because he had been seen drinking some gasoline "drying agents" with his beer a day earlier. He had been hospitalized for a methanol ingestion about a year ago.

Laboratory investigation confirmed the suspicion of a metabolic acidosis and directed the differential diagnosis to a severe, elevated anion gap, nonketotic, osmolal gap metabolic acidosis with an entirely normal urinalysis. Combined with the initial history of alcohol ingestion, abdominal pain, and papilledema, it appeared the patient's problems were secondary to methanol ingestion. This was supported by the phone conversation with the member of the patient's family. The ethanol ingestion by the patient had been metabolized by the time he returned to the emergency department. The time lag in onset of severe symptoms may have been extended secondary to the initial ingestion of both methanol and ethanol. The preferential degradation of ethanol over methanol served as a temporary protective mechanism, inhibiting the formation of methanol's toxic metabolites.

> *The laboratory confirmation of methanol ingestion at a cost of several hundred dollars was somewhat more expensive than the cost of the phone call. After immediate supportive care had been accomplished, it was necessary to correct the acidosis and to prevent the production of additional acids.*

UNCERTAIN DIAGNOSIS

Acid-base disorders can present as complex double or triple metabolic and/or respiratory problems. A careful clinical assessment and adequate laboratory testing usually allow a tentative answer, and consistently following the previously listed steps is important in monitoring a working knowledge of acid-base disorders. Most uncertain diagnoses reflect a clinician's uncertainty in how to approach the problem. If the patient's status is unclear after the correct analytical steps are followed, early consultation with an internist or nephrologist is recommended.

DISPOSITION AND FOLLOW-UP

Admission

Essentially all patients with significant acid-base disorders are admitted for further evaluation and treatment.

Admission to Critical Care Unit

Many patients admitted to the hospital will be monitored and have serial laboratory and clinical assessments in a critical care unit. Conditions appropriate for this setting include, but are not limited to, the following:

1. Any finding of organ dysfunction, causing or resulting from the acid-base imbalance (e.g., altered mental status, hemodynamic instability, or renal insufficiency)
2. Extremes of age
3. Initial laboratory values of pH less than 7.1 or more than 7.6 or HCO_3^- value less than 10 mEq/L. Elevated HCO_3^- levels are usually the result of chronic compensation for Pco_2 retention. Acute increases of HCO_3^- over 35 to 40 mEq/L are appropriate for admission. These increases are almost always due to vomiting.
4. Ingestion of exogenous toxins

Discharge

Rarely, a patient with a known underlying disorder causing a recurrent acid-base imbalance may be treated and discharged from the emergency department. This might include a patient with a mild (pH > 7.2) diabetic ketoacidosis or alkalosis associated with diuretic use requiring volume and potassium repletion only.

At the time of discharge:

1. The primary physician should be contacted and an appointment made for follow-up care.
2. The patient should have a basic understanding of what happened and how any medications may either help or be harmful.
3. A support system should be in place to enable a check on the patient's status between the time of discharge and the primary physician appointment.

CASE *Study*

An ethanol bolus and infusion are started, and the nephrologist is contacted for dialysis plans. A methanol level of 50 mg/dL was received after the patient had been transferred to the intensive care unit.

The delay in therapy began with an inadequate history during the first visit to the emergency department. The setting of chronic alcoholism plus police custody may result in a less than complete evaluation. Unfortunately, these patients are the ones requiring the most attention, including outside phone calls for additional information. The care during the second visit was appropriate, although the ethanol infusion might have been started earlier. The severity of the acidosis and history pointed to a metabolized toxin causing the problem. Methanol and ethylene glycol were the most likely sources

FINAL POINTS

- Patients with acid-base disorders often present with nonspecific symptoms. Frequently, the only clue to the presence of an acid-base disturbance is an abnormality of the vital signs.
- The diagnosis of an acid-base disturbance depends on recognition of the clinical settings in which it may occur. Confirmatory laboratory studies are then required to support the clinical impression.

- A consistent stepwise analysis of the laboratory data is the best method for understanding these disorders.
- The adequacy of respiratory compromise in metabolic acidosis can be evaluated using the formula

$$\text{Expected } P_{CO_2} = [1.5 \times (HCO_3^-)] + 8 \pm 2.$$

- The limit of respiratory compensation is approximately 10 mm Hg.
- The differential diagnosis of metabolic acidosis can be divided into groups based on the state of unmeasured anions (normal or elevated). The anion gap equation is

$$\text{Anion gap} = Na^+ - (Cl^- + HCO_3^-)$$

- The influence of alkalemia or acidemia on the potassium level must be anticipated as corrective therapy is initiated.
- Small-molecular-weight, nonpolar toxins, such as methanol and ethylene glycol, result in an elevated anion gap, osmolal gap metabolic acidosis.
- Potassium depletion is almost universally present in metabolic alkalosis, and supplements should be administered as the chloride salt.
- When treatment is indicated in metabolic alkalosis, the saline-responsive disorders require saline and the saline-resistant disorders need to be treated with aldosterone antagonists.

Bibliography

TEXTS

Halperin HL, Goldstein MB: Fluid, Electrolyte, and Acid-Base Physiology: A Problem-Based Approach, 3rd ed. Philadelphia, WB Saunders, 1999.

Maxwell M, Kleeman L, Narins RG: Clinical Disorders of Fluid and Electrolyte Metabolism, 5th ed. New York, McGraw-Hill, 1994.

Schrier RW: Renal and Electrolyte Disorders, 5th ed. Philadelphia, Lippincott-Raven, 1997.

JOURNAL ARTICLES

Chabali R: Diagnostic use of anion and osmolal gaps in pediatric emergency medicine. Pediatr Emerg Care 1997; 13:204–210.

Fulop M: Flow diagrams for the diagnosis of acid-base disorders. J Emerg Med 1998; 16:97–109.

Gilbert HC, Vender JS: Arterial blood gas monitoring. Crit Care Clin 1995; 11:233–248.

Hanna JD, Scheinman JI, Chan JC: The kidney in acid-base balance. Pediatr Clin North Am 1995; 42:1365–1395.

Hood VL, Tannen RL: Protection of acid-base balance by pH regulation of acid production. N Engl J Med 1998; 339:819–826.

Jurado RL, del Rio C, Nassar G, et al: Low anion gap. South Med J 1998; 91:624–629.

Laski ME, Kurtzman NA: Acid-base disorders in medicine. Dis Mon 1996; 42:51–125.

Palmer BF, Alpern RJ: Metabolic alkalosis. J Am Soc Nephrol 1997; 8:1462–1469.

Purssell RA, Pudek M, Brubacher J, et al: Derivation and validation of a formula to calculate the contribution of ethanol to the osmolal gap. Ann Emerg Med 2001; 8:653–659.

Rutledge J, Couch R: Initial fluid management of diabetic ketoacidosis in children. Am J Emerg Med 2000; 18:658–660.

Smulders YM, Frissen PH, Slaats EH, Silberbusch J: Renal tubular acidosis: Pathophysiology and diagnosis. Arch Intern Med 1996; 156:1629–1636.

Acknowledgment

Acknowledgment is given for the sustained contributions of the original authors of this chapter, Dietrich Jehle, MD, and Fred Harchelroad, MD.

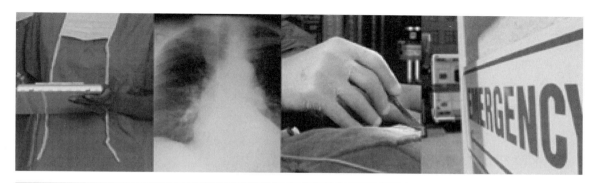

HEAD AND NECK DISORDERS

CHAPTER 22

Epistaxis

LISA CHAN

STEVEN M. JOYCE

CASE *Study*

A 30-year-old man presents to the emergency department complaining of a nosebleed of spontaneous onset. At the time of arrival there is active bleeding from his right nostril.

INTRODUCTION

Epistaxis may present a challenge for the emergency physician. If severe, it can lead to hypovolemia and shock. The patient is usually anxious and may be orthostatic from blood loss or nauseated from swallowed blood. Examining the small nasal cavity that is difficult to access must be performed expeditiously. The process is time consuming in a time-limited setting. Fortunately, most epistaxis is neither severe nor difficult to treat, but the emergency physician must always be prepared for the worst.

The exact incidence of epistaxis is uncertain, and only about 6% of patients with epistaxis seek medical attention. One estimate is that 15% of the population experiences epistaxis each year. It is more common in the winter months and is often associated with upper respiratory infection. About 10% of maxillofacial injuries are accompanied by epistaxis. Most nosebleeds are isolated incidents, but about 4% of the population has recurrent episodes in a given year. Death from epistaxis is rare. Most cases are treated with local pressure, and only a few require immediate consultation and operative intervention.

Proper management of epistaxis requires knowledge of basic nasal vascular anatomy. The blood supply to the nose originates from branches of both the external and internal carotid arteries (Fig. 22–1). The mucosa of the anterior-inferior portion of the nasal septum is the site of an anastomotic plexus of vessels supplied by the nasopalatine, descending palatine, and anterior and posterior ethmoidal arteries. This location is known as Kiesselbach's plexus or Little's area, and it is the site of 90% of anterior nosebleeds. Venous drainage parallels the arterial supply in this area. A venous plexus at the posterior portion of the inferior turbinate is a common site of posterior epistaxis. The fleshy portion of the nose beyond the nasal bones is compressible by external pressure. The posterior portion of the nasal cavity is not, making bleeding control difficult in this area. Most posterior bleeding originates from Woodruff's plexus, an area where the sphenopalatine artery emerges from its foramen.

INITIAL APPROACH AND STABILIZATION

Most patients with epistaxis are alert and able to protect their airway by expectorating blood. Most do not have significant blood loss. However, when patients are unstable, resuscitation and stabilization is necessary before a focused and detailed evaluation of the nasal cavity. When epistaxis is secondary to trauma, its evaluation and management is prioritized with other injuries (e.g., cervical spine protection).

Rapid Assessment

History. What is the duration and quantity (i.e., how many soaked washcloths or towels?) of the episode? Are there any underlying bleeding disorders?

Airway Assessment. Is the patient able to protect the airway? Airway management progresses as necessary. Is the airway compromised by pharyngeal clots? Clots may be removed manually, by suction, or by forceps.

Circulation. Incipient hypovolemic shock may be recognized by evaluation of the vital signs, mental status, skin color, and capillary refill. If the vital signs are stable and the patient can tolerate it, orthostatic pulse and blood pressure are measured.

Early Intervention

Signs of hypovolemia mandate immediate placement of an intravenous line and crystalloid infusion (see Chapter 4, Shock). Blood for hemoglobin,

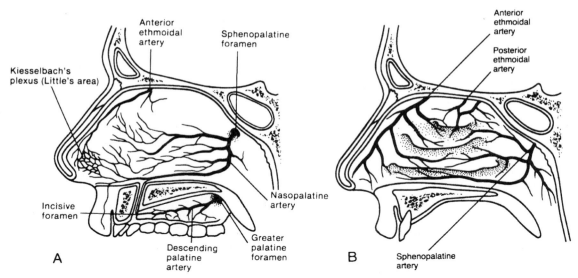

FIGURE 22–1 • *A,* Arterial blood supply to the nasal septum. *B,* Arterial blood supply to the lateral wall of the nose. (From Peretta LJ, Denslow BL, Brown CG: Emergency evaluation and management of epistaxis. Emerg Med Clin North Am 1987; 5:265–277.)

hematocrit, and transfusion cross-matching is sent to the laboratory at this time.

Anterior bleeding is best controlled by having the patient sit upright and apply manual squeezing pressure to the entire fleshy part of the nose for a full 5 to 10 minutes. This maneuver allows time for equipment to be set up and in some cases slows or stops the bleeding.

Bleeding that is not controlled by this simple maneuver may be posterior in origin. A decision is necessary at this juncture: Is the bleeding severe enough to require immediate control, or can a quick inspection for the bleeding site be made? If the former, a balloon tamponade device is placed to control the bleeding while the patient's condition is stabilized (Fig. 22–2).

CLINICAL ASSESSMENT

History

Present Illness. Was the epistaxis *spontaneous* in *onset,* or was it induced by some *mechanical trauma?* Common causes of mechanical disruption of the nasal mucosa include drying from upper respiratory infection or low humidity, fingernails or other foreign bodies, increased vascular pressure from sneezing, or a direct blow to the nose. Is this an *isolated incident,* or does the patient suffer from *recurrent epistaxis?* What *treatment,* if any, was tried at *home?*

Past Medical History. Is there a history of *blood dyscrasias, bleeding disorders,* or *easy bruising* or *bleeding?* Does the patient have gum

bleeding during teeth brushing? Has the patient had excessive bleeding with dental work or surgery? Has bleeding during menstruation been increased? *Recent illnesses,* especially upper respiratory infections, may be relevant. Is there a history of hypertension or ischemic heart disease?

Medication or Drug Use. Queries should be made about *medications* that may affect hemostasis, such as aspirin, other platelet inhibitors, anti-

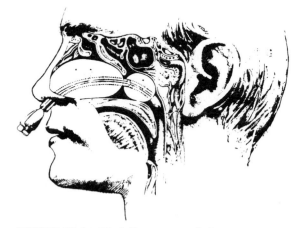

FIGURE 22–2 • The balloon tamponade device serves as both an anterior and a posterior pack. It is easily inserted and is often successful for the temporary control of posterior epistaxis in the emergency department. The balloon shown here is the Epistat balloon. (Courtesy of Xomed, Inc, Jacksonville, FL. Reproduced with permission from Abelson TI, Witt WJ: Otolaryngologic procedures. In Roberts JR, Hedges JR [eds]: Clinical Procedures in Emergency Medicine. Philadelphia, WB Saunders, 1985.)

coagulants, or alcohol. Cocaine may alter the structural integrity of the nasal mucosa.

Physical Examination

General Findings. A directed physical examination is done to search for signs of bleeding disorders—specifically, mucosal or cutaneous purpura or petechiae, lymphadenopathy, or hepatosplenomegaly.

Head, Eyes, Ears, Nose, and Throat. In cases of epistaxis caused by facial trauma, careful palpation of the orbital rims, nasal bridge, and cheekbones is performed. Extraocular muscle function and facial symmetry are assessed. Findings may suggest nasal bone fractures or other injuries, such as orbital floor blowout, tripod, or LeFort fractures.

Nasal Examination. The following equipment is needed for the examination and should be readied before the examination:

1. Protective coverings for both the physician and the patient. The nasal examination of a patient with epistaxis involves exposure to at least two body fluids. Thus, full blood precautions are indicated, including gown, gloves, a mask, and eye shield. The patient's clothes may be protected with a hospital gown, towels, or protective drape.
2. Equipment for inspection of the nasal cavity. The minimum equipment needed includes the following:
   a. Headlamp or head mirror with light source
   b. Nasal speculum of appropriate size
   c. A No. 5 to 8 Fr suction tip connected to suction at mid range
   d. Bayonet forceps
   e. Topical vasoconstrictor and anesthetic
      (1) Cocaine 4% topical solution on cotton pledget *or*
      (2) Lidocaine 4% topical solution with 1:1000 epinephrine or 0.5% to 1.0% phenylephrine added

Technique

1. The patient is positioned sitting with the emesis basin held below the chin; the face is elevated to the examiner's eye level, providing that the patient can tolerate sitting upright and the cervical spine is stable.
2. The nose is emptied of clots using suction or forceps or by having the patient blow and then inhale through the nose. The "sniff" may move a clot into the oropharynx and cause gagging.

The patient is warned of this happening, and an emesis basin is readily available (in the patient's hands).

3. A nasal speculum is used to observe the nasal septum for the presence of a septal hematoma. In external nasal trauma, the nasal bones including the septum may be fractured, causing not only epistaxis but occasionally accumulation of blood beneath the mucosa. Pressure from the hematoma may result in septal necrosis and nasal deformity if it is not recognized and drained.
4. An attempt is made to see the bleeding site by suctioning blood while holding the nostril open. The nose is examined for bleeding from the anterior septum, roof, and floor of the nasal cavity. One starts on the side from which the bleeding may have originated, but both sides are inspected.

   Often this examination will reveal a discrete bleeding site within reach of the catheter tip. If so, treatment may begin. If a discrete bleeding site is not found, a diffuse or posterior hemorrhage must be suspected. One method of differentiating a posterior hemorrhage from an anterior hemorrhage is to have the patient blow the nose, sit forward, and apply manual pressure to the nostrils while the examiner observes for blood running down the back of the patient's pharynx. Continued bleeding in the posterior pharynx with adequate anterior pressure indicates a posterior hemorrhage.
5. Vasoconstrictor and anesthetic solution saturated on cotton pledgets is applied against the suspected bleeding site. The solution decreases the bleeding, shrinks the nasal mucosa, and decreases the discomfort of the examination. Pledgets are inserted deeply into the nasal cavity, and additional pledgets are placed over them to maintain their position. The patient is asked to pinch the nose in with the pledgets in place for 5 to 10 minutes.

   Cocaine, epinephrine, and phenylephrine may be absorbed to some degree, and the patient's blood pressure is checked during this time. If a dangerous elevation in blood pressure occurs, the pledgets are removed and the blood pressure is measured again. Nasal packing is appropriate if the bleeding continues after the blood pressure has come down.
6. After 5 to 10 minutes, the pledgets are removed. Often the bleeding has ceased. The nose is reexamined to confirm the suspected bleeding site, which is usually a small defect or papule in Kiesselbach's plexus (see Fig. 22–1). Foreign bodies, tumors, and mucosal defects from fractures are more easily visualized at this

time. If the bleeding is not stopped, reapplication of pledgets, nasal packing, or balloon tamponade may be considered.

CLINICAL REASONING

Is the Site of Bleeding Located Anterior or Posterior?

Up to 90% of cases of acute epistaxis originate from the anterior nasal septum. The source of bleeding is usually visible. When the source is unclear after inspection, hematologic disorders or posterior bleeding are more likely. Posterior bleeding may be the result of tumor, elevated venous pressure, or possibly hypertension or arteriosclerosis. Different researchers have found varying degrees of correlation between the presence of hypertension and the incidence of epistaxis, varying from none to significantly high.

What Is the Most Likely Local Cause of the Bleeding?

Table 22–1 lists the causes of epistaxis. Mechanical and traumatic causes predominate in emergency department patients. Irritation of the mucosa from drying due to low humidity or high altitude, inflammation caused by upper respiratory infection, accidental scratches from a fingernail (epistaxis digitorum), and external blows to the nose with or without fracture are frequently

seen. Altered anatomy of the septum is a common cause of recurrent epistaxis.

Is This a Sign of an Underlying Systemic Problem? Especially, a Hemostatic Disorder?

Hematologic disorders comprising a deficit in primary hemostasis, such as thrombocytopenia or impaired platelet function, usually cause diffuse, bilateral mucosal bleeding. Hematologic disorders are considered in persistent or recurrent epistaxis.

DIAGNOSTIC ADJUNCTS

Laboratory Studies

In most cases, laboratory studies are not necessary. When significant blood loss or a hematologic disorder is suspected, hematocrit and hemoglobin, blood type, and crossmatch may be ordered. A platelet count, prothrombin time, and partial thromboplastin time may be indicated as well.

Radiologic Imaging

Nasal or facial bone radiographs may be indicated in patients with external trauma but may be delayed pending control of significant bleeding. In cases of suspected simple nasal fractures with-

---

TABLE 22–1. Causes of Epistaxis

Traumatic or Mechanical
    Digital (epistaxis digitorum)*
    External blow (with or without nasal or facial fracture)*
    Desiccation (winter, deviated septum, supplemental oxygen without humidification)*
    Inflammation (upper respiratory infection, allergic rhinitis)*
    Foreign body (children)
    Septal perforation (cocaine abuse, repeated cautery, submucosal hematoma)
    Barotrauma (diver's squeeze, rapid altitude gain)
    Elevated venous pressure (sneezing, Valsalva maneuver, congestive heart failure, mitral stenosis)*
Tumor (juvenile angiofibroma, sinus tumors)
Hematologic or vascular disorders
    Vascular
        Telangiectasia
        Vitamin deficiency (scurvy)
        Hypertension or arteriosclerosis
    Disorders of hemostasis
        Thrombocytopenia (drug-induced, malignancies, other)
        Platelet inhibition (aspirin, NSAIDs, von Willebrand's disease)
        Coagulopathy (hereditary, anticoagulants, liver or renal disease)
Other
    Endometriosis
    Idiopathic (accounts for about 10% of cases of epistaxis)

*Denotes a common cause.
NSAIDs, nonsteroidal anti-inflammatory drugs.

out asymmetry or obstruction, repair is often not necessary and films may not be indicated. Complex facial fractures are assessed by computed tomography.

PRINCIPLES OF MANAGEMENT

The management of epistaxis is based on a progression of maneuvers designed to stop the bleeding quickly with the least invasive method possible. Often bleeding is controlled with one or two simple maneuvers. Treating the underlying cause helps prevent recurrence. In all but the simplest cases, this requires cautery of the bleeding site or some method of tamponade. Exploring the medical basis for bleeding (e.g., hypertension or hematologic disorders) is an essential part of the management plan. It cannot be forgotten after the bleeding has stopped.

Steps to control bleeding from epistaxis may be undertaken in the following order. In cases of severe and probable posterior bleeding, early steps may be skipped in favor of expedient control.

Manual Pressure. Squeezing the fleshy part of the nose against the septum while sitting upright for 10 to 15 minutes will often control simple nosebleeds at home. Recurrence after two trials warrants examination by a physician.

Application of Topical Vasoconstrictors and Anesthetics. These may actually stop the bleeding, but this effect is usually temporary. If a mucosal bleeding site can be identified, cautery is done. If not, packing is usually necessary before the effect of the drug wears off.

Cautery. Silver nitrate is the compound most commonly used for cautery. Once hemostasis is obtained by application of topical vasoconstrictors, the bleeding point may be cauterized by touching the silver nitrate applicator to it for a few (up to 20) seconds. Some authors have recommended additional cautery of the surrounding mucosa. Overzealous cautery is avoided, however, because it may lead to septal perforation, especially after multiple applications on both sides of the septum. Cautery is not applied without prior anesthesia because it is painful and may induce sneezing. Cautery is contraindicated when a tumor is suspected because it may cause continued bleeding. It has little use in patients with epistaxis from nasal fractures. Both sides of the septum should not be cauterized at the same time because of risk of septal perforation. Repeated cauterization in the same area can also lead to septal perforation.

Anterior Packing. When the just-described measures do not control bleeding and an anterior

site is suspected, the nasal cavity may be packed under experienced supervision to tamponade the bleeding site. Several materials are available:

- *Petrolatum (Vaseline)-impregnated one-half inch gauze.* Vaseline gauze is placed using the bayonet forceps, starting at the floor of the nasal cavity and layering superiorly until the cavity is filled (Fig. 22–3).
- *Absorbable hemostatic agents.* Oxicel, Gelfoam, Surgicel, and other similar products stimulate coagulation and are absorbable. They are especially useful in patients with diffuse epistaxis that is caused by disorders of hemostasis. The mechanical irritation of gauze packing or its removal may cause recurrent hemorrhage.
- *Balloon and nasal tampon packs.* Nasal balloon packs are available commercially (e.g., Epistat) and are easily and quickly placed in position. They are not always effective. They should be coated with antibiotic ointment to make removal less traumatic (see Fig. 22–2). An alternative to balloon packs is the nasal tampon pack (e.g. Mericel, Epistat II). These devices will swell and conform to the anterior nasal cavity on exposure to moisture.

Nasal packing occludes the paranasal sinus ostia and may predispose to sinusitis. Prophylactic oral antibiotics (e.g., ampicillin) may be prescribed until the pack is removed in 48 to 72 hours. Some authorities recommend packing both sides of the nose to prevent septal displacement and loss of effective tamponade. This is an individual choice and not a medical standard.

After anterior packing, the oropharynx is visualized. If blood is seen trickling from the nasopharynx, either the anterior pack is suboptimally placed or the bleeding is from a posterior nasal source. The nasal cavity measures about 7 cm from columella to nasopharynx, so the most common error in anterior nasal packing is failure to adequately pack the posterior aspects of the anterior nasal cavity.

Posterior Packing. Only about 5% of epistaxis originates from a posterior source. When bleeding is posterior or cannot be controlled by anterior packing, the entire nasal cavity may be packed from posterior to anterior using one of several techniques:

- *Conventional gauze nasal packs.* This pack is made from a rolled gauze tampon that is drawn into the posterior nasopharynx through the mouth by means of attached silk sutures that have been tied to catheters previously passed through the nose into the pharynx. Once in place, bilateral anterior gauze packs are placed

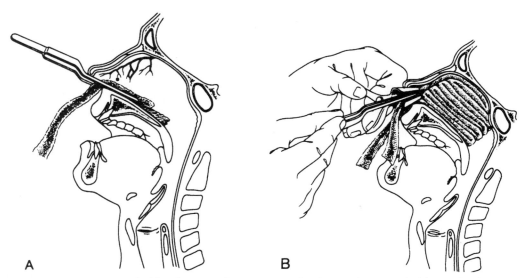

A   **B**

FIGURE 22–3 • *A*, Incorrect method for placement of an anterior nasal pack. Note that one end of the nasal packing remains inside the nasal cavity. *B*, Correct method for the placement of a layered nasal pack. (From Peretta LJ, Denslow BL, Brown CG: Emergency evaluation and management of epistaxis. Emerg Clin North Am 1987; 5:265–277.)

as previously described and the sutures are secured over padding at the nostrils. The technique is cumbersome, time consuming, and uncomfortable for the patient.

- *Foley catheter balloon pack.* A 16-Fr Foley catheter with a 30-mL balloon is passed into the pharynx, inflated with about 10 mL of saline, and withdrawn against the posterior opening of the nasal cavity. Bilateral balloons are placed for posterior epistaxis. Anterior gauze packs are placed as previously described, and the catheters are secured over padding at the nares.
- *Balloon nasal packs.* Epistat, Nasostat, and other packs tamponade the posterior and anterior nasal cavities, some with separate balloons. They are easily and quickly placed and are thus useful in patients with severe bleeding. Supplementation with gauze packing in the roof of the nasal cavity may be necessary.

The same precautions regarding prophylaxis for sinusitis apply to posterior packs as to anterior packs. In addition, posterior packs have been associated with a high rate of complications, especially hypoventilation and hypoxemia. All patients requiring posterior packing are admitted to the hospital.

Septal Hematoma. A septal hematoma must be drained by an experienced physician. If it is left untreated, pressure on the septum may result in necrosis.

Refractory Epistaxis. When bleeding cannot be controlled despite an appropriate trial of the methods just described, operative arterial ligation may be necessary. Other invasive methods such as arterial embolization have also been described. Persistent bleeding from nasal fractures may require reducing the fracture to resolve the bleeding. Admission to the otorhinolaryngology service is mandated to stabilize the patient before operation.

SPECIAL CONSIDERATIONS

Pediatric Patients

Nasal foreign bodies are a common cause of epistaxis in toddlers. Beads, toy parts, or beans may be found. A vasoconstrictor such as phenylephrine is applied. If able, the patient gently blows the nose with the other nostril occluded. If this is unsuccessful, a lubricated pediatric Foley catheter with a 5-mL balloon may be passed beyond the foreign body and the balloon gently inflated until resistance is met. The catheter is then gently withdrawn, bringing the foreign body out of the nostril. This method is probably less traumatic than the use of bayonet or "alligator" forceps and avoids the problem of aspiration if the foreign body is pushed into the pharynx. This technique, however, is used only by a physician familiar with it.

Older Hypertensive Patients

Although no causal relationship exists between hypertension and epistaxis, hypertension increases the likelihood of continued hemorrhage once bleeding starts. Therefore, duration and quantity of epistaxis may be greater in older hypertensive patients. If the diastolic blood pressure is markedly elevated, antihypertensive medication may be administered, taking care not to drop the blood pressure precipitously. Because anxiety may exacerbate the hypertension, an anxiolytic may be warranted.

Significant morbidity is associated with nasal packing in these patients, particularly those with cardiopulmonary disease. Oxygen should be administered continuously during the procedure.

DISPOSITION AND FOLLOW-UP

Discharge

Patients with uncomplicated epistaxis that has been controlled by direct pressure, vasoconstrictors, or cautery can be sent home after a short (20- to 30-minute) period of observation. Patients are warned not to mechanically irritate the nose by rubbing or blowing it for 24 hours. If drying is the suspected cause of anterior bleeding, the patient is given a petrolatum-based ointment and instructed to apply it gently inside the nares every 12 hours for 1 to 2 days. The first layer of ointment is applied before discharge. A home humidifier may be helpful in preventing recurrence.

Patients with first-time epistaxis treated with anterior packs are referred for follow-up in 24 to 48 hours. Packs are removed in 48 to 72 hours. Antibiotic coverage is maintained while the pack is present. Patients who have recurrent nosebleeds requiring anterior packing are treated in consultation with a specialist.

CONSULTATION

Displaced nasal fractures may be reduced by an experienced physician within 1 hour of occurrence. Alternatively, the patient may be referred to an otorhinolaryngologist for subsequent reduction within 5 to 7 days after the swelling has subsided.

Facial fractures associated with significant epistaxis merit otorhinolaryngologic consultation in the emergency department. These patients may be admitted or scheduled for later reduction, depending on the nature and severity of the fractures.

Hospitalization

Hospital admission is indicated for the following types of patients:

1. Patients who have lost enough blood to require transfusion until the hematocrit is stabilized.
2. Patients who develop epistaxis as a result of hematologic or coagulation disorders. Definitive diagnosis and blood product therapy should be initiated as indicated (see Chapter 4, Shock).
3. Patients with epistaxis that is refractory to nonoperative methods of treatment of underlying disorders.
4. Patients with posterior packs, who are observed for hypoventilation, hypoxia, cardiac dysrhythmias, and a failure rate up to 20%.
5. Elderly or frail patients with anterior nasal packing.

FINAL POINTS

- Epistaxis is a common problem that is often managed in the emergency department.
- The most frequent causes are trauma and mechanical factors.
- Most epistaxis originates from the anterior nasal septum.
- An ordered approach to diagnosis and treatment begins with ensuring the patency of the airway and cardiovascular stability and proceeds through identification of the bleeding site(s) and application of the least invasive treatment modality needed to achieve hemostasis.
- It is invaluable to have all the necessary equipment for diagnosis and treatment at hand before attempting management.
- Systemic causes of epistaxis, particularly disorders of hemostasis, are always considered in the differential diagnosis.

CASE *Study*

A 30-year-old man presented to the emergency department with a nosebleed that had begun spontaneously. He had active bleeding from his right nostril.

Like most patients with epistaxis, the patient is awake, alert, hemodynamically stable, and able to protect his airway. The patient is instructed to continue to apply pressure to the fleshy part of his nose.

The patient is instructed to blow his nose and clots are removed. With suctioning and a nasal speculum, an active bleeding site is found at the anterior septal mucosa. After a 10-minute application of 4% lidocaine topical solution with 1% epinephrine pledgets, the site was visible as a 2-mm papule.

Silver nitrate cautery is applied to the bleeding site on the patient's septum. After 20 minutes of observation, bleeding is still noted. An anterior nasal pack is placed; and after another observation period, the bleeding has stopped. The patient is placed on antibiotics and referred for follow-up in 24 hours.

This patient is typical of most patients with epistaxis. The key to care is methodical preparation, patient and physician protection, and a stepwise approach to evaluation and treatment. The major problems in treating epistaxis in the emergency department involve the lack of time commitment to do it right and an inexperienced examiner.

BIBLIOGRAPHY

TEXT

Woodson GE: Ear, Nose, and Throat Disorders in Primary Care. Philadelphia, WB Saunders, 2001.

JOURNAL ARTICLES

Herkner H, Laggner AN, Mullner M: Hypertension in patients presenting with epistaxis. Ann Emerg Med 2000; 35:126–130.

Neto FL, Fuchs FD, et al: Is epistaxis evidence of end-organ damage in patients with hypertension? Laryngoscope 1999; 109:1111–1115.

Pantanowitz L: Epistaxis in the older hypertensive patient. J Am Geriatr Soc 1999;47:631.

Pollice PA, Yoder MG: Epistaxis: A retrospective review of hospitalized patients. Otolaryngol Head Neck Surg 1997; 117:49.

Tan LK, Calhoun KH: Epistaxis. Med Clin North Am 1999; 83:43–56.

Viducich RA, Blanda MP, Gerson LW: Posterior epistaxis: Clinical features and acute complications. Ann Emerg Med 1995; 25:592.

Wurman LH, Sack JG, Flannerty JV, et al: The management of epistaxis. Am J Otolaryngol 1992; 13:193.

CHAPTER 23

Acute Sore Throat

ELIZABETH A. LINDBERG

CASE_Study_

A 17-year-old college student presented to the emergency department with a 5-day history of sore throat and right ear pain. It was her third visit for this chief complaint. She was seen initially at the campus health center and started on azithromycin after a rapid strep test was performed and reported as negative. She also had a "blood test," and the results were unknown to her. Two days later she was seen in the emergency department, where a throat culture was done and clindamycin was added to the azithromycin. No clinical improvement prompted the third visit to the same emergency department on the fifth day.

INTRODUCTION

Most people have been bothered by a sore throat at some time. It is the third most common complaint of patients seeking medical attention and in the top 10 chief complaints heard in the emergency department. Over $300 million dollars are spent annually on diagnosis and treatment of sore throat.

Patients seek medical attention for relief of symptoms (throat pain, difficulty swallowing, and fever) and over concerns of "strep throat." Unfortunately, many patients perceive an antibiotic is indicated to cure their sore throat, which is true in only a small percentage of cases. This seemingly simple complaint remains problematic for physicians as well. There are life-threatening complications associated with sore throat, and controversies surround both diagnosis and treatment.

Acute pharyngitis or tonsillopharyngitis is an inflammatory or infectious condition of the pharynx and tonsils. The oropharynx is composed of the soft palate, uvula, tonsillar pillars, tonsils, base of the tongue, and posterior pharyngeal wall (Fig. 23–1). Innervation of the oropharynx, larynx, middle ear, and external auditory canal arise from the ninth and tenth cranial nerves. Throat pain can be referred to or originate from any of these anatomic locations as well as the upper thorax. The pain can be perceived as sharp, burning, or scratchy.

Most cases of pharyngitis are infectious in origin, although a wide variety of causes have been identified. The infectious causes of pharyngitis are listed in Table 23–1.

The most common bacterial cause of acute pharyngitis is group A β-hemolytic *Streptococcus* (GABHS). However, streptococcal pharyngitis represents only 15% to 35% of sore throats.

GABHS remains an important etiologic agent to identify, because nonsuppurative sequelae are acute rheumatic fever and acute glomerulonephritis. Suppurative complications can arise from all types of pharyngitis and include peritonsillar and retropharyngeal abscess, Ludwig's angina, epiglottitis, cervical lymphadenitis, mastoiditis, otitis media, and sinusitis. Acute sore throat may also be the presenting symptom in serious systemic illness such as human immunodeficiency virus (HIV) infection, leukemia, neutropenia, and acute hepatitis.

Once catastrophic emergencies have been ruled out, it is important to develop clinical management strategies in the approach to sore throat that include appropriate diagnostic tests and treatment. Patient comfort, education, and satisfaction are also important goals in treating acute pharyngitis.

INITIAL APPROACH AND STABILIZATION
Priority Diagnoses

In a busy emergency department a chief complaint of sore throat may seem like a low priority. However, life-threatening complications can occur and may develop rapidly while the patient waits to be seen. The initial approach and stabilization is focused on separating those patients with serious and even life-threatening diseases from those patients with benign and self-limiting causes. Life-threatening complications are usually the result of airway compromise. Epiglottitis, retropharyngeal and severe peritonsillar abscess,

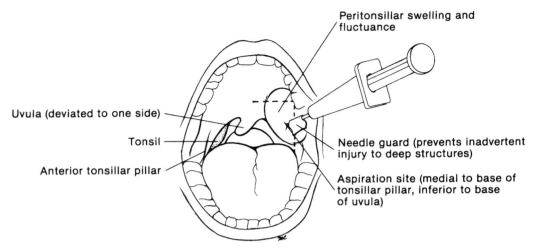

FIGURE 23–1 • Pharyngeal structures in peritonsillar abscess. Purulent aspirate confirms diagnosis. Incision and drainage follow (from same site). *Dashed line* denotes border of area for aspiration site.

TABLE 23–1. Infectious Causes of Acute Pharyngitis

Etiology	Syndrome/Disease	Estimated Importance*
Viral		
Rhinovirus	Common cold	20
Coronavirus	Common cold	≥ 5
Adenovirus	Pharyngoconjunctival fever, acute respiratory disease	5
Herpes simplex 1 and 2	Gingivitis, stomatitis, pharyngitis	4
Parainfluenza virus	Common cold, croup	2
Influenza virus A and B	Influenza	2
Epstein-Barr virus	Infectious mononucleosis	<1
Cytomegalovirus	Infectious mononucleosis	<1
Bacterial		
Streptococcus pyogenes	Pharyngitis/tonsillitis	15–35
Chlamydia trachomatis	Pharyngitis, pneumonia	0–20
Mycoplasma pneumoniae	Pneumonia, bronchitis, pharyngitis	5
Mixed anaerobic infections	Gingivitis, pharyngitis (Vincent's angina),	<1
	peritonsillitis/peritonsillar abscess (quinsy)	<1
Neisseria gonorrhoeae	Pharyngitis	<1
Corynebacterium diphtheriae	Diphtheria	<1
Arcanobacterium hemolyticum and A. ulcerans	Pharyngitis	<1

*Estimated percentage of cases of pharyngitis due to indicated organism in civilians of all ages. (Modified from Gwaltney JM: Pharyngitis. In Mandell GL, Douglas RG, Bennett JE: Principles and Practice of Infectious Disease, 3rd ed. New York, Churchill Livingstone, 1990.)

Ludwig's angina, bacterial tracheitis, and diphtheria can result in acute airway obstruction. Serious complications of sore throat include dehydration and sepsis as well as the sequelae of GABHS.

Rapid Assessment

Rapid assessment is done to seek the course and severity of the disease process, investigate the potential for airway compromise, and begin the search for systemic disease.

1. Are there signs of airway compromise such as *stridor, labored respirations, drooling, or inability to manage secretions*? Airway obstruction may be imminent, and attention is required. (See Chapter 2, Airway Management.)

2. Is the pain so severe as to significantly *limit oral intake* (dysphagia or odynophagia)? Does the patient have difficulty opening or closing the mouth (trismus)? Are there *vocal changes* such as a muffled or "hot potato" voice? The last two findings are typical of peritonsillar and retropharyngeal abscess.
3. Was the *onset* of *pain* associated with *fever*?
4. Were there any *chemical, allergic*, or *irritant exposures*?
5. Vital signs must be taken to help identify volume status, oxygenation, hypotension, and the presence of fever. Does the patient appear toxic? Airway, breathing, and circulatory status are assessed in the ill-appearing patient.

Early Intervention

1. An intravenous line is established if there are signs of hypovolemia or shock. Fluid resuscitation should be initiated with isotonic crystalloid. Blood pressure, pulse, and patient response are monitored.
2. Ongoing airway assessment is required for patients with significant symptomatology or a potentially obstructive process of the upper airway. Bringing airway management equipment to the patient's bedside is recommended.
3. Pain control with narcotic analgesia should be considered if speaking or swallowing difficulties are present. Careful titration is necessary to prevent sedation that would compromise the airway or interfere with management of secretions.
4. A tight, itchy, or sore throat may be the presenting symptom of an acute allergic reaction or anaphylaxis. Treatment should include airway management, intravenous access, epinephrine, corticosteroids, and antihistamines. (See Chapter 12, Anaphylaxis.)

CLINICAL ASSESSMENT

History

A careful history is the most important diagnostic tool in the assessment of a patient with acute pharyngitis. It is used to identify potential life-threatening emergencies and patients at risk for potential complications. The history is necessary to detect the etiology and severity of the problem as well as to establish the clinical approach to the patient.

History of Present Illness

The history of the present illness focuses on the characteristics of the sore throat.

Location and Quality of the Pain. It is important to have the patient describe the location and type of "throat" pain. Is it in the oropharynx or anatomically elsewhere? Throat pain localized only to the oropharynx is typical of GABHS. Is it sharp, stabbing, burning, or scratchy? Is it severe enough to interfere with eating, drinking, or swallowing saliva? Does it interfere with sleep? Is there a foreign body sensation along with the pain?

Onset. Was the pain gradual or sudden in onset? Trauma or acute bacterial infection is usually associated with sudden onset of pain. Viral sore throats develop more gradually.

Radiation of Pain. Does the pain radiate anywhere, or is it confined to the throat? Ear pain is often referred from the throat. Is there a change of pain with swallowing? What is the impact of swallowing on the pain, especially with or without food. Odynophagia is common in sore throat, but it may be caused by laryngeal or esophageal lesions.

Duration of Symptoms. How long has the patient had a sore throat? Deep infections such as peritonsillar abscess take 48 to 72 hours to develop. The timing of antibiotic therapy is important in GABHS pharyngitis.

Associated Symptoms. Are there any systemic symptoms such as fever, headache, malaise, nausea and vomiting, abdominal pain, or rash? The presence of cough, coryza, and hoarseness are seen more commonly in viral infections.

Family Contacts. Are there ill family members or close contacts? What is the nature of their illness? Exposure to "strep throat" infection in the previous 2 weeks increases the likelihood of GABHS. It is important to identify infectious causes as well as to determine if there are household members at risk for rheumatic fever if GABHS pharyngitis is diagnosed.

Exposure. Has there been a recent exposure to chemical or environmental irritants?

Past Medical History

Has the patient been diagnosed with "strep throat" in the past? If so, how was it diagnosed? Recurrent infection is a problem for some patients and can predispose the patient to suppurative complications such as peritonsillar abscess. Has the patient ever had infectious mononucleosis? It is unusual to get recurrent acute infectious mononucleosis. Is there any history of rheumatic fever or rheumatic heart disease? Is there a history of seasonal allergies or allergic rhinitis? What is the patient's immune status? Is there any history of HIV infection, diabetes, or cancer?

Surgical History. Has the patient had a tonsillectomy? Has the patient had a splenectomy?

Social History. Is the patient a smoker? Tobacco and marijuana use are common causes of chronic sore throat.

Sexual History. Does the patient have a vaginal or urethral discharge? Has there been any recent orogenital sexual activity? Is there any history of sexually transmitted infections?

Medication History. Is there a history of any medication allergies? It is important to inquire about the type of allergic reaction such as nausea, rash, or anaphylaxis. Is the patient currently taking any medications, including over-the-counter medications? Has the patient taken any medications for this illness? Often patients have taken antibiotics (theirs or someone else's) before being seen. As few as two doses of an antibiotic may alter culture results. What has the patient tried at home for symptomatic relief?

Immunizations. Is the patient currently up to date on immunizations? Diphtheria immunizations are part of the diphtheria/pertussis/tetanus (DPT) series.

Physical Examination

The physical examination complements the history. A simple inspection of the throat is not adequate. Important components of the physical examination are listed in Table 23–2. The age of the patient influences the preexamination probability of strep throat. For example, 25% to 35% of children with suspected GABHS have positive cultures, whereas in adults the range of positivity is from 5% to 29%.

Bedside Testing

Throat Culture. Important factors in a successful throat culture include the proper swabbing (it is a palatine sweep, including both tonsillar pillars—optional culture medium), preferably at the bedside, and laboratory capabilities.

Aspiration of Suspected Peritonsillar Abscess. Aspiration of a suspected peritonsillar abscess can be both diagnostic and therapeutic. With the patient sitting in an upright position, the area of greatest fluctuance is located. Topical (Cetacaine) or infiltrative (lidocaine) anesthesia is used. An 18-gauge needle with a 10-mL syringe is appropriate for most abscesses (see Fig. 23–1). Penetrating deep pharyngeal tissue is to be avoided. Suction with a tonsil suction tip should be available. If no purulent material is obtained, a second attempt can be made 1 cm below the first site.

CLINICAL REASONING

After initial data gathering and stabilization, the physician develops an initial differential diagnosis by answering the following questions.

Is There Evidence of a Catastrophic, Life-Threatening, or Serious Condition Requiring Immediate Attention?

If the patient demonstrates signs of respiratory distress, inability to manage secretions, or severe pain limiting jaw excursion (trismus) or has unstable vital signs indicative of respiratory or circulatory compromise, then identification of one of the six priority diagnoses should be made (Table 23–3).

Does the Patient Have an Infectious Cause of Pharyngitis? Is It Group A β-Hemolytic *Streptococcus*?

Once life-threatening and potentially serious conditions requiring immediate attention have been ruled out, a more in-depth history and specific findings in the physical examination help the physician identify the likely etiology of acute pharyngitis.

Although it can occur at any age, the peak incidence of GABHS is in the pediatric population in children aged 4 to 15 years. It is uncommon in children younger than 3 years of age. Males and females are equally affected. Most cases are seen in late fall and winter, although clusters of outbreaks can be seen throughout the year. GABHS pharyngitis is spread by means of respiratory droplets, and the incubation period is 2 to 5 days.

Special attention is given to identify GABHS pharyngitis because of the nonsuppurative sequelae of acute rheumatic fever and acute glomerular nephritis. Also, early identification and treatment may decrease the likelihood of suppurative complications. The ability to identify "strep throat" by clinical examination is inconsistent, and even the reliability of clinical assessment between observers has been questioned. High-yield findings are listed in Table 23–4. Several scoring systems have been developed in an attempt to improve diagnostic accuracy and influence treatment choices (Table 23–5).

Does the Patient Have a Noninfectious Cause of Acute Pharyngitis?

Burns. Ingestion of hot food or liquid or thermal inhalation can cause acute pharyngitis. This is usually elicited in the history, and treatment is

TABLE 23–2. Focused Physical Examination of Patients Complaining of Sore Throat

Area of Examination	Important Component	Comments
General appearance	Toxic vs. nontoxic Respiratory distress	Initial presentation and appearance will allow the physician to assess the degree of toxicity or distress.
Vital signs	Quality of voice	Muffled tone, hoarseness, or difficulty speaking should be noted.
	Heart rate/pulse Blood pressure	Tachycardia (>95 beats per minute), fever, hypertension and hypotension are not diagnostic but may represent the degree of systemic illness. Pain and increased sympathetic tone may also increase pulse and blood pressure.
	Temperature Respiratory rate Pulse oximetry	Tachypnea, stridor, labored respirations, excessive drooling, and low pulse oximetry are indicative of acute airway problems.
Skin	Presence of a rash	A fine maculopapular erythematous rash may be seen in GABHS (scarlet fever) or may be a viral exanthem.
Lymph nodes	Anterior and posterior cervical lymph nodes	The neck should be palpated for the presence of enlarged or tender lymph nodes. Axillary, supraclavicular, and inguinal nodes may also be included.
Abdomen	Palpation	Hepatomegaly or splenomegaly may be present in infectious mononucleosis, HIV, or other malignancies. Abdominal pain may be the presenting symptom in small children with streptococcal infections.
Oropharynx	Inspection of the tonsils, uvula, hard and soft palate, tonsillar fossa, and gingiva	Using a good light and tongue depressor and having the patient say "Ahhh" elevates the uvula and soft palate. Observe the tonsils for size, position, and symmetry. The uvula should be midline. Note the appearance of erythema, edema, and exudate on tonsils or pharynx. Observe any petechiae on soft palate or the presence of any ulcerative lesions. A bright red "strawberry" tongue may be seen in GABHS.
	Palpation	Palpation of the peritonsillar area may identify an area of fluctuance or induration seen in peritonsillar abscess or cellulitis.
Heart/lung	Auscultation	Note the quality of breath sounds and air movement. Listen for upper airway sounds such as stridor (usually audible without a stethoscope). Note any wheezes, rales, or rhonchi. Cardiac examination may reveal a murmur.
Genitourinary	Inspection	Only necessary if history of urethral or vaginal discharge.

GABHS, group A β-hemolytic streptococci; HIV, human immunodeficiency virus.

TABLE 23–3. Serious Illness Presenting as Acute Sore Throat

	Presentation	Associated Symptoms	Supportive History	Physical Examination	Useful Test	Management
Retropharyngeal Abscess	Usually children aged 4–5 years. Also seen in adults. Severe sore throat, dysphagia, stridor/drooling with toxic appearance	Difficulty breathing, painful or stiff neck, refusal to move neck; trismus or "hot potato" voice is common; new-onset snoring in adults	History of recent upper respiratory infection. History of recent trauma or instrumentation of throat, swallowed foreign body (e.g., fish bone) Use of crack cocaine	Fever, enlarged cervical lymph nodes, limited cervical motion, fullness of posterior pharynx Fluctuance in oropharynx and hypopharynx	1. Lateral soft plain radiographs of neck may reveal thickening of prevertebral soft tissues. Air may be present in soft tissue 2. CT may delineate extent and location of abscess	1. Airway control 2. ENT consult 3. Antibiotics
Epiglottitis	Usually children aged 2–8 years. Toxic appearing, drooling Adults: severe sore throat, odynophagia, dysphagia	Respiratory distress with stridor, suprasternal and intercostal retractions, restlessness; anterior neck pain, hoarseness, occasionally short of breath	Usually history of upper respiratory prodrome	Fever, muffled voice, tachycardia, tachypnea, cherry red epiglottis; tripod posturing Oropharynx may appear normal, tachycardia, tender anterior cervical lymph nodes	1. Lateral soft tissue x-rays of neck will reveal characteristic "thumb print" sign of swollen epiglottis. Neck films may be less specific in adults. Indirect laryngoscopy is safer owing to larger airway in adults 2. CBC 3. Blood cultures	1. Airway control 2. ENT consult 3. Antibiotics: parenteral cephalosporins (ceftriaxone is first choice). Use clindamycin for known allergies.
Peritonsillar Abscess	Usually toxic-appearing adolescent or young adult with severe throat pain, odynophagia, dysphagia	Trismus secondary to spasm of jaw muscles, unilateral pain often referred to the ear; "hot potato" voice	Possibly recent sore throat or even diagnosed strep throat on antibiotics. Over 48% to 72%: tonsillitis → undiagnosed peritonsillar cellulitis → abscess	Fever, unilateral swelling and erythema of soft palate and tonsillar pillar; uvula may be deviated away from the affected side; ipsilateral tender anterior cervical lymph nodes; tonsils may appear normal	1. Throat culture or rapid strep may be of limited usefulness 2. CT may delineate cellulitis from abscess or identify deeper space abscess 3. Aspiration of abscess	1. Aspiration of abscess 2. ENT consult 3. Antibiotics 4. If less than 72 hours, antibiotic trial with follow-up in 24–48 hours may differentiate cellulitis (resolution) from abscess (persists)
Severe Tonsillar or Uvular Edema/Ludwig's angina	Severe sore throat, tight throat, odynophagia, dysphagia, respiratory distress, stridor	Drooling, intercostal retractions, wheezing	Recent upper respiratory infection with sore throat and fever Exposure to allergen such as bee sting or ingestion of peanuts Known dental disease	Fever, tachycardia, tachypnea, erythema of tonsils and uvula Pressure of exudate on tonsils Severe tonsillar or uvular swelling; tender enlarged anterior and posterior nodes	1. Throat culture or rapid strep 2. Mono spot 3. CBC 4. Soft tissue radiograph of neck	1. Airway control 2. ENT consult 3. Corticosteroids 4. Antibiotics 5. If allergic origin, consider treating for anaphylaxis
Diphtheria	Adult or child: severe sore throat, odynophagia, dysphagia, stridor, respiratory distress; uncommon, 5–10 cases per year	Drooling, intercostal retractions, often foul odor to breath	History of upper respiratory syndrome Not current on immunizations (e.g., recent immigrants)	Fever, tachycardia, tachypnea, tender enlarged anterior cervical lymph nodes Gray membrane on tonsils and pharyngeal tissues. If removed, it will reveal a bleeding surface	1. Culture on Loeffler's medium 2. ECG (toxic myocarditis)	1. Airway control 2. Diphtheria antitoxin 3. Antibiotics
Bacterial Tracheitis	Croupy cough, toxic appearing, similar to epiglottitis; slower course and less drooling	Same as epiglottitis	History of upper respiratory infection prodrome	High fever, rhonchi or wheezing on lung examination	1. Soft tissue neck radiograph—subglottic narrowing, opaque streaks, or irregular margins	1. Airway control 2. Antibiotics 3. ENT consult

CBC, complete blood cell count; CT, computed tomography; ECG, electrocardiogram; ENT, ear, nose, and throat.

TABLE 23–4. Clinical Presentation of Group A β-Hemolytic Streptococcal Tonsillopharyngitis

Symptoms	Signs
Sudden onset localized sore throat	Tonsillopharyngeal erythema
Pain with swallowing	Tonsillopharyngeal exudate
Fever > 38.5°C (101°F)	Palatal petechiae (no vesicles or ulcers)
Headache	Beefy red, swollen uvula
Abdominal pain/anorexia	Tender anterior cervical lymphadenopathy
Nausea/vomiting	Scarlatiniform rash (blanches, sandpaper feel)
No associated coryza, conjunctivitis, or myalgia	

TABLE 23–5. McIsaac Modification for the Centor "Strep" Score

1. Add Up Points for Patient

Symptom or Sign	Points
History of fever or measured temperature >38°C	1
Absence of cough	1
Tender anterior cervical adenopathy	1
Tonsillar swelling or exudates	1
Age > 15 yr	1
Age ≥ 45 yr	–1

2. Find Risk of "Strep" Throat

Points	Likelihood Ratio	% with "Strep" (Patients with "Strep"/Total)
–1 or 0	0.05	1 (2/179)
1	0.52	10 (13/134)
2	0.95	17 (18/109)
3	2.5	35 (28/81)
4 or 5	4.9	51 (39/77)

Data from a group of 167 children aged ≥ 3 years and 453 adults in Ontario, Canada. Baseline risk of "strep" throat 17% in this population.

supportive and symptomatic. Ingestion of caustic chemicals or substances by toddlers can also present as acute pharyngitis. Clues may include the appearance of blisters, erythema, or ulcers on the lips or oral mucosa. Chemicals such as alkalis can cause liquefaction or coagulation necrosis.

Gastroesophageal Reflux Disease. This is similar to a chronic caustic exposure in severe cases. History related to timing with meals, body position, and improving/worsening factors should be explored.

Smoking. Tobacco and marijuana use can commonly cause chronic sore throat.

Trauma. Penetrating trauma can lead to retropharyngeal abscess. Local pain and dysphagia are common symptoms. An unexplained trauma history is most common in children.

Neoplastic Disorders. Nasopharyngeal carcinomas can present as acute pharyngitis. Leukemia and lymphoma may present as an acute sore throat with ulcerative or exudative oral findings. Other systemic symptoms such as prolonged fever or significant lymphadenopathy may be present.

Allergic Rhinitis. Seasonal allergic postnasal drainage can cause sore throat. Symptoms are usually worse in the morning.

Subacute Thyroiditis. Findings of a normal-appearing oropharynx and tender thyroid gland may be suggestive.

DIAGNOSTIC ADJUNCTS

Laboratory Studies

A number of laboratory tests may be useful in determining the cause of acute pharyngitis and who needs antibiotic therapy. The decision about which test to use depends on several factors, including age of patient, prevalence of streptococcal infection, immune status, history of rheumatic fever, and the likelihood of follow-up. A reasonable approach to laboratory decision making is summarized in the algorithm in Figure 23–2.

Throat Culture. The throat culture remains the "gold standard" for the diagnosis of GABHS. A sterile cotton swab should be rubbed over the tonsils, tonsillar fossa, and posterior pharynx. The swab is usually sent to the microbiology laboratory in transport media. A blood agar plate is inoculated with the swab and a bacitracin-A disc is applied. β-Hemolysis about the disc identifies GABHS. Cultures are usually read at 24 to 48 hours. A positive throat culture does not identify the carrier state. A blood agar plate costs about 60 cents. The patient charge for a throat culture varies but is generally more than $50.

Rapid Strep Test. Many commercially available rapid strep kits are available. These tests detect the presence of group A strep antigen using latex particle agglutination or enzyme

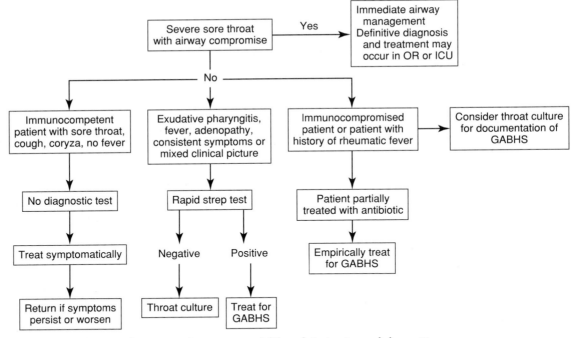

FIGURE 23–2 • Strategy for testing and treating group A β-hemolytic streptococcal pharyngitis.

immunoassay techniques. The test can be performed in approximately 30 minutes by any trained health care professional and does not need to be performed in the laboratory. The sensitivities of the kits range from 76% to 87%, and specificities range from 90% to 96%. The cost of a rapid strep test kit is about $5.

In the patient with high-yield clinical findings, a negative rapid strep test should be followed by a throat culture to avoid missing GABHS.

Newer optical immunoassay tests have also been developed. Studies indicate the optical immunoassay techniques may be more sensitive than throat culture on blood agar for identifying GABHS. Routine use of these in the future may obviate the need for throat cultures.

Radiologic Imaging

Lateral Soft Tissue View of Neck. A lateral radiograph may be useful in the diagnosis of retropharyngeal abscess, epiglottitis, and Ludwig's angina (see Chapter 27, Stridor). It is usually obtained as a portable film taken in the emergency department.

Computed Tomography. Computed tomography may be necessary to identify the presence and size of deep tissue abscesses (e.g., retropharyngeal) and may be used to differentiate abscess from cellulitis. The patient may go to the

radiology area accompanied by an individual skilled in airway management with the proper equipment.

Chest Radiograph. Although rarely indicated in most patients, chest posteroanterior and lateral views may be obtained if a retropharyngeal abscess is present. Complications of retropharyngeal abscess extension include mediastinitis and aspiration.

EXPANDED DIFFERENTIAL DIAGNOSIS

Infectious causes of a sore throat include viruses, bacteria, and fungal infections.

Viruses (50% to 80% of causes)

Adenovirus/Rhinovirus

Adenoviruses and rhinoviruses are among the most common viral causes of pharyngitis. Other tissues in the respiratory tract are affected, resulting in symptoms including cough, coryza, conjunctivitis, sneezing, and laryngitis. The pharynx and tonsils are usually mildly erythematous, and exudates are rare. Other systemic symptoms include malaise, headache, fatigue, and low-grade fever. Symptoms are usually mild and self-limited.

Epstein-Barr Virus/Cytomegalovirus
(1% to 10% of causes)

Epstein-Barr virus and, less commonly, cyto-megalovirus cause infectious mononucleosis. It is spread by means of respiratory droplets and saliva and is nicknamed the "kissing disease." Symptoms include severe sore throat, tender lymph nodes, fatigue, malaise, headache, fever, nausea, vomiting, and abdominal pain.

On physical examination, there is pronounced erythema and swelling of pharyngeal and tonsillar tissue, often accompanied by marked exudate. Tender anterior and posterior cervical lymphadenopathy is typically present. Hepatosplenomegaly is part of the disease complex, but it is often missed. Once diagnosed, it is recommended that these patients avoid contact-type activity (e.g., football), because of the significant potential of splenic rupture. Occasionally, a fine erythematous rash may later develop or become more prominent in patients treated with amoxicillin but does not indicate a drug allergy. Clinically, infectious mononucleosis may be indistinguishable from GABHS pharyngitis. Interestingly, up to 33% of patients with infectious mononucleosis may have concomitant GABHS. Symptoms may last 2 to 6 weeks. Diagnosis is made using the monospot test, which detects heterophil antibodies. Patients are usually ill 1 to 2 weeks before the test becomes positive. A complete blood cell count with differential may show a lymphocytosis with greater than 10% atypical lymphocytes. A throat culture or rapid strep test is usually part of the assessment.

Herpes Simplex Virus

Primary infection with herpes simplex virus may also produce a clinical picture similar to that of GABHS, with tonsillar erythema and exudates, fever, and cervical lymphadenopathy. Microvesicular lesions and painful shallow ulcers with surrounding erythema are seen on the soft palate, gums, lips, and buccal mucosa and may help distinguish herpes simplex from other causes. Diagnosis is made clinically and with the aid of viral cultures.

Coxsackievirus

Acute pharyngitis caused by the presence of multiple small 1- to 2-mm vesicles on the tonsils, tonsillar pillars, uvula, and soft palate suggest herpangina caused by coxsackievirus A. Most cases are seen in the late summer and spring. Coxsackievirus A16 is the major cause of hand-foot-and-mouth disease, in which similar lesions and vesicles develop in the oropharynx, hands, and feet. The diagnosis is made clinically.

Acute Retroviral Syndrome

This clinical syndrome has become increasingly recognized as a manifestation of primary HIV infection. Symptoms include fever, nonexudative pharyngitis, and lymphadenopathy, with arthralgia, myalgia, lethargy, and a maculopapular rash occurring in 40% to 80% of patients. Although clinically similar to infectious mononucleosis, it lacks tonsillar exudate and hypertrophy and has more of an acute onset. Assays for HIV type I RNA will be positive, but HIV antibodies are usually not present. Antiretroviral agents are recommended.

Bacteria

Streptococcus pyogenes—Group A (GABHS)
(15% to 35% of causes)

GABHS causes a localized inflammation of the oropharynx. It is a self-limited infection usually lasting 5 to 10 days. The organism produces many extracellular toxins, including a pyrogenic exo-toxin that produces the rash of scarlet fever. It also produces (1) a streptolysin O toxic to erythrocytes and leukocytes and (2) four types of DNAase, including streptokinase (important in thrombolytic therapy). The typical clinical presentation of GABHS is summarized in Table 23–4.

Unfortunately, many of these findings are not specific and can occur in other respiratory infections. Signs and symptoms *not* associated with GABHS include cough, coryza, hoarseness, diarrhea, conjunctivitis, anterior stomatitis, and discrete ulcerative lesions.

Clinical diagnosis alone can result in the unnecessary use of an antibiotic. This practice can lead to an increase in the likelihood of allergic reactions and promote bacterial resistance. Studies of physicians diagnosing GABHS pharyngitis on clinical presentation alone have resulted in as high as 81% overestimation on the positive side. The scoring system example in Table 23–5 is an attempt to improve on clinical accuracy and has demonstrated some benefit.

The carrier state of GABHS is seen most commonly in children and ranges from 15% to 30%. Carriers may be ill with viral infections, which makes appropriate diagnosis often difficult. The carrier state has rarely been associated with acute rheumatic fever, is rarely contagious to others, and is not associated with a rise in antibody levels (antistreptolysin O).

Acute rheumatic fever is carried by a cross-reactivity of antibodies to the M protein of the streptococcus. Clinical manifestations include carditis, valvular involvement, arthritis, subcutaneous nodules, and chorea. Acute rheumatic fever has been on the rise in certain areas of the United States and is being seen more commonly in middle-income families. Treatment of GABHS prevents acute rheumatic fever; unfortunately, most patients with acute rheumatic fever were never ill with pharyngitis. During rare epidemic situations, up to 3% of untreated streptococcal infections will result in acute rheumatic fever.

Acute glomerulonephritis is also a late sequela of a streptococcal infection. Antibiotic therapy directed at GABHS does not prevent acute glomerulonephritis. Clinical signs include hypertension, edema, proteinuria, and hematuria. Overall rate of poststreptococcal acute glomerulonephritis is 0% to 3%. Treatment is supportive and aimed at fluid and blood pressure control.

β-Hemolytic Group C and G

These Lancefield groups also cause the acute pharyngitis that is seen most commonly in adolescents and young adults. Group C has been associated with the same suppurative complications of GABHS, and most studies recommend treatment to shorten the clinical course and prevent suppurative complications. The role group C and G streptococci play in acute rheumatic fever and acute glomerulonephritis is less clear.

Commercial laboratories identify and subtype Lancefield groups B, C, F, and G via culture methods. Reporting of these specific groups on routine throat cultures varies among facilities. Current rapid strep test kits do not differentiate these agents from GABHS.

Chlamydia (C. pneumoniae, possibly C. trachomatis) and Mycoplasma pneumoniae
(2% to 5% of causes)

Pharyngitis caused by these bacteria is usually seen in association with other symptoms such as headache and cough. They are more commonly seen in adolescents and young adults and in crowded living situations, such as dormitories or military barracks. Usually, they are infections of limited duration and clinical findings. Diagnosis is made using special culture media or serologic tests, neither of which is used routinely in the emergency department.

Neisseria gonorrhoeae (1% to 2% of causes)

Gonococcal pharyngitis is seen after orogenital sexual activity with an infected partner. The presence of a urethral or vaginal discharge or a history of sexually transmitted infections should raise the index of suspicion. Pharyngeal ulcers, exudate, erythema, and cervical lymphadenopathy are common.

Diagnosis is made by doing a throat culture with a rayon swab and culturing on Thayer-Martin (chocolate agar). Specific urethral or vaginal cultures should be performed if clinically indicated. This diagnosis in children is highly suggestive of child abuse.

Arcanobacterium haemolyticus

Previously known as *Corynebacterium haemolyticus*, this organism produces a clinical illness indistinguishable from GABHS. It is most commonly seen in adolescents and young adults. Seventy percent of patients develop oropharyngeal or tonsillar exudates, 50% develop anterior cervical lymphadenopathy, 40% have fever up to 102.6°F (39.2°C), 33% have a scarlatiniform, pruritic rash, and a variable percentage (up to 67%) have a nonproductive cough. Palatal petechiae and strawberry tongue are not found. The incidence of infection with *A. haemolyticus* may be as high as GABHS in a given population.

Diagnosis depends on finding the typical pharyngitis with negative routine testing for GABHS. *A. haemolyticus* can be cultured on blood agar, but it is slow growing and β-hemolysis occurs after 48 hours.

Anaerobes/Borrelia (less than 4% of causes)

Borrelia vincentii may cause Vincent's angina. Definite diagnosis is made by anaerobic culture or visualization of spirochetes by darkfield microscopy, but usually it is a clinical diagnosis.

Oral anaerobes such as *Fusobacterium* and *Bacteroides* species can produce pharyngitis with foul breath and purulent exudates on tonsils and pharynx. There is usually underlying gingivitis, and a pseudomembrane may be present. Malnutrition, leukopenia, and immunodeficiency predispose to this disease.

Fungi

Candida albicans (Thrush) (up to 4% of causes)

Pharyngitis caused by *Candida* is most commonly seen in immunocompromised patients. It is characterized by white plaques that are usually coalesced on an ulcerative base seen on the buccal mucosa, pharynx, and tongue. In undiagnosed patients, its presence should raise the suspicion of HIV infection or a neoplastic disorder. It is commonly seen in normal infants because breast milk and formula may alter oral flora and enhance yeast growth. Diagnosis is made by the presence of hyphae with potassium hydroxide under microscopy.

Unusual Causes of Acute Pharyngitis

Tularemia can present as severe, painful lymphadenopathy and exudative pharyngitis. Rabbits and ticks are the major source of infection. Diagnosis is made on serologic testing. Treatment is with tetracycline or gentamicin.

Yersinia infection usually presents as fever, diarrhea, malaise, chills, and an ulcerative pharyngitis. Animals including rodents and swine are the reservoirs. Diagnosis is based on isolation of the organism from stool, throat, or blood culture.

The usual presentation of *Kawasaki syndrome* is fever, conjunctivitis, and erythema of oropharynx, lips, and tongue. A polymorphous rash is seen, and there is usually a solitary anterior cervical node. Erythema and edema of the hands and feet may occur. It is a disease of infants and toddlers. Diagnosis is based on fulfilling specific clinical criteria. The treatment is intravenous γ-globulin and aspirin.

PRINCIPLES OF MANAGEMENT

The management of a patient with an acute sore throat depends on the diagnosis. The management of emergent conditions is generally addressed in the initial stabilization phase and includes airway control, rehydration, and consultation with an ear, nose, and throat specialist (see Table 23–3). The management of non–life-threatening acute pharyngitis is aimed at symptomatic relief and appropriate antibiotic therapy.

Analgesia

Symptoms of acute pharyngitis can be mild to severe. Treatment options include anesthetic sprays, lozenges, salt water gargles, acetaminophen, nonsteroidal anti-inflammatory drugs such as ibuprofen, and a mild narcotic (acetaminophen with codeine derivative).

Corticosteroids

Oral prednisone has been used as an inflammatory modulator for the pain and inflammation associated with infectious mononucleosis. Studies have shown a short course of oral prednisone or a one-time intramuscular injection of dexamethasone can significantly reduce pain and inflammation in acute pharyngitis caused by other infections as well.

Antibiotics

Antibiotics are given to selected patients based on the presumed etiology of the pharyngitis. More than 50% of adults are treated with antibiotics by primary physicians. There has been a disturbing trend toward the use of nonrecommended antibiotics in undiagnosed cases (e.g., macrolides and fluoroquinolones) during the past decade.

Group A β-Hemolytic Streptococcal Pharyngitis

Treatment of GABHS will help with resolution of the severity or duration of symptoms, decrease the duration of infectivity, and decrease the likelihood of suppurative complications. The main treatment goal, however, is to eradicate GABHS to prevent rheumatic fever. Antibiotics need to be started within 9 days of symptoms.

Penicillin remains first-line therapy for GABHS in nonallergic patients. Resistance to penicillin has never been documented in vitro, but a 10% failure rate for initial therapy has been stable for several decades. Penicillin failures do occur and may be attributable to colonization with co-pathogens such as *Staphylococcus aureus* that produce β-lactamases, inactivating penicillin. The overall eradication rates with cephalosporins are 4% to 6% higher than with penicillin, but cephalosporins may cost 3 to 10 times more than penicillin.

The duration of treatment with penicillin remains 10 days. Twice-a-day dosing has been shown to be as efficacious as dosing four times a day. However, if patients miss one of the two doses, treatment is inadequate. A new dosing regimen of a single daily dose of amoxicillin has been shown to be as effective as multiple daily doses of penicillin. However, this finding needs to be confirmed before routine clinical use is begun. Because patients with GABHS pharyngitis are often symptomatically better in a few days, they need to be educated about the importance of completing therapy to prevent sequelae. Specific therapies are summarized as follows:

First-Line Therapy
Benzathine penicillin G: for patient weighing less than 27 kg: 600,000 units IM; for patient weighing more than 27 kg: 1.2 million units IM, *or*

Oral penicillin V: child, 250 mg two or three times a day for 10 days; adult, 500 mg two or three times a day for 10 days; adolescent, 500 mg two or three times a day for 10 days

If Penicillin Allergic
Erythromycin estolate: 20 to 40 mg/kg two to four times a day for 10 days, *or*

Erythromycin ethylsuccinate: 40 mg/kg two to four times a day for 10 days

Alternative Therapy
Amoxicillin

Amoxicillin/clavulanate

Azithromycin (for 5 days, with once-a-day dosing)

Clarithromycin
Cephalosporins (e.g., cefadroxil, cefaclor, cefixime)

Up to 15% of patients allergic to penicillin will be allergic to a cephalosporin. If there is a history of anaphylaxis to penicillin, a cephalosporin should not be used. In patients in whom compliance is an issue, an intramuscular injection of benzathine penicillin is the treatment of choice. Amoxicillin is preferred by many pediatricians because of taste. Also, the frequency of dosing, especially with children, will affect compliance. Once-a-day dosing antibiotics such as azithromycin are preferred by parents. Cost and compliance issues should be taken into account. Tetracycline and sulfonamides are not recommended.

Group C Streptococcal Pharyngitis

Most studies advocate treating group C *Streptococcus* because it can lead to suppurative complications. The same antibiotics as for group A *Streptococcus* are indicated.

Gonococcal Pharyngitis

The following regimens may be effective:

Ceftriaxone, 125 to 250 mg intramuscularly, plus azithromycin or doxycycline, *or*

Ciprofloxacin, 500 mg, plus azithromycin or doxycycline

Ofloxacin, 400 mg, plus azithromycin or doxycycline

Anaerobic Pharyngitis

Penicillin and clindamycin are used.

Arcanobacterium haemolyticus Pharyngitis

Erythromycin, clarithromycin, or azithromycin is used. Penicillin is probably not adequate.

Candidal Pharyngitis

Fluconazole, itraconazole, nystatin, clotrimazole, and ketoconazole are effective.

Herpes Simplex Pharyngitis

Acyclovir and other antiviral agents are administered.

UNCERTAIN DIAGNOSIS

An uncertain diagnosis is common in patients with sore throat. There are many ways to approach such patients. Figure 23–2 outlines an approach to minimize excess testing and antibiotic use (see Table 23–5). Errors are common, and clear instructions for follow-up or return if there is limited improvement are necessary. Persistent sore throat should prompt consideration of noninfectious causes.

SPECIAL CONSIDERATIONS

Immunocompromised Patients

Patients with AIDS can have a number of oral conditions that may present as an acute sore throat. These include acute retroviral syndrome, mucosal candidiasis, herpes gingivostomatitis, giant aphthous ulcers, and hairy leukoplakia ulcers. Severe odynophagia may be caused by candidal epiglottitis and esophagitis. Kaposi's sarcoma may be seen as violaceous lesions that can ulcerate. Non-Hodgkin's lymphoma can cause ulcerative lesions or nodular lesions of the tongue and oropharynx. Diagnosis is made on biopsy. Non-Hodgkin's lymphoma is the second most common neoplasm in patients with AIDS.

Splenectomized patients may be especially susceptible to streptococcal sepsis. Only mildly symptomatic patients who are reliable and close to a hospital for careful, close follow-up are treated as outpatients.

Leukopenic or leukemic patients are evaluated for adequate granulocyte counts before outpatient treatment is considered. Close follow-up is essential.

Diabetic patients and corticosteroid-dependent patients may require close supervision during any intercurrent illness, and admission is a viable option.

DISPOSITION AND FOLLOW-UP

Admission

Patients with obvious airway compromise who are intubated or patients with the potential to develop airway compromise are admitted to the ICU. Patients with a retropharyngeal abscess may go directly to the operating room. This decision is made with ENT consultation.

Patients who are not able to take oral fluids and require extended intravenous treatment may need admission to an unmonitored bed ward for supportive treatment.

Observation

Patients who need initial fluid resuscitation, intravenous therapy, inhaled aerosols, or the initiation of corticosteroids to manage partial airway obstruction secondary to edema or tissue swelling may be observed in the emergency department for several hours before a decision for disposition can be made.

Discharge

Patients should demonstrate they can take oral fluids in the emergency department before they can be discharged. This is especially important in children and infants.

Patients with a peritonsillar abscess that was aspirated in the emergency department can usually go home if they can manage secretions and take oral fluids. They should follow up in the emergency department or with an ENT specialist in 24 hours. Patients with suspected peritonsillar cellulitis who are given antibiotic therapy require similar close follow-up.

If a throat culture was performed, patients need clear instructions as to how and when those results will be given to them. Most patients are asked to call back in 24 to 48 hours.

Reasons to return to the emergency department must be clearly understood by the patient and family. These include the following:

- Difficulty breathing
- Increasing pain
- Inability to manage secretions or take fluids
- Increasing fever or new or worsening symptoms

FINAL POINTS

- Evaluation and management of acute sore throat is a complicated decision process. This is not an easy "treat and street" situation.
- Be aware of serious complications and sequelae in the patient with a simple sore throat (e.g., peritonsillar abscess).
- Although a less common cause of sore throat, GABHS commands attention in diagnosis because of its potentially serious sequelae: abscesses, rheumatic fever, glomerulonephritis.
- In patients with clinically high-yield findings, follow a negative rapid strep test with a throat culture.
- Select antibiotic therapy wisely, to minimize expense and risk to the patient.
- It is essential to educate patients about antibiotic use, including the importance of completing a course of prescribed antibiotics and why viral upper respiratory infections do not respond to antibiotic therapy.
- Patients seek medical attention with certain perceptions, and it is important to have them leave satisfied with your care. Even simple viral infections can be bothersome to patients, and prescribing symptomatic care based on symptoms (e.g., cough syrup with codeine for night time) is appreciated and may be more appropriate than the antibiotic they requested. Pain management is an essential part of treating the patient with a sore throat.

CASE *Study*

A 17-year-old college student presented to the emergency department with a 5-day history of sore throat and right ear pain. It was her third visit for this complaint. She had been seen at the campus health center and started on azithromycin after a rapid strep test was performed and found negative. She also had a "blood test" with results unknown to her. Two days later in the emergency department a throat culture was done and clindamycin was added. There was no clinical improvement, which prompted this visit on the fifth day.

The patient complained of sore throat but was able to eat and drink normally. No cough, coryza, or eye symptoms were noted. She complained of tender lymph nodes in her neck. Her review of symptoms is negative. She has a history of strep in the past but no history of infectious mononucleosis.

She has no medication allergies, is a nonsmoker, and lives in a college dormitory. Immunizations are up to date. Current medications were azithromycin, clindamycin, and acetaminophen with hydrocodone.

Her physical examination included vital signs of temperature, 99.1°F (37.3°C); blood pressure, 120/74 mm Hg; pulse, 82 beats per minute; and respirations, 20 breaths per minute. She was an alert, talkative female in no apparent distress. Her HEENT examination reviewed clear tympanic membranes and enlarged, erythematous tonsils in the oropharynx with gray-green exudate. There were no palatal petechiae or ulcerative lesions. Tender anterior and posterior lymph nodes were present. The remainder of the physical examination was normal, including a gentle examination for hepatosplenomegaly.

The campus health center was called for results. The rapid strep test was negative, and no throat culture was performed. Her white blood cell count (WBC) with differential was 8000/mm^3, with 38 neutrophils, 60 lymphocytes, and 0 atypical lymphocytes. No monospot test was performed.

On her second visit in the emergency department 2 days later, a throat culture was performed and clindamycin was added to azithromycin. There was no review of the campus health center visit at this time.

During this current visit, her repeat WBC was 9200/mm^3, with 38 neutrophils, 53 lymphocytes, 8 monocytes, and 9 atypical lymphocytes. A Monospot test was positive, and a strep screen was negative.

Unfortunately, this patient was started on a very expensive antibiotic when she had no allergy to penicillin. Also, the negative strep test was not followed up with a confirmatory culture before the antibiotic was started. She had 2 days of antibiotic therapy when a culture was done, so the negative result was unreliable. It was unclear whether the patient had only mononucleosis or if she had partially treated strep throat as well. This necessitated her taking a full course of antibiotics. The azithromycin was continued, but the clindamycin was stopped. The patient was also given a 5-day course of oral prednisone for symptomatic relief and specific instructions about infectious mononucleosis.

The patient was given two rather expensive antibiotics when neither one may have been necessary. Also, a throat culture performed after antibiotic therapy is begun is unreliable and an added expense.

Summary of Approximate Costs for Three Visits

Campus health visit (CBC, rapid strep)	
(most health fees paid with tuition):	$ 19.75
Azithromycin:	48.69
Vicodin (#20):	17.69
Emergency department visit #1	
Level I visit:	150.00
Physician fee:	49.00
Throat culture:	55.00
Clindamycin:	33.69
Emergency department visit #2	
Level I visit:	150.00
Physician fee:	49.00
WBC:	18.00
Monospot:	26.00
Prednisone:	5.99
TOTAL:	**$622.81**

Costs of Potentially Ideal Care

Campus health visit with rapid strep screen:	19.75
Throat culture due to high risk:	55.00
Symptomatic relief without antibiotics	
(e.g., gargles, acetaminophen):	5.00
Call back after negative throat culture	
and reexamination:	19.75
Monospot (may need to be repeated):	26.00
Prednisone:	6.00
TOTAL:	**$131.50**

Bibliography

TEXTS

Adams G, Boise L, Hilger P: Fundamentals of Otolaryngology, Philadelphia, WB Saunders, 1998.

American Academy of Pediatrics, Section 3—Summaries of Infectious Diseases. In Peter G (ed): 1997 Red Book: Report of the Committee on Infectious Diseases, 24th ed. Elk Grove, IL, American Academy of Pediatrics, 1997.

JOURNAL ARTICLES

Bisno AL: Acute pharyngitis. N Engl J Med 2001; 344:205–211.

Dajani A, Taubert K, Ferrieri P, et al, Committee on Rheumatic Fever and Endocarditis, Kawasaki Disease Council on Cardiovascular Disease in the Young, American Heart Association: Special statement—treatment of acute streptococcal pharyngitis and prevention of rheumatic fever: Statement for health professionals. Pediatrics 1995; 96:758–764.

Del Mar CB, Glaziou PP, Spinks AB: Antibiotics for sore throat. Cochrane Database Syst Rev 2000; (4):CD000023.

Ebell MH, Smith MA, Barry HC: Does this patient have strep throat? JAMA 2000; 284:2912–2918.

Harris R, Paine D, Wittler R, Bruhn F: Impact on empiric treatment of group A streptococcal pharyngitis using optical immunoassay. Clin Pediatr 1995; 34:122–127.

Linder JA, Stafford RS: Antibiotic treatment of adults with sore throat by community primary care physicians. JAMA 2001; 286:1181–1186.

McIsaac WJ, Goel V, Tot R, et al: The validity of a sore throat score in family practice. Can Med Assoc J 2000; 163:811–815.

Nawaz H, Smith DS, Mazhari R, et al: Concordance of clinical findings and clinical judgment in the diagnosis of streptococcal pharyngitis. Acad Emerg Med 2000; 7:1104–1109.

Pichichero ME: Group A beta-hemolytic streptococcal infections. Pediatr Rev 1998; 19:291–302.

Pichichero ME: Group A streptococcal tonsillopharyngitis: Cost-effective diagnosis and treatment. Ann Emerg Med 1995; 25:290–303.

Shulman ST: Evaluation of penicillins, cephalosporins, and macrolides for therapy of streptococcal pharyngitis. Pediatrics 1996; 97:955–959.

Stewart C: "Killer" sore throat: Prompt detection and management of serious and potentially life-threatening causes of pharyngeal pain. Emerg Med Rep 2001; 22(10):103–118.

Stewart MH, Siff JE, Cydulka RK: Evaluation of the patient with sore throat, earache, and sinusitis: An evidence based approach. Emerg Med Clin North Am 1999; 17:153–187.

Thomas M, Delmar C, Glasziou P: How effective are treatments other than antibiotics for acute sore throat? Br J Gen Pract 2000; 50:817–820.

CHAPTER 24

Earache

RONALD M. SALIK
NICHOLAS BENSON

CASE *Study*

A 66-year-old woman was brought by her daughter to the emergency department. The daughter stated that her mother had had intense pain in her left ear for several hours and was "not acting right."

CASE *Study*

A mother brought in her 6-year-old daughter because she had noticed a foul-smelling, cream-colored fluid coming out of the child's left ear for the past 2 days. The child said that her ear hurt "a little."

INTRODUCTION

Earache is a common complaint of patients coming to the emergency department. It can originate from a variety of sites in and around the ear. Otogenic causes include problems with the mastoid, middle ear, or external canal, although involvement of the temporal bone or inner ear also occurs. The ear is innervated by sensory branches of the vagus nerve (cranial nerve X), glossopharyngeal nerve (IX), auriculotemporal branch of the trigeminal nerve (V), facial nerve (VII), and branches of cervical nerves 2 and 3. Pathologic conditions, including infection and malignancy, of the upper respiratory or digestive tract (oropharynx, larynx, hypopharynx) and the teeth or mandible can cause referred pain to the ear.

The ear canal and temporal bone surrounding the middle and inner ear structures provide a relative barrier against infectious agents and trauma. Most infectious agents arrive by means of the communication between the middle ear and the posterior pharynx through the eustachian tube. The tympanic membrane is the boundary between the middle and the external ear. It is made up of squamous, fibrous, and mucosal layers. Each layer may be involved in a pathologic process specific to its cell type, although most problems are either infectious or secondary to rapid shifts in air pressure between the external and middle ear. The external canal, lined with squamous epithelium and open to the environment, is vulnerable to all forms of skin disorders and environmental pathogens.

Most earaches are caused by an acute infection or inflammation of the middle ear (otitis media) or the external ear canal (otitis externa). Otitis media is the most common cause of ear pain seen in the emergency department. It occurs most often in infants and young children, with peak incidences occurring between 6 and 36 months of age and between 4 and 6 years of age. At least 15% to 20% of all infants will develop acute otitis media. Although these infections can occur year round, the incidence is highest in the winter and early spring.

Acute otitis externa occurs in all age groups and in a variety of conditions. Certain conditions predispose to its development, such as exposure of the external ear canal to water (as with swimming, hair washing, or irrigating the canal); trauma to the canal (usually self-inflicted during attempts to remove cerumen); and a congenitally small external auditory meatus. Otitis externa persisting for more than 2 months is considered chronic external otitis. Malignant otitis externa occurs in diabetic and other immunocompromised patients and is potentially devastating.

INITIAL APPROACH AND STABILIZATION

Priority Diagnoses

Most patients with earaches are triaged to the nonacute area of the emergency department. Most cases associated with an acutely serious etiology are not otic in origin. The four priority diagnoses include malignant otitis externa, perforated tympanic membrane with dislocation of the ossicles, extension of an infectious process beyond the external and middle ear, and pain referred to the ear from outside serious causes (e.g., peritonsillar abscess).

Rapid Assessment

1. *Pain.* The rapidity of onset and severity of pain are assessed. Is the pain radiating, dull, or sharp?
2. *Associated symptoms.* Particular attention is given to complaints of shortness of breath, headache, or systemic malaise.
3. *General appearance.* The patient may have a fever, toxic appearance, or respiratory compromise.
4. *Mouth and throat.* If respiratory compromise is suggested, the oropharynx is examined for signs of a retropharyngeal abscess or a peritonsillar abscess.
5. *Neck.* The neck is checked for suppleness or a finding of meningismus.

Early Intervention

1. Any patient with a fever, toxic appearance, or respiratory compromise is moved to the acute care area of the emergency department.
2. If the patient has not taken analgesics, acetaminophen (15 to 20 mg/kg/dose) or ibuprofen (5 to 10 mg/kg/dose) is administered. Drug allergies or sensitivities to these drugs should be ascertained before their administration.
3. Antipyretics (e.g., acetaminophen) may be administered for temperature greater than 102°F (38.5°C).
4. Airway management equipment is moved near the patient if there is acute respiratory distress.

CLINICAL ASSESSMENT

History

The history is directed toward the details of the pain, any associated complaints, and predisposing factors. Most earache is related to ear, neck, or mouth problems. Because of the pediatric prevalence among patients with this complaint, the source of the history is often someone other than the patient.

Pain

Onset and Duration. Most ear pain is acute in onset, although a dull pressure often precedes the increase in pain from infectious causes. Most patients do not wait a long time (less than 24 hours) before seeking medical care.

Location. Most earache is unilateral; bilateral ear pain may suggest an infectious cause.

Pattern of Pain. Constant pain is consistent with pain of ear origin; intermittent pain or pain with highly variable intensity more often arises from extraotic sites. A sudden decrease of pain is typical of tympanic membrane rupture.

Character or Quality. Most ear pain is sharp or stabbing with associated pressure and throbbing. Dull aching pain is uncommon in patients who present with acute pain.

Severity. Interpreting severity of the pain may be impossible in children. In adults, pain of infectious origin is usually intense and moderately severe. The phrase, "the worst pain I've had in my life" is not usually heard.

Factors That Relieve or Worsen Pain. Pain that increases with biting or chewing may arise from the teeth, temporomandibular joint, or external canal.

Treatment to Date. There are many over-the-counter or "home remedies" for earache. Treatments before the emergency department visit may influence presentations or clinical findings.

Associated Symptoms

Effect on Hearing. Otitis externa can cause a significant decrease in hearing acuity by blocking the canal, whereas otitis media usually "muffles" the sound. Tympanic membrane injury with ossicle dislocation presents as acute unilateral deafness.

Discharge or Drainage. Discharge or drainage is characteristic of otitis externa or otitis media with tympanic membrane rupture.

Upper Respiratory Symptoms or Sore Throat. These symptoms are common with middle ear infections. Referred pain from an oropharyngeal lesion should also be considered (e.g., peritonsillar abscess).

Extra Sounds. Ringing is rare, but crackling or popping is common. Painful buzzing may be heard when an insect enters the ear canal.

Dizziness or Vertigo. Dizziness is a rare symptom in otitis media and suggests inner ear involvement. Labyrinthitis or a deep temporal bone infection is considered in such cases.

Precipitating Factors

Barotrauma is a frequent precipitant, and questions about recent airplane flights, underwater diving, or possible trauma from a blow or a slap on the ear are important. Blunt trauma often occurs from attempts to "clean" the ear. Frequent attempts at "wax" removal can increase external canal injuries. Rarely, the tympanic membrane may be damaged.

Past Medical History

Inquiries are made about any previous history of ear problems, particularly infections, and any treatment received. Any underlying medical problems, especially diabetes mellitus, are clarified. Queries about recent travel or vacation may point toward possible barotrauma.

Questions Specific to Patients Who Cannot Give Their Own History

- Is there a change in *affect*, *mood*, or *attention*?
- If the patient is an infant, has *ear pulling* been noted?

Physical Examination

Physical examination is done to (1) assess the general status of the patient; (2) identify potential sites of referred pain, such as the mouth, throat, teeth, and temporomandibular joint; and (3) view the external canal and tympanic membrane.

Vital Signs. Tachycardia may be a sign of significant pain, fever, dehydration, hypoxia, or septicemia. Fever is more common in patients with otitis media than in those with otitis externa.

General Appearance. Patients with uncomplicated infections do not look toxic.

External Ear Examination. The external ear and periauricular areas are inspected, looking for drainage, trauma, or edema. Gentle pressure on the tragus and gentle traction on the pinna are painful to patients with external otitis but should not cause any pain in those with otitis media. Preauricular sinus tracts or pits, which may be tender, erythematous, or draining, are rarely seen.

The Ear Canal. The largest-sized speculum that will fit easily in the canal is inserted. Traction on the external ear in the superior and posterior directions may help straighten out the canal. In infants, traction in the inferior direction may provide better results. If insertion of the speculum causes pain, acute otitis externa is suggested. The entire canal is inspected for erythema, edema, bleeding, discharge, and foreign bodies.

Cerumen in the canal can limit the examination of the canal and eardrum. Careful removal of any obstructing material with gentle irrigation is very helpful. Removal may be aided by instilling a topical solution of benzocaine, antipyrine, and glycerin (Auralgan) or 1 mL of docusate sodium (Colace) 15 minutes before irrigation. Cerumen spoons are reserved primarily for cooperative patients.

The Tympanic Membrane. After the canal has been inspected, the tympanic membrane is examined. The normal appearance has a characteristic topography with a shiny pearly gray color. Specific findings relative to the eardrum may include the following:

- Serous air-fluid in the middle ear can cause the membrane to be yellow or amber, and a fluid level may be seen.
- Blood in the middle ear appears as a blue or purple discoloration behind the tympanic membrane.
- Purulence in the middle ear causes a white or chalky appearance and associated bulging of the tympanic membrane.
- Erythema of the membrane is often seen in infants who have a fever or are crying and resisting examination. Erythema in a quiet infant with ear pain and a mild fever is suggestive of otitis media but not pathognomonic.
- With serous otitis, the membrane can appear dull and retracted.
- Numerous prior ear infections may cause a fibrotic white tympanic membrane.
- A bullous lesion on the eardrum is often caused by an infection with either *Haemophilus influenzae* or *Mycoplasma pneumoniae*.
- Visualizing a perforation of the eardrum requires a close examination, especially in the posteroinferior corner.

Pneumatic Otoscopy. An often neglected, but important, examination is a test of the mobility of the tympanic membrane with the pneumatic apparatus of the otoscope (Fig. 24–1). Loss of or limited movement is an early sign of otitis media and is often the only finding in serous otitis. It is useful in assessing a reddened tympanic membrane in the crying or febrile infant. Scarring from multiple infections may decrease mobility.

Hearing Acuity. In general, attempts to test hearing acuity will be successful only with cooperative adults. Most children are unable or unwilling to truly discriminate with which ear they hear something. Both otitis media and otitis externa may produce a conductive hearing loss.

A tuning fork can be used for Weber's and Rinne's tests. They can differentiate between hearing loss caused by disorders of the middle and external ear and disorders of the neural apparatus. In Weber's test the sound radiation from a tuning fork placed on the patient's forehead is toward the ear with a conductive hearing loss and away from one with a sensorineural loss. Rinne's test assesses air conduction versus bone conduction by comparing sound transmitted through the mastoid process with sound transmitted through air. In otitis media, bone conduction may last longer than air conduction.

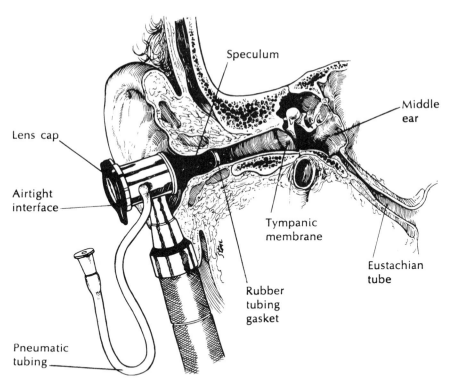

FIGURE 24–1 • Pneumatic otoscopy. (From Schwartz RH: New concepts in otitis media. Am Fam Physician 1979; 19:91–98. Published by the American Academy of Family Physicians.)

The Extraotic Examination. Even if the source is "obvious," it is best to briefly examine other sites that might explain the patient's ear pain:

1. The postauricular (mastoid) areas are palpated for tenderness or lymph node swelling.
2. The temporomandibular joint and muscles of mastication are checked for soreness, crepitus, or trismus.
3. The anterior and posterior cervical lymph nodes are palpated to determine if there is swelling or tenderness.
4. The tonsils and pharynx are examined for erythema, edema, and exudates.
5. The teeth, sinuses, and salivary glands are examined for tenderness, occult infections, or inflammation.

CLINICAL REASONING

At this point in the assessment, five questions are addressed.

Is a Serious Disease Process Present?

The patient's level of consciousness and vital signs supply major clues about the possibility of the presence of a serious disease. If the patient is alert and oriented, the fever is under control, and the airway is safe, then the risk of life-threatening disease is limited. If there is any doubt, steps are taken at once to place the patient in an environment where close observation is guaranteed and aggressive airway interventions can be instituted as necessary. In the group at risk, malignant external otitis has potentially life-threatening complications. It is a diagnosis that should not be missed.

Is the Earache of Otic Origin, or Is It Referred Pain from Another Source?

The basic physical examination of the external canal and tympanic membrane, coupled with the initial information obtained from the history, should give enough data to confirm or refute the presence of otogenic disease. Focal causes of ear pain are more common in children. The incidence of referred pain increases with age.

Does the Patient Have One of the Three Most Common Causes of Ear Pain?

The three common causes of pain of otic origin are otitis media, otitis externa, and a foreign body in the external canal. Although they have been introduced earlier in this chapter, Table 24–1 lists their distinguishing points.

Does the Patient Have an Uncommon Cause of Otogenic Ear Pain?

Less common causes of otogenic ear pain are considered if the patient does not readily fit into the diagnosis of otitis media, otitis externa, or foreign body in the external canal. Table 24–2 list these diseases with their typical characteristics.

Does the Patient Have a Nonotogenic Cause of Ear Pain?

When the ear canal and tympanic membrane are normal, referred pain is the most likely cause of earache. The ear has an extensive nerve supply, and pain may radiate to the ear from a number of structures in the head and neck. These patients are usually older, and about 80% of the complaints are caused by cervical spine lesions, dental disorders, or temporomandibular joint dysfunction. Table 24–3 lists the most common causes of referred pain and their characteristics.

DIAGNOSTIC ADJUNCTS

In most patients with earache, diagnostic adjuncts are unnecessary. Few ancillary tests are useful for reaching a diagnosis. However, in the patient with a severe middle ear or external ear infection, and in the diagnosis of referred pain, specific assessment may be beneficial.

Laboratory Studies

Complete Blood Cell Count. A complete blood cell count with white blood cell differential count, although not diagnostic, may assist the physician in determining possible patient toxicity.

Serum Glucose. A random sample for serum glucose determination may add to the suspicion of underlying diabetes mellitus in patients with severe infection.

Cultures. For patients with resistant or frequent otitis media and in neonates or immunosuppressed patients with middle ear infections, tympanocentesis with Gram's stain and culture may be diagnostically useful. This procedure is performed by an experienced physician. The majority of middle ear fluid cultures, in acute suppurative otitis media, will grow *Streptococcus pneumoniae* or nontypable *H. influenzae*. The pneumococcus is the most common agent, causing up to 50% of cases. *H. influenzae* is the second

most common agent, especially in infants and young children. *Streptococcus, Mycoplasma pneumoniae,* and *Moraxella catarrhalis* account for most of the remaining cases.

In patients with either acute or chronic otitis externa, cultures of the exudate of the canal tend to grow *Staphylococcus aureus, Pseudomonas aeruginosa,* or both. Fungus is recovered from the canal less often than bacteria. Cultures are needed in patients with resistant infection or suspected malignant otitis externa to guide antibiotic therapy.

Radiologic Imaging

Diagnostic imaging techniques are rarely needed in the workup of a patient with an earache. However, in unusual instances they may be helpful.

Plain Films. Plain films of the ear canal and mastoid may demonstrate a radiopaque foreign body in the canal (in the rare case in which uncertainty remains after the physical examination) or clouding of the mastoid air cells, which can be a complication of acute otitis media in children. A lateral soft tissue film of the neck may demonstrate disease in the retropharyngeal soft tissue space. Temporomandibular joint views may show joint erosion indicating temporomandibular disease.

Computed Tomography. Patients with malignant otitis externa or suspected bony spread of otitis media may require computed tomography or tomography of the temporal bone. Consultation is advised.

Nuclear Medicine. Bone scan or gallium scan may be indicated in patients with malignant otitis externa. These tests can monitor the efficacy of the treatment.

Audiometric Testing

Evaluation of a patient's hearing may play a role in the diagnosis and management of resolving or chronic otitis but is usually not available in the emergency department. Simple bedside hearing tests with a wristwatch or Rinne's and Weber's tests are sufficient for testing gross hearing acuity.

PRINCIPLES OF MANAGEMENT

Therapy for acute otitis media centers around antibiotic therapy, decongestants, and pain relief. Otitis externa is managed with topical therapy and analgesia. Appropriate methods for removal of foreign bodies are reviewed later in this section.

TABLE 24–1. Three Common Causes of Otogenic Ear Pain

Diagnosis	Prevalence	History	Physical Examination	Comments
Otitis media	Most common in children; first peak occurs at 6–36 months, second peak at 7 years; 65%–95% of children have one episode by age 7. More common in males, whites, lower socioeconomic levels, premature infants, and infants who are bottle fed	Prior URI, often prior infections; usually rapid onset of sharp throbbing pain without major associated symptoms. Sense of pressure, "fullness" in ear, and decreased hearing occur. Child may be tugging at ear, irritable, sleeping poorly, or screaming in pain. Pain and fever resolve often in 1–2 days with treatment.	Patient is usually febrile; experiences no pain on movement of ear lobe. Depending on stage, TM may be slightly red with poor movement to very red and bulging. If condition is superimposed on a scarred, retracted TM, it may be difficult to diagnose. TM takes up to 8 hours to change after onset of early symptoms. Canal has purulent drainage if there is spontaneous perforation. This can be cultured. Occasionally mastoid tenderness occurs (50% of cases are bilateral).	Usually there is extension of viral infection through eustachian tubes. Common bacteria are *Streptococcus pneumoniae* (35%), *Haemophilus influenzae* (25%), and *Moraxella catarrhalis* (15%); may spread to mastoid, intracranial area, and soft tissues of neck.
Otitis externa (external otitis)	Most common cause in older children and adults	Varies from mild itching to severe pain with purulence; sense of congestion and often decreased hearing.	Erythematous canal, drainage or debris. Movement of auricle (ear lobe) is painful, often out of proportion to findings. Canal may be edematous and swollen.	Originates from damage to protective waxy coating by dryness, wetness, or treatment. Organisms include *Proteus*, *Staphylococcus*, and *Streptococcus*. Extreme form, malignant otitis externa, occurs in elderly diabetics. *Pseudomonas* invades deep tissue.
Foreign body	More common in children. Beads, pebbles, beans, and paper are common. In adults, insects such as cockroaches are most frequent.	Children: ear pain, which may be more chronic; drainage, foul odor. Adults: acute onset of pain, fullness, and altered hearing acuity. If TM is perforated, bleeding, marked hearing loss, and vertigo may be present.	Children: Foreign body is usually more difficult to locate because children are less cooperative. Adults: Foreign body is usually easily seen, next to TM; may need to anesthetize or suffocate live insect. Check hearing status.	An otic microscope may be necessary for removal. After removal, reexamine patient for injury to canal or TM. About 10% of foreign bodies will not be removable in emergency department. Limit the time devoted to the procedure.

URI, upper respiratory infection; TM, tympanic membrane.

TABLE 24-2. Less Common Causes of Otogenic Ear Pain

Diagnosis	Pathophysiology	History	Physical Examination	Comments
Aerotitis	Sustained pressure imbalance between middle ear and environment; often due to eustachian tube blockage secondary to URI	Previous URI, associated with recent descent from altitude or ascent from underwater diving. Pain is severe and persistent with associated "popping" and internal pressure; may be temporarily decreased by yawning or blowing nose.	TM retracted; may be hemorrhage behind ear drum or in canal; poor TM mobility	Suggest patient prevent condition with nasal spray before descent or ascent if URI is present.
Bullous myringitis	Reaction of epithelium to viral or *Mycoplasma* infection	Acute onset pain, similar to that of otitis media	Hemorrhagic or serous blebs on TM and in auditory canal; hearing is not impaired.	Blebs resolve with treatment; needs to be distinguished from herpes zoster otitis
Trauma	Direct injury from ear picking, attempts to "clean out ear." Hemotympanum occurs from head injury and basal skull fracture. Blunt trauma to mandible can directly injure ear canal. TM ruptures with blow to external ear.	"Cleaning out" ears; trauma to face, head, mandible, or ears; "slap" on ear or side of head	Ranges from minor abrasion and excoriation to disruption of external canal and tympanic membrane. Other signs of head and mandibular trauma are present.	Minor trauma far more common. Ear examination is part of all head and facial trauma assessment. If TM perforation covers more than 20% of surface, referral is necessary. Significant hearing loss or vertigo is uncommon; if present, it points to more serious injury.
Impacted cerumen	Direct pressure on TM by inspissated cerumen	Occurs more often in elderly; associated with attempts to "clean out wax" while actually impacting it. Symptoms may range from severely to slightly decreased hearing; usually a long-standing recurrent problem.	External canal occluded by cerumen, which may be almost black. TM is not visible. Increased pain occurs with attempts to remove outer layers manually.	Prior softening may be necessary before removal is possible.
Herpes zoster otitis (Ramsay Hunt syndrome)	Herpes zoster infection of geniculate ganglion	Prodrome of malaise and fever; deep severe ear pain	Vesicular rash in ear canal; facial paralysis	Treatment is supportive and symptomatic.
Cholesteatoma	Cyst of squamous epithelium within middle ear	Progressive hearing loss	Mass in middle ear	Bony destruction may occur. Prompt surgical intervention is indicated.

URI, upper respiratory infection; TM, tympanic membrane.

TABLE 24-3. Common Causes of Pain Referred to the Ear

Diagnosis	Nerve Supply and Pathophysiology	History	Physical Examination	Comments
Cervical spine lesions	Cervical nerves II and III; rarely arises from disk, more often from bony impingement	Pain is often chronic and may be severe, with continual aching or burning; may worsen with neck flexion	Usually normal; pain may increase with neck flexion.	Radiographs may be inconclusive. Referral is necessary.
Sinusitis	Cranial nerve V; infection of maxillary sinus	URI symptoms, dull facial pain; increased pressure when leaning head forward; nasal congestion	Tenderness over sinus; opacification of sinus on transillumination	Radiograph may confirm; often overdiagnosed
Dental disorders Impacted third molars (wisdom teeth)	Cranial nerve V; third molar lodges against second molar. Inflammation may occur in gingiva.	Common in the 15- to 30-yr age group	Partial eruption may be visible. Gingiva may be red and tender.	May be accompanied by pericoronitis, an inflammation of gingiva surrounding the crown; dental radiographs may confirm diagnosis.
Dental caries/periapical abscess of mandibular or maxillary molars	Cranial nerve V; destruction of enamel; process extends into dentin.	Pain may not be apparent at tooth; may worsen with biting on hot or cold foods	Caries is usually visible. Tapping suspected tooth may induce pain.	
Temporomandibular joint dysfunction	Damaged articular surface due to malocclusion, teeth grinding, or arthritis	Pain is intermittent, may be worse in AM or PM depending on timing of bruxism (teeth grinding); may be associated with vertigo, tinnitus, headache, and jaw click	Joint may be tender or click with chewing. Trismus or muscle pain while biting may be seen.	Evaluation is complex and referral necessary.
Retropharyngeal abscess	Cranial nerve X; infection of retropharyngeal space	Occurs more often in children; usually accompanied by fever, sore throat	Erythema, fullness in oropharynx	Airway at risk; early consultation
Peritonsillar abscess	Cranial nerve IX; complication of tonsillitis, primarily *Streptococcus*	Occurs at any age; sore throat, odynophagia, "hot potato" voice	Usually obvious swelling to side of tonsil, pushed toward midline	Airway seldom at risk; may aspirate or treat with close follow-up
Malignancy of oropharynx and larynx	Cranial nerves VII, IX, and X; cancerous involvement of nerves supplying involved organ	Usually occurs in elderly; may have dysphagia, hoarseness, odynophagia, or mass sensation. Systemic symptoms are rare.	Suspicion requires full examination including palpation and laryngoscopy.	Patient is usually referred, and extensive radiologic assessment is necessary.

URI, upper respiratory infection

411

Otitis Media

Antibiotics. Although antibiotics have been the cornerstone of treatment for acute otitis media for many years, the imprudent use of antibiotics has resulted in drug-resistant strains of bacteria. The emergency physician should clinically discriminate between acute otitis media and otitis media with effusion. Given the high rate of spontaneous resolution, it may be appropriate at times to withhold antibiotics in children with mild, uncomplicated, first time, acute otitis media if good follow-up is available. About 80% of untreated patients experience resolution of symptoms by 7 to 14 days, compared with 95% of treated patients. Older children and those with mild and/or unilateral disease may also be suitable candidates for observation and analgesic therapy. A risk stratification approach for antibiotic therapy is given in Figure 24–2.

Most treatment regimens last 10 days, although several studies have demonstrated the effectiveness of therapy at 5 days.

Several treatment options are available for acute otitis media caused by drug-resistant *S. pneumoniae*. It has been suggested that higher doses of amoxicillin, 80 to 90 mg/kg/day in two to three divided doses, effectively treat half of the intermediately resistant pneumococcal strains and one third of highly resistant strains. If drug-resistant *S. pneumoniae* is recovered, other oral agents to consider include amoxicillin-clavulanate, clindamycin, macrolides, and combination therapy with rifampin.

Patients who fail amoxicillin treatment after 3 days may benefit from a change to a β-lactamase–resistant antibiotic, such as amoxicillin-clavulanate covering β-lactamase–producing *H. influenzae* or *Moraxella catarrhalis*. Parenteral ceftriaxone may be used to treat possible β-lactamase–producing strains or highly drug-resistant *S. pneumoniae*.

Respiratory syncytial virus has been identified as the principal virus invading the middle ear before the development of acute otitis media. This finding opens a potential opportunity for vaccine-based preventive treatment.

Analgesia. Most patients will benefit from analgesics. Acetaminophen or ibuprofen, with or without codeine derivatives, in tablet or liquid form may be beneficial for the first 24 to 48 hours. The mild sedation may also be useful. A slightly warmed topical anesthetic can assist with pain relief, especially in infants. The most common preparation is a solution of the anesthetics antipyrine and benzocaine with glycerin (Auralgan).

Decongestants. This adjunctive treatment is no longer routinely recommended. Decongestants have not been demonstrated to be efficacious in the treatment of most ear infections.

Tympanocentesis. Needle puncture of the tympanic membrane with (or without) conscious sedation was common in the preantibiotic era. There are disposable kits (e.g., Tymp-Tap). Serious complications (ossicle disruption, facial nerve paralysis) are avoidable when the anatomy is understood. This is not a routine procedure in the emergency department, but it may return in some role with the increasing frequency of bacterial resistance to antibiotics.

Otitis Externa

For patients with acute otitis externa, treatment consists of removing debris, reducing edema, and treating inflammation and infection. Debris may be suctioned from the canal. If suction is not effective, irrigation of the canal or manual removal of debris with a cerumen spoon may be necessary. Irrigation requires an intact tympanic membrane, and use of a cerumen spoon requires care, adequate lighting, and visualization of anatomy.

Once the canal is as clean as possible, ear drops containing a combination of antibacterial, antifungal, and corticosteroid preparations (Table 24–4) are instilled every few hours for 7 to 10 days. If the canal is occluded by edema, such that the debris cannot be removed or the drops are not guaranteed to reach the length of the canal, a wick of cotton or narrow gauze is inserted carefully. The ear drops are then placed on the wick and allowed to remain for 12 to 24 hours. If there is suspicion that the tympanic membrane is perforated, or if myringotomy tubes are in place, a suspension is used instead of weak acid solutions. Patients with cellulitis or systemic signs are given both topical and systemic antibiotics. Otitis externa usually clears in 10 to 14 days. Recurrence may be avoided by avoiding further trauma or exposure to wetness.

Foreign Body

A foreign body lodged in the canal is removed expeditiously to ease pain and to prevent the common sequelae of otitis externa. All methods of removal are variations of suction, irrigation, or direct instrumentation. The technique used depends on the physician's experience and equipment. The least invasive technique, irrigation, is tried first unless a perforated tympanic membrane is suspected. If the foreign body in the

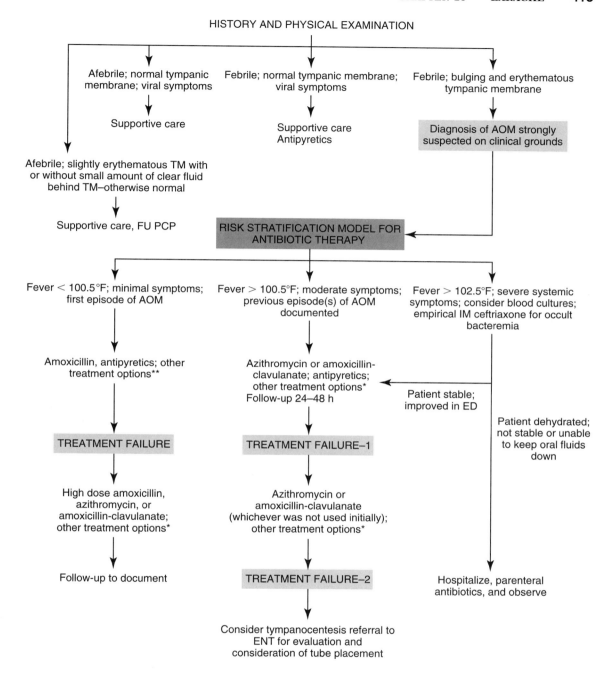

HISTORY AND PHYSICAL EXAMINATION

Afebrile; normal tympanic membrane; viral symptoms → Supportive care

Febrile; normal tympanic membrane; viral symptoms → Supportive care Antipyretics

Febrile; bulging and erythematous tympanic membrane → Diagnosis of AOM strongly suspected on clinical grounds

Afebrile; slightly erythematous TM with or without small amount of clear fluid behind TM–otherwise normal → Supportive care, FU PCP

RISK STRATIFICATION MODEL FOR ANTIBIOTIC THERAPY

Fever < 100.5°F; minimal symptoms; first episode of AOM → Amoxicillin, antipyretics; other treatment options** → TREATMENT FAILURE → High dose amoxicillin, azithromycin, or amoxicillin-clavulanate; other treatment options* → Follow-up to document

Fever > 100.5°F; moderate symptoms; previous episode(s) of AOM documented → Azithromycin or amoxicillin-clavulanate; antipyretics; other treatment options* Follow-up 24–48 h → TREATMENT FAILURE–1 → Azithromycin or amoxicillin-clavulanate (whichever was not used initially); other treatment options* → TREATMENT FAILURE–2 → Consider tympanocentesis referral to ENT for evaluation and consideration of tube placement

Fever > 102.5°F; severe systemic symptoms; consider blood cultures; empirical IM ceftriaxone for occult bacteremia

Patient stable; improved in ED

Patient dehydrated; not stable or unable to keep oral fluids down → Hospitalize, parenteral antibiotics, and observe

* Ceftriaxone IM, clarithromycin, cefprozil, cefuroxime
** TMP-SMX

FIGURE 24–2 • Treatment of acute otitis media (AOM) in a patient older than 6 months of age. ED, emergency department; TM, tympanic membrane; TMP-SMX, trimethoprim-sulfamethoxazole. (Modified from Bosker G: Acute otitis media. Emerg Med Rep 2000; 21:85–95, with permission.)

TABLE 24–4. Commonly Used Otic Drops

Preparation Name	Principal Agents	Dosage
Coly-Mycin S Otic	Colistin Neomycin Hydrocortisone	3–4 drops 3–4 times/day
Cortisporin otic solution Cortisporin otic suspension	Polymyxin B Neomycin Hydrocortisone	3–4 drops 3–4 times/day
Otic Domeboro	Acetic acid in aluminum acetate	4–6 drops q2–3 h
VōSol Otic	Acetic acid in propylene glycol	5 drops 3–4 times/day
VōSol HC Otic	Acetic acid hydrocortisone in propylene glycol	5 drops 3–4 times/day
Floxin Otic	Ofloxacin	
TobraDex	Tobramycin/dexamethasone	Used as otic drops; may be effective when Cortisporin fails

canal is made of vegetable material, irrigation is not recommended. Fluid may cause the object to swell and make extrication more difficult. If the object is an insect and the tympanic membrane is intact, mineral oil or 2% lidocaine solution can be placed in the ear to kill the insect before removal. Lidocaine is preferred.

All patients who have foreign bodies removed are presumed to have an early, unrecognized otitis externa and are started on therapy with combined antibiotic-corticosteroid ear drops. It is unusual for an object to be caught in the canal and subsequently removed without some degree of damage to the canal epithelium.

If attempts to remove a foreign body are unsuccessful in the emergency department, the patient is referred to an otolaryngologist within 24 hours. Appropriate warnings are given to the patient and family in an attempt to prevent a recurrence.

UNCERTAIN DIAGNOSIS

The cause of earache is usually revealed after careful history and examination. In those rare situations in which the diagnosis remains unclear, the emergency physician should attempt to rule out serious underlying disease (e.g., retropharyngeal or peritonsillar abscess with referred pain to the ear) and consider the less frequent causes of acute ear pain (see Tables 24–2 and 24–3). If the pain can be relieved by analgesia in the emergency department, and no other source is found, the patient may be discharged with follow-up arrangements to a primary physician or otolaryngologist. If the pain cannot be relieved, or the emergency physician is uncomfortable about discharging the patient, consultation with an otolaryngologist is recommended.

SPECIAL CONSIDERATIONS

Hearing-Impaired Patients

Patients who wear a hearing aid may develop an external otitis that impedes their ability to benefit from the device. After initial treatment, these patients are referred to an otologist for further care. The goal is to optimize their ability to use the hearing aid.

Diabetic or Immunocompromised Patients

Patients with diabetes mellitus and those who are immunosuppressed are considered at risk for malignant otitis externa. This invasive infection begins in the ear canal and spreads to the adjacent soft tissue, bone, nerves, vessels, and central nervous system. The signs of extensive inflammation are generally obvious, and antibiotic therapy with referral is necessary.

DISPOSITION AND FOLLOW-UP

Discharge

The patient with a routine ear infection can be sent home with treatment and can be seen by a primary care physician in several days. The patient is instructed to seek care sooner if the symptoms fail to resolve in 24 to 48 hours. Patients with small eardrum perforations require close follow-up, generally by a specialist, although most problems heal over time without any difficulty.

Routine follow-up in 2 weeks is important in any patient with acute otitis media to ensure that any middle ear effusion is gone. Lingering effusion can signal a latent infection that may cause damage if allowed to smolder. Patients with an underlying chronic illness, recurrent ear disease, or resistant ear infections should be seen either by their primary care physician or by a specialist within 48 to 72 hours of the emergency department visit.

Consultation / Admission

Consultation with an otolaryngologist while the patient is in the emergency department is indicated if any of the following signs or symptoms are present: excruciating pain, significant bloody discharge, granulation tissue in the ear canal, complete absence of hearing, vertigo, or other unusual problems. Patients with disruption of greater than 20% of the surface area of the tympanic membrane or with significant hearing loss or vertigo are discussed with a specialist before discharge. Whenever the emergency physician has a suspicion of malignant otitis externa, the patient should be seen by an otologist in the emergency department.

FINAL POINTS

- The history will provide most of the diagnostic information.
- The physical examination usually allows the cause of the pain to be classified as otic or nonotic.
- Regional structures are examined to include sources of pain referred to the ear and to rule out the few life-threatening disease processes.
- Most otogenic earaches are caused by otitis media, otitis externa, or a foreign body.
- Most nonotogenic earaches originate from either temporomandibular joint dysfunction, dental problems, or cervical spine problems.
- Foreign bodies of the ear canal can be missed unless the examiner specifically looks for them.
- Elderly patients with diabetes mellitus and all immunosuppressed patients are at risk for a potentially lethal malignant infection of the external ear.

CASE *Study*

A 66-year-old woman was brought by her daughter to the emergency department. The daughter said that her mother had been experiencing intense pain in her left ear for several hours and was "not acting right." The patient was extremely uncomfortable from the ear pain and had to rely on her daughter to answer many of the questions. She was an insulin-dependent diabetic and was recently discharged from the hospital with a diagnosis of pneumonia.

This woman's recent hospitalization for a major infection is strong evidence that her diabetes mellitus places her in the immunosuppressed category. To compound the situation, she may have been exposed to nosocomial pathogens during her hospital stay. Finally, the mild alteration in her mental status, evidenced by her reliance on her daughter during the history taking, suggests a systemic component. She was moved to an acute care area of the emergency department.

The daughter stated that her mother had had ear pain and drainage for the last 3 days. The pain had increased significantly that day. She said that her mother "didn't seem right" and noted "a lot of redness" around her left ear. The

patient was in fair health and took 60 units of NPH insulin daily. Vital signs were blood pressure, 170/100 mm Hg; heart rate, 100 beats per minute; respirations, 20 breaths per minute; and temperature, 102°F (38.9°C). Cellulitis and granulation tissue were noted around the opening of the left ear canal. The tympanic membrane could not be visualized. The patient had some "droop" in the left side of her face, including her eyelid.

The history and physical findings are consistent with a rapidly spreading infectious process, most likely extending beyond the external auditory canal. The patient's slightly altered mental status and seventh cranial nerve involvement also point to serious disease.

It was apparent that this patient was seriously ill and at high risk for malignant otitis externa. Early consultation with an otolaryngologist was necessary while the patient was being more extensively evaluated.

The patient was seen by an otolaryngologist and admitted to the hospital for radiologic studies and intravenous therapy with antibiotics.

CASE *Study*

A mother brought in her 6-year-old daughter because she had noticed a foul-smelling cream-colored fluid coming out of the child's left ear for the past 2 days. The child said her ear hurt "a little."

On examination, the little girl had no tenderness when her outer ear was moved. However, she strongly resisted efforts by the examiner to look inside the canal of her left ear with an otoscope. With her mother's assistance, she was held still. Otoscopy showed a moderate amount of purulent fluid and a shiny, bright red, round object about halfway down the canal.

Children may place things in their ears, nose, and other orifices. These objects cause local irritation and possible infection. The prudent physician, faced with an uncooperative child with symptoms of an acute infectious otitis externa, should complete the physical examination before treatment. The presence of a foreign object cannot be ruled out unless the canal is well visualized.

The little girl finally remembered that she stuck "something" into her ear 3 days ago (but could not remember what it was). The emergency physician was concerned about the unknown foreign body and considered ordering soft tissue radiographs to determine its size and shape.

Although it is wise to recognize that not all information concerning the nature of this foreign body is available, it is appropriate to attempt simple methods of removal before obtaining imaging studies. A radiograph is of questionable utility and significantly adds to the cost of the visit.

The patient was given conscious sedation and the foreign body removed by suction. She was started on Cortisporin Otic drops with follow up in 2 days by her primary physician.

Bibliography

TEXT

Practical ENT for Primary Care Physicians (e-text). 2002. Available at www.Medic8.com

Schuller DE: DeWeese and Saunders Otolaryngology—Head and Neck Surgery, 8th ed. St. Louis, CV Mosby, 1994.

JOURNAL ARTICLES

Block SL: Tympanocentesis: Why, when, how. Contemp Pediatr 1999; 16:103–127.

Bluestone CD: Pathogenesis of otitis media: Role of eustachian tubes. Pediatr Infect Dis J 1996; 15:281– 291.

Bosker G: Acute otitis media year 2000 update. Emerg Med Rep 2000; 21(pt 1):75–84, 21(pt 2):85–94.

Cohen R, Navel M, Grunberg J, et al: One dose ceftriaxone vs ten days of amoxicillin/clavulanate therapy for acute otitis media: Clinical efficacy and change in nasopharyngeal flora. Pediatr Infect Dis J 1999; 18:403–409.

Congeni BL: Therapy of acute otitis media in an era of antibiotic resistance. Pediatr Infect Dis J 1999; 18: 371–372.

Dowell SF, Marcy SM, Philips WR, et al: Otitis media—principles of judicious use of antimicrobial agents. Pediatrics 1998; 101:165–171.

Faden H, Duffey L, Boeve M: Otitis media: Back to the basics. Pediatr Infect Dis J 1998; 17:1105–1113.

Klein JO: Review of consensus reports on management of otitis media. Pediatr Infect Dis J 1999; 18:1152–1155.

McCracken G N Jr: Diagnosis and management of acute otitis media in the urgent care setting. Ann Emerg Med 2002; 39:413–421.

Rosenfeld RM: An evidence-based approach to treating otitis media. Pediatr Clin North Am 1996; 43:1165–1181.

Takata GS, Chan LS, Shekelle P, et al: Evidence assessment of management of acute otitis media: I. The role of antibiotics in treatment of uncomplicated otitis media. Pediatrics 2001; 108:239–247.

CHAPTER 25

The Red Painful Eye

DAVID S. HOWES

MARY KAY HINKEBEIN

CASE_Study_

A 30-year-old man presented to the emergency department with a feeling of left eye irritation and redness that had lasted for 1 day.

INTRODUCTION

Of the 2% to 3% of all emergency department visits that are for ophthalmologic disorders, the red eye is one of the most common. Most of these cases have an infectious cause and can be safely treated by an emergency physician. Many conditions are responsible for these symptoms; some are relatively innocuous, whereas others endanger visual function.

The emergency physician must be aware of the several true ocular emergencies. Almost all result from inflammation of one or more of the anatomic structures of the eye.

The eye has only a few ways of responding to noxious stimuli, infection, or vascular or neurologic insult. It can become painful, the vision can be disturbed, or the conjunctiva can become red. A clear understanding of the anatomy of the eye is essential to accurate diagnosis and treatment.

Anatomy

The _sclera_ or "white of the eye" is covered by a thin, translucent mucous membrane called the _bulbar conjunctiva_. The palpebral conjunctiva lines the inner aspect of the eyelids. Conjunctival inflammation (conjunctivitis) is characterized by vasodilation (redness), fluid exudation (swelling and tearing), and cellular migration (discharge). Conjunctivitis is the most common cause of the red eye. It is not associated with disturbance of vision or significant ocular pain.

The _cornea_ has well-developed sensory fibers. It responds to infectious, inflammatory, or traumatic injury with intense pain. Corneal edema often accompanies this process and results in blurred vision. Corneal inflammation (keratitis) is a common cause of an acute symptomatic red eye. An intense foreign-body sensation differentiates keratitis from other causes of the painful red eye.

Between the cornea and the iris is the _anterior chamber_. The ciliary body secretes the aqueous humor, which flows into the anterior chamber through the pupillary opening. The anterior chamber drains through Schlemm's canal in the limbic area. In addition, the ciliary muscle allows accommodation of the lens. The choroid is the vascular layer of the posterior three fifths of the eye that nurtures the adjacent retina. The uvea consists of the iris, ciliary body, and choroid.

The _iris_, ciliary body, and anterior choroid share a common blood supply and therefore tend to be involved in the same inflammatory processes, broadly termed _uveitis_. The patient will experience blurred vision, owing to aqueous flare or increased protein, and photophobia, secondary to cells in the aqueous humor, with accompanying ciliary body spasm. Pupil size and response to light are affected because of involvement of the iris.

The _posterior chamber_ is the space just behind the iris that ends with the crystalline lens and ciliary body. The posterior elements of the eye include the _vitreous humor_, a transparent medium that occupies the interior of the eye, thereby allowing light transmission to the photosensitive _retina_. Disorders of the posterior structures produce visual disturbance, usually without eye pain or redness. Figure 25–1 is an overview of the anatomy of the surrounding tissues and globe of the eye.

INITIAL APPROACH AND STABILIZATION

Priority Diagnoses

Patients presenting to the emergency department with complaints of a painful red eye must be triaged properly. It is essential that the following true ocular emergencies are immediately brought to the attention of the emergency physician:

- Sudden visual loss
- Chemical injury
- Vision-threatening trauma

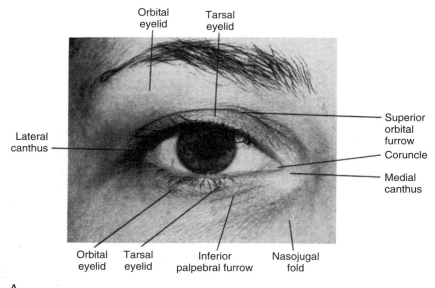

Orbital eyelid
Tarsal eyelid
Lateral canthus
Superior orbital furrow
Coruncle
Medial canthus
Orbital eyelid
Tarsal eyelid
Inferior palpebral furrow
Nasojugal fold

A

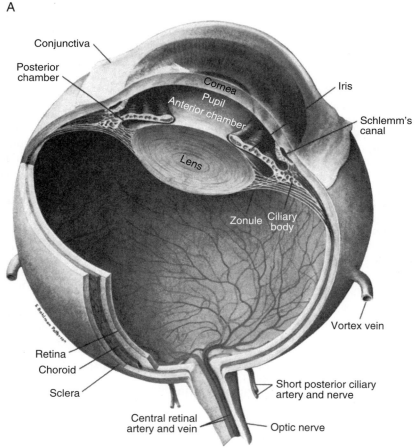

Conjunctiva
Posterior chamber
Cornea
Pupil
Anterior chamber
Iris
Schlemm's canal
Lens
Zonule   Ciliary body
Vortex vein
Retina
Choroid
Sclera
Short posterior ciliary artery and nerve
Central retinal artery and vein
Optic nerve

B

FIGURE 25–1 • *A* and *B,* Ocular anatomy. (From Newell FW: Ophthalmology: Principles and Concepts, 6th ed. St. Louis, CV Mosby, 1986.)

Visual Loss

Sudden visual loss constitutes a true ocular emergency in all patients. There are many causes of acute visual loss, and a broad differential diagnosis is necessary. Elderly patients presenting with sudden onset of painless loss of vision should be evaluated for possible central *retinal artery occlusion*, a rare but treatable ocular emergency that requires immediate attention from the emergency physician. Questioning should be limited to asking about the patient's usual visual acuity and determining the timing and nature of onset of the visual loss. In this type of patient visual acuity is likely to be poor. The patient may be able to count fingers or perceive light or may be completely blind. The pupil will react to consensual light stimulus but reacts minimally or not at all to direct light.

Central retinal artery occlusion is a time-dependent ischemic insult that is graphically apparent on funduscopic examination. The retina appears very pale with few or no retinal arteries visible. Other findings include an intact fovea, which allows the choroid vessels to be seen, presenting a "cherry-red spot" on funduscopy. Occasionally, one notes a retinal artery with a "boxcar" appearance in which there are segments of blood interspersed with atheromatous material within the vessel. When involvement is limited to a branch of the retinal artery, the corresponding findings on physical examination and loss of vision reflect the distribution of that branch.

Treatment of central retinal artery occlusion centers on efforts to promote cerebral vasodilation. This is readily accomplished by having the patient rebreathe his or her expired air by means of a paper bag for 20 minutes each hour. When available, Carbogen R (95% oxygen, 5% carbon dioxide) is used in the same manner. To lower the intraocular pressure an oral osmotic agent (β blocker), eye drops (Timolol), and intravenous acetazolamide (a carbonic anhydrase inhibitor to decrease aqueous humor production) are administered rapidly. Intermittent gentle massage of the globe may be helpful.

Endophthalmitis is an intraocular infection that may cause acute visual loss and requires immediate consultation with an ophthalmologist.

Chemical Injury

The patient with a chemical burn is self-identified by the chief complaint. Further evaluation, including evaluation of visual acuity, is delayed until initial therapy is accomplished. This includes immediate irrigation with copious amounts of fluid. Anesthetic eye drops may facilitate this treatment. Care is taken to determine the nature, concentration, and length of untreated exposure of the contaminating material. Prognosis is inversely related to the delay between injury and successful decontamination. After irrigation, a normal "non-hazy" cornea is a good prognostic sign.

Vision-Threatening Trauma

The patient with eye trauma that jeopardizes vision is brought promptly to the emergency physician's attention. Nursing and ancillary staff are instructed to handle the injured eye in a gentle manner to prevent further injury. The eye with evidence of extensive bruising and soft tissue swelling or obvious penetrating injury or irregularly shaped pupil has a potentially disrupted globe. No pressure should be applied to the globe; a metal shield is placed over the eye to protect it until the patient is examined by a physician.

Rapid Assessment / Early Intervention

Visual Acuity Testing

Visual acuity testing is performed in all patients presenting with eye complaints. The Snellen eye chart is generally used to evaluate visual acuity and is read from a distance of 20 feet (6 meters). A 20/100 reading can be interpreted as being measured at 20 ft (numerator) and representing the smallest print a patient with normal vision could read at 100 feet. Legally blind is defined as a visual acuity of 20/200 or greater. If the patient normally wears glasses, the test is conducted with them in place. If the patient's glasses are not available, a pinhole occluder may be used to approximate the lens correction. Although a Snellen eye chart is preferable, any printed material will do as long as the examiner documents the nature of the testing material, such as large newsprint at 2 feet. The patient with a severe visual deficit may be unable to read printed material. In this case, perception of fingers at a noted distance or perception of light may be all that can be recorded.

Patients are often initially unable to comply with visual acuity testing, because of ocular pain. This problem can usually be easily solved by instilling topical anesthetic drops. Intense pain from foreign bodies, corneal abrasions, keratitis, or penetrating trauma can cause severe tearing and lid spasm. Not only does anesthesia allow the best possible assessment of visual acuity, it also helps gain the patient's cooperation for the remainder of the examination.

CLINICAL ASSESSMENT

The history and physical examination are directed toward determining the degree of visual loss and the symptoms surrounding the chief complaints.

History

Background. What are the *circumstances* surrounding the *complaint*? A brief background of the problem is necessary. This includes timing and onset of the problem, as well as therapies used to date.

What is the *occupation* or *avocation* of the patient? Has the patient been hammering or striking metal objects, grinding metallic or granular surfaces, or working with overhead objects that may shed particulate matter? Exposure to the ultraviolet radiation of arc welding is an obvious problem, but it should not be forgotten that reflected sunlight, for example, with skiing in snow, prolonged time on the beach, or use of a sun lamp may also be a cause of significant injury. A history of *contact lens use* is sought.

Visual History

1. Has the patient sustained *visual impairment*? If so, what is its *character*? Blurred vision that does not improve with blinking implies a serious disease (e.g., keratitis, glaucoma).
2. Was this a *sudden, dramatic loss* or a *progressive loss*, or does the *vision wax and wane*?
3. Is the *whole visual field* affected, or are there *specific areas of loss*? Total visual loss (inability to perceive light) has a grave prognosis. It can result from opacification along the visual axis, retinal damage, or optic nerve injury.
4. Are *one* or *both eyes affected*?
5. Severe *photophobia* can result from superficial injury to the cornea or iris or from a pathologic process of the ciliary body.
6. Visual *"flashes of light"* or the perception of a hazy area in the visual field may represent symptoms of retinal detachment.

Pain History

1. What is the *severity, duration,* and *progression of ocular pain?*
2. Does the discomfort feel *superficial,* or is there a *deep* ocular lesion? The gritty, scratching, or burning sensation of conjunctivitis is more superficial in nature than the deep, burning, severe eye discomfort of acute narrow angle-closure glaucoma. Because of the pain fibers, even minor irritation of the cornea can be very painful.
3. Is there *photophobia?* This is an abnormal sensitivity to light that accompanies iritis. Although many patients complain of sensitivity to light, few have true photophobia. A distinction is made between those patients who find light uncomfortable and those who find light unbearable.

Appearance

1. Is there *redness*? When did it appear in the context of other symptoms? The most common change in appearance of an eye is redness.
2. Is there *swelling*? Patients may feel a "sense of fullness" with significant physical findings. The bulbar and palpebral conjunctivae are primary sites.
3. Is there *exudate* or *"matter"*? Eye secretions can be characterized as scant, copious, watery, or frankly purulent. Often on waking, the patient's eyelids are stuck together, because of the discharge drying overnight.

Trauma History

1. Is there *trauma associated* with the redness or pain? The patient who presents with a swollen "black eye" usually can relate the mechanism of injury. Trauma to the eye can be sustained from less obvious causes. A dust-filled environment or a windy day can be the cause of a foreign body in the eye.
2. Does the traumatic event carry a *high risk for penetrating the globe*? Penetrating injuries can be catastrophic to the eye. This must be considered in the traumatic setting, even from a more subtle cause such as a grinding-wheel spark.

Systemic Complaints. Are there *associated systemic complaints* such as fever, arthritis, skin eruption, upper respiratory infection, urethritis, or neurologic deficit?

Eye History. Has the patient ever had *previous symptoms* or *complaints* similar to those of the current problem? Is there a history of *prior eye disease* or *ocular operation*?

Ocular Medications. Were any *medications* put in the eye for *relief of symptoms*? This should include previously prescribed medications, borrowed eye medications, and over-the-counter preparations.

Past Medical History. Are there *underlying medical illnesses,* such as diabetes mellitus, collagen vascular disorder, hypertension, or conditions that would render the patient an immunocompromised host?

Physical Examination

All patients presenting with ocular complaints require a thorough eye examination. This is best accomplished by approaching the eye anatomically starting anteriorly and working posteriorly. The complete eye examination consists of visual acuity, visual fields, external examination, extraocular muscles, pupillary response, intraocular pressure, funduscopic examination, and slit lamp examination with fluorescein stain. Often patients cannot comply with visual acuity testing because of pain, swelling, or other problems. *Visual acuity testing and intraocular pressure readings should be considered the vital signs of the eye* and obtained whenever the chief complaint is ocular. If the patient cannot comply with visual acuity testing or the eye examination, the physician should instill anesthetic drops. Systemic disorders may manifest as ocular complaints; therefore, the physical examination is extended to the rest of the body, as necessary.

Eyelids and Adnexa. The eyelids and adnexa or surrounding structures of the eye are observed for symmetry, swelling, discharge, or erythema, followed by gentle palpation of the soft tissue of the orbit, lids, and zygoma.

The history of a foreign body sensation requires inspection of the lids; eversion of the upper lid is necessary. This can be accomplished by applying gentle upward and outward traction on the lashes while asking the patient to look downward. Foreign bodies such as soft contact lenses and organic materials can hide in the temporal cul-de-sac of the upper lid.

Expression of purulent material from the lacrimal sac located inside the lower inner orbital rim can establish a diagnosis of dacryocystitis. A well-circumscribed inflammation of the lid margin, especially when associated with a discharge of purulent material, is suggestive of a hordeolum (stye).

Redness, swelling, and tenderness of the lids involving the periorbital areas suggest periorbital cellulitis. This is often associated with paranasal sinus infection or previous trauma.

Pupils. The pupils are normally equal in size, are round, and react briskly to direct and consensual light. Approximately 10% of the population have anisocoria or a difference in pupil size, typically 1 mm or less. A previous picture of the patient (e.g., a driver's license picture or a parent's wallet picture of a pediatric patient), when closely examined with an ophthalmoscope at the 20+ setting, may reveal preexisting inequality of the pupils.

In evaluating pupils of unequal size, it is helpful to remember that the abnormal pupil is less reactive to light. Mydriasis or pupillary extraocular muscle dysfunction may be caused by trauma or pharmacologic agents placed in the eye. Both pupils should be approximately the same size and should constrict when light is shone in either eye. This dual response is the normal direct and consensual response. Decreased constriction response to light may represent local injury, an efferent pupillary defect commonly arising from an intracranially compressed third cranial nerve ("blown pupil"), or the less commonly diagnosed relative afferent pupillary defect (RAPD). The latter is also called a Marcus Gunn pupil and represents retinal or prechiasmal optic nerve injury. It is tested by placing the patient in a darkened room and shining a penlight into the unaffected eye. This should cause constriction of both pupils, the normal response of direct and consensual effects. Swinging the light to the affected eye normally maintains the direct and consensual constriction. If the afferent tract is injured, the presence of light is not effectively transmitted and the pupil in the affected eye dilates. The test is sufficiently sensitive to be positive in patients with near-normal (20/30) visual acuity. The pupil with local damage or with an efferent defect does not respond to either direct or consensual reflexes. Findings in the normal eye exposed to direct and consensual light and in one with efferent and afferent defects are illustrated in Figure 25–2.

The awake patient with a dilated pupil, drooping eyelid (ptosis), and extraocular motion abnormality is likely to have a third nerve palsy as a result of a space-occupying lesion, such as an intracranial aneurysm. The comatose patient with a suspected head injury with a dilated pupil needs immediate and aggressive intervention because this anisocoria may be a sign of third nerve compression caused by cerebral herniation.

A small or miotic pupil is characteristic of iritis. Iritis can be a sequela of trauma or medical illness. The red painful eye of iritis remains uncomfortable even after the instillation of a topical anesthetic. A painful response to both direct and consensual light is characteristic.

Cornea. The cornea is an avascular structure that appears optically clear. Corneal abrasions and foreign bodies are the most common types of injuries seen in the emergency department. Fluorescein is a valuable agent in the diagnosis of foreign bodies, abrasions, and inflammations of the cornea (Fig. 25–3). Defects of the corneal epithelium may be demonstrated by instillation of a small quantity of fluorescein. Areas of disruption or retained foreign body stain a brilliant green. Fluorescein is best applied by wetting a dry fluorescein strip with a sterile isotonic eye solution

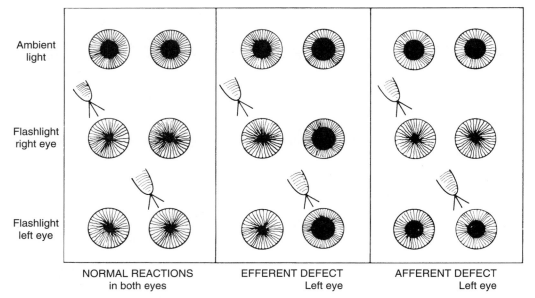

Ambient light

Flashlight right eye

Flashlight left eye

| NORMAL REACTIONS in both eyes | EFFERENT DEFECT Left eye | AFFERENT DEFECT Left eye |

FIGURE 25–2 • Pupillary reactions to penlight illumination. Note that an eye that has an efferent defect will not respond to either a direct or consensual light stimulus whereas an eye with an afferent defect will constrict when the contralateral eye is illuminated and then dilates when the penlight is swung to the involved eye. (From American Academy of Ophthalmology: Ophthalmology Study Guide. San Francisco, American Academy of Ophthalmology, 1982.)

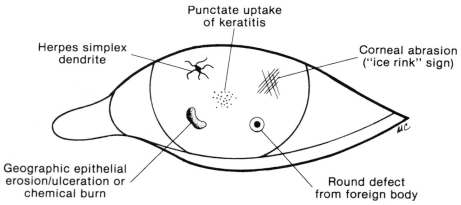

Punctate uptake of keratitis

Herpes simplex dendrite

Corneal abrasion ("ice rink" sign)

Geographic epithelial erosion/ulceration or chemical burn

Round defect from foreign body

FIGURE 25–3 • Identifying corneal epithelial staining defects. (Modified from Demartini DR, Vastine DW: Corneal abrasion and burn. In Callaham M, ed: Current Therapy in Emergency Medicine. Toronto, BC Decker, 1987, p 243.)

or topical anesthetic and dropping the formed bead into the lower conjunctival sac. Fluorescein will stain soft contact lenses, so they must be removed before instillation of this agent.

The cornea is a structure that is exquisitely sensitive to pain. Severe pain, lacrimation, and lid spasm (blepharospasm) are characteristic of severe or diffuse corneal injury. Immediate pain relief after the administration of a topical anesthetic may be diagnostic of a corneal process.

Visual inspection of the cornea reveals a smooth, regular, and mirror-like surface. Corneal edema produces a diffuse ground-glass appearance. In the patient with a red painful eye, blurred vision, and a poorly reactive pupil with a hazy cornea, acute narrow angle-closure glaucoma is highly suggested.

Anterior Chamber. The anterior chamber is a space that extends from the cornea to the iris and is an optically clear zone. Blood present in this chamber (hyphema) will layer out and cause a meniscus in the upright patient that is usually identifiable by direct inspection. A large number of inflammatory cells that layer out in a similar fashion is termed a *hypopyon,* which is generally caused by inflammation of the uveal tract.

If iritis or uveitis is suggested, the anterior chamber should be examined with a slit lamp for the presence of "flare and cell." The "flare" is caused by the release of rich plasma protein into the anterior chamber and appears as a solid beam of light extending from the back of the cornea to the iris. The "cell" is caused by the release of white blood cells into the anterior chamber and appears as tiny floating specks within the beam. The appearance of flare and cell is similar to that caused by a beam of sunlight coming into a dark, dusty room (Fig. 25–4).

Lens. The lens is rarely considered in the general examination of the eye. In general, it becomes apparent only by its opacification or absence, as when a sudden dramatic change in visual acuity occurs secondary to a lens subluxation. Ophthalmoscopy reveals a distant-appearing retina, such as one would find in the aphakic patient who has had a cataract extraction.

Vitreous. The vitreous is a gel-like substance that fills the space between the retina and the lens. Spontaneous hemorrhage may occur into the vitreous from abnormal vasculature or retinal detachment in patients with diabetes mellitus, sickle cell disease, or hypertension. The patient complains of diminished vision. Dark red or black spots and the absence of the red reflex when the fundus is viewed with an ophthalmoscope are characteristic of vitreous hemorrhage.

Retina. Most causes of the red painful eye will not include diseases of the retina. However, a complete examination of the eye includes evaluation of the fundus with attention paid to the optic nerve, arteries, and veins as well as to the background appearance of the retinal surface. The typical findings of central retinal artery occlusion have been previously discussed. Retinal vein occlusion produces a "blood and thunder" pattern in the fundus. This is generated by the extensive engorgement of the venous system and frank hemorrhage.

The diabetic patient is likely to exhibit abnormal findings on funduscopy. Although up to 70% of all diabetics have some form of retinopathy, only about 2% develop significant visual loss. This is usually caused by frank retinal hemorrhage in an area of neovascularization or proliferative new blood vessel formation.

Retro-orbit and Optic Nerve. This area is assessed indirectly by the position of the eye in the orbit (enophthalmos versus exophthalmos), the range of extraocular motion, and the visual field testing. The conduction of the prechiasmal portion of the optic nerve is specifically tested using the "swinging flashlight" or Marcus Gunn pupil test, discussed previously.

General Physical Examination

The red painful eye can often be the result of systemic diseases. The exophthalmic ocular "stare" of hyperthyroidism is best appreciated from a distance. Joint pains or rashes may identify collagen vascular or rheumatic diseases. A latent or even active urethritis may not be volunteered by an embarrassed patient who believes that this has nothing to do with his or her red painful eye. Beware of the pediatric patient who may present with a bilateral bulbar conjunctivitis as one of the earliest manifestations of Kawasaki syndrome. Acute angle-closure glaucoma can be the result of anterior uveitis.

Special Tests

Response to Topical Anesthetic. A few drops of topical anesthetic can serve as a reliable diagnostic aid to differentiate between superficial (corneal and conjunctival) and deeper sites of pain. An almost total absence of pain after a topical anesthetic strongly suggests a superficial site.

Fluorescein Staining. Applications of a moistened fluorescein-impregnated strip to the lower conjunctiva and use of a cobalt blue light will reveal corneal defects where the chemical fluoresces. This is an important part of the routine examination of any patient with a traumatic eye injury. In a special examination, the Seidel test, fluorescein is applied to a suspected corneal laceration. If aqueous humor is leaking from the laceration, a stream of clear liquid diluting the

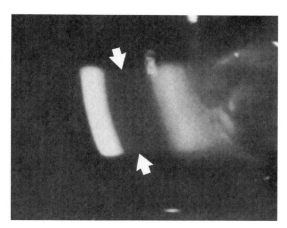

FIGURE 25–4 • A short, narrow slit beam illuminates the flare and cell of acute iritis *(arrows).* (From Lubeck D, Greene JS: Corneal injuries. Emerg Med Clin North Am 1988; 6[1]:73–94.)

fluorescein will be noted. Note that a negative result on the Seidel test does not always exclude a corneal laceration because small lacerations may seal quickly.

Slit Lamp Examination. A slit lamp is a binocular ophthalmic examining microscope. The light source projects a slit of light that illuminates a thin section of the cornea and lens. When the light source is placed at an angle to the microscope, the examiner can recognize the depth at which abnormalities occur. It is especially useful for examining the cornea, anterior chamber, lens, and ocular adnexa. The slit lamp examination is an important part of the complete eye assessment. The emergency physician must have ready access to this equipment and be familiar with its operation and interpretation of findings. Most slit lamps have both white and cobalt blue light sources so that fluorescein staining can be evaluated. Common findings include vertical linear fluorescein staining "scratches" caused by an upper eyelid foreign body or diffuse corneal fluorescein stippling caused by chemical or ultraviolet light keratitis (see Fig. 25–3). The lamp can be used to inspect the lens for possible subluxation or lens opacification resulting from cataract formation. Also, the lamp can focus a small beam of light through the anterior chamber to search for a "flare." Flare occurs when leukocytes and protein are present in the aqueous humor secondary to intraocular inflammation (see Fig. 25–4).

Tonometry. Tonometry allows the emergency physician to measure the intraocular pressure of the globe. In patients with ocular pain, nausea, vomiting, photophobia, and a poorly reactive midpoint or larger pupil, the intraocular pressure is measured to diagnose or rule out acute glaucoma. Pressures may be measured with a Schiøtz tonometer, electronic pressure gauge (Tonopen), or an applanation tonometer. The Schiøtz device is usually readily available in the emergency department. After the instillation of topical anesthesia, the tonometer is gently applied to the cornea to measure the eye pressure. Normal intraocular pressure is 10 to 20 mm Hg, which is shown by a reading of more than 3 with a 5.5 g weight using the Schiøtz tonometer. The lower the reading on the scale, the more intraocular pressure is suggested and the harder the surface of the globe. Patients with acute glaucoma may have readings greater than 40 to 60 mm Hg. Tonometry is not performed in patients in whom perforation or keratitis is present.

Mydriasis. Dilation of the iris is rarely part of an ocular examination in the emergency department. Mydriasis and cycloplegia are commonly done as part of management.

CLINICAL REASONING

After the history and physical examination, the emergency physician can classify the painful red eye into emergent, urgent, and nonurgent categories:

- *Emergent* conditions are marked by sudden visual loss, chemical eye injury, or severe eye trauma. These entities are reviewed earlier in "Initial Approach and Stabilization." They include sudden visual loss, chemical injury, and severe trauma.
- *Urgent* conditions are characterized by decreased visual acuity and moderate to severe pain. Acute glaucoma, keratitis, and uveitis are diseases that deserve prompt attention.
- *Nonurgent* conditions are characterized by normal visual acuity and mild ocular discomfort. Conjunctivitis and hordeolum are nonurgent causes of a painful red eye.

DIAGNOSTIC ADJUNCTS

Laboratory Studies

Cultures. Not all cases of suspected external ocular infection require a culture. Most bacterial and viral infections are self-limiting. Cultures are indicated, however, if there is clinical evidence of corneal involvement, if symptoms are prolonged, or if initial antimicrobial therapy has failed. Cultures should be taken in both eyes separately even if the irritation is unilateral. Cultures can help determine the normal flora present in the noninflamed eye.

Gram's stain of the exudate is especially important in identifying the acute, severe, purulent conjunctivitis caused by *Neisseria gonorrhoeae*. This infection occurs in newborns who are infected during passage through the birth canal and in adults contaminated from acute gonorrheal urethritis. Microscopic examination reveals gram-negative intracellular diplococci. Confirmatory culture is important.

Chlamydia Testing. Use of newer immunofluorescent antibody tests is helpful in identifying chlamydial conjunctivitis. Direct fluorescent antibody staining is useful for identifying the organism obtained from any appropriate body site. There are specific guidelines for obtaining conjunctival specimens.

Eosinophils. Ocular exudate may be examined for the presence of eosinophils. A finding of one or more eosinophils on material prepared with Wright's stain or a simple wet prep examination that demonstrates dark or green granulated white blood cells is considered highly suggestive of allergic conjunctivitis.

Other Laboratory Tests. Other laboratory tests are rarely of use in management of eye problems. One important exception might be the use of the erythrocyte sedimentation rate in patients with loss of vision. Among the causes of amaurosis fugax are the vasculitis syndromes, including temporal arteritis. Temporal arteritis is suggested by an elevated erythrocyte sedimentation rate.

Radiologic Imaging

In general, radiography is not helpful in the evaluation of the patient with visual loss, chemical injury, or a nontraumatic cause of a red, painful eye. However, special circumstances necessitate the use of radiographs. The patient with suspected orbital cellulitis may benefit from a computed tomogram of the orbit. Plain radiographs are useful in the localization of penetrating foreign objects.

EXPANDED DIFFERENTIAL DIAGNOSIS

After a thorough history, physical examination, and performance of diagnostic adjuncts, a diagnosis can be reached in most patients. The remainder of this chapter focuses on the six most serious and common causes of a painful red eye:

1. Infectious and allergic conjunctivitis
2. Iritis
3. Keratitis
4. Herpetic infection
5. Corneal abscess
6. Acute glaucoma

Table 25–1 highlights key differential points in making the diagnosis. Subconjunctival hemorrhage is a common cause of painless red eye. Unless severe or recurrent, it is a benign condi-

tion. More complex causes include hypertension and hemostatic disorders (Fig. 25–5A).

Conjunctivitis

Conjunctivitis encompasses a broad spectrum of ocular entities that give rise to conjunctival inflammation. The causes are multiple and range from bacterial, viral, traumatic, and systemic to allergic. Most infectious and allergic conjunctival irritations are self-limited or respond well to topical antimicrobial or anti-inflammatory agents. Other causes may have a detrimental effect on the patient's vision and possibly lead to permanent damage. A thorough history and physical examination is essential to the evaluation and treatment of conjunctivitis. Most cases of acute conjunctivitis do not alter visual acuity or cause significant eye discomfort.

Infective Conjunctivitis. Conjunctivitis frequently is the result of bacterial or viral infection, and it is often difficult to differentiate the two on physical examination. Bacterial conjunctivitis is usually associated with thick purulent discharge and minimal to no itching. Viral conjunctivitis (e.g., adenovirus) is usually not purulent and has a watery discharge, and the patient frequently has a history of recent upper respiratory infection. It is usually highly contagious, beginning in one eye and moving to the other. Both bacterial and viral conjunctivitis may give rise to crusting of the eyelids, and patients may awaken in the morning to eyes sealed shut with dried secretions. Generally the differentiating factor is the purulence.

Bacterial conjunctivitis is caused by a wide range of gram-positive (predominant) and gram-negative organisms. Cultures are usually not warranted because most infective conjunctivitis is a self-limited illness that responds to a broad range of topical antibiotics. Exceptions include any conjunctivitis in the neonate (ophthalmia

TABLE 25–1. Features That Differentiate Causes of the Red Painful Eye

	Acute Conjunctivitis	Iritis, Uveitis, Iridocyclitis	Corneal Trauma and Inflammations (Keratitis)	Acute Glaucoma
Incidence	Common	Common	Common	Uncommon
Pain	None–moderate	Moderate	Moderate–severe	Severe
Vision Affected	No	Slight	Moderate–severe	Severe
Discharge	Yes	No	Yes	No
Photophobia	No	Moderate	Moderate	Severe
Injection	Diffuse (+ lid)	Circumcorneal	Diffuse	Diffuse
Cornea	Clear	Clear	Abrasion, foreign body, ulceration, punctate stain	Cloudy
Pupil: Size, Response	Normal	Small	Normal	Large
	Normal	Poor to normal	Normal	Poor
Intraocular Pressure	Normal	Normal	Normal	Elevated

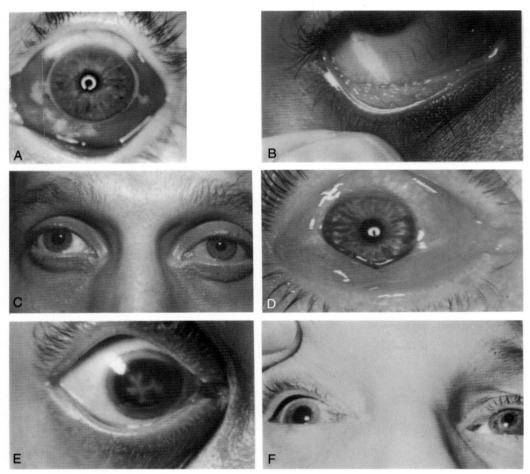

FIGURE 25–5 • External signs of eye pathology. *A,* Subconjunctival hemorrhage. *B,* Ocular allergy, enlarged lid follicles. *C,* Acute iritis. *D,* Acute epidemic keratoconjunctivitis showing corneal infiltrates and chemosis. *E,* Herpes simplex (dendritic keratitis). *F,* Narrow angle-closure glaucoma showing dilated pupil, loss of corneal luster, and red eye. (From Scheie HG, Albert DM: Textbook of Ophthalmology, 9th ed. Philadelphia, WB Saunders, 1977.)

neonatorum), severe cases, and all conjunctivitis that does not respond to empirical therapy. Neonatal conjunctivitis is always a concern and should be evaluated for possible infection with *Neisseria gonorrhoeae* and *Chlamydia.* The former is marked by a hyperacute conjunctivitis with profuse purulent exudate. Gonorrhea may also cause a severe hyperacute, painful conjunctivitis in the adult patient. An inflammatory membrane may appear on the conjunctiva. Hyperacute conjunctivitis demands an immediate workup and aggressive therapy, because corneal perforation can occur in up to 10% of cases of *Neisseria*-associated conjunctivitis. Gonorrhea needs to be considered in the sexually active adolescent as well as the sexually abused child who presents with a markedly purulent conjunctivitis and a purulent genital discharge.

C. trachomatis leads to the clinical syndromes of trachoma and adult inclusion conjunctivitis. Adult inclusion conjunctivitis caused by *Chlamydia* begins as an acute disease that is often indistinguishable from viral infection. It is most common in young adults in the sexually active years and may occur in combination with other types of venereal disease. A significant number of patients with chlamydial inclusion conjunctivitis also harbor asymptomatic gonorrheal infection. Up to 60% of men will report associated genitourinary symptoms. Findings suggestive of chlamydial infection include association with venereal symptoms and a history of chronic conjunctivitis that is unresponsive to topical antimicrobial therapy.

Newborns can be infected with chlamydia while passing through the birth canal and develop an acute conjunctivitis after an incubation period of 5 to 14 days. Infants who have received appropriate antichlamydial prophylaxis at birth may later become infected from mothers who have chlamydial cervicitis and practice poor hygiene in relation to the neonate's care. Infants with partially treated chlamydial infection are at risk for chlamydial pneumonia. Because of the frequent association of *N. gonorrhoeae* with concurrent chlamydial venereal disease (up to 33%), patients diagnosed with gonococcal conjunctivitis and their sexual partners should also receive treatment with oral antibiotics for chlamydial infection.

Allergic Conjunctivitis. Ocular allergy is a common cause of conjunctivitis. Patients may be allergic to many substances, including airborne allergens (pollen, animal dander), drugs, cosmetics, and contact lens products. In many cases the causes are never identified. Marked itching with bilateral conjunctival irritation, tearing, and nasal congestion that is chronic and recurrent strongly suggest allergic conjunctivitis. Itching is not a prominent feature of other ocular diseases.

The pale pink conjunctivae typical of ocular allergy may be accompanied by localized swelling or angioneurotic edema. This chemosis may assume alarming proportions. The lids may swell as well. If the presentation is uniocular, one should consider a reaction to insect protein as from gnats and other flying insects that lodge as conjunctival foreign bodies. This is a common problem in the summer.

A recurrent bilateral hypersensitivity often found in children with a history of family atopy is vernal conjunctivitis. This typically occurs in the spring or fall and is characterized by huge cobblestone papillae under the upper lid (see Fig. 25–5B). The discharge is characteristic in that several times a day the child may pull a ropy, thick strand of yellow material from beneath the eyelids.

Iritis (Anterior Uveitis)

The patient with acute iritis usually presents with monocular pain, redness, and photophobia. There is no discharge as with conjunctivitis, and the inflammation typical of iritis is much deeper, especially around the limbus. The pain is usually described as a deep ache, like that of a toothache. The globe itself is sore to the touch. Iritis can be a recurring condition; thus, the patient may relate having had a similar experience in the past.

The pupil in patients with iritis is small (miotic) and is poorly reactive to light (see Fig. 25–5C).

The intraocular pressure is low, and a careful examination, including fluorescein staining, will confirm the absence of foreign body or corneal abrasion as a cause of the patient's symptoms. As previously discussed, a slit lamp examination reveals cells and protein exudation (flare) in the anterior chamber. Pupillary dilatation and ciliary muscle relaxation with a mydriatic-cycloplegic medication will often decrease the pain significantly.

Keratitis

Corneal injury, whether caused by trauma or infection, may also present as accompanying conjunctival injection (see Fig. 25–5D). This is why the cornea is carefully examined in all cases of red eye. The corneal nerve endings are quite sensitive; therefore, injury from a variety of causes will present as moderate to severe pain, depending on the amount of epithelial disruption present. Vision is affected variably after corneal injury. A small central corneal abrasion or mild corneal swelling caused by overwear of a contact lens may reduce visual acuity dramatically. In contrast, a more peripheral corneal injury may affect vision minimally except for blurriness resulting from increased lacrimation.

Increased tearing is a reflex caused by the irritated corneal nerve endings, as is blepharospasm. Photophobia may also occur after corneal injury. Disruption of the optical surface causes light to be scattered within the eye. This causes bright light sources to create glare and discomfort. In addition, deep corneal injury may inflame the iris sphincter, causing a mild iritis that leads to pain and aversion to light. These responses occur to varying degrees with most corneal injuries and further reduce vision as well as limit the ease of examination.

Occasionally, symptoms of keratitis occur in the absence of an identified insult. This may be caused by corneal erosion and represents spontaneous loss of corneal epithelium. This sloughing of epithelium in an area of previous abrasion or injury probably results from a lack of complete, tightly adherent healing of the epithelium to the underlying layers of the cornea.

A similar condition occurs in the contact lens wearer who leaves the lens in place for excessively long periods. The drying effect of this overuse causes lens adherence to the cornea, and subsequent removal will cause extensive corneal damage. The patient typically awakens with severe eye pain several hours after contact lens removal. Infection secondary to contact lenses may also cause keratitis.

Excessive exposure to ultraviolet light sources such as sunlight, a sun lamp source, or an arc-welding instrument may cause diffuse corneal injury. This may be demonstrated as fine punctate fluorescein staining of the cornea that is best appreciated by slit lamp examination and is suspected based on the history.

Herpetic Infection

Symptoms of herpetic infection of the cornea may mimic those of corneal abrasion. Therefore, it is necessary to check corneal sensation if there is doubt about the cause of injury. Gentle stroking of the cornea with a drawn-out cotton swab may reveal a diminished response and may suggest herpetic infection. In early herpetic infection, superficial punctate erosions or a single vesicle of the cornea may be all that is apparent. Eventually, a typical dendritic or branching pattern of the corneal injury will be apparent on fluorescein staining (see Fig. 25–5E). An early herpetic infection can sometimes be mistaken for conjunctivitis, corneal abrasion, iritis, or even allergic conjunctivitis.

Other infectious organisms capable of causing corneal injury include herpes zoster virus and gonorrhea. Typically, bacteria invade the cornea of the immunocompromised host. Zoster infection is characterized by typical lesions in the distribution of the trigeminal nerve. Involvement of the tip of the nose (nasociliary nerve) suggests corneal involvement.

Corneal Abscess

The patient with prolonged eye redness and discharge who presents with ocular pain and diminished vision may develop an invasive corneal infection. A flocculent area of corneal exudate that cannot be removed by means of irrigation suggests that ulceration has occurred. Slit lamp examination will reveal the depth and extent of corneal injury.

Acute Glaucoma

Glaucoma refers to a number of conditions that result in an increase in intraocular pressure. It remains the leading cause of reversible blindness in the world. If the rise in intraocular pressure is constant, it will result in damage to the optic nerve, giving rise to permanent visual loss. Acute glaucoma requires immediate treatment by the emergency physician and should be considered in all patients presenting with a painful red eye. Primary open-angle glaucoma accounts for approximately 70% of the primary glaucomas. It is

most prevalent in middle to older ages and is more common in females. It can be an insidious disease and may be best diagnosed on eye examination rather than with tonometry. The classic findings are a visual field loss and pathologic cupping of the head of the optic nerve.

Acute angle-closure glaucoma results from closure of the angle in the anterior chamber. It is a relatively rare cause of glaucoma. This angle is located at the point where the cornea meets the sclera and the trabecular mesh and canal of Schlemm are located. Angle closure occurs when the iris sticks to the lens, causing a blockage and resulting in a buildup of aqueous humor in the posterior chamber. There are several causes of secondary glaucoma that may present acutely. These include inflammatory or particulate origins, angle recession injury, and a complication of corticosteroid use.

Classically, the patient with acute glaucoma notes a relatively rapid onset of a unilateral deep, severe, boring type of globe pain and appears acutely ill. Constitutional symptoms of headache, nausea, and vomiting often accompany this condition. In contrast to the small pupil seen in iritis, the pupil in the patient with acute glaucoma is usually mid-dilated and nonreactive. There is a loss of corneal luster; the cornea may appear quite hazy (see Fig. 25–5F). Cupping of the optic nerve head is commonly noted, if the fundus is visible. The diagnosis of acute glaucoma is made by the finding of an elevated intraocular pressure by tonometry.

PRINCIPLES OF MANAGEMENT

The general management of patients with a red painful eye includes relief of pain and inflammation.

Pain Control

Ocular pain may be controlled with local anesthetics, mydriatics, cycloplegics, and oral analgesics. Topical anesthetics such as 0.5% proparacaine are frequently applied during the physical examination. Relief of superficial ocular pain occurs immediately but wears off in 15 minutes. Repeated use of local anesthetics can retard healing and cause corneal injury. Therefore, local anesthetics should not be given to patients for home use. Table 25–2 lists the characteristics of commonly used anesthetics.

Muscle spasm is thought to play a role in the ocular pain of many conditions. Mydriatics paralyze the pupillary constrictor muscle, causing dilation, whereas cycloplegics affect the ciliary

TABLE 25–2. Topical Anesthetics*

Drug	Concentration (%)	Onset	Duration	Reactions	Comments
Cocaine	2–10	Immediate	20 min	Possible local ischemia, tachycardia, hypertension, restlessness. Excitation infrequent	Mydriatic (rarely used in emergency department)
Benoxinate hydrochloride (Dorsacaine)	0.4	1–2 min	10–15 min	Infrequent side effects	Compatible with fluorescein
Proparacaine hydrochloride (Ophthaine)	0.5	20 sec	10–15 min	Transient local symptoms, allergic reactions rare	Least irritating and toxic; anesthetic of choice
Tetracaine hydrochloride (Pontocaine, Ancel)	0.5	4 min	30–40 min	Drowsiness	Stings on instillation

*One or two instillations of these medications can be used for short-term examination and procedures. Prolonged use may delay healing.
From Zun L, Mathews J: Formulary of commonly used ophthalmologic medications. Emerg Med Clin North Am 1988; 6(1): 121.

muscle. Combinations of cycloplegics and mydriatics are frequently used for relief of ocular pain. Because pupillary dilation occurs, the patient is warned about driving an automobile or going out in the sunlight without eye protection. Mydriatics and cycloplegics are contraindicated in patients with known narrow-angle glaucoma. Table 25–3 lists the characteristics of common mydriatics and cycloplegics. Effective duration of these medications is influenced by the degree of iris pigmentation. Patients with lighter shades (blue) generally have longer durations of effect.

Patients with moderate to severe ocular pain may require oral or parenteral narcotic analgesics for relief of pain.

Relief of Inflammation

Topical vasoconstrictors and decongestants are used by some physicians to help control the inflammatory symptoms of conjunctivitis. They are especially useful for the treatment of allergic symptoms. Topical ketorolac (Toradol) is available for ophthalmic use. A discussion with an eye consultant is best before prescribing it. Ophthalmic corticosteroids *are not* given unless the emergency physician has consulted an ophthalmologist.

Specific Conditions

The specific management of the painful red eye depends on the diagnosis. Table 25–4 summarizes the management of specific conditions.

Infective Conjunctivitis. Conjunctivitis is the most common cause of a red eye and is not associated with visual disturbance or significant eye discomfort. Differentiating a bacterial from a viral cause is not essential in most cases because both types of infections are self-limited. Because antibiotics are believed to improve rates of early clinical and microbiologic remission, current treatment in either instance consists of a brief course (5 to 7 days) of a topical antibiotic such as 10% sulfacetamide (Sulamyd). Table 25–5 lists the characteristics of available topical antibiotics. The preferred antibiotics for initial therapy are erythromycin, sulfacetamide sodium, and aminoglycosides (usually more severe infections). If chlamydial infection is suspected, confirmatory immunofluorescent testing is performed. A prolonged course of oral and topical therapy with erythromycin is given for these infections. Hyperacute conjunctivitis requires early referral and immediate administration of a topical antibiotic and systemic parenteral coverage for gonorrhea (e.g., 1 g ceftriaxone intramuscularly). Other potential sexually transmitted diseases should be considered.

Allergic Conjunctivitis. Ocular allergy is best treated by removing the offending agent, especially inappropriately self-prescribed eye drops. Topical or oral antihistamine or decongestant medications such as levocabastine HCl (0.05% solution) or the over-the-counter combination product of naphazoline and antazoline (Vasocon-A) may be given for treatment of mild symptoms. Mast cell stabilizers (e.g., cromolyn, lodoxamide) take up to 2 weeks to act and are not used acutely. Although corticosteroid eye drops are extremely effective for allergic conditions, their use is deferred to the ophthalmologic consultant. Treating an unsuspected herpetic infection with corticosteroids can have a devastating effect on the patient's outcome.

Iritis. The initial therapy for acute iritis is directed at dilating the pupil. This promotes

TABLE 25–3. Mydriatics/Cycloplegics

Drug	Concentration (%)	Duration	Effects/Uses	Contraindications	Adverse Reactions	Notes
Mydriatic						
Phenylephrine hydrochloride (Neo-Synephrine)	2.5–10.0 (solution)	2–3 hr	Pupillary dilation, treatment of uveitis, decongestant, vasoconstriction, refraction	Narrow-angle glaucoma; hypertensive, cardiac, or patients with aneurysms	Pain on instillation, blurred vision, glare in sunlight; possible cardiovascular collapse with large dose	No cycloplegic effect; sensitive to air, heat, and light
Mydriatic cycloplegic						
Atropine sulfate	0.25–2.0 (solution) 0.5–1.0 (ointment)	2 wk	Long duration, pupillary dilation. Use for treatment of uveitis	Narrow-angle glaucoma, hypersensitivity	Possible systemic absorption, photophobia, dry mouth, loss of accommodation	Produces mydriasis and cycloplegia for refraction
Cyclopentolate hydrochloride (Cyclogyl)	0.5–2.0 (solution)	24 hr	Pupillary dilation for refraction and funduscopy	Narrow-angle glaucoma	Anticholinergic behavioral changes in older adults and children	
Homatropine hydrobromide	2–5 (solution)	10–48 hr	Long duration, pupillary dilation. Use for treatment of uveitis and for refraction in children	Narrow-angle glaucoma	2–4 day loss of accommodation, dry mouth, and photophobia	Anticholinergic. Moderate to long-acting sensitivity. Side effects are rare. Drug of choice in emergency department
Scopolamine hydrobromide (Hyoscine)	0.25 (solution)	2–7 days	Cycloplegia, treatment of uveitis, refraction in children. Use in postoperative cataract patients	Narrow-angle glaucoma	Dizziness and disorientation in elderly; tachycardia	Effective cycloplegic. Rarely used in emergency department
Tropicamide (Mydriacyl)	0.5–1.0 (solution)	6 hr	Pupillary dilation, cycloplegia, uveitis, refraction, fundus examination	Narrow-angle glaucoma	Loss of accommodation, photophobia, dry mouth, behavioral disturbances; cardiorespiratory collapse reported in children	Most useful for ophthalmoscopy. Weak cycloplegic, effective mydriatic

From Zun L, Mathews J: Formulary of commonly used ophthalmologic medications. Emerg Med Clin North Am 1988; 6(1): 122.

TABLE 25–4. Management of the Red Painful Eye

	Acute Conjunctivitis	Iritis, Uveitis	Corneal Trauma	Corneal Infection	Acute Glaucoma
Initial Emergency Department Phase	*Infectious causes:* Topical antibiotics Oral erythromycin or tetracycline (not in children) for *Chlamydia* *Allergic causes:* Antihistamine-decongestant, oral or topical	Cycloplegics Corticosteroids may be necessary but should be given by eye consultant	Foreign body removal Consider cycloplegic if lesion is deep or extensive Topical antibiotics Patching	Topical antibiotics Penicillin or cephalosporin IV for gonorrheal infection Topical antiviral agents for herpetic infection	Miotic agent, pilocarpine 2% drops Timolol, a topical β-blocking agent Latanoprost, a prostaglandin analogue Hyperosmolar agents: (a) glycerol PO, (b) mannitol IV Dorzolamide, a topical carbonic anhydrase inhibitor Acetazolamide IM or IV (less commonly used) Pain relief, usually systemic narcotics
Acute Consultant Intervention	None	Telephone consultation	None (unless perforation is suspected)	Corneal abscess requires immediate intervention by consultant	Consultant should assist in management begun by emergency department personnel
Disposition and Follow-Up	If not improved in 48 hours	Arranged with eye consultant in 24–48 hours	Arrangement is made for prompt removal by consultant if necessary Otherwise, follow-up is dependent on severity of injury	Hospitalization for abscess or gonorrhea Prompt referral for remainder of cases	Per consultant's direction Beware of systemic side effects in topical agents

TABLE 25–5. Topical Ophthalmic Antibiotics

Drug	Preparation	Use	Comments
Bacitracin	500–1000 μg/mg ointment	Most gram-positive organisms	Limited ophthalmic uses. Combined with polymyxin as Polysporin to add gram negatives
Chloramphenicol (Chloromycetin, Chloroptic, Econochlor, Ophthochlor)	0.5% solution, 1% ointment	Gram-positive and some gram-negative and anaerobic organisms	Bacteriostatic. Aplastic anemia has been reported from topical usage
Erythromycin (Ilotycin)	0.5% ointment	Chlamydia and Staphylococcus	Chlamydial infections need topical and oral treatment for at least 2 weeks
Fluoroquinolones (Ciprofloxacin, Ofloxacin)	0.3% solution	Broad spectra, resistant Streptococcus	Reserve for severe infections
Gentamicin sulfate (Garamycin, Genoptic)	3 mg/mL solution 3 mg/g ointment	Gram-negative organisms	Effective anti-infectives, generally indicated for serious ocular infections and corneal ulcers
Neomycin	2.5% mg/mL solution 5 mg/mL ointment	Limited number of gram-negative and gram-positive organisms	About 6% of the North American population can be sensitized to neomycin. Usually combined with polymyxin and bacitracin as Neosporin
Sulfacetamide sodium (Bleph-10, Cetamide, Sulamyd, Vasosulf)	10%–30% solution 10% ointment	Gram-positive and gram-negative organisms	Initial therapy for conjunctivitis; low cost, low allergenicity. Stinging on instillation
Sulfisoxazole (Gantrisin)	4% solution 4% ointment	Same as for sulfacetamide	Same as for sulfacetamide sodium. Avoid if allergy.
Tetracycline (Aureomycin)	1% solution and ointment	Chlamydia	Treatment for Chlamydia infections topically and systemically
Tobramycin (Tobrex)	0.3% solution and ointment	Same as for gentamicin	Same as for gentamicin

comfort by paralyzing the ciliary body, thus eliminating the painful ciliary spasm. A listing of mydriatic and cycloplegic agents is provided in Table 25–3. Homatropine is the drug of choice before referral. Because iritis is an inflammatory condition, a corticosteroid may be necessary. It is prescribed by the ophthalmologic consultant after confirmation of the diagnosis.

Acute Glaucoma. In acute angle-closure glaucoma, the goal of therapy is to constrict the iris away from its point of contact with the peripheral portion of the cornea. In the dilated position, it occludes the normal drainage mechanism for the aqueous humor. This is best accomplished by constricting the pupil with a miotic agent such as 1% pilocarpine. Unfortunately, even short periods of increased intraocular pressure cause ischemia of the iris and render it unresponsive to stimulation. Therefore, medication is given to lower the intraocular pressure, thus restoring circulation to the sphincter muscle so that a miotic agent will work. The first-line drug is the β-adrenergic blocker timolol 0.5%. It reduces the production of aqueous humor. If therapy fails, a hyperosmotic agent is given to increase the osmolarity of the intravascular compartment. Increased osmolarity leads to a bulk flow of water from the extravascular compartment (including the eye), thereby reducing the volume of fluid inside the eye and the intraocular pressure. Oral glycerol will suffice unless the patient is nauseated or vomiting; in this instance, mannitol is given intravenously. In addition, some authors recommend acetazolamide given parenterally to further reduce the pressure. This drug can cause severe potassium loss, so close monitoring is necessary. Topical dorzolamide has a similar action (carbonic anhydrase inhibitor) and fewer side effects. The most important treatment from the patient's perspective is adequate analgesia. Parenteral narcotics are commonly employed.

As the intraocular pressure falls, the iris sphincter will respond to the miotic agent; the peripheral iris will be stretched sufficiently to pull it away from the chamber angle. Usually this medication approach successfully terminates an attack. As the intraocular pressure falls, the corneal edema will resolve within several hours. It is emphasized that an ophthalmologist should be contacted early in the treatment phase. In addition to assisting in medical management of the attack, the ophthalmologist may perform a laser iridectomy immediately after resolution of the acute event.

Invasive Keratitis. When corneal invasion from infection is suspected, immediate consultation with an ophthalmologist is necessary. All patients are given intense topical antibiotic therapy. Patients with suspected gonorrheal infection or evidence of abscess formation are admitted to the hospital. These patients will require intensive ocular irrigation with frequent application of a topical antibiotic. In addition, intravenous antibiotic therapy may be directed by the consultant.

Endophthalmitis. This severe intraocular infection or inflammation is usually preceded by a history of recent (< 2 to 3 days) trauma (penetration) or intraocular surgery. There is marked infection of the conjunctiva, increased intraocular pressure, purulent material in the anterior chamber (hypopyon), and a significant decrease in visual acuity to basic levels (e.g., hand motion, light perception). This is a true ophthalmologic emergency requiring immediate consultation with a specialist.

Special Considerations

Pediatric Patients

A reddened eye in a neonate or infant is always abnormal. It is usually caused by infection, and chlamydial conjunctivitis is of concern. Congenital glaucoma is also considered and may be difficult to diagnose; therefore, all patients younger than 6 months of age need ophthalmologic follow-up.

Elderly Patients

The older adult frequently has coexisting medical problems. Hypertension and atherosclerosis predispose to vascular catastrophe; diabetes mellitus may be the setting in which a simple conjunctivitis has progressed to an invasive infectious keratitis with corneal abscess formation. As with children, baseline visual acuity may be more difficult to assess, and the elderly patient may have a less impressive inflammatory response.

UNCERTAIN DIAGNOSIS

Uncertain diagnosis is relatively common in patients with red eye seen in the emergency department. Once the most serious eye-threatening causes, such as those listed under "Priority Diagnoses," are ruled out, the key to appropriate management is timely follow-up. Discharge from the emergency department with analgesics as necessary and a scheduled ophthalmologic appointment is reasonable care in most cases. Any suspicion of underlying significant disease requires ophthalmologic referral while the patient is in the emergency department.

DISPOSITION AND FOLLOW-UP

The following categories are useful guidelines for ophthalmologic consultation:

- *Immediate*
  - Acute glaucoma
  - Corneal abscess
  - Central retinal artery occlusion
  - Perforation of globe
  - Herpetic keratitis
- *Urgent*
  - Iritis
  - Most keratitis, including superficial infections
- *Follow-up examination required*
  - Conjunctivitis
  - Ocular allergy

Most patients with acute conjunctivitis will improve regardless of the cause; thus, acute consultant intervention is not necessary. It is important to emphasize to the patient that if the problem has not improved in 48 hours further ophthalmologic examination is necessary. This is especially important in the patient who has a loss of visual clarity or increasing eye pain during the follow-up period.

The management of patients with acute iritis or keratitis is discussed on the telephone with the ophthalmologist; arrangements for a follow-up visit within 24 to 48 hours should be made.

Patients with invasive corneal infection, acute glaucoma, central retinal artery occlusion, or perforation of the globe need to be seen immediately by an ophthalmologist. Prompt hospitalization is indicated in most instances.

FINAL POINTS

- The eye responds to noxious stimuli in three primary ways, resulting in redness, pain, or diminished vision.
- Sudden loss of vision indicates an emergent condition that needs immediate attention.
- Visual acuity is the best indicator of eye function and must be documented in all cases.
- Corticosteroids should never be given by the emergency physician unless instructed by an ophthalmologist and herpetic infection is ruled out by fluorescein and slit lamp examination.
- Pain that is relieved by local anesthetics generally indicates superficial inflammation.
- The main differential diagnoses concerned in the red painful eye are conjunctivitis, keratitis, herpetic infection, iritis, trauma, and glaucoma.

CASE *Study*

A 30-year-old man with left eye irritation and redness for 1 day also noted slight blurring of vision and photophobia. He was otherwise healthy and denied a history of trauma, foreign-body sensation, or occupational or environmental exposure to injurious agents. He did not wear contact lenses and denied use of eye medications.

This history does not point to an immediate eye-threatening condition.

The patient's visual acuity was 20/50 in the affected eye and 20/20 in the other. He described normal vision on a recent eye examination done for employment screening. Diffuse conjunctival injection that was especially striking around the cornea was noted. The left pupil was 2 mm smaller than the right, and both direct and consensual light responses were painful for the patient. The cornea was clear, fluorescein staining was negative for abrasion, and there was no foreign body. The fundus was normal. No pain relief occurred on instillation of a local anesthetic.

The fact that the local anesthetic did not relieve the pain indicates intraocular pathology that is deeper than the cornea and conjunctiva. The conjunctival injection around the cornea is consistent with a limbic flush found with deeper eye inflammation.

The blurry vision, eye redness, a small pupil, and photophobia findings on physical examination suggested iritis. Slit lamp examination demonstrated the classic flare and cell findings associated with this disorder.

Slit lamp examination is an important skill for the emergency physician. It is almost impossible to see the classic "headlight beam in the rain" pattern without it.

The patient was given a mydriatic-cycloplegic, homatropine. It was decided not to give him a corticosteroid at this time because of the danger of undiagnosed early herpetic infection. The patient was referred to the ophthalmologist, who saw him the next day.

Bibliography

TEXTS

Rhee DJ, Pyfer MF: The Wills Eye Manual: Office and Emergency Room Diagnosis and Treatment of Eye Disease, 3rd ed. Philadelphia, Lippincott, 1999.

Trobe JD: The Physician's Guide to Eye Care, 2nd ed. San Francisco, American Academy of Ophthalmology, 2001.

JOURNAL ARTICLES

Alteveer JY, McCans KM: The red eye, the swollen eye, and acute vision loss: Handling non-traumatic eye disorders in the ED. Emerg Med Pract 2002; 4:1–28.

Alward WL: Medical management of glaucoma. N Engl J Med 1998; 339:1298–1308.

Cuculino GP, Di Marco CJ: Common ophthalmologic emergencies: A systematic approach to evaluation and management. Emerg Med Rep 2002; 23:163–178.

Kaiser PD: A comparison of pressure patching versus no patching for corneal abrasions due to trauma or foreign body removal. Ophthalmology 1995; 102:1936–1942.

Knoop K, Trott A: Ophthalmologic procedures in the emergency department. Acad Emerg Med 1994; 1:408–412 and 1995; 2:144–150, 224–230.

Leibowitz HM: The red eye. N Engl J Med 2000; 343:345–356.

LeSage N, Verreault R, Rochette L: Efficacy of eye patching for traumatic corneal abrasions: A controlled clinical trial. Ann Emerg Med 2001; 38:129–134.

Markoff DD, Chocko D: Common ophthalmic emergencies: Examination, differential diagnosis, and targeted management. Emerg Med Rep 1999; 20:1–12.

Scott JL, Ghezzi KT: Emergency treatment of the eye. Emerg Med Clin North Am 1995; 13:521–701.

Sheikh A, Hurwitz B, Cave J: Antibiotics for acute bacterial conjunctivitis (Cochrane Review). Cochrane Library, Issue 2, 2000.

Shingleton BJ, O'Donoghue MW: Blurred vision. N Engl J Med 2000; 343:556–562.

Sklar DP, Lauth JE, Johnson DR: Topical anesthesia of the eye as a diagnostic test. Ann Emerg Med 1989; 18:1209–1211.

Torok PG, Mader TH: Corneal abrasions: Diagnosis and management. Am Fam Physician 1996; 53:2521–2529, 2532.

Wightman JM, Hurley LD: Emergency department management of eye injuries. Crit Decisions Emerg Med 2000; 12(7):1–11.

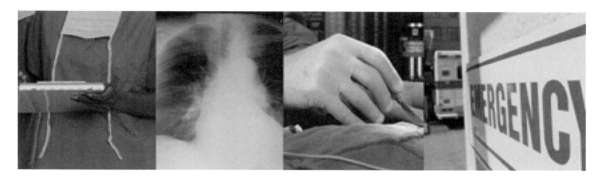

INFANCY AND CHILDHOOD DISORDERS

CHAPTER 26

Febrile Infants

JONATHAN I. SINGER

CASE_Study_

An 18-month-old girl is brought to the emergency department with a 1-day history of temperature to 103.1°F (39.5°C) associated with rhinorrhea. In triage, she cried vigorously while her rectal temperature was being confirmed. Her skin color and hydration appeared to be normal.

INTRODUCTION

Fever is defined as an elevation of body temperature in response to a pathologic stimulus. The most widely used definition of fever is a rectal temperature equal to or greater than 100.4°F (38°C). Pediatric temperature assessments by liquid crystal thermometer strips, palpation, axillary placement of mercury thermometers, and tympanic thermography are unreliable yet frequently used for screening in the emergency department. (See also Chapter 14, Febrile Adults.)

Fever is the single most common chief complaint made to physicians who evaluate ambulatory children. About 20% of all pediatric patients presenting to the emergency department have fever. Fever is most commonly seen in children as a response to infection. However, fever may also be caused by immune-mediated disease, collagen vascular disease, malignancy, and environmental factors such as a hot environment or heavy exertion. Importantly, fever may be a side effect of drug ingestion.

The likelihood of a child becoming febrile with an infectious disease depends both on the age of the child and the disease. In the first few months of life, temperature elevation with infectious disease is inconsistent. Only half of infants with superficial infections become febrile. Fewer than three fourths of newborns develop fever with deep infections. Hypothermia, with a temperature less than or equal to 97.6°F (36.5°C), may be seen with an equal or higher frequency than fever in the course of septicemia in the young child. Children of all ages with chronic, debilitating diseases who may be taking corticosteroids or antimetabolites may not consistently generate a febrile reaction.

During infection, moderate fever is probably beneficial because it enhances host defense reactions. Rapidly rising fevers and hyperpyrexia, defined as a core temperature of more than 106°F (41.1°C), are associated with several complications. Rapidly rising fever will precipitate febrile convulsions in approximately 5% of children. Importantly, a single febrile seizure does not make a child more likely to have a serious bacterial illness. Hyperpyrexia may lead to central nervous system damage and rhabdomyolysis.

The majority of children who present with fever to the emergency department are younger than 3 years of age. The severity of their illness and likelihood of serious infection may be proportional to the degree of temperature elevation, but this is not a consistent correlation. The febrile episodes are usually brief, self-limited, and uneventful. The physician must rule out serious illness and identify infectious diseases that may be benefited by specific treatment.

INITIAL APPROACH AND STABILIZATION

The ability to recognize when a febrile child looks sick or "toxic" is a necessary skill for all individuals who care for acutely ill children. For nursing as well as physician staff this necessary judgment of toxicity is a learned skill. The assessment should be done by the examiner in a noninvasive fashion.

Priority Diagnoses

In most children younger than 3 years of age, the serious causes of fever are infections, primarily bacterial. Meningitis, sepsis, pneumonia, septic arthritis, osteomyelitis, and urinary tract infection are all priority diagnoses.

Rapid Assessment/Early Intervention

Children who appear seriously ill on observation are brought directly into the treatment area for immediate evaluation and stabilization as follows:

1. Continuous monitoring of vital signs is done.
2. Supplemental oxygen with an appropriate nonrebreathing mask and a reservoir bag is given at 10 to 15 L/min.
3. Respirations are assisted by a bag-mask-valve device if ventilation is inadequate. Oropharyngeal secretions are suctioned as needed.
4. An intravenous or intraosseous line is established. Intravenous access may be difficult in infants. For the child who emergently requires fluids, intravenous access is attempted for no longer than 90 seconds, after which an intraosseous line is established.
5. A fluid bolus of 20 mL/kg of isotonic crystalloid is administered if there are signs of shock. Mottled extremities and delayed capillary refill are characteristic of shock. This bolus may be repeated up to three times, followed by clinical assessment.
6. Hypoglycemia (less than 50 mg/dL) is treated with intravenous 25% glucose (0.5 to 1.0 g/kg).
7. Intravenous antibiotics are indicated for children who have serious bacterial illness (e.g., meningitis or sepsis) (see "Principles of Management").
8. Antipyretic administration should be considered for children with temperatures of 104°F to 106°F (40.0°C to 41.1°C). A cooling blanket may be necessary for children whose temperatures exceed 106°F.

For patients outside this urgent category, initial measures include

- Recording an accurate temperature.
- Vital signs: respiratory rate and pulse rate. Pulse oximetry may be useful.
- A history of antipyretic use: the most recent dose and the time it was taken.
- Acetaminophen or ibuprofen administration as determined by recent use. Children with temperatures of 102.2°F (39°C) or more should receive an antipyretic. Children who have received less than 10 mg/kg of an antipyretic in the last 2 hours are given an additional dose of 10 mg/kg.

Early Severity Index Scoring

Nelson prospectively studied large numbers of pediatric patients in the triage setting and developed a severity scoring system using five variables: Respiratory effort, color, activity, temperature, and play (Table 26–1). Nelson's Severity Index Scoring System has applications for examiners in the triage setting. Alternately, the triage staff can derive information about toxicity from observation of a febrile child's hydration, color, playfulness, alertness, and consolability. The triage and the physician staff can utilize the six-item Yale Observation Scale as a predictive model for the presence of serious illness (Table 26–2). The scale looks at the child's response to various stimuli before a traditional physical examination is carried out. Children with a score of more than 16 on this scale have a 92% probability of being seriously ill, whereas children with a score of less than 10 have only a 2% to 3% chance of serious illness.

The application of the Yale Observation Scale presents difficulties for infants younger than several months of age. The limited repertoire of behaviors in this population may inhibit accurate prediction of toxicity. In particular, infants younger than 8 weeks of age inconsistently achieve sustained eye contact or a sociable style.

CLINICAL ASSESSMENT
History

The history is taken from the person in attendance who knows about the present illness, usually the mother. Observing the infant while taking the his-

---

TABLE 26–1. Severity Index Scoring System*

Variable	Point Value		
	0	*1*	*2*
Respiratory effort	Labored or absent	Some distress	No distress
Color	Cyanotic	Pale, flushed, mottled	Normal
Activity	Delirium, stupor, coma	Lethargy	Normal
Temperature†	≤97.4°F or ≥104°F	101.1°F–104°F	97.4°F–101°F
Play	Refuses to play	Decreased	Normal

*A patient's score is derived by summing the scores of the individual items. A score ≤7 identifies children who should receive transportation to a health care facility for immediate attention.
†97.4°F = 36.3°C; 101.0°F = 38.3°C; 104.0°F = 40°C.
From Nelson KG: An index of severity for acute pediatric illness. Am J Public Health 1980; 70:803, with permission from the American Public Health Association.

TABLE 26–2. Yale Observation Scale*

Observation Item	Point Value		
	1 (Normal)	**3 (Moderate Impairment)**	**5 (Severe Impairment)**
Quality of cry	Strong with normal tone or content and not crying	Whimpering or sobbing	Weak or moaning or high pitched
Reaction to parent stimulation	Cries briefly, then stops or content and not crying	Cries off and on	Continual cry or hardly responds
State variation	If awake stays awake or if asleep and stimulated, wakes up quickly.	Eyes close briefly if awake or awakes with prolonged stimulation	Falls to sleep or will not rouse
Color	Pink	Pale extremities or acrocyanosis	Pale or cyanotic or mottled ashen
Hydration	Skin normal, eyes normal and mucous membranes moist	Skin and eyes normal and mouth slightly dry	Skin doughy or tented and dry mucous membranes or sunken eyes
Response (talk, smile) to social overtures	Smiles or alert (≤2 mo)	Brief smile or alert briefly (≤2 mo)	No smile; face anxious, dull, expressionless or no alerting (≤2 mo)

*A patient's score is derived by summing the scores of the individual items. Only 2.7% of patients with a score ≤ 10 have a serious illness; 92.3% with a score ≥ 16 have a serious illness.
From Pediatrics 1982; 70: 806, with permission.

tory is an essential technique for quantifying and clarifying the symptoms, which may have different meanings for the historian and the examiner.

1. When did the *illness begin* and *what is its relationship to the fever*? Moderate fevers of short duration with mild or no symptoms are often self-limited and need only supportive therapy. A fever that begins well after the start of an illness may indicate an extension of the primary infection or secondary bacterial infection.

2. *How high was the temperature* and *what has been used to treat it*? The incidence of bacterial disease increases with the height of the temperature. Measures used to control the fever such as antipyretic medication or sponging assess the parents' knowledge of fever and may reveal inappropriate treatment, such as bundling a febrile child in warm clothes or sponging with alcohol. The response to antipyretics is not an indicator by which to differentiate the cause of febrile illnesses in children. This response does not discriminate between viral and bacterial infections nor distinguish between children who are at risk for invasive infection.

3. How *"ill" does the child seem* to the caregiver? Interest in feeding and playing, general activity, and overall well-being may occasionally provide information relative to the severity of illness. Simultaneous observation of the infant will help the clinician quantify the degree of projected parental concern and perform an early risk assessment (see Tables 26–1 and 26–2).

4. What *other symptoms* has the child had? Associated symptoms may be either specific, suggesting a focus of infection, or nonspecific, associated with a variety of illnesses.
   a. *Upper respiratory symptoms.* The combination of mild rhinorrhea, cough, and pharyngitis suggests viral upper respiratory infection. Acute otitis media is often superimposed on these symptoms. Older infants with otitis media may rub or pull the affected ear.
   b. *Respiratory difficulty.* Respiratory problems are often described as "chest congestion." Rapid, noisy, and difficult breathing are separate symptoms that can be quantified by simultaneous observation. Difficult breathing can be partially quantified by asking whether the infant can nurse or take a bottle in the usual way.
   c. *Vomiting* and *diarrhea.* Vomiting and diarrhea may be either specific symptoms of gastroenteritis or nonspecific symptoms associated with illness outside the gastrointestinal tract, such as otitis media, urinary tract infection, or bacteremia. Both vomiting and diarrhea are quantified as to frequency, number of episodes in a given period, relation to feeding, and presence of blood, mucus, or pus. Abdominal pain is not a common finding in gastroenteritis, and a child who screams and draws up the legs is evaluated for other significant abdominal problems.
   d. *Hydration* and *intake.* Fluid intake is assessed for all febrile infants, not only

those at obvious risk of dehydration from vomiting or diarrhea (see Chapter 28, Dehydration). The amounts and type of fluid ingested are quantified by asking how many 4- or 8-ounce bottles the infant has drunk in the past 24 hours. The frequency of wetting of diapers can be used as an estimate of urine output, but this is not useful if the child has diarrheal stools with every diaper change.

e. *Rash.* Typical exanthems may confirm the clinical diagnosis of a number of childhood diseases. A petechial rash in a febrile child is considered an associated finding of invasive infectious disease until proved otherwise (see Chapter 11, Rash).

f. *Pain* and *swelling* in the *soft tissues or extremities.* Cellulitis of the face, orbit, or elsewhere is an obvious source of fever, whereas deeper soft tissue infections are often occult. A febrile infant who cries each time the diaper is changed or refuses to walk should be suspected of having bacterial arthritis (see Chapter 30, Swollen and Painful Joints), iliopsoas abscess, or osteomyelitis of the hip or lower extremity.

5. Has the child been *exposed* to a *known illness?* Similar symptoms in household members or day-care contacts may raise suspicion of a specific illness. Contact with confirmed *Neisseria meningitidis, Haemophilus influenzae,* or *Streptococcus pneumoniae* requires close evaluation and possible antibiotic prophylaxis. Secondary spread has been reported with these organisms.

6. What *medicines* is the child taking? Parents often independently start treatment with an antibiotic remaining from a previous illness. Current or recent antibiotic use may alter both the typical symptoms of illness and the sensitivity of bacterial organisms. Allergies and undesirable side effects, commonly rash and gastroenteritis, may be symptoms of antibiotic use rather than infection.

7. Are *immunizations* "up-to-date"? Immunization status is a general measure of the caregiver's ability to provide for the child's basic health care. Immunizations may also be the cause of the "illness." Examples are febrile events after diphtheria-pertussis-tetanus (DPT), measles-mumps-rubella (MMR), and *Haemophilus influenzae* type b (Hib) immunizations. Patients who have not received the relatively new *Streptococcus pneumoniae* vaccine also may be at increased risk for a serious bacterial infection.

8. Is the child *usually healthy?* Screening questions about other medical problems and previous overnight hospitalizations will quickly elicit this information. Chronically ill and immune-compromised children are at significantly greater risk of serious infection. A developmental history is generally not necessary in an otherwise normal child with an acute febrile illness. In children who appear to have chronic illness, questions about birth weight, number of days in hospital after delivery, and developmental milestones will help to clarify their medical problems.

Physical Examination

The physical examination consists of a general assessment to determine the probability of serious illness and a detailed examination to detect a specific focus of infection. Of the two, the general assessment is more important in determining the course of action.

General Assessment. The Yale Observation Scale for febrile children (see Table 26–2) is a useful guide for identifying children who appear ill. The items on this scale address the child's consolability and response to stimulation in addition to skin color and hydration.

The child is first observed in the company of the parent. If he or she is crying, the vigor of the cry and the response to the parent's attempts to console the child are noted. In children described as "irritable," maternal rocking and cuddling often calm the infant. However, in the presence of central nervous system inflammation, rocking the infant may result in increased (paradoxical) irritability, an observation that is highly sensitive for meningitis. In contrast, a "smiling and playful" child is usually not seriously ill.

The physician must deliberately observe a sick infant's interest in drinking fluids, the infant's interest (judged by eye contact and gestures) in interacting with the caregiver, and any curiosity about the environment. The infant's interest may be piqued by a bright finger puppet or penlight or by offering a tongue blade to hold. The same object can be used to persuade the infant to look down, while checking for a supple neck, or to follow the light with his or her eyes.

Specific Examination for Focus of Infection. A detailed physical examination in a febrile infant is made in an attempt to determine the source of the fever. The information obtained in the history may be used to guide the examination, but all febrile infants require a complete examination. A thorough examination will prevent missing a focus such as otitis media, for which nonspecific symptoms such as vomiting or diarrhea might otherwise be attributed to gastroenteritis.

Assessment and auscultation of the heart, lungs, and abdomen are best done when the child is quiet. Maneuvers that typically provoke crying, such as inspecting the ears and oropharynx, are done last.

Vital Signs. A knowledge of the range of normal and abnormal parameters is essential for accurately assessing the degree of illness. Normal values for age are listed in Tables 26–3 and 26–4.

Respirations. Children have a variability of respiratory rates, especially infants younger than 6 months old, who often exhibit periodic breathing. For this reason a period of 60 seconds should be chosen. Alternately, two separate 30-second periods can be summed. During the timing, respirations can be counted by observation or by stethoscope. The physician should confirm the rate independently recorded by triage personnel.

Several observations hold true in various studies concerning children's respiratory rate:

1. There is a decrease in respiratory rate with increasing age seen in both awake and asleep infants. The decline is much faster in the first few months of life.
2. The respiratory rates tend to be higher in children evaluated in an emergency setting.
3. Children exhibit increased respiratory rate with fever. For each degree centigrade of fever the baseline respiratory rate may be increased from 2.5 to 7 breaths per minute.

Any patient with an unusually high respiratory rate should have the respiratory rate reassessed.

TABLE 26–3. Pediatric Respiratory Rates

Age	Afebrile	(SD)	Febrile	(SD)
0–2 mo	47	(17)	50	(15)
3–6 mo	45	(15)	48	(15)
7–12 mo	41	(14)	46	(14)
1–2 yr	27	(12)	40	(10)
3–6 yr	24	(10)	28	(8)
7–12 yr	18	(6)	24	(6)

SD, Standard deviation.

TABLE 26–4. Pediatric Heart Rates and Blood Pressure

Age	Heart Rate (beats per minute)	Blood Pressure (breaths per minute)
Newborn	90–150	60–80/palp
1 year	100–130	80/40–105/70
5 years	80–110	90/50–110/80

The presence of a fixed tachypnea may indicate a respiratory pathologic process and on occasion can be the only sign of pneumonia during childhood.

Heart Rate. Pediatric supine heart rates increase in a standing position, and changes may be as great as 30 beats per minute in healthy individuals. Fever typically increases the heart rate. The cardiac output is dependent on the heart rate, and rates up to 200 beats per minute are not unusual. Heart rates of more than 220 beats per minute are more likely to be caused by a cardiac problem and may require treatment. Bradycardia signifies decompensation, most often secondary to hypoxia.

Blood Pressure. Blood pressure varies with age. Low blood pressure in the presence of tachycardia signifies shock secondary to volume depletion. The following guidelines can be used to estimate the normal lower limit for systolic blood pressure: newborn, 60 mm Hg; 1 to 12 months, 70 mm Hg; and older than 12 months, 80 mm Hg plus two times age in years. Normovolemic pediatric patients may have a fall of 10 to 20 mm Hg in blood pressure on going from the supine to the upright position. The presence of fever does not alter blood pressures.

Body Measurements. Body length or body weight can be used to guide fluid therapy and drug dosages. When accurate comparisons are available, premorbid body weight and morbid body weight are sensitive for quantifying dehydration. A Broselow tape is a precalculated measurement device that links the child's body length to a variety of data points (Fig. 26–1).

Head. The anterior fontanelle is assessed when the infant is quiet and is in a sitting position. A tense or bulging anterior fontanelle may be seen as a nonspecific response to fever. The presence of a bulging fontanelle can be a manifestation of meningitis. A depressed fontanelle indicates dehydration. The fontanelle closes at between 12 and 18 months of age.

Eyes. Conjunctival injection and discharge indicate conjunctivitis, either as an isolated finding or associated with upper respiratory tract findings. Periorbital redness or swelling in a febrile state suggests dacryocystitis, ethmoidal sinusitis, or periorbital or orbital cellulitis. Bilateral conjunctival injection without discharge or pain may suggest Kawasaki syndrome if seen with certain other clinical symptoms.

Ears. Otitis media is a common diagnosis in the febrile infant regardless of other symptoms. Criteria for diagnosis are discussed in Chapter 24, Earache.

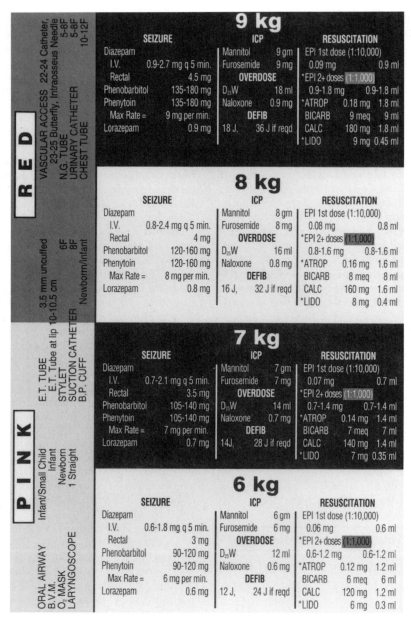

FIGURE 26–1 • The Broselow Pediatric Resuscitation Tape. Color-coded sections based on body length provide the practitioner with appropriate dose information and equipment size. (Reproduced with permission.)

Nose. Mucosal edema and drainage signify upper respiratory involvement. Nasal flaring is a sign of respiratory distress.

Oropharynx. Swelling, inflammation, and mucosal lesions suggest specific infectious causes discussed in Chapter 23, Acute Sore Throat.

Neck. Stiffness and refusal to move the head and neck are significant signs when present, but their absence does not rule out meningitis in infants younger than 12 months of age. Active voluntary neck flexion is more reliable than passive flexion.

A few small, mobile, nontender lymph nodes in the anterior triangles of the neck are common. Large, tender anterior nodes and palpable posterior nodes indicate active infection. The axillary and inguinal areas are also palpated for nodes.

Chest. Signs of respiratory pathology include the patient's position (a fixed upright posture leaning forward or a tripod fixation of the arms), grunting, intercostal retractions, nasal flaring, and accessory muscle use of respirations. The presence of stridor (see Chapter 27, Stridor) suggests a partial upper airway obstruction, and wheezing with prolongation of expiratory phase suggests a lower airway obstruction. Auscultation of the chest for quality of breath sounds is helpful to assess both airway function and the presence of alveolar or interstitial chest disease.

Abdomen. The anterior abdominal area should be inspected, percussed, palpated, and auscultated. The examination can be carried out with the child in the parent's arms and then repeated on the examining table. The inguinal, genital, and perianal areas also are assessed. Tenderness may be difficult to gauge or localize in infants.

Skin. The skin elasticity and turgor are assessed. The delayed return of skin to its original state after it is pinched into folds suggests significant dehydration. Capillary refilling time varies with the amount of pressure applied, the location of pressure application, the ambient temperature, and nutritional status of the patient. Normal refilling times are less than or equal to 3 seconds. The skin also is examined for the presence of rash.

Extremities and Spine. Observation of the child's active use and range of motion of each extremity during crawling, walking, or reaching for objects can rapidly exclude significant pathologic processes. Abnormal use of an extremity requires a detailed examination of the skin, soft tissues, and joints.

CLINICAL REASONING

After the initial assessment, history, and examination, the physician forms a preliminary differential diagnosis and develops management priorities by considering the following questions.

Does the Child Appear Ill?

The seriously ill-appearing child (Table 26–2: Yale Observation Scale score of more than 16) is identified in the initial assessment. After stabilization, these children should be presumptively managed for a serious bacterial infection. Serious bacterial infections include cellulitis, osteomyelitis, pyarthrosis, pneumonia, bacterial enteritis, urinary tract infection, meningitis, bacteremia, and septicemia.

The child who appears marginally ill (Yale Observation Scale score of 11 to 15) requires a period of observation. The fever itself may cause this degree of illness. Reassessment after lowering

of the temperature may clarify the child's appearance as continuing ill or improved.

Is There a Specific Focus of Infection?

The child may have an obvious focus of infection after history of present illness and physical examination. Common infectious foci found in 7% to 10% of young children include otitis media, pharyngitis, and pneumonia. Superficial soft tissue infections may be seen with less frequency. Rare but potentially harmful infections include those that invade muscle, fascia, bone, joints, and meninges.

Is There Currently an Extension of Disease Beyond the Readily Apparent Focus?

Nontoxic children with a readily apparent focus of infection rarely have extension of their infection to other body locales. On occasion, a moderately ill youngster will have a hematogenous spread to a distant body part, including the meninges.

If There Is No Focus of Infection, How Likely Is the Patient to Have Serious Bacterial Infection?

Nontoxic children without apparent focus of infection may have a bacterial pathogen recovered from a blood culture. This condition is referred to as occult bacteremia. Clinical judgment is not predictive of occult bacteremia. However, clinical judgment is typically predictive of the other serious bacterial infections.

If There Is No Focus of Infection and the Patient Is at Low Risk for Serious Bacterial Infection, Are Laboratory Studies Necessary?

The well-appearing nontoxic child with no apparent focus of infection who has nonspecific symptoms usually can be managed without diagnostic investigations. Selected laboratory studies may be of use in nontoxic children when certain clinical characteristics are met. The most significant parameter is magnitude of fever. Children with temperatures of 104°F (40°C) or higher (hyperpyrexia) have an increased likelihood of having significant bacterial disease, including occult bacteremia. This is an inconsistent correlation. Figure 26–2 shows one possible clinical approach to the 3- to 36-month-old child who has a fever without a source.

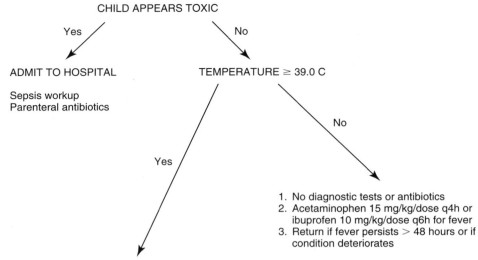

1a. Urine leukocyte esterase (LE) and nitrite or urinalysis and urine culture:
   All males ≤ 6 months and uncircumcised males 6–12 months
   All females < 12 months
   If urine screening test positive: Outpatient antibiotics (oral third-generation cephalosporin)
1b. Urine LE and nitrite or urinalysis and hold urine culture:
   Circumcised males 6–12 months and all females 12–24 months
   If urine screening test positive: Send urine culture and outpatient antibiotics (oral third-generation cephalosporin)
2. For infants and children who have not received the conjugate *S. pneumoniae* vaccine:
   Temperature ≥ 39.5° C: Obtain WBC count (or ANC) and hold blood culture
   If WBC count ≥ 15,000 (or ANC ≥ 10,000):
      Send blood culture
      Ceftriaxone 50 mg/kg up to 1 g
3. Chest radiograph: If SaO_2 < 95%, respiratory distress, tachypnea, rales, or temperature ≥ 39.5 C and WBC count ≥ 20,000 (see above)
4. Acetaminophen: 15 mg/kg/dose q4h or ibuprofen 10 mg/kg/dose q6h for fever
5. Return if fever persists > 48 hours or condition deteriorates

---

FOLLOW-UP OF CHILDREN TREATED AS OUTPATIENTS WITH POSITIVE CULTURE RESULTS:

Blood culture positive (pathogen):	Admit if febrile or ill-appearing Outpatient antibiotics if afebrile and well
Urine culture positive (pathogen):	Admit if febrile or ill-appearing Outpatient antibiotics if afebrile and well

---

FIGURE 26–2 • Algorithm for the management of a previously healthy child (3 to 36 months) with fever without a source. WBC, white blood cell; ANC, absolute neutrophil count. (From Barraff LJ: Management of fever without source in infants and children. Ann Emerg Med 2000; 36:602–614, with permission.)

Is the Patient Younger than 3 Months Old?

Febrile patients younger than 3 months old who appear toxic or septic are at high probability for invasive bacterial disease. These infants should be treated for sepsis and admitted to the hospital. Infants younger than 3 months old who are not toxic cannot be reliably excluded from serious bacterial infection on the basis of examination alone. These young children, particularly those younger than 1 month of age, lack the behavioral functions that physicians judge, such as eye contact, interaction with the examiner, response to surroundings and parents, as well as social smile. Figure 26–3 outlines one possible clinical approach to such a patient.

DIAGNOSTIC ADJUNCTS

Several laboratory procedures widely available to emergency physicians have proved to be valuable for the management of febrile pediatric patients. The following selected laboratory techniques may be adjunctive tools for evaluating febrile children.

Laboratory Studies

Complete Blood Count (CBC) with Differential Cell Count. The CBC is a satisfactory adjunct to bolster a subjective impression based on history and physical examination for the clinical disease states of leukemia (blasts), Kawasaki syndrome

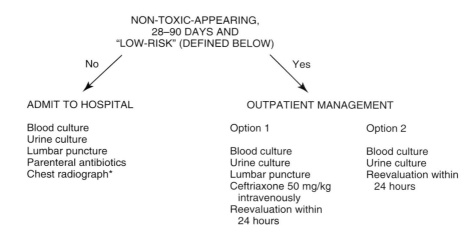

NON-TOXIC-APPEARING,
28–90 DAYS AND
"LOW-RISK" (DEFINED BELOW)

No / \ Yes

ADMIT TO HOSPITAL | OUTPATIENT MANAGEMENT

Blood culture
Urine culture
Lumbar puncture
Parenteral antibiotics
Chest radiograph*

Option 1

Blood culture
Urine culture
Lumbar puncture
Ceftriaxone 50 mg/kg
  intravenously
Reevaluation within
  24 hours

Option 2

Blood culture
Urine culture
Reevaluation within
  24 hours

* Chest radiograph if signs of pneumonia: respiratory distress, abnormal breath sounds,
tachypnea, pulse oximetry < 95%

FOLLOW-UP OF LOW-RISK INFANTS TREATED AS OUTPATIENTS WITH POSITIVE CULTURE RESULTS:

Blood culture positive (pathogen) | Admit for sepsis evaluation and parenteral antibiotic therapy pending results

Urine culture positive (pathogen) | Persistent fever: Admit for sepsis evaluation and parenteral antibiotic therapy pending results

Outpatient antibiotics if afebrile and well

LOW-RISK CRITERIA FOR FEBRILE INFANTS:

Clinical criteria:
  Previously healthy term infant with uncomplicated nursery stay
  Nontoxic clinical appearance
  No focal bacterial infection on examination (except otitis media)
Laboratory criteria:
  WBC count 5–15,000/mm^3, < 1,500 bands/mm^3, or band/neutrophil ratio < 0.2
  Negative Gram stain of unspun urine (preferred), or negative urine leukocyte esterase and nitrite, or < 5 WBCs/hpf
  When diarrhea present: < 5 WBCs/hpf in stool
  CSF: < 8 WBCs/mm^3 and negative Gram stain (option 1 only)

FIGURE 26–3 • Algorithm for the management of a previously healthy infant (birth to 90 days) with a fever without a source with a temperature of 100.4°F (38°C) or greater. (From Barraff LJ: Management of fever without source in infants and children. Ann Emerg Med 2000; 36:602–614, with permission.)

(thrombocytosis), Epstein-Barr virus infection (atypical lymphocytosis), shigellosis (excess bands), *Bordetella pertussis* infection (lymphocytosis), and *Chlamydia trachomatis* infection (eosinophilia).

The CBC is not a reliable tool to differentiate between bacterial and nonbacterial infections in children. However, various quantitative and qualitative changes in the leukocyte series may be used to assess risk for bacteremia in children. Investigators have found a threefold to fourfold risk of bacteremia in febrile children who have a total white blood cell (WBC) count greater than or equal to 15,000/mm^3. Some investigators have found that an absolute neutrophil count greater than or equal to 10,000/mm^3 may be more useful than the total

leukocyte count. More than 1,500 band counts in the newborn may suggest an increased risk of bacteremia. More than 500 band counts in children between 1 month and 2 years of age may increase the likelihood of bacteremia. Several authors endorse the acquisition and interpretation of a CBC to aid in the decision to obtain a blood culture.

Sedimentation Rate. The erythrocyte sedimentation rate (ESR) measures the free-fall of erythrocytes over either 1 hour (classic) or 30 minutes (shortened). The test indirectly measures fibrinogen levels, which is one of several proteins that increase shortly after an infectious or inflammatory insult (acute-phase reactant). The ESR has been used as a screening procedure to identify children with occult bacteremia or aid in the evaluation of potentially septic patients, particularly newborns. It has been suggested as an aid in the decision to obtain a blood culture.

Blood Culture. A blood culture is indicated in any pediatric patient who appears toxic or who has an identifiable, serious bacterial illness. Rates of recovery from blood cultures in the patient with sepsis or meningitis approach 80% to 90%. Patients with cellulitis have a wide range of recovery of from 7% to 70%. Patients with urinary tract infection, pneumonia, and bacterial enteritis have rates of recovery that are less than 10%.

Acquisition of a blood culture may be of use in a febrile pediatric patient without apparent focus of infection. The greatest unexpected yield of positive blood cultures is found in individuals between 6 and 24 months of age without apparent focus of infection who have temperatures less than or equal to 104°F (40°C).

Urinalysis. Urinary tract infection should be a diagnostic consideration in febrile children without apparent focus of infection. This is especially true for infants of both sexes younger than 1 year of age. Abnormal urine and positive urine cultures may occur in up to 5% of febrile infants younger than 1 year of age. Because the technique used for collecting urine has a major impact on the incidence of urinary tract infection (too great a contamination rate with bag urine specimens), urine samples should be acquired by straight catheterization in the non–toilet-trained child.

Rapid *Streptococcus* Screen. A rapid screening technique may be beneficial to confirm a clinical suspicion of pharyngitis from group A β-hemolytic *Streptococcus*. Positive rapid screens predict a disease state. Because false-negative results occur in up to 20% of patients, the child with a clinically suggestive streptococcal pharyngitis and negative screen should have a throat culture plated. The incidence of streptococcal pharyngitis in children older than 2 to 3 years of age supports the acquisition of a screen for streptococcal infection when there is fever without focus. The incidence of streptococcal pharyngitis in children younger than 2 to 3 years is low, such that rapid screening and culture may not be warranted.

Cerebrospinal Fluid (CSF) Analysis. The decision to perform a lumbar puncture and examine the CSF must be tailored to the clinical situation. Patients at increased risk for intracranial infection include febrile children younger than 3 months; toxic-appearing children of all ages; children whose febrile illness is accompanied by seizure, nuchal rigidity, petechial rash, or an immunocompromised state; and children with recently confirmed bacteremia.

A conservative approach is to perform a lumbar puncture in all children younger than 12 months of age who have a seizure associated with fever. Older children with febrile seizure may be evaluated by the same criteria used for any febrile child.

CSF examination can be delayed in the febrile patient who is unstable. Febrile patients at high risk for meningitis are considered unstable when their airway is unprotected, or they have generalized seizure activity, tenuously low or elevated blood pressure, or delayed capillary refilling time. In these circumstances, lumbar puncture may be associated with hypoxemia, apnea, or bradycardia. If a delay in obtaining CSF is anticipated, it is prudent to acquire a blood culture and administer antibiotics empirically after the initial resuscitation.

Radiologic Imaging

Chest Radiograph. A chest radiograph is frequently obtained in the febrile pediatric patient despite a low incidence of pneumonia in febrile children with no signs or symptoms of any respiratory illness. It is appropriate to obtain a radiograph primarily when there is clinical suspicion of pneumonia. Respiratory distress, a pulse oximetry of less than 95%, rales, and tachypnea are reasonable predictors of pneumonia in infancy or childhood. However, nontoxic patients, especially those younger than 1 year of age, can be febrile without tachypnea, cough, or rales and have "silent" pneumonia. Thus, a chest radiograph is a consideration in a well-appearing young child who is febrile to at least 103°F (39.5°C), especially if there is a WBC count of greater than or equal to 15,000/mm^3.

A chest radiograph should be obtained in the toxic-appearing child without an apparent focus of infection. In this circumstance radiography may disclose an occult (pleural, parenchymal, or pericardial) focus of infection.

Other Tests

Joint Aspiration and Synovial Fluid Analysis. Arthrocentesis is indicated in children with symptoms and signs of joint inflammation. The hip is the most common site of septic arthritis in young children, and arthrocentesis is performed in conjunction with orthopedic consultation. Synovial fluid studies and interpretations are discussed in Chapter 30, Swollen and Painful Joints.

EXPANDED DIFFERENTIAL DIAGNOSIS

After diagnostic testing, the physician may have a firm diagnosis in mind (focus of infection) and enough evidence to categorize the infection as serious or not serious. By combining clinical and, when indicated, diagnostic results, patients usually can be classified into one of three groups:

1. *"Ill or toxic" with presumed serious bacterial infection.* The ill-appearing child, as identified previously, may not have a focus of infection after clinical examination and diagnostic testing. However, the child's ill appearance alone warrants a presumptive diagnosis of serious bacterial disease. These patients generally warrant additional diagnostic testing and immediate treatment.
2. *"Nontoxic" with apparent focus of infection.* The child who appears well and has a recognized focus of infection on clinical examination need not necessarily have diagnostic testing.
3. *"Nontoxic" without apparent focus of infection.* The last group of children are those who appear well and have no apparent focus of infection. The majority of these children will recover without further treatment. However, 2% to 3% of febrile children younger than 2 to 3 years of age are bacteremic at the time of the physician encounter. If a bacteremic child is discharged from an emergency department visit, the overall risk of persistent fever is estimated to be 35%. Persistent bacteremia has an estimated occurrence of 12%. Persistently bacteremic infants and children remain febrile and may develop an extracranial focus of infection. Of greatest concern, 4.4% to 7% of untreated patients who have been documented to be bacteremic at an initial patient encounter will develop bacterial meningitis. The meningitis risk varies with the infecting organism. *N. meningitidis* has a factor of 86, *H. influenzae* a factor of 12, and *S. pneumoniae* a factor of 1.

Occult Bacteremia

Bacteremia, defined as a positive blood culture, is an expected finding in invasive or deep bacterial infections such as meningitis, sepsis, epiglottitis, septic arthritis, osteomyelitis, myositis, and fasciitis. Bacteremia is less frequently found in well-appearing febrile children with no focus of infection. When bacteremia occurs in this setting, it is termed *occult*. The most common organism isolated in unexpectedly positive blood cultures is *S. pneumoniae. N. meningitidis, Salmonella* species, and group A β-hemolytic *Streptococcus* occur far less frequently. Since the introduction of

H. influenzae type b vaccine, *H. influenzae* bacteremia is now a rarity. With the advent of the *S. pneumoniae* conjugated vaccine, it is expected that bacteremia from this organism will decline as well.

In the absence of apparent sepsis, clinical judgment is not predictive of occult bacteremia. The young patient with unsuspected *S. pneumoniae* bacteremia (pneumococcemia) may appear well or have a seemingly minor illness associated with upper respiratory tract symptoms or diarrhea that is not bloody. Only the presence of a rarely occurring cystic oral lesion predicts pneumococcemia. It may become ulcerative or necrotic, allowing *S. pneumoniae* to be recovered from the gingival lesion and the blood. Transient gingival or cheek swelling may accompany the lesion at its onset. Occult bacteremia caused by other organisms does not have pathognomonic physical findings.

All socioeconomic groups are equally affected by occult bacteremia. Children at greatest risk are those between 6 and 24 months, with temperatures of 104°F (40°C) or more.

Various changes in the CBC, ESR, and other laboratory investigations may correlate with occult bacteremia. The most often quoted factors are a peripheral WBC count of 15,000/mm³ or higher, an absolute neutrophil count greater than or equal to 10,000/mm³, and an ESR greater than or equal to 30 mm/hr by the Wintrobe method. Occult bacteremia can occur outside these clinical and laboratory parameters but with far less frequency. When analyzed on the basis of age and degree of fever, the frequency of bacteremia increases up to age 2 (Table 26–5) and with higher recorded temperatures (Table 26–6).

TABLE 26–5. Age and Occult Bacteremia

Age	Frequency (%)
≤ 1 mo	≤ 1
1–2 mo	1–3
2–3 mo	2–3
3–6 mo	2–3
6 mo–2 yr	4–7
≥ 2 yr	2–3

TABLE 26–6. Body Temperature and Occult Bacteremia

Temperature		Frequency (%)
°F	°C	
98.6	37	1–2
100.4	38	2–3
102.2	39	3–5
104	40	5–7
106	41	10–12

Several clinical studies have examined whether complications of bacteremia can be prevented by treating young febrile children with antibiotics at the initial patient encounter ("expectant treatment"). It appears that expectant treatment reduces fever, the length of illness, and the likelihood of extracranial infection but does not reduce the likelihood of meningitis. Recent clinical guidelines from the American College of Emergency Physicians and American Academy of Pediatrics are referenced in the Bibliography. The latter guidelines stratify management options into hospitalization, outpatient treatment with or without antibiotics, and observation with careful follow-up.

Sepsis

Sepsis is the presence of viable bacteria in the blood (bacteremia) with systemic toxicity. By definition, sepsis can be diagnosed only when infection is confirmed. However, the term a *septic-appearing child* is used to describe the youngster with a profound illness accompanied by a toxic appearance (looks "septic"). Typically, septic-appearing infants and children have significant tachycardia and tachypnea. Often, there is evidence of hypoperfusion and multiple organ dysfunction.

The organisms associated with occult bacteremia and septicemia in children have remained relatively constant (Table 26–7). In the past decade, *H. influenzae* septicemia has been reduced and group A β-hemolytic streptococcal invasive diseases have resurged.

PRINCIPLES OF MANAGEMENT

Immediate management of the seriously ill child was discussed earlier in the section "Initial Assessment and Stabilization." General principles of management for the febrile child include fever therapy, hydration, and antibiotic therapy.

Management of Fever

Fever of 100.4°F (38°C) or more is uncomfortable. The primary aim of lowering fever is to increase patient comfort. Lowering the temperature also permits clinical observations when the child is most comfortable and may clarify the appearance of an "irritable" child. Treating the fever does not obscure disease processes. Fever is no more or less likely to decrease with antipyretic therapy in a mild than in a serious illness; therefore, defervescence cannot be used to judge the seriousness of the underlying illness.

Fever is treated pharmacologically with acetaminophen, ibuprofen, or a combination of both. Aspirin has not been used to control fever in children since the 1980s because of concerns of the association with Reye syndrome and aspirin use. Acetaminophen is typically administered as a 15-mg/kg dose for acute fever control. Up to five doses may be administered in a 24-hour time frame. Acetaminophen is available in a number of preparations, including pediatric infant drops (80 mg in 0.8 mL), pediatric elixir (160 mg in 5 mL [1 tsp]), and children's chewable tablets (80 mg).

Ibuprofen's antipyretic effect is dose dependent in children. A 10-mg/kg dose administration

TABLE 26–7. Bacteriology of Occult Bacteremia and Sepsis*

| Age | Isolates | |
	Occult Bacteremia	Sepsis
Birth–3 months	Group B *Streptococcus*	*Escherichia coli*
	Escherichia coli	*Streptococcus*, groups B, D, A
	Klebsiella species	*Staphylococcus* species
	Salmonella species	*Listeria monocytogenes*
	Staphylococcus species	*Streptococcus pneumoniae*
	Streptococcus pneumoniae	Gram-negative rods
Older than 3 months	*Streptococcus pneumoniae*	Group A β-hemolytic
	Neisseria meningitidis	*Streptococcus*
	Salmonella species	*Neisseria meningitidis*
	Shigella species	*Staphylococcus aureus*
	Haemophilus influenzae	*Haemophilus influenzae*
	Group A *Streptococcus*	*Streptococcus pneumoniae*
		Gram-negative rods

*Organisms are listed in descending order of prevalence.

produces antipyresis that is longer acting than that from acetaminophen. Four doses are maximally administered in a 24-hour time frame. Ibuprofen is available as infant drops (50 mg/1.2 mL) and elixir (100 mg in 5 mL).

In circumstances in which inadequate fever relief is obtained with either 15 mg/kg of acetaminophen or 10 mg/kg of ibuprofen, concomitant or alternating dosing of acetaminophen and ibuprofen may be suggested. Although the antipyretic effects may be synergistic, either medicine has the potential for toxicity; when combined, there may be increased toxicity, especially to the kidneys.

Nonpharmacologic techniques such as tepid water can be used in conjunction with acetaminophen or ibuprofen to lower the temperature. Tepid water sponging is most useful for rapidly decreasing very high temperatures of more than 105.8°F (41°C). For temperatures of less than 105.8°F (41°C), sponging is an optional measure and is guided by patient comfort. Alcohol and cold or ice water sponging is not recommended; they may result in systemic toxicity and hypothermia, respectively.

Hydration

Fever increases fluid loss, and all febrile children are encouraged to increase their fluid intake above normal. Oral hydration is appropriate for all but very ill children. Parents are informed that lack of interest in eating is normal but that adequate fluid intake is essential.

Antibiotics

If the clinician chooses to treat the febrile pediatric patient presumptively for occult bacteremia, two parenteral agents are suitable. They are aqueous penicillin G and ceftriaxone (Rocephin). Ceftriaxone has beneficial tissue penetration and pharmacokinetics and is active against a majority of the organisms associated with bacteremia. Ceftriaxone also has limited toxicity, making the antibiotic an optional choice for presumptive therapy of occult bacteremia.

For presumed sepsis in children older than 3 months of age, empirical treatment should include cefotaxime or ceftriaxone, with or without vancomycin, depending on the prevalence of resistant strains of *Staphylococcus epidermidis* or *Streptococcus pneumoniae* in the area.

UNCERTAIN DIAGNOSIS

The majority of this chapter has discussed the clinical approach to children with fever. If a source is not identified, and the patient is ill enough to require admission, the workup for the source can be continued as an inpatient procedure. Otherwise, fever without source can be followed up by the patient's primary provider.

SPECIAL CONSIDERATIONS

Immunocompromised Children

Immunocompromised children are characterized by (1) increased susceptibility to infectious agents, (2) inability to respond to infection, and (3) failure to develop typical signs and symptoms of infection. In the immunocompromised child, signs of infection that would usually be considered trivial require aggressive evaluation, paying special attention to areas affected by opportunistic and unusual infections, such as the oral and perianal areas, joints, bone, and skin.

Sickle Cell Disease and Asplenia. Children younger than 5 years of age with sickle cell disease are extremely vulnerable to overwhelming sepsis (*S. pneumoniae*, *H. influenzae*). Surgical asplenia from trauma, hereditary spherocytosis, Hodgkin's disease, and idiopathic thrombocytopenia purpura result in similar risk. Fulminant sepsis can evolve over hours and carries a high mortality.

Cancer and Leukemia. Immune system compromise may be caused by the disease itself, by chemotherapy, or by corticosteroid use. Serious infection occurs with the usual bacterial pathogens, usually benign viruses (varicella) or opportunistic organisms from endogenous skin and gut flora. The height of fever correlates with the severity of infection; children with temperatures of more than 102.2°F (39°C) have a 25% incidence of positive blood cultures. Normal or low temperatures may, however, occur in the presence of sepsis. Neutropenia, an absolute neutrophil count of less than 500/mm^3, increases the risk of infection significantly.

Acquired Immune Deficiency Syndrome. Most infants with acquired immune deficiency syndrome (AIDS) present with a triad of hepatosplenomegaly, chronic interstitial pneumonia, and failure to thrive. In addition to opportunistic infections, the child with AIDS is also susceptible to recurrent infections with the common childhood bacterial organisms.

Corticosteroid Therapy. Prolonged high-dose therapy (more than 4 weeks) significantly increases the risk of both common and opportunistic infection. Even after short parenteral treatment, oral therapy, or inhalation therapy, pediatric patients may exhibit increased risk for opportunistic infection. Corticosteroid therapy from any route may mask the usual signs of infection.

Chronic Illness. Children with congenital heart disease, lung disease, cystic fibrosis, nephritic syndrome, and other chronic illnesses are at increased risk of various infections.

DISPOSITION AND FOLLOW-UP

Admission

Which febrile children are admitted to the hospital?

- Children with documented serious bacterial disease and all high-risk infants younger than 3 months of age
- The child who appears ill despite an unclear diagnosis
- Children who need therapy that cannot be provided at home (e.g., oxygen, intravenous fluids, or antibiotics)
- Children whose families cannot be relied on to observe the patient or return for repeat evaluation or therapy

A relative indication includes children with immunocompromise or chronic illness.

Admission to Intensive Care Unit

Which patients should be admitted to the intensive care unit?

- Any child who requires high-flow oxygen, ventilation, or fluids for initial resuscitation or continued management of compromised vital functions
- Children with bacterial meningitis or sepsis

Discharge

Which patients can go home?

- The "well" febrile child with a reliable caregiver, who clearly understands instructions for follow-up and available follow-up, is able to comply with the indicated therapy (oral antibiotics, fluids), and will follow up on cultures and other testing (e.g., chest radiograph).

The plan for the patient who goes home should include

1. Acetaminophen or ibuprofen for fever control
2. Oral hydration
3. Antibiotics as indicated
4. Explanation of anticipated course of illness
5. Clear timing of expected follow-up with primary caregiver
6. How to obtain the final result of any cultures (blood or urine)
7. Indications for a repeat assessment should the patient's condition deteriorate

FINAL POINTS

- The goal in the initial approach to the febrile infant is to determine whether the child appears ill. Objective scales such as the Yale Observation Scale can assist in this assessment.
- Febrile infants who are lethargic and poorly responsive are presumed to be septic, and intravenous antibiotics are administered early in their emergency department course.
- Simultaneous observation of the child while obtaining a history from the caregiver allows the examiner to clarify the reported behavior and symptoms of the child.
- Physical examination will help to determine the probability of serious illness as well as detect a specific focus of infection.
- The general condition of the child, age, height of the fever, underlying medical problems, and exposures determine the need for diagnostic investigations.
- Blood culture is warranted in circumstances in which children satisfy criteria for risk of occult bacteremia, especially when 6 to 24 months old with temperatures higher than 104°F (40°C).
- Evaluation of the child with a simple febrile seizure emphasizes determining the cause of the fever.
- Intracranial infection should be considered in a child who experiences a seizure after a febrile illness.
- Management of a febrile illness in children consists of providing therapy for the fever, hydration, and appropriate antibiotic therapy, which is usually based on the likely bacterial organism rather than on culture results.
- Febrile children discharged from the emergency department need reliable caregivers who are adequately instructed on indications for follow-up examination.

CASE*Study*

An 18-month-old girl is brought to the emergency department with a 1-day history of temperature to 103°F (39.5°C) and rhinorrhea. She cried vigorously while her rectal temperature was being confirmed. Her skin color and hydration appeared normal.

The historian provided additional history that there were two episodes of nonbilious vomiting accompanying the child's fever. By the physician's examination, the child did not appear toxic and was without an apparent focus of infection.

The 18-month-old child with a maximal temperature of 103°F (39.5°C) who had no apparent form of infection and does not look toxic may be managed without any diagnostic interventions. The hydrated child without underlying medical problems may be managed presumptively as having a viral infection. Supportive care should be rendered and arrangements made for follow-up care within 24 hours.

An alternate concept is to recognize that the child has a small risk for occult bacteremia, urinary tract infection, or pneumonia. Many

practitioners would suggest acquisition of relevant laboratory studies.

The child was catheterized, and urinalysis showed a specific gravity of 1.015, no leukocytes, and no bacteria. A CBC and blood culture were obtained. The WBC count was 16,700/mm^3 with a left shift. The child was presumptively treated for occult bacteremia: 50 mg/kg of ceftriaxone (Rocephin) mixed with lidocaine was administered intramuscularly. A chest radiograph was not performed because there were no respiratory signs or symptoms. Arrangements were made for a repeat examination within 24 hours.

The physician documented the following: "Diagnosis—fever without localizing signs; leukocytosis: rule out bacteremia." The mother understood that blood culture results were pending. She indicated willingness and ability to have the child reassessed at the primary physician's office within 24 hours. The primary physician was contacted and concurred with management.

Bibliography

TEXTS

Cantor RM, Santamaria JP: Pediatric Emergency Guide. Dallas, American College of Emergency Physicians, 1997.

Strange GR: Pediatric Emergency Medicine: A Comprehensive Study Guide. American College of Emergency Physicians. New York, McGraw-Hill, 1996.

JOURNAL ARTICLES

American College of Emergency Physicians: Clinical policy for the initial approach to children under the age of two years presenting with fever. Ann Emerg Med 1992; 22:628–637.

Bachur R, Perry H, Harper MB: Occult pneumonias: Empiric chest radiographs in febrile children with leukocytosis. Ann Emerg Med 1999; 33:166–173.

Baraff LG: Management of fever without source in infants and children. Ann Emerg Med 2000; 36:602–614.

Bass JW, Steele RW, Wittler RR, et al: Antimicrobial treatment of occult bacteremia: A multicenter cooperative study. Pediatr Infect Dis J 1993; 12:466–473.

Dagan R, Sofer S, Phillip M, et al: Ambulatory care of febrile infants younger than two months of age classified as being at low risk for having serious bacterial infections. J Pediatr 1998; 112:355–360.

Fleisher GR, Rosenberg N, Vincei R, et al: Intramuscular versus oral antibiotic therapy for the prevention of meningitis and other bacterial sequelae in young febrile children at risk for occult bacteremia. J Pediatr 1994; 124:504–512.

Heubi JE, Bine JP: Acetaminophen use in children: More is not better. J Pediatr 1997; 130:175–177.

Kramer MS, Shapira ED: Management of the young febrile child: A commentary on recent practice guidelines. Pediatrics 1997; 100:128–133.

Kramer MS: The young febrile child: Evidence-based diagnostic and therapeutic strategies. Emerg Med Pract 2000; 2(7):1–24.

Singer J, Vest J, Prince A: Occult bacteremia and septicemia in febrile children less than two years of age. Emerg Med Clin North Am 13:381–416, 1995.

Slater M, Krug S: Evaluation of the infant with fever without source: an evidence based approach. Emerg Med Clin North Am 1999; 17:97–126.

Yamamoto LG, Worthley RG, Melish ME, et al: A revised decision analysis of strategies in the management of febrile children at risk for occult bacteremia. Am J Emerg Med 1998; 16:193–207.

Zerr D, Del Becarro MA, Cummings P. Predictors of Physician Compliance with a Published Guideline on Management of Febrile Infants. Pediatr Infect Dis J. 18:232–238, 1999.

CHAPTER 27

Stridor

TERESITA MORALES-YURIK
GARY R. STRANGE

CASE *Study*

A 3-year-old boy was well until he awoke from sleep at 3 AM with a high fever. His mother brought him to the emergency department because he was unable to lie down, had noisy respirations, and was drooling saliva.

INTRODUCTION

Stridor is a harsh, high-pitched, raspy sound made as air passes through a partially obstructed upper airway. The upper airway begins with the pharynx and includes the trachea and main bronchi. Anatomically, it can be divided into three main areas: (1) the supraglottic airway (above the vocal cords); (2) the glottic and subglottic airway; and (3) the intrathoracic airway. Depending on the location of the obstruction, disorders that cause stridor have different clinical features and varying tendencies to develop complete obstruction. Stridor from supraglottic obstruction is generally heard primarily on inspiration. Obstruction of the glottic and subglottic airway leads to stridor that may occur during inspiration or expiration. Intrathoracic airway obstruction causes stridor that is loudest on expiration because intrathoracic pressure rises on expiration and tends to cause airway collapse.

Upper airway obstruction in children may be caused by infection, inflammation, foreign body, or congenital abnormality. Ninety percent of cases are due to infection. The same processes occur in the adult population but only rarely result in clinically recognizable obstruction, largely because of anatomic differences.

The pediatric airway (Fig. 27–1) differs in several important ways from that of the adult:

1. The tracheal cartilage of the child is relatively soft and pliable. During inspiration, negative intratracheal pressure results in narrowing of the supraglottic and subglottic airway, whereas during expiration, the airway widens. Inspiratory stridor is more common than expiratory stridor at these levels.

2. The epiglottis of the infant or small child is relatively long, and the aryepiglottic folds are redundant. The mucous membranes are softer and looser, and the lymphoid tissue is abundant. Swelling of these tissues can be marked and may lead to obstruction.

3. The epiglottis and larynx lie higher in the infant, at the level of C2 or C3. In the adult, they are found at the level of C5 or C6. This more cephalad position of the glottic opening makes intubation of the infant more difficult.

4. The diameter of the trachea in the infant and child (3 to 5 mm) is far smaller than that in the adult (7 to 8 mm). Foreign bodies or edema that causes only partial blockage in the adult airway may result in complete obstruction in children. Airway resistance is inversely proportional to the fourth power of the radius. Therefore, a reduction in the radius of the trachea by half causes a 16-fold increase in resistance. Clearly, small amounts of edema can result in marked obstruction of air flow.

5. The cricoid ring is the only circumferential support of the upper airway in the child, and it represents the narrowest portion. An endotracheal tube that fits through the glottic opening will be snug in the subglottic region. This obviates the need for cuffed endotracheal tubes in children younger than 8 years of age. Because the cricoid is the only circumferential support for the pediatric airway, injury to it by pressure from a cuffed tube or by surgical disruption during cricothyrotomy must be avoided.

Although most children with stridor do not present with a compromised airway, some childhood infectious diseases may progress to complete airway obstruction very rapidly and present a great challenge to the emergency physician. Accurate clinical diagnosis and definitive airway stabilization can prevent a devastating outcome.

INITIAL APPROACH AND STABILIZATION

All patients with stridor are brought immediately into the acute area of the emergency department

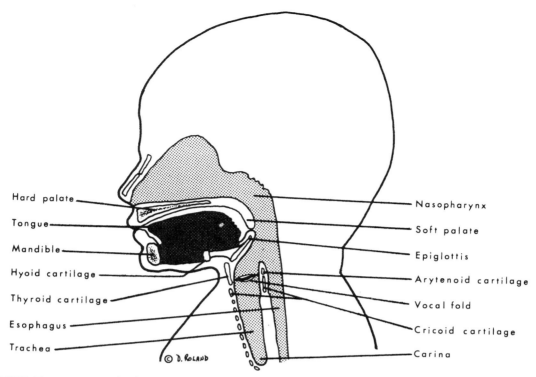

FIGURE 27–1 • Anatomy of pediatric airway. (From Lumpkin JR: Airway obstruction. Topics Emerg Med 1980; 2[1]:16.)

and are seen by a physician. The first priority when presented with a child with stridor is to determine the adequacy of ventilation and oxygenation. This information guides airway management and the need for respiratory support. The physician must stabilize and evaluate the respiratory system in a systematic way and anticipate the need for definitive airway management.

Priority Diagnoses

The four priority diagnoses to consider initially are the ones that have the potential for sudden deterioration of the child's condition and the need for emergent airway management:

1. Acute epiglottitis
2. Croup (viral laryngotracheobronchitis)
3. Foreign body aspiration
4. Retropharyngeal abscess

Rapid Assessment

During the initial assessment and stabilization, important questions arise:

1. What sort of breathing difficulty has the child been having and when did it begin? What are the airway sounds like?

2. Is the child able to speak or cry?
3. Is the child able to swallow? Has he or she been drooling?
4. Is there a known or possible foreign body aspiration?
5. Is there a history of neck trauma?
6. Has the child had any home therapy?
7. Has there been any change in his condition during the transport to the emergency department?

Simple observation of the child in the arms of the parent is an important aspect of the evaluation. It may provide useful information and the child will not find it threatening.

1. The position the child assumes spontaneously is noted.
2. Does the child feel feverish or look toxic?
3. Are there intercostal or supraclavicular retractions?
4. Is the child cyanotic, lethargic, or poorly responsive?
5. The respiratory rate is recorded, and the rest of the vital signs, cardiac monitoring, and pulse oximetry placement may be deferred if they are upsetting to the child.

Early Intervention

Immediate stabilization decisions must be made:

1. As long as the child is conscious, moving air, and able to talk, the following interventions are indicated, followed by a more complete history and physical examination:
   a. Oxygen is given by blow-by technique or mask if tolerated. Oxygen flow is 6 to 8 L/min.
   b. The child is allowed to assume a position of comfort and not forced to lie down in case complete obstruction may result.
   c. All unnecessary disturbances are eliminated. No intravenous lines are placed, arterial blood gas samples taken, or laboratory specimens collected until absolute need is determined.
2. If the child is in marked respiratory distress and there is frank or impending respiratory failure, ventilatory support is instituted immediately. Impending respiratory failure is recognizable when the following signs are observed:
   a. There is increased work of breathing with tiring.
   b. There is increasing tachypnea (more than 40 breaths per minute is an initial cutoff).
   c. There is increasing tachycardia (varies with age of child, more than 130 beats per minute may be initial limit, under 6 years of age).
   d. Onset of bradycardia, which may be abrupt.
   e. Cyanosis is noted. (Anemic children may not develop obvious cyanosis.)
   f. Lethargy is marked or the child is unresponsive.
3. Interventions then include the following:
   a. Ventilation with a bag-valve-mask unit and 100% oxygen is attempted. High pressures may be necessary to force oxygen past an upper airway obstruction, and this is best generated with an adult-sized bag. Endotracheal intubation is likely to be difficult, especially with supraglottic infections.
   b. If adequate ventilation is achieved by bagging, moving the child to the operating room for attempted intubation by an anesthesiologist, with a surgeon standing by to perform a tracheostomy if intubation is unsuccessful, is the best approach.
   c. If inadequate ventilation is obtained with bagging, endotracheal intubation is attempted in the emergency department. If it is unsuccessful, needle cricothyrotomy and positive-pressure ventilation are performed by the physician most skilled in these techniques.

CLINICAL ASSESSMENT

A complete history and physical examination allow the causes of upper airway partial obstruction to be differentiated, thereby guiding proper management.

History

The parents' description of the cause of illness and sounds they have heard will assist in categorizing the problem.

1. *Onset. Severity of onset and associated factors are very significant.* Had the *child been well* before the onset of stridor? Were there symptoms of an *upper respiratory infection* or *sore throat* before the onset? Abrupt onset of stridor with maximal distress from the beginning suggests foreign body aspiration. Rapidly progressive distress is characteristic of epiglottitis, whereas slow or "sputtering" progression is consistent with viral laryngotracheobronchitis.
2. Has the child had *similar problems* before? Congenital airway problems can lead to recurrent episodes of distress.
3. Has the child had *pain on swallowing*? Has the child been drooling? Supraglottic obstructions give rise to dysphagia. The child may drool to avoid swallowing.
4. Is there known or possible *foreign body aspiration* or exposure to *caustic agents*? Where the child was found and objectives of play or food being eaten are important areas to explore.
5. Has the child had a *cough* or *hoarseness*? A harsh, brassy cough, often described as a croupy cough, is suggestive of subglottic infection. Hoarseness results when there is interference with the precise, symmetric approximation of the vocal cords from a pathologic process in the larynx.
6. Has the child had a *fever*? What was the *temperature*? Although fever may be associated with any of the causes of stridor, high fever is more common with supraglottic infections.
7. Are the child's *immunizations* up to date? With aggressive immunization programs, diphtheria has practically disappeared. Sporadic resurgences do occur, however. With the introduction of an effective vaccine against *Haemophilus influenzae* type b, the incidence of all diseases caused by this organism has dropped dramatically.
8. The past medical history is explored to include
   a. Congenital conditions
   b. Current medications
   c. Known allergies
   d. Trauma history

Physical Examination

Initial Respiratory Assessment. The degree of respiratory distress is assessed as described under "Initial Approach and Stabilization." Parameters to be considered are respiratory rate, respiratory effort, skin color, and mental status.

Vital Signs. Respiratory rate, pulse rate, and temperature are obtained. In addition to initial measurements of pulse and respirations, the trend in these parameters is followed closely because they correlate with the child's improving or deteriorating respiratory status. One study comparing heart rate, respiratory rate, and degree of stridor with arterial blood gases in children with croup found that the respiratory rate was the best indicator of hypoxemia. Table 27–1 lists the normal respiratory rates by age group for comparison.

The temperature may be helpful in differentiating the causes of upper airway obstruction. A normal temperature is evidence, although not conclusive, against infectious causes. Foreign bodies of the upper airway are not associated with fever in the acute situation. Those that have passed the carina may present subacutely as atelectasis, infection, and fever. High fever and toxic appearance are highly suggestive of supraglottic infection in the child with stridor. Obtaining an oral or rectal temperature in this setting is contraindicated, but a tympanic temperature may be obtained if the procedure does not disturb the child.

Auscultation of the Chest. Breath sounds are assessed both in a quiet state and during crying, when this is possible. The forced air flow during crying may reveal abnormal sounds not appreciated when the child is quiet. In the infant, the nose may be the source of loud transmitted air flow sounds. Suctioning the nares will facilitate assessment of air flow in the rest of the upper airway, but suctioning is not attempted if epiglottitis is suspected.

Body Position. The position the child assumes can be quite characteristic for the type of obstruction. Patients with respiratory distress often prefer the upright position. Subglottic obstruction (as with viral laryngotracheobronchitis) is an exception because position has minimal effect on the airway in this area. These patients frequently remain recumbent.

Supraglottic obstructions are greatly affected by position. Children with retropharyngeal abscess often assume a position with their elbows on a table, head supported on their hands, and neck hyperextended. The classic position of the child with epiglottitis is sitting upright with an open mouth, chin forward, and head extended as in the anatomic "sniffing position," which maximizes air entry.

Visualization of the Pharynx and Epiglottis. Direct visualization of these structures may be considered in diagnosing the cause of a child's stridor. The cephalad position of the epiglottis in the infant makes its visualization much simpler than it is in the adult. Successful visualization, by simply asking the patient to open the mouth and shining a light in, has been reported in up to 80% of cases of epiglottitis. The tip of the erythematous, edematous epiglottis is seen in these circumstances. Sometimes the epiglottis cannot be visualized using that technique. Until recently, direct visualization of the hypopharynx and use of a tongue blade were thought to induce laryngospasm and bradycardia, leading to complete obstruction and cardiac arrest. Several studies have evaluated the safety of direct laryngoscopic visualization in children with suspected epiglottitis. They reported that direct laryngoscopic visualization, with care not to touch the epiglottis and hypopharynx, was uniformly safe. These series suggest children who are stable will usually tolerate careful laryngoscopy or application of a tongue blade to the mid or anterior tongue. As a rule, only clinicians who are comfortable with all aspects of pediatric airway management should perform these techniques. Equipment should be available to intervene if stridor worsens or laryngospasm occurs. In general, it is best to use these techniques in children with moderate or low suspicion of epiglottitis who are clinically stable. In patients with strongly suspected epiglottitis, instrumentation to improve visualization is not indicated.

In viral laryngotracheobronchitis, the mucous membranes are erythematous, with only slight edema, and the epiglottis, if visualized, is normal.

Foreign bodies may be seen, but an inability to visualize them directly does not rule out their presence.

A retropharyngeal abscess may be visualized as a midline or unilateral erythematous swelling in the posterior pharynx.

TABLE 27–1. Normal Afebrile Pediatric Respiratory Rates

Age	Rate (breaths per minute)
Neonate	35–65
1–6 mo	30–50
6–12 mo	30–50
1–2 yr	25–35
3–6 yr	20–25
7–12 yr	14–22
Over 12 yr	12–16

Palpation of the Neck. The cervical lymph nodes are frequently enlarged and tender in patients with a retropharyngeal abscess. Tenderness evoked by external pressure on the larynx is seen with epiglottitis in older children and adults. Cervical spine precautions must be maintained in the patient with stridor who has a suggested traumatic etiology.

Allergic Signs. Laryngeal edema and laryngospasm from allergies may present as stridor. Frequently, the finding develops rapidly. Other features such as a rash, hypotension, and wheezing should raise the suspicion that an allergic reaction is present.

CLINICAL REASONING

An initial differential diagnosis is developed by answering the following questions.

Is Stridor Present?

Stridor is differentiated from other airway sounds, such as wheezing or rhonchi, on physical examination. The presence of stridor points to upper airway obstruction.

If Stridor Is Present, Is Immediate Airway Management Necessary and Is the Obstruction Supraglottic or Subglottic?

Subglottic obstruction results in a harsh stridor and is frequently associated with a similarly harsh cough. Supraglottic obstruction results in a softer stridor, which is associated with a muffled voice and cough. Dysphagia may be a prominent associated finding.

Is the Most Likely Cause One of the Four Life-Threatening Diseases Requiring Immediate Intervention?

These are acute epiglottitis, croup (viral laryngotracheobronchitis), foreign body aspirations, and retropharyngeal abscess. Figure 27–2 gives a diagnostic approach to stridor, depending on the location of the obstruction and the propensity to develop complete obstruction. The four priority diagnoses are discussed later in this section.

Who Should Be Managing the Airway and What Techniques Should Be Used?

The most experienced physicians should be in charge of airway management decisions. Airway management techniques are discussed in Chapter 2, Airway Management.

Priority Diagnoses

Epiglottitis

Epiglottitis is especially important because the natural history of the disease is acute onset with rapid progression to respiratory compromise. The initial complaint is usually sore throat and pain on swallowing. This is accompanied by fever and an often toxic appearance. As the edema and infiltration of the supraglottic structures increase, muffling of the voice, low-pitched stridor, and drooling of saliva develop. At this point, the child typically assumes an upright posture, holding the neck extended and the jaw forward. These patients are usually apprehensive and fearful but sit quietly and give their full attention to holding the airway open and breathing. As the obstruction progresses, intercostal and supraclavicular retractions and use of accessory muscles are seen. The diagnosis is confirmed by direct or radiographic visualization of the edematous epiglottis.

Acute epiglottitis has diminished in frequency since 1990. With the introduction of an effective vaccine against *H. influenzae* type b, the incidence of all diseases due to this organism has dropped considerably. The average annual incidence of epiglottitis declined from 10.9 per 10,000 admissions before 1990 to 1.8 per 10,000 admissions from 1990 to 1992. Despite significant reduction in incidence because of immunization practices, epiglottitis remains a dangerous airway infection.

Viral Laryngotracheobronchitis (Croup)

Approximately 90% of children presenting with stridor have croup. It is the most common infectious cause of acute upper airway obstruction in pediatrics, accounting for approximately 20,000 hospital admissions per year. Croup is an infection of the subglottic trachea and, to a lesser extent, the bronchi by parainfluenza or respiratory syncytial viruses. It occurs in children younger than those affected by epiglottitis, most commonly between the ages of 6 months and 3 years. There is usually a preceding upper respiratory infection, and the child will have been ill for several days before the onset of stridor. Fever may be present but is usually low grade. Because of the tracheal involvement, there is hoarseness, and the subglottic obstruction results in a characteristic "barking cough" as well as the higher-pitched stridor. These children do not appear toxic and in spite of

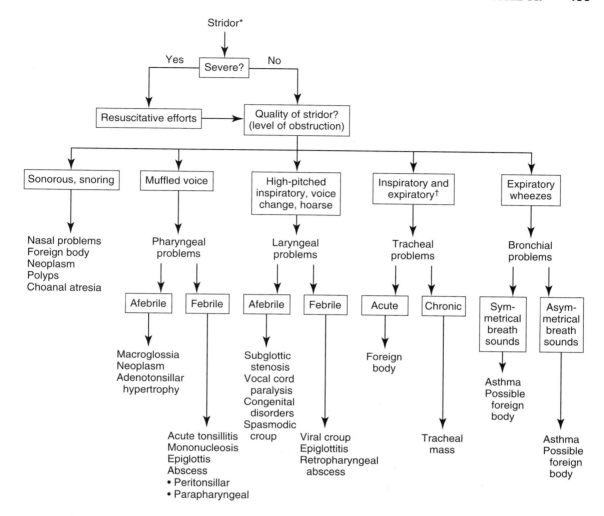

*The age of the patient must be considered in making a specific diagnosis.
†Laryngeal problems are quite frequently associated with inspiratory and expiratory stridor.

FIGURE 27–2 • Diagnostic approach to stridor. (Adapted from Handler SD: Stridor. In Fleisher GR, Ludwig S [eds]: Textbook of Pediatric Emergency Medicine. Baltimore, Williams & Wilkins, 1993, p 477, with permission.)

noisy respirations are often playful and active. Occasionally, croup can be very severe and can result in significant respiratory compromise. Croup scores (Table 27–2) have been developed to assist the physician in determining the degree of compromise and therefore the need for intervention.

Foreign Bodies

Sudden onset of stridor and respiratory distress with no antecedent or associated signs or symptoms suggests the potential of foreign-body aspiration or ingestion. This is the leading cause of home-related deaths in the United States for children younger than 6 years old, with 2000 deaths

occurring each year. It can occur in any age group but is most common in infants and younger children, who frequently put any object they encounter in their mouths. Fewer than 50% of children who have aspirated foreign bodies present within 24 hours of the initial aspiration. Generally, those with upper respiratory foreign bodies present more acutely than those with foreign bodies that have lodged in the lower respiratory tract.

Large foreign bodies are most likely to lodge in the supraglottic area or to enter the esophagus, where they may result in compression of the posterior tracheal wall. Complete obstruction may result. Smaller foreign bodies may pass through the glottis and come to lie in the trachea

TABLE 27–2. Croup Score

	0	1	2	3
Stridor	None	Mild	Moderate at rest	Severe on inspiration and expiration
Retraction	None	Mild	Moderate	Severe
Air entry	Normal	Mild decrease	Moderate	Marked decrease
Color	Normal	Normal (0 score)	Normal (0 score)	Dusky, cyanotic
Level of consciousness	Normal	Restless when disturbed	Anxious, agitated, restless when disturbed	Lethargic, depressed

Score: 4–5 mild, 5–6 mild-moderate, 8 severe (or any sign of severity).
From Davis HW, et al: Acute upper airway obstruction, croup, and epiglottitis. Pediatr Clin North Am 1981; 28:4.

(Fig. 27–3) or may pass into the bronchi. The child may be in marked distress and unable to speak in the former situation but may be surprisingly asymptomatic in the latter. Bronchial foreign bodies may exist for some time before they cause symptoms and may be diagnosed in the setting of unilateral atelectasis, hyperinflation, or pneumonia.

Retropharyngeal Abscess

Retropharyngeal abscess usually develops as an extension of a pharyngeal infection. However,

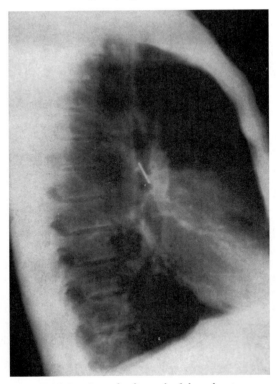

FIGURE 27–3 • Lateral radiograph of chest showing aspirated coin in tracheal air column. (From Pons P: Foreign bodies. In Rosen P, et al [eds]: Emergency Medicine: Concepts and Clinical Practice, 2nd ed. St. Louis, CV Mosby, 1988.)

penetrating trauma, iatrogenic instrumentation, and foreign bodies are other important causes. These are usually mixed aerobic and anaerobic infections, with group A streptococci predominating. This infection occurs most frequently in very young children (younger than the age of 1 year and almost always before age 6) before atrophy of retropharyngeal lymph nodes.

Sore throat and fever have usually been present for a few days, with eventual seeding of the retropharyngeal lymph nodes by bacteria. Early on, midline or unilateral swelling of the posterior pharynx is present. With the spread of the bacterial infection an abscess forms, and children develop fever, stridor, drooling, and respiratory distress. The presentation is similar to that of epiglottitis except for a slower progression of disease and a younger age group. The cervical lymph nodes are usually tender and enlarged.

Other than airway obstruction, complications include aspiration if the abscess ruptures, mediastinitis if it dissects into the mediastinum, and sudden death if the abscess erodes into vascular structures.

DIAGNOSTIC ADJUNCTS

If the specific diagnosis is not clear, laboratory and radiographic evaluations are used to further refine the differential diagnosis. Radiographic visualization of the upper airway is the most useful adjunct after the history and physical examination.

Radiologic Imaging

Soft tissue *neck radiographs* in the stridorous child are not always necessary. When the diagnosis is unclear, they can be very helpful. At no time should a stridorous child be sent to the radiology department unattended. The safest alternative is a portable upright film taken in the emergency department. An appropriate lateral film of the soft tissue of the neck requires that the film be obtained with the child's neck extended during the terminal phase of inspiration. Poor extension of the neck during these films causes a "bunching up" of the pharyngeal soft tissue that often is mistaken for a retropharyngeal mass or abscess.

In patients with epiglottitis, the lateral neck film demonstrates the enlarged epiglottis, thickened aryepiglottic folds, and ballooning of the hypopharynx (Fig. 27–4). These findings may not be obvious in all cases of pediatric epiglottitis. As many as 70% of all children with epiglottitis have radiographs that were initially read as negative by the radiologist.

In patients with viral laryngotracheobronchitis, radiography is usually unnecessary. The lateral view is usually normal. An anteroposterior view may reveal subglottic narrowing. The trachea in this view has been described as having the appearance of a steeple. Radiographs are indicated when there is no response to the standard management of croup, when a patient's symptoms worsen, for recurrent or persistent stridor, or for a clinical presentation of laryngotracheobronchitis during an atypical time of the year.

Retropharyngeal abscess is a difficult diagnosis clinically. To confirm a clinical suspicion of retropharyngeal abscess, the initial diagnostic study is a lateral radiograph of the soft tissue of the neck, with the neck in extension. A bulging in the posterior pharynx is highly suggestive of retropharyngeal abscess, but there is abundant prevertebral soft tissue in the child and this tissue is even more prominent during expiration. If the radiograph appears normal and an abscess is highly suggested, computed tomography of the neck is definitive in establishing the diagnosis. The diagnosis is made when the width of the retropharyngeal space at the level of the second cervical vertebra is twice the diameter of the vertebral body. This criterion has a 90% sensitivity.

Foreign bodies may be radiopaque and easily visualized (see Fig. 27–3) or radiolucent and give rise only to secondary changes that suggest their presence. In addition to tracheal foreign bodies, esophageal foreign bodies can produce respiratory compromise by compressing the posterior tracheal wall. When a foreign body is suspected, lateral and anteroposterior views of the neck and chest are obtained. If the films are negative, then inspiration and expiration films should be obtained. If the child cannot or will not cooperate for these views, right and left lateral decubitus views can be obtained, to search for the phenomenon of air trapping. The patient's condition determines when and where these radiographs are taken.

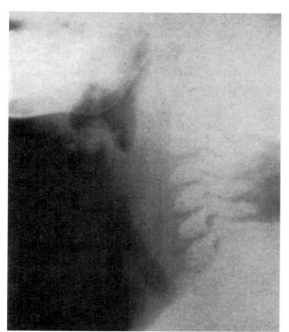 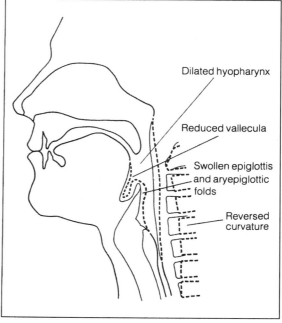

FIGURE 27–4 • The classic "thumb sign" of an edematous epiglottis is evident in this lateral neck film. The schematic illustrates the findings to look for in a lateral film in a patient with suspected epiglottitis. Such films are superfluous in a child with the classic history, signs, and symptoms of epiglottitis; they can be of tremendous help, however, in the diagnosis of mild or questionable cases—particularly when explaining to parents the need for aggressive treatment. (From Ashenoft C, Steele R: Epiglottitis. J Respir Dis 1998; 9:31.)

Laboratory Studies

Laboratory tests may be supportive of a specific diagnosis or can be used to evaluate the patient's clinical status and progress during treatment. Specimens are not obtained from the stridulous child until airway control is ensured.

Arterial or Capillary Blood Gas Analysis. Arterial or capillary blood gases are not indicated early in the evaluation of patients with upper airway obstruction because the trauma of obtaining the specimen can precipitate struggling and further airway compromise. Furthermore, in this situation, the initial diagnosis of respiratory failure is made on clinical grounds. In severe cases and after initial diagnosis and management, blood gas analysis may be used to follow the patient's respiratory status.

Complete Blood Cell Count and Differential. A complete blood cell count may be useful in supporting the diagnosis made on clinical and radiographic grounds. A high white blood cell count with a shift to the left is consistent with a diagnosis of bacterial infection, such as epiglottitis or bacterial tracheitis. The white blood cell count with croup and foreign bodies is usually normal.

Cultures. Specimens of blood or purulent drainage from the site of infection are obtained for culture. In children with epiglottitis, blood cultures may be positive for *H. influenzae*. In patients with retropharyngeal abscess, cultures of blood, posterior pharyngeal secretions, or abscess are obtained. Both aerobic and anaerobic organisms are sought.

Special Tests

Pulse oximetry and capnography have been evaluated as tools for assessing the severity of a child's stridor. Pulse oximetry is a noninvasive tool for monitoring hypoxemia in the setting of upper airway obstruction. It should be routinely obtained on all children with stridor, except if it is disturbing to the patient with possible epiglottitis. Capnometry, the measurement of exhaled end-tidal carbon dioxide levels, has emerged as a noninvasive measure of cardiopulmonary circulation. Whereas hypoxia signifies fatigue and impending airway obstruction, hypercarbia (detected by capnometry) has been found to be an earlier predictor of clinical deterioration and the need for intubation in children admitted to an intensive care unit.

EXPANDED DIFFERENTIAL DIAGNOSIS

Once the initial assessment, clinical examination, stabilization, and response to therapy information is evaluated, the physician takes into consideration the four preliminary diagnoses and selects the most likely specific diagnosis. Specific management for that problem is started.

Table 27–3 and Figure 27–2 list less common causes of upper airway obstruction that are considered when the presentation is atypical and the diagnosis remains unclear.

PRINCIPLES OF MANAGEMENT

General Principles

The therapeutic approach to the pediatric patient with upper airway obstruction will vary depending on the precise cause. The therapeutic principles that may apply depend on the specific cause and include the following:

1. Mechanical maintenance of an open airway
2. Provision of an enriched oxygen content for inhalation
3. Provision of humidified oxygen or mist for inhalation
4. Vasoconstriction and bronchodilatation through inhaled racemic or L-isomer epinephrine
5. Early antimicrobial therapy for suspected infectious causes
6. Endoscopic removal of foreign bodies

Specific Principles

Each of the four most common and priority causes has specific therapies.

Epiglottitis

The diagnosis of epiglottitis is confirmed by direct or radiographic visualization. When the diagnosis is clinically evident and the patient is maintaining air flow, the recommended approach

---

TABLE 27–3. Uncommon Causes of Upper Airway Obstruction in Children

Congenital anomalies	Trauma
Vascular ring	Blunt laryngeal
Tracheoesophageal fistula	Penetrating neck
Tracheal web	Ingestions
Tumors	Caustics
Subglottic hemangioma	Chemical fumes
Infections	Smoke inhalation
Bacterial tracheitis	Allergic laryngeal edema
Mononucleosis	
Cervical osteomyelitis	
Tetanus	
Botulism	
Diphtheria	

is direct visualization by an anesthesiologist in the operating room. Optimally, a team, which may include a senior pediatrician, the emergency physician, an anesthesiologist, otolaryngologist, and general surgeon, is quickly mobilized. After visual confirmation of the diagnosis, endotracheal intubation is attempted. If this is unsuccessful, an attending otolaryngologist performs a tracheostomy. Once the supraglottic obstruction is bypassed by either of these techniques, the patient is usually able to ventilate adequately. Sedation and restraints are necessary to prevent the patient from accidentally or intentionally removing the tube.

Once the airway is secured, blood cultures are obtained and intravenous antibiotics are administered. These should be effective against *H. influenzae* type b and other common organisms that cause epiglottitis. Second- and third-generation cephalosporins, specifically cefuroxime, ceftriaxone, and cefotaxime, have emerged as the antibiotics of choice for treatment of acute epiglottitis. These agents have a wide therapeutic to toxic ratio, do not require monitoring of serum drug levels, and are useful particularly for patients allergic to penicillin.

Corticosteroid therapy is used by some, but there is no conclusive evidence of its benefit in epiglottitis.

When the diagnosis is less evident, radiologic visualization of the epiglottis is performed. Once the diagnosis is confirmed, the protocol just outlined is again recommended. All children with epiglottitis require intubation under controlled circumstances to prevent sudden airway obstruction. In the past, children who were expectantly managed without intubation in intensive care units had a mortality rate greater than 5%. In contrast, mortality in intubated children is less than 1%.

Viral Laryngotracheobronchitis (Croup)

The management of viral croup is guided by the use of a clinical croup score like the one outlined in Table 27–2.

- Patients with croup scores less than 6: Humidified oxygen/mist therapy.
- Patients with croup scores of 7 to 8: Humidified oxygen/mist therapy, racemic epinephrine.
- Patients with croup scores of more than 8: Racemic epinephrine; intubation is considered.

An experienced clinician's evaluation may be more accurate than any scoring system for evaluating the degree of airway compromise. Features suggestive of impending airway obstruction have

been identified, including age younger than 6 months, stridor at rest, cyanosis, decreased level of consciousness, hypoxia, and hypercarbia. Humidified mist (air or oxygen) is the mainstay of treatment of croup. Theoretically, the benefits are derived from providing moisture to the inflamed mucosa, preventing drying and crusting, and increased mobilization of secretions. This may be achieved at home or in the emergency department using a cool mist humidifier. Humidified oxygen is used in more severely ill children to improve hypoxemia. Croup tents are effective in this respect but restrict observation of the patient. For this reason, their use is limited.

Adequate hydration is necessary to loosen inspissated secretions. It is best accomplished orally, with parental assistance. Intravenous fluids become necessary in the very ill child if oral hydration is not possible.

Fever control with acetaminophen or ibuprofen provides comfort and reduces metabolic rate and oxygen consumption.

Aerosolized racemic epinephrine has been demonstrated to be beneficial in the treatment of croup. Its effects result from vasoconstriction of the subglottic mucosa and submucosal capillaries and bronchodilator actions in the smooth muscle of the lower respiratory tract. It is indicated in moderate and severe croup exacerbations and/or stridor at rest. Racemic epinephrine is composed of equal amounts of D- and L-isomers of epinephrine. The L-form is essentially the only active isomer in the racemic mixture. Direct comparisons of racemic epinephrine to an equal amount of the L-isomer have shown no differences in outcome for the treatment of croup, including croup scores, side effects, heart rate, blood pressure, and respiratory rate. Racemic epinephrine is not available as a pharmacologic preparation in many other countries, nor in some general hospitals in the United States that predominantly treat adults. The L-form is less expensive, is more readily available, and does not carry the risk of additional adverse effects.

Racemic epinephrine is administered by diluting 0.5 mL (2% solution) in 2.5 mL of sterile water or saline and delivering this mixture by nebulizer. The administered dose for the L-isomer is 0.25 mL of the 1:1000 solution for children younger than 6 months and 5 mL of the 1:1000 concentration for older children (both prediluted with normal saline). Although treatment with racemic epinephrine has not been shown to alter the natural course of the disease, it is a temporizing intervention that offers relief from acute respiratory distress and may decrease the need for an artificial airway.

The half-life of epinephrine is only 1 to 2 hours. Within 2 hours of treatment patients may return to a croup score equivalent to that on presentation. This is an infrequent occurrence. Based on these data the general practice has been to observe any child who received racemic epinephrine as therapy for croup for 2 to 3 hours. After observation, most children may be discharged, if improvement has been sustained.

The efficacy of corticosteroids in the treatment of croup has been demonstrated. Dexamethasone sodium phosphate (Decadron) has been the corticosteroid most frequently studied in the management of croup. It is quickly absorbed when given orally or intramuscularly, achieving high plasma levels within 15 minutes. Its relative anti-inflammatory potency is 25 times that of hydrocortisone. Its half-life varies from 36 to 72 hours so that a single dose may be all that is required to get the patient past the initial severity stage.

A meta-analysis including over 1200 children with croup from 10 studies found that intramuscular dexamethasone (0.6 mg/kg) decreased croup scores and intubation rates in admitted children. More recently, another study demonstrated that the use of dexamethasone in the outpatient management of moderately severe croup was associated with a reduction in severity of illness within 24 hours after treatment. There is no experimental evidence demonstrating one formulation of corticosteroid is superior to another. Corticosteroids are absorbed similarly whether they are given parenterally or by mouth. Nebulized steroids have demonstrated no clinical advantage, and administration my be upsetting to the child. No study investigating the role of corticosteroids in the management of croup has reported adverse effects from their use. The efficacy of corticosteroids in mildly ill children who do not require aerosolized epinephrine treatment remains unanswered.

Several studies (retrospective and prospective) have concluded that selected children presenting with croup and significant distress may be effectively treated with racemic epinephrine and corticosteroids. They can be safely discharged home if after being observed for 2 to 3 hours they do not have stridor or retractions, have reliable caregivers, and have access to appropriate follow-up care.

Foreign Bodies

A patient with a partial obstruction from a foreign body is allowed initially to maintain a clear airway by coughing while preparations for possible intubation, bronchoscopy, and tracheostomy are made. If this is not effective or if the patient's condition is deteriorating, abdominal thrusts are recommended in the adult and older child. In smaller children and infants, a combination of back blows and chest thrusts is recommended. If this is unsuccessful, direct laryngoscopy with removal of visualized foreign bodies using Magill forceps is recommended. For subglottic foreign bodies, bronchoscopy is necessary for removal.

Esophageal foreign bodies may result in airway obstruction by compressing the posterior tracheal wall. Endoscopy is the preferred technique for their removal.

Retropharyngeal Abscess

For the unstable child with significant respiratory distress or altered mental status, diagnostic studies are deferred until the child's airway has been secured. Once the airway is secured and the diagnosis has been confirmed, intravenous antibiotic selection should include coverage for β-lactamase–producing organisms, gram-negative rods, and anaerobes. This combination will frequently involve clindamycin and a third-generation cephalosporin or nafcillin and a third-generation cephalosporin.

Consultation with an otolaryngologist is obtained to evaluate the need for surgical drainage of the abscess. Although surgical drainage is the mainstay of treatment, its role has been challenged by reports of therapeutic success without incision and drainage.

Elective intubation for stable children with a patent airway is not recommended, unless there is going to be a prolonged interhospital transport.

UNCERTAIN DIAGNOSIS

If after the initial assessment and stabilization, clinical evaluation, radiographs, and laboratory results the diagnosis remains uncertain, the patient can be further observed while a consultation with a pediatrician is obtained.

SPECIAL CONSIDERATIONS
Infants Younger than 2 Years of Age

In infants younger than 2 years of age, the "classic presentation" of epiglottitis is not seen. The progression of the disease in infants is not as rapid as that in older children, and frequently an upper respiratory infection has preceded it. Recumbency does not seem to produce the expected increase in respiratory obstruction, and drooling is rarely noted. A harsh cough may be present, making differentiation from croup even more difficult.

Infants with retropharyngeal abscess have a presentation similar to that of the infant with epiglottitis except for a slower progression of the disease, a younger age group, and a tendency to lie on the side with the neck hyperextended.

Older Children and Adults

With the introduction of the vaccine for *H. influenzae* type b, patients with epiglottitis tend to have disease caused by organisms other than *H. influenzae* type b (particularly group A β-hemolytic *Streptococcus*) and tend to be older (the median age has risen to 7 years), with adolescents, teenagers, and even adults more frequently affected.

DISPOSITION AND FOLLOW-UP

Immediate Consultation

It is the recommendation for the child with clinically evident epiglottitis to confirm the diagnosis, secure the airway, and start antibiotic therapy. It is also the recommendation for a child with subglottic or esophageal foreign bodies that have caused complete airway obstruction or require removal to avoid complete airway obstruction.

Admission

The following patients are admitted to a general pediatric floor for treatment or observation:

1. Children with viral laryngotracheobronchitis who show initial improvement after epinephrine administration but have recurrent stridor or obstruction during the 2- to 3-hour observation period
2. Children with dehydration and inability to keep down fluids
3. Children who live far from the hospital or who have unreliable caregivers
4. Children from whom a foreign body has been removed when observation is indicated
5. Children with retropharyngeal abscess after drainage

The following patients are admitted for monitoring in the intensive care unit:

1. Children with epiglottitis after intubation and all children with a toxic appearance
2. Those with viral laryngotracheobronchitis who do not respond to treatment with racemic epinephrine

3. Children with a foreign body before its removal
4. Children with retropharyngeal abscess before drainage

Discharge

The following patients may be discharged with close follow-up by their pediatrician or other primary care physician:

1. Those with viral laryngotracheobronchitis who respond to mist therapy alone.
2. Those with moderate croup who respond to nebulized epinephrine and corticosteroids in the emergency department and do not have recurrent stridor or rebound obstruction after 2 to 3 hours of observation. Data from one study shows that in addition to the psychosocial benefits of not hospitalizing all patients presenting with croup who receive nebulized racemic epinephrine, there are also economic benefits. Only 1 day of hospitalization for croup was $1,115.00. When extrapolated to the nation as a whole and to current health care costs, the cost benefit would be enormous.
3. Those with foreign body with uncomplicated removal.

On discharge, the parents are instructed in the use of humidification at home, if this is appropriate, and are given criteria for determining the need to return to the emergency department. Close observation for recurrence of respiratory distress is essential; and if the parents give any indication of inability to provide close monitoring, admission is recommended.

FINAL POINTS

- Stridor is a high-pitched, raspy sound made as air passes through a partially obstructed airway.
- The pediatric airway is particularly susceptible to obstruction because of its small diameter and flexibility. Resistance to air flow is inversely proportional to the fourth power of the radius of the airway. Therefore, small decreases in airway diameter greatly increase air flow resistance.
- Infection is the most common cause of upper airway obstruction in the pediatric age group. Viral laryngotracheobronchitis and epiglottitis account for 95% of cases.
- The onset and rapidity of progression of symptoms and the prodromal and associated symptoms will help to differentiate the cause of the obstruction.

- When supraglottic obstruction is strongly suspected, the patient is not disturbed and is allowed to stay upright. If instrumentation is considered, the physician must be prepared to secure the airway by endotracheal intubation; if that is unsuccessful, needle cricothyroidotomy is done.
- When viral laryngotracheobronchitis is treated with racemic epinephrine, improvement may be temporary; recurrence of obstruction after 2 to 3 hours may occur.
- An alert patient with a partially obstructed airway is allowed to continue to try to clear the airway by coughing before attempts are made to remove a foreign body.
- Early oral or parenteral corticosteroid therapy has a demonstrated benefit to laryngotracheobronchitis.

CASE *Study*

A 3-year-old boy was well until he awoke from sleep at 3 AM with a high fever. His mother brought him to the emergency department because he was unable to lie down, had noisy respirations, and was drooling saliva.

On arrival, the child was sitting upright with his neck extended and his head held forward. Saliva was drooling from his mouth, and he had quiet, muffled speech and a low-pitched stridor. He was alert and had good skin color, a respiratory rate of 30 breaths per minute, and a heart rate of 140 beats per minute. The patient was brought into the acute care area and the physician was notified.

Observation of the patient on arrival to the emergency department is a very important aspect of the initial evaluation that is often overlooked. Without threatening the patient, the physician can notice if the patient looks toxic, the degree of respiratory distress, and if there is a potential for rapid deterioration and a need for emergent airway management.

Stabilization is essential while evaluating the respiratory system. Oxygen is administered by blow-by technique while the child is allowed to sit on his mother's lap. The rate, depth, and pattern of respirations are noted, and evidence of fatigue is sought. The child is observed for anxiety, altered level of consciousness, position of comfort, and any abnormal chest configuration or retractions. In the small child, "head bobbing" with each breath is suggestive of severe distress.

The presence of stridor is a clue to the presence of partial upper airway obstruction. This distinction narrows the diagnostic possibilities significantly. Dysphagia and drooling may coexist with stridor and if present are suggestive of epiglottitis, peritonsillar abscess, retropharyngeal abscess or hematoma, foreign body aspiration, or diphtheria.

This presentation is consistent with a supraglottic obstruction, and complete obstruction is possible at any time. The staff is instructed not to lay the child down or disturb him in any way.

No further pertinent history was obtained. Physical examination was limited to observation of the child's general appearance and respiratory status. The temperature, obtained tympanically, was 104°F (40°C). The emergency physician attempted to visualize the epiglottis by asking the child to open his mouth wide, but nothing was seen.

The guiding principle in the initial approach to the stridulous child is to avoid disturbing or upsetting the child. In most children with partial airway obstruction, particularly epiglottitis, the child is usually anxious but quietly concentrating on maintaining an open airway and breathing. Any disturbance can lead to marked worsening of this condition, even to inducing complete airway obstruction. Manipulation of the upper airway to confirm the diagnosis is unnecessary.

Oximetry is a useful, relatively noninvasive way to estimate oxygenation but should be used only if it does not disturb the patient. No venous or arterial punctures or radiographs are done that will dangerously delay definitive intervention.

While the operating room team and other consultants are being assembled, the emergency physician should be prepared for emergent airway stabilization by having available the following equipment:

- *Bag-valve-mask (adult size) connected to oxygen*
- *Endotracheal tube with stylet*
- *Cricothyroidotomy set*

This patient was transported to the operating room, where an anesthesiologist and an otolaryngologist were standing by. The anesthesiologist visualized the epiglottis by direct laryngoscopy. It was fiery red and markedly swollen. The tissue was so swollen that the glottic opening could not be identified. Pressure on the chest caused some egress of air through this swollen tissue, but an attempt at intubation was unsuccessful. A tracheostomy was rapidly performed, and the patient was ventilated.

Even under the most controlled circumstances, intubation in the setting of epiglottitis may be very difficult. It is not attempted in the emergency department unless necessitated by patient decompensation.

After tracheostomy, intravenous antibiotics were administered and the child was transported to the intensive care unit.

Each hospital and emergency department must have a preplanned protocol for the management of patients with acute airway obstruction, taking into account available personnel, their skills, and facilities.

Bibliography

TEXT

Fleisher GR, Ludwig S: Textbook of Pediatric Emergency Medicine, 4th ed. Baltimore, Williams & Wilkins, 2000.

JOURNAL ARTICLES

Ausejo M, Saenz A, Pham B, et al: Glucocorticoids for croup (Cochrane Review). In: Cochrane Library, Issue 2. Oxford, Update Software, 2000.

Bank DE, Krug SE: New approaches to upper airway disease. Emerg Med Clin North Am 1995; 13:473–478.

Cressman W, Myer C: Diagnosis and management of croup and epiglottitis. Pediatr Clin North Am 1994; 41:265–276.

Cruz MN, Stewart G, Rosenberg N: Use of dexamethasone in the outpatient management of acute laryngotracheitis. Pediatrics 1995; 96:220–223.

DeLorenzo R, Singer J, Matre W: Retropharyngeal abscess in an afebrile child. Am J Emerg Med 1993; 11:151–154.

Kairys SW, Olmstead EM, O'Conner GT: Steroid treatment of laryngotracheitis: A meta-analysis of the evidence from randomized trials. Pediatrics 1989; 83:683–693.

Ledwith C, Shea L, Mauro RD: Safety and efficacy of nebulized racemic epinephrine in conjunction with oral dexamethasone and mist in the outpatient treatment of croup. Ann Emerg Med 1995; 25:331–337.

Mancker AJ, Petrak EM, Krug SE: Contribution of routine pulse oximetry to evaluation and management of patients with respiratory illness in a pediatric emergency department. Ann Emerg Med 1995; 25:36–40.

Nagy M, Backstron J: Comparison of the sensitivity of lateral neck radiographs and computed tomography scanning in pediatric deep-neck infections. Laryngoscope 1999; 109:775–779.

Pendergast M, Jones JS, Hartman D: Racemic epinephrine in the treatment of laryngotracheitis: Can we identify children for outpatient therapy? Am J Emerg Med 1994; 12:613–616.

Santamaria JP, Schafermeyer R: Stridor: A review. Pediatr Emerg Care 1992; 8:229–234.

CHAPTER 28

Dehydration

WILLIAM AHRENS
JONATHAN I. SINGER

CASE *Study*

A 3-month-old boy is brought to the emergency department by his parents with a history of 2 days of vomiting and diarrhea. They note he is less active than usual and is beginning to refuse to take his bottle.

INTRODUCTION

Fluid balance is maintained if oral intake of water and electrolytes is sufficient to replace ongoing insensible (respiration, sweat), urinary, and any additional losses. In childhood, many diseases may diminish or interrupt normal fluid intake. Others cause abnormal fluid losses from the skin, respiratory tract, gastrointestinal tract, and urinary system.

Dehydration is one of the most common medical conditions affecting children. The majority of cases are mild and easily managed on an outpatient basis. Moderate dehydration, which may require an observation room or inpatient care, is commonly encountered in the United States during winter epidemics of viral gastroenteritis. Severe dehydration is a relatively rare occurrence in the United States but is the leading cause of infant mortality worldwide, accounting for the deaths of approximately 5 million infants a year. Severely dehydrated children die as a result of diminished delivery of oxygen and energy substrate to the brain, heart, and kidneys.

Pediatric patients are much more likely to suffer morbidity and mortality from dehydration than are adult patients. This is partly because they are more commonly afflicted with diarrheal illnesses. However, differences in physiology, especially in the first year of life, account for much of the increased vulnerability to the loss of fluids and electrolytes.

The daily turnover of free water in an infant may be three to four times that of an adult. There is a direct correlation among metabolic rate, caloric requirements, and free water requirements. The high caloric demand of a growing infant necessitates a substantial amount of free water. This physiology can account for the increased vulnerability to fluid and electrolyte loss in infants and children. In addition, infants have increased free water insensible loss from their skin and respiratory tract and have less ability to concentrate urine. They lose a greater volume of water with excreted waste products. Infants have a proportionately greater amount of body water contained in the intravascular space than adults. This makes them vulnerable to vascular collapse when challenged by an acute loss of a large amount of fluid.

The presentation of dehydration varies depending on the relative loss of water and sodium. When there is a proportionate loss of both water and sodium, the serum sodium level remains in the normal range and the result is *isotonic dehydration*. This is the most common form of dehydration, occurring in 70% to 80% of dehydrated children. *Hypertonic dehydration* (Na > 145 mEq/L) occurs when there is a greater loss of water than of sodium or when isotonic dehydration is treated with high-sodium replacement fluids such as chicken soup. This form occurs in 10% to 15% of dehydrated children and is more common in children younger than the age of 6 months. The hypertonic serum results in fluid shifts out of the cells. Intracellular dehydration is poorly tolerated by the brain, and lethargy, coma, or seizures frequently result. *Hypotonic dehydration* (Na < 130 mEq/L) occurs when there is a greater loss of sodium than of water or when hypotonic fluids such as water are used exclusively for rehydration. Seizures and cardiovascular collapse are early and prominent features of hypotonic dehydration.

INITIAL APPROACH AND STABILIZATION
Priority Diagnoses

Burns, hyperglycemia, febrile states, illnesses associated with increased respiratory rates, and gastrointestinal derangements associated with vomiting or diarrhea cause abnormal fluid losses, leading to dehydration. Gastroenteritis is by far the most common cause. Viral agents (usually a rotavirus) are the most frequent offenders. Bacteria are the second leading cause, with the usual agents being *Shigella, Salmonella, Escherichia coli, Yersinia enterocolitica,* and *Campylobacter fetus.*

Rapid Assessment

The most important aspect of the initial approach is to assess cardiovascular stability and resuscitate unstable patients. Children brought to the emergency department with complaints of vomiting, diarrhea, and poor oral intake are immediately assessed with regard to the adequacy of respiratory, circulatory, and central nervous system function. Unless other problems coexist, the *airway* and the *ventilatory status* are usually adequate. Physical assessment of the patient's *circulation* is done by noting the following signs:

- *Skin signs*
  - Decreased capillary refill
  - Pallor or cyanosis
  - Mottling
  - Decreased turgor
- *Head, eyes, ears, nose, and throat signs*
  - Depressed fontanelle
  - Absence of tears
  - Dry mucous membranes
  - Soft, sunken eyeballs
- *Vital signs*
  - Tachycardia
  - Tachypnea
  - Hypotension

The *rapid neurologic assessment* includes assessment of responsiveness, which may be graded as alert and interactive, lethargic or poorly interactive, responsive only to pain, or unresponsive. Seizures may be focal or generalized.

Early Intervention

Mild dehydration, evidenced by normal vital signs and minimal evidence of dehydration, such as decreased tearing and dry mucous membranes, does not require immediate intervention.

More severely dehydrated children, who present with signs of hypovolemia (tachycardia) or mental status changes, will benefit from immediate fluid administration.

Vascular Access. Establishment of a peripheral line is attempted. In severe dehydration, if this is unsuccessful in 2 to 3 minutes or with two attempts, an intraosseous infusion is used.

Fluid Administration. Patients who are severely volume depleted are given a bolus infusion as rapidly as possible of 20 mL/kg of isotonic crystalloid solution. Such an infusion may be carried out even if the pulse and blood pressure are normal for age. A second bolus is required if the patient remains in shock. On occasion, 60 to 80 mL/kg may be required to restore perfusion. Early shock may be difficult to detect in young infants. Any suspicions should be responded to with an initial fluid bolus.

Patients who have dehydration combined with seizures, marked lethargy, or coma may have a hypertonic form of dehydration. Initial treatment is the same, but subsequently slow rehydration with gradual return of the serum sodium concentration to normal is undertaken. Too rapid a drop in serum sodium level can result in cerebral edema and seizures. Seizures are treated with diazepam if they are persistent or recurrent. The airway and the ventilatory status are carefully monitored, and endotracheal intubation is accomplished if the respiratory status is marginal or inadequate.

CLINICAL ASSESSMENT

In a patient with an adequate airway, ventilation, circulatory status, and vital signs, evaluative procedures can precede therapeutic interventions.

History

The history is directed toward determining the kind and amount of fluid loss, the kind and amount of fluid administered to correct the loss, the cause of the fluid loss, and the patient's usual state of health.

1. *When* did the child *become sick?* The duration of illness is important because it represents the opportunity for greater fluid loss.
2. *How much vomiting* or *diarrhea* has occurred? What do these *fluids look like?* Stool consistency and odor as well as the presence of mucus or blood are noted. Emesis is examined for color and content, especially blood.
3. Is the child *tolerating oral fluid?* What *oral fluids* have been *given* and in what *amounts?* Feeding without vomiting suggests less potential for severe dehydration. High-solute fluids (boiled milk, soups) and low-solute fluids (gelatin or water, colas) can lead to hypernatremia and hyponatremia, respectively.
4. *When* did the child *last urinate* or have a *wet diaper?* Decreased frequency of urination is highly suggestive of significant dehydration.
5. Has the child had a *fever?*
6. Has the child been *unusually sleepy* or *poorly responsive?* Behavioral changes are important

to assess. Interaction and emotion reflect the final clinical impact area of fluid loss.

7. Are there *other children* at home, in school, or in day care with *similar problems*? If others are asymptomatic, did this child eat anything different from the others? Viral, bacterial, and protozoan enteric organisms can be transmitted through contaminated food, water, or direct contact with fecal material. Person-to-person transfer is quite prevalent in day-care centers. Enteric disease is commonly found in other family members.

8. Does the child have *preexisting medical problems*? Endocrine, metabolic, and renal diseases are particularly pertinent in assessing the cause of dehydration. Recent antibiotic use arouses suspicion of pseudomembranous colitis as a cause for diarrhea. Acute or chronic use of salicylates, acetaminophen, or nonsteroidal anti-inflammatory drugs should be considered in acidotic, dehydrated patients. Infants with cystic fibrosis are at greater risk for insensible losses. Inquiries about preexisting disease states should include queries on prior hospitalizations and pertinent family history.

9. *When* was the *last time* the child was *weighed* and *what was* the *weight*? Comparing the premorbid weight with the present weight is the best way of estimating the degree of dehydration.
   - Previous weight – current weight = weight loss (in kilograms).
   - Percent of weight loss = fraction of weight loss × 100.
   - Current weight (in kilograms) × fraction of weight loss = fluid deficit (in liters).
   - An alternative calculation can be used based on the total body water (TBW): TBW = 0.6 × weight (in kilograms).
   - Fluid deficit = (premorbid weight – morbid weight) × 0.6.

Physical Examination

The physical examination allows the physician to

- Estimate the magnitude and type of fluid and electrolyte imbalance that is present.
- Focus on systemic toxicity associated with dehydration.
- Confirm the history in seeking specific potential disease processes.

A complete examination is performed. Emphasis is placed on the following areas.

Vital Signs. Supine pulse and blood pressure measurements are traditionally recorded. Orthostatic vital signs are of limited usefulness in pediatric patients, because typical changes may be absent in dehydration. Also, normovolemic children may have an increase of 30 to 40 beats per minute on standing and variable blood pressure changes. Tachycardia is consistently found in patients with significant dehydration, but hypotension is usually a late finding, occurring only after the child's marked capacity for compensation is exhausted. With hypotonic dehydration, hypotension occurs earlier and is more prominent.

An accurate measure of the respiratory rate is necessary in that substantial water loss can occur through the lungs during marked hyperventilation. Deep Kussmaul ventilations suggest metabolic acidosis.

Elevated temperature also increases the insensible loss of fluid through the skin. Water requirements increase by 7 mL/kg/24 hr for each degree of temperature elevation beyond 99°F (37.2°C) measured rectally.

The child's current weight is obtained. If there is a known previous weight, this is obtained in comparable clothing.

Hydration Status. The physical examination is instrumental in assessing the status of hydration regardless of the cause of dehydration. Signs and symptoms of dehydration result from extracellular volume depletion. When interstitial fluid is depleted, there may be loss of skin elasticity, with tenting and altered skin turgor (doughy or rubbery skin with hypernatremia), reduction of retro-orbital tissue fluid (creating sunken eyeballs), and intraocular fluid (causing soft eyeballs) or reduction of cerebrospinal fluid volume, manifested by a flattened fontanelle. Dehydrated patients also have depressed tear formation, thickening of saliva, and drying of mucous membranes.

Intravascular volume depletion leads to reduction in urine volume and peripheral vasoconstriction, with cold, mottled, and poorly perfused skin. A limited indicator of hydration status in children is the capillary refill time. After 5 seconds of cutaneous pressure or squeezing of the nail bed, release of pressure allows the patient's capillary beds to reperfuse. The compressed tissues normally refill within 2 to 3 seconds. A capillary refill time of more than 3 seconds is suggestive of dehydration.

Other abnormalities seen with dehydration include decreased spontaneous motor activity, tachycardia, tachypnea, altered consciousness, and, as a late phenomenon compared with adults, depressed blood pressure. Decreased urine volume manifested by infrequent urination or diaper wetting during assessment and early observation is commonly seen in moderate to severe dehydration.

Altered Consciousness. Infants may have poor glycogen stores and with poor oral intake may become hypoglycemic. Irritability, obtundation, and seizure may result. Similar manifestations may occur with hypernatremic dehydration, secondary to brain desiccation.

General Physical Examination. In the pursuit of metabolic, infectious, neoplastic, or toxicologic derangement, the clinician searches for focal neurologic abnormalities, nuchal rigidity, petechiae, abdominal guarding, rebound tenderness, abdominal mass, a "surgical" abdomen, and rectal tenderness or mass.

CLINICAL REASONING

Once the data are gathered, they are collated to assist in management decisions.

What is the Estimated Degree of Dehydration?

By convention, dehydration is expressed as mild, moderate, or severe, based on clinical findings (Table 28–1). Patients with mild dehydration have lost between 1% and 5% of body weight. With the possible exception of decreased tearing or dry mucous membranes, their physical examination results are normal. Patients with moderate dehydration have lost 5% to 10% of body weight. Moderate dehydration is manifested by a sunken fontanelle, sunken eyes, dry mucous membranes, dry lips, and minimal loss of skin elasticity. The loss of skin elasticity can be demonstrated over the abdomen, if the skin tents or remains in a sharp fold when picked up. Patients with severe dehydration have lost more than 10% of their body weight. They will have intense vasoconstriction, with cold, mottled, poorly perfused skin, delayed capillary refill, and definite loss of skin turgor. They have altered motor activity, altered consciousness, a rapid, thready pulse, and collapsed vessels. These events may be followed by a precipitous drop in blood pressure.

What is the Probable Cause of Fluid Loss?

The major causes of dehydration are decreased ingestion, increased kidney excretion or respiratory loss, and increased excretion from abnormal mechanisms (e.g., vomiting, diarrhea, excessive sweating). After the clinical assessment, the cause of the child's condition can usually be placed in one or more of these categories.

Sometimes the cause will be obvious from information obtained in the history and on physical examination. An acute onset of vomiting and diarrhea without blood or mucus, associated with fever and occurring in a setting where other children are ill with a similar problem, almost certainly represents viral gastroenteritis. In other cases, the cause will not be so obvious and diagnostic testing will be necessary to define the exact cause. Another approach to the initial differential diagnosis is to categorize the disorder by the primary organ systems involved (Table 28–2).

Table 28–1. Estimation of Dehydration

	Mild	Moderate	Severe
Weight loss—infants	1%–5%	5%–10%	10%–15% or more
Weight loss—children	3%–4%	6%–8%	10%
Pulse	Normal	Slightly increased	Very increased
Blood pressure	Normal	Normal to orthostatic, > 10 mm Hg change	Orthostatic to shock
Behavior	Normal	Irritable, more thirsty	Hyperirritable to lethargic
Thirst	Slight	Moderate	Intense
Mucous membranes*	Normal	Dry	Parched
Tears	Present	Decreased	Absent, sunken eyes
Anterior fontanelle	Normal	Normal to sunken	Sunken
External jugular vein	Visible when supine	Not visible except with supraclavicular pressure	Not visible even with supraclavicular pressure
Skin (less useful in children > 2 yr)	Capillary refill <2 sec	Slowed capillary refill, >2–4 sec (decreased turgor)	Very delayed capillary refill (> 4 sec) and tenting; skin cool, acrocyanotic, or mottled*
Urine specific gravity	1.015–1.020	>1.020; oliguria	Oliguria or anuria

*These signs are less prominent in patients who have hypernatremia. From Jospe N, Forbes G: Fluid and electrolytes—clinical aspects. Pediatr Rev 1996; 17:397.

TABLE 28–2. Causes of Dehydration by Organ System

Gastrointestinal	Nephrogenic diabetes insipidus
	Renal tubular acidosis
Infants	Sickle hemoglobinopathy
Carbohydrate malabsorption	
Duodenal atresia	**Endocrine**
Annular pancreas	
Pyloric stenosis*	Cystic fibrosis
Necrotizing enterocolitis	Diabetic ketoacidosis*
Neural crest tumors	Central diabetes insipidus
Short bowel syndrome	Adrenogenital syndrome
Intussusception	Adrenal hemorrhage
Children	Addison's disease
Viral gastroenteritis*	Hypothalamic disorders
Bacterial gastroenteritis	Thyrotoxicosis
Pseudomembranous colitis	
Giardiasis	**Iatrogenic**
Cryptosporidiosis	
Entamoeba	Salicylates
Hirschsprung's disease	Ipecac
Midgut volvulus	Diuretic abuse
Peritonitis	Mannitol
Adolescents	Glycerol
Food poisoning*	High solute intake*
Pancreatitis	Nasogastric suctioning
Regional enteritis	
Ulcerative colitis	**Mixed**
Anorexia nervosa	
Bulimia	Hemolytic uremic syndrome
Scleroderma	Reye's syndrome
Cardinoid	Stomatitis
	Burns*
	Stevens-Johnson syndrome
Renal	Hyperthermia
	Interstitial spacing fluid*
Renal dysplasia	
Nephrogenic diabetes	

*Most common causes.

Is There Likely to Be an Electrolyte Abnormality?

Most dehydrated infants do not have electrolyte abnormalities requiring intervention other than appropriate rehydration. Children with severe dehydration, prolonged courses of illness, and home rehydration methods that have hypotonic or hypertonic replacement potential should have their electrolyte levels measured.

DIAGNOSTIC ADJUNCTS

Laboratory adjuncts may aid diagnostic reasoning or facilitate management decisions in those patients who have moderate to severe dehydration (>10% volume loss). Maximum information will be derived from the urinalysis, blood chemistries, and hemogram. Other testing, such as radiologic imaging, is tailored to the clinical setting.

Laboratory Studies

Urinalysis

Specific Gravity. Urine specific gravity is also an indirect indicator of hydration status. As intravascular volume decreases, renal perfusion decreases and increased free water is reabsorbed from the renal tubules, resulting in increasingly concentrated urine and thus a rise in specific gravity. Young infants, however, have a diminished capacity to concentrate urine, and thus can have a normal specific gravity despite relatively severe dehydration. A random specific gravity of between 1.010 and 1.020 indicates clinical fluid balance, whereas 1.020 or higher suggests an absolute or relative water-restricted state in a child with mature kidneys. Diluted urine in an apparently dehydrated child should raise the suspicion of adrenal insufficiency, aldosteronism, or chronic renal disease.

Glucose Concentration. The presence of glucose implies overload of the renal tubular reabsorptive capabilities and mandates measurement of the serum glucose level.

Protein. Proteinuria, if transient, is benign and nondiagnostic.

Ketones. Ketonuria is commonly found in patients with uncontrolled diabetes mellitus. It is more often present in pediatric nondiabetic patients with any anorexic state and with many febrile illnesses.

White Cells. Pyuria, defined as a leukocyte count greater than or equal to $10/mm^3$ in uncentrifuged urine, may reflect a renal parenchymal reaction to the presence of bacteria or may simply be an inflammatory response to an extrarenal lesion. Sterile pyuria is common in patients with viral gastroenteritis and many febrile illnesses associated with dehydration.

Bacteria. The presence of bacteria in an uncentrifuged, high-power microscopic examination suggests a urinary tract infection, which during infancy can cause vomiting, diarrhea, and abdominal distention without micturitional complaints.

Serum Electrolytes

Patients with mild dehydration rarely warrant serum electrolyte measurement. With moderate to severe dehydration, physiologic derangement of sodium, potassium, chloride, and bicarbonate (HCO_3^-) often occurs. Serum electrolyte measurements provide information on acid-base status and are essential for calculating replacements of electrolyte deficits.

The serum sodium is primarily altered by the tonicity of the fluids used to rehydrate and maintain fluid balance in the patient. As previously noted, little or no free water repletion results in hypernatremic states. Too much free water repletion causes a hyponatremic condition.

In most patients who are significantly dehydrated, serum HCO_3^- is low. Most of the time this results from the loss of HCO_3^- through diarrhea, and then the HCO_3^- level is slightly decreased. Starvation ketosis can contribute in patients who cannot tolerate oral feedings. In this situation, HCO_3^- may be moderately low. In patients in shock, lactic acidosis may be present and severe metabolic acidosis can result.

In some patients, the serum potassium value is low, which usually reflects losses from vomiting and diarrhea. The vast majority of the time hypokalemia is clinically insignificant. In patients on diuretic therapy who develop severe diarrhea, however, hypokalemia can become severe and cardiac and neurologic abnormalities can result.

Blood Urea Nitrogen and Creatinine

Determinations of blood urea nitrogen (BUN) and serum creatinine are of value in helping to ascertain the adequacy of renal function in a clinically dehydrated patient. The two determinations are best viewed in concert, observing their absolute values as well as their relation to one another. BUN and creatinine ratios of greater than 20:1 are seen in patients with severe dehydration.

As whole-body water and thus intravascular volume are lost, renal perfusion decreases and BUN and creatinine values rise. Although an increase in BUN and creatinine levels almost always indicates significant dehydration, both values can be normal in the presence of volume deficit, especially in young infants.

Glucose

Many infantile illnesses may be accompanied by poor oral intake, decreased gluconeogenesis, and depressed glycogen stores, leading to symptomatic hypoglycemia. In dehydrated patients with altered mental status, the blood glucose level should be rapidly estimated by reagent strip testing while awaiting formal laboratory confirmation.

Complete Blood Cell Count

Hemoglobin/Hematocrit. Reduced intravascular fluid volume without a corresponding loss in red cell mass leads to hemoconcentration. This finding may be a useful means of confirming dehydration.

White Blood Cell Count and Differential. The peripheral leukocyte count and peripheral smear may help to bolster the subjective impression of a diarrheal illness caused by either *Shigella* or *Campylobacter*. The presence of more than 10% immature neutrophils (bands), particularly when associated with a normal or low leukocyte count, suggests an infection by either of these enteric pathogens.

Blood Gas Analysis

A capillary or arterial blood gas analysis provides specific information about the respiratory, circulatory, and metabolic state of the dehydrated patient. Many laboratories report the pH and Pco_2 from the venous specimen submitted for other chemical analyses.

EXPANDED DIFFERENTIAL DIAGNOSIS

After laboratory evaluation, the likely origin of dehydration can be established. The history of the present illness is most likely to aid in determining whether dehydration is caused by a gastrointestinal disorder, endocrine disturbance, chronic renal disease, iatrogenic disorder, or multisystemic affliction (see Table 28–2). The physician interprets the historical information within the framework of an epidemiologic trend. The physical examination may confirm the clinical suspicion. Laboratory studies are helpful in establishing a metabolic derangement that may be occult on the basis of the physical examination.

Gastrointestinal diseases are the most common causes of water loss in all pediatric age groups. Acute diarrheal states far exceed any other gastrointestinal disorder in causing water and electrolyte imbalance. Recognition of the mechanism and etiologic agent responsible for excessive stool losses may be improved with characterization of stool patterns (Table 28–3).

Following gastrointestinal disease, the most common causes of total body water loss are the febrile illnesses characteristic of early childhood. These problems are predominantly viral in origin and often lead to multisystemic dysfunction, poor feeding, and low fluid intake. Hyperpnea and hyperpyrexia may exaggerate insensible water loss. Fortunately, these childhood afflictions are short-lived, and only mild to moderate states of dehydration ensue.

Acute salicylate ingestion leads to hyperpnea, hyperthermia, vomiting, and increased excretion of an excessive solute load, imposed by the accumulation of organic acids. Dehydration follows if the condition is untreated. Other dehydrating entities that may present with altered mental status, acidosis, and altered carbohydrate metabolism include sepsis, diabetes mellitus, uremia, and intoxications with ethanol, methanol, isopropyl alcohol, chloral hydrate, ethylene glycol, and isoniazid.

PRINCIPLES OF MANAGEMENT

The therapeutic principle for managing dehydration is to restore perfusion and cellular function by providing rehydrating fluids and electrolytes while monitoring the patient's progress. The type of fluid given, necessary supplemental electrolytes, route of fluid administration, and speed of administration rest with the initial assessment of the degree and type of dehydration.

Severely dehydrated patients who are in hypovolemic shock need airway management, oxygen, ventilation, and intravenous access. Two intravenous lines are placed using the largest cannulae that can be inserted into the peripheral veins. Failure to cannulate in two attempts over 90 seconds is an indication for intraosseous infusion, venous cutdown, or central line placement. Isotonic crystalloid solution is infused at 20 mL/kg, ideally over a period of no more than 5 minutes. After the initial fluid bolus has been given, the child is assessed for improvement by noting the sensorium, capillary refill time, pulse rate, and blood pressure. If there is no improvement, the 20-mL/kg bolus is repeated. After the third bolus (total 60 mL/kg), if there is still no improvement, central venous pressure measurement is required in an intensive care setting to monitor further fluid therapy.

Under less severe circumstances, management of dehydration in the emergency department is directed toward the following:

1. Deficit correction by replacing estimated percentage of volume lost
2. Correction of ongoing losses using electrolyte solutions based on origin of losses
3. Estimating maintenance requirements
4. Determining the therapeutic route: oral versus parenteral
5. Refining the estimates based on the patient's progress or analysis of laboratory results

Estimating Fluid and Electrolyte Composition Under Circumstances of Loss

In general, fluid loss that occurs rapidly will resemble extracellular fluid in its composition (sodium: 140 mEq/L), whereas fluid loss that occurs insidiously resembles intracellular fluid (potassium: 150 mEq/L).

If stool loss can be quantitated, it is known that a liter of diarrheal stool contains 45 to 50 mEq sodium, 10 to 80 mEq potassium, and

TABLE 28–3. Characteristics of Diarrhea

Stool Descriptors	Disease
Watery, without mucus or blood	Infection with *Giardia, Cryptosporidium, Escherichia coli,* or *Aeromonas;* viral infection; food poisoning
Watery, with mucus or blood	*Campylobacter, Shigella, Yersinia*
Loose, slimy, with variable mucus or blood. Particularly foul odor.	*Salmonella*
Loose, mixed with blood, "currant jelly" appearance	Intussusception

10 to 100 mEq chloride. If one can accurately determine the volume lost by diarrheal stools, electrolyte losses can be projected based on body weight. In the usual case of acute diarrhea, 9 mEq/kg of sodium is lost and 10 mEq/kg of potassium is lost.

Gastric fluids contain 10 to 80 mEq sodium, 10 to 20 mEq potassium, and 100 to 150 mEq chloride per liter.

Establishing Maintenance Levels of Fluid and Electrolytes

The major losses of water by the body occur through insensible evaporation of water from the lungs and skin and through excretion of urine and feces. Maintenance levels of fluids and electrolytes are best estimated using the surface area method (Fig. 28–1). Insensible water loss amounts to 500 mL/m^2/day. Hence, the obligatory water replacement for the pediatric patient ranges from 950 to 1300 mL/m^2/day.

The normal intake of sodium is between 30 and 80 mEq/m^2/day. The amount of 50 mEq/m^2/day is widely prescribed for calculating maintenance regimens. The daily intake of potassium is 40 mEq/m^2/day.

Two other methods for estimating maintenance amounts are the "4:2:1" rule and the use of the Broselow Pediatric Resuscitation tape. The "4:2:1" rule is a method for rapid calculation of hourly pediatric fluid requirements. The fluid is dextrose 5% in water (D_5W) with at least 30 mEq/L sodium chloride.

4 mL/kg/hr for the first 10 kg *plus*
2 mL/kg/hr for the second 10 kg *plus*
1 mL/kg/hr for every kg over 20 kg

For example, a 24-kg child would receive 64 mL/kg/hr of maintenance fluid (40 mL/hr for first 10 kg, plus 20 mL/hr for second 10 kg, plus 4 mL/hr for 4 kg over 20 kg). To simplify, once the child weighs more than 20 kg, that weight (in kilograms) plus 40 mL equals the hourly maintenance rate.

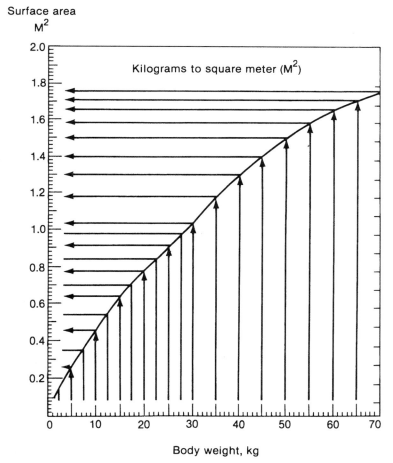

FIGURE 28–1 • Body weight to surface area nomogram. (From Sinkinson CA: Simplifying the complexities of pediatric dehydration. Emerg Med Rep 1989; 10[7]:53.)

The Broselow Pediatric Resuscitation tape was developed by an emergency physician in the late 1980s. The tape is divided into sections (different colors) for each increment of weight based on length. The tape gives maintenance fluid requirements, drug dosages, and sizes of emergency equipment for each section (increment) of length. (See Ch. 26) These estimates of weight by length have been within 15% of patient weight 80% of the time and serve as a useful starting point for pediatric care. The tape measures up to 60 inches.

Therapeutics: Oral Versus Parenteral

Oral glucose-electrolyte rehydration solutions (ORS) have been shown during the past decade to be highly effective in the treatment of dehydration, especially dehydration secondary to acute diarrhea. This therapy is based on the physiologic observation that active glucose absorption in the small bowel promotes the absorption of sodium. Oral rehydration therapy has had a dramatic impact on the morbidity and mortality of diarrheal disease in the developing world. There has been less acceptance of oral rehydration therapy as a primary treatment for dehydrating diarrhea in the developed world. The reservation is not justified. Similarly, several marketed pharmaceutical preparations with sodium concentrations ranging from 45 to 75 mmol/L (Pedialyte RS, Pedialyte, Lytren, Resol, Infalyte) have proved to be a safe and cost-effective means of treating dehydrated children in the United States.

Intravenous fluids historically have been the main form of pediatric rehydration, even in milder cases. However, intravenous fluids can now be reserved for patients with moderate to severe dehydration who need rapid restoration of intravascular volume. Intravenous fluids are also given to those patients who do not respond to oral rehydration attempts.

Therapeutics Based on Type of Dehydration

Isonatremic Dehydration. For most patients with isonatremic dehydration, rehydration is accomplished over 24 hours. Half of the estimated volume deficit is delivered over the first 8 hours, and the remaining half occurs over the next 16 hours. It is important to add the daily maintenance requirements to the volume deficit. Acceptable replacement fluid is dextrose 5% (D5) in 0.2 normal saline (NS). The addition of glucose provides some calories and diminishes further catabolism.

Hypernatremic Dehydration. The key to the management of hypernatremic dehydration is to lower the serum sodium level by no more than 10 to 15 mEq/L per 24 hours. If the sodium level falls too rapidly, cerebral edema can result as free water is drawn into brain cells "protected" by idiogenic osmols. Patients who are unstable are resuscitated by 20-mL/kg boluses of 0.9 NS until cardiovascular stability is restored. Although there is no universal agreement on the composition of subsequent fluid, D5/0.45 NS is usually adequate and probably less likely to result in a rapid fall in serum sodium than D5/0.2 NS. In contrast to isonatremic dehydration, the correction of the deficit is spread over 48 to 72 hours. Electrolytes are monitored closely. In cases of severe hypernatremia, it is reasonable to consult a pediatric intensivist or nephrologist.

Hyponatremic Dehydration. The goal of managing hyponatremic dehydration is to restore the volume deficit and correct sodium losses. Patients who are significantly dehydrated receive an initial bolus of 20 mL/kg of 0.9 NS. Sodium replacement in milliequivalents can be calculated using the formula

$$(\text{Sodium desired} - \text{sodium actual}) \times \text{Weight (kg)} \times 0.6$$

The factor 0.6 reflects the fractional distribution of sodium. In general, replacement is undertaken slowly to avoid overcorrection. Usually the sodium value is raised only 5 mEq/L to a level that stops seizures. A rapid rise in sodium level has been associated with central pontine myelinolysis in both adult and pediatric patients.

Patients with hyponatremia-induced seizures or significant altered mental status often respond to an initial 20-mL/kg bolus of 0.9 NS, which raises the serum sodium level sufficiently to improve neurologic function. In some cases, it may be necessary to intravenously administer 3% NS at a dose up to 4 mL/kg.

Refined Estimates Based on Patient Progress

The rate of fluid administration is largely influenced by the length of time the patient will remain under the care of the emergency physician. Suggested emergency department regimens include the following:

1. *Therapy for 3 to 6 hours:* Up to 30 mL/kg given over 30 minutes, followed by 10 mL/kg/hr.
2. *Therapy for 6 to 8 hours:* Bolus of 10 to 20 mL/kg given over 30 minutes, followed by 1500 to 2000 mL/m^2 given over 24 hours (maintenance rate); goal is to correct at least 50% of the projected deficit.

3. *Therapy for 12 hours:* Bolus, followed by maintenance rate and correction of 75% to 100% of the deficit.
4. *Therapy for 24 hours:* Bolus, followed by replacement of half the deficit and one third of the maintenance requirements in the first 12 hours, followed by half the deficit and two thirds of the maintenance needs in the remaining 24 hours.

Fluids are continued for at least 8 hours in the patient who presents with a serum sodium level less than 130 mEq/L or greater than 145 mEq/L, a potassium concentration of less than 3 mEq/L, and an HCO_3^- value less than or equal to 14 mEq/L or acidosis (pH less than 7.10). Fluids are given until there is a urinary output of at least 1 mL/kg/hr. Vital signs are recorded at 1-hour intervals at a minimum, and examination is repeated at 2-hour intervals, if possible.

DISPOSITION AND FOLLOW-UP

Admission

The decision to admit a severely dehydrated patient to the hospital is usually made based on the history and physical examination. In cases of mild to moderate dehydration, the decision to admit is delayed until the response to initial therapies is observed. A decision on disposition is based on the age of the patient, the underlying disease state, the past medical history, an estimate of parental compliance, and the availability of holding unit facilities.

Admission to the hospital for dehydrating illness is considered in the following circumstances:

- *Etiology.* Hyperpyrexic (temperature of more than 104°F [40°C]) children younger than 6 months of age known to have *Shigella* or *Salmonella* gastroenteritis are admitted for treatment with intravenous antibiotics.
- *Age of patient.* Patients younger than 2 months of age with any degree of dehydration are admitted.
- *Degree of dehydration.* All patients with severe dehydration are admitted to the hospital.
- *Blood chemistry abnormalities.* Admission is warranted for patients with levels of sodium less than 125 mEq/L or more than 150 mEq/L, potassium levels less than 2.5 mEq/L or more than 6 mEq/L, HCO_3^- levels less than 10 mEq/L, pH less than 7.0, BUN values more than 30 mg/dL, and creatinine values more than 1 mg/dL at presentation.
- *Past medical history.* Patients with underlying malnourishment, diabetes mellitus, chronic renal disease, or hemoglobinopathy are best rehydrated as inpatients.
- *Parenting.* If the managing physician is not assured of parental or patient compliance with plans for continued outpatient management, rehydration is carried out on an inpatient basis.
- *Facilities.* Attempts at outpatient rehydration in the emergency department may not be possible if there are inadequate personnel or physical facilities to address the patient's needs. Short-stay units may be an acceptable alternative for care in most cases of uncomplicated dehydration secondary to gastroenteritis.
- *Efficacy of prior treatment.* Patients with persistent electrolyte or acid-base imbalance, despite attempts at oral rehydration, are admitted for further therapy.

Discharge/Follow-up

The patient evaluated for a dehydrating illness may be discharged when the managing physician is confident of the diagnosis, degree of dehydration, adequacy of parenting skills, and availability of follow-up arrangements.

Instructions. Compliance is likely to be improved when the family is given explicit written instructions that are verbally reinforced by both the physician and the nursing staff. Such written instructions indicate both preferred and prohibited fluids.

- For the child with isolated diarrhea, parents are encouraged to provide one of the 45 to 50 mEq sodium/L proprietary oral glucose solutions on an ad lib basis.
- For patients who have been vomiting, parents are advised to administer small volumes of fluid at frequent intervals to minimize gastric distention. Volumes may be increased, and intervals between feedings can be advanced gradually.
- After 24 hours of clear fluid replacement (isotonic fluid preferred), infants are returned to dilute formula and advanced slowly to full-strength formula during 2 to 3 days. Strict regimens of clear liquids are not encouraged for longer than 24 hours.
- Reintroduction of partial-strength formula (especially nonlactose products) or bland solids such as rice, cereal, and potatoes (nonlactose carbohydrate foods) may prevent or minimize the deficit of calories and may promote the repair of the intestinal mucosa.
- Breast-fed infants are not discouraged from suckling in the presence of any dehydrating illness.
- After a 24-hour clear liquid regimen, older children may be fed a high-carbohydrate, low-fat

diet, which can be provided by bananas, rice, applesauce, and toast or saltines (BRAT diet).

Follow-up. Parents are encouraged to seek medical attention if their child cannot tolerate the just-described dietary regimen or shows signs and symptoms of dehydration. Emergency department reassessment is recommended for unexplained fever, abdominal discomfort, irritability, seizure, neck stiffness, or nonblanching rash. When possible, an appointment with the patient's primary physician is arranged within 24 hours of emergency department discharge. If he or she is not available, the emergency department can fulfill the need for monitoring the patient's progress. The follow-up physician will adapt the graduated feeding regimen to the child's needs.

FINAL POINTS

- The problem-solving approach in the emergency department attempts to establish the clinical estimate of fluid loss and underlying disease process responsible for dehydrating illness.

- The clinician establishes by history and physical examination the magnitude and type of fluid and electrolyte imbalance.
- Extremes of age increase susceptibility to developing dehydration and decrease tolerance to its effects.
- A patient may be hemodynamically stable but significantly dehydrated.
- Major causes of dehydration include decreased ingestion, increased kidney excretion or respiratory loss, and increased excretion by abnormal mechanisms (vomiting, diarrhea).
- Therapy is directed toward increasing plasma volume immediately, followed by giving therapeutic fluids and electrolytes that correct deficits, provide maintenance, and replete ongoing losses.
- Tolerating oral fluids is *not* the same as oral rehydration. Oral rehydration therapy is safe and cost effective.
- Intravenous or intraosseous routes are used when life-threatening vascular deficits exist.
- Any patient with significant dehydrating illness who is volume resuscitated and released requires explicit discharge instructions and timely follow-up examination.

CASE *Study*

A 3-month-old boy is brought to the emergency department by his parents with a history of 2 days of vomiting and diarrhea. They state he is less active than usual and is beginning to refuse to take his bottle.

Further questioning reveals that the infant is vomiting after every feeding. He is taking Enfamil, 4 ounces, every 3 hours. He has had at least 10 watery, nonbloody stools in the past 12 hours. He has also had a low-grade fever. Because of the watery consistency of the stools, the parents are not sure when he last urinated. The patient was a full-term infant and was completely well until the present illness.

On physical examination, the infant's temperature is 101°F, the respiratory rate is 40 breaths per minute, the heart rate is 175 beats per minute, and blood pressure is 86/48 mm Hg. Weight is 8.5 kg. He is listless but easily arousable. His skin color is good, peripheral pulses are normal, and capillary refill is good. His eyes do not appear sunken, his anterior fontanelle is flat, and his mucous membranes are moist. His heart, lung, and abdominal examinations are normal.

Key questions to answer in the course of care include the following:

- *Is the infant stable?*
- *Is the infant significantly dehydrated?*
- *Does the infant need laboratory studies?*
- *If the infant is dehydrated, how should he be rehydrated?*
- *Does the infant require admission?*
- *If the infant is discharged, what instructions should the parents receive and what kind of follow-up is necessary?*

The infant was assessed as stable because of adequate peripheral perfusion and normal blood pressure. Because of his young age and listless appearance, a glucose oxidase test strip, complete blood cell count (CBC), blood culture, urinalysis, urine culture, and serum electrolytes were obtained. While the laboratory tests were being done, the infant was given a 4-ounce bottle of Pedialyte, which he took eagerly.

The CBC was normal. The urinalysis showed no red or white blood cells, and the specific gravity was 1.006. The serum electrolytes revealed sodium, 140 mEq/L; potassium, 4 mEq/L; chloride, 111 mEq/L; and

HCO_3^-, 13 mEq/L. The blood glucose level was 96 mg/dL.

The infant did not vomit the Pedialyte and had no stools during his 2-hour emergency department visit. He appeared to become more alert and was discharged home. The parents were instructed to give Pedialyte, 4 ounces every 4 hours, and to follow up in the clinic the next day.

The parents did not keep the clinic appointment. They returned in 2 days to the emergency department, stating that while the vomiting had stopped the infant's diarrhea continued and that he was "not acting right." His oral intake had decreased, as had the frequency of his wet diapers.

On examination, the infant was extremely lethargic. His heart rate was 195 beats per minute, temperature was 97°F (36.1°C), and blood pressure was 60 mm Hg by palpation. Weight was 7.0 kg. The peripheral pulses were thready. The heart, lungs, and abdomen were normal.

The combination of altered mental status, poor peripheral perfusion, and marginal blood pressure indicates that the infant is in impending shock. The history of gastroenteritis makes it most likely that he is severely dehydrated and that shock is therefore caused by hypovolemia. By weight, the infant has lost more than 15% of fluid volume and was probably down from the usual weight on the first admission. The first priority of management is to deliver sufficient fluid to restore adequate perfusion and to prevent complete cardiovascular collapse.

After two attempts, an intravenous line is started and 20 mL/kg of 0.9% NS was delivered as a rapid bolus. The infant became more alert, but the heart rate remained at 190 beats per minute and the peripheral pulses remained thready. Consequently, another 20-mL/kg bolus of 0.9% NS was administered as rapidly as possible.

After this, the infant's color improved, the heart rate decreased to 175 beats per minute, the skin color became pink, and the peripheral pulses became regular. Electrolytes obtained during the resuscitation revealed sodium, 146 mEq/L; potassium, 3.5 mEq/L; chloride, 118 mEq/L; and HCO_3^-, 8 mEq/L.

In isonatremic dehydration, the serum sodium concentration is within its normal range. After the patient is stabilized, rehydration can be accomplished over the next 24 hours. Half of the estimated volume deficit is delivered over the first 8 hours, and the remainder occurs over the next 16 hours. Although it is difficult to calculate exactly the volume deficit, it is reasonable to assume that any severely dehydrated patient has lost at least 10% to 15% of total body water. It is important to recognize that in addition to correcting fluid losses, the patient must also receive the required daily maintenance of water and electrolytes. In patients with continuing severe diarrhea, water lost in the stool may also need to be replaced.

In this case, the 3-month-old infant weighs 7 kg and the estimated free water deficit is at least 10%. That amounts to 700 g, which equals 700 mL of water. Fluid therapy would consist of the following:

- Maintenance: 100 mL/kg × 7 kg = 700 mL/day. When given intravenously over 24 hours this is about 30 mL/hr.
- The deficit is 700 mL. Half, or 350 mL, is given over the first 8 hours, which equals about 44 mL/hr.

Thus, for the first 8 hours fluid therapy consists of:

- Maintenance 30 mL/hr + Deficit 44 mL/hr = 74 mL/hr × 8 hours.

The remaining deficit of 350 mL is replaced over the next 16 hours at a rate of 22 mL/hr. Added to the maintenance rate of 30 mL/hr, this equals 52 mL/hr for 16 hours.

Appropriate replacement fluid is D5/0.2 NS or D5/0.45 NS, which contains enough sodium to provide the required 2 to 4 mEq/kg/day. After the patient urinates, 40 mEq/L of potassium may be added to the fluid, to supply the daily requirements and correct losses. The glucose in the solution provides some calories and minimizes further catabolism.

This patient demonstrates the difficulty in assessing the hydration status in young infants and the tendency to underestimate the volume deficit.

Bibliography

TEXTS

Adelman RD, Solhung MJ: Pathophysiology of body fluids and fluid therapy. In Behrman RE, Kliegman RM, Jenson HB (eds): Nelson Textbook of Pediatrics, 16th ed. Philadelphia, WB Saunders, 2000, pp 188–227.

Chameides L, Hazinski MF (eds): Pediatric Advanced Life Support. Dallas, American Heart Association and the American Academy of Pediatrics, 1997, chapters 2 and 6.

Rudzinski JP, Wolanyk D, Mackey M: Fluids and electrolytes. In Strange GR, Ahrens WR, Lelyveld S, Schafermeyer RW (eds): Pediatric Emergency Medicine: A Comprehensive Study Guide. New York, McGraw-Hill, 1996, pp 337–349.

JOURNAL ARTICLES

American Academy of Pediatrics Provisional Committee on Quality Improvement, Subcommittee on Acute Gastroenteritis: Practice parameter: The management of acute gastroenteritis in young children. Pediatrics 1996; 97:424–435.

Cohen MB, Mezoff AG, Laney DW, et al: Use of a single solution for oral rehydration and maintenance therapy in infants with diarrhea and mild to moderate dehydration. Pediatrics 1995; 95:639–645.

Gorelick MH, Shaw KN, Murphy KO: Validity and reliability of clinical signs in the diagnosis of dehydration in children. Pediatrics 1997; 99:1–6.

Hellerstein S: Fluid and electrolytes: Clinical aspects. Pediatr Rev 1993; 14:103–115.

Holliday M: The evolution of therapy for dehydration: Should deficit therapy still be taught? Pediatrics 1996; 98:171–177.

Lubitz DS, Seidel JA, Chameides L, et al: A rapid method for estimating weight and resuscitation drug dosages from length in the pediatric age group. Ann Emerg Med 1988; 17:576.

Luten RC: Rapid rehydration in pediatric patients. Ann Emerg Med 1996; 17:399–403.

McConnochie KM, Conners GP, et al: How commonly are children hospitalized for dehydration eligible for care in alternative settings? Arch Pediatr Adolesc Med 1999; 153:1233–1241.

Nolpe J, Forbes G: Fluids and electrolytes—clinical aspects. Pediatr Rev 1996; 17:399–403.

Reid SR, Bonadio WA: Outpatient rapid intravenous rehydration to correct dehydration and resolve vomiting in children with acute gastroenteritis. Ann Emerg Med 1996; 28:318–323.

Teach SJ, Yates EW, Feld LG: Laboratory predictors of fluid deficit in acutely dehydrated children. Clin Pediatr 1997; 36:395–400.

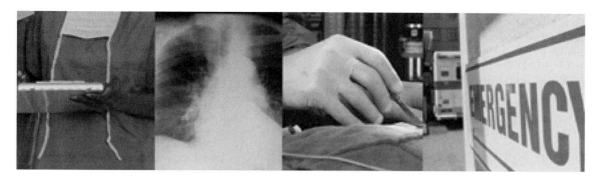

MUSCULOSKELETAL DISORDERS

CHAPTER 29

Acute Low Back Pain

MARK D. WRIGHT

CASE *Study*

A 44-year-old construction worker noted severe, acute low back pain (ALBP) after lifting a heavy object while on the job. Pain was immediate, localized to the right lower lumbar area, and made worse with movement of the back and leg on the affected side. He stopped working and notified his supervisor, who recommended he seek immediate evaluation at the local emergency department.

INTRODUCTION

Presentations of acute low back pain (ALBP) in the emergency department can range from truly emergent, life-threatening conditions (ruptured abdominal aortic aneurysm, ectopic pregnancy) to the completely benign, such as an asymptomatic patient simply requesting a note to return to work. The emergency physician must possess a thorough understanding of this common and debilitating clinical entity as a basis for appropriate management.

Definitions

ALBP is considered one of many common *musculoskeletal syndromes*. ALBP, simply defined, is pain localized to the lumbosacral region of the spine, often including the buttocks and legs. The sensation of ALBP may originate from nonspinal conditions. Pain, defined as an unpleasant sensory and emotional experience, can be categorized by duration, as *acute* (up to 3 months) or *chronic* (longer than 3 months). This distinction is essential for the formulation of management strategies. Pain *severity*, although subjective, can be helpful in monitoring progress of therapy. ALBP may be also defined as *occupational* (work related) because many back injuries occur on the job. The focus in this chapter is on the problem of ALBP (less than 3 months' duration) in adults.

Epidemiology

ALBP is one of the most common clinical problems encountered in emergency medicine. Most adults (60% to 80%) will experience some form of ALBP during their lifetime. Ten to 20 percent of adults will have one episode of ALBP each year. It is the most common cause of disability for adults younger than age 45. Most episodes are categorized as simple mechanical pain and will resolve within 1 month with little intervention; however, a portion (10%) will go on to have chronic symptoms. A smaller group will present with potentially serious signs or symptoms ("red flags") necessitating emergent treatment. Approximately 1% of the U.S. population is chronically disabled by low back problems. Economic estimates for the total cost associated with this condition, although difficult to assess precisely, may approach $75 to $100 billion annually. Low back pain has been called "the most expensive benign condition in industrialized countries."

Anatomy/Physiology/Pathophysiology

The lumbosacral spine is a complex biomechanical structure. Anatomically, it consists of bones (five lumbar vertebrae, the sacrum and coccyx), intervertebral discs, joints (facet joint, sacroiliac joint), nonneural soft tissues (muscles, tendons, fascia, ligaments), nervous tissue (spinal cord, nerve roots), and vascular tissue. Each vertebral "unit" has a three-part articulation made up of two facet joints and the intervertebral disc.

The ligaments of the lumbar spine provide mechanical stability (Fig. 29–1). There are two groups of supporting ligaments:

1. Anterior ligamentous complex: anterior and posterior longitudinal ligaments and the annulus fibrosus (fibrous covering of the disc)
2. Posterior ligamentous complex: ligamentum flavum, interspinous ligament, supraspinous ligament, and facet joint capsule

The spinal cord terminates at the L1–L2 interspace. Below this, nerve roots from the lumbar and sacral cord make up the cauda equina.

483

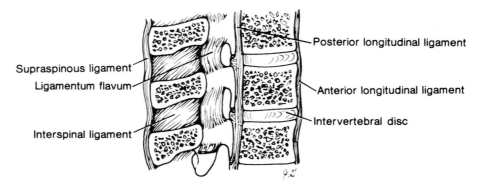

FIGURE 29–1 • Lateral view of the lumbar spine demonstrating the ligaments that support the anterior (anterior longitudinal, posterior longitudinal) and the posterior (supraspinous, intraspinous) elements of the vertebrae. Note the position of the ligamentum flavum forming a smooth posterior wall of the neural foramen. (From Borenstein DG, Wiesel SW: Low Back Pain: Medical Diagnosis and Comprehensive Management. Philadelphia, WB Saunders, 1989.)

Injuries below the terminus of the cord (L1) may damage the roots of the cauda equina only, with no cord involvement. Vascular supply to the cord is from the anterior and posterior spinal arteries.

The intervertebral discs are composed of the nucleus pulposus (colloidal gel, about 80% water) and the surrounding fibrous annulus fibrosus. The posterior longitudinal ligament is much narrower than the anterior component, allowing posterior disc herniations into the region of nerve roots of the cauda equina. Herniations usually occur to one side or the other of the posterior ligament with potential for nerve root impingement. Greater motion at the L4–L5 and L5–S1 articulations allows for increased risk of herniations and joint degeneration at these levels. The outer third of the annulus contains fine nerve endings that register pain.

The exact anatomic correlates and mechanisms of pain generation in the lumbar spine are complex and not clearly understood. Patients with minimal degenerative changes on radiographs may present with severe pain, whereas patients with severe degeneration may have minimal symptoms. Biomechanically, the vertebral unit is susceptible to forces of shear, compression, distraction, and torsion (twisting) and vibration (usually occupational). With repeated trauma, mechanical breakdown is presumed to occur. The progressive degeneration of spinal structures, in particular intervertebral discs and facet joints, is believed to play a central role in development of pain.

Many anatomic elements of the lumbosacral spine have potential to cause pain. Distinct qualities of pain are associated with specific structures in the spine. Primary low back pain consists of pain originating from the spine, spinal column, or peripheral nerves. It is divided into three cate-

gories based on the source of the pain: superficial somatic, deep somatic, and radicular.

Superficial somatic pain results from processes involving the skin or subcutaneous tissues. It is usually sharp or burning (e.g., herpes zoster).

Deep somatic (spondylogenic) pain results from processes involving the vertebral column, surrounding muscles, attaching tendons, ligaments, fascia, dura, or vertebral venous plexus. It is perceived as a deep, dull ache. Its most common cause is strain with avulsion of tendinous attachments of muscles or rupture of muscle fibers or sheaths. Muscle pain may also occur without overt injury when there is persistent use of a specific muscle group or when reflex spasm develops secondary to inflammatory or degenerative processes. Other spondylogenic contributors to ALBP include mechanical disruption of bones, joints, and ligaments; inflammation of joints and ligaments; neoplasm of bone; infections of bones and joints; distention of the vertebral venous plexus; and compression of the spinal dura.

Radicular pain results from stimulation of the proximal spinal nerves. It is typically lancinating, sharp, or burning. Mechanical disruption and degeneration are the most common processes leading to radicular pain, most commonly resulting from herniated intervertebral discs or spinal stenosis.

Although most cases of ALBP are related to lumbosacral musculoskeletal disorders, a number of pelvic, retroperitoneal, and abdominal structures can be the source of pain referred to the lower back. It is important to diagnose these causes of referred or "secondary" back pain because their management differs markedly from that for primary ALBP. Additionally, some of these problems can be life threatening. The goals of the emergency department evaluation are to determine the likely cause of the patient's pain, to rule out life-threatening and debilitating conditions, to initiate appropriate therapeutic interventions, and to ensure appropriate referral for further evaluation and treatment.

INITIAL APPROACH AND STABILIZATION

Priority Diagnoses (Red Flags)

A number of serious clinical conditions can present as either isolated low back pain or low back pain combined with additional signs and symptoms:

- *Ruptured aortic aneurysm*: the triad of severe ALBP, hypotension, and abdominal pain with pulsatile abdominal mass heralds this condition. Pain typically radiates to the back, abdomen, and flank and can radiate to the thigh and chest. Risk factors include advanced age and smoking. Pain of rupture is often excruciating and described as "tearing" or "ripping." The patient may have a history of aneurysm or aortic graft repair.
- *Ruptured ectopic pregnancy*: Cardinal signs and symptoms include amenorrhea, abdominal or pelvic pain, and irregular vaginal bleeding. Back pain is typically referred to the lower back. Ectopic pregnancy is the most common cause of maternal death.
- *The cauda equina syndrome*: This condition can result from trauma, infection, or a space-occupying lesion in the region of the cauda equina. Typically, injury or compression of one or more nerve roots causes hyperesthesia progressing to anesthesia in a characteristic "saddle" distribution. Distally, various motor and sensory deficits can occur depending on the nerve roots involved. Urinary and bowel dysfunction with incontinence may occur with lower sacral root involvement.
- *Neoplastic disease*: Patients with a new or metastatic neoplastic disease may present with a chief complaint of ALBP. Patients with new neurologic defects, especially if bilateral symptoms or multiple nerve roots are involved (e.g., from compression by tumor bulk), are at high risk. Systemic signs, such as weight loss that is unintentional, emaciation, fatigue, fever, night sweats, anorexia, and urinary or fecal dysfunction, are actively sought in patients with suspected neoplasm.

Rapid Assessment

"Red flags" that suggest priority diagnoses can appear in three different areas of the assessment. Any of these findings should raise the potential of a serious etiology.

- *Presenting complaint*: Trauma, writhing pain, night pain, bilateral radiculopathy, perianal or saddle numbness/paresthesia (cauda equina syndrome), change or loss of bowel/bladder function, and progressive neurologic deficit need to be evaluated.
- *History*: A history of cancer, a disorder with risk of infection or hemorrhage, an older patient with new onset of back pain, a patient with unexplained weight loss, and a woman with a possible pregnancy are suggestive.
- *Physical examination*: Vital signs may reveal hemodynamic instability or fever. A brief abdominal and neurologic examination may give an indication of an emergent condition. A pulsatile abdominal mass with or without abdominal pain or a neurologic deficit not explained by monoradiculopathy must be promptly evaluated, with further testing and early consultation considered.

Early Intervention

Rapid assessment and institution of basic life support (the ABCs) should begin as clinical conditions warrant. Most cases of ALBP do not require early intervention, other than analgesics.

Patients with severe, incapacitating musculoskeletal pain often have severely limited range of motion. They need reassurance, careful movement, and early examination. Analgesics (usually parenteral narcotics) may be administered if the patient has a history of onset with strain, exertion, unaccustomed activity, previous similar episodes, and the finding of localized lumbosacral tenderness of muscle spasm combined with normal vital signs (or mild to moderate tachycardia and hypertension consistent with severe pain). A more comfortable patient will be able to cooperate with the data gathering to follow.

CLINICAL ASSESSMENT

History

The initial history includes questions to rapidly assess the presence of a serious underlying condition and to place the symptoms in the context of the patient's work and daily activity.

1. *Where is the pain located?* This is critical for differential formulation. Unilateral, localized pain can help identify possible structures involved (e.g., sacroiliac joint, paraspinal muscles). Diffuse pain localized to the lumbar area often suggests a mechanical musculoskeletal cause but is not specific. Generalized pain can

be associated with various rheumatologic conditions. Original location of pain, even with radiation, can suggest pain source (e.g., hip bursitis radiating to lumbar area).

2. *How did the pain start?* Is there a specific injury associated with onset of pain? Did the pain start suddenly with activity such as lifting (suggesting a mechanical etiology)? Did the pain develop slowly with other constitutional symptoms (suggesting a possible infectious, neoplastic, or rheumatologic cause)?

3. *Does the pain radiate?* Pain radiation pattern, in a nerve root distribution, suggests nerve root compression. Common ALBP radiation patterns include lumbar area to buttocks or posterior or lateral thigh (sciatica). Back pain radiating into the scrotal area may be seen in renal calculi or abdominal aortic aneurysm.

4. *How severe is the pain?* Pain severity can suggest certain "red flag" conditions (dissecting or leaking abdominal aortic aneurysm).

5. *What makes the pain better or worse?* Modifying factors often suggest the etiology: lumbar pain made better sitting suggests spinal stenosis. Pain with sudden increase in intrathoracic pressure (as occurs with cough or sneeze) may suggest disc herniation.

6. *What has the patient done for pain relief?* The patient's efforts toward pain relief may offer insight into their understanding of the underlying processes. Medications taken may influence medications given in the emergency department, and assist in gauging the patient's degree of pain and tolerance.

7. *Are there symptoms related to other systems,* particularly urinary, reproductive, cardiovascular, and gastrointestinal symptoms? These symptoms suggest secondary, nonmusculoskeletal causes of low back pain. Endocrinopathies, malignancies, and metabolic bone disease may directly affect the lumbosacral structures. Rheumatic and connective tissue disorders may also have a direct effect, and arthritides associated with psoriasis and colitis may involve the lower back. Previous cardiovascular disease may be important in suggesting secondary causes, such as abdominal aortic aneurysm.

8. *Has there been loss of bowel or bladder function?* These ominous signs suggest possible cauda equina syndrome from low sacral nerve root compression, requiring an immediate assessment and intervention.

9. *Is there a prior history of back problems?* History of previous injury or surgery is important. Chronic or recurring pain can pose a significant challenge: Is this a new process or exacerbation of the old? Previous injury or

occupational risk for back injury can accelerate the degenerative process. Development of certain conditions (e.g., spinal stenosis) may occur in individuals with a long history of low back problems.

10. *Did the injury or problem occur on the job?* A topic often neglected, a work-related injury necessitates special consideration regarding legal and insurance requirements.

11. *What is the patient's work, social, and past medical history?* These questions are valuable to better understand the context and life impact of the back pain on the patient.

Physical Examination

Examination of the spine includes inspection, palpation, range of motion, and neurologic assessment for the lumbar spine, sacrum, coccyx, and adjacent structures. Examination of other structures depends on the history and suspicion of "red flags."

The physical examination of the patient with low back pain is conducted with the patient in four positions: standing, sitting, supine, and prone. The examination includes passive maneuvers (performed with the patient remaining still) and active maneuvers (requiring the patient's involvement and cooperation). Although the entire examination may not be possible in the severely ill or very uncomfortable patient, the initial examination is as complete as possible. Sensory, motor, and strength components are assessed. Depending on the patient's chief complaint, the physical examination is expanded to include other organ systems.

Standing

1. The patient's posture and any abnormal spinal contour are noted. Scoliosis may result from leg-length differences, assessed during the supine examination. Kyphosis or excessive lumbar lordosis may be noted.

2. The lumbar paravertebral muscles are palpated for tenderness or spasm. Tenderness localized over the sacroiliac joint is identified. Trigger points may be detected during palpation.

3. Active range of motion is assessed by asking the patient to flex and extend the spine and bend laterally (to each side). Normal range of motion is 90 degrees of flexion, 15 degrees of extension, and 45 degrees of lateral bending.

4. Normal gait is observed, and the ability to walk on heels and toes is tested. The ability to heel-and-toe walk is an indication of good lower extremity strength and tests the L4–L5 and L5–S1 areas (Table 29–1).

TABLE 29–1. Examination for Nerve Root Compression

Site of Disc Herniation	Nerve Root Involved	Reflex Changes	Motor Changes	Pain Distribution and Sensory Changes	Comment
L3-L4	L4	Decreased knee jerk	Weakness of quadriceps	Anterolateral thigh, across knee, and down anteromedial leg	Uncommon site for disc herniation
L4-L5	L5	Usually not associated with reflex changes; occasionally knee jerk is decreased	Weakness of anterior tibial, peroneal, and extensor hallucis longus muscles (weak dorsiflexion of foot and big toe)	Posterolateral thigh, anterolateral leg, and dorsal foot and big toe. Occasionally numbness of heel and bottom of foot	Trouble with heel walking
L5-S1	S1	Decreased/absent ankle jerk	Weakness of gastrocnemius and soleus muscles (weakness of plantar flexion)	Posterior thigh, posterior leg, and lateral foot (fourth and fifth toes)	Trouble with toe walking or standing on tiptoes
Cauda equina	S2, S3, S4, S5 Possibly lower lumbar roots	Decreased rectal tone, loss of bulbocavernosus reflex and anal wink	Diffuse motor weakness in lower extremities may progress to paraplegia	Perineal or "saddle anesthesia"	Bowel and bladder problems—especially urinary retention—may present with bilateral sciatica

From Roberts JR: In focus: Sciatica and disc disease. Emerg Med Ambulatory Care News, May, 1989. Reprinted with permission.

5. The stoop test is performed by having the patient go from a standing position to a squatting position. In the squatting position, intrathecal pressure is increased and the cerebrospinal fluid reduces skeletal pressure on the spinal cord. In patients with central spinal stenosis, squatting will result in reduced pain (increased cerebrospinal fluid around the cord in the narrowed canal).

Supine

1. A thorough abdominal examination is performed, with particular attention to the presence of any organ enlargement or masses that are present. A diligent search for a pulsatile mass, abdominal bruit, or abnormal femoral pulse is essential, especially in patients who are at a greater risk of developing an abdominal aortic aneurysm. On selected patients, rectal examination is performed, looking for evidence of a mass, bleeding, abnormal rectal tone, or abnormal prostate.
2. Passive straight-leg raising (PSLR) is performed. This test is positive if pain radiates down the posterior or lateral aspects of the thigh. Increased pain in the back is *not* a positive result of this test. Increased pain without radiation is most consistent with a muscular origin of the pain, but radiation indicates stretching of nerve roots over a herniated disc, resulting in pain along the nerve root course. The nerve root is actually stretched when the angle of the raised leg reaches 30 degrees. Pain from the beginning of PSLR is suggestive of malingering.
3. Crossed straight-leg raising (CSLR) is a variation of PSLR that has been found to be highly spe-

cific for lumbar disc herniation. In this test, the asymptomatic leg is raised. If pain is increased in the contralateral leg (with the asymptomatic leg raised), the result of the CSLR test is positive. This finding has been shown to correlate with disc herniation in a high percentage of cases.

4. Leg-length differences are measured from the anterior-superior iliac spine to the superior aspect of the medial malleolus. Discrepancies greater than 1.5 cm are considered significant for scoliosis or other structural abnormalities.
5. The quadriceps and calf muscles are evaluated for atrophy. Muscle weakness and neurologic deficit over a period of weeks will cause atrophy. Lack of atrophy in the presence of long-term complaints of weakness is suggestive of malingering.
6. Motor strength is assessed by checking dorsiflexion and plantarflexion of the great toe against resistance (see Table 29–1).
7. Sensation is checked over the lower extremities by evaluating perception of light touch, pinprick, and sharp-dull discrimination. The corresponding dermatomes are compared in each leg (see Table 29–1).
8. Patellar (knee-jerk) and Achilles (ankle-jerk) reflexes are checked.
9. A palm-heel test is conducted by the examiner, placing his palms under the patient's heels. The patient is then asked to raise the leg while keeping it straight, first on one side and then on the other. When the patient is cooperating and attempting to raise one leg, the opposite heel should press firmly on the examiner's palm. If it does not, the patient is not exerting adequate effort and this suggests malingering.

Prone

(A pillow can be placed beneath the abdomen to reduce lumbar lordosis and increase patient comfort.)

1. The patient is asked to localize the pain again. Localization of pain in different locations with changes in position suggests malingering.
2. Palpation for tenderness is repeated. Tenderness of the costovertebral angles and spinous processes is noted, as well as paravertebral muscle tenderness and spasm.
3. Reverse straight-leg raising (the bow-string test) is performed by hyperextending each leg posteriorly. Pain radiating into the thigh is a positive result of this test, indicating nerve root stretching over the herniated disc.
4. The sensory examination is completed. The perineal and perianal areas are included because they are affected by compression of nerve roots in the cauda equina.

Sitting

1. A motor examination of the quadriceps is performed by having the patient extend each lower leg, actively and passively.
2. The hidden straight-leg raising test is performed as follows: With the patient in the sitting position, the lower leg is extended at the knee, giving 90 degrees of flexion at the hip. This action gives the same result as the straight-leg raising test performed with the patient in the supine position. Results are positive if the pain radiates along the sciatic nerve distribution on the affected side. A discrepancy between this test and the supine PSLR suggests malingering.
3. Deep tendon reflexes (of the patellar and Achilles tendons) are rechecked.
4. Muscle strength testing, by dorsiflexion and plantarflexion of the foot against resistance, is repeated.

Clinical Reasoning

On completion of the history and physical examination, the physician is usually able to address the following questions.

Is the Back Pain a Symptom of a Life-Threatening Problem That Requires Immediate Intervention?

Problems such as abdominal aneurysm and ectopic pregnancy that may result in hemorrhagic shock are generally identified, and early management is started at the time of the initial patient evaluation. At times, the patient presentation is less obvious and the diagnosis is more difficult to make. Close monitoring of the patient's vital signs and clinical course is essential because deterioration may occur at any time. If a patient remains stable, studies to confirm these serious diagnoses are performed (Table 29–2). Early surgical consultation is advised because emergent intervention may be necessary if the condition deteriorates before test results are available.

Is There an Immediate Risk of Long-Term Neurologic Impairment?

The majority of the primary musculoskeletal back pain syndromes are managed conservatively; however, two problems may require expeditious intervention to prevent permanent neurologic deficits: the cauda equina syndrome and spinal cord compression.

The cauda equina syndrome is an uncommon but very serious complication of lumbar disc disease. Patients typically present with ALBP, unilateral or bilateral radiation, perineal anesthesia, motor weakness of the lower extremities, and bowel or bladder dysfunction (usually urinary retention). Onset may be acute, but often signs and symptoms of disc herniation precede cauda equina syndrome for some time. Classically, surgical intervention within 6 hours of the onset of symptoms is considered the essential therapy to prevent permanent paralysis and bladder dysfunction.

Acute spinal cord compression may present as ALBP with lower extremity, bowel, or bladder deficits. Immediate intervention is required to prevent permanent neurologic abnormalities. Spinal cord compression can be caused by central disc herniation, abscess, tuberculoma, arteriovenous malformation, hematomas, expanding tumor mass, or displaced fracture fragments.

Is the ALBP from a Musculoskeletal, Mechanical Cause?

Mechanical low back pain, the most common presentation in the emergency department, comprises up to 98% of all low back problems. Almost 70% are related to dysfunction of the disc, facet joints, and sacroiliac joints. Mechanical problems can be placed into five groups: (1) strains/sprains (nonspecific), (2) intervertebral disc herniation (with or without sciatica), (3) osteoarthritis, (4) spinal stenosis, and (5) spondylolysis/spondylolisthesis.

Lumbar strains/sprains usually occur in the soft tissues surrounding the vertebral unit. These

---

TABLE 29–2. Diagnostic Imaging to Provide Anatomic Definition of Acute Low Back Pain (ALBP)

Plain Radiographs

- Plain films are not recommended for routine evaluation of patients with ALBP within the first month of symptoms unless a "red flag" condition is suspected (see below) [B].
- Plain films of the lumbar spine are recommended for ruling out fractures when any of the following "red flags" are present: recent significant trauma (any age), recent mild trauma (age > 50), patient > 70 years, osteoporosis and history of prolonged steroid use, and ankylosing spondylitis [C].
- Plain films in combination with complete blood cell count and erythrocyte sedimentation rate may be useful in ruling out infection or tumor in patients with ALBP and the following "red flags": history of cancer, recent infection, history of tuberculosis, fever > 100°F, IV drug abuse, prolonged steroid use, ALBP worse with rest, unexplained weight loss [C].
- The use of imaging studies such as bone scan, CT, or MRI may be indicated in the presence of red flags for tumor or infection (even if plain films are negative) [C].
- Routine use of oblique lumbar views is not recommended for adults owing to increased radiation exposure [B].

CT, MRI, Myelography, and CT-myelography

- In the presence of "red flags" suggesting cauda equina syndrome or progressive motor weakness, prompt use of CT, MRI, myelography or CT-myelography is recommended. Consideration for surgical consultation is recommended [C].
- When clinical findings suggest tumor, infection, fracture, or other space-occupying lesion of the spine, use of special studies is recommended as well as specialist consultation [C].
- Routine spinal imaging tests are not recommended in the first month of symptoms (except in the presence of "red flags"). After 1 month, imaging is acceptable when surgery is considered [B].
- For patients with prior back surgery and ALBP, MRI with contrast medium enhancement appears to be the imaging test of choice to distinguish disc herniation from scar tissue [D].
- Myelography and CT-myelography are invasive tests with increased risk of complications. These tests are only indicated in special situations for preoperative planning [D].
- MRI provides the greatest detail of anatomy, especially the area within the vertebral canal, and the spinal cord.

Discography (Intervertebral Disc Imaging)

- Discography is invasive and is not recommended for assessing ALBP [C].
- Because of increased potential risks, CT-discography is not recommended over other imaging studies (CT, MRI) for assessing suspected nerve root compression due to disc herniation [C].

Rating system from AHCPR Clinical Practice Guidelines: Rating of scientific evidence supporting the recommendation: A, strong; B, moderate; C, limited; D, did not meet inclusion criteria.

---

include muscles, fascia, and ligaments. These commonly occur with lifting activities. Pain is usually well localized and reproducible. In healthy, young individuals these injuries often resolve spontaneously in 2 to 6 weeks, with minimal intervention.

Intervertebral disc herniation generally occurs as the last step in the degenerative process of the intervertebral disc (Fig. 29–2). Movements such as bending, flexion, and extension compress the disc and stretch fibers of the annulus. Over time, tears in the annulus fibers develop with extrusion of disc contents posteriorly toward the cord and the cauda equina. Symptomatic herniations may not be associated with a single traumatic event but rather accumulated trauma. Small herniations may be asymptomatic. There is no clear relationship between extent of disc protrusion and severity of symptoms. *Sciatica* is radicular nerve pain or pain radiating along the course of the sciatic nerve. It is thought to be the result of nerve root compression and inflammation of surrounding tissues. Painful sciatica may be present with a minimal neurologic deficit. Conversely, severe

radiculopathy with development of paralysis may occur without pain.

When herniation is suspected and diagnostic studies are performed (i.e., computed tomography or magnetic resonance imaging), it is important for the clinician to correlate the study findings (if any) with the location and distribution of symptoms. It is not uncommon for a frank herniation to be visualized on one side but with symptoms on the opposite side! When peripheral neurologic symptoms are absent, radicular pain symptoms may improve with conservative treatment. Persistence of symptoms and neurologic findings may require definitive surgical treatment.

Osteoarthritis occurs most commonly in middle age and elderly patients, preferentially affecting the cervical and lumbar spine. It often manifests as morning stiffness with limited range of motion. Pain often worsens throughout the day. As in disc herniation, radiographs of the lumbar spine may not correlate with the severity of symptoms.

Spinal stenosis is a narrowing of the spinal canal. Patients with this condition are older and

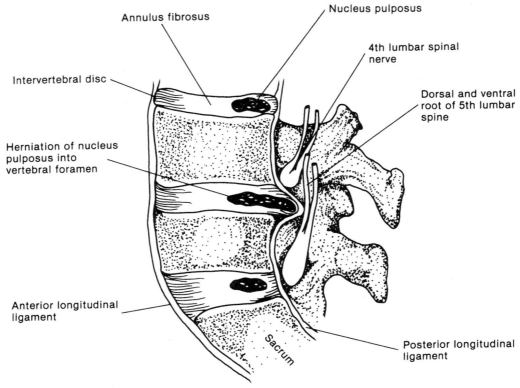

FIGURE 29–2 • Anatomy of a herniated intervertebral disc. Note that the annulus is thinner in the posterior region, predisposing the patient to posterior herniation. As noted, an L4-L5 disc causes compression of the fifth lumbar nerve root. Central or massive herniation may compress the cauda equina. (From Roberts JR: In focus: Sciatica and disc disease. Emerg Med Ambulatory Care News, May 1989.)

usually have a long-standing history of back problems. Often, osteoarthritis and disc degeneration are also present. Patients often describe aching pain and heaviness in the legs. In contrast to disc disease, this pain is usually worse with extension and improved with flexion or sitting. Computed tomography and magnetic resonance imaging are the preferred diagnostic adjuncts for assessing the anatomic detail of the central canal.

Spondylolysis is suspected to be stress or fatigue fractures occurring at the pars interarticularis. This condition is most commonly encountered in young, athletic individuals (see also "Special Considerations"). The cause is attributed to repeated stress, especially hyperextensions, and immaturity of the posterior vertebral arch (in young individuals). Initially, one side of the vertebral arch incurs repeated stress and microfracture, followed by complete fracture. Finally, increased stress occurs on the remaining intact side, with subsequent fracture resulting.

Spondylolisthesis is forward slippage of an upper vertebral body on a lower vertebral body, secondary to spondylolysis of the intervening pars articulation. The incidence is 2% to 5%.

Spondylolisthesis most commonly occurs at the L5–S1 level (anterior slippage of L5) with possible involvement of L5–S1 nerve roots. Four grades of displacement are recognized: grade I, 0% to 25%; grade II, 25% to 50%; grade III, 50% to 75%; and grade IV, 75% to 100%. As with many conditions of the low back, degree of pain does not necessarily correlate with degree of slippage. Other pain sources such as disc herniation may contribute to an otherwise low-grade spondylolisthesis.

Is the Pain Due to a Nonmechanical, Musculoskeletal Cause?

Although the majority of patients seen with ALBP will have mechanical causes, other nonmechanical causes frequently present as low back pain symptoms.

Rheumatologic

The seronegative spondyloarthropathies presenting as ALBP include ankylosing spondylitis (most common), psoriatic arthritis, Reiter's syndrome, and enteropathic spondylitis (Crohn's disease and ulcerative colitis). These related disorders often present as back pain especially involving the sacroiliac joints. Pathogenesis is not clearly understood. HLA-B27–positive individuals (4% to 8% of the white population) have a 2% to 10% chance of developing ankylosing spondylitis. Clinical features include morning stiffness, age younger than 40 years, insidious development, peripheral joint involvement, and improvement with exercise. On examination there is symmetric restricted range of motion. Peripheral features include costochondritis, plantar fasciitis, and Achilles tendonitis.

Polymyalgia rheumatica and fibromyalgia, two conditions believed to be nonarticular, often have generalized pain and aching and may have low back pain symptomatology.

Neoplastic

Primary tumors are generally rare. Multiple myeloma is a common primary bone marrow malignancy in adults. Back pain is the presenting symptom in a third of cases. It usually occurs after age 40. Urine and serum electrophoresis for light chains is diagnostic for the condition. Osteoid osteoma is a benign neoplasm.

Metastatic tumors are 25 times more common than primary tumors of the vertebrae. They may comprise 30% to 50% of the vertebrae before being visible on plain radiographs. These tumors often require bone scan or magnetic resonance imaging to be observed. Common malignancies that metastasize include those of breast, lung, prostate, lymphoma, melanoma, colon, and kidney. Metastases to the spine are found in up to 70% of all patients with primary tumors, and back pain is present in 90%. Epidural cord compression occurs in 5% of cancer patients. Neoplastic infiltration of the meninges may also present as ALBP during diagnostic maneuvers for meningitis (neck flexion and straight-leg raising).

Infections/Inflammations

Infectious causes should be entertained, especially in the intravenous drug user, patients with recent spinal procedures, the immunosuppressed, and children (see "Special Considerations"). Osteomyelitis, discitis, and associated epidural abscesses are included in the differential diagnosis. Changes on plain radiographs may not be evident early in the disease, and computed tomography or magnetic resonance imaging is necessary if these diagnoses are considered. Epidural abscess may progress rapidly, and the diagnosis should be aggressively pursued to avoid spinal cord compromise or cauda equina syndrome.

Other infections with associated back pain include pilonidal cyst abscess and perirectal abscess.

Meningitis, more commonly associated with fever, headache, and neck stiffness, can present as low back symptoms often elicited by nerve root stretching during straight-leg raising and neck flexion.

Transverse myelitis is a rare, often postviral complication that may present with ALBP and neurologic findings. MRI assessment is diagnostic.

Vascular/Hematologic

Arteriovenous malformation is a congenital lesion that may spontaneously hemorrhage, causing an acute compressing hematoma within the spinal canal. Epidural hematoma may also present as ALBP, especially in patients on anticoagulant medication and those with recent spinal procedures or trauma. Low back pain with hip extension may suggest a psoas muscle hemorrhage secondary to trauma. Hemoglobinopathies (thalassemias, sickle cell) may be associated with bone infarcts, manifesting as ALBP during periods of low tissue oxygenation.

Endocrine/Metabolic

Osteoporosis is the most common metabolic condition causing low back pain. It is responsible for 70% of spinal fractures in women older than age 45. Risk factors include white race, thin body habitus, smoking, alcohol use, sedentary lifestyle, and postmenopausal age group. Up to one half of vertebral compression fractures are asymptomatic. Most occur spontaneously or from minimal trauma. Pain, initially severe, often resolves spontaneously over many weeks. Paget's disease (osteitis deformans) is characterized by excessive bone resorption and formation, with unclear cause (but is possibly virus mediated). Alkaline phosphatase levels are often elevated, representing increased osteoblast activity. The spine and pelvis are often affected, producing localized pain or neural compression.

Is the Back Pain Secondary to a Disease Process in a System Other than Musculoskeletal?

The history and physical examination are usually sufficient to differentiate primary musculoskeletal from secondary back pain. Diagnostic studies in the emergency department do not often add significant information but are usually necessary to confirm secondary causes (see Table 29–2).

Referred Pain

Nearly all abdominal and pelvic organ disorders may have ALBP as a symptom. Common presentations include the following:

- *Gastrointestinal*: Biliary colic, diverticulitis, gastric or duodenal ulcers (especially the posterior duodenal wall), and pancreatitis (often refers pain to the thoracic/upper lumbar area with associated epigastric pain) may present as ALBP.
- *Urinary*: Nephrolithiasis ("kidney stone") with renal colic (classically flank pain radiating to the groin), pyelonephritis, cystitis, and prostatitis are examples.
- *Gynecologic*: Back pain is not a frequent symptom associated with gynecologic disorders, but clinicians should consider pelvic inflammatory disease, endometriosis, ovarian cyst rupture, and tumors (including rupture and torsion).
- *Nonspinal, musculoskeletal*: Hip pain and trochanteric bursitis are examples.

DIAGNOSTIC ADJUNCTS

Laboratory Studies

Blood and urine tests are generally not necessary for most presentations of ALBP. However, certain diagnostic considerations will be aided by the following laboratory tests:

Complete Blood Cell (CBC) Count. The CBC count is helpful in establishing an infectious cause, either intrinsic (i.e., osteomyelitis, discitis, abscess) or from a referred source (i.e., pyelonephritis), although the white blood cell count is nonspecific for infection. Patients with risk factors for infection (immunocompromise, diabetes, malignancy, and intravenous drug abuse) are especially important to assess. The CBC can determine the hematologic status of patients with known or suspected malignancy (absolute neutrophil counts, thrombocytopenia).

Erythrocyte Sedimentation Rate (ESR). This test can be useful in evaluation of suspected inflammatory conditions, including rheumatologic disorders and infections. It should be ordered when there is concern for malignancy or infections in ALBP cases, although it *cannot* rule them out.

Coagulation Studies. These studies are important especially for "red flag" presentations of abdominal aortic aneurysm rupture, ectopic pregnancy, and known or suspected malignancy.

Urinalysis. Urinalysis is helpful to determine a potential referred source of ALBP, such as nephrolithiasis (red blood cells, crystals); urinary tract infection (red blood cells, leukocytes, leukocyte esterase, bacteria); or occult urinary malignancy (red blood cells, malignant cells).

Pregnancy Test. This is useful when evaluating for possible ectopic pregnancy and before the use of radiologic studies in women of childbearing age.

Other Tests. Other tests that are ordered less often include rheumatologic studies (HLA-B27 for ankylosing spondylitis, rheumatoid factor), acid phosphatase (prostatic cancer), alkaline phosphatase (metastatic disease, Paget's disease, osteomalacia, hyperparathyroidism), calcium, and phosphorus.

Radiologic Imaging

Studies to Provide Anatomic Definition

In accord with Agency for Health Care Policy and Research (AHCPR) Clinical Practice Guidelines, Table 29–2 lists the format recommendations for the use of special studies. Plain radiographs are often considered by the clinician and frequently expected by patients. However, for most presentations of ALBP, radiographs are not immediately indicated. The guideline panel evaluated commonly employed methods of evaluation and treatment and provides a rating system based on the strength of the scientific evidence supporting the recommendation: A, strong; B, moderate; C, limited; D, did not meet inclusion criteria. This system was the basis for (1) recommendations for, (2) recommendations against, or (3) options (situations in which evidence for potential benefits is weak but potential costs and harm are small).

Other Tests for Evidence of Physiologic Dysfunction

A *bone scan* involves the use of intravenous radioactive compounds that localize to metabolically active bone. Bone scanning is recommended to evaluate ALBP when tumor, infection, or occult fracture is suggested. Bone scans have a low specificity and may be best for occult fracture or combined with the ESR in cases of possible spine metastasis or myelitis. They are contraindicated during pregnancy.

Electrophysiologic tests are sometimes employed in the evaluations of patients to assess physiologic function of the spinal cord, nerve roots, and peripheral nerves. Most, however, are not helpful in the assessment of acute low back symptoms and are seldom used by the emergency physician. Tests include the following:

- Needle electromyography (EMG): to assess acute and chronic nerve root dysfunction, spinal cord dysfunction (myelopathy), and muscle dysfunction (myopathy)
- H-reflex: sensory conduction through nerve roots

- F-wave response: motor conduction through nerve roots to assess proximal neuropathies
- Nerve conduction studies: to assess acute and chronic nerve entrapment

PRINCIPLES OF MANAGEMENT

The primary role of the physician in the evaluation and treatment of ALBP is to screen for those conditions requiring immediate intervention, to initiate treatment, and to facilitate follow-up by the patient's primary physician or a consultant. As noted earlier, treatment of ALBP encompasses many fields of medicine. To provide consistent, state-of-the-art treatment for this condition, clinical practice guidelines have been developed. Although not universally accepted, guidelines provide the clinician with a comprehensive analysis of the current evidence for evaluation and management of ALBP.

Guidelines for the initial assessment and treatment of ALBP are shown in Figures 29–3 and 29–4. The key element is the recognition of "red flags," which were defined previously.

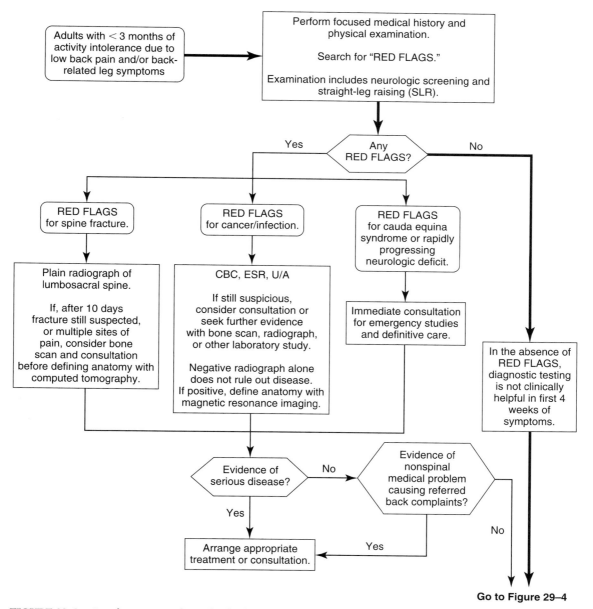

FIGURE 29–3 • Initial assessment of acute low back symptoms. CBC, complete blood cell count; ESR, erythrocyte sedimentation rate; U/A, urinalysis.

Initial Visit

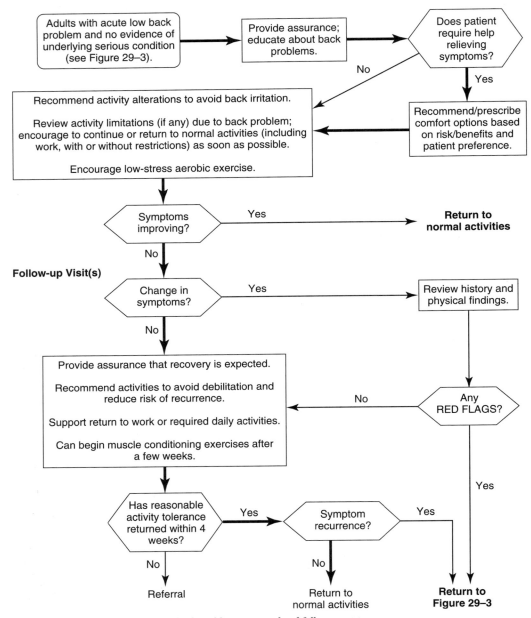

FIGURE 29–4 • Treatment of acute low back problems on initial and follow-up visits.

Symptom Management

The following four tables, adapted from the AHCPR Clinical Practice Guideline, summarize current treatment strategies:

- Table 29–3: Medications
- Table 29–4: Physical Treatments
- Table 29–5: Injection Therapy
- Table 29–6: Activity Modification

Patient Education

Accurate information about low back pain found to be of benefit to patients includes

- Expectation of rapid recovery and recurrent nature of low back problems
- Effective and safe symptom control methods
- Activity modification recommendations

TABLE 29–3. Medications for Acute Low Back Pain (ALBP)

Nonsteroidal Anti-inflammatory Drugs (NSAIDs) and Acetaminophen

- NSAIDs are acceptable for treating patients with ALBP [B].
- NSAID use should be guided by side effect risk (gastrointestinal irritation), cost, comorbidity, and patient/provider preference [C].
- Acetaminophen is acceptable and reasonably safe for treating ALBP [C].
- Phenylbutazone is not recommended for use based on increased risk for bone marrow suppression [C].

Muscle Relaxants

- Muscle relaxants are an option in the treatment of ALBP but have not been shown to be more effective than NSAIDs.
- No additional benefit is gained by using muscle relaxants with NSAIDs vs. NSAIDs alone [C].
- When considering the use of muscle relaxants, potential for drowsiness should be weighed against the patient's intolerance of other agents (up to 30% of patients experience drowsiness and other side effects) [C].

Opioid Analgesics

- Opioid use should be guided by consideration of potential complications vs. other options. Opioids are an option for treatment of ALBP when used for time-limited courses [C].
- Opioids appear to be no more effective in relieving ALBP than safer analgesics such as acetaminophen, aspirin, and other NSAIDs [C].
- Clinicians should be aware of opioid side effects (drowsiness, decreased reaction time, clouded judgment), which lead to discontinuation by as many as one third of patients [C].
- If opioids are used, patients should be warned of potential physical dependence and dangers of driving or operating heavy equipment [C].

Oral Steroids

- Oral corticosteroids are *not* recommended for the treatment of ALBP [C].
- The use of oral corticosteroids for extended periods or in high doses for short periods has potential for severe side effects [D].

Colchicine

- Colchicine is *not* recommended for treatment of ALBP based on conflicting evidence of effectiveness and potential for serious side effects [B].

Antidepressant Medications

- Antidepressants are *not* recommended for the treatment of ALBP [C].

Rating system from AHCPR Clinical Practice Guidelines; A, strong; B, moderate; C, limited; D, does not meet inclusion creteria.

- Lack of need for special studies or investigations unless serious signs and symptoms present
- Risks and benefits of commonly available diagnostic evaluations and treatment when symptoms persist

Surgical Management

Surgical management may be considered, especially in the patient with unremitting symptoms. Patients should be made aware of all risks, benefits, and alternative treatment options before surgery (Table 29–7).

UNCERTAIN DIAGNOSIS

When the initial complaint, on presentation to the emergency department, is back pain, assessment for critical, urgent, and nonurgent status is a first step. After critical and urgent causes are ruled out, or have an extremely low probability, nonurgent causes may be sought. When a clinician has completed an evaluation for back pain, often the etiology remains unclear. Patient pain status and hemodynamic status are reevaluated at this time.

If pain is well controlled and the patient's condition is stable, discharge is recommended with 24- to 72-hour follow-up with a primary physician. The patient and preferably caregiver at home should clearly understand discharge instructions. Patients need to return if a condition worsens.

If pain is not controlled, patients need to be admitted and treated with parenteral analgesics. If the etiology is unclear and the patient's condition is not stable, admission is required. Consultations for spinal surgery (often

TABLE 29–4. Physical Treatments of Acute Lower Back Pain (ALBP)

Physical Agents and Modalities

- The use of physical agents and modalities (ice, heat, ultrasound, cutaneous laser, electrical stimulation *excluding* TENS) in the treatment of ALBP is of insufficiently proven benefit to justify their cost. *Option*: Patients may be taught self-application of heat or cold at home [C].

Transcutaneous Electrical Nerve Stimulation (TENS)

- TENS is *not* recommended in the treatment of ALBP [C].

Shoe Insoles and Shoe Lifts

- Shoe insoles may be effective for patients with ALBP who stand for prolonged periods of time, given the low cost and low potential for harm [C].
- Shoe lifts are *not* recommended for treatment of ALBP when lower limb length difference is < 2 cm [D].

Lumbar Corsets and Back Belts

- The use of lumbar corsets and support belts have *not* been proven beneficial for treatment of ALBP [D].
- Lumbar corsets, used preventively, may reduce lost work time from low back problems in individuals doing frequent lifting [C].

Spinal Traction

- Spinal traction is *not* recommended in the treatment of patients with ALBP [B].

Spinal Manipulation

- Spinal manipulation can be helpful for ALBP without radiculopathy when used within the first month of symptoms [B].
- In patients with symptoms longer than 1 month, manipulation therapy is probably safe but efficacy is unproved [C].
- There is insufficient evidence to recommend manipulation therapy in patients with radiculopathy [C].
- Manipulation therapy should be avoided when findings suggest progressive or severe neurologic deficits. Diagnostic assessment should be performed to rule out serious neurologic conditions [D].
- If manipulation therapy has not resulted in symptomatic improvement allowing increased function within 1 month, manipulation should be stopped and the patient reevaluated [D].

Biofeedback

- Biofeedback is *not* recommended for treatment of ALBP [C].

Rating system from AHCPR Clinical Practice Guidelines: A, strong; B, moderate; C, limited; D, does not meet inclusion criteria.

TABLE 29–5. Injection Therapy for Acute Low Back Pain (ALBP)

Trigger Point and Ligamentous Injections

- Trigger point injections are invasive and *not* recommended in the treatment of ALBP [C].
- Ligamentous and sclerosant injections are invasive and not recommended in the treatment of ALBP [C].

Facet Joint Injections

- Facet joint injection is invasive and *not* recommended in the treatment of ALBP [C].

Epidural Injections

- There is no evidence to support the use of invasive epidural injections of corticosteroids, local anesthetics and/or opioids as a treatment for ALBP without radiculopathy [D].
- Epidural corticosteroid injections are an option for short-term relief of radicular pain after failure of conservative treatment and as a means of avoiding surgery [C].

Acupuncture

Invasive needle acupuncture and other dry needling techniques are not recommended for treatment of ALBP [D].

Rating system from AHCPR Clinical Practice Guidelines: A, strong; B, moderate; C, limited; D, does not meet inclusion criteria.

Table 29–6. Activity Modification for Acute Low Back Pain (ALBP)

Activity Recommendations

- Patients with ALBP may be more comfortable by temporarily limiting or avoiding specific activities known to increase mechanical stress on the spine, such as prolonged unsupported sitting, heavy lifting, and twisting the back while lifting [D].
- For the employed patient, activity recommendations need to take into consideration the patient's age, general health, and physical demands of the job [D].

Bed Rest

- A gradual return to normal activities is more effective than prolonged bed rest for ALBP [B].
- Prolonged bed rest for more than 4 days may lead to debilitation and is not recommended for treatment of ALBP [B].
- Most patients with ALBP will not require bed rest. *Option*: Bed rest for 2 to 4 days for severe initial symptoms or primarily leg symptoms [D].

Exercise

- Low-stress aerobic exercise can prevent debilitation owing to inactivity during the first month of symptoms and thereafter may help return patients to their highest level of functioning [C].
- Aerobic (endurance) exercise programs, which minimally stress the back, can be started during the first 2 weeks for most patients with ALBP (walking, biking, swimming) [D].
- Conditioning exercises for the trunk muscles (especially back extensors), gradually increased, are helpful for ALBP, especially if symptoms persist. During the first 2 weeks, these exercises may aggravate symptoms due to mechanical stress more than endurance exercises [C].
- Back-specific exercise machines provide no apparent benefit over traditional exercise in the treatment of ALBP [D].
- There is no evidence to support stretching back muscles in the treatment of ALBP [D]. Recommended exercise quotas, gradually increased, result in better outcomes than advising patients to stop exercising if pain occurs [C].

Rating system from AHCPR Clinical Practice Guidelines: A, strong; B, moderate; C, limited; D, does not meet inclusion criteria.

Table 29–7. Surgical Information for Acute Low Back Pain (ALBP)

Surgery for Herniated Disk

- Clinicians are advised to discuss alternate treatment options with the sciatica patient after 1 month of conservative therapy. Specialist referral should be considered when (1) sciatica is severe and disabling, (2) sciatica symptoms persist or progress, and (3) there is evidence of nerve root compromise [B].
- Standard discectomy and microdiscectomy are of similar efficacy in those patients with herniated disk and nerve root involvement [B].
- Chemonucleolysis (chymopapain) is an acceptable treatment but less efficacious than standard diskectomy or microdiskectomy. Allergic sensitivity testing should be considered before use to reduce the incidence of anaphylaxis [C].
- Percutaneous diskectomy and other new methods of lumbar disk surgery are less efficacious than chymopapain and are not recommended until controlled trials have proven their efficacy [C].
- Patients with ALBP and no findings suggestive of nerve root compression or "red flag" conditions do not need surgical consultation [D].

Surgery for Spinal Stenosis

- Conservative management can be considered for elderly patients with spinal stenosis who can adequately function in activities of daily living. Surgery should not be considered in the first 3 months of symptoms. Treatment should take into consideration other medical problems, lifestyle preferences, and risks of surgery [D].
- Surgery decisions should take into consideration degree of neurologic claudication symptoms, associated limitations, and detectable neurologic compromise as well as imaging tests [D].

Spinal Fusion

- The use of spinal fusion is not recommended in the first 3 months of symptoms in the absence of fracture, dislocation, infection, or complications of tumor [C].

Rating system from AHCPR Clinical Practice Guidelines: A, strong; B, moderate; C, limited; D, does not meet inclusion criteria.

neurosurgery and/or orthopedics) are recommended for these patients.

Certain diagnostic maneuvers (confusion tests) can be helpful in separating out organic versus nonorganic causes of low back pain (Table 29–8).

SPECIAL CONSIDERATIONS

Patients with Occupational Low Back Injuries

Low back injuries on the job comprise over 50% of all occupational musculoskeletal injuries and up to 25% of all workplace injuries. However, each year 10% of the back injuries account for 80% of back injury costs and 30% of all musculoskeletal injury costs. Each year approximately 2% of employees will have a compensable back injury. Risk factors for occupational back injury include repetitive and heavy lifting, vibration from vehicle operation, and previous back injury. Nonmechanical risk factors include smoking, poor job rating by supervisors, short duration of employment, younger age, and poor job satisfaction (which may be the single most important factor).

The work-related low back injury is commonly encountered in the emergency department. Although approached and often treated identically to other ALBP, special considerations are warranted. Specific attention to the job duties and return-to-work (RTW) status must be addressed. Many clinicians simply take the worker off work for varying time periods. This may be necessary for a few days for symptom control; however, RTW with modified duty should be considered as soon as possible.

Modified duty is usually any work available at the patient's place of employment that satisfies work restrictions. Work restrictions can include office work with minimal lifting and avoidance of prolonged standing or excessive sitting. This benefits both employer and employee, avoiding lost wages for the employee and lost productivity for the employer. Many employers provide for modified duty, and the clinician may call and discuss plans for off-duty time and modified duty for the patient.

The use of narcotic analgesic medications needs to be carefully discussed. Written precautions at discharge are advisable, and workers with hazardous duties should avoid the use of these drugs while on the job. All patients using these medications should avoid driving.

As with non–work-related back injuries, most occupation-related injuries resolve spontaneously. However, prolonged back pain should prompt clinicians to consider other causes (as noted in the differential diagnosis). A chronic work injury that is not acute should be referred to the primary physician or an occupational medicine specialist.

Pediatric Patients

Back pain in children is actually common but not frequently brought to a physician's attention. Lifetime prevalence among school-aged children is approximately 34%. Most back pain is associated with activity or specific injuries. Sports involving hyperextension, twisting, bending, and axial loading are the most likely to result in injuries. These include gymnastics, football, tennis, cycling, weightlifting, and volleyball. Up to one half of cases of sports-related back problems involve a fracture of the pars interarticularis (spondylolysis) with or without spondylolisthesis (anterior displacement of the vertebral body secondary to spondylolysis). Children often describe vague, nonlocalized back pain while walking or during activity. Clinical findings tend to be less prevalent than those in adults, and only 10% of children have motor, sensory, or reflex deficits.

TABLE 29–8. Maneuvers to Diagnose Organic versus Nonorganic Causes of Low Back Pain

Maneuver	Findings
Hoover test (patient states unable to raise leg off table). In a supine position, patient is asked to raise the affected leg while examiner holds hands cupped under both heels. Normally, when attempting to lift the affected leg, downward pressure should be felt on the opposite heel.	Downward pressure from the opposite foot is not appreciated, suggesting minimal effort to raise the affected leg.
Superficial palpation of the lumbar area	Unusual sensitivity to light touch (unusual with lumbar complaints; possible exception: herpes zoster—shingles)
Straight-leg raising: performed in sitting and supine positions	Pain should occur in both positions.
Hip flexion	Pain should not be increased with passive vs. active flexion.
Axial loading (light pressure to top of head)	This should not increase lumbar symptoms.

Pediatric back pain causes include

- *Spondylolysis:* A stress fracture at the pars interarticularis generally occurs between ages 5 and 20. This fracture is best seen on oblique radiographs of the lumbar spine as a radiolucency at the "neck" of the commonly described "Scottie dog."
- *Spondylolisthesis* (see earlier description): This disorder has a familial predisposition (up to 40% in Native Americans and Eskimos).
- *Scheuermann's osteochondritis (adolescent round back):* This manifests as increased kyphosis in the thoracolumbar region. There is an increased incidence of spondylolisthesis. The cause is unknown but is thought to possibly result from repetitive and excessive mechanical stress.
- *Disc herniation:* This is relatively rare in children. It occurs most often in adolescence. Sciatica may or may not be present. Diagnosis often requires computed tomography or magnetic resonance imaging because disc space narrowing is not common.
- *Discitis:* This infection of the intervertebral disc often presents as fever, disc space narrowing on radiography, and an elevated sedimentation rate. It may be associated with other systemic symptoms such as an upper respiratory tract infection or pharyngitis. Young children may present with refusal to stand or walk. Treatment involves rest, pain control, and antibiotics.
- *Benign tumors:* Osteoblastoma, aneurysmal bone cyst, and osteoid osteoma often present as pain (especially night pain) and stiffness. *Primary malignant neoplasms* (rare) include Ewing's sarcoma, lymphoma, and leukemia. *Metastatic lesions* often occur at multiple sites and commonly present as intractable pain, weight loss, and fever. These include neuroblastoma, rhabdomyosarcoma, and, less commonly, retinoblastoma, Wilms' tumor, and teratoma-teratocarcinoma.

Elderly Patients

Back pain in the elderly should arouse suspicion for a structural pathologic process, especially in the patient with no prior history of back problems. Problems include osteoporosis and fractures. Radiographs should always be considered early in the assessment of a patient. Nonvertebral diagnoses include abdominal aortic aneurysm and malignancy.

Patients with Chronic Low Back Pain

Although not the main focus of this chapter, chronic low back pain (more than 3 months duration) is frequently encountered in the emergency department. This may be because of inadequate access to primary care services or from psychological and emotional factors. It is estimated that up to one half of patients with chronic back pain are disabled because of psychiatric factors.

The management of these individuals is best done with a primary physician and consultation with a pain management specialist. It is wise to avoid providing opiates for more than a few days, if at all, until the patient is seen by the regular physician. Most state licensing boards have specific guidelines for the use of chronic opiate therapy.

Malingerers

Malingering is considered the willful and deliberate falsification of signs or symptoms with secondary gain (e.g., monetary gain, time off work) as the motive. The malingerer may present with unusual symptomatology:

- Inconsistent response to light and deep palpation (i.e., excessive grimacing)
- Unusual nonradicular sensory deficits inconsistent with common neurologic patterns (stocking-type numbness)

Malingering should not be confused with *somatoform disorders, which* are conditions expressed as physical disease, often without an organic basis, linked to psychological dysfunction (and are *not* deliberate). Table 29–2 lists some physical examination maneuvers that may assist in determining nonorganic pain.

DISPOSITION AND FOLLOW-UP

Admission

Admission should be considered for all patients with presentations of "red flag" symptomatology (see "Priority Diagnoses"). Immediate consultation with one or more specialty services may be necessary. Other conditions that may warrant admission include

- Acute infectious conditions (especially with immunocompromise or immunosuppression)
- Spinal fractures that may have occult associated injuries (especially in the elderly)
- Patients with intractable pain
- Patients with neurologic deficits at risk for progression (frail, elderly)

Discharge

Most patients with ALBP can be discharged after appropriate therapy. Specific written instructions are given and discussed with the patient or family member providing care.

Precautions for worsening signs or symptoms should be clearly communicated, and patients should be asked to verify their understanding of the instructions. Patients are advised to contact their physician and arrange for follow-up.

The self-limited course of most episodes of ALBP should be emphasized. Medications are used judiciously with consideration of documented effectiveness and side effects. Strict bed rest is no longer advocated, and patients can be as active as tolerated, with restrictions including no lifting, minimal twisting (rotation) and bending of the spine, and avoidance of prolonged standing or sitting.

Work status should be assessed and work duties modified to avoid injury aggravation. In the acute phase, many patients will benefit from a few days off work. If the injury was work related, arrangements should be made for follow-up with either the primary provider or an occupational medicine physician.

Final Points

- Acute low back pain (ALBP) is a common clinical problem seen in the emergency department.

A thorough understanding of, and rapid assessment for, rare but potentially serious conditions ("red flags") are important and treatment must be instituted promptly, including specialty consultation as needed.

- Patients are advised that most cases of low back pain are benign, require minimal use of diagnostic studies, and often resolve with conservative treatment (90% resolve in 6 weeks).
- Clinical practice guidelines exist to assist in the management of ALBP, providing literature-supported therapies and minimizing continued use of costly, unproved treatment modalities.
- Many cases of ALBP seen by the emergency physician will be work related and require appropriate follow-up and consideration for the safe return to work.
- An understanding of the less common causes and presentations of ALBP in special circumstances (children, the elderly) is essential to facilitate appropriate follow-up.

CASE *Study*

A 44-year-old construction worker noted severe, acute low back pain after lifting a heavy object on the job. Pain was immediate, localized to the right lower lumbar area, and made worse with movement of the back and leg on the affected side. He stopped working and notified his supervisor, who advised him to seek immediate evaluation at the local emergency department.

Initial assessment of the patient showed normal vital signs except for a temperature of 100.6°F (38.1°C). The patient appeared in moderate distress and had difficulty sitting on the examination room table. He indicated significant moderate to severe pain localized to the right lumbar area with some radiation only to the right buttock. He specifically denied pain or numbness radiating to the legs and had no loss of bowel or bladder control. Pain was partially relieved by avoiding movement. He denied any associated abdominal or urinary tract symptoms. The past medical history was hypertension, well controlled with a β blocker. Review of systems noted no history of back problems or injury and no kidney, urinary, or gastrointestinal problems. There was no family history of musculoskeletal disorders (e.g., arthritis).

Examination revealed a moderately obese male. The lumbar area appeared grossly normal

without scars, swelling, deformity, or other lesions. Pain was reproduced in the right lumbar paraspinal muscle region with some palpable spasm. There was no costovertebral angle tenderness. The range of motion of the spine was limited on lateral bending and rotation to the right. A brief, general physical examination revealed only mild nasal congestion. Lower extremity assessment revealed no focal neurologic deficits, and pain was elicited with straight-leg raising (both sitting and supine).

The patient was noted to have a low-grade fever on presentation. Despite mild upper respiratory symptoms, a CBC, an ESR, and urinalysis were ordered. The CBC was normal, the ESR was normal at 10 mm/hr, and results of urinalysis were normal.

The patient requested radiographs of his back. After history and examination, it was determined that radiographs were not indicated at this time. The thought process and decision making were explained to the patient.

Differential diagnosis at this juncture is primarily focused on acute soft tissue strain of the lumbar area. The presence of pain radiating into the buttock on the affected side has the possibility of early sciatica. With a low-grade fever, a possible infectious cause was considered; however, normal laboratory test results were reassuring.

The algorithm (see Figs. 29–3 and 29–4) was used to reassure the patient regarding the benign, although certainly bothersome, nature of his injury. "Red flag" signs and symptoms were discussed, and the patient was told to watch for any worsening of his condition.

The patient was advised about the nature of the illness and the expected course. Recommendations included rest at home for the next 24 to 48 hours and avoidance of all lifting, bending or twisting at the waist, and prolonged standing or sitting (patient had planned a long car drive the coming weekend and was advised to make alternate plans).

The patient requested pain medication and was given an intramuscular dose of ketorolac, 30 mg, and two oral tablets of acetaminophen, 500 mg, with hydrocodone, 5 mg. He was observed in the emergency department for 30 minutes and had excellent pain relief. Medication at home included ibuprofen, 600 mg orally every 6 to 8 hours with food, and acetaminophen/ hydrocodone, one to two tablets orally up to every 4 hours for additional pain relief. He was warned regarding possible allergy, drowsiness, and gastrointestinal upset and constipation with the medications. He was advised to avoid driving or operating machinery/equipment while taking the medications and to avoid drinking alcohol while on the hydrocodone preparation.

This patient had his injury on the job (occupational injury). This is important, because most private insurers specifically exclude work injuries from coverage. Many physicians forget this, and it can cause difficulties for the patient regarding return to work (RTW) and, if the problem does not resolve rapidly, problems obtaining temporary benefits for lost work time. It is imperative that the clinician address RTW because many employees can return to modified duty and do not aggravate their condition. Sometimes, no other work that fits restrictions is available and the patient is to be off work until symptoms resolve, for safe return. Many employers prefer their employee to RTW at modified duty if it is safe for them to do so.

The injured worker was given a work excuse recommending no work for 2 days to stabilize pain and observe for any worsening signs. After this time, the employee was advised to have a reexamination by his personal physician or an occupational medicine specialist. He was advised to return should he have any acute worsening of symptoms (increasing pain, further radiation of pain into the lower extremity, loss of bowel or bladder function, and fever) before transfer of care to his regular physician. A family member arrived to drive the patient home.

This clinical case, although simple, illustrates several important points. The initial presentation of an occupational acute back injury is often seen by the emergency department physician. Appropriate evaluation, treatment, and disposition (taking RTW into consideration) are essential to avoid delay in further treatment, lost wages to the employee, and lost productivity for the employer.

Bibliography

TEXTS

Anderssen GBJ: The Epidemiology of Spinal Disorders. The Adult Spine: Principles and Practice. New York, Raven, 1997.

Bigos S, Bowyer O, Braen G, et al: Acute Low Back Problems in Adults. Clinical Practice Guidelines No. 14. AHCPR publication No. 95–0642. Rockville, MD, Agency for Health Care Policy and Research, Public Health Service, U.S. Department of Health and Human Services, December 1994.

Hoppenfeld S. Orthopaedic Neurology: A Diagnostic Guide to Neurologic Levels. Philadelphia, Lippincott-Raven, 1997.

JOURNAL ARTICLES

Anderson GBJ, Lucente T, Davis AM: A comparison of osteopathic spinal manipulation with standard care for patients with low back pain. N Engl J Med 1999; 34:1426–1431.

Argoff CA, Wheeler AH: Spinal and radicular disorders. Neurol Clin 1998; 16:833–849.

Della-Ciustina DA: Back pain: Cost effective strategies for distinguishing between benign and life-threatening causes. Emerg Med Pract 2000; 2(2):1–24.

Deyo RA, Weinstein JN: Low back pain. N Engl J Med 2001; 344:363–370.

Edlow JA, Bosher GA: The challenge of acute back pain. Emerg Med Rep 1999; 20(pt I):193–200; (pt II): 201–210.

Haldeman S: Diagnostic tests for the evaluation of back and neck pain. Neurol Clin 1996; 14:103–117.

Hashemi L, Webster BS, Clancy EA: Trends in disability duration and cost of workers' compensation low back pain claims (1988–1996). J Occup Environ Med 1998; 40:1110–1119.

Lurie JD, Gerber PD, Sox NC: A pain in the back. N Engl J Med 2000; 343:723–726.

Nikkanen HE, Brown DFM, Nadel ES: Low back pain. J Emerg Med 2002; 22:279–283.

Payne WK III: Common orthopedic problems: Back pain in children and adolescents. Pediatr Clin North Am 1996; 43:899–917.

Schiff D, Batchelor T, Wen PY: Neurologic emergencies in cancer patients. Neurol Clin 1998; 16:449–483.

Swenson R: Lower back pain, differential diagnosis: A reasonable clinical approach. Neurol Clin North Am 1999; 17:43–63.

Teoh D, Krug SE: Back pain in children and adolescents. Pediatr Emerg Med Rep 1999; 4:115–126.

Van Tulder MW, Koes BW, Bouter LM: Conservative treatment of acute and chronic nonspecific low back pain: A systematic review of randomized controlled trials of the most common interventions. Spine 1997; 22:2128–2156.

The author wishes to acknowledge the work of Herbert Sutherland and Gary Strange in the writing of this chapter for the first edition of this book.

CHAPTER 30

The Swollen and Painful Joint

ARTHUR B. SANDERS

CASE *Study*

A 20-year-old woman presented with a 2-day history of aching in her left wrist. She complained of pain and swelling in her left knee associated with a low-grade fever. She had noted some new "spots" on the extensor surfaces of her distal forearms and shins.

INTRODUCTION

The skeletal articulations in the body are designed to facilitate movement. Their mobility ranges from immovable to freely movable. Syndesmoses, such as the tibiofibular attachment and the sutures of the skull, are immovable and rarely affected by inflammation. The cartilaginous joints include the epiphyseal plates in growing bone, the intervertebral discs, and the pubic symphysis. These have a slightly increased risk of problems. The freely movable, diarthrodial joints, which make up nearly all of the joints of the extremities, are the most prone to inflammation. These joints are composed of an articular cartilage that covers the weight- or stress-bearing surfaces and a fibrous joint capsule lined by synovium. Articular cartilage is distinguished by a low concentration of cells and a lack of blood vessels, lymphatic channels, and nerves. Nourishment is obtained from synovial fluid that is produced by the synovial lining. The synovial lining is highly vascular and richly innervated by branches from the nerve roots that innervate muscles crossing the joint. Inflammation or irritation of the synovial lining produces pain and increased fluid. The synovium is thrown into folds at the margin of the articular cartilage but does not cover the weight-bearing surfaces. These folds allow the lining to be stretched with motion. The joint cavity contains a small amount of highly viscous fluid that lubricates the joint surfaces. Synovial fluid is composed of a transudate of plasma plus mucin, a complex macromolecule added by the type B cells in the synovial lining. Mucin is responsible for the high viscosity of this extremely effective lubricating fluid.

The articulation is additionally supported by ligaments, tendons, and muscles. Some diarthrodial joints, such as the knee, radiocarpal, and sternoclavicular joints, contain intra-articular fibrocartilaginous menisci that act as stress-reducing washers, allowing the opposing articular surfaces to glide freely past each other. The menisci are attached at their periphery to the fibrous capsule.

These complex joint structures may be affected by inflammatory processes, which usually have an immunologic, crystalline, or infectious origin. Inflammation is a pathologic process involving white blood cells, enzymes, and physiologically active substances. The end result is tissue damage, particularly to the articular cartilage. The inciting agent may be unknown (e.g., rheumatoid arthritis) or recognized (e.g., gout). Trauma is the most common cause of the swollen, painful joint. Previous injury is a predisposing factor in nontraumatic causes as well.

INITIAL APPROACH AND STABILIZATION

Joint pain and swelling is not a life-threatening problem. Patients are triaged and evaluated in turn, based on their acuity. They belong in the "urgent" category because they may have severe pain and can suffer permanent joint damage if they are not evaluated appropriately and treated promptly. Analgesia may be given after the physician's initial evaluation.

CLINICAL ASSESSMENT

The history and physical examination provide information that will allow the physician to determine the most likely cause for the patient's problem and the need for further diagnostic testing.

History

Patients presenting with joint pain or swelling often carry the self-diagnosis of "arthritis." An effort is necessary to avoid accepting this self-diagnosis and possibly precluding a thorough assessment.

The following information is obtained:

1. *How long* have the *symptoms* been *present?* Arthritic symptoms of less than 6 weeks' duration are considered acute; those of over 6 weeks' duration are considered chronic.
2. Did the problem *develop gradually* or *suddenly?* Rapid onset of joint swelling or pain is typical of trauma, crystalline-induced disease, and infection. Normally, the joint space is small and the capsule is poorly compliant; therefore, it takes only a small amount of increased synovial fluid to cause pain.
3. Has it been *steadily* getting *worse,* or do the symptoms *wax and wane?*
4. Are *other joints* involved at any time? Symptoms may be migratory (moving from joint to joint with complete resolution in the first joints) or additive, with new joints becoming involved (while the first joints still hurt).
5. Has there been any *recent trauma* to the area or any *known injury* to the joint in the past?
6. Is there a *prior history* of arthritis, joint pain, or surgery? Joints with previous involvement or damage are the most susceptible to infection.
7. Does the patient take *medications* or a *drug of abuse?*
8. Is the patient *sexually active?* If male, has there been a penile discharge or urinary symptoms? If female, what is the menstrual history? Has there been a recent vaginal discharge or pelvic pain?
9. Has the patient had a *rash* anywhere on his/her body?
10. Has the patient been *traveling* to an *area endemic for Lyme disease?* Arthritis can be a late manifestation of Lyme disease, which is prevalent in the northeastern United States as well as in several western and midwestern states. Questions about tick bites, a rash, and other symptoms within 6 months of travel may be appropriate.

Physical Examination

The physical examination is important to ascertain objective criteria for arthritis, to determine the pattern of joint involvement, and to seek extra-articular signs of a causal process.

Joint Examination. Any involved joint is evaluated in a systemic fashion.

Inspection. Erythema of the overlying skin is commonly associated with gout and septic arthritis. Swelling may represent an effusion or edema of the surrounding tissue. In the knee, elbow, and distal joints, intracapsular fluid causes a symmetric swelling and can be palpated as a "bogginess" or "fluctuant" feeling of the joint capsule. Periarticular swelling is usually more localized. The two findings may be combined, complicating the differentiation. Deformity may represent chronic bony changes or acute fracture or dislocation.

Palpation. Warmth is usually noted first. It is best to begin proximally and move distally over the joint to determine the skin temperature. Tenderness is often exquisite, and a gentle examination is essential. Pain is often diffuse in the joint with intra-articular disease but usually more localized with extra-articular problems. Palpation will usually differentiate effusion from tissue edema.

Motion. Without inducing too much pain, it is important to determine the range of motion in all joint directions. Patients with pain and limitation of motion in all directions are more likely to have intra-articular disease processes. Note should be made of any difference in active or passive range of motion of the joint. Patients with extra-articular disease usually have pain on active but not passive motion.

Other Joint Involvement. In addition to the joint initially identified by the patient, other joints may be involved. A complete joint examination, including the temporomandibular joint and vertebral column, is important to determine the number of joints involved and assist in narrowing the differential diagnosis.

General Examination. In addition to the joint examinations, other systems may provide valuable clues to the etiology.

Vital Signs. Fever is present in more than 50% of cases of septic arthritis and may be present in other forms of arthritis as well.

Skin. There may be a number of cutaneous findings:

1. Petechial rash is associated with arthritis in vasculitis and systemic lupus erythematosus.
2. Pustulovesicular skin lesions on the extremities are characteristic of disseminated gonococcal infection.
3. Subcutaneous nodules are seen in rheumatoid arthritis.
4. Erythema chronicum migrans is seen with Lyme disease.
5. Erythema marginatum is seen with acute rheumatic fever.
6. Pitting of the fingernails is associated with psoriatic arthritis.
7. Needle tracks suggest intravenous drug abuse, which can be a precipitating factor for septic arthritis.

8. Tophi (uric acid crystals in subcutaneous tissue) are associated with gout but are rare.
9. Buccal or genital ulcers are associated with lupus, Reiter's syndrome, or Behçet's disease.

Eyes. Conjunctivitis and iritis in association with arthritis are part of the presentation of Reiter's syndrome and ankylosing spondylitis.

Chest. Auscultation may reveal pleural or pericardial friction rubs owing to inflammatory reactions found in rheumatic diseases such as systemic lupus erythematosus.

Abdomen. An enlarged or tender liver may indicate infectious hepatitis, which may cause arthritis.

Pelvic and Genital Area. A genital examination with a culture for gonococci is indicated when septic arthritis is a possibility.

CLINICAL REASONING

On completion of the history and physical examination, it is useful to make three important diagnostic decisions.

Is the Pain Articular (from the Joint) or Extra-articular (from Tendons, Bursae, or Other Periarticular Structures)?

Pain from articular and synovial surfaces worsens with both active and passive movement, whereas nonarticular pain worsens with active movement much more than with passive motion. The degree of tenderness of the periarticular tissue and pain localized to this area point to problems outside the joint capsule.

Are there Objective Criteria for Inflammation ("Arthritis"), or Is There only Subjective Pain ("Arthralgia")?

Important criteria for arthritis include (1) joint pain on passive movement, (2) swelling consistent with joint effusion, (3) limitation of motion of the joint, (4) warmth emanating from the joint, and (5) erythema over the joint. The first four criteria are the most useful in diagnosis.

How Many Joints Are Involved?

Monoarticular (one joint) and oligoarticular (two to four joints) diseases possess a similar list of diagnostic possibilities, whereas polyarticular (more than four joints) disease usually is due to other causes (Table 30–1).

Once the diagnosis of acute arthritis is made, the patient's clinical picture and the number of joints involved can usually provide a "ballpark" diagnosis. Systemic disease of immunologic origin most often causes polyarticular disease. Monoarticular disease is of particular importance to the emergency physician because of the possibility of a septic joint, which can rapidly destroy the joint surface.

Can a Specific Diagnosis Be Made?

One can use the clinical history, physical examination, and diagnostic adjuncts in consideration of the serious and common diseases that present as joint pain (Table 30–2). It is most important in the emergency department setting to rule out septic arthritis as the cause of acute monoarticular

TABLE 30–1. Common Causes of Acute Arthritis

Monoarticular or Oligoarticular	Polyarticular
Infection Bacterial Granulomatous	**Infection** Viral
Crystal-Induced Gout Pseudogout	**Inflammatory** Small joint pattern Rheumatoid arthritis Systemic lupus erythematosus Polymyositis Progressive systemic sclerosis
Traumatic Hemarthrosis Synovitis	Large joint pattern Rheumatoid variant Ankylosing spondylitis Reiter's syndrome
Nontraumatic Hemarthrosis Inherited coagulopathy Anticoagulant-induced	Psoriatic arthritis Rheumatic fever Lyme disease
Degenerative Joint Disease	**Degenerative Joint Disease**

TABLE 30–2. Diagnosis and Management of Major Types of Acute Monoarticular Arthritis

Diagnosis or Class	Laboratory	Radiography	Synovial Fluid	Treatment
Septic	Elevated WBC, ESR, possible cultures from other sites	Soft tissue swelling, osteopenia, joint space narrowing, subchondral erosions	WBC >50,000 PMN >85% Glucose <50 mg/dL Gram stain positive in 65% of cases Culture positive	Admission IV antibiotics Splinting Drainage
Gout	Serum uric acid elevated 70%–90%	Soft tissue swelling, tophi	WBC 2,500–50,000 PMN 40%–90% Urate crystals	Oral NSAIDs Colchicine, IV or PO
Pseudogout		Soft tissue swelling, chondrocalcinosis	WBC 2,500–50,000 PMN 40%–90% Calcium pyrophosphate crystals	Oral NSAIDs Colchicine, IV or PO
Inflammatory joint disease	ESR elevated in 60%–80%	Soft tissue swelling, erosions	WBC 10,000–50,000 PMN 65%–85%	Oral NSAIDs
Degenerative joint disease		Joint space narrowing, marginal osteophytes, subchondral sclerosis	WBC < 5,000 PMN < 25%	Oral NSAIDs
Traumatic		Soft tissue swelling	Bloody WBC <10,000 Fat droplets (usually represent a fracture)	Aspiration Compression Splint

ESR, erythrocyte sedimentation rate; IV, intravenous; NSAIDs, nonsteroidal anti-inflammatory drugs; PMN, polymorphonuclear neutrophils; PO, orally; WBC, white blood cells.

arthritis. Polyarticular disease may be impossible to diagnose specifically in the emergency department, requiring extended follow-up and testing to arrive at the underlying cause.

Septic Arthritis

Acute bacterial arthritis has the potential to destroy a joint in only 3 to 4 days. No joint is immune, but the knee is the most common site (about 50% of cases), followed by the hip (13%), shoulder (9%), wrist (8%), ankle (8%), and elbow (7%). Hematogenous spread is the most common means by which bacteria infect a joint, but direct inoculation into the joint or spread from adjacent structures is also possible. Risk factors for septic arthritis include recent joint surgery or procedure, a prosthetic joint, patients with compromised immune systems (e.g., patients with human immunodeficiency virus infection, the very young or old), intravenous drug abusers, patients taking immunosuppressive drugs, or patients with chronic diseases. *Staphylococcus aureus* is the most common bacterial cause. Gram-negative organisms and anaerobes are becoming more common. Children are at risk for *Escherichia coli* and *Haemophilus influenzae* joint infections as well as for *S. aureus*. Patients with sickle cell disease can have *Salmonella* arthritis. In sexually active patients *Neisseria gonorrhoeae* can cause a

monoarticular or polyarticular arthritis. Tuberculosis is a rare infectious cause. Viral arthritis is typically polyarticular.

Disseminated gonococcal infection complicates about 0.2% of gonococcal genitourinary infections. Arthritis is one of its most frequent manifestations. Fever is present in about 90% of such cases, and skin lesions are found in about 50%. The most commonly affected joints are the knee and ankle, although the hip and phalangeal joints are also vulnerable. Polyarticular, often migratory arthralgia is seen in about 75% of cases of disseminated gonococcal infection, usually preceding the arthritis. Most studies report that more women are affected than men.

Crystal-Induced Arthritides

Gouty attacks have an acute onset with escalation of symptoms over 12 to 24 hours. The symptoms are monoarticular or oligoarticular and most commonly involve the metatarsophalangeal joint at the base of the first toe, the ankle, the dorsum of the foot, the wrist, or the knee. Usually there is associated soft tissue inflammation that resembles cellulitis. Gout is predominantly a disease of men. Women are affected usually only after menopause. The process is produced by an inflammatory reaction to uric acid crystals in the joint and periarticular tissues. The serum uric acid level is not necessarily elevated during an acute attack.

Pseudogout is an acute monoarticular arthritis caused by calcium pyrophosphate crystals in the joint fluid. Pseudogout usually occurs in older patients and affects men and women equally. The knee is the most common site. The radiographic finding of chondrocalcinosis (Fig. 30–1) means the patient is at risk for attacks of pseudogout; however, there is little correlation with the radiographic findings and clinical course.

Traumatic Synovitis or Hemarthrosis

Acute injury to a joint may result in immediate swelling (less than 2 hours after injury) or delayed effusion within 12 to 24 hours. Immediate swelling, with marked effusion and pain, is usually secondary to bleeding into the joint (hemarthrosis). Because of its exposed position, the knee is the joint most commonly involved with traumatic hemarthrosis, and in 90% of cases there is associated intra-articular disruption or damage. Meniscal or anterior cruciate ligament tears are the most frequent injuries. Although acute joint instability may not occur, significant long-term disability can result after this type of injury. Traumatic synovitis is a less serious injury and is infrequently associated with internal joint damage. The usual outcome is full recovery.

Nontraumatic Hemarthrosis

Bleeding into a joint is common in patients with inherited coagulopathies and occasionally occurs in patients being treated with anticoagulants.

Polyarticular Arthritides

Patients with rheumatoid arthritis, spondyloarthropathies ("rheumatoid variants"), and other collagen vascular diseases may occasionally present to the emergency department with complaints of joint pain. Although these problems are usually polyarticular, pain in an isolated joint can be out of proportion to the others. It is important to consider the need for arthrocentesis to determine if infection is the cause of the more painful or inflamed joint. If infection is excluded to a reasonable degree, the patient is treated for the underlying disease.

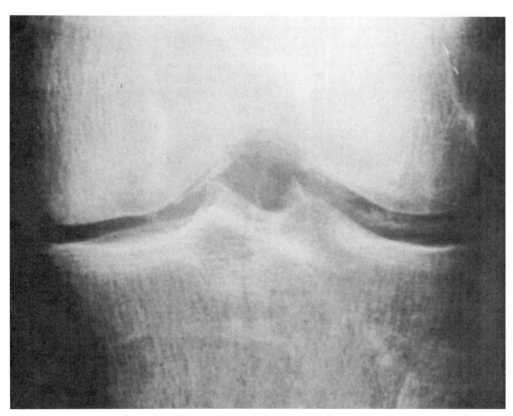

FIGURE 30–1 • The radiographic findings of chondrocalcinosis in the knee joint.

Inflammatory polyarthritis has two common patterns. One is the small joint or symmetric pattern typical of rheumatoid arthritis but also seen in systemic lupus erythematosus, polymyositis, and progressive systemic sclerosis and transiently in some viral infections such as rubella and hepatitis B. The other pattern is the asymmetric large joint or axial skeletal involvement characteristic of ankylosing spondylitis, Reiter's syndrome, psoriatic arthritis, enteropathic arthritis, acute rheumatic fever, and Lyme disease. This latter pattern of joint involvement and group of diseases is sometimes termed the *rheumatoid variant(s)*.

Degenerative Joint Disease

Degenerative joint disease is a disease of age and overuse. Ninety percent of elderly patients have some degree of degenerative joint disease in their hands, and 30% to 50% have involvement of their hips by age 65. Symptoms are usually mild, but acute exacerbations with swelling and evidence of inflammation may occur. Stiffness is the most common complaint, and joint pain usually increases over the course of the day. Physical examination shows enlargement of bone and limitation of motion. Radiographs will demonstrate osteophytes, joint space narrowing, and bony deformity.

Periarticular Syndromes

Bursitis is inflammation of a closed space that is adjacent to but isolated from the synovial cavity. The prepatellar, olecranon, and subdeltoid bursae are most frequently affected. Idiopathic bursitis occurs in young, healthy individuals and is probably caused by overuse or repetitive injury. It does not have associated systemic symptoms. Septic bursitis is more common in older individuals with predisposing disorders such as diabetes.

Tendonitis is inflammation of a tendon, usually caused by repetitive injury or overuse. Common locations are the biceps tendon of the shoulder, the extensor tendon inserts at the elbow, and the extensor pollicis at the thumb. There is associated tenderness and pain, especially with active movement, but little swelling and no systemic manifestations.

Osteomyelitis is bacterial infection of bone and may occur adjacent to or spread to involve a joint. Systemic manifestations of infection are usually present. Radiographic changes take up to 3 weeks to appear.

DIAGNOSTIC ADJUNCTS

Laboratory Studies

Laboratory tests of blood are not usually helpful in the diagnosis of the acutely painful joint. A leukocyte count, erythrocyte sedimentation rate (ESR), and serum uric acid level occasionally confirm the clinical impression but are not routinely recommended. In the majority of proved cases of septic arthritis, leukocyte counts are within the normal range and elevated counts may arise from a number of different causes. An elevated ESR indicates inflammation, but the test is nonspecific and the overlap between patients with and without various inflammatory diseases is great. The serum uric acid level does not correlate with gouty attacks and can be within the normal range in up to one third of cases of acute gouty arthritis. Tests such as serum complement, rheumatoid factor, and antinuclear antibodies have no diagnostic value in the emergency department.

Radiographic Imaging

Radiographic changes due to arthritis require weeks to develop, and therefore initial radiographs have limited diagnostic value. For most joints, standard radiographic views are adequate, but occasionally weight-bearing or stress views are necessary to gauge joint stability in patients with traumatic arthritis.

The radiographic assessment of joints includes inspection of alignment, bones, cartilage, and soft tissues. Specific abnormalities that appear after several weeks may be remembered by using the mnemonic SECONDS:

> **S**oft tissue swelling is almost universal and nonspecific.
> **E**rosions classically occur at the cartilage-synovial junction in patients with rheumatoid arthritis (symmetric "punched out" erosions without bony overgrowth) and chronic gout (asymmetric lesions with an overlying thin rim of bony overgrowth).
> **C**alcification can be intra-articular (indicating a fracture or degenerative fragment) or periarticular (indicating tendonitis or bursitis).
> **O**steopenia is most pronounced near the involved joint in osteomyelitis, rheumatoid arthritis, and septic arthritis.
> **N**arrowing of the joint space indicates loss of articular cartilage and is found early in individuals with rheumatoid arthritis.
> **D**eformity is due to chronic destructive changes of whatever cause.

Stippling refers to early chondrocalcinosis that produces punctate radiodensities in hyaline cartilage (see Fig. 30–1). Subchondral cysts and sclerosis are seen in people with advanced degenerative joint disease.

The most common plain film finding in acute monoarticular arthritis is a normal joint with soft tissue swelling. At present, computed tomography, nuclear medicine techniques, and magnetic resonance imaging do not contribute significantly to the emergency department diagnosis of the swollen and painful joint. However, magnetic resonance imaging has supplanted the arthrogram as the procedure of choice for evaluating soft tissue injuries of most joints.

Special Tests

Arthrocentesis

Arthrocentesis and appropriate analysis of synovial fluid are necessary to help the physician arrive at a specific diagnosis for acute monoarticular arthritis in the emergency department. Although synovial fluid can be analyzed in many ways (Table 30–3), it is diagnostic only in patients with bacterial and crystal-induced arthritis. Clinical analysis in the emergency department is directed toward diagnosing these disorders.

The most important function of arthrocentesis is to exclude bacterial infection. No other technique differentiates septic arthritis from other causes of inflammatory arthritis. It is appropriate to perform arthrocentesis at the initial presentation of a patient with acute arthritis. Because different types of arthritis can coexist, it is worthwhile to obtain synovial fluid during an exacerbation ("flare") in a patient with known arthritis, especially if the exacerbation is atypical for the patient's known disease.

Arthrocentesis is a safe procedure and has a low complication rate and few contraindications. It is not performed when the joint space might be seeded by passage through infected tissue or when the results would not influence therapy. When obviously infected skin is avoided, the risk of bacterial arthritis resulting from arthrocentesis is less than 1 in 10,000. When necessary, arthrocentesis can be safely performed in a patient with bleeding disorders, although in such cases it would be prudent to treat the hemorrhagic diathesis before arthrocentesis.

Elements of Synovial Fluid Analysis (Table 30–3)

General Appearance. Normal joint fluid is clear and light yellow. Clouding of joint fluid is caused by the presence of fibrin and leukocytes. Pink or bloody joint fluid, especially with a "fat sheen" on the surface, represents some disruption in the articular surface (intra-articular fracture), synovial lining, cartilage, or ligaments.

Viscosity. Normal joint fluid has a high viscosity, primarily related to mucin, a complex of protein and hyaluronic acid. With inflammation, mucin is denatured and viscosity decreases. Normal joint fluid will "string" 1 to 2 inches when a drop is placed between the gloved thumb and forefinger and the digits are quickly separated. The mucin clot test using 3% acetic acid is the traditional test for intact mucin, but the string test done at the bedside gives immediate results and is almost as good.

Polarized Microscopic Examination. Examining a drop of fluid with a polarizing microscope is necessary to detect monosodium urate (gout) and calcium pyrophosphate dihydrate (pseudogout) crystals. Polarizers are placed above and below the specimen and then turned 90 degrees to each other so that no light can reach the examiner's eye unless it has been affected by an object between the polarizers. This specific property is called birefringence, which means that the plane

---

TABLE 30–3. Synovial Fluid Analysis

Routine for the Emergency Department	**Not Indicated in the Emergency Department**
General appearance	Mucin clot (acetic acid) test
String test	Spontaneous clot
Polarized light microscopic examination for crystals	Protein
Gram's stain	Acid-fast (mycobacteria) stain
Aerobic culture	Anaerobic, mycobacterial, and fungal culture
Gonococcal culture	Lactate, other organic acids

Occasionally Useful in the Emergency Department

Leukocyte count
Glucose

of polarized light passing through such an object is rotated. Thus, light passing through a birefringent object is also able to pass through the polarizer in front of the observer's eye, causing the object to appear to glow against the black background (Fig. 30–2). The direction in which the birefringent crystal rotates the plane of polarized light is determined by use of the first-order red compensator. Urate crystals have negative birefringence, resulting in a gold-yellow color when the axis of the compensator is parallel to the crystal. Calcium pyrophosphate crystals have positive birefringence, giving a blue color when the axis of the compensator is parallel to the crystal. The use of a compensator is not mandatory because the appearance of these two crystals is very different. Urate crystals are usually needle shaped, numerous, and strongly birefringent, glowing brightly. Calcium pyrophosphate crystals are smaller, rhomboid shaped, fewer in number, and weakly birefringent. Other objects or crystals sometimes found in joint fluid may be birefringent, but they can be differentiated from these crystals by shape and size.

Leukocyte Count. Normal synovial fluid has a leukocyte count of less than 200 cells/mm^3, with a differential that includes 10% to 60% polymorphonuclear cells. Inflammatory fluid has more than 5000 cells/mm^3. With increasing inflammation, the number of leukocytes and the percentage of polymorphonuclear cells increase, but the overlaps are too great for single values to be diagnostic of a specific disease (see Table 30–2). Synovial fluid protein and glucose values are of little diagnostic value and are not routinely recommended.

Gram's Stain. Gram's staining of synovial fluid can be diagnostic. Bacteria can be seen in 70% to 90% of culture-proven bacterial arthritides caused by gram-positive bacteria, in about 50% caused by gram-negative bacteria, and in 20% to 30% from gonococci.

Cultures. Cultures for bacteria including gonococci are required. Synovial fluid cultures for tuberculosis and viruses may be useful later in the workup if bacterial cultures are negative. Blood cultures are useful because they are positive in about half of patients with gram-positive bacterial arthritides and in 10% to 20% of those with arthritis from gram-negative bacterial causes. Vaginal, cervical, rectal, penile, and pharyngeal cultures are useful when gonococcemia is suspected.

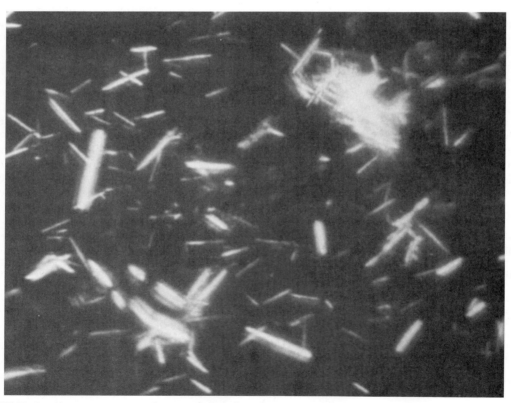

FIGURE 30–2 • Numerous urate crystals seen with the polarized microscope. Note the characteristic needle-like shape and strong birefringence.

PRINCIPLES OF MANAGEMENT

The therapeutic approach to acute arthritis depends on the specific diagnosis. Available treatment modalities include

- Aspiration of the joint fluid
- Antibiotics
- Anti-inflammatory medications
- Splinting and pressure dressings
- Intra-articular injections

The goals are joint rest, decreasing inflammation, and aggressive treatment of intra-articular infection. Specific treatments are discussed here and listed in Table 30–2.

Septic Arthritis

Antibiotics. The key to successful treatment of bacterial arthritis is initiation of appropriate antibiotic therapy as early as possible after the onset of symptoms. Therefore, early diagnosis and presumptive selection of antibiotics are essential. Antibiotics may be chosen based on Gram's stain findings from the synovial fluid. A second- or third-generation cephalosporin with an aminoglycoside can be used empirically. Vancomycin may be necessary in cases of methicillin resistance.

Joint Drainage. In most patients with septic arthritis, the joints are adequately drained by repeated arthrocentesis. Initially, they may require two or three aspirations per day. Most patients require between six and nine arthrocenteses before resolution of the effusion. The process is slightly more successful if it is initiated within 3 days of the onset of symptoms. Occasionally, open drainage is required in patients in whom needle drainage cannot remove the fluid owing to the presence of intra-articular adhesions or marked thickness of the fluid. Patients with septic arthritis of the hip cannot easily undergo repeat arthrocentesis, so they are often treated by open drainage.

Splinting. Splinting of the involved extremity is important and should be done soon after the initial arthrocentesis.

Analgesia and Anti-inflammatory Agents. Septic arthritis can be very painful. Analgesia and anti-inflammatory agents are given in proportion to pain.

Crystal-Induced Arthritis

Nonsteroidal Anti-inflammatory Drugs (NSAIDs). NSAIDs are effective in hastening the resolution of acute attacks of gout and have a lower incidence of side effects than the traditional treatment with colchicine. Indomethacin has been used most often in this regard, but other NSAIDs are probably just as effective if given in high doses for short periods of time. Most attacks resolve within a few days, and therapy is rarely indicated for longer than 1 week. NSAIDs that selectively inhibit the cyclooxygenase-2 enzyme such as celecoxib are very effective in treating the inflammatory response without the harmful gastrointestinal side effects of most nonselective NSAIDs. These medications remain relatively expensive, but they should be considered in patients who have risk factors for gastrointestinal problems.

Colchicine. Colchicine is the traditional agent used for the treatment of acute gout, with a response rate of about 70% within 48 hours compared with a spontaneous resolution rate of 30% to 40%. Colchicine is also effective in acute pseudogout, with a response rate of about 40%. Colchicine is administered orally or intravenously in small doses until (1) clinical improvement begins, (2) early gastrointestinal toxicity develops with nausea or diarrhea, or (3) the maximum safe dose is reached. A common protocol is an oral dose of 1 mg initially followed by 0.5 mg every 2 hours until one of the three endpoints is reached. For intravenous use, the initial dose is 1 to 2 mg with repeat doses of 1 mg every 4 to 6 hours. There are limits in dosing for elderly patients and those with impaired renal function. The therapeutic margin of colchicine is extremely narrow, and significant toxicity can occur with single doses as low as 6 mg orally or 4 mg intravenously. For this reason, NSAIDs are the drugs of choice.

Aspiration. Complete aspiration of the involved joint is occasionally followed by resolution of the inflammation. Intra-articular injection of corticosteroids is effective in attacks of gout and pseudogout but is recommended only for physicians experienced in their use.

Analgesics. Acute gout can be exquisitely painful. Narcotic analgesics may be required for 24 hours until the anti-inflammatory medications take effect.

Traumatic Hemarthrosis

The most important point concerning the acute management of traumatic hemarthrosis is its frequent association with significant intra-articular damage. An acute traumatic hemarthrosis of the knee is associated in approximately 90% of cases with significant intra-articular disruption. Almost two thirds of such injuries are ligamentous or meniscal tears. The 5- to 10-year follow-up studies of these injuries indicate that about 80% of patients will have continued problems after a single traumatic hemarthrosis of the knee.

The role of aspiration in the management of an acute traumatic hemarthrosis is unsettled. Some clinicians are advocates of always aspirating and some are proponents of never aspirating. Three reasons favor routine aspiration: (1) reducing swelling relieves the patient's pain, (2) blood in the synovial space is an irritant and may lead to further cartilage damage, and (3) the presence of fat globules in the synovial fluid is highly predictive of a significant intra-articular disruption. The argument advanced against routine aspiration is usually the risk of infection or further joint damage from arthrocentesis.

Whether aspiration is performed or not, the involved joint is placed in a compression dressing, splinted, elevated, and treated with intermittent ice for at least 24 to 36 hours. Analgesics such as acetaminophen with or without narcotics are preferred rather than aspirin or NSAIDs, which may inhibit platelet function and retard cartilage healing.

Nontraumatic Hemarthrosis

An occasional patient may present with an acute nontraumatic hemarthrosis. Patients with an inherited coagulation factor deficiency and those using anticoagulant drugs have an obvious reason for bleeding. In rare patients, bleeding into a joint may occur for no obvious reason. When investigated, some of these patients may turn out to have a synovial pathologic process. Blood within the synovial space is irritating, and repeated joint hemorrhages produce chronic changes in the synovium, leading to localized degenerative joint damage. It is appropriate to remove the irritating blood from the joint with arthrocentesis. This can be done safely in most patients, even those with prolonged coagulation times. Consultation is recommended before this invasive procedure.

Other than rest and splinting, these patients do not require specific therapy unless it is necessary to adjust their anticoagulant dose or administer a deficient coagulation factor. The use of aspirin and NSAIDs may impair platelet function and exacerbate bleeding.

Polyarticular Arthritis

For patients presenting with inflammatory polyarticular arthritis, the emergency physician must first exclude bacterial infection. If this can be done to a reasonable degree, symptomatic treatment can begin with oral NSAIDs. Intra-articular corticosteroids are not recommended as a treatment for the first presentation of inflammatory arthritis. Although rheumatoid arthritis and the "rheumatoid variants" are usually polyarticular, they may present initially with monoarticular involvement. The polyarticular pattern usually becomes evident within 6 months.

Degenerative Arthritis

Management of degenerative joint disease is complicated by the fact that there is no specific treatment that reverses joint damage or halts further progression. The physician's role is to educate the patient, stress the avoidance of further joint abuse, and use medications and physical modalities to maximize patient function. Acetaminophen may be useful to control pain. Aspirin provides anti-inflammatory effects. NSAIDs are often used, although there is some evidence that NSAIDs may impede cartilage repair.

Intra-articular Injections

Arthrocentesis and intra-articular injections may be used for a variety of arthritic problems. Simple arthrocentesis may markedly relieve symptoms, especially in the setting of a tense, tender effusion caused by trauma. Instillation of local anesthetics can provide further relief, but, particularly in weight-bearing joints, continued ambulation during the anesthetic period can result in further joint injury.

UNCERTAIN DIAGNOSIS

Infectious and crystalline origins are the primary goals of the differential diagnostic effort in the emergency department. Other diagnoses include prodromes of diseases such as hepatitis and infectious mononucleosis. Early referral, including telephone consultation with an internist, rheumatologist, or orthopedist, and close follow-up should be pursued in the patient with an uncertain diagnosis of an acutely inflamed joint.

SPECIAL CONSIDERATIONS
Patients with Previously Damaged Joints

Previously damaged joints, especially from rheumatoid arthritis, are the most susceptible to infection. The tendency to ascribe joint pain and edema to the underlying rheumatoid arthritis may cause the physician to miss an active bacterial infection or inflammation secondary to gout or pseudogout. New-onset monoarticular arthritis or an unusual pattern of a joint flare in a patient with rheumatoid arthritis should encourage strong consideration for joint aspiration and evaluation. In addition, the possibility of recent injury to the joint or penetrating or blunt trauma must be explored. The patient should be asked about recent needle aspiration of the joint or injections of corticosteroids into the joint.

Patients with Prosthetic Joints

Prosthetic joint infections may be a consequence of local infection, such as intraoperative contamination (60% to 80% of cases) or bacteremia (20% to 40% of cases). Eventually, the implanted hardware will become less susceptible to infection by hematogenous spread because the pseudocapsule develops around it. Compared with people with infections of native joints, most patients with an infected prosthesis exhibit a prolonged low-grade course with gradually increasing pain. Usually, no significant fever or swelling occurs. Thus, a high index of suspicion is needed for identification of prosthetic joint infection. Physical findings usually are minimal in an infection of the prosthetic joint, and swelling usually is slight. The most distinctive finding is a draining sinus, presumed to originate in the underlying infected prosthetic joint. Successful treatment of an infected implanted joint requires appropriate antibiotic therapy combined with removal of the hardware.

Elderly Patients

Forty-five percent of people with septic arthritis are older than age 65 years. The elderly are predisposed to septic arthritis, mainly for their increased likelihood to have the disorders discussed earlier.

Pediatric Patients

Common causes of limp in the toddler are infections (e.g., septic arthritis, osteomyelitis). Because of significant sequelae, which may result from a diagnostic delay, especially in children younger than 1 year of age, it is imperative that the emergency physician consider these diagnoses when dealing with a febrile child with bone or joint pain or refusal to bear weight on an extremity.

Immunosuppressed Patients

A number of conditions that have an adverse effect on the host's defenses (e.g., liver disease, diabetes mellitus, lymphoma, solid tumors, complement deficiencies [C7, C8], immunosuppressive drugs, hypogammaglobulinemia) are noted increasingly in patients with septic arthritis. The possible contribution of these diseases to the clinical presentation must be determined.

DISPOSITION AND FOLLOW-UP

Admission

Patients with septic joints are admitted to the hospital for intravenous antibiotic therapy and possible surgical drainage. Patients with incapacitating acute arthritis of other causes are admitted for medical and physical therapy to restore functional ability.

Discharge

Most other patients can be discharged with outpatient follow-up. Before patients are discharged from the emergency department, the following conditions are met: (1) synovial fluid Gram's stain shows no bacteria, (2) the involved joint is splinted or immobilized and the patient has crutches or supports, (3) the patient has received a first dose of medication, and (4) the patient understands the diagnosis and the importance of follow-up.

Referral and Follow-up

The patient with an inflammatory joint in whom the possibility of infection exists is rechecked in 24 hours. Patients with gout and other inflammatory conditions are rechecked within 3 to 5 days. Patients with joint injury are rechecked after the swelling has diminished, usually in 5 to 7 days.

Discharge instructions stress resting the joint, avoidance of weight bearing on the large joints of the leg, use of elevation and ice to reduce edema, and recommendations to return if the pain is not improved in 24 to 48 hours.

FINAL POINTS

- The cause of acute monoarticular arthritis can be found in many cases by careful history, physical examination, and use of diagnostic tests in the emergency department.
- The most important task for the emergency physician, when presented with a patient who has acute arthritis, is to diagnose or exclude septic (bacterial) arthritis.
- Arthrocentesis is the only definitive means of diagnosing bacterial arthritis.
- When the diagnosis is determined in the emergency department, specific therapy is initiated. If the diagnosis remains unclear, symptomatic treatment with analgesics and immobilization is used. In either case, appropriate follow-up is arranged for further evaluation and treatment.

CASE *Study*

A 20-year-old woman presented to the emergency department with a 2-day history of aching in her left wrist. She complained of pain and swelling in her left knee and a low-grade fever. She mentioned some new "spots" on the extensor surfaces of her distal forearms and shins.

The patient had no previous history of joint problems. Physical examination demonstrated an erythematous, hot, swollen left knee. The knee was tender to both active and passive range of motion. The "spots" are three to four small, distal ulcers with erythematous bases. She is sexually active but has no genitourinary symptoms.

The findings are consistent with a monoarticular arthritis. Because of the rapidity of onset, physical findings, and age group, she was at high risk for septic arthritis, a process that can rapidly destroy a joint.

An arthrocentesis of the left knee obtained 3 mL of cloudy yellow fluid. The white blood cell count in the synovial fluid was 70,000/mm³ with 90% polymorphonuclear leukocytes. The analysis was negative for crystals, and Gram's stain showed no bacteria.

Purulent synovial fluid with a high leukocyte count and an overwhelming preponderance of polymorphonuclear leukocytes points to bacterial infection. The Gram stain is very helpful if it is positive, but a negative result does not exclude a septic joint, especially one caused by gonococci. The history, clinical findings, and results of the joint fluid analysis all pointed to septic arthritis secondary to disseminated gonococcal infection with the arthritis dermatitis syndrome. The patient was admitted to the hospital for treatment. The patient's left leg was immobilized after arthrocentesis, and intravenous ceftriaxone was started.

Bibliography

TEXTS

Kelley WN, Harris ED, Ruddy S, et al: Textbook of Rheumatology. Philadelphia, WB Saunders, 1997.

Schumacher HR (ed): Primer of the Rheumatic Diseases. Atlanta, Arthritis Foundation, 1993.

JOURNAL ARTICLES

Cucurull E, Espinoza LR: Gonococcal arthritis. Rheum Dis Clin North Am 1998; 24:305–322.

Felter RA, Venglarcik J: Bone and joint infections in children: Diagnosis and treatment. Pediatr Emerg Med Rep 1999; 4(3):21–23.

Freed JF, Nies KM, Boyer RS, et al: Acute monoarticular arthritis: A diagnostic approach. JAMA 1980; 243: 2314–2316.

Goldenberg DL, Reed JI: Bacterial arthritis. N Engl J Med 1985; 312:764–771.

Lawrence LL: The limping child. Emerg Med Clin North Am 1998; 16:911–929.

Pioro MH, Mandell BF: Septic arthritis. Rheum Dis Clin North Am 1997; 23:239–258.

Rose CD, Eppes SC: Infection-related arthritis. Rheum Dis Clin North Am 1997; 23:677–695.

Stimler MM: Infectious arthritis: Tailoring initial treatment to clinical findings. Postgrad Med 1996; 99:127–139.

Till SH: Assessment, investigation, and management of acute monoarthritis. J Accid Emerg Med 1999; 16:355–361.

The author wishes to acknowledge the work of J. Stephan Stapczynski in the writing of this chapter for the first edition of this book.

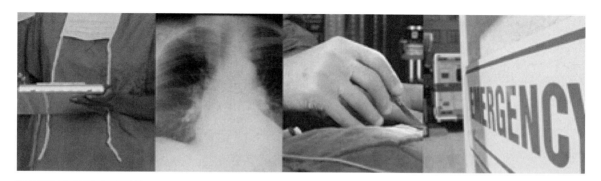

NERVOUS SYSTEM DISORDERS

CHAPTER 31

Altered Mental Status

SIDNEY STARKMAN
STEWART WRIGHT

CASE *Study*

A 50-year-old man was found unconscious in a downtown park. He appeared disheveled and smelled of alcohol. Bystanders called the rescue squad.

INTRODUCTION

Definitions

The term *altered mental status* (AMS) describes a change from the "normal" mental state. The term *level of consciousness* indicates the patient's state of awareness and arousal. Awareness represents the ability of the patient to relate to self and the environment. *Arousal* is used interchangeably with the terms *alertness* or *wakefulness.*

Depression in the level of consciousness is one way in which mental status is commonly altered. Other alterations manifest themselves as disturbances in behavior, appearance, orientation, memory, mood, affect, judgment, language, and thought content. Abnormal mental status can be caused by an organic, functional (psychiatric), or mixed disorder. Organic illnesses are recognized as having a structural, biochemical, or pharmacologic basis, e.g., brain tumors, Alzheimer's disease, or a toxic ingestion. Functional illnesses, for decision-making in the emergency department, are considered as having no clearly defined pathophysiologic basis. They include disorders such as paranoid schizophrenia, manic-depressive states, and hysterical conversion reactions.

This chapter focuses on two major forms of AMS: depressed consciousness and delirium. The emphasis is on depressed consciousness, since this is most commonly encountered. Except during sleep, the normal level of consciousness is alert and aware.

Coma is the term used to describe the deepest depression in the level of consciousness. Patients who are comatose are unresponsive and have no useful speech. *Drowsiness*, *lethargy*, *stupor*, and *obtundation* are imprecise terms used to describe progressively deeper decreases in the level of consciousness on the continuum from aware and alert to coma. When these terms are used, because there are no universal definitions, they are best accompanied by a brief description of the patient's behavior, both spontaneous and in response to external stimuli. For example, "the patient is lethargic" means that the patient is at rest with the eyes closed and in response to his or her name being called, opens the eyes, looks around, says some unintelligible words, and then immediately closes the eyes again.

Patients with a depressed level of consciousness, who are still arousable, have difficulty maintaining attention to stimuli or tasks when aroused. Because there is a decrease in alertness, these patients are unlikely to be able to think clearly about internal or external stimuli. This inability to maintain a coherent stream of thought or action is called *confusion*. Most patients with a depressed level of consciousness tend to exhibit confusion, and determining its presence on physical examination is part of an AMS assessment.

Delirium is the term used to describe patients in an agitated confusional state. Delirium is often associated with autonomic hyperactivity and a heightened awareness of stimuli. Classic examples are cocaine intoxication and the abstinence syndromes associated with alcohol withdrawal.

Physiology

Coma (or unconsciousness) is defined as a condition in which neither arousal nor awareness is present. Arousal (alertness or wakefulness) is dependent on an intact reticular activating system that runs through the brain stem from the pons and projects to the thalami and then to both cortical cerebral hemispheres. Awareness depends on the proper functioning of the cerebral cortex. Coma can be induced if either the reticular activating system or both cerebral hemispheres are structurally damaged or chemically depressed by an endogenous or exogenous agent. Typically, a unilateral cerebral hemispheric lesion will not produce coma until it causes significant distortion of the brain stem and suppresses the reticular activating system. Identifying whether the cerebral hemispheres or brain stem is the site of processes altering mental status assists in directing the physical examination and differential diagnosis. An altered level of consciousness may indicate a primary brain disorder or systemic disease. Most structural lesions of the brain that cause coma compress the brain stem, whereas systemic disease produces coma by affecting the ascending reticular activating system and/or both cerebral hemispheres.

Epidemiology

AMS is a common presentation in the emergency department. Depending on the patient population served, 5% to 10% of patients may present with some degree of this finding. Approximately 80% of patients presenting with AMS have systemic or metabolic disorders. Drug ingestions are the most common cause. Structural lesions account for nearly 20%. Depressed level of consciousness accounts for more than 70% of patients with AMS. Delirium is seen in about 10% of the group. Acute confusional status and dementia make up most of the remainder.

The full range of AMS, and its numerous causes, must be unraveled in a relatively short time, while continuously protecting the patient from further insult or injury. Sources of AMS often overlap in their clinical presentation, and a precise diagnosis is not always made in the emergency department. Nonetheless, the management principles applied are useful in protecting the patient and identifying or excluding the most serious causes.

INITIAL APPROACH AND STABILIZATION

The initial assessment of patients with AMS involves stabilizing basic life functions, protecting the patient from further injury, and promptly treating reversible causes.

Priority Diagnoses

Potentially rapidly reversible causes of AMS include hypoglycemia, hypothermia/hyperthermia, opioid overdose, shock states, hypoxemia, and hypertensive encephalopathy.

Life-threatening causes include meningitis, an intracranial mass lesion, renal/hepatic failure, sepsis, toxins (e.g., cyanide, carbon monoxide), and acid-base disorders.

Rapid Assessment

1. *What is the basic history of this illness? Who is giving the history?* The prehospital history is reviewed with the rescue squad or relatives. Were there any *bottles or medication containers* at the scene and brought to the hospital? Was there anything notable about the *environment* in which the patient was found?
2. Were there *others in the vicinity in a similar state? A history of trauma, seizures, diabetes, or other medical problems?* How long has the patient had altered consciousness? *When was the patient last observed as "normal"?*
3. Were clothes pockets examined for *identification, suicide notes, and drug bottles?* Is the patient wearing a *medical alert bracelet?* Telephone calls are initiated to obtain background information or history relating to the patient's present illness.

Early Intervention

Certain interventions are performed simultaneously while performing the examination and assessing the level of consciousness. The essential elements of early intervention are addressed here.

Airway/Breathing. The airway is managed while maintaining cervical spine immobilization. A nasopharyngeal airway, oropharyngeal airway, or endotracheal tube is placed, depending on the patient's airway patency and protection. Endotracheal intubation is performed in patients who cannot protect their airway (e.g., those who are comatose and not rapidly becoming more alert or those who were initially lethargic and are becoming more obtunded).

Oxygenation. Pulse oximetry is obtained and monitored in all patients. Supplemental oxygen is provided, particularly for patients with pulse oximetry of less than 92%.

Spine Stabilization. The comatose patient or patient with depressed consciousness may have a head injury and complicating cervical spine injury. The injury could be the initiating event or secondary to a fall while the patient was becoming unconscious. In these cases, a cervical spine fracture is always assumed to be present and the cervical spine is immobilized.

Vital Signs. Vital signs, including temperature, are obtained and monitored. Hyperthermia or hypothermia and hypertension or hypo tension necessitate instituting an appropriate early intervention.

Intravenous Access. Intravenous access is established with one or more lines, depending on the patient's hemodynamic status. An isotonic crystalloid is the initial therapeutic fluid of choice. The rate is dependent on the patient's vital signs and the clinical estimate of adequate perfusion.

Before infusion, blood samples are drawn and sent for analysis.

Initial Laboratory Data. Initial screening laboratory tests are usually ordered early during the patient's care. These include a complete blood cell count; determination of levels of electrolytes, serum glucose, blood nitrogen, and creatinine; and urinalysis. Arterial blood gases are obtained in patients with respiratory compromise and who are intubated. Blood and urine samples are saved for other tests.

Glucose. The blood glucose level is rapidly determined with a bedside test strip measurement. Hyperglycemia may be associated with worse outcome in acute brain injury. Therefore, glucose is administered only to treat hypoglycemia. Patients who are hypoglycemic with a glucose level below 60 mg/dL are treated with intravenous infusion of 50 mL of 50% dextrose. This should raise the glucose level 50 to 75 mg/dL. The laboratory serum glucose measurement confirms the bedside test. In children, 2 mL/kg of 25% dextrose is used. When vascular access cannot be obtained rapidly, glucagon may be administered intramuscularly. The response to glucose administration is noted and recorded.

Thiamine. Thiamine is given to suspected alcoholics or other undernourished patients because of the potential for a glucose load to aggravate an underlying thiamine deficiency. The dose of thiamine is 100 mg administered intravenously. It is usually given concurrently to the glucose bolus.

Naloxone. When an opiate overdose is possible, 2 mg of naloxone is administered intravenously. If the patient is suspected of narcotic overdose, the first dose is decreased to 0.4 mg (one ampule) or less. The dose is repeated depending on the patient's response. The response to naloxone is noted and recorded. Emergency department personnel must prepare for the patient with a narcotic overdose who awakens in response to the naloxone and then becomes combative and resists further medical evaluation. Avoiding acute opiate withdrawal is an important therapeutic goal.

Cardiac Monitoring. Cardiac monitor leads are attached and the cardiac rhythm is observed. Treatment is instituted for significant dysrhythmias as necessary.

Level of Consciousness. In the patient who is not alert, arousal is assessed using voice, touch, or noxious stimuli, such as pressure to the sternum or to the nailbed of the middle finger of each hand. In patients who may have a spinal cord injury, pressure is applied to the supraorbital nerve as it exits its foramen. The patient's response is observed and recorded using the mnemonic AVPU (*A*lert, responds to *V*oice, responds to *P*ain, or *U*nresponsive).

The Glasgow Coma Scale (GCS) is commonly used to gauge the degree of AMS (Table 31–1). The GCS was originally devised to quantify the degree of depression in level of consciousness in patients with head trauma but has demonstrated applicability in a variety of disease states. The highest score on the GCS is 15, and the worst possible score is 3. A score of 8 or less typically corresponds to coma. Higher scores correspond to sequentially higher levels of consciousness. Patients with GCS scores greater than 8 may harbor equally life-threatening diseases. The score for the motor response is based on the best response. Therefore, a hemiplegia on one side and a normal response on the other side are scored as 6.

Both the AVPU and the GCS assessments serve as valuable comparative standards to monitor subsequent deterioration or improvement in the patient's level of consciousness. In addition, they improve communication among health care providers as the patient's course of care progresses.

Pupillary Responses. The direct and consensual pupillary responses to light are evaluated. Asymmetry, extremes of dilation or constriction, or poor reactivity is each a sign of a potentially serious central nervous system (CNS) process.

Seizure Precautions. The patient is observed for seizure activity. A rhythmical twitching of some of the digits of either hand or a rhythmic,

---

TABLE 31–1. Glasgow Coma Scale

Eye Opening

Spontaneously	4
To verbal command	3
To pain	2
No response	1

Best Motor Response

Obeys commands	6
Localizes to pain	5
Withdraws to pain	4
Abnormal flexion	3
Abnormal extension	2
No response	1

Best Verbal Response

Oriented, converses	5
Disoriented	4
Inappropriate words	3
Incomprehensible sounds	2
No response	1

small-amplitude horizontal jerking of the eyes may be the only clue the patient is in status epilepticus. If the patient is seizing and does not respond to the aforementioned treatments, the seizures are controlled with intravenously administered diazepam or lorazepam (see Chapter 33, Seizures). Further assessments of mental status are obviously influenced by the addition of a sedative.

Suspected Meningitis. If meningitis is suspected, a lumbar puncture is performed early in the patient's care. AMS and fever raise the possibility of meningitis in any patient. If there are signs of increased intracranial pressure or focal deficits on examination, the lumbar puncture is delayed pending results of computed tomography (CT) of the head. Appropriate antibiotics are initiated early in the course of care (e.g., before CT) if there is a high suspicion for meningitis.

Elevated Intracranial Pressure. If the patient with a decreased level of consciousness has a unilaterally dilated pupil that is sluggishly responsive or unresponsive to light, cerebral herniation is suggested. The patient is intubated and the P_{CO_2} brought to a level of about 30 mm Hg, intravenous mannitol, 0.25 to 0.50 g/kg, is administered, and a CT of the head is obtained emergently. The neurosurgical consultant is notified immediately. More information is given in Chapters 34, Stroke, and 48, Head and Neck Trauma.

Urine Output. An indwelling catheter is placed if necessary to monitor urine output. A urine specimen is obtained for urinalysis and for screening for drugs of abuse and pregnancy testing when appropriate. Urine is checked for myoglobin in patients with rhabdomyolysis, for example, in cocaine intoxication.

CLINICAL ASSESSMENT

The patient in an altered state of consciousness often arrives in the emergency department with no one able to give a medical history. The patient may not be able to give a history or often not a reliable one. It is then necessary to seek information from other sources, including paramedics and police. If only an address is available, the police may be asked to go to the site for information. A conscientious effort in data gathering outside the emergency department can have a significant return in unraveling the cause of the AMS.

History

1. *Did the patient verbalize any complaints or concerns before the onset of the change in men-*

tal status? Patients with headache before their change in mental status are suspected to have an intracranial hemorrhage. Headache is also common in carbon monoxide poisoning. Patients who express feelings of depression are at risk for having taken an overdose of medications.

2. *When was the patient last seen in a normal state of mental health? What is the normal state?* The time elapsed before being discovered is important because other conditions, such as dehydration, can complicate the original cause of the change in mental status. Patients may have a baseline level of confusion that must be considered during the evaluation.

3. *Was there a gradual or abrupt deterioration of mental status?* Abrupt changes are usually the result of more serious and catastrophic disorders. Rapid onset of coma is seen in aneurysmal subarachnoid hemorrhage, intracerebral hemorrhage, and acute obstructive hydrocephalus caused by intraventricular extension of intracerebral hemorrhage. A patient with change in mental status over hours usually has a metabolic problem. Hypoglycemia and intoxication are commonly found. Nonmetabolic causes are infection and intracranial hemorrhage resulting from head trauma.

4. *Has the condition changed since it was initially recognized?* Serial monitoring of the patient's status is critical. Rapid deterioration in mental status may be indicative of increasing intracranial pressure or a worsening metabolic process. Meningitis can have a rapid downhill course from both spreading infection and an increase in intracranial pressure.

5. *What is the patient's past medical history? Has the patient ever had a similar episode?* It is necessary to know the patient's underlying medical illnesses and whether the patient has recently been ill. Diabetes, hypertension, cerebrovascular disease, alcoholism, and depression are common concurrent disorders.

6. *What are the patient's current medications?* Many medications, as well as drugs of abuse, can alter mental status. The most common are amphetamines, cocaine, sedative hypnotics, opiates, and antidepressants.

7. *Is the patient an alcoholic or other substance abuser?* In many patients in the emergency department, alcohol or substance abuse is a complicating factor. The difficulty is differentiating abuse as a primary cause of the patient's condition versus being a contributor to another process. Unfortunately, this group of patients is more susceptible to a number of disorders causing AMS, such as trauma, infection,

uncontrolled hypertension, and diabetes mellitus.

Physical Examination

A thorough physical examination will (1) assess vital functions, (2) discover systemic causes of AMS, (3) determine whether focal neurologic signs are present, and (4) more accurately characterize the mental status changes. Another aspect is the thorough examination of the patient's clothing, pockets, and accompanying items (wallet, purse) to identify potential etiologies, or sources of information.

Vital Signs and Systemic Evaluation

Blood Pressure. Hypotension is rarely due to intracranial causes except as a terminal event. When hypotension is present, volume loss, redistribution from venodilatation, or cardiac insufficiency is the probable cause. Cushing's triad of hypertension, bradycardia, and bradypnea is a late finding associated with markedly increased intracranial pressure. Severe hypertension with diastolic blood pressures exceeding 120 mm Hg may induce encephalopathy. Hypertensive encephalopathy may present as AMS, rarely coma. Most patients in a coma with significantly elevated blood pressure have an intracranial hemorrhage (see Chapter 10, Hypertension).

Respirations. Altered ventilatory patterns can provide clues to causes. Cheyne-Stokes respirations are characterized by periodic breathing of alternating episodes of hyperventilation and hypoventilation. This may occur from acidosis or from various brain lesions. The localizing value of this pattern is poor. Hyperventilation is common and may come from hypoxia, acidosis, drug toxicities, or midbrain reticular formation lesions. Again, the localizing value is nonspecific. Apneustic breathing is characterized by a pause at the end of the inspiration. It is rare but is associated with lesions of the mid to caudal pons resulting from a focal stroke, meningitis, hypoglycemia, or hypoxia. Ataxic breathing is completely without pattern and suggests damage to the medulla and lower pons. Depressed respiratory rate may be caused by toxins (e.g., opiates and benzodiazepines).

Temperature. Fever is found primarily in infectious disorders but can occur after prolonged seizures, producing coma at temperatures exceeding 42°C (108°F). Hyperthermia may indicate neuroleptic malignant syndrome (AMS, muscle rigidity, and fever). Environmental hyperthermia is also seen when weather conditions are appropriate. Hypothermia may be subtle and con-

tribute to a depressed mental status, with the appearance of coma at about 20°C (68°F). All patients with fever and AMS must be considered as potentially having underlying meningitis.

Pulse. While heart rate by itself does not cause mental status changes, dysrhythmias of all types can cause blood pressure abnormalities and secondary depressed consciousness.

Head, Ears, and Nasopharynx. The skull is inspected for external signs of trauma. Ecchymoses of the mastoid (Battle's sign) and hemotympanum are indicative of a basilar skull fracture. The breath odor is noted for alcohol, ketones, or odors associated with toxins (e.g., cyanide).

Eyes. The eye examination is especially important in evaluating the patient with AMS. Its major value is in the comatose or consciousness-depressed patient.

Lids. The lids offer some information. Partial unilateral ptosis especially with elevation of the lower lid and small pupil suggest Horner's syndrome. Severe unilateral ptosis is usually caused by third nerve palsy. Active resistance to eye opening suggests a functioning cortex and an uncooperative patient.

Pupillary Size, Symmetry, and Reactivity. The reactivity of pupils is a key differentiator between structural lesions and metabolic disorders. In most metabolic disorders, reactivity is maintained. Bilateral pupillary constriction (pinpoint pupils) is seen in patients with opiate overdose or in pontine lesions. Pupillary asymmetry of 1 to 2 mm with reactivity can be seen in 10% of normal people. Pupillary asymmetry or unilateral dilation of a pupil without reactivity can be caused by uncal (or transtentorial) herniation. Besides a decreased level of consciousness, this pupillary dilatation is classically the earliest sign of uncal herniation, indicating lateral displacement of the medial temporal lobe against the third cranial nerve. Parasympathetic fibers run on the outside of this oculomotor nerve, so pressure on the oculomotor nerve causes a loss of parasympathetic tone, resulting in the finding of an ipsilateral dilated and nonreactive pupil (Fig. 31–1). Bilateral unreactive and fixed pupils are an ominous finding, indicative of central herniation, hypoxic injury, or brain death. The use of mydriatic eye drops can confound interpretation of pupillary responses.

Corneal Reflexes. Corneal stimulation will produce a blink response if the fifth (sensory) and seventh (motor) cranial nerves are intact. It is another measure of brain stem function.

Extraocular Movements. In the patient with coma or a significant depression of

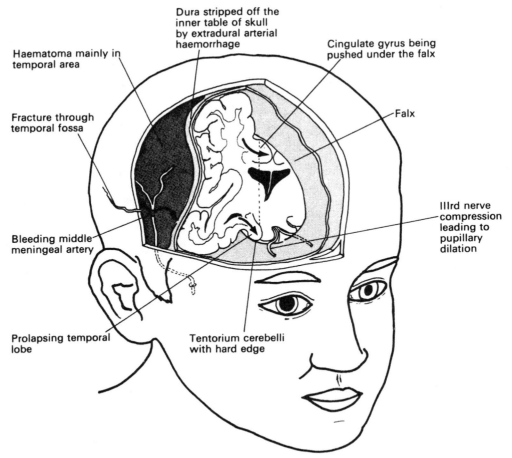

FIGURE 31–1 • Uncal herniation causing compression of third cranial nerve and ipsilateral pupillary dilation in a patient with an epidural hematoma. A subdural hematoma from torn bridging veins can have the same effect. (From Patten J: Neurological Differential Diagnosis. New York, Springer-Verlag, 1977.)

consciousness, brain stem function can be evaluated by testing for extraocular muscle function. Brain stem function represented by cranial nerves III through VIII is preserved if the "doll's eyes" sign is present. This sign is meant to represent that the eyes move conjugately with full range laterally and medially. The term comes from mechanical dolls whose eyes appeared to roll up or down when the head of the doll was tilted down or up.

The movement of the eyes in response to rotation of the head in the opposite direction is the *oculocephalic reflex*. In the patient who is fully awake, the eyes rotate with the head movement, staying relatively in the same position within the head, looking forward (negative "doll's eyes"). In the unconscious patient with an intact brain stem and extraocular movement system, when the head is rapidly rotated horizontally to one side, the patient's eyes fully rotate conjugately in the opposite direction (negative "doll's eyes"). The patient with a suppressed (e.g., barbiturate) or damaged brain stem responds with the eyes rotating with the head movement. Conjugate or dysconjugate incomplete rotation of the globes during oculocephalic testing indicates disruption of the central or peripheral extraocular motor system, usually owing to focal brain stem dysfunction or symmetric drug-induced suppression. Oculocephalic testing is not performed in the patient who may have sustained a cervical spine injury.

The *oculovestibular* (cold caloric test) is a more powerful means to evaluate the extraocular motor system in the unconscious patient. The semicircular canals are stimulated with cold-water irrigation of the ears (Fig. 31–2). Before irrigation, the tympanic membranes are noted to be intact and the head is flexed 30 degrees from supine. In the comatose patient with intact brain stem function, the eyes will deviate conjugately and fully toward the side of the stimulus.

Funduscopic Examination. Subhyaloid (preretinal) hemorrhages are associated with sub-

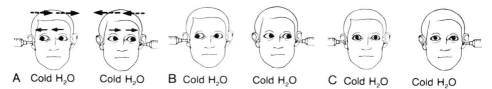

FIGURE 31–2 • Response to caloric stimulation of the vestibular apparatus with the head placed in 30 degrees of flexion. *A*, Awake or psychogenic coma. *B*, Indicates coma with brain stem intact. *C*, Severe brain stem injury or deep toxic-metabolic depression. (Adapted from Plum F, Posner JB: The Diagnosis of Stupor and Coma, 3rd ed. Philadelphia, FA Davis, 1980.)

arachnoid hemorrhage. The intracranial blood leaks out the lamina cribrosa of the optic nerve and layers out between the retina and the vitreous membrane. The presence of papilledema usually indicates increased intracranial pressure that has been present for more than 12 hours.

Neck. The presence of meningismus (nuchal rigidity) indicates inflammation of the meninges from meningitis or a subarachnoid hemorrhage. If there is any potential of trauma, the cervical spine is placed in appropriate immobilization.

Cardiopulmonary. Dysrhythmias, valvular disorders, and heart failure can be responsible for, contribute to, or complicate the AMS condition. Respiratory insufficiency, infection, or metastasis from pulmonary cancer can cause mental changes.

Abdomen/Back. The abdomen and back are examined for signs of infection, mass lesions, or renal or hepatic pathology. An enlarged liver may represent hepatic congestion from heart failure or infiltration of the liver by some other process. A firm nodular liver or a caput medusa usually indicates underlying cirrhosis. An enlarged spleen may be the first clue to sequestration from sickle cell disease or blast crises in the patient with leukemia. Abdominal infections that lead to sepsis may be discovered by noticing localized abdominal pain or a diffusely rigid anterior wall. Periumbilical ecchymosis (Cullen's sign) and flank ecchymosis (Grey Turner's sign) are late findings indicative of hemorrhagic pancreatitis. The rectal examination may reveal melena or the cancerous source of a brain metastasis. Lack of bowel sounds and distention may indicate ileus or obstruction.

Extremities. The examiner should look for petechiae, ecchymoses, presence or absence of sweating, skin changes, or needle marks. Observation of position is important: an out-turned leg may be caused by hemiparesis or a hip fracture.

Skin. Just as the eyes are the windows to the brain, the skin can be the window to the metabolic system. This largest of all organs should not be overlooked during the examination. Diabetes causes a number of skin changes, including hyper-

pigmented atrophic macules on the shins and intertriginous candidiasis or erythrasma. Less commonly, diabetics can have localized fat atrophy or the pink and yellow plaques of lipoidica diabeticorum. Hypertriglyceridemia can cause eruptive xanthomatosis, which is most commonly seen around the eyes.

Uremic frost, a fine white powder seen on a sallow complexion, may be seen on severely uremic patients. Hepatic disease leads to spider angiomas, palmar erythema, and jaundice.

Thyroid disease may present as coma. The classic description of myxedema coma includes periorbital swelling; pale, cool, dry skin; and loss of eyebrows. Thyrotoxicosis can lead to moist, warm skin; nail bed separation; and pretibial edema.

Varicella zoster has a typical ulcerative crusted lesion. Herpes simplex, a potentially devastating cause of encephalopathy, also has a characteristic vesicle on an erythematous base and occasional dimpling before ulceration.

Toxins can also lead to skin coloration. Prolonged exposure to significant levels of carbon monoxide in the blood can cause a characteristic cherry-red color of the mucous membranes. Lead-intoxicated children may have darkened gingival margins.

Neurologic Examination

Level of Consciousness. The Glasgow Coma Scale is applied periodically to monitor the progress or deterioration of the patient. Abnormalities in speech and language are sought. Aphasic speech localizes to the dominant hemisphere.

Cranial Nerves. Facial movement is evaluated as well as other lower cranial nerve functions, including the gag reflex. Generally, eye movement is the most useful of the cranial nerve assessments.

Motor/Sensory Responses. Asymmetry of movement is carefully sought. It may indicate a hemiparesis. Finger twitching may be the only residua of ongoing seizure activity. Purposeful avoidance of painful stimuli denotes an intact corticospinal tract and a nearly awake patient. Spontaneous flexion (decorticate posturing) of the arms at the elbows and wrists indicates damage at the level of the hemispheres. Arm extension with internal rotation (decerebrate posturing) is the result of lesions or a metabolic effect in the midbrain area. Flaccidity, despite a painful stimulus, is an ominous finding. Care must be taken in interpreting the patient without motor responsiveness, because severe hypothermia or a massive overdose of sedative/hypnotics can mimic a death-like state.

Deep Tendon and Pathologic Reflexes. These are tested to assist in localizing lesions as to upper motor neuron (spinal cord and above), lower motor neuron (peripheral nerve), unilateral, or bilateral. They also assess symmetry of responsiveness.

Cerebellar Function, Station, and Gait. These features may not be adequately evaluated with depressed level of consciousness.

Mental Status Examination (MSE). A patient may be able to cooperate with a basic MSE, depending on the state of wakefulness. Confusion may be integrated into an AMS, appearing as abnormal awareness. There are many way to assess the "awareness" component of consciousness. Most are not applicable for rapid use in the emergency department. The Quick Confusion Scale (QCS) can be applied in less than 2 min and has demonstrated comparable efficacy in revealing an altered awareness as the Mini-Mental State Examination (MMSE) (Tables 31–2 and 31–3). The MMSE takes more than twice the time to administer. The QCS is administered to patients who score 15 (normal) on the GCS. It can serve as a discriminator of cognitive function. Scores less than 11 support an abnormal cognitive function. Educational level is thought to influence the scoring and must be considered.

TABLE 31–2. The Quick Confusion Scale

Item	Score (No. correct)	× (weight)	=	(Total)
1. What year is it now?	0 or 1 (score 1 if correct, 0 if incorrect)	×2	=	—
2. What month is it? Present memory phrase: "Repeat this phrase after me and remember it: *John Brown, 42 Market Street, New York.*"	0 or 1	×2	=	—
3. About what time is it? (Answer correct if within 1 hour)	0 or 1	×2	=	—
4. Count backwards from 20 to 1.	0, 1, or 2	×1	=	—
5. Say the months in reverse.	0, 1, or 2	×1	=	—
6. Repeat memory phrase (each underlined portion correct is worth 1 point).	0, 1, 2, 3, 4, or 5	×1	=	—
Final score is the sum of the totals			=	—

From Huff JS, Farace E, Brady WJ, et al: The quick confusion scale in the ED: Comparison with the mini-mental state examination. Am J Emerg Med 2001; 19:461–464.

TABLE 31–3. Explanation of Scoring Quick Confusion Scale

Quick Confusion Scale scores (highest number in category indicates correct response; decreased scoring indicates increased number of errors)
Item 1. "What year is it now?"
  Score 1 if answered correctly, 0 if incorrect.
Item 2. "What month is it?"
  Score 1 if answered correctly, 0 if incorrect.
Item 3. "About what time is it?"
  Answer considered correct if within 1 hour; score 1 if correct, 0 if incorrect.
Item 4. "Count backwards from 20 to 1."
  Score 2 if correctly performed; score 1 if one error, score 0 if 2 or more errors.
Item 5. "Say the months in reverse."
  Score 2 if correctly performed: score 1 if one error, score 0 if 2 or more errors.
Item 6. Repeat memory phrase
  John Brown, 42 Market Street, New York
Each underlined portion correctly recalled is worth 1 point in scoring; score 5 if correctly performed; each error drops score by 1.
Final score is sum of the weighted totals; Items 1, 2, and 3 are multiplied by 2 and summed with the other Item scores to yield the final score. The highest score is 15. Score a less than 11 suggest cognitive dys-function.

From Huff JS, Farace E, Brady WJ, et al: The quick confusion scale in the ED: Comparison with the mini-mental state examination. Am J Emerg Med 2001; 19:461–464.

CLINICAL REASONING

After the history and physical examination, decision priorities are established and the preliminary differential diagnosis is constructed by asking the following questions.

Is the Cause of the AMS Life Threatening?

Most causes of AMS requiring immediate attention are cardiopulmonary. The priorities of advanced life support are instituted in these patients. Stabilization of the airway and oxygenation comes first, then evaluation of cardiac dysrhythmias and volume status. Additional causes include the following (see also "Priority Diagnoses"):

- *Substrate deficiency.* Oxygen, thiamine, and glucose are either measured or administered early in the course of care.
- *Abnormalities of temperature regulation* (hypothermia and hyperthermia)
- *Poisoning* (carbon monoxide, cyanide)
- *Infection* (meningitis)
- *Causes of raised intracranial pressure,* particularly herniation syndromes from focal lesions (mass lesions, post-traumatic brain injury). All these can be lethal and are reversible.

Is the AMS Caused by a Primary CNS Disease, or is it the Consequence of a Systemic Illness?

Differentiating between primary or secondary CNS diseases is based primarily on the presence or absence of focal abnormalities on the neurologic examination. Focal findings strongly suggest the presence of a specific lesion in the CNS. Systemic problems, such as a lack of nutrients (glucose, oxygen), metabolic problems (sodium, calcium), or an accumulation of toxins (carbon dioxide, carbon monoxide, alcohol) causes diffuse CNS dysfunction manifesting as AMS. Occasionally, hypoglycemia, hyponatremia, hepatic encephalopathy, or nonketotic hyperosmolar coma can present as focal neurologic signs. In all cases of focal neurologic signs, a search for a structural intracranial lesion is initiated. As noted in the pupillary reactivity discussions, preserved reactivity is characteristic of a systemic process. The absence of focal findings does not rule out a primary CNS process.

Is the Presentation Consistent with one of the Causes of AMS Frequently Seen in the Emergency Department?

The most common treatable sources of AMS may be remembered by the mnemonic AEIOU-TIPS ("TIPS on the VOWELS"). Table 31–4 illustrates how the mnemonic is used. The majority of these cases present as confusion with depressed consciousness or coma.

Alcohol. Alcohol intoxication is the most common cause of AMS seen in the emergency department. The odor of alcohol is usually detectable on the patient's breath. The level of intoxication depends on the patient's tolerance to alcohol. Patients with altered states of consciousness may have multiple processes simultaneously. The intoxicated patient can fall and hit his or her head, resulting in primary brain injury and a secondary complication such as a CNS hemorrhage. A difficult decision in clinical emergency medicine is whether to attribute the patient's clinical state to alcohol intoxication or to search for alternative causes (see Chapter 16, Alcohol Intoxication). Some general guidelines include the following:

- Is the patient's clinical status consistent with the blood alcohol level? Although the individual patient's tolerance to alcohol varies, a blood alcohol level of less than 250 mg/dL rarely causes true coma.
- Is the patient's mental status improving with time? Decreased mental status caused by ethanol intoxication should improve gradually as the alcohol metabolizes. A worsening condition, as observed by a changing neurologic examination, prompts the need to find another cause.
- Focal neurologic deficits are not attributable to alcohol intoxication.
- When in doubt, search for other sources.

Epilepsy, Encephalopathy. Seizures cause an AMS during the ictal and postictal phases. They may be due to a known seizure disorder, primary CNS diseases such as meningitis or intracranial hemorrhage, or a secondary systemic problem (e.g., hypoxia). The postictal phase of a seizure usually lasts minutes to hours and shows gradual

---

TABLE 31–4. Mnemonic for Treatable Causes of Altered Mental Status

Alcohol	**T**rauma
Epilepsy, electrolytes, encephalopathy	**I**nfection
	Psychiatric
Insulin, intussusception	**S**hock, subarachnoid
Opiates/overdose	hemorrhage, snake bite
Urea (metabolic)	

clearing. The emergency department approach to seizures is discussed in Chapter 33, Seizures. Marked elevations in blood pressure may signify hypertensive encephalopathy with diastolic pressure typically greater than 130 mm Hg or in response to an intracranial catastrophe (e.g., intracerebral hemorrhage). Hypertensive encephalopathy occurs at relatively lower levels but is higher than expected in the peri–term pregnancy period of the patient with eclampsia. Eclampsia manifests itself as depressed level of consciousness and sometimes seizures. Magnetic resonance imaging reveals reversible edema of the posterior hemisphere.

Insulin. Hypoglycemia is usually secondary to diabetes and insulin treatment or to depleted liver glycogen stores and inadequate diet. It is diagnosed by portable glucose measurement and the usually extremely rapid improvement in mental status after the administration of intravenous dextrose (usually 25 g). Intravenous administration of dextrose in the patient with coma caused by hypoglycemia should not be delayed while waiting for laboratory confirmation of the portable glucose level. Hyperglycemia and accompanying hyperosmolarity represent the other extreme of glucose metabolism causing AMS. It almost always presents as depressed consciousness. Diagnosis is confirmed by laboratory testing (see Chapter 20, Diabetes, for more information on hypoglycemia and hyperglycemia).

Opiates/Other Overdose. Opiates cause respiratory depression, decreased mental status, and symmetric pinpoint pupils. Patients may have needle tracks if intravenous injection is used. The opiate antagonist naloxone provides very rapid reversal of coma and can be diagnostic. In narcotic addicts, naloxone may trigger a withdrawal syndrome and vomiting. Other exogenous toxins can cause coma or AMS. A history of drug abuse, suicide attempt, or depression may help elucidate specific toxins. Laboratory studies may demonstrate a metabolic acidosis or increased anion gap. Toxicology screen usually reveals the presence of medications or drugs of abuse (see Chapter 15, The Poisoned Patient).

Urea. Urea represents several metabolic (including electrolyte and endocrine) disorders. Renal insufficiency is a relatively rare cause of AMS. Creatinine levels over 7 mg/dL or a blood urea nitrogen value over 100 mg/dL can contribute to mental changes directly or by decreased excretion of renal metabolized substances. Other metabolic causes include endogenous toxins, such as are found in hepatic failure and bowel ischemia. Electrolytes are primarily represented by changes in sodium and calcium. Table 31–5

TABLE 31–5. Electrolyte Abnormalities Resulting in Altered Mental Status

Electrolyte Disorder	Lethargy	Stupor	Coma
Hypernatremia	+	+	+
Hyponatremia	+	+	+
Hyperkalemia	-	-	-
Hypokalemia	+	-	-
Hypercalcemia	+	+	+
Hypocalcemia	+	Rare	-
Hypermagnesemia	+	-	Rare
Hypomagnesemia	+	-	-
Hypophosphatemia	+	+	+
Hypoglycemia	+	+	+
Hyperglycemia	+	+	+

lists the electrolyte abnormalities that can cause AMS. Myxedema coma is caused by severe hypothyroidism; thyroid storm of hyperthyroidism often presents as delirium.

Trauma. Head trauma can result in primary brain parenchymal injury, or it can produce CNS hemorrhage. Focal neurologic signs are often seen, and there may be associated increased intracranial pressure. CT of the head rapidly diagnoses the sites of intracranial and intracerebral bleeding (see Chapter 48, Head and Neck Trauma).

Infection. Infections of the CNS can produce AMS or coma. Herpes simplex is a frequent cause of encephalitis, whereas *Streptococcus pneumoniae, Neisseria meningitidis,* and *Haemophilus influenzae* most commonly cause bacterial meningitis. Viruses, fungi, and carcinoma can cause aseptic meningitis. Although antibiotics may be started empirically, a cerebrospinal fluid analysis is necessary to diagnose meningitis. Infection in other sites (e.g., lung or urinary tract), with associated bacteremia or sepsis, often results in mental status changes. This is most often seen at the extremes of age.

Psychiatric. Psychogenic coma or depressed consciousness is sometimes seen in the emergency department. Usually it resolves with patience and support. A common form of psychogenic AMS is pseudoseizures (psychogenic seizures), which can sometimes be extremely difficult to diagnose, requiring video and electroencephalographic telemetry monitoring for confirmation. Clues to the diagnosis of a pseudocoma (psychogenic, hysterical, or malingering coma) are the presence of eyelid fluttering, Bell's phenomenon (elevation of the globes when eyelid opening is resisted by the patient), and absence of a postictal phase after generalized seizures. The patient may be observed to look away from the examiner when the patient's eyelids are opened and the examiner's face is extremely close. These clues to psychogenic causes of coma or depressed consciousness are not definitive in excluding an organic cause. In *psychogenic amnesia*, patients often forget who they are and perhaps where they are but otherwise know the day and date and have normal memory function. This is typically inconsistent with the organic disease processes as described earlier. The neurologic examination is otherwise normal. In *hysterical coma*, performance of ice-water calorics produces ipsilateral deviation of the eyes with fast-phase nystagmus in the opposite direction. This fast-phase is not seen in truly comatose patients. Because of the intensity of the stimulus and the associated nausea and unpleasant vertiginous sensation, the patient may be unsteady and vomit. In a patient suspected of hysterical coma, caloric testing is used only as a last resort.

Shock (Including Temperature). Inadequate cerebral perfusion is a common cause of AMS. The vital signs may reflect inadequate cardiac output, respiratory failure, or hypoxia. Typically, a systolic blood pressure below 80 mm Hg is required to cause a decrease in the level of consciousness in an adult (see Chapter 2, Airway Management). Severe hypothermia (<30°C) can cause coma. Heat stroke with hyperthermia greater than 41°C (105°F) is associated with confusion and delirium.

DIAGNOSTIC ADJUNCTS

The sequence of ordering laboratory tests depends on the history and physical examination. The first three tests that follow are ordered for the majority of patients with AMS. The remaining tests are selected on the basis of the patient's findings.

Laboratory Studies

Complete Blood Cell Count (CBC) and Differential. A CBC is obtained to measure the hemoglobin and hematocrit, particularly if anemia is suggested. An elevated white blood cell count and, in particular, a differential count with a left shift support the presence of underlying infection.

Serum Chemistries. Serum glucose, electrolytes, blood urea nitrogen, creatinine, calcium, and magnesium assess most of the metabolic causes of altered states of consciousness. Hepatic function tests are ordered if warranted by the clinical presentation. Table 31–5 lists the types of electrolyte abnormalities that can cause AMS.

Alcohol and Toxicologic Screen. An alcohol screen and ethanol level may be useful in patients in whom confirmation of alcohol intoxication is needed to explain the clinical picture.

Screening for other toxicologic substances may be necessary when drug ingestion is suspected but cannot be accurately confirmed by other means. Drug levels are useful when specific antidotes or interventions are available and necessary (e.g., acetaminophen, salicylates).

Arterial Blood Gas Analysis. Arterial blood gas measurements are useful when hypoxia, hypercapnia, or metabolic acidosis/alkalosis is considered. In general, arterial blood gases are measured in comatose patients or those needing ventilatory support.

Carboxyhemoglobin Level. This test is obtained in all patients with a suspected exposure to carbon monoxide.

Radiologic Imaging

Chest Radiographs. A chest radiograph may help elucidate pulmonary causes of an AMS, such as pneumonia or congestive heart failure. Rarely, a source of brain metastases may be found.

Skull Radiographs. These studies are usually not indicated in evaluating the patient with AMS unless skull fracture is suspected clinically. If a skull fracture is suggested, computed tomography is a more useful test.

Computed Tomography. A head CT is ordered under the following circumstances in the presence of AMS: (1) suspected trauma, (2) suspected intracranial hemorrhage, (3) presence of unexplained focal neurologic deficits, (4) papilledema, (5) if other nonintracranial causes of coma have been ruled out, and (6) AMS that is unexplained after emergency department evaluation.

Magnetic Resonance Imaging. At present, this valuable test is becoming more commonly used in the emergency setting. In general, it is used after the patient is stabilized and other causes of AMS have not been found.

Electrocardiogram

An electrocardiogram identifies dysrhythmias, cardiac ischemia, and drug effects, such as a widened QRS complex from tricyclic antidepressants and other anticholinergic drugs. Metabolic effects on the electrocardiogram are seen in severe hyperkalemia. Prolongation of the QT interval due to drugs, hypocalcemia, or the long QT syndrome may be found.

Special Tests

Lumbar Puncture. A lumbar puncture is indicated in any patient in whom meningitis is suspected. It can be done safely in patients without papilledema or other evidence of raised intracranial pressure (e.g., deepening of coma, changes in respiratory pattern, decorticate or decerebrate posturing) and in whom neurologic examination reveals no focal deficits. If meningitis is suspected but a lumbar puncture is contraindicated, then appropriate antibiotics in doses appropriate to treat meningitis are administered before the patient is transported for CT of the head.

Electroencephalogram. Patients who have a history of epilepsy, had a generalized motor seizure as part of the presentation, or have rhythmical movements of the digits or eyes should be considered to be continuously seizing with subtle motor signs or without motor signs (nonconvulsive status epilepticus). The patient who is intubated and has received paralytic agents will not be able to manifest motor signs of continuing seizure activity. An electroencephalogram may be diagnostic of status epilepticus.

EXPANDED DIFFERENTIAL DIAGNOSIS

Depressed Level of Consciousness. Table 31–6 lists some of the more common causes of depressed levels of consciousness.

Delirium. Table 31–7 outlines the criteria recommended for making the diagnosis of delirium. Table 31–8 lists the major etiologies of delirium.

PRINCIPLES OF MANAGEMENT

The basic general principles of management include the following (Fig. 31–3).

Prompt Empirical Treatment of Reversible Metabolic Causes

As discussed in "Initial Approach and Stabilization" earlier, empirical treatment with

---

TABLE 31–6. Differential Diagnosis of Depressed Level of Consciousness

Cerebrovascular Ischemia

    Basilar artery migraine
    Brain stem infarction
    Cerebral sinovenous thrombosis
    Large cerebral infarction

Drug/Toxin-Related

    Alcohols, anticonvulsants
    Carbon monoxide
    Cellular toxins: carbon monoxide, cyanide, hydrogen
       sulfide
    γ-Hydroxybutyric acid
    Heavy metals
    Opiates
    Sedative/hypnotics
    Tricyclic antidepressants

Endocrine

    Addison's disease, Cushing's disease
    Hypernatremia, hyponatremia
    Pituitary apoplexy
    Thyrotoxicosis or myxedema coma

Environmental

    Hypothermia, hyperthermia
    Neuroleptic malignant syndrome

Infections

    Brain abscess
    Encephalitis
    Meningitis
    Sepsis

Intracranial Hemorrhage

    Epidural hematoma
    Intracerebral hemorrhage
    Subarachnoid hemorrhage
    Subdural hematoma

Metabolic/Substrate Deficiency

    Acidosis, alkalosis
    Hepatic failure
    Hypercalcemia/hypocalcemia
    Hypoglycemia
    Hypoxia or respiratory insufficiency
    Ketoacidosis/hyperglycemia
    Uremia
    Wernicke's encephalopathy (thiamine deficiency)

Pediatric emphasis

    Intussusception in children
    Reye's syndrome

Trauma

    Traumatic diffuse axonal injury

Tumor/mass

    Benign-large
    Malignant-metastasis
    Malignant-primary

Other

    Conversion reaction (pseudocoma)
    Epilepsy (status epilepticus)
    Hypertensive encephalopathy
    Shock

TABLE 31–7. Criteria for Delirium

A. Reduced ability to maintain attention to external stimuli, e.g., questions must be repeated because attention wanders, and to appropriately shift attention to new external stimuli, e.g., perseverates answer to a previous question
B. Disorganized thinking, as indicated by rambling, irrelevant, or incoherent speech
C. At least two of the following:
   1. Reduced level of consciousness, e.g., difficulty keeping awake during examination
   2. Perceptual disturbances: misinterpretations, illusions, or hallucinations
   3. Disturbance of sleep-wake cycle with insomnia or daytime sleepiness
   4. Increased or decreased psychomotor activity
   5. Disorientation to time, place, or person
   6. Memory impairment, e.g., inability to learn new material, such as repeating the names of several unrelated objects 5 minutes after learning them, or to remember past events, such as history of current episode of illness
D. Clinical features develop over a short period of time (usually hours to days) and tend to fluctuate over the course of a day
E. Either (1) or (2):
   (1) Evidence from the history, physical examination, or laboratory tests of a specific organic factor (or factors) judged to be etiologically related to the disturbance
   (2) In the absence of such evidence, an etiologic organic factor can be presumed if the disturbance cannot be accounted for by any nonorganic mental disorder, e.g., manic episode accounting for agitation and sleep disturbance

From Diagnostic and Statistical Manual of Mental Disorders, 4th ed, rev. Washington, DC, American Psychiatric Association, 1994, with permission.

TABLE 31–8. Delirium

Abstinence States

Alcohol
Barbiturates
Benzodiazepines

Drug-related

Cocaine
Amphetamine
PCP (phencyclidine)
Atropine derivatives
Ergotamine

Cerebrovascular

Ischemia to temporal lobes or upper brain stem
Cerebral contusion
Subarachnoid hemorrhage
Postical state
Postconcussion

Infections

Bacterial/tubercular/viral meningitis
Encephalitis (e.g., herpes simplex)
Typhoid fever
Pneumonia
Sepsis
Rheumatic fever

Others

Thyrotoxicosis
Postoperative states

oxygen is given immediately to all patients with AMS.

1. Glucose is given if the patient is hypoglycemic.
2. Thiamine is administered before glucose to potentially malnourished patients and to patients who have symptoms consistent with Wernicke's encephalopathy (triad of AMS, extraocular movement impairment, and ataxia).
3. Naloxone is administered to patients suspected of a narcotic overdose (meiotic pupils, shallow respirations, decreased level of consciousness).
4. Flumazenil may be considered in isolated overdose of a benzodiazepine, presenting as a decreased level of consciousness, depressed respiratory rate, and access to benzodiazepines. This condition may be the result of iatrogenic administration of a benzodiazepine. Although flumazenil is a specific benzodiazepine antagonist, its use is avoided when there is the possibility of a mixed overdose because flumazenil may be a proconvulsant and cause seizures in patients who have taken other drugs (e.g., tricyclic antidepressants and cocaine).

Support of Vital Signs

Abnormalities in the vital signs are immediately addressed. Endotracheal intubation may be needed to control the airway, prevent aspiration,

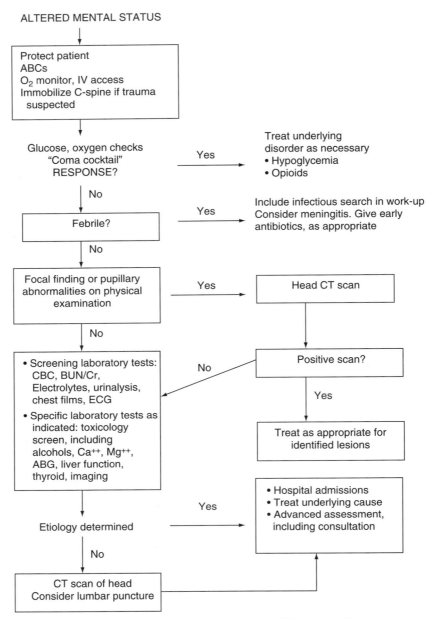

FIGURE 31–3 • Management outlines for altered mental status. ABG, arterial blood gas analysis; CBC, complete blood cell count; ECG, electrocardiogram.

and support ventilation. Shock is treated with crystalloids initially. Correction of blood loss and pressor agents may be used as needed once the cause is determined. Severe hypertension (diastolic pressure greater than 120 to 130 mm Hg) is treated with antihypertensives (see Chapter 10, Hypertension). Hyperthermia or hypothermia is appropriately corrected.

Prevention of Complications or Further CNS Damage

1. Patients with signs of increased intracranial pressure (e.g., transtentorial herniation causing ipsilateral pupillary dilatation) are treated with controlled ventilation and osmotic diuresis using mannitol.

2. Active seizures can be controlled with a benzo-diazepine, followed by phenytoin to prevent further seizures.
3. The cervical spine is immobilized in all coma-tose patients until a cervical spine fracture can be ruled out. More information on preventing secondary complications is given in Chapter 48, Head and Neck Trauma.

Definitive Specific Therapy Based on the Determined Etiology

The history, physical examination, and diagnostic tests will give a definitive diagnosis in most patients with AMS.

Patients with drug overdoses or toxic expo-sures are decontaminated and treated specifi-cally.

CNS hemorrhage is evaluated for neurosurgical evacuation (see Chapter 34, Stroke). Meningitis is treated with antibiotics. Psychotherapy is initiated in patients in psychogenic coma (see Chapter 35, Behavioral Disorders).

UNCERTAIN DIAGNOSIS

Often the diagnosis remains unclear despite the most thorough history and physical, laboratory, and radiographic examinations. A logical approach to this type of patient is essential. The following steps may help to find a disposition and treatment plan:

1. Reassess the information. The patient's his-tory may be obtained from late-arriving or found relatives or friends. All of the labora-tory values should be viewed together with any calculated values such as anion and osmo-lal gap.
2. Reassess the patient. The physical examina-tion may change during the emergency department stay and lend further clues. Further treatment and diagnostic possibilities may be found.
3. Discuss the case with the patient's primary physician and look through any available medical records from previous admissions. Admission records from other hospitals should also be obtained.
4. Consult with an internist or a neurologist. Other possibilities may become obvious through this discussion.
5. If the patient remains with AMS, admission from inpatient observation and treatment is necessary. Many diagnoses may become clear with the luxury of time.

SPECIAL CONSIDERATIONS
Pediatric Patients

Head injuries in children differ in several ways from those in adults. Children in traumatic coma more often do not have a surgically correctable lesion, although one is always sought. After seizures, the postictal state in children occasion-ally can be prolonged.

Reye's syndrome, a postviral illness associated with specific enteroviruses and influenza viruses, is a cause of AMS in children. The use of salicy-lates during the viral illness has been associated with an increased risk of the development of Reye's syndrome.

Elderly Patients

Dementia is most commonly seen in this group. It represents the deterioration of multiple cognitive functions that may precede a decreased level of consciousness. The Quick Confusion Scale may help reveal significant changes. More detailed testing may be necessary for subtle findings. Progressive dementias include vascular dis-ease ("mini-strokes"), Alzheimer's disease, and Parkinson's disease. Delirium is also common in this population, and the differential diagnosis is consistent with that shown in Table 31–8.

Medical problems and injury can commonly present as AMS in older patients. Cerebrovascular disease is primarily a disease of older individuals. Chronic subdural hematomas present much more commonly in the elderly. Only about half the time, a history of head trauma in the prior several weeks is obtained. The head trauma may be quite minor. Metabolic deficiencies, such as hypo-glycemia and hypothyroidism, are also more fre-quent in this age group. The elderly patient can be very sensitive to medications. These are often the cause of AMS. A recent change in medication, dosage, or confusion about medications to be taken must be pursued during the data gathering. Sedative-hypnotic medications, amantadine, his-tamine antagonists, nonsteroidal anti-inflamma-tory drugs, salicylates, neuroleptics, digitalis, β blockers, and fluoroquinolone antibiotics can result in AMS even when taken in therapeutic dosages. Furthermore, the elderly patient may intentionally or accidentally, because of memory impairment, take an overdose of drugs.

Psychiatric conditions may be caused by med-ical problems, or masquerade as such. Depressive syndromes can significantly affect cognitive func-tion. Major life changes (moving, retirement, death of a loved one) may promote a progressive and disabling depression. A psychiatric history should be part of the AMS assessment in the elderly.

DISPOSITION AND FOLLOW-UP

The disposition of patients with AMS depends on the specific diagnosis made, the clinical course in the emergency department, and the patients' support system at home.

Admission

All patients who continue with a depressed consciousness need admission, monitoring, and neurologic and/or neurosurgical consultation along with their emergency management and diagnostic regimen. Patients with heightened AMS (delirium) are admitted for diagnosis and therapy.

Patients with seizures or AMS caused by hypoglycemia are usually admitted for observation and reevaluation of their diabetes management. Patients with hypoglycemia from long-acting oral hypoglycemic agents are admitted because of the high potential for recurrence of the hypoglycemic state.

The patient with a narcotic overdose may awaken in response to naloxone, become combative, and resist further medical evaluation. Because the naloxone duration of action is 1 hour and the opiate taken (e.g., methadone or propoxyphene) may have a much longer half-life, the narcotic overdose patient tends to be admitted to the hospital and observed. Possible complications (e.g., aspiration pneumonia) that occurred during the comatose state are evaluated.

Discharge

Patients with depressed consciousness from alcohol intoxication are observed and monitored until they fully recover to their usual baseline state. Psychologic or social worker intervention regarding the problem of alcoholism is addressed before discharge.

Patients presenting with AMS from ingestion of drugs can be discharged if the drugs do not have delayed absorption and after the patients are toxicologically decontaminated. Discharge should be delayed until a "normal" mental status is observed. Any patient with suicidal attempts or gestures is evaluated psychiatrically before discharge. Selective early discharge of opioid overdose patients after several hours of observation may be appropriate.

Patients with less severe AMS secondary to seizures or hypoglycemia may be discharged only if they have returned to normal and fully compre-

hend the possible consequences of another episode. They are discharged optimally to a support system of family or friends. Follow-up with their primary physician is arranged.

Patients presenting in psychogenic coma can be discharged if they have "fully recovered" and the diagnosis is confirmed, preferably with consultation by neurology. If patients persist in "coma" or have any residual deficit, they require neurologic and psychiatric consultation. Similarly, if patients appear to be malingering or are diagnosed as hysterical conversion reaction, consultation is obtained, especially if any signs or symptoms of neurologic disorder persist.

On discharge from the emergency department, all patients and their family members are informed that the patient should return immediately if there is any recurrence of symptoms. It is important to arrange follow-up for these patients in 24 to 48 hours and to have a back-up plan for the people in the patient's support system should the patient refuse appropriate follow-up. Specific disposition depends on the underlying cause of the AMS.

FINAL POINTS

- Coma is at the extreme of findings manifested by depressed levels of consciousness.
- Delirium is AMS with increased psychomotor activity.
- When a person loses the sense of orientation owing to an organic illness, it is usually in the sequence of time, place, and, finally, person.
- Patients with an organic cause of their AMS are usually disoriented, whereas patients with a psychogenic cause are not disoriented.
- A mixed presentation of AMS caused by organic and functional disorders is relatively common. Admission may be necessary to differentiate the primary cause of AMS.
- The Glasgow Coma Scale is a clinical tool to quantify changes in the patient's level of consciousness.
- Pupillary reflexes and eye motor function are important clinical signs in assessing function of the CNS, particularly the brain stem.
- Patients with AMS may have multiple causes at the same time. Serious life-threatening diseases are always considered and ruled out first.
- AMS is empirically treated to cover reversible causes without waiting for diagnostic tests.
- The most common treatable causes of AMS may be remembered by the mnemonics AEIOU and TIPS.
- Whenever meningitis is suggested, antibiotics are given immediately. CT should not delay the first dose.

A 50-year-old man was found unconscious in a downtown park. He appeared disheveled and smelled of alcohol. Bystanders called the rescue squad.

The paramedics arrived and found the patient comatose. His Glasgow Coma Scale score was 7 (no eye opening = 1; unintelligible sounds = 2; nonspecific withdrawal movements = 4). His breathing was noisy but improved with a jaw-thrust maneuver. His gag reflex was intact but weak. He was placed on a backboard with spine precautions. Vital signs were blood pressure, 140/90 mm Hg; pulse, 90 beats per minute; respiratory rate, 24 breaths per minute. He was given thiamine, glucose, and naloxone with no response. An empty bottle of wine was found in his jacket, along with a nearly full bottle of phenytoin capsules dated 2 weeks earlier. A companion stated that his friend had complained of headaches for about 2 weeks. The patient reeked of alcohol, and his pants were stained with urine. His right pupil was 6 mm and did not appear reactive. The left pupil was 3 mm and reactive.

Although the patient is a known alcoholic and appears to be in an alcoholic stupor or possibly in a postictal state, the history and physical point to a more urgent situation. The pupil asymmetry and nonreactive state are particularly troublesome and suggest that the coma is caused by a structural rather than metabolic condition. Rapid transport is indicated, with early hospital notification. Although the airway is patent, the gag reflex is weak; and the patient may benefit from controlled ventilation (true coma, focal finding). Therefore, an orotracheal tube is put in place, with the head and neck immobilized, before transport, and the patient's ventilation is controlled.

On arriving at the emergency department, the rescue squad's findings were confirmed. The patient remained comatose with a Glasgow Coma Scale score of 7 and a nonreactive, 6-mm-dilated right pupil. The vital signs were unchanged. However, the patient's respirations had become somewhat irregular. Old scars were noted on his forehead, and a more recent wound with encrusted sutures was found. In response to noxious stimuli, his left side moved much less than his right. The placement of the orotracheal tube was checked by direct visualization. Ventilation was continued with 100% oxygen. A ventilator was requested from respiratory therapy. A second intravenous line was placed.

There was no response to the glucose, thiamine, and naloxone given in the field. Mannitol, 25 g, was given intravenously. Blood for laboratory tests, including arterial blood gas analysis, was drawn. The patient was transported for CT of the head and other radiologic studies. The neurosurgeon was called and the operating room staff notified. The patient's belongings were searched for phone numbers to call. Prior medical records were requested.

The patient's physical findings are consistent with increased intracranial pressure and uncal herniation. Emergency treatment to reduce intracranial pressure by controlled ventilation and osmotic agents is indicated. Preparations for urgent neurosurgical intervention are begun. The entire emergency department team is mobilized and motivated to maximize the efficiency and effectiveness of the patient's care.

The CT showed a large, right parietofrontal chronic subdural hematoma. Fresh blood within the subdural hematoma probably explained his recent deterioration. His alcohol level was only 50 mg/dL.

The patient's alcohol level does not account for a significant AMS, much less outright coma. When the mismatch is a low alcohol level and a high degree of mental status impairment, then other serious conditions must be aggressively sought. In this case, findings consistent with uncal herniation prompted a rapid diagnostic effort.

The patient was taken immediately to the operating room to have the subdural hematoma evacuated. He remained stable. After successful evacuation, he was transported to the recovery unit in stable condition.

Even in the presence of cerebral herniation, early intubation and measures to reduce intracranial pressure can successfully, but temporarily, stabilize a patient so that proper resuscitation and diagnosis can be carried out before surgical intervention.

After evacuation of the subdural hematoma, the patient had an uneventful course and recovered with a slight residual weakness. He swore he would give up his drinking habit.

This patient was successfully treated because the life-threatening process was recognized early. The obvious distraction of this patient being alcoholic was properly interpreted as a risk factor, rather than a convenient means of explaining his symptoms.

Bibliography

TEXTS

Plum F, Posner JB: The Diagnosis of Stupor and Coma, 3rd ed. Philadelphia, FA Davis, 1982.

Taylor RL: Distinguishing Psychological from Organic Disorders, 2nd ed. New York, Springer, 2000.

JOURNAL ARTICLES

American College of Emergency Physicians: Clinical policy for the initial approach to patients presenting with altered mental status. Ann Emerg Med 1999; 33:251–280.

American Psychiatric Association Work Group on Delirium: Practice Guidelines for the Treatment of Patients with Delirium. Am J Psychiatry 1999; 156(May Suppl):1–20.

Ashton CH, Teoh R, Davies DM: Drug-induced stupor and coma: Some physical signs and their pharmacological basis. Adverse Drug React Acute Poisoning Rev 1989; 8(1):1–59.

Bates D: The management of medical coma. J Neurol Neurosurg Psychiatry 1993; 56:589–598.

Brady WJ: Life-threatening syndromes presenting with altered mentation and muscular rigidity. Emerg Med Rep 1999; 20(6):51–60.

Diringer MN: Early prediction of outcome from coma. Curr Opin Neurol Neurosurg 1992; 5:826–830.

Doyon S, Roberts JR: Reappraisal of the "coma cocktail": Dextrose, flumazenil, naloxone, and thiamine. Emerg Med Clin North Am 1994; 12:301–316.

Feske SK: Coma and confusional states: Emergency diagnosis and management. Neurol Clin 1998; 16:237–256.

Giacino JT: Disorders of consciousness: Differential diagnosis and neuropathologic features. Semin Neurol 1997; 17:105–111.

Huff JS, Farace E, Brady WJ, et al: The quick confusion scale in the ED: Comparison with the Mini-Mental State Examination. Am J Emerg Med 2001; 19:461–464.

Hustey FM, Meldon SW: The prevalence and documentation of impaired mental status in elderly emergency department patients. Ann Emerg Med 2002; 39:248–253.

Murphy B: Delirium. Emerg Med Clin North Am 2000; 18:243–252.

O'Keefe KP, Sanson TG: Elderly patients with altered mental status. Emerg Med Clin North Am 1998; 16:701–715.

Patterson CJ, Gauthier S, Bergman H, et al: The recognition, assessment and management of dementing disorders. Can Med Assoc J 1999; 160(12 Suppl):S1–S15.

Samuels MA: The evaluation of comatose patients. Hosp Pract (Off Ed) 1992; 28(3):165–182.

Schneider SM: Altered mental status in the elderly: Current assessment and management strategies for a complex clinical syndrome. Emerg Med Rep 1996; 17(5):43–54.

CHAPTER 32

Headache

VIRGIL DAVIS

CASE *Study*

A 45-year-old man told the triage nurse that he had a headache for 2 days and had come to the emergency department to find out why.

INTRODUCTION

Headache is a patient complaint encountered daily in the emergency department. It accounts for 1% to 6% of total visits depending on the site. Approximately 90% of the population will experience headache at some time in their lives. It may represent a simple short-lived event or a chronic emotional difficulty, or it may herald an intracerebral catastrophe. The majority of headaches managed in the emergency department do not represent medically serious conditions. Depending on the patient population, up to 15% of headaches are caused by serious underlying conditions. The primary goal of the emergency physician is to distinguish those patients presenting with headache due to potentially serious conditions from those with benign causes.

The term *headache* technically refers to any head pain including pain in the face, neck, and ears, but it is generally used to describe pain perceived in the scalp and cranium. Pain-sensitive structures in this area include

- The structures between the epidermis of the scalp and periosteum of the skull
- The venous sinuses and their branches within the cranium
- The structures at the base of the brain, including the dura mater
- The arteries of the dura mater
- The cranial nerves

The parenchyma of the brain, most of the meninges, and the skull are not pain sensitive. Thus, headache is not a sensitive indicator of serious intracranial pathologic processes.

Tension and traction of pain-sensitive structures, vascular changes, and inflammation cause pain in the head. Tension results from constriction of neck and scalp muscles from cervical arthritis, irritating lesions, or emotional distress. Traction may be due to an intracranial mass and may be felt at the base of the head, before a rise in intracranial pressure. Vascular distention or dilation manifests as the throbbing pain characteristic of migraine and cluster headache. Inflammation is associated with meningitis, arteritis, or sinusitis. It is usually infectious but may be caused by intracerebral irritants such as blood.

The International Headache Society (IHS) has developed a classification system for headaches that divides this complaint into primary and secondary headaches. Primary headaches include migraine, tension, and cluster headaches. These are considered to be benign, recurrent events that account for 90% of the headaches seen in the emergency department. Secondary headaches are a symptom of an underlying disease.

Although there are a large number of secondary causes of headache, the emergency physician is generally concerned with a discrete set of common complaints or deadly disorders. The priority in the emergency department is to exclude the life-threatening secondary headaches. Once this occurs, symptomatic treatment and disposition can follow. Generally, definitive diagnosis and management will occur in the outpatient system.

INITIAL APPROACH AND STABILIZATION

Priority Diagnoses

The initial assessment of the patient with headache is focused on whether the patient has an emergent cause for the pain, including

- Intracranial hemorrhage
- Infectious meningitis
- Hypertensive encephalopathy
- Hypoxic conditions
- Mass lesion in the brain

If any of these conditions are suggested, the workup of the patient proceeds immediately with diagnostic studies until the diagnosis is made or the condition is ruled out.

Rapid Assessment

History

Severity and Onset of Pain. In patients who describe the "worst headache of their lives" or have a sudden onset of pain, it is likely to be of vascular origin. Intracranial bleeding, particularly a subarachnoid hemorrhage (SAH), is of paramount concern for the emergency physician in these cases.

Prior History of Headaches. Many headache patients have a history of a primary headache disorder, such as migraine. Although the most likely reason for emergency department visits will be benign headaches, these patients have an equal risk for serious causes when compared with the general population. A significant departure from the pattern and character of previous headaches should lead to thorough neurologic examination and the strong consideration of neuroimaging, with cerebrospinal fluid (CSF) evaluation if indicated.

History of Head Trauma. Acute or subacute intracranial bleeding (e.g., subdural hematoma or SAH) may be preceded by head trauma. A period of 3 to 4 weeks is discussed, because of the potential for a subacute process. In the elderly or patients with coagulopathies, even minor head trauma requires diagnostic tests to rule out a central nervous system (CNS) hemorrhage.

Human Immunodeficiency Virus (HIV) Infection or Immunosuppression with New-Onset Headaches. These patients are at high risk for meningitis (often without meningeal signs or fever), brain abscess, and intracranial mass lesions. Opportunistic CNS infections are much more common in AIDS patients (82%) versus normal, healthy patient populations (4%).

Physical Examination

Blood Pressure. A diastolic pressure of greater than 120 to 130 mm Hg can indicate hypertensive encephalopathy or cerebrovascular response to a mass lesion. Prompt examination of the optic disc for papilledema is indicated to assess for elevated intracranial pressure. Significant hypertension associated with headache merits computed tomography (CT) and possible CSF evaluation, if the history is suggestive of SAH.

Tachypnea. Mild to moderate hypoxia can cause headaches. A particularly important cause is carbon monoxide (CO) poisoning. Pulse oximetry will have normal readings in the patient with CO poisoning. A patient with a history of possible CO exposure or unexplained tachypnea and headache should be put on 100% oxygen until arterial blood gases, including CO level, are determined.

Fever. Infections such as meningitis, encephalitis, or brain abscess must be considered when a patient is febrile. Headache may be part of a "nonspecific" viral illness. Lumbar puncture (LP) should be promptly considered in patients with fever and headache.

Meningismus. Meningismus represents the clinical manifestation of meningeal irritation. This is most often seen as nuchal rigidity to flexion. The presence of a stiff neck, fever, and headache alerts the physician to the possibility of meningitis. Pain with neck flexion or pain/stiffness in other directions of head and neck movement (e.g., rotation) is less diagnostic of meningeal involvement.

Mental Status. Is the patient oriented and responding appropriately? Altered level of consciousness generally indicates a serious intracranial pathologic process such as stroke, intracranial hemorrhage, or meningitis. Mental status changes mandate prompt CT and laboratory evaluation for metabolic abnormalities, including electrolytes, glucose and calcium levels, renal and liver function tests, CO level, CSF studies, and urine toxicology.

Neurologic Evaluation. Focal neurologic deficits indicate potentially serious disease processes and require prompt workup. A rapid assessment of symmetric motor strength and extremity movement is sufficient screening.

Early Intervention

Tachypnea. Patients with suspected oxygenation or respiratory problems are placed on 100% oxygen. Blood samples for measurement of arterial blood gases and CO levels are drawn.

Blood Pressure. Patients with hypertensive encephalopathy (papilledema, mental status changes, and diastolic blood pressure of more than 130 mm Hg) need to have their blood pressure regulated with intravenous antihypertensive agents. The arterial pressure is closely monitored, with a goal reduction of 15% to 20% within 60 to 120 minutes.

Altered Mental Status (AMS). Patients with headache and AMS may be given 100 mg of thiamine. A blood glucose level is checked by bedside glucose strip test, or glucose is empirically administered if the glucometer is unavailable. Naloxone may be given intravenously if there is concern for narcotic overdose (depressed mental status, respiratory depression, pinpoint pupils) and can be titrated from 0.2 to 2 mg. Some chronic headache sufferers are narcotic addicted, and care must be taken to avoid precipitating narcotic withdrawal with naloxone. Headache with altered mental status must raise concern about a potential serious underlying cause, especially the priority diagnoses listed earlier.

Fever and Meningismus. If there are no signs of increased intracranial pressure, an LP is performed and, pending findings, appropriate broad-spectrum antibiotic therapy is given. Antibiotic coverage may be narrowed after CSF studies are completed. Antibiotic therapy is given before any delay caused by imaging studies.

Seizures. Seizure activity indicates a significant intracranial pathologic process. Lorazepam is the benzodiazepine of choice to terminate an active seizure, and phenytoin or phenobarbital may be added to prevent further seizure activity (see Chapter 33, Seizures).

Intracranial Pressure. Increased intracranial pressure secondary to hemorrhage, trauma, or tumor may be controlled with osmotic diuresis. This may be achieved with mannitol and/or brief hyperventilation (for imminent herniation only). These interventions are considered for patients with evidence of impending herniation and are of unclear long-term benefit.

CLINICAL ASSESSMENT

The history and physical examination are focused to corroborate the patient's description of pain and to elicit signs and symptoms of focal neurologic deficits. A search for systemic disease findings that may cause headache is also part of the assessment.

History

Key points in the history will distinguish an acute from a chronic process causing the headache.

Age. *Age older than 55 years* is associated with an increased risk of headache secondary to a serious cause. Studies report age older than 65 years to be associated with a 15% risk of serious conditions, whereas patients younger than 65 years had only a 1% to 2% chance of serious causes. SAH, tumor, cerebrovascular accident, and temporal arteritis are all more likely in those older than age 55 years. The new onset of primary headache is also considered relatively unlikely in this group. Any patient older than 50 to 55 years of age with a new-onset headache should undergo evaluation for secondary causes.

Nature of Pain. Is the pain characterized as *sharp, dull, aching,* or *throbbing*? A patient with a severe headache caused by an SAH may be unable to characterize the pain except for "the worst in my life." Vascular headaches are usually perceived as throbbing, whereas muscle contraction headaches may be felt as a band or a tightening around the head.

Onset. Is this a *new headache*? Has it *occurred before*? Does it fit a pattern of *chronic or recurrent headaches*? Time of onset is determined. Migraines begin in the early morning hours, and cluster headaches occur at night. Both may awaken the patient. Headaches of vascular origin are usually acute in onset. Chronic headaches with no change in pattern or intensity are very likely benign and do not require extensive evaluation.

Location. Is the headache *localized* or *generalized*? *Migraine* is derived from the Greek hemikrania, an affliction of half of the cranium. The majority of migraine sufferers will report headaches that present on either side in subsequent attacks, although one side is often affected more frequently. Additionally, 20% of migraine attacks will begin bilaterally and then localize to one side. A generalized headache may represent increased intracerebral pressure or a psychogenic disease. Occipital headaches more often originate from tension or traction.

Duration. *How long* has the headache *lasted*? Migraines may last hours to days. Cluster headaches may last minutes to hours. Progressive mass lesions cause headaches of increasing intensity and duration. A constant headache of long duration is rarely caused by an acute medical condition.

Severity/Psychologic and Physiologic Importance. Intense pain may represent an SAH or vascular headache. Tension headaches are usually dull and persistent and do not wake the patient. An important part of the examination is to assess how the pain has affected the patient's life. Incapacitating headache is an urgent or emergent problem no matter what the underlying diagnosis.

Prodrome. Visual, tactile, or, rarely, olfactory auras may precede migraine pain. This classic migraine (aura preceding headache) occurs in 20% of migraine patients.

Associated Symptoms. Associated symptoms may include nausea, vomiting, dizziness, loss of consciousness, weakness, eye problems, and neck stiffness. Meningeal symptoms and signs are commonly associated with SAH and meningitis. Focal motor paresis can indicate a cerebrovascular accident, subdural hemorrhage, mass lesion, or migraine. Nausea and vomiting may accompany a migraine, hypertensive, or fever-associated headache. It may also be secondary to increased intracranial or intraocular pressure.

Precipitating Factors. A history of trauma, recreational drug use, exertion, fatigue, alcohol use, or sexual activity preceding the headache may help elucidate the cause. Fatigue, stress, menstruation, and ingestion of specific foods may precipitate migraines. Emotional stress and depression are important contributors to headache. Sleep, appetite, and sexual disturbances may suggest headache secondary to psychogenic factors. Any headache with rapid onset during strenuous activity, Valsalva maneuver, or sexual intercourse is of concern for SAH or vascular origin.

Family History. A family history of migraine is positive for 60% of migraine sufferers. SAH and cerebral aneurysm have been found to be familial.

Medical and Medication History. Alcoholism, recent trauma, bleeding disorders, and use of anticoagulant medication are all associated with an increased risk of subdural hematoma. Acute traumatic head injury suggests cerebral edema or focal hemorrhage.

Medical conditions such as hypertension, hypercapnia, hypoxia, hypothyroidism, metastatic malignancies, acute anemia, hypoglycemia, and steroid deficiency can all result in headache. HIV infection poses risk for cerebral toxoplasmosis, cryptococcosis, and lymphoma. Pregnant and postpartum patients are at risk for sagittal sinus thrombosis. Exposure to nitrates may trigger headaches, and oral contraceptives may exacerbate migraines.

Medications used for head pain in the past, as well as their efficacy, serve as a guide for the evaluation and treatment of the current headache. A patient who has taken ergotamine in the past and has experienced headache relief probably has migraine headache.

Travel History. Patients who travel to regions endemic for tick populations may develop Lyme disease with aseptic meningitis or a variety of other tickborne encephalitides.

Toxic Exposures. Has the patient been exposed to any toxic gases, such as chlorine or CO? Do other people in a similar environment have headaches? Two or more family members presenting with headache should raise the suspicion of CO poisoning in the home.

Physical Examination

The physical examination emphasizes the neurologic assessment, and a search is made for any focal abnormalities or systemic signs to explain the headache's origin.

Vital Signs. Abnormal vital signs in patients with headache often suggest serious illness.

1. Fever without meningismus may indicate a systemic illness causing the headache.

2. Hypertension rarely causes headache unless the diastolic blood pressure is greater than 120 to 130 mm Hg. Often, mild hypertension is secondary to pain.
3. Tachycardia and tachypnea may occur with a headache secondary to hypoxia, anemia, or CO poisoning. More often, tachycardia reflects severe pain.

General Appearance. Is the patient in severe distress, agitated, or anxious? Conversely, is the patient resting comfortably, speaking with family or friends? Is the patient resting silently in a darkened room? The latter is typical of a patient with migraine headache, SAH, or any other cause associated with photophobia.

Head and Neck. The head, face, and neck are inspected for evidence of trauma or other abnormalities.

1. The head is palpated for scalp swelling or hematoma. The sinuses and teeth are examined for tenderness, representing a periapical abscess. Tender scalp or neck muscles may indicate a muscle contraction headache or irritation secondary to another cause. The temporal arteries are palpated for firmness or tenderness in all patients older than 50 years of age.
2. Auscultation for carotid bruits may indicate stenosis or an arteriovenous malformation.
3. Meningismus is assessed carefully. Many patients with tension headaches may have a "stiff neck." Meningismus is a reflex flexion (nuchal) rigidity with pain. It may result from meningitis, encephalitis, or SAH. The patient whose neck is stiff on rotary or lateral motion is less likely to have serious disease.
4. The ears are inspected for hemotympanum or infection.

Neurologic Examination
1. Mental status. A directed mental status examination includes evaluation of orientation, memory, concentration, and speech (see Chapter 31, Altered Mental Status). Marked alteration in level of consciousness indicates a true medical emergency. Delirium and dementia may result from meningitis, cerebral anoxia, hypercarbia, or trauma. Personality changes may indicate frontal lobe pathology. Speech deficits may indicate a mass lesion or cerebrovascular accident.
2. The ocular examination is important in patients with headache. A "steamy" cornea may be seen in patients with acute glaucoma. An irregular pupil causing pain on examination with direct or consensual light indicates iritis. A unilateral dilated pupil, unreactive to direct

and consensual light, coupled with a decreased level of consciousness indicates imminent temporal lobe herniation. A visual field deficit may indicate a pituitary adenoma, brain tumor, stroke, or arteriovenous malformation. The funduscopic examination allows visual access to the small vasculature of the body and to the optic nerve tract, both of which have a close anatomic relationship to the meningeal coverings and the subarachnoid space. Funduscopy may show papilledema caused by increased intracranial pressure. This finding usually takes hours to days to develop. Retinal hemorrhages may be seen, suggesting intracerebral or subarachnoid hemorrhage. Vascular spasm, flame hemorrhage, and exudate consistent with malignant hypertension also may be found.

3. Motor and sensory examinations, of cranial and peripheral nerves, are imperative. Localized weakness or abnormal sensation may be due to mass lesions, hemorrhage, cerebrovascular accident, or migraine.

4. Gait examination and rapid alternating movements assess cerebellar function. Dyscoordination and ataxia may be the only signs of a posterior fossa mass or hemorrhage.

5. Testing the bicep, patellar, and Achilles deep tendon reflexes, plus the Babinski reflex, is standard. An asymmetric response may be the only localizing finding.

Selected Examinations. The history, vital signs, and general appearance can indicate the presence of system disease. A screening physical examination including cardiovascular, pulmonary, and abdominal examinations is recommended. Potential high-yield sources of infection (the ears, nose, and throat area, the lungs, and the genitourinary tract) are explored in the patient with fever.

CLINICAL REASONING

After the history and physical examination are complete, a distinction is made between emergent, urgent, and nonurgent cases of headache. These categories are defined by how quickly the diagnoses must be made, or treatment initiated, to prevent diminished function and loss of life. A number of pathologic processes are classified in this manner in Table 32–1. A prioritized differential diagnosis is constructed by answering three questions.

Is a Potentially Catastrophic Disease Process Occurring?

The signs and symptoms reviewed in the previous sections indicate the presence of catastrophic illness (Table 32–2). Emergent causes of headache are often dynamic, and these signs and symptoms may develop at any time during the evaluation.

TABLE 32–1. Common Causes of Headache Presenting in the Emergency Department

Emergent Causes

Intracranial hemorrhage—subarachnoid hemorrhage; subdural, epidural, or intracerebral hematoma
Meningitis or encephalitis
Severe hypertension with encephalopathy
Disorder of oxygenation or respiration: hypoxia, hypercarbia, carbon monoxide poisoning

Urgent Causes

Vascular—migraine, cluster, cerebrovascular accident, arteriovenous malformation, altitude sickness, giant cell arteritis
Mass—brain tumor, abscess, arteriovenous malformation
Potential head trauma or chronic subdural hematoma
Secondary to systemic disorder, hypoglycemia, fever, hypothyroid, anemia
Miscellaneous—glaucoma, benign intracranial hypertension

Less Urgent Causes

Muscle contraction (tension)
Secondary to diet or medications
Fatigue, post exertion, post coital
Post trauma
Post lumbar puncture
Sinusitis without complications
Myofascial pain syndrome

TABLE 32–2. Characteristics of Emergent Causes of Headache

Cause	Affected Population	History	Associated Symptoms	Physical Examination	Diagnostic Adjuncts	Management Principles
Subarachnoid hemorrhage	Adults, 20–50 years old. May occur during strenuous activity (e.g., lifting, sexual intercourse). Account for 1% of headaches seen in emergency department.	50%–60% of patients have a "sentinel bleed." Pain is abrupt in onset, throbbing, and often described as "the worst headache of my life." The pain may radiate to the neck or back.	Commonly nausea, photophobia, and neck and back pain. May have diplopia, vomiting, transient loss of consciousness, or seizure. Increased pain with standing.	Nuchal rigidity common. May see seizure (10%), focal neurologic deficit, or depressed level of consciousness.	Head CT is sensitive in over 90%. Lumbar puncture will show either RBCs or xanthochromia in 99% of true subarachnoid hemorrhage.	These patients are kept quiet and calm and admitted to intensive care. Neurosurgeon is consulted early in their care.
Bacterial meningitis	Most often seen in infants and elderly. Causes 1% of headaches seen in emergency department.	Prodrome is highly variable. Usual onset of severe diffuse pain over hours. Seldom has precipitating factors, although another site of infection (e.g., otitis media) may be present.	Almost always occurs with complaint of neck pain, malaise, photophobia. More severely affected patients are confused and have vomiting.	Patients have fever (90%), nuchal rigidity. Often depressed or agitated level of consciousness. Skin may show hemorrhagic or petechial rash.	Lumbar puncture definitive, characteristically elevated WBCs >50/hpf, elevated protein, normal or decreased glucose. Immunologic cerebrospinal studies may help.	All patients are taken to intensive care. Early treatment with antibiotics is top priority.
Hypertensive with encephalopathy	Primarily in patients with long-standing hypertension. 4% of headache presentations in emergency department.	Onset of pain is usually rapid and may awaken patient from sleep. Pain is severe, global, and throbbing. May have headache history or poorly controlled hypertension; often poor medication compliance.	Patients are often confused; may have chest pain or shortness of breath. Can present with seizure activity.	Diastolic blood pressure usually above 130 mm Hg (>80% of patients). Funduscopic changes including vasospasm, hemorrhage, and papilledema. Patients often have depressed level of consciousness, becoming comatose with intracerebral hemorrhage.	Renal insufficiency is common with elevated protein level in urine. Also evaluate the heart (ECG, enzymes).	Parenteral blood pressure control is essential. Decrease blood pressure by 10%–20% over 1 hour.

CT, computed tomography; ECG, electrocardiogram; RBCs, red blood cells; WBC, white blood cells.

Emergent Causes

Subarachnoid hemorrhage is a true medical emergency and accounts for approximately 1% of persons with headache seen in the emergency department—approximately 25,000 per year. Most bleeding occurs from rupture of a saccular aneurysm. Arteriovenous malformations are a common source of SAHs in those younger than 20 years of age. Forty to 50 percent of these patients die before reaching the hospital. Approximately one half of SAH patients die within 1 month of their hemorrhage, and one third of the remaining survivors will have severe neurologic sequelae. The clinical picture with SAH varies from asymptomatic, to patients with syncope, to those who are comatose. Most patients experience a sudden onset of a severe diffuse headache. Occasionally, the vascular lesion may present in a less acute manner, with worsening of a previous headache pattern, associated with nausea, vomiting, dizziness, and nuchal rigidity. This is the pattern of a sentinel hemorrhage, or early warning of impending aneurysm rupture. Sentinel bleeding occurs in 50% of SAH patients. Subhyaloid or pre-retinal hemorrhages, with blood layered between the retina and vitreous sac, may be seen on funduscopic examination of patients with SAH.

Risk factors for SAH are not completely elucidated. Smoking is clearly a risk factor. Familial SAH carries an increased relative risk of four times. Collagen vascular diseases such as polycystic kidney disease, coarctation of the aorta, abdominal aortic aneurysm, Ehlers-Danlos and Marfan's syndromes, fibromuscular dysplasia, and hereditary telangiectasia are strong risk factors. Other risk factors include Graves' disease and sickle cell disease. Any patient with a headache and one of these risk factors deserves serious evaluation for SAH. Possible risk factors include increasing age, female gender, alcohol and stimulant drug abuse, and birth control pills.

Meningitis is the cause of headache in approximately 1% of patients. The most common causative organisms in adults are *Streptococcus pneumoniae* and *Neisseria meningitidis*. Clinical signs include fever, meningismus, nausea and vomiting, and abnormal mental status. Diagnosis is made by clinical examination and CSF analysis. Immediate antibiotic therapy is crucial, with broad-spectrum coverage and the ability to cross the blood-brain barrier.

Severe hypertension is the cause of headache in approximately 4% of emergency department patients. The pain is diffuse and throbbing, is worse in the morning, and may awaken the patient from sleep. If the headache is associated with diastolic pressures greater than 120 to 130 mm Hg, with altered mental status and papilledema, hypertensive encephalopathy is diagnosed (see Chapter 10, Hypertension).

If Emergent Processes Can Be Ruled Out, What Urgent Processes Must Be Considered? (Table 32–3)

Migraine and cluster headaches are often diagnosed by their characteristic histories. The history of giant cell arteritis is less specific, but a tender temporal artery and elevated erythrocyte sedimentation rate (ESR) require treatment. Cerebrovascular accidents (CVAs, stroke) usually result in objective neurologic abnormalities (see Chapter 34, Stroke). The history and stigmata of head trauma lead the physician to investigate this possibility (see Chapter 48, Head and Neck Trauma).

An intracerebral mass without abnormal neurologic findings is difficult to diagnose, but the progressive nature of the headache or a slowly evolving neurologic finding is significant. If the pain has interrupted the patient's ability to lead a normal life, it is an urgent problem, and both the underlying pathology and the severity of symptoms have a role in the categorization.

Urgent Causes

Migraines are diagnosed in approximately 20% of patients who complain of headache. Although the precise cause is unknown, migraines are associated with decreased cerebral blood flow and extracerebral vasodilatation. Fifty percent of migraine patients have their first episode by age 20. Classic migraines are associated with an aura and premonitory sensory, motor, or visual symptoms (present in only 20% of migraine patients). This is followed by a throbbing unilateral headache with associated nausea, vomiting, and photophobia. Some patients have focal neurologic findings as part of the migraine. Migraines may be precipitated by a number of factors, including stress, menstruation, oral contraceptives, physical exertion, certain foods, and lack of sleep. Common or atypical migraines have similar symptoms, although an aura does not occur and the head pain is only unilateral.

Cluster headaches are less common than migraines. They usually occur in men between the ages of 20 and 50. Cluster headaches are characterized by an abrupt onset of intense unilateral periorbital pain. The pain peaks in a few minutes and lasts for 45 minutes. Attacks tend to come at

TABLE 32–3. Characteristics of Urgent Causes of Headache

Cause	Affected Population	History	Associated Symptoms	Physical Examination	Diagnostic Adjuncts	Management Principles
Migraine	Sixty percent of patients are female. May begin in childhood, usually before age 40.	Dull ache evolves to a severe throbbing over minutes to hours. Usually affects the same hemicranium. Onset occurs in the morning and has a recurrent pattern lasting hours to days. In some patients (35%), scotomas, flashing lights, paresthesias, and hallucinations occur as prodrome; more often there is no prodrome. Precipitated by stress, fatigue, diet, hormonal changes. Family history in 60%.	Photophobia, nausea, vomiting.	Patients usually rest in dark, with eyes closed. Uncomfortable from pain. Affected hemicranium may be tender. Rare to find neurologic or funduscopic abnormalities.	No useful tests. May respond to parenteral phenothiazines.	Outpatient treatment unless intractable vomiting. Pain relief sought because prophylactic medications (e.g., β blockers, ergotamine) do not work by time patient appears in emergency department.
Cluster	Eighty percent of patients are male, between 20 and 40 years of age. Not commonly seen in emergency department. Patients often aware of the pattern.	No prodrome. Pain is a burning, often severe sensation. Commonly periorbital. Occurs at night and in clusters lasting weeks to months. Usual duration is 15 min to 4 hr. Often occurs after ethanol ingestion or use of vasodilators. Family history rare, but patients are often heavy smokers.	Nasal congestion, rhinorrhea, tearing, conjunctival flush.	Patients are uncomfortable from pain. Face may be flushed or blanched. Increased secretions from eye and nose. Horner's syndrome sometimes seen.	None	Once diagnosed, management is prophylactic. Pain can be decreased occasionally with oxygen or ergotamine. Primary treatment is analgesia.
Giant cell (temporal) arteritis	Almost always over 55 years. Females comprise 60% of patients.	No prodrome. Pain is a deep, aching, throbbing, and burning. Can be moderate to severe. May be very slow or rapid in onset. Usually located over temples, often unilateral. Seldom has precipitating factors. Family history positive on occasion.	Pain may also be in ear, teeth, or temporal area with mastication. Visual scintillation or fleeting loss of vision (amaurosis fugax) noted in up to 10% of patients. This is a serious complication.	Tenderness over temporal artery most common finding. Visual changes are usually gone by time of examination, but careful testing is important. Some patients experience relief with pressure on the carotid artery.	Almost always elevated erythrocyte sedimentation rate. Anemia is common.	Early corticosteroid use in high doses (at least 60 mg of prednisone). Delayed diagnosis or therapy can lead to permanent vision deficits.
Space-occupying lesion (tumor, abscess, hemorrhage)	Only 30%–50% of patients with mass lesion have pain. It usually occurs after intracranial pressure has increased.	Pain is without prodrome and is deep, dull, and aching. Intensity ranges from moderate to severe. Location is typically bifrontal or occipital. It is worse in early morning, but rarely awakens patient from sleep. Increased by straining or exertion. Pain may last weeks to years and often steadily progresses in severity. Abscess may be preceded by ear or sinus infection. History may point to origin of metastases.	Aching in neck muscles. Nausea and vomiting. Seizures, altered mental status.	Up to 50% of patients have neurologic abnormalities, most often focal findings or changes in funduscopic examination (e.g., papilledema). Altered mental status is common.	Radiographic imaging with computed tomography and magnetic resonance imaging is diagnostic.	Must be suspected in patients with recurrent headache. Early referral and intracranial pressure control is goal in emergency department.

the same hour each day for several weeks and then disappear for months. There are often associated symptoms of lacrimation, conjunctival injection, ptosis, nasal stuffiness, rhinorrhea, and Horner's syndrome. During the active period, ethanol can precipitate attacks.

Cerebrovascular accidents can cause headaches. Invariably, there are associated focal symptoms with a CVA, usually weakness. The history, physical examination, and CT scan usually give the diagnosis (see Chapter 34, Stroke).

Giant cell arteritis is an uncommon disease characterized by painful inflammation of the temporal artery and other arteries. It is highly associated with polymyalgia rheumatica and occurs primarily in patients older than 55 years of age. Systemic symptoms such as fever, malaise, and weakness occur, in addition to localized tenderness over the superficial temporal artery. The erythrocyte sedimentation rate is typically elevated. The clinical diagnosis is confirmed by a temporal artery biopsy. It should be noted that 50% will not have tenderness of the temporal artery, and 28% will have a headache in a location other than temporal. Any patient older than the age of 55 with an elevated ESR merits a neurology consultation.

Intracranial mass lesions, including tumor, hematoma, or abscess, account for approximately 3% of people with headaches seen in the emergency department. The headaches usually recur, with progressive increases in frequency and intensity. The pain is more intense in the morning and may awaken the patient from sleep. Personality and mental status changes may occur. A CT scan of the head is usually necessary to make this diagnosis. If the patient has had the headache for longer than 10 weeks, without signs of increased intracranial pressure, a tumor is very unlikely.

Acute angle-closure glaucoma can cause intense periorbital pain, nausea, and vomiting, secondary to increased intraocular pressure. Physical examination reveals a cloudy cornea, a mid-range and poorly reactive pupil, and a firm, tense globe, secondary to marked elevation of the intraocular pressure (see Chapter 25, The Red, Painful Eye).

HIV infection and immunosuppression put patients at risk for a variety of atypical causes of headache. Eleven to 55 percent of HIV patients will have headaches, and 80% have an identifiable secondary cause. Patients may have an aseptic meningitis associated with seroconversion. *Toxoplasma gondii* causes multiple brain abscesses with or without focal deficits. B-cell lymphomas are common in HIV patients. Cryptococcal meningitis affects 10% of patients with AIDS. Most HIV-infected and AIDS patients do not display meningeal signs and may

not have significant metal status changes. All patients with HIV infection, immunosuppression therapy, or strong risk factors for HIV with a new headache should have a CT scan and LP. The CT should be done with and without contrast medium enhancement to evaluate for lymphoma and cerebral abscess.

Is a Less Urgent Process Occurring?

Characteristics of these conditions are given in Table 32–4. There is a considerable overlap between migraine-like symptoms and underlying tension/traction headaches. Nausea, throbbing unilateral pain, and scalp muscle tenderness occur frequently in tension headache, and migraine headaches do not always fit the classic pattern. In this context, the emergency physician can only treat the headache relative to its severity and strive to differentiate the true emergent and urgent causes from the less urgent ones.

Less Urgent Causes

Muscle contraction or tension headaches account for one third of all patients with headache coming to the emergency department. The headache is usually bilateral and is described as dull, pressing, or band-like. It varies with intensity during the day and decreases with sleep. There is clinical overlap of symptoms with migraine headaches, and some patients with tension headache have nausea, vomiting, photophobia, and lightheadedness. The patient will generally give a history of similar headaches in the past.

Acute sinusitis accounts for less than 1% of complaints of headache in emergency departments. The pain is localized over the involved sinus and is described as a constant ache or pressure. This sensation is accentuated by bending forward. The headache is more intense in the morning and may be associated with rhinorrhea, fever, chills, and postnasal drip. The involved sinuses are tender to percussion. Radiographs show air-fluid levels in acute sinusitis and cloudiness with chronic inflammation.

DIAGNOSTIC ADJUNCTS

There are no routine laboratory tests for the patient with headache. Results of the history and physical examination guide the appropriate diagnostic tests.

Laboratory Studies

Erythrocyte Sedimentation Rate. An ESR is indicated in patients older than 55 years of age

TABLE 32–4. Characteristics of Less Urgent Causes of Headache

Cause	Affected Population	History	Associated Symptoms	Physical Examination	Diagnostic Adjuncts	Management Principles
Muscle contraction (tension)	Patients aged 20–60. Females affected more than males.	Pain begins without prodrome. Mild to moderately severe, steady ache, constricting "band" or "vice" around head. May appear in forehead or temple but most often in neck and occiput. Onset insidious at varying times of day. Lasts for hours to years. Precipitated by fatigue and stress. Patient may have history of depression or "headache-prone" family member.	Anxiety, sadness, depression, insomnia.	Normal neurologic examination. Muscles tender over area of pain, particularly neck and occiput.	No specific test.	A frustrating problem for both patient and physician. Oral analgesia and nonsteroidal anti-inflammatory medication are mainstays of treatment. Majority of care given by primary physician. Important to avoid complacency and monitor for changing symptoms.
Post-traumatic	Seen in up to one third of patients who have been hospitalized for head trauma. Can follow even minor head injury.	No prodrome. Pain is dull, mild to moderate in severity. Onset occurs hours to days after injury. May last for years. Prior history of trauma.	Sense of disequilibrium, fatigue, memory and attention deficits. Mood swings can occur.	Normal.	Head computed tomography considered to rule out subacute or chronic subdural hematoma or contusion.	May be difficult to treat. Oral analgesia is best choice. Early referral to neurologist or neurosurgeon important.
Sinusitis	Any age.	No prodrome. Pain is due to pressure and fullness in frontal area. Pressure increases with leaning forward. Pain can be mild to severe and is constant; can last for years. Often initiated by upper respiratory infection, dental infections. Patient may have history of allergies, rarely some element of immunocompromise (diabetes mellitus).	Nasal congestion, postnasal drip. May have nasal obstruction.	Low-grade fever, tenderness over involved sinus.	Sinus films may show air-fluid levels or mucosal thickening.	Broad-spectrum, gram-positive oriented antibiotic and decongestant therapy initiated in emergency department. ENT referral if persistent. May be a subtle cause of headache.

with pain in the region of the temporal artery. Almost all patients with temporal arteritis have an elevated ESR, and a normal result virtually rules out arteritis. An ESR greater than 55 mm/hr with the appropriate clinical presentation generally merits treatment for temporal arteritis and neurologic consultation.

Complete Blood Cell Count with Differential. This test has low yield in the headache patient. It may be considered in patients with fever, meningismus, or suspected anemia. Both the white cell count and the differential are nonspecific indicators of infection or inflammation and neither diagnose nor exclude any specific disorders.

Carboxyhemoglobin. Determining the carboxyhemoglobin level is indicated in patients who were confined in a closed environment and exposed to smoke or a faulty heater or when several people from the same environment complain of headache. There is a 7% prevalence of unsuspected CO poisoning.

Arterial Blood Gas Analysis. Arterial blood gas measurements are ordered in any patient with signs, symptoms, or situations suggestive of risk for hypoxia or acidosis.

Radiologic Imaging

Computed Tomography. CT is often used in the patient with headache. Because headaches are a frequent complaint in the emergency department, a large amount of health care resources are used for CT in this population. Although CT is certainly an appropriate test in certain groups of headache sufferers, the vast majority of patients do not require CT. Physician clinical judgment plays an important role in these decisions. Indications for CT include the following:

- First or worst headaches, new headache older than age 50 years
- New headache in patients with cancer or immunosuppression, including HIV infection
- Headache associated with mental status changes
- Headache associated with fever or meningeal signs
- Headache associated with focal deficit
- Migrainous pain and no prior diagnosis of migraine with aura
- Headache associated with anticoagulant use or preceding trauma
- Headache associated with evidence of increased intracranial pressure

CT for other presentations has a very low yield and should not be routinely ordered. The scan is usually done without contrast medium enhancement. Contrast medium is used to enhance small neoplasms and abscesses, but, in general, adding contrast medium to a CT scan has been shown to increase both cost and risk of side effects but not alter management. In the subset of the population with known malignancy, HIV infection, or immunosuppression, obtaining a CT with and without contrast medium enhancement is reasonable.

CT is often used to diagnose SAH. Although this is a useful modality, limitations do exist. Third-generation CT scanners have a significantly higher sensitivity than older models. CT performed within 12 hours of onset of headache has a sensitivity of 95% to 100% for SAH. After 12 hours the sensitivity decreases to 80% to 90%, at 3 to 5 days it is 75% to 85%, at 1 week it is 50%, and at 2 weeks scanning is 30% sensitive. By 3 weeks, the bleeding is undetectable. A clinician's pretest probability for SAH must be taken into account along with the headache time frame. In general, a physician with very high suspicion for SAH will perform an LP if CT is negative. If the suspicion is moderate, but CT is done 12 to 24 hours after pain onset, an LP is performed. Patients who present within 12 hours and have a low risk of SAH, or patients with a low risk presenting within 24 hours, do not always require LP.

Radiography. Sinus radiographs are not required in patients with a history and physical examination consistent with sinusitis, as they may be treated empirically. In patients with an unclear diagnosis or with a history of possible intracranial extension of infection, imaging is required. CT of the sinuses has a higher yield and makes diagnosis of deep (sphenoidal and ethmoidal) sinusitis easier. The relative charges for sinus radiographs and CT scans are institution dependent but are often similar.

Skull radiographs are rarely indicated to evaluate patients with headache.

Angiography. Angiography is obtained in patients who have a positive CT for SAH, a negative CT and positive LP, or a classic history for SAH and a negative evaluation. Angiography can be falsely negative, and 1% of angiograms repeated within 2 weeks (classic history and initial negative angiogram) will demonstrate an aneurysm.

Magnetic Resonance Angiography. This may be substituted for angiography; however, the current indications are unclear, and this study should be pursued in consultation with either a neurosurgeon or neuroradiologist.

Special Tests

Lumbar Puncture. The LP is performed early in the evaluation of a patient with fever and meningismus to diagnose meningitis. The CSF is analyzed for white blood cell count and differential, red blood cells, and glucose and protein levels. Gram's staining is performed, and a culture is done for bacteria, viruses, or fungus. Turbid CSF, elevated opening pressure, high white blood cell and protein levels, and a low glucose level are consistent with bacterial meningitis. CSF analysis is also done on patients suspected of having SAH, when the head CT is negative (see earlier). The diagnosis is confirmed by finding blood in the CSF or by the presence of xanthochromia, representing hemorrhage of more than 6 to 12 hours old, with red blood cell breakdown. Xanthochromia is not evident if the LP is performed within 4 hours of the onset of bleeding, and early LP may have false-negative results. If increased intracranial pressure is possible, a CT of the head is obtained before LP. The LP is performed after the CT interpretation. If the CT is abnormal, a discussion with the radiologist and neurosurgeon occurs before LP. A complication of LP is the post-LP headache, secondary to CSF hypotension (hypovolemia), occurring in 5% to 30% of patients requiring LP. Patients are advised to remain supine for 30 minutes after the procedure to lower the risk.

PRINCIPLES OF MANAGEMENT

The principles of management include

- Prompt attention to life-threatening signs and symptoms
- Pain control
- Volume replacement if anorexia and vomiting are significant symptoms associated with headache
- Treatment of specific diseases

Prompt attention to life-threatening signs and symptoms includes airway management, blood pressure control, and observation for seizures or increased intracranial pressure. Immediate management was discussed earlier.

Analgesia for headache usually depends on the diagnosis. Patients with structural lesions such as tumors, abscesses, or bleeding may be given parenteral narcotics such as meperidine (Demerol) or morphine. These are often given in combination with antiemetics (Phenergan, Vistaril) for relief of the acute headache. These medications have the side effect of decreased level of consciousness, and patients are closely monitored.

Studies indicate that patients with severe headaches, especially migraines, can often be treated successfully in the emergency department with intravenous phenothiazines. Chlorpromazine is given, 5 to 10 mg over 3 minutes, and can be repeated, to a total of 30 mg. Prochlorperazine, 10 mg intravenously over 3 minutes, can be given as a single dose. Side effects of these medications include postural hypertension and extrapyramidal signs. If extrapyramidal signs appear, they are treated with an antihistamine (diphenhydramine), with relief for up to 75% of patients.

Patients with acute headaches need relief and often require narcotics. Unfortunately, there are subsets of patients, with chronic headaches or pain syndromes who abuse the medical system to obtain narcotics. Additionally, there are also patients with chronic headaches who are at risk for narcotic addiction if given multiple narcotics in the emergency department. Caution is advised for outpatient use of narcotics for headaches. In selected circumstances, and preferably after speaking to the primary physician, a limited number of oral narcotic-containing compounds (e.g., Tylenol No. 3, Vicodin, or Percodan) may be prescribed. Nonnarcotic medications (nonsteroidal anti-inflammatory agents [NSAIDs]) are the most commonly prescribed drugs for outpatient analgesia. Many emergency departments have developed clinical protocols to better manage patients with chronic pain, in conjunction with primary physicians. Often, protocols require that patients who are identified with recurrent visits to the emergency department for pain-related complaints enter into pain contracts with the emergency department and primary physician. Such contracts specify the frequency and amount of narcotics dispensed by each physician. Patients who exceed these amounts, or who do not enter into such contracts, are often offered only nonnarcotic analgesia in the emergency department.

Specific Treatment

Emergent Causes

Subarachnoid hemorrhage is associated with significant morbidity and mortality. The prognosis for patients with SAH varies with the initial presentation. Morbidity and mortality secondary to SAH are caused by the initial hemorrhage, rebleeding at 24 hours and at 1 month, and cerebral vasospasm after bleeding. Forty to 60 percent of patients with SAH will survive only 1 month in spite of treatment. Medical management includes bed rest and hypertension control. Nimodipine, a calcium channel blocker, has been shown to decrease morbidity and mortality in noncomatose patients with SAH. This improvement is postulated to be from the control of cerebral vasospasm, an important cause of secondary injury in SAH. The head of the bed is raised slightly (about 30 degrees). Anticonvulsant treatment, antifibrinolytic therapy, and volume control are controversial and may be instituted after discussion with the neurology or neurosurgical consultant. Prompt neurosurgical consultation is indicated to assess the need for emergency surgery or ventriculostomy.

Bacterial meningitis has a mortality of approximately 18%. Patients can present with headache, but systemic symptoms including fever and tachycardia are also present. The classic triad is altered mental status, nuchal rigidity, and fever. Patients may have confusion, meningismus, and lethargy, and their condition may deteriorate clinically during observation. In a recent review, 95% of patients with bacterial meningitis had two of the three triad signs. If a high suspicion for meningitis is present, the patient requires immediate antibiotic therapy to prevent further neurologic damage. LP can follow the first antibiotic dose, without deleterious effect on the results. If focal neurologic findings are present, and suspicion for meningitis remains, antibiotics should be given, CT completed, and LP then attempted. *S. pneumoniae* and *N. meningitidis* are the two most common bacterial agents causing meningitis in the adult population. Broad-spectrum antibiotics are recommended initially, and a narrowed spectrum is used when susceptibilities return. Cefotaxime given intravenously is typically a first choice, with the addition of ampicillin (for *S. pneumoniae*) and rifampin (for *N. meningitidis*). If drug-resistant *S. pneumoniae* is endemic, vancomycin is added.

Hypertensive encephalopathy is diagnosed after entities such as ischemic, thrombotic, or hemorrhagic stroke, intracranial mass, and SAH have been ruled out with CT, magnetic resonance imaging, or LP. Altered mental status signifies end-organ damage secondary to hypertension, and blood pressure management is crucial. When the mean arterial pressure is beyond the ability of the cerebral vasculature to autoregulate, ischemia and encephalopathy occur. The goal pressure is not a single "normal" number but a 10% to 25% decrease in the initial mean arterial pressure over 1 to 3 hours. Rapid drops in pressure may lead to worsening ischemia in watershed areas of brain tissue (those still perfused because of collateral circulation, risking loss of flow as pressure drops). Nitroprusside and labetalol are agents typically used, because they have reliable short-acting effects and are parenteral, allowing for rapid titration. (See Chapter 10, Hypertension.)

Urgent Causes

Migraine Headaches. First-line therapy for migraine headache includes

- Nonnarcotic analgesics (aspirin, acetaminophen, NSAIDs, parenteral ketorolac)
- Antiemetics and phenothiazines (metoclopramide, chlorpromazine, prochlorperazine)
- Triptans (sumatriptan, zolmitriptan, rizatriptan)

The nonnarcotic analgesics are often the first therapy initiated by patients, and lack of pain relief is often what triggers their visit to the emergency department. If these medications have not been used, they may be given in the emergency department. Intramuscular use of ketorolac has been studied and may be the most tolerated (parenteral dosing). The addition of prochlorperazine may relieve nausea and have up to 75% efficacy for relief of migraine pain. A dopaminergic pathway has been hypothesized as the therapeutic mechanism. Metoclopramide and chlorpromazine also relieve nausea, although their effectiveness for primary migraine relief is much less.

The "triptan" medications (serotonin agonists) have been studied extensively for the acute management of migraine headaches. The first to be on the market, sumatriptan has been shown to be effective in 70% to 80% of migraine sufferers when given within the first 2 hours of pain onset. If patients experience relief with these medications in the emergency department setting, outpatient preparations (subcutaneous, intramuscular, sublingual, oral, nasal spray) are available and may be prescribed. Patients must be aware that recurrent headaches (within 24 hours) can occur with these medications, in spite of initial relief (up to 40% of cases). Recurrent pain is milder and typically responds to a second medication dose. Sumatriptan causes cranial vessel vasoconstriction but does not cross the blood-brain barrier (vascular changes only). Triptans and ergot alkaloids both cause vasoconstriction and should not be given within 24 hours of each other (prolonged spasm). These drugs continue to be underutilized in the emergency department. Triptans should be avoided in patients with coronary artery disease, uncontrolled hypertension, and peripheral vascular disease.

Ergot alkaloids (ergotamine, dihydroergotamine) have a long history of use for migraine pain relief and are second-line therapeutic agents. They are also serotonin agonists and cause vasoconstriction. Ergotamine has peripheral vasculature effects, causes serious ischemic events and severe nausea and gastrointestinal effects, and is not used in acute headache care. Patients should be asked if they use this drug for home therapy. Dihydroergotamine has minimal peripheral effects and has fewer gastrointestinal effects. Nausea secondary to migraine may be worsened by dihydroergotamine, and antiemetics should be given. Dihydroergotamine is contraindicated in patients with uncontrolled hypertension and peripheral or coronary vascular disease and is also absolutely contraindicated in pregnancy.

Droperidol has been studied for migraine relief and has demonstrated symptomatic relief as a single agent (80% of study patients) as well as successfully relieving pain in resistant migraines. Intramuscular and intravenous preparations of droperidol are available. Recently, concerns have been raised about cardiac complications related to this drug.

Narcotic agents are often the final pathway in the regimen of migraine therapy. Patients may become narcotic habituated, and rebound pain occurs after cycles of chronic use. Meperidine has been repetitively studied, with variable results: pain relief in some and recurrent pain (rebound) because of its short half-life in others.

Preventative therapy for migraine headaches is directed by the patient's primary physician or by a neurologist. Medications may include β blockers, tricyclic antidepressants, valproic acid, caffeine, and NSAIDs. The patient is asked for a complete list of the medications being used.

Cluster headaches respond to inhaled oxygen (non-rebreather 6 to 10 L/min), which may produce cerebral vasoconstriction and some relief in approximately 15 minutes.

Triptans (by oral or subcutaneous route) have been shown to abort cluster headaches, as has dihydroergotamine. They must be taken early in the headache cycle.

Giant cell arteritis is treated with high doses of oral corticosteroids (60 to 80 mg). The major morbidity of temporal arteritis is blindness associated with extension of the arteritis to involve the ophthalmic artery. Corticosteroids result in an initial improvement in 80% to 90% of cases, although vision loss is not reversible. Emergency department physicians should initiate therapy based on clinical suspicion, and close follow-up should be arranged with a neurologist.

A *mass lesion* such as a tumor or abscess is treated symptomatically. If there are signs of elevated intracranial pressure, initial measures including hyperventilation, osmotic agents, and corticosteroids are started, with consultation by a neurosurgeon.

Acute glaucoma is treated with miotics (pilocarpine), topical β-blocking agents (timolol), carbonic anhydrase inhibitors (acetazolamide), and osmotic diuretics (mannitol, glycerol, or sorbitol). Antiemetics and systemic analgesia provide some comfort for the patient as well. Ophthalmologic consultation is obtained in the emergency department. (See Chapter 25, The Red, Painful Eye.)

Less Urgent Causes

Muscle contraction and posttraumatic headaches can generally be managed with nonnarcotic analgesics such as acetaminophen, aspirin, or ibuprofen. A short course of muscle relaxants is sometimes useful. Chronic symptoms may be treated by antidepressants, relaxation training, or biofeedback. Persistent posttraumatic headache requires thorough assessment, including CT of the head.

Acute sinus headache is treated with topical vasoconstrictors, antibiotics, and analgesics. Consultation with an otolaryngologist is appropriate if the frontal sinuses are chronically involved or the infection does not resolve quickly.

UNCERTAIN DIAGNOSIS

In approximately 30% of patients who present to an ambulatory care setting with headache, no definitive diagnosis can be made. Often the headache corresponds to features found with several types of headache. At a particular stage in development, a headache caused by a mass lesion or trauma might easily be confused with a muscle contraction headache. A headache may have the combined features of a viral meningitis, migraine, and muscle contraction headache. Diagnostic testing, such as CT or LP, may help solve some of these dilemmas but cannot resolve all of them. The emergency physician has several options in this situation. It is less important to make a specific diagnosis than to formulate a rational plan that anticipates catastrophic illness and protects the patient from the consequences:

1. There should be clear identification and treatment of life-threatening symptoms and conditions.
2. The patient is observed serially for complications or development of relevant signs and symptoms. These observations may be made during a several-hour stay in the emergency department or during follow-up in 24 to 48 hours at the primary physician's office.
3. Depending on the level of physician concern, careful instructions are given as to what poten-

tial problems to anticipate, the signs and symptoms that should prompt return, and when and where to follow up. If data point to less serious causes of headache, the patient is given non-narcotic analgesics and is asked to keep a headache diary.

4. If the patient is discharged, he or she should understand that a definitive diagnosis has not been made. The differentiation between headache types may be made several weeks later after follow-up.

Special Considerations

Pediatric Patients

Headache is a common presenting complaint in children. It is estimated that 40% of 7-year-olds and 75% of 15-year-olds will experience headache. Any headache accompanied by fever, lethargy, meningeal signs, or other neurologic abnormality must be considered meningitis until proved otherwise. Most of the causes of adult headache (see Table 32–1) also cause headache in children. Up to 40% of pediatric headaches may be caused by viral infection of the upper respiratory tract. Muscle contraction, migraine, and sinusitis are also common causes of acute headache. Migraine variants are more common in children than in adults and include cyclic vomiting, cyclic abdominal pain, familial hemiplegic migraine, and other rare types. Sinusitis should be suspected in children with respiratory symptoms and an acute or chronic headache. Resolution of the headache should parallel improvement in the systemic illness. Primary CNS tumors account for 20% of cancers in children. Tumors may present as acute pain (awaken from sleep), abnormal neurologic examination, vomiting, confusion, or intermittent headaches over several months. CT or magnetic resonance imaging should be done for these patients.

Elderly Patients

Headache is less common in elderly people than in other adults, with a prevalence of 5% to 50%. This statement applies particularly to muscle contraction and tension headaches. Although all causes of headache listed (see Table 32–1) can result in headache in the elderly, some entities are relatively of more concern. In those patients with headache who are older than 65 years of age, 15% of the headaches are due to serious causes, versus 1% to 2% in those younger than age 65. CVAs are common in the elderly. In patients with cerebral thrombosis or infarction the headache rarely pre-dominates, whereas in those with intracranial hemorrhage it may be a prominent symptom. Approximately 20% of patients with stroke have headache as a presenting symptom, with neurologic abnormality. Giant cell arteritis is considered in any patient who is older than 55 years old. Primary CNS tumor or metastasis often results in a persistent and progressive headache that increases with activities that increase intracranial pressure, such as cough or straining with bowel movements.

DISPOSITION AND FOLLOW-UP

In addition to the acuity of the condition, the patient's disposition is influenced by home support system, emergency physician's level of comfort in considering discharge, pain status at the time of discharge, and available follow-up care.

Admission

All patients with emergent causes of headache are admitted for definitive care, and consultation with a neurologist or neurosurgeon is arranged (see Table 32–1). Among those with urgent causes of headache, a patient with a CVA, giant cell arteritis, mass lesion, head trauma, or glaucoma is admitted. Admission is considered in patients with frontal sinusitis and high risk of spread to the CNS.

Discharge

Patients with cluster, tension, mild to moderate posttraumatic headache, sinusitis, and vascular headaches may be discharged to home. The majority of patients with migraine-type headaches are treated and discharged by their primary physician or neurologist before complete resolution of the pain. All patients leaving the emergency department are given discharge instructions that include when and where to follow up and symptoms that mandate a return to the emergency department. Patients must understand their diagnosis and the dose, indications, and side effects of the prescribed medications. If narcotic analgesia is given, the patient is advised not to drive or drink alcohol. Transportation is arranged to help the patient get home.

Patients are asked to return to the emergency department if the headache

• Becomes significantly worse from the pain level at time of discharge
• Changes in character
• Causes a change in mental status

- Triggers multiple episodes of vomiting
- Is accompanied by new neurologic deficit

FINAL POINTS

- Headache may represent a catastrophic illness or a minor problem.
- A meticulous history and neurologic examination are important to distinguish serious from less serious causes of headache.
- The sudden onset of a headache in a patient who does not normally have headaches may indicate a serious intracranial pathologic process.
- Depending on the delay in presentation, many patients with SAH will have normal head CT scans. An LP is necessary in this group.
- Migraine and muscle tension headaches are the most common causes of headaches treated in the emergency department.
- Management often coexists with and response influences the diagnosis. The patient's condition may change at any time.
- Although a definitive diagnosis cannot always be made, a serious pathologic process should be ruled out and the patient given clear follow-up instructions.
- In up to 30% of patients there may not be a clear diagnosis of the headache after their evaluation in the emergency department.

CASE *Study*

A 45-year-old man told the triage nurse that he had a headache for 2 days and had come to the emergency department to find out why.

This patient was from Mexico and was in the United States on business for his trucking company. He presented with a headache for the previous 2 days and was vague regarding how or when the headache began. His head throbbed and his back ached. He had not seen a doctor in many years. His mother had migraines.

The patient's symptoms were worrisome. His headache must have seemed significant to interrupt business and seek medical care in a foreign country. The headache did not fit any typical pattern.

On physical examination, the patient's vital signs were normal. He was in mild to moderate distress and was waiting patiently for the examination to be conducted. He was alert and oriented. The results of the physical examination, including the neurologic examination, were completely normal. He reported no head trauma and had no signs of systemic disease. A muscle contraction headache from tension was considered.

It did not appear that this patient's headache was emergent or urgent. The headache did not fit into any typical headache pattern. He had none of the symptoms of migraine or cluster headache. He was younger than the usual age group that has giant cell arteritis. The short duration (2 days) was unlikely for intracerebral mass.

The case is difficult, and more information is necessary. A second, more detailed history revealed that the patient was under a great deal of stress with acquisition of a second trucking company and insufficient drivers to staff the vehicles.

An ESR was done to rule out giant cell arteritis, and a CBC was done to screen for anemia or infection. Both test results were normal. A head CT scan was not ordered because the patient did not have abnormal neurologic signs, a sudden onset of a severe headache, or associated head trauma. A lumbar puncture was considered, but neither fever nor meningismus was present.

Patients with headache often present with diagnostic dilemmas. The emergency physician must do everything possible to rule out serious illness. An extra effort in obtaining additional data, observation of the patient, and consultation with other physicians is often necessary.

The patient was discharged with an NSAID. He was asked to return in 1 to 2 days for a repeat evaluation. He returned 2 days later with neck and back stiffness and his headache was worse. A different physician obtained a second history of headache onset during sexual intercourse. The patient had not felt comfortable giving this information to the initial physician who examined him. A head CT scan was read as positive for blood in the subarachnoid spaces.

Although diagnostic adjuncts have clear indications, it is very important to have a thorough history and physical examination. The first physician did not obtain a clear history of the onset and character of the headache. It is important to specifically ask the patient if the onset was sudden and what he was doing during this time. If the patient is vague or a poor historian, CT should be considered. If the patient's history is worrisome, CT is usually the most helpful study. An ESR in a patient younger than age 55 years is of low yield. A CBC is rarely helpful.

The same headache process may present as different in progression or severity. Reevaluation is a valuable tool when a diagnosis is uncertain. Be aware of cultural, sexual, and religious factors. Most patients with SAH present with obvious neurologic symptoms, but 10% have minimal signs and symptoms. A high index of suspicion is necessary when headaches do not fit a typical pattern.

Bibliography

TEXTS

Diamond ML, Solomon GD (eds): Diamond and Dalessio's The Practicing Physician's Approach to Headache, 6th ed. Philadelphia, WB Saunders, 1999.

Olesen J, Tfelt-Hansen P, Welch KMA: The Headaches, 2nd ed. Philadelphia, Lippincott Williams & Wilkins, 2000.

JOURNAL ARTICLES

American College of Emergency Physicians, Clinical policy: Critical issues in the evaluation and management of patients presenting to the emergency department with acute headache. Ann Emerg Med 2002; 39:108–122.

Attia J, et al: Does this adult patient have acute meningitis? JAMA 1999; 282:175–181.

Edlow JA, Caplan LR: Avoiding pitfalls in the diagnosis of subarachnoid hemorrhage. N Engl J Med 2000; 342:29–36.

Field AG, Wang E: Evaluation of the patient with nontraumatic headache. Emerg Med Clin North Am 1999; 17:127–152.

Godwin SA, Villa J: Acute headaches in the ED: Evidence-based evaluation and treatment options. Emerg Med Pract 2001; 3(6):1–32.

Ignatoff WB, Grim P: Migraine headache: Evidence-based treatment guidelines for emergency management. Emerg Med Rep 1999; 20:257–248.

Miner JR, Fish SJ, Smith SW, et al: Droperidol vs. prochlorperazine for benign headaches in the emergency department. Acad Emerg Med 2001; 8:873–879.

Morgenstern LB, Luna-Gonzales H, Huber JC, et al: Worst headache and subarachnoid hemorrhage: Prospective, modern computed tomography and spinal fluid analysis. Ann Emerg Med 1998; 32:297–304.

New "triptans" and other drugs for migraine. Med Lett 1998; 40:97–100.

Pitetti RD: Pediatric headaches. Pediatr Emerg Med Rep 1999; 4:127–138.

Smetana GW, Shmerling RH: Does this patient have temporal arteritis? JAMA 2002; 287:92–101.

Vinson DR: Treatment patterns of isolated benign headache in US emergency departments. Ann Emerg Med 2002; 39:215–222.

The author wishes to acknowledge the work of Judith Brillman in the writing of this chapter for the first edition of this book.

CHAPTER 33

Seizures

SHAWNA LANGSTAFF

CASE *Study*

The rescue squad radioed the emergency department from the scene where a 50-year-old man was observed to have a grand mal seizure while waiting to purchase a bottle of wine at a local liquor store. The squad members reported he was well known to them as a chronic alcoholic and emergency department "frequent flyer."

INTRODUCTION

A seizure is the sudden disorderly discharge of many neurons in the brain. The physical manifestations of this event are different depending on the anatomic origin and spread of the discharge within the brain. For example, a focal discharge may be represented by tonic movements of one extremity (motor cortex), sensory hallucinations (sensory cortex), auditory or vertiginous sensations (superior temporal cortex), or olfactory and gustatory hallucinations (mesial temporal cortex). A more global discharge of the entire cerebral cortex may result in a generalized tonic-clonic seizure.

Epilepsy, a Greek word meaning "to seize upon" or "to take hold of," is often used interchangeably with *seizure* by the layperson. Epilepsy actually defines a clinical condition in which a person has recurrent seizures secondary to an abnormal focus of electrical activity within a specific part of the brain. This abnormal focus may be the result of a congenital or an acquired structural defect. The current definition of *status epilepticus* is seizure activity lasting 30 minutes or repetitive seizures without the return to full consciousness between episodes. This is a serious condition that requires emergent therapy to avoid hypotension, hypoglycemia, hyperthermia, metabolic acidosis, and irreversible brain injury.

Seizures cause significant morbidity. Ten percent of adults living to 80 years of age will have one seizure during their lifetime. Seizures have a bimodal frequency, with the highest incidence being in those younger than 11 years of age and older than 60 years of age. First-time unprovoked generalized seizures account for 1% to 2% of all emergency department visits. It is estimated there are 50,000 to 250,000 episodes of status epilepticus annually. Status epilepticus has a 2.7% mortality rate if terminated before 30 minutes but a 32% mortality if persisting beyond 60 minutes. The most frequent causes of adult status epilepticus are stroke, withdrawal from anticonvulsant therapy, withdrawal from alcohol, anoxia, and metabolic disorders. In children, the most common causes are systemic infection, congenital anomaly, anoxia, metabolic derangement, withdrawal from anticonvulsant therapy, central nervous system (CNS) infections, and trauma.

Pathophysiology

Several factors contribute to the pathogenesis of seizures. The permeability of the blood-brain barrier is altered by hypoxia, infection, or aberration of the cerebral autoregulation of blood flow. This allows toxins to enter the brain and directly induce seizures. Electrolyte abnormalities may further predispose the brain to seizures. Increased extracellular potassium decreases neuronal hyperpolarization, which increases the risk of seizures. Low extracellular calcium and magnesium concentrations increase synaptic excitability and may also lead to seizures. Cerebral edema from trauma, diabetic ketoacidosis, or metabolic abnormality causes the space between cells to decrease, predisposing the brain to seizures. An imbalance between the excitatory and inhibitory neurotransmitters can also cause seizures. Increased concentrations of glutamate or aspartate (excitatory amino acids) may occur after a hypoxic insult; or depletion of γ-aminobutyric acid (GABA), an inhibitory neurotransmitter, may lead to seizures.

The mechanism for irreversible neuronal injury in prolonged status epilepticus is not completely understood. The oxygen and glucose utilization in the brain increases significantly. The body is able to compensate for this higher metabolic activity for about 30 minutes. At this time, demand outweighs supply and the brain begins to suffer permanent injury secondary to a relative insufficiency of both oxygen and glucose. Autoregulation of cerebral blood flow fails, and perfusion becomes dependent on mean arterial blood pressure. As blood pressure begins to drop or normalize, in turn lowering the cerebral perfusion pressure, the flow to the brain becomes compromised.

In addition to being harmful to the CNS, status epilepticus can produce life-threatening systemic effects. The body can usually supply the increased energy requirements demanded by this condition for 20 to 30 minutes. During this time, the patient becomes tachycardic and hypertensive while catecholamine levels rise. Patients become hyperglycemic as a result of increased circulating catecholamines and cortisol. The rigorous muscular contractions cause the lactate level to rise, induce hyperthermia, and may lead to rhabdomyolysis. Blood flow to skin slows, and the core body temperature may become dangerously high. Carbon dioxide excretion slows while production continues to increase, and the patient develops a metabolic and respiratory acidosis. This acidosis may cause hyperkalemia, which can have further effects on the myocardium and propagate seizure activity. The patient may develop respiratory compromise from airway obstruction or aspirations (secretions and/or emesis) and irregular diaphragmatic contractions. Patients may develop neurogenic pulmonary edema and severe hypotension with prolonged uncontrolled seizures. Compression fractures of the spine and posterior shoulder dislocations have been noted after seizure activity.

Classification

Petit Mal. Usually, petit mal seizures are brief, lasting only a few seconds. The patient becomes unaware or suddenly loses consciousness. This type of seizure may consist of eye twitching or staring into space. There is no postictal period, and the person's activity resumes immediately after the seizure.

Grand Mal. These seizures usually begin with abrupt loss of consciousness and motor tone. Then patients drop to the floor and have tonic-clonic movements. Tongue biting is common, and patients are often incontinent. The postictal period consists of sustained altered mental status and lasts several minutes to an hour.

Partial Seizures. These seizures are caused by electrical discharges in specific areas of the brain and often suggest a locally impacting structural lesion in the brain. They are characterized by unilateral tonic-clonic movements of an extremity and sensory, visual, olfactory, or gustatory hallucinations and are usually preceded by an aura. Consciousness and mentation are not affected. Partial seizures may progress to generalized seizures.

Complex Partial Seizures. These are focal seizures usually involving the temporal lobe. Consciousness and mentation are affected, and patients present with bizarre thinking or behavior.

Generalized Seizures. These seizures begin with an abrupt loss of consciousness, followed by tonic-clonic movement, tongue biting, incontinence, and extended postictal period. They are thought to originate from electrical stimulation of the entire cortex.

INITIAL APPROACH AND STABILIZATION

Many patients with seizures are initially evaluated by paramedics at the scene of their seizure. The paramedics can stabilize the patients, begin treatment, and provide crucial information that may help determine the cause of the seizure. Prehospital personnel are instrumental in obtaining history from bystanders and collecting evidence such as empty pill bottles, evidence of alcohol usage, drug paraphernalia, or findings of trauma. Most importantly, they protect the patient from further harm, such as potential airway compromise, and treat reversible causes of seizure, such as hypoglycemia and hypoxia. Finally, they can initiate antiseizure therapy such as administration of a benzodiazepine. If there is no prehospital care, these steps occur during the initial assessment in the emergency department.

Priority Diagnoses

The potentially life-threatening or the reversible causes of seizure are considered first after the patient's arrival. These include hypoglycemia, hypoxia, cardiac dysrhythmia, drug or poison ingestion, intracranial hemorrhage, meningitis, and eclampsia.

Rapid Assessment

The following questions need to be answered:

1. What was the patient doing before the event?
2. How long did the seizure last?
3. What parts of the body were moving?
4. Did tongue biting or incontinence occur?
5. Was the patient confused after the event?
6. Does the patient have a seizure disorder? If so, what medications does the patient take?
7. Is there a chance of pregnancy?

8. Was there evidence of drugs, alcohol, or trauma? Does the patient have a history of traumatic head injury?

9. Was there chest pain, shortness of breath, and vomiting before the event?

10. What other medical problem does the patient have? Does the patient take medications?

11. How is the patient's airway, breathing, and circulation status? Vital signs are recorded.

12. Does the patient respond to verbal or painful stimuli? What is the Glasgow Coma Score? (See Chapter 31, Altered Mental Status, and Chapter 48, Head and Neck Trauma.) Most seizure patients experience a period of confusion after the seizure called the postictal phase. This lasts anywhere from minutes up to an hour. If the postictal phase does not resolve, the patient should be assumed to be in nonconvulsive status epilepticus, which should be treated aggressively to avoid permanent neuronal damage.

Early Intervention

Airway Control. If possible, the patient is placed in the left lateral decubitus position to prevent possible aspiration. A nasopharyngeal airway may be needed with supplemental oxygen via nasal cannula. The padded bite blocks are no longer recommended. Endotracheal intubation is not attempted if the patient is actively seizing, but it may be attempted after administration of benzodiazepines.

Intravenous Catheter. An intravenous catheter is placed as soon as possible. This will enable the emergency physician to administer antiseizure medication, to treat hypoglycemia and hypotension, and to prepare for rapid sequence intubation if necessary.

Cervical Spine. Cervical spine immobilization is attempted. Although difficult in an actively seizing patient, immobilization is important in the setting of trauma, because a cervical spine injury can occur from a fall from a standing position.

Cardiac Monitoring. The patient is monitored for any possible dysrhythmias or metabolic causes for the seizure.

Hypoglycemia Prophylaxis. When the intravenous line is placed, a drop of blood is tested using blood glucose strips to screen for possible hypoglycemia. This is the most common metabolic cause for seizure. If the patient is hypoglycemic, 50 mL of a 50% glucose solution should be administered, with 100 mg of thiamine. The dose for children is 2 mL/kg of a 25% glucose solution.

Anticonvulsant Therapy. This is administered for seizures lasting longer than 5 to 7 minutes or for recurrent seizures without conscious periods between seizures. Lorazepam is recommended by neurologists as the first-line anticonvulsant in a dose of 0.1 mg/kg. Eighty percent of seizures are terminated with benzodiazepines.

CLINICAL ASSESSMENT

The history and physical examination allow the physician (1) to determine whether the event was a true seizure or something that mimics seizures and (2) to look for clues indicating whether the seizure was primary or secondary to another disease process.

History

Obtaining an accurate history is often the most challenging part of the workup in a patient with a seizure. Several different sources may be used to obtain information, including the patient, friends and family, the paramedics, and a previous chart (if available). Key points in the history include the following:

1. A detailed description of *exactly what happened before, during, and after the event.* Was there an aura, onset in specific muscles, loss of consciousness, tongue biting, or incontinence? Was there a *postictal state?* What was the time course of the event? Were there any *precipitating events,* such as stress, fatigue, or lack of sleep?

2. What *type of seizure* was it? Seizures may be classified by distinguishing generalized seizures (bilaterally symmetric and without local onset) from partial (focal) seizures (seizures that begin locally). Knowledge of the type of seizure allows the part of the brain that is responsible to be localized.

3. Does the patient have a *history of a seizure disorder?* If so, how frequently does the patient have seizures? How compliant is the patient in taking his or her medications? One of the most common reasons patients with seizures come to the emergency department is a subtherapeutic level of an anticonvulsant drug.

4. A complete list of the *medications* being taken by the patient is important. Seizures can represent toxic drug effects (Table 33–1).

5. Is the seizure secondary to a *traumatic event?* The approach to a seizure secondary to head trauma is similar to that used for a nontraumatic seizure, and some additional precautions must be taken (see Chapter 48, Head and Neck Trauma).

TABLE 33–1. Etiology of Seizures

Primary (idiopathic)	
Secondary	
Hypoxia	Multiple causes, including impaired respiration, circulation, and oxygen-carrying capacity of blood
Toxic	Intoxication with cocaine, amphetamines, tricyclic antidepressants, theophyllines, penicillin, lidocaine, physostigmine, oral hypoglycemics, isoniazid, phenothiazines, pentazocine, lithium, lead, mercury
	Withdrawal from alcohol, barbiturates, hypnotics
Traumatic	Concussion, contusion, hemorrhage
Neoplastic	Primary or metastatic
Infections	Meningitis, encephalitis, brain abscess, toxoplasmosis, neurocysticercosis, neurosyphilis,
Vascular	Cerebrovascular accident, hemorrhage, arteriovenous malformation, vasospasm, hypertensive encephalopathy
Metabolic	Hyponatremia, hypoglycemia, uremia, hepatic failure, hypercarbia, hypoxia, hypocalcemia, hypomagnesemia, diabetic ketoacidosis, hyperosmolar states
Endocrine	Addison's disease, hypothyroidism, hyperthyroidism
Obstetric	Eclampsia

6. Does the patient have a history of *drug* or *alcohol abuse*? Grand mal seizures are common when people addicted to alcohol, barbiturates, or sedative-hypnotics suddenly abstain or go through withdrawal.
7. Has the patient been in a usual *state of health* or has there been a *recent illness* (e.g., fever, headache, stiff neck, lethargy, or vomiting)?

The past medical history/review of systems includes the following:

- *Cardiac disease.* Is there a history of coronary or valvular heart disease? Are there known cardiac dysrhythmias? Is the patient taking cardiac medications such as quinidine?
- *Pulmonary disease.* Does the patient have chest pain or shortness of breath? Any disease that causes significant hypoxia may lead to seizures.
- *Endocrine diseases.* Does the patient have diabetes, thyroid disease, or parathyroid hyponatremia or thyrotoxic storm? All may present as a seizure.
- *Renal disease.* Does the patient have a history of kidney disease? Does the patient require dialysis? Uremia can lead to seizures.
- *Oncologic diseases.* Is there any history of cancer? Metastasis to the brain is common, and frequent sites of origin are the lung, breast, skin (melanoma), and gastrointestinal tract. Tumors also affect electrolyte balance with paraneoplastic syndromes and the syndrome of inappropriate secretion of antidiuretic hormone (SIADH).
- *Immunocompromised patient.* Patients who are immunocompromised, such as those with AIDS, may have a variety of parasitic, fungal, viral, and bacterial infections, as well as neoplastic diseases, that cause seizures.

Family history is important and may reveal the presence of epilepsy in other family members. Although it is most significant in patients with classic petit mal seizures, heredity plays an important role in many types of seizure disorders.

Physical Examination

A systematic and thorough examination of the patient from head to toe is important to elicit possible causes of the seizure.

Vital Signs. Vital signs are reassessed, including temperature and pulse oximetry. An elevated temperature may be a sign of prolonged seizure activity as well as infection. Temperature is lowered with rectal antipyretics.

Head, Eyes, Ears, Nose, and Throat. A thorough examination of the head is important to rule out signs of trauma, such as contusions, lacerations, raccoon eyes, or Battle's sign. Both tympanic membranes are examined for hemotympanum or otitis media. Extraocular motions, pupils, and optic discs are examined. Tongue lacerations are documented. Gingival hyperplasia may be a clue for ongoing phenytoin therapy.

Neck. The cervical spine is palpated for tenderness, crepitus, or "stepoffs." The neck is examined for signs of meningismus and bruits, which may be an indication of possible cerebrovascular disease.

Chest. The chest wall is examined externally for any signs of trauma, including subcutaneous emphysema. The lungs are auscultated for evidence of rales, rhonchi, or other pulmonary sounds.

Cardiovascular. Auscultation is accomplished to detect evidence of atrial fibrillation, murmurs, or rubs.

Spine. The patient is log-rolled to allow inspection and palpation of the back area. Cervical, thoracic, and lumbar spine precautions are maintained. Vertebral compression fractures are associated with seizures, and such injury may be noted only during the back examination.

Extremities. The extremities are checked for any evidence of trauma. Seizure is the most common cause of posterior shoulder dislocation.

Neurologic Examination. This portion of the physical examination is repeated serially as the patient recovers from the postictal period. The purpose of the neurologic examination is to find any possible focal deficit that may indicate a structural lesion in the brain. A reliable neurologic assessment cannot be obtained in a patient younger than 18 months of age. Some patients with epilepsy experience *Todd's paralysis* during the postictal phase, which is a temporary deficit usually consisting of focal hemiparesis, aphasia, or a facial droop. This typically resolves in less than 24 hours but can last several days.

The neurologic examination consists of the following components:

- Mental status examination. This should be rechecked frequently as patients recover from their postictal period.
- Cranial nerve function
- Motor strength and symmetry in all four extremities
- Reflexes, including deep tendon reflexes and Babinski testing
- Sensory examination
- Cerebellar function
- Gait and stance

CLINICAL REASONING

Was this Event, In Fact, A True Seizure?

When not witnessed by the physician, this determination must be based largely on the details of the history.

Factors that tend to support a diagnosis of seizures include

- A history of similar events
- A precipitating cause, such as sleep deprivation, stress, or fatigue
- The presence of an aura just before the event
- The description of tonic-clonic movement and loss of consciousness
- The postictal state
- Tongue biting
- Incontinence of bowels or bladder

When observed, a generalized (grand mal) seizure is usually easy to identify. It begins as a *tonic extension* of the truck and extremities. There is usually no preceding focal activity or aura, and consciousness is lost immediately. After several seconds of tonic extension, fine vibration of the extremities indicates the *clonic extension* phase of the seizure. This cycle repeats itself, giving rise to the term *tonic-clonic* seizure. Some generalized seizures begin with a partial seizure. This initial focality then generalizes to a tonic-clonic seizure and is highly suggestive of a structural lesion.

The information obtained is compared with the characteristics of other conditions that may mimic seizure activity.

Cerebrovascular Insufficiency. Patients with transient ischemic attacks may have episodes that mimic seizures. Vertebrobasilar insufficiency results in decreased blood flow to the brain stem. Patients may complain of cranial nerve symptoms, such as diplopia, slurred speech, and vertigo followed by syncope. There is generally no tonic-clonic movement or postictal state.

Syncope. Patients with syncope experience a sudden, transient loss of consciousness and collapse. Forty percent of patients will experience convulsive syncope in which there is a degree of muscle twitching or tonic contractions. There is usually no tongue biting or postictal phase. The etiology of syncope includes dysrhythmias, hypovolemia, vasovagal abnormalities, metabolic abnormalities, and primary neurologic diseases (see Chapter 9, Syncope).

Cataplexy. After stress or excitement, some patients with narcolepsy develop a sudden loss of muscle tone, resulting in a fall. These episodes may resemble myoclonic seizures. Physicians should be concerned about cataplexy in patients with a history of narcolepsy.

Hyperventilation. In response to stress, many patients hyperventilate, causing a respiratory alkalosis. The metabolic changes can result in carpopedal spasm, muscle twitching, and circumoral paresthesias. There is typically no loss of consciousness.

Dissociative States. Patients with severe psychiatric disturbances may present in trance-like states that resemble petit mal, absence, or temporal lobe seizures. Patients with dissociative states usually are able to mentally function. Electroencephalography may assist in the diagnosis.

Pseudoseizures or Factitious Seizures. These are behavioral episodes in which patients purposefully or unconsciously display seizure-like activity with no organic basis. It is estimated that up to 20% of patients treated for seizure disorders have pseudoseizures. Some patients who have an organic basis for seizures may have pseudoseizures on occasion. Factitious seizures can be difficult to diagnose even by an experienced observer. Most patients exhibit abnormal limb or trunk movements, but the orderly tonic-clonic sequence is not usually present. Attacks generally occur in the presence of a crowd to gain attention. The patient is unhurt by falling, tongue biting and incontinence are rare, and there is frequently no postictal period. The patient may respond to direct questioning or diversion tactics or may purposefully move an ammonia capsule away from the nose, all the time maintaining the seizure activity.

If the Patient had a True Seizure, What is the Cause?

Thirty-five to 40 percent of seizures have no clear source and are thus termed *idiopathic*. Table 33–1 lists the major causes of seizures. The emergent causes of seizures to be considered in the emergency department are discussed next.

Hypoxia. Hypoxic encephalopathy after suffocation or respiratory failure is a serious cause of seizures that must be immediately addressed. Supplemental oxygen is always administered, and the potential causes for hypoxia are reviewed. If the patient is cyanotic or has abnormal findings on pulmonary examination, a chest radiograph and arterial blood gas analysis are obtained immediately. In clinically relevant circumstances (e.g., fire, suicide attempt), a carbon monoxide level is obtained. When the carboxyhemoglobin concentration is greater than 50%, seizures are likely to occur. Definitive airway management may be necessary in some patients to support their oxygenation.

Hypoglycemia. Hypoglycemia is the most common metabolic cause of seizure. A fingerstick blood glucose level is immediately tested after stabilization of the ABCs. If a glucometer is not available, it is prudent to treat the patient empirically with 25 g of glucose in a 50% glucose solution.

Cardiac Dysrhythmias. Ventricular fibrillation can lead to seizures and can cause hypoxic encephalopathy. It is important to put the patient on an electrocardiographic monitor immediately.

Intracranial Hemorrhage. Seizures occur in 16% of patients within cerebrovascular events. In fact, up to 25% of subarachnoid hemorrhage, 20% of hemorrhagic strokes, and 6% of ischemic strokes present as first-time seizures.

Tumor. Approximately 30% of primary brain tumors present as a first-time seizure. In addition, 18% of metastatic brain tumors present as a first-time seizure. Computed tomography (CT) of the head is an important initial imaging study to elicit the extent of an intracranial pathologic process. In some patients, magnetic resonance imaging (MRI) may be warranted later in the workup.

Trauma. Patients with a history of traumatic head injury have a 16% chance of developing an acquired seizure disorder. Acutely, trauma is associated with a 0.4% to 30% incidence of seizures depending on the duration of loss of consciousness. Patients with penetrating head injuries have a 30% to 50% risk of developing seizures.

Infection. Meningitis, cerebral abscesses, and viral meningitis are all associated with seizures. As many as 25% of patients with meningitis have seizures. In the southwestern United States and in developing countries, neurocysticercosis presents and is associated with 50% of new-onset seizures. In patients with human immunodeficiency virus (HIV) infection, toxoplasmosis and cryptococcal meningitis are the most common cause of seizures. Any patient who has a fever, headache, vomiting, and/or stiff neck associated with a seizure should have an aggressive workup.

Metabolic. Metabolic abnormalities account for 9% of acute onset seizures. Hypoglycemia is the most common correctable metabolic abnormality causing seizures. Hyponatremia or hypernatremia and hypocalcemia or hypercalcemia should be considered in seizure patients. Hypomagnesemia can cause seizures in alcoholics and should be corrected. Uremia also causes seizures, usually 2 to 3 days after the patient has become anuric.

Drugs/Toxins. Ingestion of a wide variety of toxins may present clinically as seizure activity. Although supportive therapy alone is the primary treatment for many of these agents, specific antidotes must be considered for the following drugs: cyanide, tricyclic antidepressants, meperidine, penicillin, theophylline, methanol, and ethylene glycol. Lead poisoning in children and mercury poisoning in adults must be considered. Isoniazid decreases GABA synthesis in the CNS, which leads to seizures. Cocaine, amphetamines, heroin, and 3,4-methylenedioxymethamphetamine (MDMA "ecstasy") also can cause seizures.

Alcohol. Alcohol withdrawal seizures may occur between 6 hours and 7 days after the cessation of sustained alcohol ingestion. Alcohol is a contributing factor in 50% of adults presenting to the emergency department with seizure activity. It acts as a CNS depressant and anesthetic and exhibits anticonvulsant properties. When the alcohol is withdrawn, the brain becomes hyperexcitable and seizures are likely to occur.

Pregnancy. Eclampsia causes seizures in the peripartum period or immediate postpartum period. Eclampsia occurs when a pregnant woman has hypertension, proteinuria, and edema and finally seizes. This usually occurs in the third trimester, but it may occur up to 2 weeks post partum. Patients require assessment of vital signs, intravenous magnesium, and, most importantly, the delivery of the child.

Epilepsy. Epilepsy is a condition that causes recurrent seizures. These seizures may increase in frequency during times of stress or hormonal changes.

The differential diagnosis of seizures also varies with the age group of the patient. Table 33–2 lists the most common causes in each age group. Many of these diseases require laboratory studies to help make the diagnosis.

DIAGNOSTIC ADJUNCTS

Diagnostic tests are performed to help determine the etiology of secondary seizures. There are few areas of medicine in which more unnecessary tests are ordered than in the workup of a seizure patient. It is neither cost effective nor practical to order tests for every patient. The patient's medical history and physical examination findings dictate the selection of laboratory tests.

Laboratory Studies

Complete Blood Cell Count with Differential. The white blood cell count with differential is ordered when an infectious etiology is suspected. It should be noted that 33% of patients with seizures will have an abnormal white blood cell count, in the absence of infection, secondary to demargination. Many authors believe this test does not assist with management of seizure patients. The hemoglobin level will indirectly reflect the oxygen-carrying capacity of the blood.

Serum Electrolytes. Serum electrolytes are important studies to order when evaluating seizures. Correctable metabolic abnormalities are responsible for approximately 9% of seizures. Hyponatremia and hypernatremia can cause seizures, and both are easily corrected. Electrolytes are especially important in patients with first-time seizures. Electrolytes are also obtained for patients taking diuretics and in those who present with signs or symptoms of neoplastic disease, renal failure, or endocrine abnormalities (e.g., hypoadrenalism, hypothyroidism, or hyperthyroidism).

Serum Glucose. A glucose level is indicated in all patients who suffer seizures. A bedside blood glucose test strip determination can be used as a screening device for hypoglycemia as a cause of seizures. Hypoglycemia is easily reversed by providing glucose solution intravenously.

Calcium and Magnesium. Calcium and magnesium levels are obtained in patients with muscle spasms, twitching, or a positive Chvostek's or Trousseau's sign. Magnesium is an especially important test in malnourished patients, patients with abnormal sodium or potassium levels, or chronic alcoholics.

Toxicology Screen. This test is used in patients who are suspected of overdosing on medications or who are known illicit drug abusers with seizures.

Anticonvulsant Drug Levels. Anticonvulsant (typically phenytoin, phenobarbital, and carbamazepine) levels are indicated in all patients who have been prescribed or who state they are taking anticonvulsant medications. These test results are reasonably accurate and are available in most laboratories.

Arterial Blood Gases. Profound alterations in acid-base status can occur immediately after a

---

TABLE 33–2. Causes of Seizures in Different Age Groups

Age at Onset	Probable Cause
Neonatal	Congenital anomaly, birth injury, anoxia, metabolic disorder (e.g., hypoglycemia, hypocalcemia, vitamin B_6 deficiency, phenylketonuria)
Infancy (3 mo – 1 yr)	As above; infantile spasms
Early childhood (1–3 yr)	Infantile spasms, febrile convulsions, birth injury and anoxia, infections, trauma, metabolic disorders
Childhood (3–10 yr)	Perinatal anoxia, injury at birth or later, infections, thrombosis of cerebral arteries or veins, metabolic, idiopathic epilepsy
Adolescence (10–18 yr)	Idiopathic epilepsy, trauma, recreational drugs
Early adulthood (18–25 yr)	Idiopathic, trauma, neoplasm, drug or alcohol withdrawal
Middle age (35–60 yr)	Trauma, neoplasm, vascular disease, alcohol or drug withdrawal
Later life (over 60 yr)	Vascular disease, tumor, degenerative disease, trauma

Adapted from Adams RD, Victor M: Principles of Neurology, 6th ed. New York, McGraw-Hill, 1997.

single grand mal seizure. The pH may drop to as low as 7.05. The significant lactic acidosis that occurs after a single grand mal seizure usually resolves spontaneously within 40 to 60 minutes after cessation. Serum potassium elevation does not accompany the lactic acidosis. If arterial blood gas levels are significantly abnormal after a seizure, a repeat test is recommended in 40 to 60 minutes to uncover persistent acid-base disorders that may have caused the seizure (e.g., isoniazid ingestion, theophylline toxicity).

Radiologic Imaging

Computed Tomography of the Head. CT has evolved into an important imaging tool used for the emergency department workup of seizures. It is indicated for patients with focal neurologic findings, first-time seizures, suspected head trauma, or CNS tumors. About 7% of patients with subarachnoid hemorrhage have no abnormal findings on CT. If a subarachnoid hemorrhage is suggested despite a negative CT of the head, a lumbar puncture should be performed, looking for red blood cells or xanthochromia. Most acute cerebrovascular infarctions are not detected on the initial CT, with changes evolving over 12 to 24 hours. CT is recommended for patients on anticoagulation therapy, HIV-positive patients, those with traumatic injury, cancer patients, alcoholic patients, and patients with meningeal signs.

Skull Films. These studies are of limited value, and more information is obtained from a CT.

Magnetic Resonance Imaging. MRI may be useful as part of the neurologic workup but is not usually part of the acute emergency department workup of the patient with seizures. MRI may be the preferred imaging examination in pediatric patients, to best evaluate the posterior fossa and temporal lobe regions.

Electrocardiogram

A 12-lead electrocardiogram is useful in patients suspected of seizure or seizure-like activity from hypoxia, hypotension, dysrhythmia, or acute myocardial infarction.

Special Tests

Lumbar Puncture. Lumbar puncture is critical for patients with fever, headache, and nuchal rigidity. Cerebrospinal fluid analysis can identify meningitis or subarachnoid hemorrhage, and elevated spinal fluid pressures may be quantified.

Electroencephalography. This is a useful test in the workup of a patient with a seizure disorder but is seldom ordered in the emergency department. It may help differentiate true seizures from pseudoseizures. An electroencephalogram (EEG) also may uncover nonconvulsive status epilepticus.

EXPANDED DIFFERENTIAL DIAGNOSIS

Once the history, physical examination, and ancillary tests are completed, the emergency physician is generally able to limit the differential diagnosis to one or two major categories (see Table 33–1). If the ancillary tests do not reveal a specific etiology of the seizures, the patient is considered to have idiopathic epilepsy.

A simplified classification of seizures by clinical type is presented in Table 33–3. Seizures can be either generalized or partial. Generalized seizures involve the whole body and occur in 20% to 40% of patients with epilepsy. Generalized absence or petit mal seizures can be difficult to diagnose. There is no aura, loss of posture, incontinence, or postictal confusion. The attack rarely lasts more than 20 seconds. Absence seizures invariably start in childhood, and patients are rarely brought to the emergency department for this problem. Tonic-clonic or grand mal generalized seizures occur in both children and adults. There may be a brief aura followed by loss of consciousness and rhythmic tonic-clonic movements lasting 1 to 5 minutes. Tongue biting, cyanosis, and bowel or bladder incontinence may occur. Postictal confusion lasts from minutes to hours.

Partial seizures occur primarily in adults and represent abnormal electrical activity in one area of the brain, causing motor, sensory, or autonomic dysfunction. Partial seizures are considered complex if the focal discharge spreads and causes altered consciousness or combines with motor, sensory, and autonomic dysfunction. Psychomotor or temporal lobe seizures are a type of complex partial seizure. Presentations are consistent for single individuals but extremely variable overall.

PRINCIPLES OF MANAGEMENT

The management of patients with seizures follows these basic principles.

General Supportive Measures

All seizure patients immediately receive three general supportive measures.

TABLE 33–3. Classification of Epileptic Seizures According to Clinical Type

I. Partial (Focal and Local) Seizures
   A. Simple partial seizures (consciousness not impaired)
      1. With motor symptoms
      2. With somatosensory or special sensory symptoms (simple hallucinations, such as tingling, light flashes, buzzing)
      3. With autonomic symptoms or signs (e.g., epigastric sensation, pallor, sweating, flushing, piloerection, and pupillary dilatation)
      4. With psychic symptoms (disturbances of higher cerebral function, e.g., déjà vu, fear, distortion of time perception)
   B. Complex partial seizures (impairment of consciousness and often automatisms)
      1. With simple partial onset followed by impairment of consciousness
      2. With impairment of conscious onset
   C. Partial seizures evolving to secondarily generalized seizures (e.g., generalized tonic-clonic seizures)
      1. Simple partial seizures evolving to generalized seizures
      2. Complex partial seizures evolving to generalized seizures
      3. Simple partial seizures evolving to complex partial seizures and further evolving to generalized seizures
II. Generalized Seizures (Convulsive or Nonconvulsive)
   A. Absence seizures (impairment of consciousness alone or with mild clonic, atonic, or tonic components and automatisms)

Modified and abbreviated from the Commission on Classification and Terminology of the International League against Epilepsy.

1. Airway protection and supplemental oxygen. A nasal or oral airway may be placed to ensure airway patency.
2. An intravenous line is established to give anticonvulsant medications as needed.
3. Seizure precautions. Many emergency departments have protocols specifying protective measures to be used for patients who may seize. Bed rails are placed up, and hard surfaces are padded. Clothing and dentures are removed. During an active seizure the patient is placed in the left lateral decubitus position to avoid aspiration. In the postictal phase, these patients may be difficult to manage, but they generally should not be restrained.

Eliminate Causal Factors of Seizure

Prompt attention is given to the search for life-threatening causes of seizures. These include hypoxia, cardiac dysrhythmias, hypoglycemia, meningitis, eclampsia, hyponatremia, intracranial hemorrhage, and specific toxins. Specific therapies depend on the cause of the disease.

Pharmacologic Control of Active Seizures

Antiseizure medications are indicated if the patient has had more than one seizure or is having a single seizure that has lasted more than 5 minutes. Benzodiazepines are first-line therapy followed by anticonvulsants. The treatment protocol for status epilepticus is noted in Table 33–4.

Benzodiazepines. This class of drugs controls seizures in up to 80% of patients. It potentiates the GABA response and strengthens the inhibition of neuron firing. *Lorazepam* is the current drug of choice for the initial treatment of seizures. The usual dosage is 0.1 mg/kg. It is given in 2-mg/min intravenous boluses, up to 4 mg. It has a high affinity for the benzodiazepine receptor in the brain, a low lipid solubility, and a small volume of distribution, and it provides a longer duration of action (4 to 14 hours) than diazepam (20 minutes). Lorazepam is rapidly metabolized in the liver and does not have an active metabolite. Mean time to seizure cessation for lorazepam is 3 minutes. Intramuscular lorazepam has stopped seizures when intravenous access is not achieved, and there are case reports of rectal lorazepam being successful in treating seizures in pediatric patients.

Diazepam is frequently given intravenously or rectally. The intravenous dose is 2 to 5 mg/min, up to a maximum of 20 mg. Diazepam is highly lipophilic so it rapidly accumulates in the brain, typically within 1 to 2 minutes. Within 20 minutes it redistributes to the other fatty parts of the body. Diazepam is degraded in the liver and has an active metabolite (N-dismethydiazepam). Total elimination from the body may take up to 24 hours. Many authors believe that diazepam has more cumulative depressant properties than lorazepam. Studies have shown that approximately 10% of patients using either drug have significant respiratory depression.

Midazolam (intravenously or intramuscularly) also has been used to treat seizures. It is highly lipophilic, and its onset of action is extremely rapid. Seizures are usually terminated within 1 minute. Midazolam is rapidly metabolized by

TABLE 33–4. Treatment of Status Epilepticus

Time (minutes)	Procedure
0	Institute basic life support (ABCs)
	Place nasopharyngeal airway
	Oxygen via nasal cannula/mask
	Place on cardiac monitor and initiate pulse oximetry; monitor vital signs
	Establish intravenous line and check blood for glucose
	Obtain laboratory evaluation
	Check anticonvulsant levels
	Electrolytes
	Blood urea nitrogen
	Arterial blood gases
	Electrocardiogram
	Urine toxicology screen
5	If hypoglycemic, thiamine, 100 mg IV, and dextrose in water 50%, 50 mL IV push
10	Lorazepam, 0.1 mg/kg IV at 2 mg/min up to 4 mg total dose, *or*
	Diazepam, 0.2 mg/kg IV at 5 mg/min, repeat q4–5 min up to 20 mg
	Diazepam must be followed by loading fosphenytoin or phenytoin.
15	Fosphenytoin IV, 150 mg/min, at 18 mg/kg; *or* phenytoin, 50 mg/min, at 20 mg/kg
	Monitor blood pressure and cardiac rhythm.
30	If status continues, give additional fosphenytoin or phenytoin at 5 mg/kg until a maximum of 30 mg/kg.
	If status persists, start endotracheal intubation using rapid sequence intubation.
	Phenobarbital,* 100 mg/min, at 20 mg/kg
	Establish general anesthesia with pentobarbital, midazolam, or propofol.
	Vasopressors may be required.

*Phenobarbital may be used before phenytoin if (1) previous control with phenobarbital has been used, (2) there are severe cardiac conduction problems, (3) patient is allergic to phenytoin, or (4) patient is younger than 6 years old.

Adapted from Willmore LJ: Epilepsy emergencies: The first seizure and status epilepticus. Neurology 1998; 51(S4): S34–S38.

the liver and as a result is very short acting. Refractory status epilepticus has been successfully treated with a midazolam drip.

Phenytoin. Phenytoin (Dilantin) is effective in terminating up to 90% of seizures. Although brain concentrations of the drug peak in 6 to 10 minutes, the physical properties of the drug necessitate relatively slow infusion. Phenytoin is insoluble in water and therefore is solubilized in a basic solution of 40% propylene glycol, 10% ethanol, and sodium hydroxide (a pH of 12). As a result, it is highly toxic to veins and causes necrosis if it infiltrates into the subcutaneous tissue (from the intravenous catheter). Phenytoin can cause hypotension and cardiac dysrhythmias (widening of the QT interval) and should not be given faster that 50 mg/min. The dose is 20 mg/kg. The standard "gram of Dilantin" may be an inadequate dose of medication for any patient weighing more than 50 kg, and an inadequate dose may allow the progression of convulsive status epilepticus to nonconvulsive status epilepticus (only identified by electroencephalography, which often delays definitive measures to terminate the seizures).

Fosphenytoin. This is a water-soluble prodrug of phenytoin. Once it enters the blood, it is rapidly converted to phenytoin. It can be given intramuscularly (peak levels in 30 minutes) or intravenously (peak levels in 6 minutes). Fosphenytoin, 1.5 mg, is equivalent to 1 mg of phenytoin, and the loading dose is 18 mg/kg. Unlike phenytoin, fosphenytoin can be given at a faster rate, up to 150 mg/min. It does not cause any respiratory depression and is an ideal drug to treat seizures in the emergency setting. Pruritus and paresthesias are the most common side effects, but fosphenytoin may cause hypotension and the infusion should be closely monitored.

Phenobarbital. This medication is not as lipophilic as the benzodiazepines. It enters the brain within 3 minutes, and its effects last for several hours. The half-life ranges from 50 to 150 hours. Drug excretion is reduced in patients with renal or liver failure. Sedation, respiratory depression, and hypotension are side effects. Careful monitoring of the patient is necessary during drug administration, which is usually no faster than 100 mg/min, with a total dosage of 20 mg/kg.

Pentobarbital. Pentobarbital anesthesia is usually reserved for refractory cases of status epilepticus. Endotracheal intubation is required because the amount of respiratory depression is significant. In addition, all motor activity is suppressed and continuous EEG monitoring is required (to determine when the seizure activity stops). The loading dose is 5 mg/kg at 50 mg/min intravenously, followed by a continuous infusion of 0.5 to 3 mg/kg/hr. Hypotension is common and may require vasopressors.

Propofol. This is a very short-acting intravenous anesthetic that is rapidly degraded by the liver. It is given as a continuous infusion, with a loading dose of 1.5 mg/kg followed by an infusion at 6 to 10 mg/kg/hr. This agent can cause respiratory and CNS depression, which may require active airway management. Hypotension is a frequent side effect and may limit the dose given.

Etomidate. This intravenous anesthetic produces anesthesia within 1 minute. It is given as a continuous infusion with continuous electroencephalographic monitoring. Corticosteroids also must be given during and after long-term administration of this drug because etomidate causes adrenal suppression.

Attention to Complications of Seizures

Complications of seizures include aspiration, acidosis, dislocations, and fractures. Aspiration pneumonia may not be obvious on the initial radiograph, but arterial blood gas determination will often show hypoxia. Occasionally, loose teeth are aspirated, causing bronchial obstruction. Patients who aspirate are treated with antibiotics such as penicillin that cover oral anaerobes. If bronchial obstruction is present, bronchoscopy must be considered for removal of a foreign body.

The lactic acidosis after seizures can be severe; however, it usually corrects itself. Bicarbonate treatment is generally not indicated unless the arterial pH is less than 7.0, and this level of severity is usually due to other causes.

Patients with seizures may have musculoskeletal injuries such as fractures or lacerations. Posterior dislocation of the shoulder occurs from intense muscular contractions during tonic-clonic seizures and requires prompt reduction. Musculoskeletal injuries and lacerations are addressed and specifically treated.

UNCERTAIN DIAGNOSIS

The evaluation of an emergency department patient with first-time unprovoked seizure includes metabolic and electrolyte studies, observation, a CT or MRI, and a search for an infective source. The history should address familial seizure disorders, trauma, medical illness, alcohol or drug use/withdrawal, and prior seizure events. In spite of the evaluation and history, in an otherwise healthy individual the unprovoked seizure may be isolated and will have no discernible cause. These patients are referred for further evaluation.

Electroencephalographic testing is a very important part of the workup and diagnosis of seizure. The characteristics of the spikes *during the event* are what define the seizure; however, most studies are done between or after seizure events.

Patients are counseled that approximately 10% of people will have one seizure in their lifetime (not related to acute illness). Development of epilepsy has only a 3% incidence, with emphasis on the fact that not all seizures lead to epilepsy. Factors that may predict a high likelihood for second seizure (risk of 65% within 2 years) include brain lesion, brain injury, and an abnormal EEG. Recurrence risk is low (24% within 2 years) in patients with normal brain, normal EEG, and no family epilepsy history. When a second seizure does occur, the risk of subsequent events is greater than 80% and reliably indicates epilepsy.

SPECIAL CONSIDERATIONS

Pediatric Patients

Three to 5 percent of children have febrile seizures. These usually occur after 6 months of age and most commonly between 9 and 24 months, but they can occur up to 5 years of age. This condition is benign, is more common in males, is often familial, and usually presents as a brief grand mal seizure. Simple febrile seizures last less than 15 minutes and have a short postictal period. Complicated febrile seizures last longer than 15 minutes, may have a focal onset, and have a longer postictal period. An extensive diagnostic workup may not be necessary in children older than 18 months of age who have not been receiving antibiotics. In children younger than 18 months, a clinical neurologic examination may not be reliable, with clinical signs of meningitis more difficult to assess. If no source of the fever is identified in those younger than 18 months of age, a septic workup, including a lumbar puncture, is considered.

Children with febrile seizures recover completely, and there are no long-term sequelae. Approximately 33% of children with one febrile seizure will go on to have another one. However, only 5% of these children develop epilepsy in the future. No further treatment is usually necessary, although parents are asked to be aggressive about monitoring and lowering the child's temperature during illness.

Elderly Patients

Seizures in the geriatric age group are primarily reactive, occurring secondary to anatomic abnormality (scarring or stroke), progressive abnormality (degeneration of cortical regions), or transient abnormality (abnormal electrolytes, hyperosmotic states, or hypoxia).

In patients 60 years of age or older presenting to the emergency department with acute seizure, a 26% mortality exists. In 54% of elderly patients with new-onset seizure, cerebral infarction or hemorrhagic stroke is found to be the cause. Although the majority of seizures in this group are general, focal seizure may occur with arteriovenous malformations and unruptured cerebrovascular aneurysm, as adjacent brain is compressed.

Degenerative disorders of the brain increase seizure risk. The degeneration may be caused by normal aging, primary brain neoplasm, encephalomalacia after trauma or stroke, or demyelinating disease. Alzheimer's dementia is also thought to be a significant risk factor in seizure development in the elderly.

There are multiple transient metabolic abnormalities that may trigger seizure activity, including hypoglycemia, hypernatremia, hyperosmolar nonketotic coma, and hypomagnesemia. Seizures from these causes are most responsive to return of metabolic baseline and stability.

The medical management of seizures in the elderly population is also complicated by many factors. Altered drug metabolism and clearance occurs secondary to hepatic and renal insufficiency. Polypharmacy increases the risk of medication interactions, and patients may have trouble with outpatient regimens, leading to subtherapeutic or toxic drug levels.

DISPOSITION AND FOLLOW-UP

The disposition of patients with seizures depends on making a reasonable determination of the etiology and ruling out serious disease processes.

Admission

Patients with the following types of seizures are generally admitted to the hospital:

- Status epilepticus
- Seizures secondary to infectious etiology
- New-onset seizures in patients older than 50 years of age
- Eclampsia
- Seizures due to intracranial hemorrhage or tumor
- Seizures due to hypoxia, hyponatremia, hypoglycemia, cardiac dysrhythmias, or drug toxicity

Patients who have not regained full consciousness, and those who have metabolic or hemodynamic abnormalities requiring close monitoring, are admitted to an intensive care unit. Hospital admission is also considered in (1) patients who have alcohol or drug-withdrawal seizures and appear stable, (2) children with complex febrile seizures, and (3) young patients with new-onset seizures. Admission depends on the reliability of the parents and caregivers to encourage follow-up and return visits as needed.

Neurology Consultation

Consultation with a neurologist is indicated under the following circumstances: (1) all patients admitted, (2) patients with new-onset seizures, (3) breakthrough seizures in a patient with therapeutic anticonvulsant drug levels, and (4) all patients with an uncertain diagnosis who are referred for further evaluation.

Discharge

Patients with a known seizure disorder and subtherapeutic drug levels may be sent home after anticonvulsant supplementation. All patients who are sent home are given clear discharge instructions and instructions to follow up with their primary physician or their clinic. Patients are also instructed not to drive an automobile or operate machinery (a danger for themselves and others if they were to have another seizure). Anticonvulsant levels should be rechecked in 1 to 2 weeks by their primary physician. Patients with first-time seizures who are sent home are not typically started on antiseizure medication. The evaluation and discharge of these patients can have many medicolegal issues. This group is instructed to follow up with the consulting neurologist for further assessment.

FINAL POINTS

- The workup of a seizure patient is as easy or as difficult as one makes it. By obtaining a careful history and ordering laboratory tests judiciously, most patients are well managed.
- Any potentially life-threatening diseases, specifically cardiac dysrhythmias, hypoglycemia, hyponatremia, toxic ingestions, and meningitis, are assessed and ruled out or treated.
- The best observer account of what actually took place before, during, and just after the event is obtained and documented.
- Other conditions, such as syncope, factitious seizures, and cataplexy can mimic seizures.

- Precautions are taken to prevent further seizures.
- Status epilepticus is associated with significant morbidity. It is treated in a rational stepwise manner.

- The history and physical examination dictate the need for ancillary tests.
- Complications of seizures include aspiration, acidosis, lacerations, fractures, and dislocations.

CASE *Study*

The rescue squad radioed the emergency department from the scene where a 50-year-old man was observed to have a grand mal seizure while waiting to purchase a bottle of wine at a local liquor store. The squad members reported he was well known to them as a chronic alcoholic and emergency department "frequent flyer."

The patient was having a generalized seizure when the rescue squad arrived. From bystander reports it was determined that the seizure had lasted about 8 minutes. The patient had a pulse, but blood pressure could not be measured. He was placed on oxygen and a cardiac monitor, and an intravenous line was started with difficulty. Thiamine and glucose were administered intravenously without any change in condition. The paramedics requested an order for an anticonvulsant drug. The emergency physician ordered 5 mg of intravenous diazepam, which terminated the seizure in 2 to 3 minutes. Transport time to the hospital was 5 to 10 minutes.

Alcohol withdrawal seizures generally terminate spontaneously and do not need anticonvulsant therapy. Even before the patient arrives, the emergency physician should be thinking of other causes for this patient's seizures.

The patient arrived in the emergency department lethargic and purposefully responsive to painful stimuli only. The rescue squad had no other medical history. They believed that the patient was improving and repeated the history of chronic alcohol abuse. The patient was breathing spontaneously, with an intact gag reflex. A bedside glucose test strip showed a glucose concentration of 140 mg/dL. Supplemental oxygen was continued at 4 L/min. The cardiac monitor showed a sinus tachycardia, with a heart rate of 120 beats per minute. The patient was afebrile and without meningeal signs.

Many major catastrophic problems have been ruled out in this patient. Intracranial hemorrhage is still a significant possibility, as is drug or poison ingestion. Assessment of meningeal signs before clearing the cervical spine in a patient without a history of significant trauma is appropriate.

The patient was gradually waking up and complained of a bad headache. He stated that he had been on a drinking binge for the past several days to relieve the headache pain. He had "rum fits" several years ago when he was jailed following a brawl and drinking binge. The physical examination revealed no focal findings, although the patient remained slightly lethargic. The patient's alcohol level was 285 mg/dL. A CT scan of the head was done, revealing a small subdural hematoma.

Even though this patient had no focal findings, several aspects of his course were sufficient to warrant the CT of the head: (1) he required anticonvulsant medication to stop his prolonged seizures, (2) he had had a bad headache before his seizure, and (3) his alcohol level was very high when he had the seizure. Alcohol withdrawal seizures occur when there is an abrupt fall in ethanol level. They may last more than 5 minutes and may require short-term anticonvulsant treatment. Alcoholics often fall and hit their heads and may not have obvious signs and symptoms of trauma.

The patient was taken to surgery for evacuation of the subdural hematoma.

The emergency physician must always have a high index of suspicion for intracranial hemorrhage in alcoholic patients. Symptoms of altered mental status cannot be attributed solely to acute alcoholism or withdrawal.

Bibliography

TEXT

Adams RD, Victor M: Principles of Neurology, 6th ed. New York, McGraw-Hill, 1997.

Journal Articles

American College of Emergency Physicians: Clinical policy for the initial approach to patients with a chief complaint of seizure who are not in status epilepticus. Ann Emerg Med 1997; 29:706–724.

American College of Emergency Physicians: Practice parameter: Neuroimaging in the emergency patient presenting with seizure (summary statement). Ann Emerg Med 1996; 28:114–118.

Bradford JC, Kyriakedes CG: Evidence-based emergency medicine evaluation and diagnostic testing: Evaluation of the patient with seizures: An evidence-based approach. Emerg Med Clin North Am 1999; 17:1–20.

Consensus statements: Medical management of epilepsy. Neurology 1998; 51(Suppl 4):S39–S43.

Delanty N, Vaughan CJ, French JA: Medical causes of seizures. Lancet 1998; 352:383–390.

Devinsky O: Patients with refractory seizures. N Engl J Med 1999; 340:1565–1570.

Diaz-Arrastia R, Agostini MA, Van Ness PC: Evolving treatment strategies for epilepsy. JAMA 2002; 287:2917–2920.

Freeland ES, McMicken DB: Alcohol-related seizures: I and II. Pathophysiology, differential diagnosis, and evaluation. J Emerg Med 1993; 11:463–473, 605–618.

Gold CR, Peirog J: A rational approach to pediatric seizures. Pediatr Emerg Med Rep 2000; 5:121–132.

Holland KD: Efficacy, pharmacology, and adverse effects of antiepileptic drugs. Neurol Clin 2001; 19:313–345.

Jagoda A, Colucciello SA: Seizures: Accurate diagnosis and effective treatment. Emerg Med Pract 2000; 2:1–24.

Payne TA, Bleck TP: Update on neurologic critical care: Status epilepticus. Crit Care Clin 1997; 13(1):17–38.

Pellock JM: Treatment of seizures and epilepsy in children and adolescents. Neurology 1998; 51(Suppl 4):S8–S14.

Roth HL, Drislane FW: Neurologic emergencies: Seizures. Neurol Clin 1998; 16:257–284.

Terndrup TE: Clinical issues in the acute childhood seizure management in the emergency department. J Child Neurol 1998; 13(Suppl 1):S8–S10.

Willmore LJ: Epilepsy emergencies: The first seizure and status epilepticus. Neurology 1998; 51(Suppl 4):S34–S38.

The author wishes to acknowledge the work of Marc Nelson in the writing of this chapter for the first edition of this book.

CHAPTER 34

Stroke

ARTHUR B. SANDERS

CASE *Study*

A 66-year-old man was brought to the emergency department by the rescue squad with sudden onset of right arm and leg weakness and inability to speak.

INTRODUCTION

Stroke is the third leading cause of death in the United States after heart disease and cancer. It is the most lethal and disabling of the neurologic diseases. There are 700,000 to 750,000 strokes each year in the United States. Almost 5% of the U.S. population older than 65 years of age has had a stroke at one time in their lives. As the population ages, stroke will be an increasing problem that emergency health care professionals will encounter. From an economic and functional standpoint, stroke is one of the most devastating problems in medicine. Over the past decade, our approach to patients with acute stroke has radically changed with our ability to intervene and minimize the patient's neurologic injury and improve the eventual functional outcome. However, the acute management of stroke, at the present time, remains largely supportive for many patients, with a select few meeting criteria for thrombolysis. Anticoagulation has a more clearly defined role but is generally reserved for large, acute strokes, with evolving neurologic deficits.

A stroke is a sudden neurologic deficit that results from the disruption of the blood supply to a distinct region of the brain. The two major causes of stroke are ischemia and hemorrhage.

Ischemic strokes occur when a cerebral blood vessel becomes occluded. Seventy-five percent to 80% of strokes are ischemic.

Hemorrhagic strokes account for 20% of strokes and are caused by the rupture of a cerebral vessel.

Ischemic strokes most commonly result from thrombosis in an atherosclerotic artery. Less common causes of ischemia include vasculitis, dissection, hypercoagulable states, polycythemia, and infections. About 20% of ischemic strokes are caused by emboli, most often from the bifurcation of the carotid arteries. Emboli also can be of cardiac origin: left ventricular mural thrombus, atrial mural thrombus, valvular heart disease, or septal defects.

Hemorrhagic strokes are caused by the rupture of an intracranial blood vessel, which results in an intracerebral hemorrhage or in bleeding on the surface of the brain, which is usually a subarachnoid hemorrhage. The most common hemorrhagic stroke is an intracerebral hemorrhage from a ruptured arteriole, often secondary to chronic hypertension. Intracerebral hemorrhages also occur in patients who are anticoagulated or have a bleeding diathesis, and they have been associated with cocaine use. In older patients, amyloid angiopathy may predispose to intracranial hemorrhage. Subarachnoid hemorrhage from the rupture of an aneurysm can cause a stroke. Arteriovenous malformations account for about 5% of subarachnoid hemorrhages and are more common in younger populations.

The blood supply to the brain comes from four vessels arising off the aortic arch: two carotid and two vertebral arteries. Figure 34–1 illustrates the pertinent anatomy of the cerebral blood supply. The common carotid artery bifurcates into internal and external carotid arteries at the level of the hyoid bone. Only the internal carotid artery enters the skull through the carotid canal. At the cavernous sinus the internal carotid artery gives rise to the ophthalmic arteries and then trifurcates into the anterior and middle cerebral arteries and posterior communicating artery. The vertebral arteries ascend through the foramina in the cervical vertebral transverse processes and enters the skull at the foramen magnum. The two vertebral arteries join at the level of the upper medulla to form the basilar artery, which divides at the midbrain to form the two posterior cerebral arteries. Anastomosis between the anterior and posterior cerebral vessels by means of the anterior and posterior communicating arteries creates the circle of Willis. This circular arterial linkage lies at the base of the brain, surrounding the optic chiasm and pituitary stalk. Strokes can be classified based on

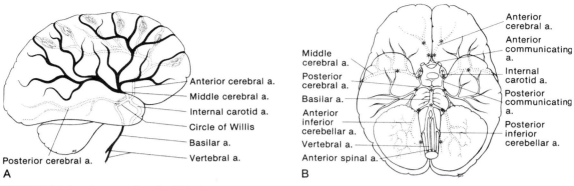

FIGURE 34–1 • Anatomy of cerebral blood supply. *A,* Lateral view. *B,* Basal view. *Asterisks* denote common areas for atheroma.

their anatomic distribution. Strokes of the anterior circulation involve the carotid artery distribution, whereas strokes of the posterior circulation involve the vertebrobasilar system.

INITIAL APPROACH AND STABILIZATION

Prehospital Care

The emergency medical services (EMS) system is a key element in the treatment of patients with acute stroke. Because of the 3-hour time window from symptom onset to the administration of thrombolytics, symptoms suggestive of stroke must be regarded as a true emergency, similar to those of acute myocardial infarction. Patients need to be educated about the warning signs and symptoms of stroke and the need for calling the emergency squad. EMS units must be dispatched promptly to the scene when a call is received about a possible stroke, and medics must ensure rapid transport to a hospital capable of delivering thrombolytics to stroke victims. Such hospitals often have stroke protocols that allow for emergent computed tomography (CT) with definitive readings, laboratory evaluation, and administration of thrombolytics.

Information gathering in the field directed toward possible causes, potential complications, and a brief past medical history including medications and allergies follows a standardized format to be applied quickly and uniformly. Some EMS systems have developed standardized stroke scales that can be easily used by medics in evaluating patients. The Cincinnati Stroke Scale consists of the evaluation of three physical findings: facial droop, arm drift, and speech. Abnormalities on these tests would indicate a possible stroke and initiate prompt transport to the hospital.

In the emergency department, all patients in whom acute cerebrovascular disease is suspected

are brought immediately to a monitored bed and need emergent attention.

Priority Diagnoses

The earliest diagnostic concerns relate to the complications of the presenting "stroke." Airway, breathing, and circulation status are the initial focus of care. Assessing the underlying causes and their potential reversibility is the next step in care.

Rapid Assessment

1. What are the patient's symptoms? When did they begin, and how long have they lasted? Have they changed since onset?
2. Is there a significant history of known diseases predisposing to stroke (e.g., diabetes or hypertension)?
3. What medications is the patient taking?
4. The airway status and adequacy of ventilation are assessed.
5. The vital signs and general appearance of the patient are noted. Temperature measurement is important. Hyperthermia may worsen an acute stroke and give clues to its etiology.
6. Level of consciousness is either described or measured according to the Glasgow Coma Scale.
7. Pupil size, equality, and reaction to light are noted.
8. A description of the weakness present is given, including any abnormal responses to stimulation (e.g., posturing).
9. Facial droop: the patient is asked to smile or show the teeth, and any asymmetry is reported.
10. Arm drift: the patient closes the eyes and holds both arms out in front. Any drift of one arm down indicates possible weakness.

11. Speech: the patient is asked to repeat a phrase such as "You can't teach old dogs new tricks." Any slurring, use of inappropriate words, or word finding difficulty is noted.

Early Intervention

Oxygen. Supplemental oxygen is given by either nasal cannula or mask as tolerated, 4 to 6 L/min; 1 to 2 L/min is given initially if obstructive pulmonary disease is present.

Intravenous Access. Vascular access is obtained early in anticipation of medication administration or fluid resuscitation. The infusate is usually normal saline at a TKO rate because overhydration may worsen cerebral edema and elevated intracranial pressure.

Cardiac Monitor/Pulse Oximetry. A cardiac monitor allows the out-of-hospital providers to describe and observe the cardiac rhythm in transit. Up to 30% of patients with a new neurologic insult have an abnormal cardiac rhythm.

Bedside Blood Glucose Test. A finger stick blood glucose test is done to assess the patient's blood glucose level. Hypoglycemia and hyperglycemia can worsen neurologic deficits and may need emergent treatment.

Complications

The complications of acute cerebrovascular disease are anticipated.

Airway Compromise. If the stroke victim is having respiratory difficulties or cannot protect the airway, intubation should be done.

Dysrhythmias. Ventricular dysrhythmias are to be anticipated. Treatment with defibrillation is appropriate in an unstable patient with ventricular tachycardia or fibrillation.

Hypertension. Hypertension is often seen in patients presenting with acute cerebrovascular disease. In acute situations, hypertension may be physiologic, allowing adequate cerebral perfusion if intracranial pressure is elevated. An acute lowering in pressure may result in failure of perfusion of a stenotic or thrombosed cerebral vessel, leading to neuronal ischemia in the tissue supplied by that vessel. Therefore, mild to moderate hypertension in stroke does not require treatment. Severe hypertension, greater than 220 mm Hg systolic or 120 mm Hg diastolic, or hypertensive encephalopathy may be treated initially with labetalol or nitroprusside to lower the pressure gradually. Precipitous drops in the blood pressure can decrease cerebral blood flow and worsen the stroke. The blood pressure is gradually reduced to approximately 180/110 mm Hg while the patient is closely monitored.

Cerebral Edema or Herniation Syndrome. Acute herniation is uncommon in the early hours of a cerebrovascular accident. It is caused by brain edema, mass effect, and uncal herniation through the tentorial notch. Management aims to reduce intracranial pressure. Treatment is controversial and may include intubation and mild hyperventilation to a PCO_2 of 30 to 35 mm Hg, elevating the head of the bed, fluid restriction, and osmotic diuretics.

CLINICAL ASSESSMENT

The history and physical examination can differentiate a cerebrovascular occlusion from other causes of stroke, establish the initial extent of the neurologic deficit, and identify complications. It is important to repeat the initial examination serially during the course of care to detect changing neurologic signs and symptoms.

History

1. How did the *symptoms evolve*? The patient or family is asked to describe the *exact time of onset and progression* of the *symptoms*. If the patient woke with the symptoms or is found unable to provide history because of aphasia or altered mental status, the last time he or she was at his or her baseline is considered the time of stroke occurrence.
2. What is the *nature* of the symptoms? The type of weakness, speech impediment, vision impairment, gait change, and changes in level of consciousness are identified. What can't the patient do now that he or she could do before?
3. Are there *associated symptoms*? Is there numbness, tingling, vertigo, syncope, nausea or vomiting, chest pain, or palpitations? Cardiac symptoms, significant weight loss, or fever may point to pathologic processes causative for stroke.
4. Has the patient had *similar symptoms before*? Prior reversible presentations of cerebrovascular disease consistent with a diagnosis of transient ischemic attack (TIA) are harbingers of impending stroke.
5. In evaluating patients with chronic medical problems and impairments (i.e., a nursing home patient who may have had a stroke), an attempt is made *first to establish a "functional baseline"* from information given by the caretaker. What were the *patient's capabilities before* the *acute event* (i.e., dressing, eating, bathing, transferring independently)? Changes from the baseline are explored.

6. Does the patient have any *risk factors* for stroke (Table 34–1)?
7. *Current medications* and any *known* allergies are noted.
8. *Past medical history*, including hospitalizations, surgical procedures, and chronic illnesses are noted. The cardiac history, valvular disease, and any prior neurologic presentations are emphasized.

Physical Examination

In the physical examination the physician seeks evidence of cardiac or atherosclerotic vascular disease, increased intracranial pressure, or herniation syndrome and establishes a neurologic and functional baseline for future comparisons. Table 34–2 lists the pertinent elements of the physical examination in the patient with suspected stroke.

The fleeting nature of neurologic findings in patients with stroke syndromes is often frustrating. The physical examination is used not only to establish the extent of the deficit but also to seek possible causes of the signs or symptoms. The physician should not be dissuaded by the patient who states that the neurologic symptoms that brought him or her to the emergency department are now resolved. A careful examination is still necessary to avoid missing subtle findings.

Neurologic symptoms can be further assessed by the use of the National Institutes of Health (NIH) Stroke Scale (Table 34–3). This scale allows physicians to objectively assess how severe the stroke is, which correlates with long-term outcome. The scale evaluates level of consciousness, visual assessment, motor function, sensation and neglect, and cerebellar function. Maximum deficit is 42, and normal neurologic examination is zero. Patients can be objectively followed over time by serial examinations with different observers using the NIH Stroke Scale and with deficits serving as implications for treatment. Patients with NIH Stroke Scale scores of less than 4 are usually not candidates for emergent thrombolytic treatment because the risks may outweigh the benefits. Patients with severe deficits (NIH Stroke Scale

score > 22) are at increased risks for bleeding with the use of thrombolytics.

CLINICAL REASONING

After data gathering, the emergency physician addresses four questions.

Are the Findings Due to a Noncerebrovascular Cause That May Mimic a Stroke Syndrome?

Noncerebrovascular diseases to consider include the following:

- *Subdural and epidural hematoma.* Both forms may manifest with lateralizing signs. Subdural hematoma is more likely to be confused with stroke (see Chapter 48, Head and Neck Trauma).
- *Postictal state with Todd's paralysis.* This condition is preceded by a history or physical findings consistent with seizure; it usually lasts 2 to 3 hours and has a rapidly improving neurologic pattern.
- *Occult neoplasm.* Rarely the onset may be acute if a hemorrhage occurs within the tumor. More often there is an insidious onset associated with systemic symptoms (e.g., anorexia, weight loss).
- *Drug toxicity.* Although lateralizing deficits are rare, stroke can be caused by abuse of narcotics or sedative-hypnotics. This diagnosis is usually supported by a characteristic toxidrome (see Chapter 15, The Poisoned Patient). It can also be a complication of abuse because intravenous drug use increases the potential for brain abscess, septic emboli, and thrombotic stroke.
- *Metabolic encephalopathy.* Stroke syndromes rarely occur in patients with hypoxia, hypoglycemia, hyperthermia, or nonketotic hyperosmolar coma. Data gathering usually gives clues to these systemic diseases.
- *Central nervous system infections.* Meningitis, encephalitis, and brain abscess rarely present as a stroke. Other signs of infection such as fever, elevated white blood cell count,

---

TABLE 34–1. Risk Factors for Stroke

Age > 50 years	History of transient ischemic attacks
Male sex	Atherosclerotic cardiovascular disease
Hypertension	Other cardiovascular disease (e.g., atrial fibrillation, congestive heart
Diabetes mellitus	failure, aortic valvular disease)
Cigarette smoking	Hypercoagulable state, can be associated with hematologic or gastrointestinal cancer
Hyperlipidemia	Polycythemia and sickle cell anemia
Race and heredity	

TABLE 34–2. Important Components of the Physical Examination in the Patient with Stroke Symptoms

Area of Examination	Important Components	Comments
Vital signs	Blood pressure	May be elevated, often in response to need for increased cerebral pressure
	Heart rate	Usually normal or bradycardic. The latter is due to a parasympathetic mediated baroreceptor response
		Extrasystolic beats are common and usually ventricular in origin.
	Respirations	Variable. If they slow suddenly, consider impending herniation.
	Temperature	Patient usually afebrile. Elevated temperature points to an infectious process that may be a cause or complication
General appearance	Position, movement, color, diaphoresis	Rough gauge of how the patient is tolerating the event
Eye	Conjugate deviation	May indicate frontal or brain stem lesion or visual field cut
	Pupils—asymmetry and reaction	If abnormal, consider herniation and midbrain dysfunction
	Fundi	Nicking, hemorrhage, "cotton wool" spots indicate hypertension or diabetes. Degree of capillary thickening ("silver or copper wiring") is indicative of chronic hypertension. Papilledema indicates increased intracranial pressure.
		Subhyaloid or preretinal hemorrhage may be seen in patients with subarachnoid or intracranial hemorrhage.
Neck	Carotid bruits	Direct evidence of cerebrovascular disease
Lungs	Auscultation	Signs of consolidation, rales, wheezes often due to aspiration as a complication
Cardiac	Auscultation	Irregular rhythm may indicate atrial fibrillation or extrasystoles. Murmurs suggest valvular disease (aortic stenosis is the most important lesion)
Neurologic	Level of consciousness	Progression to coma may signal impending herniation
	Speech	Poor fluency and one- to two-word phrases indicate an expressive (Broca's area) aphasia.
		Comprehension of commands is intact in expressive aphasia, lost in receptive aphasia (Wernicke's)
	Cranial nerve	Dilated and unreactive pupil may indicate uncal herniation. Central seventh nerve palsy ipsilateral to hemiparesis is consistent with hemispheric infarct. Peripheral seventh nerve palsy or other cranial nerve palsy contralateral to hemiparesis is consistent with brain stem infarct
	Motor	Assess for focal weakness. If leg is weakest, suspect anterior cerebral artery infarct. Middle cerebral artery lesions manifest as hemiplegia or face and arm weakness exceeding leg weakness. Subtle weakness of arms may be assessed by "drift" test.
		Have patient hold arms at 90-degree angle in front with eyes closed and watch for downward drifting of affected arm.
	Sensory	Check response to pain, touch, and proprioception in all extremities.
	Reflexes at biceps, knee, ankle, and foot	Reflexes are usually decreased in distribution of weakness in acute stages. Inequality of reflexes and Babinski sign (upgoing great toe) are lateralizing signs.
	Coordination, station, and gait	Gait, heel, and toe walking (if able), finger/nose and heel/knee/shin for cerebellar testing

immunosuppression, meningismus, headache, or a prodromal history may be present.

- *TIAs* have their own differential diagnosis, including focal seizures, migraine aura, syncope, and dysrhythmias.

What Type of Stroke is Present?

Table 34–4 lists the major categories of stroke, along with a description of the typical presentation, associated symptoms and risk factors, and examination findings. The emergency physician considers which time course, progression, and overall pattern best fit the clinical picture. Diagnosing a specific stroke syndrome influences the management of the patient with a stroke. Although the final answer may not be known for 24 hours, factors to consider include the following questions:

1. Are there any neurologic deficits at this time? If the deficits have resolved, the diagnosis is most consistent with a TIA.
2. Is the clinical course progressive, constant, or fluctuating?

TABLE 34–3. National Institutes of Health Stroke Scale

1a. Level of Consciousness (LOC)	0 = Alert
	1 = Drowsy
	2 = Stupor
	3 = Coma
1b. LOC Questions	0 = Answers questions on age and month correctly
	1 = Answers one correctly
	2 = Answers none correctly
1c. LOC Commands	0 = Performs eye opening and grip correctly
	1 = Performs one task correctly
	2 = Performs neither command correctly
2. Best Gaze	0 = Normal
	1 = Partial gaze palsy
	2 = Total gaze paresis or forced deviation
3. Visual	0 = No visual loss
	1 = Partial hemianopia
	2 = Complete hemianopia
	3 = Bilateral hemianopia
4. Facial Palsy	0 = Normal
	1 = Minor paralysis
	2 = Partial paralysis
	3 = Complete paralysis
5a. Left Arm Motor	0 = No drift 10 sec
	1 = Drift
	2 = Some effort against gravity
	3 = No effort against gravity
	4 = No movement
5b. Right Arm Motor	0 = No drift 10 sec
	1 = Drift
	2 = Some effort against gravity
	3 = No effort against gravity
	4 = No movement
6a. Left Leg Motor	0 = No drift 10 sec
	1 = Drift
	2 = Some effort against gravity
	3 = No effort against gravity
	4 = No movement
6b. Right Leg Motor	0 = No drift 10 sec
	1 = Drift
	2 = Some effort against gravity
	3 = No effort against gravity
	4 = No movement
7. Limb Ataxia	0 = Normal
	1 = Present in one limb
	2 = Present in two limbs
8. Sensory	0 = Normal
	1 = Mild sensory loss
	2 = Severe sensory loss
9. Language	0 = Normal
	1 = Mild or moderate aphasia
	2 = Severe aphasia
	3 = Global aphasia
10. Dysarthria	0 = Normal
	1 = Mild to moderate dysphasia
	2 = Severe dysphasia
11. Extinction and Inattention (Neglect)	0 = Normal
	1 = Partial neglect
	2 = Profound neglect

3. Are there potential sources of cerebral emboli? Most of these sources are cardiac in nature. These patients require investigation for mural thrombus, atrial fibrillation, atrial myoma, or valvular heart disease.

4. Most importantly, is intracranial hemorrhage present? Factors supporting this diagnosis are hypertension, anticoagulation therapy, headache, altered mental status, nuchal rigidity, and subhyaloid hemorrhage.

TABLE 34–4. Stroke Symptoms

	Presentation	Associated Symptoms	Risk Factors	Physical Examination	Useful Tests	Additional Aspects
Transient ischemic attack (TIA)	Sudden onset of symptoms (vision or speech change, focal weakness) Short duration—minutes to hours (maximum 24 hr)	Numbness/sensory loss Vertigo (basilar TIA) Speech change (dysarthria, aphasia) Gait change—ataxia Vision change (diplopia, field cut, monocular or bilateral vision loss)	Age Male sex Smoking ASCVD Hyperlipidemia Heart disease Hypercoagulable states	Usually normal unless attack still in progress Funduscopic changes Cardiac examination (murmur) Carotid bruits	Good HX/PE Noninvasive carotid evaluation Carotid arteriogram	20% to 50% of TIA patients have a stroke within 2–5 years
Progressive stroke	Sudden onset of symptoms Duration > 24 hr Progressive neurologic signs and symptoms	Same as above Nausea and vomiting on occasion	Same as above	Hypertension/bradycardia typical Possible dysrhythmia Neurologic examination findings are referable to involved area Funduscopic, carotid, and cardiac changes as above	Baseline laboratory studies CT scan of head Cerebral angiography (?)	Seen in 15%–25% of stroke patients
Completed stroke	Sudden onset of symptoms Duration—permanent No progression or regression of symptoms	Same as above	Same as above	Same as above	Same as above	If thrombotic, may commonly develop during sleep with symptoms perceived on awakening in the morning (resulting from low flow through a stenotic area)
Embolic stroke	Sudden onset of symptoms Duration > 24 hr	Same as above	Same, especially heart disease (e.g., atrial fibrillation and cardiac mural thrombosis)	Same—emphasis on cardiac examination	Same above	May occur at any time; often follows exertion Often responsible for hemorrhagic infarction: friable clot dissolves with perfusion through ischemic vessels May be acutely associated with seizures in up to 20% of patients
Subarachnoid hemorrhage	Sudden onset of symptoms Severe headache, syncope and nuchal pain Focal neurologic signs, including cranial nerves	Nausea and vomiting Obtundation, sometimes comatose	None (aneurysms are congenital)	Hypertension/bradycardia Nuchal tenderness and rigidity to movement Fundi—subhyaloid hemorrhage or papilledema Dilated pupil if posterior communicating artery aneurysm Neurologic examination is nonfocal	Same as above LP considered if CT scan negative and if diagnosis still suspected	One third from anterior communicating artery aneurysms One fourth from middle carotid artery aneurysms One fifth from posterior communicating artery aneurysm
Intracerebral hemorrhage	Sudden onset of symptoms (dense hemiplegia, hemianesthesia, field cut, obtundation) Duration > 24 hr usually permanent	Usually comatose Rapid progression to loss of consciousness Reticular activating system impairment	Hypertension (brain stem and basal ganglia) Anticoagulant therapy (frontal, parietal, temporal, and occipital lobes)	Usually comatose Cranial nerve findings (e.g., cranial nerve III palsy) Hemiparesis/hemisensory loss, pinpoint pupils (pontine or cerebellar) Posturing Ataxia, vertigo, vomiting (cerebellar) Upgoing Babinski sign	Same as above, except LP not done	Occurs in 10% to 20% of stroke patients

ASCVD, atherosclerotic cerebrovascular disease; CT, computed tomography; HX/PE, history and physical examination; LP, lumbar puncture.

Are Any Complications of Stroke Present or Evolving?

The patient must be reassessed and treated for the major early complications noted in the initial approach:

- Airway compromise
- Dysrhythmias
- Hypertension
- Cerebral edema or herniation syndrome

Does the Patient's History and Physical Examination Fit a Specific Stroke Location Syndrome?

The clinical assessment frequently helps to localize the site of brain injury in a stroke. Although it is preferable to analyze the findings in the context of neuroanatomy, common findings are associated with specific vascular syndromes. The syndromes most commonly seen in the emergency department are discussed here.

Internal Carotid Syndrome. This is a combination of hemiparesis, hemisensory deficit, aphasia, and hemianopsia.

Middle Cerebral Artery Syndrome. Contralateral hemiparesis or hemiplegia, contralateral impairment of sensation, dysarthria, and expressive or receptive aphasia comprise this syndrome. The face and arm are usually affected more than the leg.

Anterior Cerebral Artery Syndrome. Contralateral lower extremity paresis or paralysis, contralateral lower extremity sensory deficit, urinary incontinence, and abnormalities in behavior are the main features of this syndrome.

Vertebral Basilar Syndrome. This is a combination of hemiparesis or quadriparesis, dysarthria, dysphagia, impaired sensation, vertigo, nausea, vomiting, nystagmus, diplopia, and internuclear ophthalmoplegia.

Lateral Medullary (Wallenberg Syndrome). The Wallenberg syndrome comprises vertigo, nausea, vomiting, nystagmus, dysphagia, ataxia, ipsilateral Horner's syndrome, and impaired sensation to the ipsilateral face and contralateral body.

Lacunar Infarct Syndrome. This entity involves thrombosis of the small penetrating end arteries. Patients are usually hypertensive and manifest isolated neurologic deficits. Lesions in the internal capsule produce pure motor hemiparesis, thalamic lesions cause contralateral sensory loss, and pontine infarcts produce ataxic hemiparesis.

DIAGNOSTIC ADJUNCTS

In the patient with suspected stroke, emergent head CT is the priority. While this is in progress, several blood studies are sent to the laboratory.

Laboratory Studies

Electrolyte and glucose levels are measured and renal and liver function tests are ordered to determine if there is a metabolic component to the neurologic symptoms.

A complete blood cell count and clotting studies (prothrombin time, partial thromboplastin time, and platelets) are indicated in all patients in whom anticoagulation is being considered.

Measurement of arterial blood gases helps to evaluate patients for hypoxia and acidosis, as well as providing the P_{CO_2} level to guide possible mild hyperventilation of patients with suspected elevated intracranial pressure.

Drug screening is indicated if there is a history of drug ingestion or signs of a specific toxidrome.

Radiologic Imaging

Computed Tomography of the Head. CT is the most important diagnostic adjunct for diagnosing stroke syndromes. It has excellent sensitivity (greater than 90%) in detecting hemorrhagic or ischemic stroke. It can also differentiate between different disease processes that result in stroke symptoms (Fig. 34–2). Its advantages include its availability, simplicity, noninvasiveness, and relatively low cost. A nonenhanced head CT scan is indicated emergently in all patients with suspected stroke syndromes.

The primary reason for emergent CT of the head is to determine if the stroke is ischemic or hemorrhagic. Intracerebral hemorrhage, hemorrhagic infarctions, and up to 95% of subarachnoid hemorrhages are readily apparent on early CT scans (within 24 hours of symptom onset). However, the CT scan is often normal within the first 12 to 24 hours of an ischemic stroke, because, generally, an acute cerebral infarction is radiographically isodense to the surrounding brain. One study demonstrated only 30% of early ischemic changes on CT scans taken within the first three hours. Thus, in the acute phase, the diagnosis of an acute ischemic stroke is based on clinical judgment and the absence of hemorrhage on CT. Beyond 24 hours postinfarction, the affected area becomes hypodense and more visible on CT.

Chest Radiographs. Standard posteroanterior and lateral chest films are ordered for patients

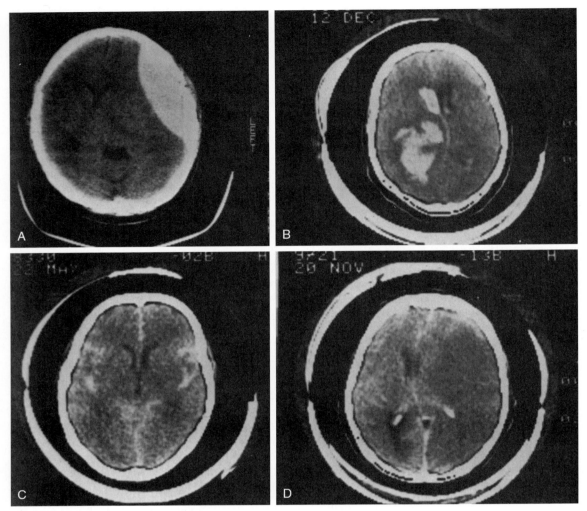

FIGURE 34–2 • Computed tomography of head. Examples of discernible lesions that may manifest as an acute neurologic deficit. *A,* Acute epidural hematoma with midline shift secondary to mass effect and edema. *B,* Right thalamic intracerebral hemorrhage with surrounding edema. *C,* Subarachnoid hemorrhage with blood visible in the sylvian fissures and intracerebral sulci. *D,* Acute left hemispheric complete stroke with edema and midline shift.

with suspected stroke syndromes to look for evidence of aspiration, pneumonia, or tumor.

Cerebral Angiography. Angiography of the four cerebral arteries is used to visualize vascular abnormalities of the brain (arteriovenous malformations, tumors, or aneurysms), to demonstrate displacement of cerebral vessels by mass effect, or, therapeutically, to occlude arteries with emboli or induced thrombi. In patients with hemorrhagic strokes, neurosurgical consultants may order angiography to better define the anatomy.

Magnetic Resonance Imaging (MRI). MRI may play a role in detecting subtle ischemic strokes; however, it is currently not superior to CT for evaluating hemorrhage. Newer MRI techniques such as magnetic resonance angiography (MRA) and diffusion-weighted MRI may play a role in the diagnostic workup of acute stroke in the future. At present, however, MRI is not a routine emergency department test for patients with acute stroke syndromes and should not delay their workup and treatment.

Electrocardiography

Electrocardiograms and cardiac monitoring are ordered for patients with stroke syndromes to identify dysrhythmias diagnosed on the cardiac monitor. Some ischemic strokes have concomitant coronary ischemia. Atrial fibrillation suggests the possibility of embolic stroke.

Special Tests

Lumbar Puncture. Examining a sample of the cerebrospinal fluid (CSF) may allow detection of blood or xanthochromia indicative of an intracranial or subarachnoid hemorrhage that is not evident on CT (occurring in 5% to 7% of patients). This is the principal indication and benefit of performing lumbar punctures in patients with acute cerebrovascular disease. It has been used to distinguish between hemorrhagic and nonhemorrhagic infarction when CT was not available; however, it has many false negatives in this role, and a decision to anticoagulate a patient based on this test is not recommended.

The procedure carries a risk of transtentorial herniation if increased intracranial pressure or a mass lesion exists. Therefore, unless meningitis is suspected, CT is obtained first. The risk of herniation is relatively small in the absence of the signs and symptoms of increased intracranial pressure (e.g., headache, papilledema, decreased level of consciousness, unilateral dilated pupil, or other evidence of herniation).

Noninvasive Carotid Evaluation: Ultrasound Imaging and Oculoplethysmography. Asymptomatic carotid bruits are initially evaluated by noninvasive means. Although expert opinions vary, most do not require carotid angiography. These imaging techniques can differentiate external carotid and subclavian bruits from those of common and internal carotid origin. The latter are of greater clinical concern and may require carotid arteriographic evaluation. Noninvasive carotid tests are generally not available in the emergency department.

PRINCIPLES OF MANAGEMENT

In patients with stroke most of the emergency physician's effort is directed toward data gathering and differential diagnostic decisions. Beyond supportive care and anticipation and treatment of complications, the most important management involves the decision about reperfusion treatments. The era of the acute management of stroke patients is changing. Over the past decade, the use of thrombolytics for patients in the first 3 hours of acute ischemic stroke has become the standard of care. Other reperfusion techniques and the emergent use of neuroprotective agents are being investigated. All these strategies are time dependent, in which the effective treatment must be provided during a narrow window of opportunity. The use of stroke centers, stroke teams, and stroke protocols has been debated in the literature as techniques to ensure the prompt

workup and management of stroke patients who are eligible for time-dependent treatment. The optimal management of the stroke patient requires a smoothly functioning interdisciplinary approach that is established in the institution and community well before the patient arrives with acute symptoms.

General Management

Assessment and support of airway and breathing are used as indicated. Supplemental oxygen is given to improve oxygenation to the brain.

Circulation is assessed and supported. Intravenous access is established in all patients. Overhydrating may worsen brain edema and should be avoided; however, judicious hydration with isotonic fluid may increase cerebral blood flow in dehydrated patients and those with poor cardiac output. In addition, it may decrease blood viscosity by hemodilution and further improve perfusion of the ischemic brain. Hypotonic solutions and 5% dextrose are generally avoided. Electrocardiographic monitoring is maintained to assess cardiac rhythm abnormalities, and treatment is instituted if indicated.

Complications are anticipated. These include airway compromise, dysrhythmias, hypertension, and cerebral edema. Emergent management has been reviewed in the section on Initial Approach and Stabilization.

Specific Treatment Issues

Glucose Control. Glucose levels are monitored and controlled as necessary. Hyperglycemia can worsen ischemic injury to the brain, secondary to anaerobic metabolism and the buildup of lactate, and should be avoided. Hypoglycemia can produce focal neurologic deficits, mimicking stroke, and may also be associated with seizure.

Fever. Temperature control is important in patients with acute stroke. Fever can worsen neurologic injury and is treated with antipyretics. The source of the fever is also ascertained.

Blood Pressure. Hypertension is the primary risk factor for stroke; however, blood pressure control in patients with acute stroke is controversial. The blood pressure is often elevated in patients with acute stroke syndromes, and it may be necessary to maintain cerebral perfusion pressure because of increased intracranial pressure due to acute stroke. Thus, aggressively lowering the blood pressure may worsen cerebral perfusion and ischemic injury. Although many patients with stroke will have hypertension, few will require emergent treatment. In most patients, the blood pressure will gradually normalize without anti-hypertensive therapy. The clinical dilemma is more complicated by the need to lower the blood pressure if the patient is a candidate for thrombolytic treatment or has a hemorrhagic stroke. Thrombolytic candidates have their blood pressure managed by a clinical protocol before, during, and after treatment. Patients with high blood pressures have a greater risk for central nervous system hemorrhage after thrombolytic treatment, and a blood pressure exceeding 185/110 mm Hg is a contraindication to thrombolytics. For nonthrombolytic candidates with ischemic strokes, patients with diastolic blood pressures greater than 105 to 120 mm Hg or systolic pressures greater than 220 mm Hg may be treated with labetalol. Diastolic pressures greater than 140 mm Hg can be treated with nitroprusside. The goal is to gradually lower the diastolic pressure to below 110 mm Hg. Agents such as nifedipine, which can cause precipitous drops in the blood pressure and extension of stroke, should be avoided (see Chapter 10, Hypertension).

Seizures. Seizures can occur secondary to stroke and must be brought under control. Emergent treatment is with diazepam or lorazepam to break the seizure, and then the patient is loaded with intravenous phenytoin to prevent further seizures (see Chapter 33, Seizures).

Thrombolytics for Acute Thrombotic Stroke. The current era of therapy for acute ischemic stroke was ushered in by the publication of the NIH trial demonstrating the improvement in functional status with the use of tissue plasminogen activator (tPA) for acute ischemic stroke using a 3-hour time window. This randomized, multicenter, double-blinded, placebo-controlled study demonstrated improvement in the neurologic deficits in patients with stroke at 24 hours and at 3 months when they received tPA versus placebo. Those receiving tPA were 30% more likely to have minimal or no disability at 3 months. There were no differences in overall mortality, and 6.4% of patients receiving tPA experienced intracerebral hemorrhage within 36 hours of treatment. Other trials have shown no benefits with the use of streptokinase and no benefits when thrombolytics were administered after 3 hours from the onset of stroke symptoms. The use of intra-arterial thrombolytics has shown benefit for certain large middle cerebral artery strokes and basilar artery strokes. The use of other agents such as ancrod and prourokinase has been shown to decrease disability and death. Investigation of the use of mechanical means of reperfusion in the clotted artery, of neuroprotective agents, and of combined regimens of intravenous and locally infused thrombolytics continues.

The use of tPA for acute ischemic stroke within 3 hours of symptoms has been approved by the U.S. Food and Drug Administration and endorsed by the American Heart Association and American Academy of Neurology. The problem is that most patients with stroke are not eligible for treatment because they present after the 3-hour time window. In addition, because of the high incidence of intracerebral hemorrhages, one must be certain of the diagnosis of ischemic stroke and not intracerebral hemorrhage. Exclusion criteria for the use of thrombolytics in adult patients include the following: evidence or suspicion of intracranial hemorrhage, minor or rapidly improving neurologic status as measured by the NIH stroke scale, active or recent bleeding elsewhere, bleeding diathesis, recent intracranial surgery, serious head trauma or stroke, major surgery within 14 days or serious trauma, myocardial infarction, pregnancy, recent arterial puncture at noncompressible site, post–myocardial infarction pericarditis, lumbar puncture within 7 days, history of intracranial hemorrhage, arteriovenous malformation or aneurysm, seizure at onset of stroke, or blood pressure greater then 185/110 mm Hg. For these reasons, the use of tPA for patients presenting with acute stroke is complicated and best initiated as part of an interdisciplinary protocol with emergency medicine, neurology, neurosurgery, and neuroradiology involvement.

The use of other anticoagulant agents in acute stroke is unproven. Heparin is frequently used by neurologists if the stroke is progressive and the patient is not eligible for thrombolytics. Low-molecular-weight heparins are also used. However, neither type of heparin has been shown to decrease disability or mortality. Aspirin, warfarin, and ticlopidine can reduce the risk of stroke in patients presenting with TIA symptoms and can reduce the risk of recurrent stroke.

Subarachnoid Hemorrhage. Priorities include placing the patient in a quiet room to reduce stimulation and vasospasm, maintaining adequate arterial blood pressure, and treating cerebral edema appropriately. Early neurosurgical consultation is key to determine if surgical intervention is indicated. Intracranial pressure monitoring may be indicated. The use of nimodipine may be of benefit.

Intracerebral Hemorrhage. The mass effect caused by the intracerebral hematoma and associated cerebral edema are treated with the selected use of hyperventilation, diuretics, and positional maneuvers. Emergent neurosurgical consultation is essential.

UNCERTAIN DIAGNOSIS

It is not uncommon to be unsure of the diagnosis of stroke or of the specific location of infarction after the initial patient evaluation. In addition, whereas CT sensitivity for acute intracranial hemorrhage approaches 100%, sensitivity for ischemic stroke is only 30% at 3 hours and 100% within 24 hours. As a result, a thorough history and physical examination and emergent diagnostic studies with CT are imperative. Specific history of prior stroke, diabetes mellitus, liver disease, and seizure disorder should be obtained. In addition, a disorder such as Bell's palsy should be considered. Finally, consultation with a neurologist and clear communication of historical data and physical findings should be made early. Generally, the majority of patients with unclear diagnoses of stroke or TIA should be admitted for observation and further workup.

SPECIAL CONSIDERATIONS

Pediatric Patients

Pediatric patients presenting with stroke usually have either an intracranial hemorrhage or a vascular occlusion. The pathophysiology of both disease processes differs from that seen in adults. Intracranial hemorrhage in children most often occurs after rupture of an arteriovenous malformation or congenital (berry) aneurysm. Less commonly, a hemostatic deficit (thrombocytopenia, hemophilia, leukemia) or occult head trauma with subdural or epidural hematoma may be seen. The clinical picture is similar to that in adults, with the exception being children younger than 2 years of age. Any significant decrease in the level of consciousness in these patients warrants early CT evaluation. Therapy is usually supportive, with embolization of arteriovenous malformations and surgical drainage of intracranial hematomas performed at the discretion of the neurosurgeon.

In contrast to adults, acute vascular occlusion is less common and may occur secondary to arterial embolization or thrombosis (e.g., acute infantile hemiplegia) or secondary to venous thrombosis of the cerebral sinuses. Acute infantile hemiplegia occurs most commonly in children between 1 and 3 years of age, but similar presentations may occur in older children. Most commonly, the disease is idiopathic, but it can be caused by other diseases such as sickle cell anemia, lupus erythematosus, congenital heart disease with embolization, polycythemia, or acute arteritis (polyarteritis nodosa, Takayasu's disease). The clinical presentation mimics that of an acute stroke. Treatment is supportive, with concomitant treatment of the underlying pathogenic condition. There is usually residual hemiparesis, spasticity, and mild intellectual or behavioral impairment after the illness, but the degree of functional recovery is usually greater than that seen in adults with stroke. Cerebral venous thrombosis usually occurs secondary to local sinus infection or dehydration. Secondary cerebral edema often results in increased intracranial pressure, obtundation, a bulging fontanelle, and seizures. The diagnosis is primarily clinical, and therapy is supportive, with concomitant treatment of cerebral edema and underlying conditions. Rarely, traumatic or nontraumatic carotid artery dissection can cause stroke in the younger patient.

Elderly Patients

To understand the special problems of stroke in the elderly, one must understand the pathophysiology of aging. Decreased functional reserve in most organ systems, decreased sensitivity to the perception of painful stimuli, decreased resistance to the pathophysiologic processes of infection and malignancy, increased likelihood of drug interactions and intolerances, and survival into the peak age range for many serious diseases all place the elderly patient at significant risk. Misdiagnosis of a treatable entity mimicking acute stroke, impaired prestroke medical and functional baselines, and a more complicated clinical course due to these factors are all commonly encountered in elderly patients. Age itself is not a contraindication to thrombolytic treatment if the patient presents with acute thrombotic stroke within the 3-hour time window, but it should be noted that older patients may have a higher prevalence of amyloid angiopathy, which can predispose to intracerebral hemorrhages.

Previously Impaired Patients

In a patient with a previous history of chronic medical diseases (e.g., the nursing home patient), the diagnosis of stroke can be exceedingly difficult. If the patient is normally obtunded, demented, has had a previous stroke, or has extreme functional impairment, the appearance of neurologic findings with acute stroke may be extremely subtle. A large number of other disease presentations may mimic that of acute stroke, may contribute to this etiology, or may complicate its clinical course. They must be considered in these patients. For example, in a patient with controlled congestive heart failure and ischemic heart disease, a routine urinary tract infection may increase demands on cardiac output, resulting in worsening heart failure, silent infarction, and development of a mural thrombus with embolic stroke. Without pain, the clinical presentation would likely be mild dyspnea, refusal to eat or ambulate, obtundation, or other functional impairment. For these reasons, evaluation of the previously impaired patient must be complete, and attention must be paid to subtle changes from the baseline level of function. A thorough search for other mimicking or complicating conditions is necessary.

Because of their decreased physiologic reserve, routine therapy may create a complicated clinical course in these patients. Tube feedings may result in hyperosmolar complications; fluid therapy may cause dehydration, overhydration, or electrolyte imbalance; catheterization for incontinence may lead to urosepsis; and prolonged bed rest may lead to bedsores, thrombophlebitis, and pulmonary embolism. These considerations are more germane during the later phases of hospital management but may be contributing factors in the patient coming to the emergency department from an extended care or convalescent center.

DISPOSITION AND FOLLOW-UP

The status of the neurologic deficit and its etiology are the primary factors in patient disposition. Patients with stroke syndromes should be seen by neurology or neurosurgery consultants.

Admission

Patients presenting with an acute stroke are admitted to the hospital. Serial monitoring of the neurologic deficit, workup for specific stroke causes, anticipation and treatment of complications, and patient comfort are all reasons for admission. Admission to the intensive care unit is required to manage patients with subarachnoid and intracerebral hemorrhage, obtunded patients, and those with complications, such as extreme hypertension or cerebral edema.

Discharge

The only subset of stroke patients who are considered for discharge are those presenting with TIAs. These patients will generally receive a neurology consult in the emergency department. Many patients with TIAs will be admitted to begin the workup and treatment. Outpatient evaluation is acceptable if the patient has completely recovered and is expected to be compliant and if arrangements for close follow-up can be made. Any early recurrence of symptoms should prompt emergent admission and expedited workup.

FINAL POINTS

- Initial patient care efforts are focused on basic stabilization and assessment of the extent of the deficit and its possible cause.
- A high index of suspicion and mental preparation is maintained for complications including airway compromise, dysrhythmias, high or low blood pressure, cerebral edema, or herniation syndrome.
- The history and physical examination help differentiate patients with cerebrovascular disease from patients with other diseases that produce stroke symptoms.
- Identification of candidates for thrombolytic therapy within the 3-hour time window from the onset of symptoms is a challenge for health care providers. Multidisciplinary teams and protocols often aid in accomplishing the goal of emergent treatment of the appropriate patient.
- Emergent nonenhanced head CT is key for distinguishing thrombotic from hemorrhagic strokes but the study has its limitations.
- Admission is usually the appropriate disposition for patients with acute stroke. Patients with new onset of obtundation, progressive neurologic findings, or complications are candidates for admission to the intensive care unit. Patients with hemorrhagic strokes are promptly evaluated by neurosurgery.

CASE*Study*

A 66-year-old man was brought to the emergency department by the rescue squad with sudden onset of right arm and leg weakness and inability to speak.

The rescue squad reported that the patient had experienced sudden right-sided weakness and inability to speak 1 hour ago. He was taking hydrochlorothiazide for hypertension and had a history of several similar transient episodes of weakness on the right side. He was alert and awake. Vital signs were blood pressure, 200/120 mm Hg; pulse, 65 beats per minute with irregular rhythm; and respiratory rate, 18 breaths per minute and adequate. There was right facial, right arm, and right leg weakness. The Cincinnati Prehospital Stroke Scale was positive in all three factors evaluated, making stroke a likely diagnosis. Oxygen by nasal cannula at 4 L/min was started, and an intravenous line of normal saline was placed at a to-keep-open rate. The cardiac monitor showed one to two unifocal premature ventricular contractions per minute. The squad reported a 5-minute estimated time of arrival to the hospital.

This patient's age, sex, previous history of transient neurologic deficit, hypertension history, and current symptoms all point to the probability of cerebrovascular disease. No dysrhythmic prophylaxis is indicated at this time. Optimally, a family member who knows the patient and his medical history well should accompany the patient. Other information, such as lists of medications, physician's name, hospital card, and any lists of diagnoses or medical records in the family's possession can be of help to the emergency physician. The onset of symptoms 1 hour before the EMS call indicates that the patient may be a candidate for emergent thrombolytic therapy within the 3-hour time window. The institutional stroke team and protocol are activated.

The patient confirmed the onset of symptoms while he was watching the local evening news on television at 6 PM. His family was there and confirms the time of onset of symptoms. He had a previous history of temporary weakness in his leg that resolved in 5 minutes. This occurred twice in the past 3 months. He had hypertension and was on hydrochlorothiazide.

On physical examination the patient was found to be alert and in acute distress. Blood pressure was 180/100 mm Hg, pulse was 60 beats per minute and irregular, respiratory rate was 18 breaths per minute, and temperature was 98.4°F (36.8°C). The rest of the examination showed the following:

HEENT (head, eyes, ears, nose, throat): Mild arteriovenous nicking and early "copper wiring" changes in the fundi, otherwise negative

Neck: No bruits or jugular venous distention

Lungs: Clear

Cardiac: No murmur, rubs, or gallops

Abdomen: Unremarkable

Extremities: Unremarkable

Neurologic: Obvious expressive aphasia; comprehends commands. Cranial nerves II to XII were intact except for mild right central seventh nerve palsy.

Motor: Right hemiparesis, greater in the upper extremity

Sensory: Decreased on right side to pain

Reflexes: Decreased on right side; Babinski reflexes positive on right

Cerebellar examination: Impaired on right side due to weakness; intact on left side

NIH Stroke Scale: The patient had a deficit of 12.

The findings are consistent with an acute stroke. The time course was within the 3-hour window for thrombolytic treatment. The stroke team and protocol were activated. Laboratory studies and an emergent CT scan were ordered. The institution was set up to ensure that an emergent stroke CT takes priority over other studies and a neuroradiologist is available to read it immediately on completion.

A head CT scan was read by the neuroradiologist as normal with no evidence of a hemorrhage. The values for the complete blood cell count, electrolytes, glucose, blood urea nitrogen, creatinine, arterial blood gases, and clotting studies were normal. The patient's blood pressure was under control, and he had no contraindication to thrombolytics. It was now 2 hours since the onset of symptoms. The risks and benefits were explained to the patient and his family, and the decision was made to treat with intravenous tPA. The patient was admitted to the intensive care unit for close monitoring of possible complications. He was discharged to a rehabilitation facility 5 days later. He was functioning independently 3 months later with mild residual deficits.

BIBLIOGRAPHY

TEXTS

American Heart Association: Stroke. In: Textbook of Advanced Cardiac Life Support. Dallas, American Heart Association, 2000.

Frankel MR, Chimowitz M: Cerebrovascular disease. In Shah SM, Kelly KM (eds): Emergency Neurology: Principles and Practice. Cambridge, UK, Cambridge University Press, 1999.

JOURNAL ARTICLES

Albers GW, Bates VE, Clark WM, et al: Intravenous tissue-type plasminogen activator for the treatment of acute stroke. JAMA 2000; 283:1145–1150.

Alberts MJ, Hademenos G, Latchaw RE et al: Recommendations for the establishment of primary stroke centers. JAMA 2000; 283:3102–3109.

Baumlin KM, Richardson LD: Stroke syndromes. Emerg Med Clin North Am 1997; 15:551–561.

Brott T, Bogousslavsky J: Treatment of acute ischemic stroke. N Engl J Med 2000; 343:10:710–722.

Duldner JE, Emerman CL: Stroke: Comprehensive guidelines for clinical assessment and emergency management: I and II. Emerg Med Rep 1997; 18:201–212, 213–222.

Johnson ES, Lanes SF, Wentworth CE III, et al: A meta-regression analysis of the dose response effect of aspirin on stroke. Arch Intern Med 1999; 159:1248–1253.

Katzen IL, Furlan AJ, Lloyd LE, et al: Use of tissue-type plasminogen activator for acute ischemic stroke. JAMA 2000; 283:1151–1158.

Kothari RU, Hacke W, Brott T, et al: Cardiopulmonary resuscitation and emergency cardiovascular care: Stroke. Ann Emerg Med 2001; 37:137–144.

Kothari RU, Pancioli A, Liu T, et al: Cincinnati prehospital stroke scale: Reproducibility and validity. Ann Emerg Med 1999; 33:373–378.

Kwiatkowski TG, Libman RB, Frankel M, et al: Effects of tissue plasminogen activator for acute ischemic stroke at one year. N Engl J Med 1999; 340:1781–1787.

Lang ES: Use of thrombolytic therapy in patients with acute ischemic stroke. Ann Emerg Med 2002; 39:296–298.

Lewandowski C, Barson W: Treatment of acute ischemic stroke. Ann Emerg Med 2001; 37:202–216.

National Institute of Neurological Disorders and Stroke rt-PA Stroke Study Group: Tissue plasminogen activator for acute ischemic stroke. N Engl J Med 1995; 333: 1581–1587.

Patel SC, Levine SR, Tilley BC: Lack of clinical significance of early ischemic changes on computed tomography in acute stroke. JAMA 2001; 286:2830–2838.

Sherman DG, Atkinson RP, Chippendale T, et al: Intravenous ancrod for treatment of acute ischemic stroke. JAMA 2000; 283:2395–2403.

Smith RW, Scott PA, Grant RJ, et al: Emergency physician treatment of acute stroke with recombinant tissue plasminogen activator: A retrospective analysis. Acad Emerg Med 1999; 6:618–625.

The author wishes to acknowledge the work of Louis Binder in the writing of this chapter for the first edition of this book.

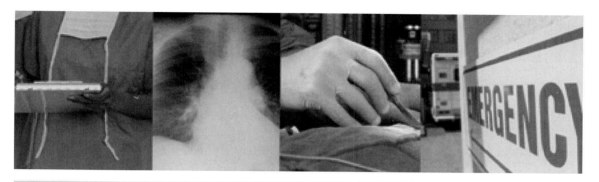

PSYCHOBEHAVIORAL DISORDERS

CHAPTER 35

Psychobehavioral Disorders

JENNIFER M. BOCOCK

KAREL ISELY

CASE *Study*

A 34-year-old man was brought to the emergency department by ambulance after apparently falling in his shower. He was awake, was slightly agitated, and occasionally spoke unintelligible words.

INTRODUCTION

A psychobehavioral disorder is defined as a disturbance in behavior, thinking, or feeling that may result in harm. Aggressive or violent acts, toward others or oneself, may result if external or internal stressors overwhelm the patient's ability to cope. Patients may present with depression, anxiety, aggression, personality changes, hallucinations, or delusions, all of which may be caused or exacerbated by medical and psychiatric conditions. Several studies show high rates of medical illness (24% to 50%) in patients presenting with apparent psychiatric symptoms. Emergency physicians are often challenged in attempting to differentiate medical from psychiatric causes of behavioral disturbances. The need to protect, diagnose, treat, and provide appropriate disposition for these patients is an essential role of emergency medicine.

Epidemiology

Primary psychiatric complaints are seen in 2% to 12% of emergency department visits. When substance abuse and psychiatric illness are included as comorbid conditions with the presenting complaint, the percentage may double.

Treatment of patients with psychiatric complaints in the emergency department is difficult because of several factors:

- Time constraints reduce the opportunity for prolonged interaction between the physician and the patient. Psychobehavioral complaints typically require an involved interview and up to threefold more staff time than purely medical encounters.

- Psychiatric patients more frequently present at night, when staffing and social resources are limited and disposition is often more difficult.
- Psychiatric patients can be uncooperative, unpleasant, and even dangerous both to staff members and to themselves. Nearly 90% of all departments report episodes of violence that have occurred within the past 2 years. In a survey of 170 teaching hospitals, there were 32 reports of the restraint of at least one patient per day, 41 claims of at least one verbal threat per day, and 23 reports of threats involving weapons once per month. A minority of hospitals provide appropriate training for the physicians, nurses, and staff who are managing violent patients.
- Bias, regarding repeat visitors ("regulars") or patients with psychobehavioral complaints, may interfere with care by staff and physicians. Patients with psychobehavioral illness are less likely to comply with follow-up care instructions and have a greater tendency to use the emergency department for their medical needs, both of which leave health care providers frustrated. One emergency department demonstrated that 3% of psychiatric patients were responsible for 20% of the total psychiatric visits.
- Patients and family members are often dissatisfied with the treatment of the patient before the emergency department visit. They may have specific demands or expectations that are either unwarranted or unrealistic.
- A significant percentage of these patients will have an underlying medical condition causing their psychobehavioral presentation, which may be life-threatening if not diagnosed and treated. Three percent to 18% of patients diagnosed with a primary psychiatric illness later had revealed an undetected medical illness contributing to their clinical findings. Elderly patients, when presenting with dementia symptoms, are found to have treatable and often reversible causes of their symptoms in up to 40% of cases. Finally, in one study, 4% of psychiatric study patients who were "medically cleared" in the emergency department required urgent medical treatment in the 24 hours after admission to a psychiatric unit.

Considerable strain and risk develop for the emergency department staff and their patients as a result of these circumstances. Realistic care plans and goals may help manage time and improve patient care in the demanding setting of the emergency department and may include the following:

1. A thorough basic evaluation including psychiatric history, physical examination, mental status examination, and selected laboratory tests
2. The recognition of potentially life-threatening medical illness
3. An organized approach to differentiate organic illness from psychiatric disease
4. The appropriate classification of psychiatric disease within broad categories, with appropriate management and disposition
5. The anticipation and management of violent patients
6. The maintenance of a perspective for patient advocacy
7. Recognition that up to one third of patients cannot be differentiated as having either underlying medical illness or a psychiatric disorder within the time frame of an emergency department visit.

INITIAL APPROACH AND STABILIZATION

Priority Diagnoses

Potentially life-threatening causes of behavioral disorders may include the following:

- Anticholinergic intoxication
- Cerebral hypoxia and hypoperfusion
- Drug or alcohol intoxication and withdrawal
- Electrolyte abnormalities
- Endocrine (thyroid, adrenal) disorders
- Hepatic/renal failure
- Hypertensive encephalopathy
- Hypoglycemia
- Intracranial hemorrhage
- Medications in therapeutic or toxic levels (especially in the elderly)
- Meningitis and encephalitis
- Wernicke's encephalopathy

Rapid Assessment/Early Intervention

1. The first priority is to determine if the patient has an immediate threat to life. Airway, breathing, and circulation are rapidly assessed, as is the level of consciousness. Abnormal vital signs are addressed, and a search for signs of overdose, significant intoxication, or evidence of

injury is initiated. Treatment with respiratory support, oxygen, and resuscitative fluids is initiated as appropriate. Naloxone, glucose, and thiamine are administered as needed for cases complicated by altered mental status.
2. Unless immediate medical intervention is required, the patient is placed in a comfortable, reasonably private room with minimal outside intrusions.
3. If suicidal tendency or violent behavior is suspected, the patient is never left unattended and any potentially dangerous items are removed from the room.
4. Security personnel are notified and are given explicit orders regarding prevention of elopement, when indicated.
5. If the patient is threatening violence or is actively violent and cannot be convinced to cooperate, physical or pharmaceutical restraint may be necessary. Restraints are used to ensure the safety of both the staff and patient and to allow for a thorough assessment and appropriate therapeutic intervention.

CLINICAL ASSESSMENT

The initial approach operates on the assumption that a medical problem is contributing to or is causing the abnormal psychobehavioral presentation. A detailed history with review of systems, past episodes, and current medication list is completed for possible clues to the etiology. Physical examination should be thorough, with special attention to abnormal vital signs. A careful neurologic examination should be completed. Interviews with family, friends, or witnesses of the current episode are recommended. These people are asked to remain in the emergency department or to provide health care provider names and telephone numbers to permit further information gathering. The patient's medical records are requested and may be the only clue to the past medical and psychiatric history, allergies, medication lists, and follow-up care access.

History

Goals when gathering history from the psychobehavioral disorder patient are to determine what the person is thinking and why the disorder is currently emergent, to obtain information about any previous psychiatric history, and to understand the structure and availability of the patient's personal support system.

The quality of the history obtained from these patients depends on the mindset of the physician, the clinical setting, and the structure of the interview. The attitude and biases of the physician greatly influence the exchange of information during the interview. The best attitude is one of "detached concern," with empathy and understanding for the patient without judgment. The setting should be quiet, reasonably private, and nonthreatening. The interview is focused on information gathering, but it also attempts to establish trust. General information questions should be addressed early, leading to more personal, potentially emotional, questions as the interview progresses. The physician specifically determines the following:

1. A description of the *current episode*, including the acuity of onset and the duration
2. A description of *behavior leading up to the current event* and any previous occurrences
3. Any *suicidal* or *homicidal ideations*
4. *Associated symptoms:*
   a. Disorientation
   b. Agitation, insomnia, anorexia
   c. Memory or thought disorders
   d. Hallucinations (visual, auditory, olfactory)
   e. Delusions, phobias
   f. Other
5. A history of *drug* and *alcohol* abuse
6. A place of *employment* and *residence (or lack thereof)*
7. The names of spouse, children, family, friends, or others involved in the *support system*
8. A history of *previous therapy programs, counselors, mental health contacts*, or *psychiatrists*
9. *Past medical or surgical history*, medications, allergies, adverse drug reactions

Mental Status Examination

After obtaining the history and performing an initial screening physical examination, the physician should perform a detailed mental status examination (MSE) on every patient with an emotional disorder. The MSE typically has six components.

Appearance and Behavior. The patient's *dress* and state of *hygiene* are assessed. Is the patient *alert*, and what is the level of *interaction with the environment*? How does the patient *respond to people*? What current *activities* is the patient engaged in?

Orientation. Orientation to *person* (name and address), *place* (name and function of hospital), *time* (day of week, month, year), and situation (evolution of events leading to hospitalization) is assessed.

Affect and Mood. The patient is asked to *describe his or her mood*. The *affect* is noted, as well as the range and any fluctuations. *Anxiety, anger, fear, depression,* and *euphoria* are all considered moods.

Thought. The patient's *thought content* is considered, and the presence of *delusions, obsessions,* or *phobias* is noted. The patient's *thought processes* also are considered ("train of thought") for *appropriateness, logic,* and *chronologic organization*.

Perceptions. The presence of hallucinations, illusions, paranoia, or unusual feelings is assessed.

Cognitive. The patient's immediate, recent, and remote *memories* are all specifically assessed. *Communication skills* are tested by noting vocabulary and language comprehension. *Insight* is screened as (1) minimal—patient acknowledges that a problem exists, (2) moderate—patient understands the nature of the problem, or (3) significant— patient understands why he or she has a problem. The ability to use insight to function in society is considered the *level of judgment*. The patient's thought content is reassessed by considering whether *concrete* or *abstract thought* is being used and by estimating the general level of intelligence.

Mental Status Examination Summary

An efficient way to perform a MSE is described as follows:

1. Introduce oneself to the patient while assessing appearance and behavior.
2. Assess orientation by asking the patient's name, address, current location, and the exact date.
3. Ask the patient to describe his or her mood and observe the affect. (You may need to furnish examples, "Are you happy? Are you angry?")
4. Ask the patient to describe what he or she is thinking as you assess thought processes.
5. Specifically ask the patient whether hallucinations, illusions, or other disorders of perception are present.
6. Start the cognitive assessment by checking the patient's memory: ask the patient to recall your name, what he or she ate for the previous meal, and who was president before the current president.
7. Assess communication and thinking by asking the patient to perform a simple arithmetic set and to explain a common proverb.

8. Assess insight and judgment by asking how the patient views the current problem and how it affects his or her role in society.

Physical Examination

A general physical examination follows the MSE. The patient is told simply and exactly what is going to be done. Undressing is left to near the end of the assessment. Rectal and pelvic examinations are deferred, unless they are indicated.

CLINICAL REASONING

Are These Findings of Medical (Organic) or Psychiatric (Functional) Etiology?

This question directs the preliminary differential diagnosis for the broad presentations of emotional disorders. The information needed to answer this question is usually found in the clinical assessment data (Table 35–1).

History

The onset of the event is the first clue to the etiology. Medical causes frequently have an acute, rapid onset of behavior changes at any age. Psychiatric causes have a more gradual buildup of symptoms, taking weeks to months to reach the point of needing emergency care, and typically begin by the second decade, continuing with the initial symptom presentation ("first break") into the mid-40s. It is extremely rare for schizophrenia or other acute psychiatric illnesses to present, for a first time, after the fifth decade.

Mental Status Examination

The MSE organizes the evaluation of the basic mental and cognitive functioning of a patient. The main elements of the examination include appearance, motor, speech, affect and mood, thought content and processes, perception, insight and judgment, and impulse control. Medical causes often leave the patient with a fluctuating level of consciousness, often accompanied by cognitive change, attention disturbances, and disorientation to time, place, or situation. Primarily, psychiatric patients will often be very alert, almost hypervigilant and, although delusions may be present and their thought processes scattered, their cognitive processing remains sharp. Patients may be anxious and display agitation, with poor immediate memory. Solitary auditory hallucinations are most commonly of psychiatric etiology, whereas visual hallucinations are typical of medical illnesses.

Physical Examination

The examination of the psychiatric patient may be difficult, complicated by the patient's agitation, violence, and inability to understand the need for cooperation. Medical illnesses may present as abnormal vital signs and neurologic abnormalities, and patients may have occult signs of trauma. Primarily, patients with psychiatric disorders often have a normal examination, have normal vital

TABLE 35–1. Clues Gathered from Data that Differentiate between Organic and Functional Causes of Behavioral Problems

Organic	Functional
History	**History**
Acute onset	Onset over weeks to months
Any age	Onset from age 12 to 40 years
Mental Status Examination	**Mental Status Examination**
Fluctuating level of consciousness	Alert
Disoriented	Oriented
Attention disturbances	Agitated, anxious
Poor recent memory	Poor immediate memory
Hallucinations: visual, tactile, auditory	Hallucinations: most commonly auditory
Cognitive changes	Delusions, illusions
Physical Examination	**Physical Examination**
Abnormal vital signs	Normal vital signs
Nystagmus	No nystagmus
Focal neurologic signs	Purposeful movement
Signs of trauma	No signs of trauma

signs, and will display a normal gait with purposeful movements.

It is useful to initially consider that a patient's behavior is caused by a medical condition, because he or she may be treated and the psychiatric condition dramatically improved or resolved. Many patients, however, have findings that will not clearly fit into the division of medical versus psychiatric etiology. Up to 30% of patients with a behavioral problem have elements of both psychiatric abnormality and medical disease. These patients are not easily separated into a single class but belong in a heterogeneous zone. The cause of their disorder is often still ambiguous at the time of disposition.

DIAGNOSTIC ADJUNCTS

Ancillary tests can help to confirm or exclude differential diagnoses of medical causes for behavioral disturbances. At times, a patient's behavior is clearly psychiatric in origin. When there is no suggestion in the clinical findings or MSE of a medical cause, ancillary tests are not necessary. More commonly, ancillary tests are necessary to clarify the origin of the patient's behavioral disturbance. Several studies suggest a more liberal testing be done for patients with new psychiatric symptoms and report a greater than 60% incidence of an apparently contributing medical cause. Patients older than the age of 40, especially the elderly population, are more likely to have an underlying medical illness and will benefit from a more liberal use of laboratory studies.

Screening tests for the medical clearance of all psychiatric patients, before their admission to a psychiatric unit, have been evaluated and have demonstrated limited utility. Careful examination by the physician should lead to appropriate testing use. History alone has been demonstrated to be up to 94% sensitive for medical illness causing behavioral disorders, whereas the use of the laboratory (complete blood cell count, chemistry tests, urinalysis, toxicologic screening, and alcohol level) detected only 20%. Abnormalities on routine screening studies did not result in significant management changes and did not *predict* the need for medical intervention after transfer to the psychiatric unit.

The following tests may be considered for the patient with a suspected medical cause or for those with equivocal signs and symptoms.

Laboratory Studies

Complete Blood Cell Count with Differential. The hemoglobin level indirectly reflects the patient's oxygen-carrying capacity. A low hemoglobin or hematocrit may reflect anemia. An abnormal white blood cell count may indicate an infectious or inflammatory process. An elevated mean corpuscular volume may reflect nutrient deficiency (vitamin B_{12}) or chronic alcohol abuse.

Serum Electrolytes. Both hyponatremia and hypernatremia may present with altered mental status. The bicarbonate level, with calculation of the anion gap, may indicate an acid-base disturbance. Electrolytes are essential in the initial evaluation of ingestion and overdose cases and are helpful for evaluating those patients on medication that may cause electrolyte disturbances.

Glucose. Glucose measurements can be rapidly determined by bedside test strip screening and are confirmed by laboratory analysis. Both hypoglycemia and hyperglycemia may present as bizarre behavior or an altered level of consciousness.

Arterial Blood Gas (ABG) Analysis. If decreased oxygen saturation is found by pulse oximetry, if there is possible exposure to carbon monoxide, or if an anion gap abnormality is calculated, ABG analysis is indicated for the patient workup. Hypoxemia commonly presents as abnormal behavior, and increased P_{CO_2} or carbon monoxide exposure can depress the level of consciousness. pH and Pa_{CO_2} values are necessary for acid-base calculations, including the assessment of physiologic compensatory mechanisms.

Blood Urea Nitrogen and Creatinine. Renal function evaluation assesses hydration status, reveals possible renal damage from ingested materials, and indicates the excretion function of the kidneys.

Urinalysis. The search for an infectious cause of behavioral changes should start with this test, especially in elderly patients. Urinary tract infections and urosepsis are common in this particular population and may present as altered mental status.

Toxicology Screen. The availability of rapid toxicologic testing has increased the usefulness of screening in the emergency department setting. However, in spite of the advances in turnaround time, the toxicology urine screen rarely changes the immediate emergency department management and may be most beneficial to the physician caring for the admitted patient.

Calcium. Hypercalcemia can present as confusion, psychosis, lethargy, or coma. Hypocalcemia can present as lethargy or emotional irritability, along with many other signs. A calcium level is typically included with basic chemistry panels and should be added for complete electrolyte evaluation in these cases.

Ammonia and Liver Function Tests. History or physical findings suggestive of liver disease or hepatic encephalopathy should trigger an evaluation of liver function (transaminases, alkaline phosphatase, total and direct bilirubin). An elevated ammonia level may present as an altered mental status. Abnormal liver function may alter the dosage or the medication choices for some patients.

Thyroid Evaluation. Thyroid disease encompasses many behavioral presentations, including depression, anxiety, agitation, or confusion. Physical clues to thyroid disease should be evident on examination (thyroid masses or nodules, bruits, abnormal vital signs, skin and hair coarsening, and myxedema). The history may reveal heat or cold intolerance, altered sleep patterns, skin or hair changes, weight change, palpitations, and energy level change (increased or decreased).

Specific Drug Levels. The ability to test for toxins and medication levels varies by institution. If the patient is on a medication with a measurable level (such as an anticonvulsant or lithium), one should be obtained. Toxins that may be abused (alcohol, acetaminophen, salicylates) should be tested for in a patient with overdose history.

Lumbar Puncture. Lumbar puncture should be considered in patients when there is suspicion of central nervous system infection (patients with altered mental status, fever, and/or meningismus) and no other explanation of symptoms. An intracranial hemorrhage also can trigger bizarre behavior. There is still debate over the necessity of computed tomography (CT) before lumbar puncture in those with suspected hemorrhages; however, any signs of elevated intracranial pressure should be documented, and it is recommended that a scan be completed and read before lumbar puncture in these patients.

Radiographic Imaging

Computed Tomography of the Head. CT is indicated if the patient's change in behavior was acute in onset, associated with trauma, accompanied by new or focal neurologic deficits, or unexplained by history, examination, or other screening laboratory tests. Patients are evaluated for signs of occult head trauma (e.g., ecchymoses, lacerations, abrasions, hemotympanum, oral or dental damage).

Chest Radiograph. A clinical examination finding or vital sign abnormality that suggests a pulmonary source (low pulse oximetry, unexplained tachycardia, fever, or tachypnea) or initial laboratory results that suggest infection (not identified elsewhere) should trigger a request for a standard chest radiograph.

Other Tests

Electrocardiogram. In elderly patients, in whom myocardial infarction, dysrhythmia, or other cardiac dysfunction can present as a change in mental status, an electrocardiogram is suggested. Evidence of electrolyte disturbances, hypothyroidism and pulmonary embolism may also be seen on the tracing and should be correlated to results of physical examination and history. The electrocardiogram should be routinely used for patients with known overdoses or unknown ingestions, to evaluate cardiotoxic effects of ingested substances, and to assess potential for cardiovascular decompensation.

Electroencephalogram. An electroencephalogram is indicated if the presentation suggests a rare, nonconvulsive status epilepticus, and it is best coordinated with the admitting service and the neurologist on call.

EXPANDED DIFFERENTIAL DIAGNOSIS

A detailed psychiatric differential diagnosis is not the goal of the emergency department assessment. The final diagnosis may take days to determine. Table 35–2 lists many medical diseases that present as psychobehavioral problems. Table 35–3 describes the characteristics of five major psychiatric categories that can be seen in the emergency department.

PRINCIPLES OF MANAGEMENT

The management principles for psychobehavioral patients include

- Establishment of rapport
- Maintenance of situational control, which may include seclusion and physical restraint
- Judicious use of medications
- Evaluation of the patient's social support system
- Maintenance of a realistic perspective of what the emergency department can accomplish

Establishing Rapport

The presenting psychiatric problem is rarely cured during a brief stay in an emergency department. A respectful approach, with genuine concern and interest, will lessen patient or family anguish and will minimize disturbance (confrontation, violence, outbursts) in the department.

TABLE 35–2. Classes of Organic Disease That May Present as Psychobehavioral Disorders

---

Medical (in order of frequency)

Neurologic (e.g., hypoxia, ischemia, mass lesions, degenerative lesions)
Infectious (e.g., sepsis [pneumonia, urinary tract infection], meningitis, endocarditis)
Endocrine (e.g., diabetes, thyroid, adrenal, pituitary)
Electrolyte (e.g., sodium, acid-base, calcium, blood area nitrogen/creatinine)
Nutrition (e.g., thiamine, vitamin B_{12})
Collagen vascular (e.g., systemic lupus erythematosus, polyarteritis nodosa)

Pharmaceutical Use (prescription or "borrowed")

Benzodiazepines	Corticosteroids
Propranolol	Digitalis
Cimetidine	Nonsteroidal anti-inflammatory drugs
Tricyclic antidepressants	Anticonvulsants

Drug Abuse or Withdrawal

Alcohol	Amphetamines
Cocaine	Barbiturates
Opiates	Phencyclidine (PCP)

TABLE 35–3. General Classes of Functional Disorders Presenting as Psychobehavioral Problems in the Emergency Department

---

Affective—Depression

1. Background: Very common; about 20% of female and 10% of male adults have had at least one episode.
2. History: Anhedonia, depressed, sad, hopeless, irritable, anorexia, insomnia, fatigue.
3. Mental status examination: Patient feels worthless or sad; has poor concentration; depressed affect; thoughts of suicide.
4. Physical appearance: Poor hygiene, tired-appearing.
5. If the physician feels sad or fatigued after evaluating this patient, the diagnosis is considered.

Affective—Mania

1. Background: Uncommon, may be difficult to diagnose because of "mask" or episodic nature.
2. History: Increased activity, restlessness, talkativeness, insomnia, euphoria; unusual or risky behavior.
3. Mental status examination: Talkative, hyperactive; flight of ideas; grandiosity; short attention span; irritable; lack of judgment; impulsive; mood lability; hallucinations or delusions.
4. Physical appearance: hyperactive; tired-appearing but still pushing.

Schizophrenia

1. Background: Prodromal, active and residual phases; lifetime prevalence is around 1%.
2. History: Decreased level of performance in some activity; unusual thinking; deteriorating personal relationships; poor volition; withdrawal; psychomotor or bizarre behavior.
3. Mental status examination: Disturbance of thought content and form; hallucinations or delusions; inappropriate and blunted affect; disturbed sense of self; unusual relation to environment.
4. Physical appearance: Disheveled; repetitive psychomotor behavior.

Personality Disorder—Borderline Personality

1. Background: Personality traits that are inflexible, maladaptive, and impair functioning. Borderline personality is common, more often in women than in men.
2. History: Instability in interpersonal behavior, mood, and self-image.
3. Mental status examination: Unpredictable behavior; dysphoric mood or feelings of anger or emptiness; affective instability; identity disturbance.
4. Physical appearance: Signs of self-damaging acts such as suicidal gestures, self-mutilation, recurrent accidents or fights.
5. If the physician feels manipulated, "pushed into a corner," or in a "lose-lose" situation, consider this diagnosis. These patients can make physicians work very hard to meet their unrealistic expectations.

Anxiety

1. Background: Common response to stressful situations.
2. History: Panic attacks, fear, apprehension; dyspnea, palpitations, dizziness.
3. Mental status examination: Apprehensive, anxious, jittery; worries, ruminates; hypervigilant; poor concentration.
4. Physical appearance: Autonomic hyperactivity, trembling, restlessness.

Patients should be made as comfortable as possible and treated respectfully during search, removal of clothing and dangerous personal belongings, and requests for the restroom or for food. No threatening or derisive terms should be allowed by the staff or tolerated from other patients. Confrontation should be kept out of the interaction if possible. Family members should be apprised of any situation changes.

Maintaining Situational Control

In acute psychiatric situations, the patient is seeking to regain control over painful emotions. The hospital environment is a controlled location, and being in the hospital by itself may provide sufficient structure and sense of control to improve the patient situation.

Physicians escalate the control mechanism to match the patient's needs and response to care. Methods of control range from simple use of voice and impersonal physical gestures ("I'm sorry, you can't get out of bed" while at the same time assisting the patient back into bed), to a show of unified force ("These three guards and I will have to help you back into bed"), to actual physical restraint ("I'm sorry you wouldn't cooperate. We must place you back in bed, and will secure you for your own safety"). Establishing control includes judicious use of ancillary personnel including security, patient representatives, social workers, mental health workers, psychologists, and psychiatrists. These workers are often key for controlling situations while patients are in the emergency department and for facilitating efficient patient disposition to other sites for definitive care.

Seclusion and Physical Restraint

The decision to seclude a patient or apply physical restraint can be difficult to make. It is usually based on the need to decrease stimuli, to ensure both staff and patient safety, or to prevent damage to the physical environment. Seclusion or physical restraint implementation criteria are then reassessed at intervals during the entire patient interaction, and the patient is physically monitored and evaluated.

Seclusion includes the placement of the patient into a room *involuntarily* and then preventing elopement by means of a guard or locked door. This may be useful for the extremely agitated patient, those who are acutely suicidal or homicidal, or those with acute psychosis. The patient must be checked frequently (every 5 to 10 minutes at a minimum) and be observed on camera if available. Seclusion may be sequentially eased as behavior improves. Conversely, seclusion may be prolonged or may progress to physical restraint if the clinical situation becomes more serious and warrants more stringent safety measures.

Physical restraint is a difficult clinical choice, because it clearly demonstrates that all previous attempts to defuse the situation have failed. The result is the patient losing control over a portion of his or her dignity. The procedure should be carried out as civilly and as quickly as possible, while assuring the patient that this is for the patient's safety. Restraints should be placed only by those who are trained, to maximize patient and staff safety.

Soft leather or durable nylon four-point restraints are the two types typically provided for use in hospitals. Five staff members are recommended, with a single team leader and a team member at each limb. Optimally, the physician is not part of the restraint team, because this can immediately compromise the physician's rapport with the patient. This situation rarely occurs. The patient should be supine and have all four limbs restrained, with arms at the sides and legs spread. Restraints should be affixed firmly to the bed frame. The circulation should not be obstructed, with one fingerbreadth of space remaining between the skin and the restraint.

Patients who are restrained require frequent patient monitoring for assessment of circulation, skin integrity, vital signs, and toileting needs. The need for continuous restraint should be reassessed by the physician and/or the team leader every 30 minutes. If there is an improvement in the condition, a first step may be taken by releasing one upper limb and then proceeding to the opposite lower limb if continued improvement occurs. Restraint orders are of a limited time duration, and reassessment and reordering are required to continue the restraint. The goal is to move toward less restrictive restraint options if sufficient patient control can be established.

Use of Medication

Pharmacologic restraint may be necessary when caring for patients with acute behavioral disorders. Medication administration may be offered in a voluntary manner or given involuntarily. Medications may be used alone or as an adjunct to physical restraint. The appropriate patient may be given the choice as to the route of administration (oral vs. intramuscular). Oral medications have no role in the case of an uncooperative, acutely psychotic patient.

The three classes of drugs typically used are the butyrophenones, the benzodiazepines, and the atypical antipsychotics. The emergency physician must have a working knowledge of pharmacologic principles, contraindications, and the side effects involved when using these medications. The few specific indications for pharmacologic restraint are

- Relief of psychotic symptoms due to medical or psychiatric illness (may obscure medial causes)
- When patient safety outweighs a delay of diagnosis of acute psychological illness
- To slow the psychological progression of the patient's process
- To stop violent behavior and threatening occurrences, such as spitting, biting, verbal threats, and self-harm by struggling with restraints, or for patient and staff safety during diagnostic procedures

Haloperidol (Haldol) is the butyrophenone antipsychotic of choice. It is indicated for treatment of psychotic behavior in patients, control of the disruptive patient unresponsive to verbal de-escalation or physical restraints, initiation of antipsychotic treatment for those with scheduled follow-up, or control of a psychotic patient transferred to another facility. The initial oral dose of haloperidol is 5 to 10 mg (1 to 2 mg for elderly patients), with onset of action in 30 minutes and a duration of 2 to 4 hours. The initial intramuscular dose is 5 to 10 mg (less for elderly patients), with onset of action in 10 to 30 minutes and a variable duration of effect. A repeat dose may be given every 30 minutes until symptom control is achieved. The average total dose recommended is 4 to 20 mg. It is necessary to reassess the target symptoms every 30 minutes. This evaluation includes level of consciousness, organization of thinking, lessening of anxiety, and cooperation with health care providers. The best target symptom is level of sedation; when the patient becomes drowsy, sufficient medication has been administered.

Droperidol (Inapsine) had been a second choice in the butyrophenone class. Intramuscular doses ranging from 5 to 20 mg have been successful for the control of agitated patients, with a typical intramuscular starting dose of 2.5 mg (or 1.25 to 2.5 mg intravenously) generally resulting in clinical effect, with reassessment and repeat dose in 30 minutes if necessary. Studies show a faster onset of action and a shorter half-life for intramuscularly administered droperidol versus intramuscularly administered haloperidol (similar onset intravenously). Droperidol primarily has sedative and antiemetic effects and does not treat psychotic features.

In 2001, the FDA issued a black box warning about the use of droperidol, because cardiac function abnormalities and dysrhythmias have occurred, with sudden cardiac deaths. QRS complex prolongation may be the basis of these findings, and a premedication electrocardiogram with 2 to 4 hours of monitored observation is currently recommended. Because of these issues, haloperidol is the better clinical choice for current patient management.

All butyrophenones are contraindicated in patients who are pregnant or lactating. They should not be used for overdose of phencyclidine (PCP) and should not be the sole agent used in treating drug or alcohol withdrawal. A theoretical risk of lowering the seizure threshold exists in patients with sympathomimetic intoxication, although clinical studies have not supported this concern. The only absolute contraindications are an anticholinergic intoxication or a true past allergy to butyrophenones. Side effects of butyrophenones include sedation, hypotension, and extrapyramidal effects (dystonia, akathisia, parkinsonism, and tardive dyskinesia). The latter group may be seen in 20% to 30% of patients receiving these drugs acutely. Extrapyramidal side effects are treated with an anticholinergic agent (benztropine, 1 to 2 mg intramuscularly) or an antihistamine (diphenhydramine, 25 to 50 mg parenterally).

The benzodiazepine of choice is *lorazepam* (Ativan), with rapid onset of action orally, intramuscularly, or intravenously; a short half-life; no clinically active metabolites; and a high level of effectiveness. It is especially effective for patients with agitation from drug and alcohol intoxication or withdrawal. A good sedative effect occurs in the acutely psychotic and the severely anxious patient. Lorazepam is dosed in 1- to 2-mg increments (0.5 mg in the elderly) and is titrated to clinical effect, with up to 120 mg (in 24 hours) reported as safe in the medical literature. Target symptoms are monitored at least every 15 minutes, with repeat dosing every 15 to 30 minutes until symptoms are controlled. The best target symptom is sedation. Respiratory depression can occur with high doses. Prolongation of effect occurs in those with hepatic or renal dysfunction. *Midazolam* (Versed) is a second benzodiazepine option, with demonstrated safety, good efficacy with intramuscular administration (less reliable effect with oral dosing), and a much shorter half-life than lorazepam.

The most important risk when using a benzodiazepine is respiratory depression; patients must be closely monitored, especially if they initially require physical restraints. Common side effects also include sedation, nausea, ataxia, confusion, and postdose amnesia.

The combination of butyrophenones with benzodiazepines is more clinically effective than use of either class of drug alone. A study comparing combined lorazepam and haloperidol with either agent used alone for the acutely psychotic patient demonstrated that the combination achieved more rapid tranquilization with fewer side effects (thought to be due to fewer required doses of either drug alone).

Atypical antipsychotics are also used for sedation of the acutely psychotic patient. The oral preparations require patient cooperation, because liquid or oral dissolving formulas predominate. Risperidone (0.5 to 2 mg), olanzapine (2.5 to 10 mg), and quietapine (25 to 100 mg) are first-line choices among oral antipsychotic medications. Chlorpromazine, loxapine, and thiothixene are also available in intramuscular preparations, but 40% to 50% of physicians in a psychiatric emergency service stated that they would not choose these medications in the acute setting.

Support Systems

Patients with psychiatric illness often isolate themselves from family, friends, and society. Alternatively, they may try to stay involved with society but may have a difficult time fitting in with "normal" societal rules and behaviors. For both of these groups, the importance of some type of a support system cannot be overlooked. There may be family members or friends who continue to care for and watch out for the well-being of the patient. Case managers or therapists may follow the needs and service schedules for patients. Religious authority figures or assisted living staff may also be important in these patients' lives and care. If permission is given by the patient, and without breaking confidentiality of the patient case, these people may be of great assistance in the scheduling of follow-up and the daily care of these patients.

Realistic Emergency Department Perspective

The emergency department is a place for the assessment and management of emergent conditions. It is also a place where decisions about hospitalization versus outpatient care must be made, because not all patients can or should be hospitalized. Family members and patients alike may not realize this perspective when they initially present with what appears to be an emergent situation. As clinical situations evolve and change, so do the needs of the patient and the resources available for their use. The use of psychiatric social workers or others extensively trained in the assessment of the acute psychiatric patient may be beneficial in the emergency department setting. They may help to care for patients and best maximize the facilities and services available in the community.

UNCERTAIN DIAGNOSIS

Despite a complete history, physical examination, and adjunctive testing, the exact etiology of a patient's psychobehavioral disorder may remain unclear. In such cases, it is prudent to err on the side of a continuing medical evaluation, assuming a medical etiology until proven otherwise. Also, continuing a combined medical and psychiatric evaluation, with concurrent treatment, is indicated for those with both causes present in the case.

A second issue of concern is that patients with primary psychiatric problems often present with additional vague somatic complaints. Patients with depression may complain of headaches, constipation, weakness, back pain, and other nonspecific maladies, while denying all psychiatric complaints. Somatization is more common among patients who do not have a stable and consistent relationship with a physician, and complaints should be assessed for possible medical cause. Follow-up for evaluation of the psychiatric component of the complaints should also be arranged.

Finally, approximately one third of psychiatric patients seen remain in a sort of "gray zone," where the etiology is unclear but the need for treatment is obvious. Most of these patients warrant admission. If the patient is found safe for discharge, continued psychiatric evaluation continues on an outpatient basis, allowing the necessary diagnostic time for a full assessment of the patient's condition and case-specific therapy.

SPECIAL CONSIDERATIONS

Violent Patients

There are thousands of assaults in hospitals each year, and the emergency department is a site of major risk. Patients can present in an agitated or aggressive state and may become progressively more aggressive and angry while they wait for evaluation. The emergency physician must be prepared to act in a definitive manner to control and secure the violent patient, while anticipating impending escalation of violence. Proactive behavior, for the protection of both the staff and the patient, is often necessary (Fig. 35–1). Anticipation of violence associated with specific clinical disorders or known behavior patterns is also important (Table 35–4).

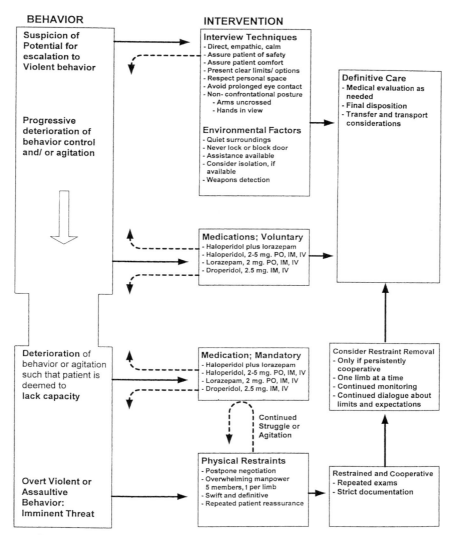

FIGURE 35–1 • Behavior intervention flowchart. *Dashed arrow* indicates refusal or incomplete response to intervention; *solid arrow* shows satisfactory response to intervention.

Verbal de-escalation is typically the physician's first tool, allowing staff to convey concern for the patient's situation and also reassuring the patient of continued safety. Both verbal and physical signals can convey the staff is professional; they want the patient to feel safe, but if necessary they will firmly control the clinical situation. The physician's speech should remain calm, nonprovocative, and empathetic. Patients should be searched for weapons and placed in a secure room that contains no potential weapons or harmful implements. When approaching a potentially violent patient, staff should not carry anything into the room that could be used by the patient as a weapon. Medical personnel should keep a safe distance from potentially violent patients (respect-

ing personal space) and not allow the patient to come between themselves and the door. A panic button or other means of staff safety alarm or monitor should always be in place. Staff members should be calm and nonconfrontational. Prolonged or intense eye contact may increase patient agitation and should not be done. It is important to avoid confrontational body language, such as crossed and folded arms.

Other useful tools for de-escalation of the agitated patient include seclusion in a quiet room, decreased length of waiting, and physical comforts, e.g., dry clothes, a blanket, a cool drink (never hot coffee). The presence of friends or family members may improve or worsen a patient's agitation. They may be included if their presence is

---

TABLE 35–4. Disorders Associated with Violence

Primary Psychiatric Disorders

Conduct disorder and oppositional defiant disorder
Dementia and delirium
Dissociative disorders
Intermittent explosive disorders
Mental retardation
Personality change because of a general medical condition—aggressive type
Personality disorders (antisocial and borderline)
Posttraumatic stress disorders
Premenstrual dysphoric disorders
Schizophrenia, paranoid type
Sexual sadism

Other Causes

Substance abuse disorders
Intracranial pathology causing dementia, delirium, affective or psychotic syndromes, or personality changes (e.g., trauma, infection, neoplasm, anatomic defect, vascular malformation, cerebrovascular accident, degenerative disease)
Medications
Seizure or seizure-like syndromes, including behaviors occurring during ictal, postictal, and interictal periods
Systemic disorders causing dementia, delirium, affective or psychotic syndromes, or personality changes (metabolic, endocrine, infectious, environmental), and other specific disorders

---

From Hill S, Petit J: The violent patient. Emerg Clin North Am 2000; 18:302.

helpful or necessarily prevented from entering until the situation has been defused.

At times, no amount of verbal redirection will render an agitated patient cooperative, and pharmaceutical or physical restraints are indicated. Intravenous or intramuscular doses of combined butyrophenones and benzodiazepines are effective means of sedating a violent patient. If a patient requires physical restraint before the physician evaluation and treatment, an experienced restraint team should be involved in the case. A patient who is struggling against restraints is at increased risk for injury and subsequent rhabdomyolysis and should receive sedation for additional protection.

Pediatric Patients

The principles that apply to adults also apply to children and adolescents presenting to the emergency department with psychobehavioral disorders. Situational crises, suicidal ideation and gestures, affective disorders, and schizophreniform illness are common in children. Medical factors, such as drug toxicity, overdose, metabolic disorders, and trauma, should also be considered in pediatric cases.

Elderly Patients

Elderly patients represent a large percentage of patients who present to the emergency depart-

ment with psychobehavioral disorders. The prevalence of affective and schizophreniform illnesses are high in these patients; however, a medical pathologic process remains the most common cause of altered mental status in the elderly. Up to 40% of elderly patients presenting with obvious cognitive impairment have treatable physical or psychological disorders causing the behavior. All patients with significant cognitive impairment should have a thorough workup, with a complete medical history including medications, physical examination, psychological testing, laboratory assessment, and radiographic analysis when clinically indicated. Table 35–5 lists many medical disorders that may present as psychiatric symptoms.

Another consideration in the elderly population is the high incidence of undiagnosed depression. Medical disease, neurobiology, and psychosocial changes all contribute to the development of depression in the elderly. Clinical symptoms do not clearly correlate with depression in this group, because multiple illnesses and complaints may be concurrent, masking depressive findings. Some sources advocate depression screening for the elderly as part of their emergency department visit, because 25% to 30% of the elderly seen in the emergency department are depressed. Suicide attempts among the elderly have a higher lethality, with a 3:1 ratio of attempted to completed suicide.

TABLE 35–5. Medical Disorders That Can Present with Psychiatric Symptoms

Medical/Toxic Effects	CNS	Infections	Metabolic/Endocrine	Cardiopulmonary	Miscellaneous
Alcohol and drug abuse	Subdural hematoma	Pneumonia	Thyroid disease	Dysrhythmias	Systemic lupus erythematosus
Drugs of abuse	Tumor	Urinary tract infection	Adrenal disease	Myocardial infarction	Vasculitis
Cocaine	Intracranial aneurysm	Sepsis	Renal disease	Congestive heart failure	Temporal arteritis
Marijuana	Hypertensive encephalopathy	Malaria	Pituitary dysfunction	COPD/asthma	Anemia
Phencyclidine	Primary CNS infection	Legionnaire's disease	Diabetic ketoacidosis,	Pulmonary embolism	
LSD	Normal pressure	Syphilis	hypoglycemia		
Heroin	hydrocephalus	Typhoid fever	Hepatic encephalopathy,		
Amphetamines	Seizure disorders	Diphtheria	Wilson's disease		
Jimson weed	Postictal nonconvulsive	Rocky Mountain spotted	Imbalances of Na$^+$, K$^+$, Ca^{2+}		
GHB	status	fever	Vitamin deficiencies		
Prescription medications		Acute rheumatic fever			
(common offenders)					
Benzodiazepines					
Digitalis					
Tricyclic antidepressants					
Corticosteroids					
Anticonvulsants					
Cimetidine					
Propranolol					

CNS, central nervous system; COPD, chronic obstructive pulmonary disease; GHB, gamma hydroxybutyrate.
From Jagoda A, Riggis S: Psychiatric emergencies. Emerg Med Clin North Am 2000; 18:193.

Patients with Suicidal Intent

Approximately 30,000 Americans commit suicide annually, with numbers continuing to rise over the last decade. Suicide is the eighth leading cause of all deaths, the third leading cause of death among those 15 to 24 years old, and the fourth leading cause for those 25 to 44 years. The 15- to 34-year-old group is the most likely to attempt suicide. It is estimated that only 50% of suicides are actually reported and that as many as 20 attempts have occurred for each reported suicide death.

Men are 4 times more likely to complete suicide, whereas women are 10 times more likely to make a suicide gesture. Suicide deaths in men are more likely to be violent, with 50% more frequent use of firearms.

One study has suggested that 50% of patients successfully committing suicide have seen one or more physicians within the preceding month. Other studies have not confirmed this percentage, but a majority of these patients have seen their physician within the past year (75% in the past 6 months). Ninety percent of patients with completed suicides had a history of psychiatric disease, most commonly alcohol abuse and major depression. Many clues should raise the suspicion of suicidal intent during the evaluation of a patient in the emergency department and should be aggressively sought (Table 35–6).

Direct patient questioning with regard to suicidal intent (possible plan and available means) is critical during patient evaluation and disposition planning. Discussing suicidal ideation and intent does not increase the likelihood of completed suicide. The best predictor of completed suicide is a history of suicide attempt. Differentiating a suicide gesture or thought from serious lethal intent is a primary goal.

A risk stratification key, developed for the nonpsychiatrist to assess the potential for a repeat suicide attempt or the need for psychiatric intervention, is the "SAD PERSONS" scale shown in Table 35–7. Patients with a score of 5 or less are considered at low risk, scores of 6 to 8 indicate a moderate risk, and a score greater than nine is considered high risk. Individuals at high risk require immediate psychiatric intervention in an inpatient setting. Approximately 50% of the moderate-risk group require hospitalization, with the remainder safe for outpatient follow-up, whereas low-risk patients can utilize outpatient psychiatric follow-up. The stratification scale has flaws, such as not controlling for the effect of intoxicants on patient responses nor requiring corroboration of the patient's story by family, friends, or other involved health care professionals. Finally, patients may have only a single risk factor, with a low score on the assessment scale, but that factor may be so dangerous that immediate intervention is required. For example, a patient with a stated future intent and access to a handgun would only score a 2 but is a high risk for completed suicide. Clinical judgment is the best indicator of the necessary disposition and follow-up in these cases. If there is any uncertainty as to a patient's potential risk, the case should be discussed with a psychiatric consultant. Protecting the patient is of the utmost importance.

DISPOSITION AND FOLLOW-UP

The disposition of patients with behavioral disorders is often challenging and may be difficult. Psychiatric disorders are chronic, the patients are often uncooperative, and their arrival in the emergency department is often at times when disposition resources are limited. Difficulties are

---

TABLE 35–6. Clues Prompting Consideration of a Patient's Suicide Potential

Single-vehicle, single-driver crash
Accidental ingestion
Risk-taking behavior (walking on freeway, dangerous activities)
Unclear reasons for seeking medical care
Stationary object accidents (e.g., striking a bridge abutment)
No evidence of avoidance attempt in crash, usually motor vehicle crash
No safety equipment used (e.g., seat belts)
Previous history of multiple injuries
Major psychiatric disease (schizophrenia)
Chronic, painful, or debilitating medical illness
Victims of violence (e.g., domestic or sexual assault)
Marked personality changes
Suicidal threats
Social disorder

TABLE 35–7. Modified SAD PERSONS Scale

Category	Points	Description
S = Sex	1	Male
A = Age	1	< 19 or > 45 years
D = Depression or hopelessness	2	Admits to depression or decreased concentration, appetite, sleep, libido
P = Previous attempts or psychiatric care	1	Previous inpatient or outpatient psychiatric care
E = Excessive alcohol or drug use	1	Stigmata of chronic addiction or recent frequent use
R = Rational thinking loss	2	Organic brain syndrome or psychosis
S = Separated, divorced, or widowed	1	
O = Organized or serious attempt	2	Well-thought-out plan or "life-threatening" presentation
N = No social supports	1	No close family, friends, job, or active religious affiliation
S = Stated future intent	2	Determined to repeat attempt or ambivalent about repeat attempt

From Hockberger RS, Rothstein RJ: Assessment of suicide potential by nonpsychiatrists using the SAD PERSON'S Score. J Emerg Med 1988; 6:99–107.

somewhat lessened by the knowledge that the emergency department is not alone in caring for these patients, and support services, mental health resources, and community programs are available for consultation. It is useful to maintain contact with mental health caregivers, to acknowledge their professional skill and the effort they put into the management of these emotionally disturbed patients, and to follow up on the efficacy of clinical referrals.

Admission

Many patients treated in the emergency department are referred to more definitive inpatient care facilities. Patients with mixed medical and psychiatric causes, or an uncertain diagnosis, are usually admitted for continued evaluation and management. Specific indications for admission include

- Initial acute psychosis
- Acute psychosis without remission
- Mania
- Suicidal or homicidal ideation
- Demented patients unable to care for themselves
- Stuporous depressed patients
- Catatonic patients
- Acute anxiety unresponsive to medications

Psychiatric Consultation

When hospitalization or close follow-up is necessary, a formal consultation with a psychiatrist is recommended, usually occurring by phone. The two components of a telephone consultation are the case presentation to the psychiatrist, followed by the assessment and consult responses.

The following information should be relayed to the psychiatrist:

1. Patient's name and vital information
2. How the patient came to the emergency department
3. Brief history of current episode and psychiatric background
4. MSE results
5. Diagnostic impression of the illness. An attempt should be made to fit the presentation into one of the five groups in Table 35–3. If unable to do so, descriptive information should be provided.
6. Resources of the patient, the family, and the emergency department

The psychiatrist should be able to:

1. Provide clarification that a psychiatric problem exists.
2. Focus on the patient's discomfort and the means needed to resolve it.
3. Provide clear communication and aid in reaching agreement on a sensible management plan, with a primary goal of patient safety.

Involuntary Commitment

Many patients with psychobehavioral disorders will not agree to be admitted to the hospital, and the emergency care physician, along with a consulting psychiatrist, will need to intervene and hospitalize the patient involuntarily (involuntary commitment). Involuntary commitment is a difficult balance between the medical need to expedite treatment and the legal right to personal freedom. The emergency care physician should know the state laws and requirements for involuntary commitment. Generally, the patient must be shown to be a danger to himself/herself or others or to be unable to care for himself/herself adequately.

Discharge

The most important factor for the discharge of a psychiatric patient is a clearly arranged follow-up appointment and plan. This information is given to the person most responsible for the patient, and a plan is developed if the patient elects not to keep the follow-up appointment. The plan usually involves the support person calling the primary physician or returning with the patient to the emergency department.

FINAL POINTS

- Known psychiatric patients may have concurrent medical conditions.
- Pure medical problems may present as emotional disorders. Differentiation of psychiatric from medical illness may be difficult.
- The major classes of psychiatric illness must be recognized and therapy begun as soon as possible.
- The cause of behavioral disorders may be psychiatric or medical, yet in up to 30% of patients the cause is mixed or of uncertain etiology. Error should be on the side of further medical evaluation in these cases.

- Although the emergency physician's role is limited, the most important function is to exclude medical causes.
- Consider the potential for suicidal intent with certain types of presentation.
- Do not leave potentially dangerous or suicidal patients unsupervised.
- Ask direct questions regarding suicidal intent, plans, and available means.
- These patients take time and resources, and care extends beyond the emergency department.
- Many of these patients are admitted, some involuntarily, and this requires special communication skills and an understanding of the law.

CASE *Study*

A 34-year-old man was brought to the emergency department by ambulance after apparently falling in his shower. He was awake, was slightly agitated, and occasionally spoke unintelligible words.

The patient was described by the rescue squad as a "known schizophrenic." The patient's mother, who lived with him, had called 911. He was "taking a shower," and she heard a loud "thud in the bathroom" and then found the patient slumped over in the tub. The paramedics noted that the patient was "awake but tired" when they arrived. They mentioned the patient's mother was an invalid and chose to remain at home. A telephone call to her revealed the patient was usually completely compliant in taking his medications. She thought he had gradually been becoming more "emotional" during the week before this apparent fall in the shower.

The gradual onset of confusion directs the investigation toward an organic cause. Trauma is certainly a potential secondary organic factor causing this patient's behavior, with paramedics reporting "awake but tired," but some process seems to be active before the fall.

The physical examination showed the patient fluctuating in and out of consciousness. While awake, he was lethargic, speaking garbled words. His pupils were equal and reactive. He had no obvious facial trauma except for one large abrasion with ecchymosis on the forehead. His neck had no obvious trauma or step offs, but he remained in the cervical collar because of his mental status. He had no obvious chest wall, back, or abdominal trauma. His lungs were clear, his heart rhythm was regular and without murmur. His abdomen was soft, with no obvious pain on examination. Bowel sounds were normal. He moved all four extremities purposefully, and they were without obvious deformity.

The physical findings in this patient are significant in that they provide clues to the possibility of a medical cause for the abnormal behavior. These findings should remove the bias that this patient may be "just another schizophrenic." Historical and physical findings point to a medical cause for the recent change in this patient, and to assume that he is presenting with a psychiatric disorder is a serious error. He did not manifest hallucinations or delusions. He now has this relatively acute incident, was found lying down in the shower, showed signs of recent head trauma, and had a reported change in behavior during the past week. He was lethargic and had no memory of how he fell. With a past history of psychiatric illness but current findings pointing to a medical cause, this patient requires further testing.

Because an organic cause of abnormal behavior was likely in this patient, with an apparent fall in the shower, the working diagnosis was intracranial trauma. The patient's cervical spine radiographs were negative. Computed tomography of the head was ordered and reported as normal.

Because the organic cause is still unexplained, the workup continues, to exclude other metabolic, toxicologic, or neurologic abnormalities.

Orders were issued for a complete blood cell count; determination of serum electrolytes, blood urea nitrogen, creatinine, calcium, and glucose; arterial blood gas analysis; and urine toxicology screen. The clinically remarkable electrolyte values were sodium, 108 mEq/L, and chloride, 85 mEq/L.

Acute severe hyponatremia could explain the patient's presentation, and a serious treatable intracranial hemorrhage was excluded.

Further workup by the admitting physician categorized the patient as euvolemic hyponatremia. Other tests (urine osmolarity, 8 mOsm/L; serum osmolarity, 230 mOsm/L) exclude the syndrome of inappropriate secretion of antidiuretic hormone (SIADH) as the cause of the hyponatremia (although it can present *after* intracranial trauma). The final diagnosis for this event is altered mental status secondary to hyponatremia, caused by psychogenic polydipsia. He was admitted by an internist, and an inpatient psychiatric consultation was arranged.

The emergency department physician telephoned the patient's mother a second time and on direct questioning she revealed that indeed her son had been gulping huge volumes of water for the past week. In fact, he had been drinking water from the shower nozzle when he slipped and fell.

This case demonstrates the mixed organic and functional disorders that may be seen in some patients. This patient's schizophrenia led to a behavior that resulted in an organic disorder, and this organic disorder presented as a psychobehavioral problem.

Bibliography

TEXTS

Allen MH, Currier GW, Hughes DH, et al: The expert consensus guideline series: treatment of behavioral emergencies. Postgrad Med Special Report 2001 (May): 1–90.

American Psychiatric Association: Diagnostic and Statistical Manual of Mental Disorders, 4th ed. Washington, DC, American Psychiatric Association, 1994.

Hyman SE (ed): Manual of Psychiatric Emergencies, 3rd ed. Boston, Little, Brown, 1994.

JOURNAL ARTICLES

Annas GJ: The last resort—the use of physical restraints in medical emergencies. N Engl J Med 1999; 341:1408–1412.

Blanchard JC, Curtis KM: Violence in the emergency department. Emerg Med Clin North Am 1999; 17: 717–731.

Drugs that may cause psychiatric symptoms. Med Lett 2002; 44:59–62.

Jagoda A, Riggio S (eds): Psychiatric emergencies. Emerg Med Clin North Am 2000; 18(2).

Jacobs DG: A 52-year-old suicidal man. JAMA 2000; 283:2693–2699.

Kao LW, Moore GP: The violent patient: Clinical management, use of physical and chemical restraints, and medicolegal concerns. Emerg Med Pract 1999; 1(6):1–24.

Karas S: Behavioral emergencies: differentiating medical from psychiatric disease. Emerg Med Pract 2002; 4:1–20.

Mann AJ: A current perspective of suicide and attempted suicide. Ann Intern Med 2002; 136:302–311.

McCourt JD, Weller JP, Broderick KB: Mandatory laboratory testing for emergency department psychiatric medical screening exam: Useful or useless? Acad Emerg Med 2001; 8(5):572.

Olshaker JS, Browne B, Jerrard DA: Medical clearance and screening of psychiatric patients in the emergency department. Acad Emerg Med 1997; 4:124–128.

Rives W: Emergency department assessment of suicidal patients. Psychiatr Clin North Am 1999; 22:779–787.

Salkin SS: Use of restraints and seclusion in the ED. ED Legal Lett 1998; 9(6):57–68.

Tintinalli JE, Peacock FW, Wright MA: Emergency medical evaluation of the psychiatric patient. Ann Emerg Med 1994; 23:859–862.

U.S. Preventive Services Task Force: Screening for depression: Recommendations and rationale. Ann Intern Med 2002; 136:760–764.

Williams JW, Noel PH, Cordes JA, et al: Is this patient clinically depressed? JAMA 2002; 287:1160–1170.

Zametkin AJ, Alter MR, Yemini T: Suicide in teenagers: Assessment, management, and prevention. JAMA 2001; 286:3120–3125.

CHAPTER 36

Domestic Violence

TERESITA HOGAN

CASE *Study*

A 23-year-old woman presents to the emergency department, at 9:30 AM, stating "I fell down a flight of stairs." She is complaining of pain in her right ribs and left forearm. Further questioning reveals she fell the previous night after losing her balance because she had "had too much to drink."

INTRODUCTION

Definitions

Domestic violence may be narrowly defined as the acute infliction of physical harm by one intimate partner to the other. A broader definition includes psychological abuse, threats, manipulation, coercion, social isolation, and physical or sexual abuse. The term *interpersonal violence* is increasingly used as a synonym for domestic violence. The word "domestic" encompasses all abuse within the extended family setting, including child physical and sexual abuse, spousal abuse, elder abuse, and sibling abuse. Domestic violence includes "family violence," which occurs in both existing and broken families. In fact, most battered women are not wives but are single, separated, or divorced and may be living apart from the batterer (Fig. 36–1).

Both domestic violence and sexual assault have at their root the intent of power, control, dominance, and degradation. The gender neutral term *domestic violence* was chosen over others (e.g., *wife abuse*) to encompass violence against men, elderly, and those in same-sex relationships. Violence against a woman by a male partner is the most common form of domestic violence.

Domestic violence is typically ongoing, extending over many years. On average, 35 battering episodes have occurred before an abused woman reports one assault. This reported event therefore represents a continuous pattern of violence, intimidation, and control over time, not a single act of assault. The intervals between assault are part of the abuse cycle, not a respite.

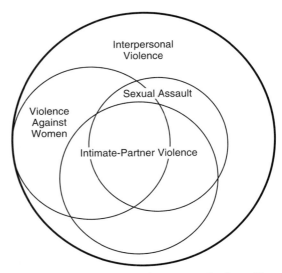

FIGURE 36–1 • Categories of interpersonal violence. Note: Because the exact proportions of these categories are unknown, the areas in the figure are not drawn to scale.

Battering syndrome (or battered woman's syndrome) is the syndrome of dominance and control by the perpetrator increasing the entrapment of the victim. This is a vicious cycle of escalating frequency and severity of recurrent abusive behavior. This pattern may culminate in the death of the victim. Battering syndrome is classified as a form of post-traumatic stress disorder.

Stockholm syndrome requires the presence of additional extreme features not seen in the battering syndrome. The hallmark of Stockholm syndrome is complete monopolization of the victim to extreme, and demonstration of affection for all others, such as children, family, or pets, is forbidden. The batterer expresses omnipotence over the victim by controlling every move, preventing sleep, or any outside contact, including medical attention. Batterers control toileting and claim to know everything the victim thinks and does.

Epidemiology

Basic prevalence and incidence data for domestic violence are difficult to determine, because authorities do not entirely agree on the definitions. Many contradictions exist in patient identification and reporting methods, which leads to an underestimation of the problem. Domestic violence is believed to be the leading cause of serious injury to women between the ages of 15 and 44 years. The annual prevalence in the United States is between 8 and 15 million events, with an annual incidence of 1.9 million women involved. The cumulative prevalence of domestic violence in all women presenting to emergency departments is as high as 54%.

The frightening escalation of domestic violence is highlighted by the following:

- Once initially assaulted, female victims subsequently average 3.1 battery episodes annually.
- Violence by an intimate is more dangerous than stranger violence. Physical injury resulted in 52% of assaults by intimates, but stranger violence resulted in physical injury in only 20% of the cases.
- A home in which any member has been hit or injured in a family fight is 4.4 times more likely to be the scene of a homicide than a violence-free home.
- Fifty-two percent of female murder victims were killed by who was a current or former partner.
- U.S. Justice Department statistics for 1996 revealed that an average of four women are murdered by domestic partners every day.
- Fifty percent of murdered female domestic violence victims are killed in their *own* home.

The lifetime pattern of assault is noted in Table 36–1.

The risk of abuse is highest in adolescents and young adult women. One of every 10 high school students experiences physical violence in a dating relationship. Adolescent girls who are pregnant or currently parenting are very susceptible to domestic violence. More than 70% of this teen population report assaults by their children's father. Date rape accounts for 60% of all reported sexual assaults, the majority occurring in women between the ages of 16 and 24.

Domestic violence affects all socioeconomic groups, ethnic groups, races, and religions. Middle class, well-educated women are frequently battered, but the diagnosis is not considered by health care providers, owing to "reverse" prejudice. Risk factors for domestic violence have been identified and are listed in Table 36–2. Studies conflict with regard to whether victims of adult domestic violence are more likely to have been abused when they were children.

Substance abuse is strongly linked to domestic violence. The strongest factor predicting injury in domestic violence is alcohol abuse by the male partner. Abuse of *both* alcohol and illicit substances is associated with a 16-fold increased risk for suicide, when compared with the risk of people abusing either alcohol or illicit drugs. Illicit drug use increases a woman's risk of dying by family violence 28 times. Approximately 50% of victims report that the abuser was intoxicated at the time of the violence. It is unclear if substance abuse is a direct or indirect factor or simply a modifier of behavior. Nonetheless, substance abuse is not an acceptable excuse for violence; acceptance of this excuse reinforces the batterer's refusal to accept responsibility for his or her actions.

Substance use and abuse can be the cause and the result of domestic violence. It may develop or worsen as an attempt to escape the reality of the violence. Any substance abuser must be questioned about the possibility of victimization, and whether the person loses control, loses his or her temper, or lashes out at others when impaired.

The most dangerous period for battered women is during attempts to end the relationship with the batterer. Women who are separating from their husbands have a 25-fold higher risk of violence against them, compared with those who maintain their marriage. This may help explain why victims are fearful of ending abusive relationships.

TABLE 36–1. Life Span of Abuse

Age of Victim (yr)	Injuries due to Abuse (%)
16–17	34
18–20	42
21–30	35
31–40	26
41–50	24
51–60	17
> 61	18

TABLE 36–2. Risk Factors for Domestic Violence

Pregnancy
Age between 17 and 28 years
Use and abuse of alcohol by either partner
Interracial or interreligious relationships
Separated, divorced, and single women
Partners who have a mental or physical disability
Partners with financial or other dependence, who require support
Wives with educational or occupational status higher than spouse
Husbands with less occupational or wage status than expected

Pertinent Psychology and Sociology

To understand domestic violence, it helps to understand the social and psychological constructs of human relationships. How do victims get into such terrible situations and why do they stay? Why do perpetrators inflict injury on someone they supposedly love? What situations create and propagate domestic violence?

Profile of the Victim

Victims of domestic violence are overwhelmingly of the female gender. The National Institute of Justice has documented that the male partner inflicts more serious injury on the female. Domestic violence is about controlling the behavior of another. Assaults without realistic chance of injury do not wield as much power over the victim as assaults where injury is likely. The lack of physical strength in most women, compared with their male partner, makes physical assault by the male an effective tool for control.

Despite an effort to define a personality type for victims of domestic violence (a person with poor self-esteem or an overly dependent personality), no personality profile is consistently sensitive or specific in predicting who is potentially a victim of domestic violence. This occurs because violence is the result of the actions of the perpetrator, not the victim.

Profile of the Abuser

Perpetrators of domestic violence are predominantly male. A history of witnessing family abuse as children is one risk factor that stands out in the background of abusers. This has been the basis of the "abuse excuse" in famous court cases. Still, domestic violence is ultimately a choice made by individuals who are inflicting systematic harm while attempting to control their partners.

Additional batterer personality traits have been found. Batterers lack assertive interpersonal skills and cannot ask for what they want, nor can they set expectations for others. They tend to externalize responsibility for their negative behaviors, and the victim is frequently blamed for "making" the abuser commit the assault.

Tactics of Abuse

There is a common and recognizable pattern for abusive behavior. Because domestic violence is about power and control, with the batterer wanting control and taking it from the victim, the first step of domestic violence is verbal abuse and destroying the victim's self-confidence. This raises the batterer's status and begins control of the victim's behavior. Verbal abuse may lead to or be a form of emotional abuse.

Emotional abuse may precede or accompany physical violence. Emotional abuse is a pattern of behaviors acted out to maintain the batterer's authority over the victim through fear and degradation. The more extreme the coercion, such as forcing the victim to behave in ways that are against personal, moral or religious principles, the more power the batterer possesses. Emotional abuse takes the form of threats of harm, physical and social isolation, extreme jealousy and possessiveness, deprivation, intimidation, lying, breaking promises, and destroying trust.

Isolation is a common tactic of abuse. The abuser systematically isolates the victim from all forms of support. Any contact between the victim and any supportive person leads to violent behavior on the part of the batterer. The victim may willingly accept isolation to prevent more violence. Anyone or anything that the victim loves can be used as a weapon. The more powerful the love felt by the victim, the more of a weapon that love becomes in the batterer's hands. Beloved pets may be abused or killed to gain control over the victim's behavior. Children are frequently used to control victims, in spite of cultural or legal controls. Court-ordered child visitations with the batterer are often used to control the victim. A woman may know her children are at risk when with a batterer, and the implied threat again imposes behavioral control.

"Cycle of violence" refers to three components common in all domestic violence:

1. Tension-building phase
2. Acute battering event
3. Decline and then absence of tension (the reconciliation or honeymoon phase)

During tension building, the victim is compliant and accommodating as an effort to avoid violence. Despite these efforts, the batterer lashes out with increasing frequency and intensity, until acute battery occurs. This is frequently followed by an interlude when the batterer is contrite, begs for forgiveness, promises an end of abuse, and demonstrates loving behavior. Paradoxically, the victim may become so anxious during the tension-building phase that she precipitates the abuse just to get to the event, ending apprehension. These stages are important to understand, because the victim is amenable to intervention during the first two stages and much less likely to end the situation during "reconciliation."

Reasons Victims Stay

It is difficult to understand why victims of domestic violence stay in these apparently intolerable situations. There are thousands of individual and collective reasons for why victims stay, grouped roughly into five categories: love, hope, dependence, fear, and learned helplessness.

Love is the primary reason initially uniting most couples. Victims often still love their batterers; therefore, the victims make excuses for the batterer, blame themselves for the abusive behavior, and repeatedly forgive the abuse. Victims view the batterer through unrealistic eyes, refusing to believe their beloved is capable of such violence without themselves having a role in prompting it.

Hope that the violence will end, that the promises of reform are real, and that the relationship will again flourish at the original happy state prevents the victims from leaving.

Dependence, emotional and financial, often links victims to their batterers. Batterers use this initial dependence and build it up to extreme levels. The batterer's behavior seeks to increase every kind of dependence to more completely dominate the victim.

Fear is a universal emotion among victims of domestic violence. Constant threats, followed by very real punishment, convince the victim that the abuser has power and will destroy all that the victim cherishes. The batterer strives to make the victim feel responsible for the abuse, therefore controlling the victim's actions.

Learned helplessness is a behavior that occurs secondary to all of the previous factors. Individuals who are tortured by inescapable negative stimuli adapt, allowing the situation to control them. Paralyzing terror occurs at the slightest sign of forthcoming abuse, and the more severe the abuse the more minimal the response becomes.

Reasons for Cover Up

Victims of domestic violence often attempt to cover up the situation, even when seeking medical attention. The reasons for this denial mirror the reasons for remaining with abusers.

- Continued love for the partner
- Fear of retribution
- Lack of other support or alternative shelter
- Immobilization due to psychological or physical trauma
- Cultural and religious values to maintain the family
- Humiliation about the situation
- Self blame and doubt about decision making

- Need to protect the partner against exposure
- Need to protect children from abuse
- Failure to understand the situation and possible danger
- Mistrust of the health care system, society, or legal system

Physician Barriers to Domestic Violence History

Another barrier to the identification of domestic violence comes not from victims or batterers but surprisingly from physicians. Physicians have demonstrated significant issues that may interfere with the discovery of domestic violence.

- *Reverse prejudice*: My patients are not "the kind" to be battered.
- *Cultural indoctrination*: leave private matters private, "what he did isn't so bad."
- *Victim bias*, or believing the patient incited the abuse or will never leave the situation, even when offered assistance.
- *Blaming the victim* is a common theme in society. It absolves the physician of responsibility to help and the batterer of responsibility for the abuse, and it perpetuates the violence.
- *Inadequate training*: failure of education/awareness.
- *Cynicism*: "I've tried this before and failed," or "It is always such an ordeal for me."

Physicians must examine their own experiences with domestic violence. As part of human society, physicians are not immune to this cultural tragedy. Thirty-one percent of female physicians and 14% of male physicians acknowledge previous abuse. Women physicians in particular must deal with their own vulnerability and fear. All physicians should understand their own personal concepts about power and control, especially in context of the family. This will allow improved clinical perspective and delivery of professional care to domestic violence victims without hindrance of personal issues.

Female physicians often identify with victims, but this can evoke a fear response that eliminates violence from the differential diagnosis. Male physicians have different issues that decrease the detection of domestic violence. Primarily, women victims are less likely to disclose the violence to a male physician. Male physicians may appear less interested in the issue and frequently do not consider it in the differential diagnosis. They hesitate to become involved because of a false or convenient belief that the victim does not want to discuss it, or that it would be too painful to discuss. Male physicians are more likely to become frustrated by perceived powerlessness at correcting the situation and the inability to rescue the patient immediately.

Physicians have to prepare to appropriately care for victims of domestic violence. This requires familiarity with the principles discussed in this chapter. Physicians must examine their own attitudes about domestic violence and overcome these biases through education. They can initiate the road to recovery or perpetuate the cycle of violence. Physicians must overcome the obstacles that typically impair an appropriate response to victims of domestic violence.

- Do business pressures prevent taking the time necessary to detect the problem?
- Is there a failure to elicit the appropriate history in spite of obvious clues?
- Is there frustration with the enormity of the task, and failure to take it on at all?
- Is there a reverse bias that inhibits discovery in the white, middle, or upper class patient?
- Does dealing with domestic violence expose personal fears or vulnerability?
- Is there a belief that the victim is to blame?
- Is there a fear of offending patients?
- Is there a fear of the inability to resolve the problem?
- Is there a belief that resolution is only a matter of the victim stopping the violence or walking out?

Education and awareness are the greatest tools physicians have available to protect patient trust and assisting victims of domestic violence.

Importance in Emergency Medicine

Domestic violence is a major cause of injury, disability, homelessness, substance abuse, suicides and suicide attempts, and homicides and homicide attempts. The first contact with the health care system that these victims will encounter is the emergency department. Emergency physicians are in a unique position to identify domestic abuse and to intervene. Battered women account for 22% to 35% of women seeking care in the emergency department. Ten to 15 percent of injured women coming to the emergency department are injured during domestic violence. The remaining 85% to 90% of domestic violence victims present with a chief complaint other than injury.

It is essential that emergency physicians identify victims of domestic violence. Once identified, victims must be treated appropriately, and we are failing on both accounts. Studies show that only 5% of victims seen in a major emergency department were correctly identified as victims of domestic violence. When the violence is identified, treatment of domestic abuse victims is substandard. The emergency physician determined the victim's relationship to the assailant in 25% of cases and assessed the victim's future safety in only 10%, 4% of victims received psychiatric consultation, only 8% received social service referral, and only 2% received information on domestic violence. Victims of domestic violence may present to the emergency department 6 to 11 times before the diagnosis of abuse is finally made. The most significant reason for missed diagnosis is simply a failure of the physician to ask about abuse and to consider the possibility.

There are over 1200 shelters in the United States for battered women. The Centers for Disease Control established the National Center for Injury Prevention and Control in 1992. The duty of this agency is to develop surveillance systems, prevention methods, communication and education programs, and coalitions to support victims of domestic violence in the United States. Most communities have domestic violence hot lines, with additional therapists, support groups, and social service workers trained specifically in this difficult area. Emergency physicians are often the first to access these services for the victims of domestic violence. Without a working knowledge of the available resources, physicians slow their patient's ability to benefit from these essential services.

INITIAL APPROACH AND STABILIZATION

Prehospital Data

Emergency medical services personnel may provide unique clues to identify problems associated with domestic violence and should be trained to look for clues in the home. It is important for emergency services personnel to report observations and suspicions to the emergency department staff and for the staff to actively pursue this information. The only clue to assist discovery of domestic abuse may come from prehospital personnel who are present at the home.

Enhanced Institutional Environment

Once a potential domestic violence victim enters the institution, support should be evident. This support system may counter the negative cultural influences that lead to fear, silence, and mistrust by victims. Evidence a supportive institution exists includes prominent posters on domestic violence in the waiting room (Fig. 36–2). Posters should be legible enough to be read from a

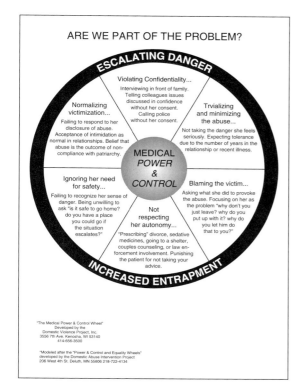

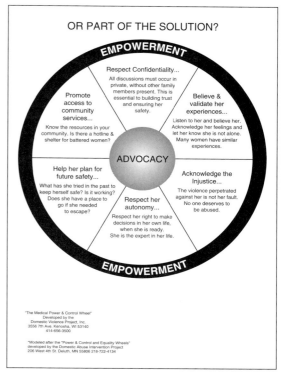

FIGURE 36–2 • Sample domestic abuse poster. (Developed by and used by permission of Pathways of Courage, the Domestic Violence Project, Inc, Kenosha, Wisconsin.)

distance, such that an accompanying batterer may not shield the victims from this information. Pamphlets on domestic violence and referral services should be placed in areas where victims may pocket them without being noticed. Many institutions place pamphlets in the bathrooms, patient care rooms, and other areas where the victim will be unaccompanied and unobserved. Referral numbers should be inconspicuous, printed within recipe cards, on child care materials, or on discharge instructions for various complaints. Ingenious methods for disseminating educational and supportive material have been devised.

Rapid Assessment

The single most effective tool to enhance the detection of domestic violence is the routine screening of all women who present to the emergency department. Domestic violence is sufficiently prevalent to justify routine screening (Fig. 36–3). Although many women will not volunteer the history of domestic violence, they expect doctors to ask about abuse and will admit to it when asked in an empathetic and nonjudgmental manner. Eighty-five percent of Americans reported

that they would tell a physician about domestic violence. Seventy-eight percent of patients surveyed favored routine domestic violence inquiry, but only 7% had ever been asked by a health care provider.

The simple recognition that domestic violence exists and is a concern can make a positive impression on a victim. An example of a supportive opening statement is "Because abuse and violence affect so many of my patients, I've begun to ask about it routinely." A physician's concern validates the victim's feelings and encourages the victim to seek help. Medical contact with the patient may be the only opportunity to stop the cycle of violence.

The Partner Violence Screen (PVS) developed by Feldhaus consists of three questions and requires 20 seconds to administer. The three PVS questions have been shown to detect 71.4% of women identified by the Conflicts Tactics Scale, the gold standard for measuring known domestic violence.

1. *Have you been hit, kicked, punched, or otherwise hurt by someone within the past year? If so, by whom?*
2. *Do you feel safe in your current relationship?*
3. *Is there a partner from your past making you feel unsafe now?*

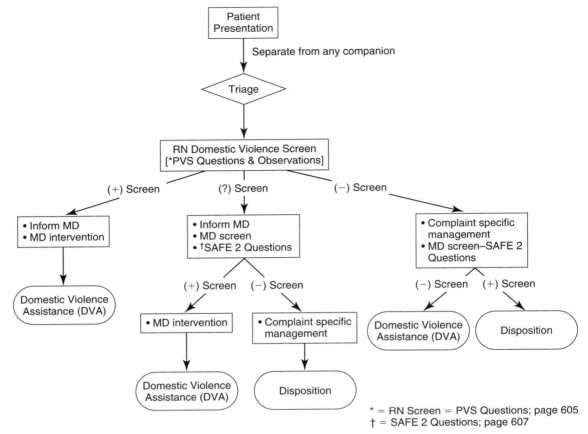

FIGURE 36–3 • Domestic violence screening.

In general, the more extensive a screening tool becomes the more likely it is to detect victims of abuse. Screens that combine questions and staff observation have greater positive predictive value. Objective screening observations (physical indicators and emotional observations) have been described as

- Injuries consistent with abuse (burns, welts, bruises, and bites)
- Defensive injuries of hands or the ulnar aspect of the forearm (blocking blows or stab injury)
- Fractures, dislocations, and other injuries inconsistent with the history of events
- Pattern injuries
- The presence of dried blood or semen
- Sites of injury including the face, throat, breasts, abdomen, genitalia, or bilateral extremities
- Drug toxicity or alcohol intoxication overdose
- A difficult or problem pregnancy
- An inexplicable fear of caregivers, companions, and hospital staff
- A patient who is withdrawn, fearful, or depressed
- Observed verbal abuse or threatening gestures toward patient, by the companion
- Suicide attempt

Screens are useful because they enforce the systematic, institutional implementation of appropriate questions for a large population of women. A screen provides the physician with a standard set of validated questions designed to detect domestic violence.

Early Intervention

Stabilization of life-threatening injuries must be provided, with initial attention to the ABCs of resuscitation. The physician must diagnose and treat physical injuries, plus any other medical, surgical, or psychiatric problems that coexist. Most victims of domestic violence present with stable vital signs and do not have immediately life-threatening injuries. Young (< age 35) female trauma patients with head, neck, and face injuries not due to motor vehicle accidents often are found to be victims of domestic violence. An astute physician is aware that domestic battery usually manifests as trauma to the central body and head, and careful evaluation for intracranial and intra-abdominal trauma should occur.

CLINICAL ASSESSMENT

History

Once the patient is assessed and all acute problems are stabilized, the emergency department staff must provide a safe environment with an opportunity for private and compassionate conversation for the disclosure of the abuse, a complete history, and appropriate interventions. Adequate time for all of this must be ensured by the physician and staff.

If a translator is required for communication, anyone accompanying the patient should not serve in this capacity. Family and friends are often the most convenient translators, but their personal involvement severely restricts patient privacy and may prevent reporting.

If it is necessary to question family members, this should be done cautiously. The batterer may be among those questioned, and other family members may be placed in danger. Questions should be direct but open ended, such as "Mary seems frightened, do you know why?"

If the physician's ability to maintain confidentiality is limited because of mandatory reporting requirements, the victim should be made aware of these requirements early in the encounter.

Domestic violence victims are often difficult to detect, presenting with a multitude of shielding complaints to cover up the abuse. Also, victims may be unaware of the physical and psychological toll caused by abuse or may be in denial about the situation. There are approximately twice as many presenting complaints relating to illness or stress versus actual domestic injury (Table 36–3).

Key Identification Questions

Questions have been developed to assist in the identification of domestic violence. Although the following list is instructive, all questions should be asked in the physician's own words, with appropriate follow-up questions for best effect and situational adaptation.

General Questions

- How are things at home?
- Do you and your partner fight?
- Does this fighting ever become physical?
- Have you been hit or harmed in the past year?
- Are you, or have you ever been, in a relationship in which you have been physically hurt or threatened by your partner?
- Are you, or have you ever been, in a relationship in which you believed you were treated badly? In what ways were you treated badly?

- Has your partner ever purposefully destroyed things that you cared about?
- Has your partner ever forced you to have sex when you didn't want to? Are you ever forced to engage in sexual activity that makes you feel uncomfortable?
- We all fight at home. What happens when you and your partner fight or disagree?
- Sometimes we see injuries like this after couples argue. Is this what happened?
- Do you ever feel afraid of your partner?
- Has your partner ever prevented you from leaving the house, seeing friends or family, getting a job, or continuing your education?
- How does your partner act when drinking or on drugs? Is your partner ever abusive verbally or physically?
- Do you ever feel upset that you or your partner abuse alcohol or drugs? Why?
- Do you have guns in your home? Has your partner ever threatened to use any weapon against you when angry?
- Is there a partner from a previous relationship who makes you feel unsafe *now*? (To ensure you don't miss victimization by a past relationship.)

A second technique is to elicit a history of domestic violence with the use of the mnemonic SAFE-2.

S: *Stress/Safety*. What stress are you under at home or with your partner? Do you feel safe?

A: *Afraid/Abused*. Do you feel afraid of anything or anyone? Do you feel abused or taken advantage of, or are you hurt emotionally or physically by anyone? (*Note:* the victim may not understand the word "abused" as intended. Make every effort to use other words or phrases that are very specific identifiers of abuse, allowing the patient to avoid using the label, because the label itself may be a barrier.)

F: *Friends/Family*. Do you have friends or family you can rely on? Do friends or family hurt you? Are you afraid for any of your friends or family?

E: *Emergency/Escape*. Do you have the ability to escape, get out of this situation, or get to a safe place? Does your partner prevent you from seeing people or doing what you need to do? Does your partner keep you isolated? Are you in an emergency or dangerous situation now? How can I help provide an escape plan for you?

TABLE 36–3. Shielding Complaints Offered by Domestic Violence Victims

---

Physical Symptoms Related to Stress

Sleep disturbances
Appetite disturbances
Fatigue
Decreased concentration
Sexual dysfunction
Chronic headaches
Abdominal and gastrointestinal complaints
Palpitations
Dizziness
Paresthesias
Dyspnea
Atypical chest pain

Vague Medical Complaints

Gastrointestinal complaints without organic basis
Any complaint unsupported by history, physical examination, or laboratory findings

Substance Abuse

Alcohol
Minor tranquilizers
Pain medications

Chronic Pelvic Complaints

Vaginal pain
Urinary tract symptoms
Dyspareunia

Psychiatric Complaints

Anxiety
Depression
Suicidal ideation

Frequent Repeat Visits

Homelessness

Pregnancy-Related Complaints

Little or no prenatal care
Preterm bleeding
Miscarriage
Self-induced abortion

Questions to Be Avoided

It is important to note the types of questions to avoid asking. These questions may lead to further isolation of the victim, imply judgment and blame that further demean the victim, and perpetuate the abuse cycle. The victim's perception of shame and worthlessness may be aggravated by using certain words, such as "domestic violence," "abused," and "battered." These words may be negative stigmata for the victim and should be avoided. Words such as "hurt," "frightened," or "treated badly" should be substituted. Do not ask:

- Why do you stay in the situation?
- Why don't you leave your partner?
- Why do you keep going back to your partner?
- What did you do to that caused your partner to hit you or want to hurt you?
- Why are you here if you aren't going to take our advice?

Danger Assessment

Once identified as a victim of violence, the patient also should be asked the following questions.

These may be addressed by other health care providers, but the emergency physician should be aware of their importance.

- What is the exact nature of the violence (physical/sexual) that occurred?
- Were any weapons involved? Is a gun accessible?
- How long has the violence been occurring?
- Is the pattern of violence changing (escalation)?
- What triggers the violence?
- Is there anything different about the violent episode today?
- When was the last act of violence or abuse?
- Is anyone else a victim or at risk of becoming harmed?
- Are children being abused or witnessing the abuse to yourself?
- What is the victim's state of mental health (any psychiatric issues)?
- What is the batterer's state of mental health (any psychiatric issues)?
- What is the victim's ability to cope with the abuse?
- Does the victim have accessible support systems?
- Does the batterer have accessible support systems?
- Does either the victim or batterer use or abuse any substances?
- What is the relationship of substance abuse to the violent events?
- Does the victim function at home and work or at school?
- What efforts has the victim made to end the abuse? Was there any effect (positive or negative)?
- Does the victim want medical, social service, clerical, law enforcement, or legal assistance?

An expanded social history should be taken addressing the relationship of the batterer to the victim, the exact living situation for each partner, and the number of residents in each household. The legal relationship between the partners and the legal status of all children in the household should be well understood by the physician and social service providers.

A substantial delay between the injury and the presentation for treatment may be a mechanism of defense for the victim or may be further coercion and abuse by the batterer. Noncompliance with treatment plan, failure to obtain or take medication, and failure to keep follow-up appointments may be evidence of continued manipulation and isolation by the batterer.

When the history of domestic violence is volunteered, the physician must respond appropriately. The patient may be in an extremely dangerous situation as the victim risks the disclosure of the situation, and physicians must understand the degree of danger that exists for the victim.

Physician Interaction with the Batterer

The physician may have to discuss the violence and battery with the abuser. It is smart to have protection available for all involved during these events. The initial approach of the discussion should be nonjudgmental. The CAGE questions, developed for alcoholic screening (see Chapter 16, Alcohol Intoxication), may be adapted for optimal dialogue with the batterer.

- Do you ever have trouble with anger?
- Have you ever done anything while you were angry that you regretted later?
- Has your anger ever gotten you into trouble?
- Have you ever tried doing something to help you deal with your anger?

Physical Examination

A complete physical examination is performed with the patient fully disrobed to uncover injuries the patient may be hiding. Too often, the diagnosis of domestic violence is missed because the focal site of the chief complaint (sprained ankle, sore wrist) is all that is examined. We accept the brief, simplified history, "I tripped," and we do not search for, or discover, the multiple other injuries that are obvious or concealed.

When a history of abuse is given, an attempt is made to correlate physical findings with the patient's history of the event. Specifically, the areas of chief complaint are examined to corroborate the patient's history and the mechanism of injury. If the patient was hit in the face, then the head, face, and neck are examined for injury from hyperextension or flexion.

A complete head-to-toe examination should be performed. The back, buttocks, and perineum are examined, and inquiries about potential sexual assault are made.

Injuries characteristic abuse patterns include

- Bilateral injuries that are symmetric of the upper and lower extremities, head, face, or torso. Upper arms and wrists are examined for restraint injuries caused by the forceful grasp of the abuser. The ulnar aspect of the forearms is evaluated for injury indicating self-defense.
- Injuries at multiple sites and varying degrees of healing, especially if not consistent with a single mechanism
- Fingernail scratches, cigarette burns, rope burns, or ligature marks

- Abrasions, minor lacerations, or welts at multiple sites
- Pattern injuries described as marks, designs, stamps, or imprints that are transferred by the force of impact from a blunt object onto the skin of the victim during a hard blow
- Contusions in the pattern of a shoe sole or heel (kicking or stomping)
- Circular contusions, particularly those that are perfectly circular
- Parallel contusions with central clearing (strikes by rods or sticks)
- Slap marks (marks suggesting the open palm or finger) and grasp marks (contusions in the pattern of a closed hand)
- Bite marks that are clearly apparent or appear as only a clear semicircular contusion or abrasion

CLINICAL REASONING

Has Appropriate Screening for Domestic Violence Been Completed?

Domestic violence screening should be a part of the evaluation of all female patients in the emergency department. The initial screen should include a series of open and nonjudgmental questions for every female patient. Partner Violence Screen (PVS) questions are validated for this purpose and may be universally asked of all women during triage. Additionally, the triage nurse should also document nonverbal and behavioral observations that may correlate with domestic violence. PVS observations include interaction between the patient and any companions, physical findings consistent with abuse or nonconsistent with the chief complaint, demeanor consistent with abuse, and any coercive or abusive behavior by the companion. An algorithm for domestic violence screening is presented in Figure 36–3.

Has the Health Care Provider Supported and Encouraged the Patient to Reveal Potential Domestic Violence?

For screening to be effective, it must be conducted in a private and safe environment. Patients should be separated from companions for the initial triage, and companions may be sent to the registration desk. Every attempt should be made to have private question and examination periods with the patient that arouse no suspicion. Possible opportunities are during physical examination, in the radiology suite, or during other evaluations and treatments.

What Are Appropriate Actions for Positive Results on Violence Screening?

Domestic violence victim assistance should be a part of the emergency department service. Even if the triage screen is negative, the physician should perform a second screening during patient evaluation. When the emergency department chart is restructured with the inclusion of specific domestic violence questions, there is a significant increase in the recognition rate of domestic violence. The PVS or SAFE-2 questions are useful tools. Screening by the nurse and physician will highlight the commitment of the system and the ability to help victims. The average patient may need to be questioned multiple times before the chance of domestic violence disclosure is forthcoming.

DIAGNOSTIC ADJUNCTS

There are no diagnostic tests for domestic violence. Do not confront a patient with studies and results or use that information in an accusative manner.

Screening examinations for pregnancy and sexually transmitted diseases are important for the continued reproductive health of these patients. The patient must be allowed the autonomy to select the services she wants provided for her benefit. Concerned physicians should discuss the health consequences of pregnancy and sexually transmitted diseases with the patient and allow her to choose evaluation and intervention that she finds appropriate. If a pelvic examination is being conducted for other medical reasons, screening for sexually transmitted diseases and pregnancy should be completed as a routine part of the examination.

Radiologic imaging may be ordered to screen for fracture patterns that are consistent with abuse, and information on both acute fracture and old healed trauma is useful. Multiple old fractures, fractures of varying ages, or poorly aligned, partially healed fractures are suggestive of abuse. These films and their findings may be used in an open and frank discussion with the patient about the strength of the examiner's suspicions, the severity of abuse, and the victim's options for assistance.

PRINCIPLES OF MANAGEMENT

General Principles

The victim's emotional status also is evaluated, and treatment is evaluated for emotional injuries. The first step is conveying the message that the victim is not at fault. It is also important to provide assurance, state that domestic abuse is not acceptable, and advise the patient about available options for care and support.

Domestic violence is a tragically common problem, affecting millions of innocent and intelligent people. Victims need to be told that they are not alone and that there are many resources and experts available to help because the problem is so common. The ability of the emergency department staff to communicate with patients may stop the victim from remaining in the violent situation and look for help and begin healing.

Appropriate intervention lowers the risk of post-traumatic stress disorder and other long-term sequelae of domestic abuse. The large prevalence of domestic violence indicates the need to provide appropriate backup services, such as after-hours social services and 24-hour hot-line help.

The role of social services in the emergency department is critical. Interventions for domestic violence situations are time intensive and require undivided attention. The emergency department staff are not able to provide victims with the time needed to initiate appropriate intervention, and social services personnel may provide the time, allowing the victim to trust the system and prevent a lost opportunity for help. Some emergency departments have enhanced success by providing emergency advocacy services, resulting in increased use of shelters and shelter-based counseling. Advocacy can provide the link between the emergency department and community services essential to the treatment of victims of abuse. When the emergency department staff partners with advocacy groups, long-term comprehensive services can be provided.

Information and evidentiary materials are collected following the appropriate chain of evidence rules. Notification and release of information to the authorities must be provided and is legally required. The patient must be aware of these notification requirements. In states where reporting is not mandated, the victim's right to refuse notification should be respected.

Documentation is especially important in cases of domestic violence. The coordination of resources for counseling and follow-up, assurance of patient safety, and involvement of the legal system all require appropriate documentation.

Photographic Evidence

Photographing visible injuries for the medical record is an important option. Photographs require a scale reference, such as a ruler, as an indicator of size. The patient's face is included in at least one picture, because it must be clear the injuries exist on this patient, specifically. Photographs follow the "chain of evidence," as does other physical evidence from the patient. Requirements specific to the institution, including documenting the evidence, tagging clothing, or completion of the sexual assault kit, should be clearly understood. All evidence collected must be appropriately labeled with the patient's name, date, time, medical record number, physician's name, and the name of a witness to any photographs.

Consents from the patient or others where appropriate should be obtained and documented.

UNCERTAIN DIAGNOSIS

In the vast majority of cases, patients do not volunteer the history of domestic violence. The dynamics of domestic violence and the emotional incapacitation it causes typically prevent the victim from volunteering this information. The physician and emergency department staff need to uncover this difficult history. The batterer may refuse to leave the patient and may insist on answering questions for the victim. The physician or emergency department staff should find a nonthreatening way to document the history of the abuse in private.

Abuse that is not identified or addressed during the emergency department encounter may increase the sense of entrapment and perpetuate victimization. Misdiagnosis of domestic violence sequelae as psychiatric illness may lead to inappropriate hospitalization and medication. The use of tranquilizers or sedative medications impairs the victim's ability to defuse an abusive situation, protect herself and her family, or flee the scene if necessary. Inappropriate prescription of medications may initiate or perpetuate drug abuse, particularly in a vulnerable population. Missing this diagnosis exposes the patient to further abuse, which may result in serious morbidity (emotional or physical damage) and higher mortality.

If the diagnosis of domestic violence cannot be confirmed, the history-taking technique should be reviewed. What questions may enhance the likelihood that an abuse history will be confirmed? How was the patient approached? Was the interview in a private setting? Did body language and appearance indicate time and interest in what the victim had to say? Was the questioning nonthreatening and nonjudgmental? What can help a patient feel safe and disclose the violence?

The following are ways the physician can attempt to help a victim of abuse:

1. Define violent behavior as unacceptable and a criminal offense.
2. Explain that the violence is solely and unequivocally the responsibility of the batterer.
3. Communicate the high prevalence of this abuse and the incidence among women of all backgrounds.
4. Communicate concern for the victim's safety.
5. Inform the victim of the many expert assistance programs that are freely available.
6. Advise the victim that the violence will not stop as long as the victim remains within the relationship.

Be patient! It is frequently enough to let victims know there is help available. The cure for domestic violence is a process that may require years to evolve and complete. It is unrealistic to expect immediate resolution or an immediate response to domestic violence. The following therapeutic messages may be beneficial:

- No one deserves to be battered.
- Domestic violence is not the victim's fault.
- Domestic violence is common and affects millions of innocent, intelligent women.
- No victim is alone; help is always available.
- Victims have options; people do care.

It is the victim's decision when it is safe to leave an abusive situation and there are sufficient emotional and economic resources to do so. It is the physician's job to provide the victim with housing options, social support, and resources she can easily access. This should be done with compassion and in a manner that ensures safety. If abuse cannot be confirmed, let the patient know that resources exist if the need ever does exist.

SPECIAL CONSIDERATIONS
Pediatric Patients

Child abuse is an intricate and involved subspecialty topic, and the focus here is limited to children in the context of domestic violence and will not include the greater topic of child abuse.

Children are often the silent victims of domestic violence. Approximately 85% of children in violent homes are direct witnesses to assault. In 30% to 54% of domestic violence cases, the children are assaulted, with 15% sustaining injury. Children of battered women often demonstrate significant behavioral problems, including acting out, poor school performance, substance abuse, learning disabilities, depression, and inappropriate withdrawal or aggression toward other children or adults.

Extending coercive tactics to include children is often part of a relationship with ongoing battery. As many as 70% of batterers will also abuse their children, which is referred to as *tangential abuse*. The batterer hurts and controls the mother through harm inflicted on the children. In 25% of abuse cases with a woman murdered by an intimate partner, the event is witnessed by a child or a child is injured or murdered. One half of these murders occurred in the home of the victim. Case reviews of abused children reveal that one half of their mothers are also abused.

Witnessing domestic violence during childhood legitimizes and reinforces this as a pattern of adult behavior, and the child adapts to this as a learned response. It is seen as an appropriate way to manage conflict, primarily interfamilial conflict, projecting a moral acceptance of hitting other family members. These children become confused about the concepts of love and violence, beneficence and pain.

Physicians must be very concerned about the safety of the mothers of abused children. Studies show that up to 60% of mothers of abused children are themselves abused, causing a severe strain on both the mother and the physician. When dealing with the issue of child abuse, both of these adults, mother and the physician, primarily care for the interests of the child. Physicians must realize there is an additional obligation to the mother. The discovery of child abuse may be a trigger for violence by the batterer, and the mother may be at extremely high risk during this time.

Elderly Patients

Many authorities prefer the term *elder mistreatment* to *elder abuse*, because this term encompasses acts of commission or deliberate abuse, as well as acts of omission, inadvertent actions, and intentional neglect that result in harm to the elder person. Unintentional mistreatment may be caused by ignorance, inexperience, and lack of ability or lack of desire to provide proper care. This term includes physical, emotional, psychological, and sexual abuse, as well as financial exploitation, neglect (intentional and unintentional), and abandonment. Careless or neglectful caregivers and children may unwittingly inflict some forms of elder abuse. Physician education about elder abuse and immediate reaction is pivotal for the identification, treatment, and prevention of elder abuse.

The extent of elder abuse is large, with an estimated 2 million persons older than the age of 60 abused annually in the United States. Neglect is the most common type of elder abuse, comprising more than one half of these cases. Elderly women report a large incidence of domestic violence. Thirty-three to 50 percent of women older than 70 years of age report they suffer some form of abuse. In the elderly, abuse escalates when victims develop illness or disability. The numbers of elderly abused patients are projected to rise dramatically with the aging of the population. One of every eight Americans is predicted to be older than age 65 by 2010. The elderly suffer abuse at the hands of their children, partner, or hired caregiver. Risk increases when family supervision of, and interaction with, the caregiver is minimal. Elders may decide living with an abusive partner is preferable to loss of independence and placement in a nursing home, thereby increasing their risk for abuse. Falls are more likely to occur in the elderly population, and this history is often accepted as fact, when the patient was actually pushed or beaten. Osteoporosis and other chronic diseases may make the frequency of poorly explained fractures easier to accept.

Cognitive status is important when considering abuse of the elderly. Mild cognitive impairment is often unrecognized in the emergency department setting, and screening for impairment with the Mini-Mental Status Examination is suggested. Once cognitive impairment is recognized, it can be classified and identified and decision-making capacity can be assessed. Patient cognitive impairment greatly increases the strain on the caregiver, predisposing abuse and decreasing the elder's ability to report abuse while raising questions about the credibility of such reports.

Physicians who care for nursing home residents have a critical role in the identification, treatment, and prevention of elder abuse. In the long-term-care setting, a number of people can inflict abuse, including employees, other residents, visitors, or intruders, thus complicating the identification of the problem. Emergency physicians must be aware that substandard care or neglect can result in declining health, deterioration, mental status, pain, and emotional trauma for the nursing home patient. When abuse is suspected, it is appropriate to discuss the plan of care with the patient's private physician to ensure that it is carried out appropriately.

Elder abuse is defined by state laws, which vary from state to state. However, in all 50 states it is mandatory that elder abuse be reported. All health care workers providing care in the homes of elderly patients should be on the lookout for behaviors that signal elder abuse. Adult protective services generally include statewide systems with the ability to immediately investigate elder abuse complaints, including emergency services, evaluation, counseling, and relocation of the individual to a safe setting. All physicians should know the resources available in their state and that every institution has access to these resources. Every state has a long-term-care ombudsman program, established by the Older Americans Act of 1978, mandating regular on-site visitation of nursing facilities, to ensure compliance with minimum standards. This act was amended in 1987, and additional nursing home reform legislation was enacted with quality of care requirements for resident health care and assessment defined (necessary for Medicaid and Medicare participation). Many states have toll-free elder abuse hot lines. When patients have additional mental or physical disabilities, a second resource may be used, the Disabled Persons Protection Commission's Abuse Reporting System, also state-based. Most states have groups that oversee issues on aging and have adult protective service agencies, which are valuable resources for the physician. State groups often accept reports on nursing homes and other institutions and conduct appropriate evaluations of the neglect or abuse allegations. A listing is available through the American Medical Association (www.ama-asso.org).

Victims of Sexual Assault

Sexual assault is a crime of control and violence, when sexual contact and sexual acts are committed against the will of the victim. The incidence of sexual assault is 1.6 per 1000 people (male and female) older than 12 years of age and 3 per 1000 females older than 12 years of age. The sexual assault of boys is much more difficult to discover and should be considered in the emergency department. It is estimated that between 3% and 5% of boys in the United States have had prepubertal sexual contact with an adult male. Assault rates were highest, per capita, among 16- to 19-year-old urban low-income women. In 75% of cases the perpetrator is a family member, intimate partner, or an acquaintance. One third of the cases are reported to the police, and in 16% of the cases a lethal weapon (gun or knife) in involved. Approximately 1 in 1000 rape victims die secondary to the assault. Of the surviving victims, approximately one third have repetitive bouts of severe depression and one third develop post-traumatic stress disorder.

The presentation of the patient in the emergency department is often the first contact with health care after the assault. All victims receive medical care, whether they decide to pursue legal recourse or prefer law enforcement not to be summoned. All evidence is preserved with a sexual assault kit, and the clothing from the attack is also included for evidence testing.

In the emergency department, the medical, psychological, social, and legal needs of the patient are addressed. A quiet and private location is found, and family or friends may remain in if the victim requests. A rape-crisis counselor or SANE (Sexual Assault Nurse Examiners) nurse may be requested to accompany and advise patients.

The history is brief, limited, and focused. The name of the patient and the person providing the history is included (especially if the patient is unable to give a history or the event was witnessed). Quotations are utilized as needed for the assault description; date, time, and location of the assault are documented.

The assailant(s) size, height, race, speech pattern or accent, clothing, and any other remarkable features are noted. All acts of the assault are described, including masturbatory or oral contact and penetration (oral, vaginal, or anal) by any body part or foreign body. Methods of control or assault are documented (restraint, physical blows, weapons, threats, or harm).

Any sites of injury or pain are described. All events or hygiene attempts, after the assault, are documented. The pertinent gynecologic history (last period, any perineal or genital injuries or surgeries, last consensual intercourse act) is documented.

Evidence collection must be preceded by a completed informed consent. Evidence for the sexual assault kit is collected methodically, to meet evidentiary standards established in 1987. All injury (bruising, bites, and lacerations) sites are documented, and a body diagram is completed. If needed, photographs should be taken before the patient leaves the emergency department.

All clothing is placed in paper bags. Nail scrapings, secretion scrapings, hair (head and pubic) samples, and foreign debris (dirt, twigs, and fabric) are collected and labeled. An ultraviolet light source may illuminate moist or dried seminal fluid on the victim's skin. Oral, genital, and rectal swabs are collected. The oral cavity, external genitalia, vagina, perineum, and rectum are examined for any injury (bruising, swelling, skin tears, and lacerations). A colposcopic examination is encouraged, improving the yield of findings on examination, and the findings are recorded for legal use, if needed.

The assault kit is sealed and packaged according to chain of custody evidence protocol. When charges are filed, the kit is documented, signed to an officer, and subsequently delivered to the appropriate crime laboratory. If the chain of custody is lost or broken, the kit cannot be used as evidence. Additionally, medical specimens (as well as legal evidence) are obtained, including tests for pregnancy, *Chlamydia* and *Neisseria gonorrhoeae* infection, human immunodeficiency virus (HIV) infection, syphilis, and hepatitis. Current prophylaxis recommendations from the CDC for sexually transmitted diseases include

- Ceftrixone, 125 mg intramuscularly
- Doxycycline, 100 mg, two times per day, orally, for 7 days
- Metronidazole, 1 g in a single oral dose
- Ethinyl estradiol/norgestrel (Ovral), 2 tablets orally, with dose repeated in 12 hours (total dose: 4 tablets) is the preferred current regimen.

Current pregnancy prevention regimens should be started within 24 hours of assault (absolutely no later than 72 hours). Side effects may include breast tenderness, nausea, and vomiting.

HIV exposure is of serious concern for these victims. HIV testing is not best completed through the emergency department for many reasons. Extensive counseling (before and after the test), confidentiality, and follow-up complaints are frequently cited. HIV prophylaxis has not been shown to be effective, because seroconversion after sexual assault has a very low occurrence rate. It is in the best interest of the patient to receive basic counseling, information on testing, and a referral to a women's health center or assault center for comprehensive care.

Physiologic and social needs are crucial to address during the emergency department encounter. Rape crisis counselors, SANE personnel, and social services provide support to victims and act as advocates with medical care providers, law enforcement agencies, and patients. Rape crisis phone numbers (and locations) and follow-up physician information are provided and reviewed. Religious organizations may have available clerical support if that is desired by the patient.

If the crisis intervention by emergency department providers, rape crisis centers, social services, law enforcement, and clerical support is handled efficiently, maximum patient support and benefit is realized. This allows for smoother transitions for the patients from the victim state, through strong coping skills, to their former lifestyle.

Legal Considerations

Physicians must be aware of their obligation to patients who are victims of domestic violence. Physicians have been successfully sued for neglect because they did not ask about domestic violence, accepted unlikely explanations for injuries, and failed to provide adequate follow-up and resources to the patient.

Duty to Warn. If a physician is aware of a patient's intent to harm a third party, the physician has the legal duty to warn the third party. Many states recognize the legal duty that physicians have toward third parties at risk of harm by the physician's patient. This has been upheld in court, even with physician breach of patient confidentiality while making such a warning. This is of importance to the physician treating a batterer, specifically when the batterer makes threatening statements regarding a victim.

Duty to Report. In some states, the reporting of domestic violence is mandatory. The duty to warn exists independently from the duty to report. Some states mandate one without the other, whereas some mandate both. The duty to report specifies that if a physician is aware of a domestic abuse incident, that physician must notify the appropriate governmental agency. Physicians may experience a serious ethical dilemma between the mandates of the state and a patient's best interests. The physician may be held liable to police or social services if the appropriate authority is not informed. Criminal reporting statutes are enacted to inform police of the occurrence of crimes, rather than protecting the victim of the crime. Physicians must be aware that the act of domestic violence reporting may place a patient at higher risk of further injury. Reports made to governmental agencies may cause the agency (or police) to contact the batterer, and governmental agencies may not have the ability to detain the batterer. The batterer may subsequently take out his rage over the report on the victim. It is critical that a physician explain mandatory reporting to the victim and make the victim aware that a report is being filed.

Reporting does not ensure the safety of competent adult victims nor connect them with actual resources to stop abuse. Mandatory reporting has been eliminated in many states. Physicians must make a calculated decision about involving governmental agencies when reporting is not mandated. When reporting is not mandatory, the victims may (out of fear) recant their complaints of domestic violence and seek legal action against the reporting physician. These cases are rare, but a well-documented chart is the best defense. The chart should reflect, in quotes, the patient's allegation of violence, the physician's reasonable belief that this is true, and the action taken to address the violence on behalf of the welfare of the patient.

Patient Rights. Charts should always reflect the request for the patient's permission to notify authorities, whether or not consent was obtained for this notification. If consent was not obtained, the patient's right to autonomy is respected, with the realization that competent patients are able to determine their own treatment. The refusal of a competent patient to notify authorities of domestic violence episodes should be respected and charted as such. Disclosure of the diagnosis of abuse to any third party should be done only with the victim's knowledge and consent. The only valid reason for not complying with the patient's wishes is if the physician believes the patient is incompetent. In that case, the patient requires a competency evaluation and may require commitment if she is unable to care for herself.

A patient has legal recourses on her own, because battery is a crime in all 50 states. Batterers may be subject to prosecution for assault, battery, aggravated assault, harassment, intimidation, stalking, attempted murder, or murder. The patient may have the batterer detained or arrested, have a temporary or permanent restraining (or protective) order enacted, or file an injunction against the batterer. She may then initiate separation, divorce proceedings, and child custody proceedings.

Legal advice is never given to the patient unless it is from an attorney. All criminal and civil actions are very complex, and the patient needs expert advice on these issues. The institution of legal action against a batterer is often an extreme trigger and may cost the victim her life. Victims should be counseled accordingly, and documentation should be made indicating the patient's understanding.

Documentation

This information is critical to a patient's legal case. Medical records provide concrete evidence of injuries and abuse that may be crucial for the successful outcome of any legal proceeding. Medical records may be admissible in court, and the documenting physician, nurse, or social worker must ensure four things:

1. The records were provided by the health care professional in question, as a part of the usual and customary patient care.
2. The records accurately reflect the course of the patient encounter at the stated time and place.
3. The records were made in accordance with routine procedures.
4. The records have been properly stored and access is limited to the professional staff.

Medical evidence is not required in the majority of legal actions, and physician testimony is required in even less. A well-documented chart may reduce the need for physician testimony, with physician involvement in court proceedings occurring in less than 5% of domestic violence cases (those who sought medical care). Although physicians should be aware of the possibility, the fear of being called into court is largely exaggerated and should not hinder the care to victims.

DISPOSITION AND FOLLOW-UP

The risk to the victim (and others in the family) must be assessed, and safe options provided for the victim and her loved ones after leaving the emergency department. Access to a shelter, legal services, and counseling services should be offered. A physician's concern for the victim's well-being and assessment of further injury or death must be clearly explained. Finally, the victim must be respected and her autonomy ensured.

Immediate Consultation

The physician must determine if immediate consultation is required. Immediate commitment may be appropriate if the victim is suicidal or unable to care for herself. Immediate psychiatric evaluation should be provided if possible.

Admission

The victim may require admission for urgent medical or psychiatric treatment. This simplifies the disposition, because it ensures a "safe harbor" for the patient during the time of hospitalization. If the patient has no safe place to go, the physician may consider overnight hospitalization for the patient's protection and to establish alternative safe housing.

Discharge and Follow-up

Disposition is ultimately determined with the patient. If the patient is discharged, the physician must first document that a safety plan has been developed by the physician or another health care worker together with the patient. The physician needs to address the patient's safety after discharge and when returning home. The immediate safety assessment must explore the victim's sense of safety after giving an accurate statement of abuse events and receiving medical care. She needs to feel safe returning home and understand that she can always return again for assistance.

The immediate injury or death risk to the patient when returning to the home environment should be assessed and frankly discussed by the physician and patient. The victim should clearly understand these issues and may be discharged if she so requests. The physician must make sure the safety plan is understood and documented and the victim has a realistic chance of following the plan after discharge. A contract with the patient is made to contact an appropriate referral at a specific date and time and provide the specific means of doing so.

Follow-up and consultation are essential, because individual cases of domestic violence are processes that may require years to end. Recent trends have improved the follow-up care offered to victims of domestic violence. Emergency departments with a recognized high incidence of domestic violence have developed hospital-based intervention programs, linking with community groups to provide ongoing support and advocacy. Many communities have solicited physician input for community-based training programs to enhance awareness of domestic violence, educating heath care workers (including physicians) and members of the community.

Counseling programs do exist for men who batter, and physicians and emergency department staff should have ready access to these resources, as well as to resources for the victim. Batterer intervention may lead to behavior modification to help end the cycle of abuse.

Other resources include the following:

- National Domestic Violence Hotline: 1-800-799-7233. (A helpful resource with availability of interpreters and a hearing-impaired TTY line [800-787-3224]).
- National Resource Center on Domestic Violence: 1-800-537-2238. This is the central site in a national network of domestic violence resources. It offers technical assistance, public education, research and analysis, and an electronic network.
- Centers for Disease Control (www.cdc.gov).

FINAL POINTS

- Use the mnemonic RADAR for the important points of domestic violence intervention.
  - **R**outine screening of all female patients is the single best method for detection of domestic violence in a population unlikely to volunteer the information. (Use the SAFE-2 questions or more extensive question sets if the SAFE-2 questions are negative and suspicion is high.)

- **A**sk direct questions, be nonjudgmental, allow time to listen, and speak to the patient in private.
- **D**ocument all findings and make sure you comply with legal directives.
- **A**ssess patient safety with a danger assessment. Both physician and patient must be aware of the risks of the victim returning home. Ensure that the patient has an escape plan.
- **R**eview the patient's options and referrals, and contract with the patient to ensure follow-up. Be patient. It may take years to break the cycle of violence.
- Optimal treatment for victims of domestic violence is achieved only when the physician has an understanding of the fundamental dynamics of the problem. The physician must acquire a sense of competency and comfort with domestic violence cases through education.
- The emergency department staff must also acquire a sense of competency and comfort with domestic violence cases through education.
- The physician must advocate the development of clear instruction guidelines to maximize care for domestic abuse victims. The optimal medical response to domestic violence is preplanned, with familiarity of institutional resources.
- Easily accessible referrals must be created, used, and evaluated for effective treatment of abuse patients. Early intervention and early referral are made to the support and advocacy groups for patient assistance.
- Physicians must be knowledgeable about the requirements and consequences in their state.
- Restructuring the emergency department chart to highlight domestic violence significantly increases the recognition and identification of victims.
- Every emergency department should have written protocols and procedures for the identification, treatment, and appropriate referral of the domestic violence victim that should make patient safety paramount.
- All patients must be screened for domestic violence in a private area without arousing the suspicions of an accompanying partner.
- Patient education or referral materials on domestic violence should be made easily accessible to all emergency department patients in a manner easily hidden from batterers.
- A contract should be made with patients for appropriate follow-up.
- The physician and staff can empower the patient by clearly explaining that the power to change the situation for the better belongs to the victim.

CASE *Study*

A 23-year-old woman presents to the emergency department, at 9:30 AM, stating "I fell down a flight of stairs." She is complaining of pain in her right ribs and left forearm. Further questioning reveals that she fell the previous night after losing her balance because she had "had too much to drink."

The patient denies loss of consciousness, headache, nausea, or vomiting. She went to bed after her fall down the stairs. She is here now because she is a little sore—"no big deal." She loudly says that she is "in a hurry to get to work so I don't get fired," and then asks, "Can we please just skip the questions and speed this up?"

When asked the above questions the patient denied all concern of injury. Unknown to staff, her boyfriend was hovering immediately outside the triage area during questioning.

The triage nurse noted a bruised and swollen left eye and jaw and that the patient was very apprehensive and nervous. She saw pattern injuries to the ulnar forearm, consistent with defensive wounds.

The nurse was careful to document her findings and spoke directly with the emergency department physician.

Physical examination reveals a thin, well-groomed woman who is anxious but in no apparent discomfort. She is sitting on the edge of the table dressed in a gown, pants, and shoes. Swelling is evident under her left eye, and bruising of the face is detected under heavy makeup.

Vital signs: Blood pressure, 116/68 mm Hg; pulse, 82 and regular; respiratory rate, 12 breaths per minute; temperature, 98.2°F tympanic.

Scalp: Atraumatic/nontender.

Face: Heavy makeup with soft tissue edema under left eye and discoloration to left zygoma and left jaw line. Pupils equal and reactive, tympanic membrane clear.

Neck: Supple, no bony stepoff or tenderness, no jugular venous distention, trachea midline.

Chest wall: Lower rib margin on the left is tender without crepitus (subcutaneous air).

Continued on following page

Lungs: Full, equal breath sounds, with significant left-sided splinting on deep inspiration.

Heart: Regular rate and rhythm, S1 and S2, no murmur.

Back: No spine tenderness. Slight left costovertebral angle tenderness. Three parallel linear contusions are noted over the left flank, each about 15 cm in length.

Abdomen: Soft, nondistended, nontender; no guarding or rebound.

No organomegaly. Positive bowel sounds.

Pelvis: Stable and nontender to stress.

Genitourinary: Normal external female genitalia; refuses speculum, bimanual, and rectal examinations.

Extremities: Four circular contusions noted in a line across the posterior upper right arm. A single circular contusion noted anteriorly on the right forearm. Two linear contusions each about 5 cm in length on the middle of the left forearm, ulnar aspect, with bony tenderness and slight soft tissue swelling, without deformity. Sensory, vascular, and motor examinations are intact on all extremities. No clubbing, cyanosis, or edema is noted.

Neurologic: No Battle's sign or raccoon eyes, no cerebrospinal fluid oto/rhinorrhea, awake and alert, oriented times 3. Pupils are equal, round, and reactive to light; extraocular motions are intact; cranial nerves II through XII are intact; strength is 5/5 in all extremities; gait is normal.

During the physical examination, the physician states "that must have been some fall down the stairs. It is hard to get all these injuries from a fall. Are you sure that is all that happened?" The patient states in a loud voice "That's what I said happened. Can you please hurry? I'll get fired if I'm late for work."

The patient is wheeled to radiology for chest and left forearm radiographs.

The technician reports that the patient and another emergency department patient were yelling at each other. The other patient is a 25-year-old man who is having a radiograph of his right hand. He says he hit a wall with his fist (and has a boxer's fracture). The physician asks the charge nurse to place the male patient at the far end of the department away from the female patient and ensure that they have no further contact.

When the patient returns from the radiology department, the physician sits down in the examination room and asks the SAFE-2 questions. Initially, the patient is very withdrawn, and the physician asks if another patient in the department is frightening her. "We are concerned that you may be afraid of this man, and he is in another part of the department and cannot hear what we are saying."

The patient states the other patient is her boyfriend. He beat her last night after he had been drinking. She has family in the area but is ashamed to tell them about her situation. They do not like her boyfriend, and she has defied them to live with him. Her boyfriend, conversely, hates her family and threatens that she has to choose "them or me."

The victim states she wants to go home with her boyfriend. She states he is always sorry whenever he hits her, and she knows he will be sorry now. She is not afraid of going home. The physician asks the danger assessment questions and carefully documents the patient's answers. The follow-up material and discharge information for her injuries include numbers for social services and other agencies that provide victim assistance. The patient refuses to see any of these individuals now but does agree to speak with a counselor on the phone. She sets up an appointment for follow-up medical care.

This case is typical of domestic abuse. In this instance, the boyfriend had severely beaten the victim and allowed her to seek help only when he sought care for his own injury. The victim was terrified of retribution and feared that the boyfriend was listening to her interaction with the physician. The boyfriend took another opportunity to intimidate the victim in radiology. When the physician compassionately explained overwhelming evidence of beating, and reassured her the boyfriend was not listening, the patient admitted to the abuse.

The boyfriend was a patient in the same emergency department with a history of drinking the previous night and getting into a fight at a bar. Only in the context of the victim did the real story became obvious. Because of the female patient's concerns, social services did not address the batterer. The batterer was asked if he had difficulty with anger and with drinking. He denied both, and treatment or counseling options through the hospital were provided.

The physician orchestrated a delay in splinting and orthopedic referral for the abuser while social service counseled the victim over the phone. With reassurance, temporary safety, and complete confidentiality, the victim discussed her situation. If the contact had not been made in the emergency department during her visit, the patient probably would not have spoken to a counselor. Subsequently, the victim was able to gain some perspective about her abuse. She heard the message that the abuse is wrong, the abuse was not her fault, and that she had options and support available. This is the closest she had ever come to dealing with the problem in more than 5 years of abuse.

She refused to press charges or notify authorities. She refused to allow social services to contact the batterer for possible intervention. She accepted contact numbers and a set appointment with counseling services. The patient insisted on going home with the abuser, waiting for him until he was discharged from the department.

Domestic violence can be very frustrating to address, especially in the emergency setting. Breaking long-term cycles of behavior often takes time and repeated attempts. The emergency physician took the appropriate steps and documented them. The patient's potential for leaving this abusive situation has been improved, and she has information on how to assist herself. This was the best available intervention at the present.

Bibliography

TEXTS

American Medical Association: Diagnostic and Treatment Guidelines on Elder Abuse And Neglect. Chicago, AMA Press, 1992.

American Medical Association: Diagnostic and Treatment Guidelines on Domestic Violence. Chicago, AMA Press, 1992.

Haywood YC, Scott JL: Domestic violence. Emerg Med Clin North Am 1999; 17(3).

Salber PR, Taliaferro E: The Physician's Guide to Domestic Violence. Volcano, CA, Volcano Press, 1994.

Stark ED, Flitcraft AH: Violence among intimates: An epidemiological review. In Hasselt VN, Morrison AS, Bellack M, Hersen VN (eds): Handbook of Family Violence. New York, Plenum, 1998, pp 293–319.

Tjaden P, Thoennes N: Prevalence, Incidence, and Consequences of Violence Against Women: Findings from the National Violence Against Women Survey. National Institute of Justice Centers for Disease Control and Prevention. US Department of Justice, Office of Justice Programs, National Institute of Justice, 1998.

JOURNAL ARTICLES

Brookoff D, O'Brien KK, Cook CS, et al: Characteristics of participants in domestic violence. JAMA 1997; 277:1369–1373.

Ciancone AC, Wilson C, Collette R, et al: Sexual assault nurse examiner programs in the United States. Ann Emerg Med 2000; 35:353–357.

Coben JH, Friedman DI: Health care use by perpetrators of domestic violence. J Emerg Med 2002; 22(3):313–317.

Dearwater SR, Coben JH, Campbell JC, et al: Prevalence of intimate partner abuse in women treated at community hospital emergency departments. JAMA 1998; 280:433–438.

Derogatis LR, Bass EB: Clinical characteristics of women with a history of childhood abuse. JAMA 1997; 277:1362–1368.

Derse AR: Family violence and the emergency physician: legal and ethical considerations. ED Legal Lett 1997; 8(5):45–54.

Duhaime AC, Christian CW, Royce LB, et al: Nonaccidental head injury in infants: The "shaken-baby syndrome." N Engl J Med 1998; 338:1822–1829.

Eisenstat SA, Bancroft L: Domestic violence. N Engl J Med 1999; 341:886–892.

Feldhaus KM, Koziol-McLain J, Amsbury HL, et al: Accuracy of 3 brief screening questions for detecting partner violence in the emergency department. JAMA 1997; 227:1357–1361.

Gremillion DH, Kanof EP: Overcoming barriers to physician involvement in identifying and referring victims of domestic violence. Ann Emerg Med 1996; 27:769–773.

Houry D, Sachs CJ, Feldhaus KM, et al: Violence-inflicted injuries: reporting laws in the fifty states. Ann Emerg Med 2002; 39:56–60.

Kyrrialou DN, Anglin D, Taliaferro E, et al: Risk factors for injury to women from domestic violence. N Engl J Med 1999; 34:1892–1898.

Leder MR, Leder MS: Emergency department evaluation and management of the sexually abused child or adolescent. Pediatr Emerg Rep 2000; 5(6):61–72.

Ross PA, Brady WJ: Evaluating pediataric sexual abuse in the emergency department. Emerg Med Reports 2002; 23(6):70–80.

Schiavone FM, Cronin KA: When intimate partner violence presents in the emergency department. Emerg Med Specialty Rep 2002; 535Z:1–8.

Sisley A, et al: Violence in America: A public health crisis—domestic violence. J Trauma 1999; 46:1105–1113.

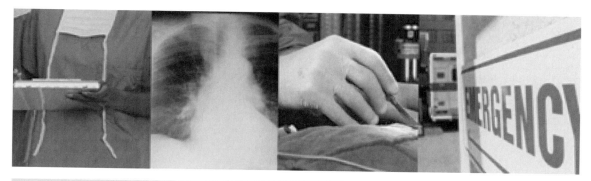

THORACORESPIRATORY DISORDERS

CHAPTER 37

Acute Dyspnea

STEVE YAMAGUCHI

JENNIFER M. BOCOCK

CASE *Study*

A 19-year-old man presented with the sudden onset of left-sided chest pain and difficulty breathing while playing basketball. He denied previous episodes of shortness of breath or any history of trauma. On arrival, he appeared uncomfortable but was in no acute distress.

INTRODUCTION

In the normal individual, breathing is a function that occurs automatically without conscious respiratory effort or discomfort. The dyspneic patient perceives the inability to breathe comfortably as an unpleasant sense of increased work of breathing. Dyspnea is perceived differently by each patient, and it is difficult to clinically quantify or even verbally express. Patients often complain "I can't get a good breath" to describe difficulty breathing or shortness of breath. Acute dyspnea is a rapid onset of these sensations or worsening of baseline respiratory insufficiency causing the patient to seek medical care.

The physiology of breathing is complex and is regulated at multiple sites in the body, including sensory receptors, chemoreceptors, and the brain stem. Sensory input, from the lungs, ventilatory muscles, and chemical receptors, is sent to the central nervous system, and the conscious awareness of dyspnea is generated. The most important chemical regulators of breathing are carbon dioxide (CO_2) and oxygen (O_2). The chemoreceptors responsible for detecting minute changes in blood pH caused by changes in CO_2 content are linked to respiratory drive centers in the brain. The carotid body plays a major role in the respiratory regulation, detecting small changes in O_2 tension, and stimulating the brain stem to alter ventilation. Small changes in CO_2 and O_2 concentrations occur secondary to many pathologic states. Other factors contributing to an awareness of breathing include respiratory muscle weakness or fatigue, loss of airway patency, changes in lung compliance, and the pleura/chest wall interface.

Two to 3 percent of all emergency department visitors have a chief complaint of respiratory distress in varying degrees. Fifteen to 25 percent of all hospital admissions include dyspnea as an admitting concern. Patients often present with multiple associated complaints, including chest pain, cough, and fever. The symptom of dyspnea must be evaluated in a systematic fashion, with all potential causes addressed.

INITIAL APPROACH AND STABILIZATION

Priority Diagnoses

Approximately 75% of all dyspneic patients will have a cardiac or a pulmonary cause for their dyspnea. Many of these patients have one of the following priority diagnoses:

- Hyperactive airway disease
- Chronic obstructive pulmonary disease (COPD)
- Congestive heart failure (CHF)
- Pneumonia
- Pulmonary embolism

Rapid Assessment

All dyspneic patients should be evaluated in a timely manner. Appropriate triage allows for rapid assessment and treatment in the acute care setting.

History

1. The patient's history and the prehospital events are obtained from the patient and rescue squad. Prolonged questioning may be counterproductive, and further details can be obtained after stabilization. Questions that need only a "yes" or "no" response ("Are you having chest pain?" and "Are you hurting anywhere?") help limit additional demand on the patient's respiratory effort.
2. What is the time course of the shortness of breath? Was there a specific precipitating factor?

3. Are there any other symptoms, such as chest pain, cough, fever, or a history of injury?
4. Does the patient take any medications? Inhaler, diuretic, nitroglycerin, or corticosteroid use should be verified and quantified.
5. Does the patient have a history of an underlying cause of the symptoms (asthma, emphysema, congestive heart failure)?

Physical Examination

1. Appearance and mental status are very important. Can the patient talk and respond appropriately to questions?
2. Is the airway patent and protected?
3. What are the vital signs, including pulse oximetry?
4. The experienced physician will develop a "sixth sense" regarding the need for endotracheal intubation and ventilatory support. Clues that the patient may require early intubation may include
   a. Altered mental status
   b. Impending patient exhaustion (inability to speak)
   c. Patient position, in particular patient tripoding (sitting upright, leaning forward on upper extremities with diaphoresis, pallor, and accessory muscle use)
5. Specific examination for cyanosis, rales, wheezing, edema, or evidence of trauma is important.

Early Intervention

Early intervention is necessary to prevent the decompensation of the dyspneic patient.

Airway. Airway patency, protection, and ventilatory status are addressed and immediately managed if necessary. Early, active airway management may be needed for the severely dyspneic or fatigued patient. Oxygenation and ventilation may be supplemented by passive (supplemental O_2) or active (bag-valve-mask or intubation) management (see Chapter 2. Airway Management).

Supplemental Oxygen. Oxygen is provided to all dyspneic patients, regardless of the etiology. Baseline room air oximetry is helpful; however, oxygen should not be withheld for this measurement.

A *nasal cannula* is simple and inexpensive, providing an F_{IO_2} of 24% to 40% and flow rates of 1 to 5 L/min. When rates exceeding 4 to 5 L/min are used, the nasal mucosa may become irritated and humidity must be added. For each liter of oxygen per nasal cannula, there is an estimated increase in the F_{IO_2} by 3% to 4%. A nasal cannula

may be used for patients with suspected acute myocardial ischemia or infarction, mild dyspnea, and a mild to moderate exacerbation of chronic obstructive pulmonary disease (COPD).

Simple masks deliver O_2 at low flow rates of 5 to 10 L/min, but precise percentages are difficult to control with the F_{IO_2}, ranging from 40% to 50%. These masks require high flow O_2, because low flow rates may allow carbon dioxide rebreathing.

The *Venturi mask* delivers a set percentage of O_2. These masks can be set to deliver 24% to 50% F_{IO_2} oxygen, with O_2 flow rates of 4 to 12 L/min. These masks are most helpful for COPD patients when a known and consistent percentage of oxygen is desired.

Non-rebreather masks have a valve that opens to an oxygen *reservoir bag* throughout inspiration and provide up to 90% F_{IO_2}. Exhalation is to the air, preventing reinhalation of the exhaled breath. This method is used for severely dyspneic patients and for preoxygenation of patients before intubation.

Intravenous Access. An intravenous line is placed in all dyspneic patients for administration of medications and fluids, as appropriate. The potential for fluid overload in the dyspneic patient should be closely monitored.

Cardiac Monitor. Monitoring is essential for cardiac dysrhythmias, respiratory status, and oximetry.

Medical Therapy. Nebulized bronchodilators are the treatment of choice for patients with acute bronchospasm. Nitroglycerin plays a major role in therapy for cardiac ischemia and for congestive heart failure. Morphine is beneficial in cardiac ischemia as an anxiolytic and as a preload reducer (relaxation of pulmonary vasculature). The use of a diuretic, for example, furosemide, will reduce the preload in patients with congestive heart failure. Cautious dosing of nitrates, morphine, or diuretics is necessary in patients with a potential for hypotension.

Needle Decompression. Tension pneumothorax requires immediate relief with anterior chest wall needle decompression. Spontaneous pneumothorax without "tension" (increased intrapleural pressure) does not need such aggressive intervention early in the course of care.

CLINICAL ASSESSMENT

History

The severely dyspneic patient often has difficulty giving an adequate history. Patient responses to a detailed history may be possible after initial stabilization, and the family or the rescue squad should be asked initial pertinent questions. The patient's previous medical record and information from the primary physician are often needed to clarify the patient's baseline medical status. Several key questions must be asked regarding any dyspneic patient:

1. *Has there been a similar event in the past?* This may be the single most important question the physician can ask. The majority of patients presenting to the emergency department with shortness of breath have an underlying disorder causing the dyspnea.
2. *How long have you been short of breath? Was the onset sudden or gradual?* The longer the evolution of symptoms, the less likely the problem can be reversed in the emergency department. Sudden onset usually represents a structural, infectious, or acute ischemic event.
3. *Does anything make it better or worse?* Did home O_2, nebulized medications, or position changes affect the shortness of breath?
4. *Are there associated symptoms?* Specifically, one should inquire about the presence of chest pain, cough, fever, sputum, hemoptysis, orthopnea, paroxysmal nocturnal dyspnea, and dyspnea on exertion.
5. *What medications are currently taken?* The patient's medication list can provide insight into underlying conditions. Home O_2, inhalers, diuretics, or cardiac medications may reveal an underlying illness.
6. *Are there medication allergies or reactions?* There is no need to exacerbate a difficult respiratory situation with an allergic reaction.
7. *What therapy has worked in the past?* Many patients know the therapeutic regimens that work for them. This information may expedite care.
8. *What is the past medical history?* Is there a history of myocardial infarction, congestive heart failure, COPD, deep vein thrombosis, asthma, or pulmonary embolism? Is there a history of any pulmonary or cardiac surgical procedures? Recent hospitalizations or prolonged immobilization?

Physical Examination

A more detailed examination is completed after the rapid assessment (ABCs) is performed and the patient is initially stabilized.

Vital Signs

Blood Pressure. The blood pressure is frequently elevated in patients with bronchospasm and congestive heart failure. Treatment of the underlying condition will usually reduce the blood pressure to the patient's normal range. Tension pneumothorax, cardiogenic shock, and volume depletion are considered in any dyspneic and hypotensive patient. Eight to 10 percent of patients with pulmonary embolism present with associated shock.

Pulse. The majority of patients with significant dyspnea are tachycardic unless using a β-blocking agent. Return of the pulse to an acceptable range (80 to 100 beats per minute) is used as an estimate of the response to therapy.

Respiratory Rate. A normal respiratory rate is 10 to 12 breaths per minute in a healthy adult. The rate should be measured for a 30-second to 1-minute interval for an accurate count. Patients with a rate consistently greater than 40 breaths per minute may require mechanical ventilation to protect against fatigue and respiratory failure. Patients with respiratory distress and a rate of less than 12 breaths per minute are also at risk for respiratory failure. A normal respiratory rate can be reassuring in some cases. Fewer than 15% of patients with pulmonary embolism have respiratory rates less than 20 breaths per minute.

Respiratory Pattern. Deep respirations (inspiratory and expiratory phase) with a sensation of air hunger can occur with metabolic acidosis. Patients with upper airway obstruction have difficulty with inspiration, are often stridorous, and cannot manage their oral secretions. Patients with lower airway disease and obstruction primarily have expiratory difficulty, with wheezing and a prolonged expiratory phase.

Temperature. The presence of fever usually indicates an infectious cause of the dyspnea. One must be cautious assuming an infectious source with low-grade fever, because many other conditions can present as low-grade fever. Oral temperatures are inaccurate in dyspneic patients; a rectal or core temperature measurement is preferred.

Pulse Oximetry. Commonly called the fifth vital sign, pulse oximetry is helpful as a screening tool when assessing the dyspneic patient. Healthy individuals have readings of 95% to 100%. A normal pulse oximetry does not rule out catastrophic disease; approximately 25% of patients with pulmonary embolism will have a normal oximetry reading. A low reading, 90% to 92%, may be the baseline for patients with chronic lung disease. Many chronic pulmonary patients may know their typical oximetry values.

Pulsus Paradoxus. Pulsus paradoxus is an exaggeration of the normal physiologic fall in systolic blood pressure during respiration. Pulsus is measured by inflating a manual blood pressure cuff above the systolic blood pressure and slowly deflating it until systolic sounds are heard during expiration. The cuff is further deflated until the sounds are heard throughout the ventilatory cycle. The pressure difference between the sounds with expiration and those with inspiration is normally less than 10 mm Hg. With pulsus paradoxus, the difference is classically elevated 20 to 30 mm Hg or more (patients with severe asthma or cardiac tamponade). This test is not particularly sensitive and can be time consuming. The emergency department ambient noise level will also make this measurement difficult.

General Assessment

Rapid Assessment. A quick and focused approach should be used for the acutely dyspneic patient. The rapid assessment of the ABCs is completed as soon as possible. Stabilization and the anticipation of catastrophe is of utmost importance in any dyspneic patient.

Ability to Speak. The patient's ability to speak and the length of the spoken phrases (single words or complete sentences) are helpful in assessing severity of dyspnea. Patients who complain loud and long about shortness of breath can be less worrisome than those who are breathless or gasp one-word answers.

Mental Status. Is the patient agitated, disoriented, or showing signs of lethargy and somnolence? These symptoms are indicators of severe hypoxia and indicate the need for aggressive interventions.

Positioning. The severely dyspneic patient usually sits bolt upright and leans forward, whereas patients who rest supine are less likely to have serious disease.

Cyanosis. There are two types of cyanosis: central and peripheral. Peripheral cyanosis (acrocyanosis) occurs when increased oxygen extraction occurs in the peripheral capillary beds of patients with preexisting vasoconstriction. Peripheral cyanosis typically has a mottled appearance of the extremities. Central cyanosis is more apparent, typically at the mouth and face, and requires a desaturation or loss of 5 g of hemoglobin. An individual with a normal hemoglobin of 15 g/dL develops central cyanosis at an oxygen saturation of less than 70%. The anemic patient may not manifest cyanosis until extreme desaturation levels occur. Both types of cyanosis represent a worsening of oxygenation and are indicators of worsening clinical status in the dyspneic patient.

Pulmonary. The patient's breathing is evaluated for accessory muscle use, splinting, or paradoxical chest movement. Percussion for dullness is frequently omitted from the pulmonary examination, but it can be very useful. Unilateral hyperresonance suggests a pneumothorax, and dullness may represent pleural effusion or consolidation. The chest is auscultated for audible stridor, inspiratory-expiratory flow ratio, wheezes, rales, rhonchi, and rubs and for evidence of consolidation (e.g., bronchial breath sounds, egophony).

Cardiovascular. The neck veins are examined for the presence of jugular venous distention, which suggests congestive heart failure, fluid overload, or impaired venous return. Emergent causes of jugular venous distention include tension pneumothorax and cardiac tamponade, and both must be ruled out. The presence of murmurs, rubs, or gallops with cardiac auscultation is helpful when assessing cardiac causes of dyspnea.

Extremities. Extremities are examined for the presence of edema, the presence and quality of pulses, and presence of peripheral cyanosis. The fingernails are examined for signs of clubbing, a finding that suggests long-term respiratory difficulty and is associated with some pulmonary neoplasms.

Neurologic. The patient's mental status and ability to cooperate are a final common pathway for assessment of oxygenation, ventilation, and circulation. Inability to provide sufficient oxygen to the brain leads to agitation, confusion, and somnolence. Fatigue also has a significant role in a patient's ability to respond; increased work of breathing rapidly depletes body energy stores.

CLINICAL REASONING

The differential diagnosis of dyspnea is extensive. The information obtained by the history and physical examination, when combined with the response to initial stabilization, helps the physician determine a prioritized approach to management. The following questions can help narrow the differential diagnosis and guide treatment of the dyspneic patient.

Is This True Dyspnea? What Is the Precise Nature of the Patient's Complaint?

The unpleasant sensation of increasing effort to breathe, or "air hunger," can be matched to the clinical scenario. Many patients are short of breath, and it is important to isolate each complaint and distinguish true dyspnea from hyperventilation, sighing respirations, and other forms of breathlessness. It is necessary to distinguish true dyspnea from limited respiration secondary to thoracic pain from pleurisy or rib fractures. The nature of the unpleasant sensation is an important distinction. The feeling of the inability to move air (in and out) is characteristic of obstructive lung disease in both upper and lower airways. A sense of suffocation is often described by patients with congestive heart failure or with weakened respiratory muscles.

Is This of Pulmonary or Nonpulmonary Origin?

Tables 37–1 and 37–2 list the differential diagnoses for pulmonary and nonpulmonary causes of dyspnea. *Pulmonary* causes are the most frequent causes of dyspnea. Respiratory symptoms including cough, sputum production, and peripheral chest pain, are components of the history and physical examination that should be elicited. Signs and symptoms indicating primary pulmonary causes of dyspnea direct the physician to a differential diagnosis based on the anatomic elements of the respiratory tract (upper airway, bronchi, bronchioles and alveoli, the interstitium including the vasculature, thoracic cage/pleural interface, respiratory muscle structures).

Nonpulmonary causes are primarily of cardiac or other nonpulmonary origin. Distinguishing between pulmonary and cardiac origins of dyspnea is difficult. Dyspnea of cardiac origin occurs when left atrial pressure is elevated, with accumulation of fluid into the interstitial spaces of the lung. Congestion leads to decreased lung compliance, increased work of breathing, reflex bronchospasm, and poor gas exchange. Patients usually have a history of cardiac disease, chest pain or discomfort, orthopnea, and paroxysmal nocturnal dyspnea.

TABLE 37–1. Pulmonary Causes of Dyspnea: An Anatomic Approach*

Upper airway
  Foreign body
  Epiglottitis
  Laryngospasm, angioedema
  Trauma
Bronchi (large and small airways)
  Asthma
  Bronchitis
  Bronchiolitis
  Bronchogenic carcinoma
Alveoli
  Pneumonia
  Pulmonary tuberculosis
  Emphysema
  Toxic inhalation (e.g., paraquat)
  Pulmonary contusion
  Adult respiratory distress syndrome

Interstitium, including vasculature
  Pneumoconiosis
  Pulmonary embolus
  Pulmonary fibrosis (restrictive disease)
Thoracic cage-lung interface
  Pneumothorax
  Hemothorax
  Effusion
Respiratory musculoskeletal structure
  Rib fracture
  Flail chest
  Guillain-Barré syndrome
  Myasthenia gravis
  Other muscular disorders, botulism, tetanus

*Some processes may occur in more than one site.

TABLE 37–2. Nonpulmonary Causes of Dyspnea

Cardiac

Acute ischemia or infarction
Cardiac valve dysfunction
Cardiac dysrhythmia
Congestive heart failure
Cardiac tamponade

Miscellaneous

Central nervous system stimulation–head trauma, mass lesion, cerebrovascular accident, aspirin, sepsis
Acid-base disorder–metabolic acidosis (MUDPILES)
Decreased O_2-carrying capacity–anemia, carbon monoxide, methemoglobinemia
Endocrine–hyperthyroidism, pregnancy
Psychogenic–hyperventilation syndrome

What Are the Common and Catastrophic Causes of Dyspnea to Be Considered in Each Patient?

Tables 37–3 and 37–4 list the most important pulmonary and nonpulmonary causes of dyspnea, with pertinent characteristics.

DIAGNOSTIC ADJUNCTS

Clinical findings reveal the cause of the dyspnea in most cases presenting to the emergency department. Diagnostic tests are frequently necessary to confirm the diagnosis, gauge the severity of the problem, screen for unexpected findings, and assess the response to therapy.

Laboratory Studies

Arterial Blood Gas Analysis. Arterial blood gas testing is performed on all severely compromised patients to evaluate the adequacy of oxygenation and ventilation and to assess acid-base status. These measurements can be used to calculate the alveolar-arterial (A – a) gradient. This is moderately useful in determining efficiency of gas exchange and measures the difference between the PO_2 in the alveoli and arterial blood:

$$A – a \text{ gradient} = [(FIO_2)(\text{barometric pressure} – 47 \text{ mm Hg})] – [(1.25)(\text{measured } PCO_2)] – (\text{measured } PO_2)$$

The PO_2 and PCO_2 are obtained from the arterial blood gas analysis. At sea level, the FIO_2 of room air is 21% and barometric pressure is 713 mm Hg. The FIO_2 is estimated while on supplemental oxygen. The A – a gradient is used to assess the shunting of oxygen-rich blood or physiologic impairment of oxygenation. The A – a gradient is typically no greater than a person's age divided by 10 plus 10. The normal range in people without lung disease is 5 to 20 mm Hg.

Assessment for CO_2 retention in the dyspneic patient is helpful in detection of impending respiratory failure. The acid-base status of the patient may reflect metabolic or respiratory sources or a combination of both (see Chapter 21, Acute Metabolic Acidosis and Metabolic Alkalosis). Compensatory changes may also be revealed by the gas results.

Complete Blood Cell Count with Differential. In the majority of patients, this test is ordered to assess the hemoglobin level. The white blood cell count and differential can suggest or support the diagnoses of infection or inflammation. Clinical correlation is always necessary in the patient with an elevated white blood cell count, because these results are not specific.

Serum Electrolytes. Assessment of the sodium, potassium, and bicarbonate concentrations in an ill patient can offer insight into the patient's toleration of the precipitating illness. These levels are helpful in moderately ill patients but are much less useful in the assessment of mild dyspnea.

Cardiac Enzymes. Creatine phosphokinase (CPK), CPK-MB, and troponin are measures that can diagnose potential of myocardial injury or infarction. Troponin levels rise and can be detected 4 to 6 hours after cardiac injury.

D-Dimer Assay. D-Dimer is a by-product of fibrinolysis and becomes elevated in patients with thromboembolism. Infection and chronic inflammatory states also cause elevations, which are false-positive results (for pulmonary embolism). The D-dimer assay is a sensitive test for thromboembolism but is not specific. Multiple types of D-dimer assay are available, primarily latex agglutination or enzyme-linked immunosorbent assay. The presence of a negative D-dimer test, with a PO_2 greater than 80 mm Hg and a respiratory rate less than 20 breaths per minute, helps rule out pulmonary embolism.

Gram's Stain of Sputum. The sputum Gram stain remains a useful diagnostic tool in selected cases of pneumonia. Acceptable specimens may be difficult to obtain; deep suction, cough stimulation, and purulent secretions have higher positive smear results.

Radiologic Imaging

Chest Radiographs. Posteroanterior and lateral radiographic views of the chest are an important adjunct in the evaluation of the dyspneic patient. The lateral view is an important component of the radiographic evaluation. Portable anteroposterior chest films should be limited to the severely ill patient. Table 37–5 describes the typical radiographic findings of the common causes of dyspnea.

Ventilation/Perfusion ($\{\dot{V}\}/\{\dot{Q}\}$) Scanning. This minimally invasive procedure is usually ordered when a pulmonary embolus is suspected. Three steps are involved: (1) The perfusion scan is performed after injection of radiolabeled albumin. A completely normal scan will rule out the diagnosis of pulmonary embolism. (2) If the perfusion scan is abnormal, the chest radiograph is reviewed. If the perfusion defect correlates with an abnormality on the radiograph, the scan is indeterminate. (3) If the region of perfusion defect appears normal on the radiograph, a ventilation scan is then completed. A radioactive inert gas is inhaled, and

TABLE 37–3. Characteristics of Common Pulmonary Causes of Dyspnea

Specific Condition	Epidemiology	Etiology	History	Physical Findings	Useful Tests
Asthma	Common in children and young adults with decreasing incidence with advancing age. Patients with adult onset usually have a worse prognosis. Frequently there is a family history of asthma	Caused by a reduction in small airway diameter. Edema, mucosal inflammation, and mucous secretion. May be related to allergic, infectious, occupational, emotional, or exercise-related causes	Most patients have a history of previous attacks. Precipitating factors usually present. The onset of wheezing is variable. Chest pain, sputum production, or fever may be present	Usually tachycardia and tachypnea. Wheezing usually present but may be absent in severe asthma. I:E ratio may be increased. Cyanosis and marked retractions are signs of severe bronchospasm	Spirometry useful for assessing severity and response to therapy. Chest radiograph and blood gas measurement may be helpful in complicated cases
Emphysema	Significant disease is almost always associated with tobacco use; rarely α_1-antitrypsin deficiency exists. Increasing incidence with advancing age. More common in men	Defined on a pathologic basis as an abnormal, permanent enlargement of the air spaces distal to the terminal bronchioles, accompanied by destruction of their walls. This is present to some extent in most people older than 50 years but is much more common and severe in tobacco users	History of previous episodes of dyspnea. Most patients have smoking history	Barrel chest. Wheezes or decreased breath sounds may be present	Blood gas measurement, chest radiograph. Blood gas: Low Po_2, normal or high Pco_2
Chronic bronchitis	Defined as daily productive cough for >3 months Seen almost exclusively in smokers, although occupational and environmental factors may play a role. More common with advancing age. More common in men	Defined clinically as a chronic condition of excess mucus secretion in the bronchial tree from hyperplasia and hypertrophy of the mucus-secreting goblet cells in the large airways. Chronic hypoxemia and hypercapnia from poor ventilation lead to polycythemia, pulmonary hypertension, and cor pulmonale. Many patients have underlying viral or bacterial infections. Many have concomitant emphysema	History of dyspnea and smoking. Copious sputum production	Often cyanotic and cachectic. Wheezes, rales, and decreased breath sounds are present	Blood gas measurements, chest radiograph, sputum Gram stain. Blood gas: low Po_2, high Pco_2, low pH in acute phase
Pneumonia	Seen in all age groups but more dangerous in the very young and very old. Seen more frequently in alcoholics, diabetics, and patients with immunodeficiency syndromes	Causative organism varies with age and underlying medical condition. Enteric organisms and *Listeria* are more common in neonates. Viral and mycoplasmal pneumonias are more commonly found in children and young adults. *Pneumococcus* is the most common cause of community-acquired bacterial pneumonia. Enteric organisms, *Haemophilus influenzae*, *Klebsiella*, and staphylococci	Fever, variable degree of toxicity. Cough, sputum production, or hemoptysis	Fever, variable degree of toxicity. Tachypnea and tachycardia	Blood gas analysis, chest radiograph, sputum Gram's stain, complete blood cell count

Continued on following page

TABLE 37–3. Characteristics of Common Pulmonary Causes of Dyspnea *Continued*

Specific Condition	Epidemiology	Etiology	History	Physical Findings	Useful Tests
		cause pneumonia in alcoholics and debilitated patients. *Pneumocystis carinii* is common in AIDS patients			
Pneumothorax	Typically occurs in patients with underlying lung disease such as asthma, chronic obstructive pulmonary disease, or malignancies. May occur in otherwise healthy people, particularly thin young males	Results from the spontaneous rupture of a pulmonary or subpleural bleb into the pleural space	Sudden onset of dyspnea and sharp pleuritic chest pain. May have history of trauma, heavy exertion, or previous pneumothorax	Unilateral decreased breath sounds. Tracheal deviation, jugular venous distention, and hypotension occur with tension	Upright chest radiograph; may need expiratory view if pneumothorax is small
Pulmonary embolus	Probably occurs much more commonly than suspected, particularly in hospitalized patients. Incidence increases with advancing age, recent surgery, malignancies, prolonged immobilization, and pregnancy	Greater than ninety-five percent of emboli arise from the deep veins of the pelvis and legs. Large emboli lodge in proximal pulmonary artery and cause hypotension and shock. Smaller emboli lodge more distally and lead to dyspnea, pleuritic pain, and hypoxia	Usually sudden onset of dyspnea (85%) with sharp pleuritic chest pain (75% of patients). Hemoptysis (30%), cough (50%), and anxiety (60%) are common. Risk factors are usually present. Syncope is a rare but important presentation (10%)	Tachycardia (40%), tachypnea (90% have >16/min), cyanosis (20%), increased pulmonic valve closure (50%), increased temperature (40%)	Chest radiograph, blood gas analysis (85%–90% with Po_2 <80 mm Hg), D-dimer levels, spiral CT of chest, ventilation-perfusion scan, pulmonary angiography

I:E ratio, inspiratory-expiratory ratio.

TABLE 37-4. Characteristics of Common Nonpulmonary Causes of Dyspnea

Specific Condition	Epidemiology	Etiology	History	Physical Findings	Useful Tests
Congestive heart failure	Incidence increases dramatically with advancing age. Most patients have a known history of cardiac disease or significant risk factors	Left ventricular dysfunction leads to elevated venous pressure and resultant fluid collection in the lung parenchyma. Common causes of heart failure include myocardial ischemia, tachydysrhythmias, increased sodium intake, and noncompliance with diuretic therapy	Variable onset of symptoms. Cough, orthopnea, paroxysmal nocturnal dyspnea, and chest pain are common. Risk factors for heart disease	Rales, wheezes, jugular venous distention, gallop rhythm, peripheral edema. Often extremely diaphoretic	Chest radiograph, blood gas, electrocardiagram B-type natriuretic peptide may have differentiating value
Myocardial ischemia/ infarction	The leading cause of death in most industrialized countries. Occurs at a younger age in men, but the difference evens out with advancing age. Risk factors include tobacco use, hypertension, diabetes, unfavorable lipid profile, and a positive family history	Usually caused by the gradual development of fixed atherosclerotic lesions in the coronary circulation leading to an imbalance between myocardial oxygen supply and demand. Arterial spasm may play a role in some patients	May have chest or epigastric pain, nausea, emesis, diaphoresis. Risk factors include diabetes, hypertension, tobacco, hyperlipidemia, family history	Usually normal; may be diaphoretic and have apprehensive appearance. May have gallop rhythm, new murmur, or signs of congestive heart failure	Electrocardiogram, cardiac enzymes, chest radiograph
Decreased oxygen-carrying capacity	Any age, trauma victim, severe anemia, toxic exposure	Either absolute loss of hemoglobin from blood loss, or functional loss from binding with toxins (e.g., carbon monoxide), or changing structure (e.g., methemoglobinemia)	Patients may have source of blood loss or other exposure. Dyspnea may be presenting complaint with toxin such as carbon monoxide. Associated weakness, fatigue	Pallor, cyanosis, source of blood loss	Complete blood cell count, clotting studies, carboxyhemoglobin, direct viewing of "brown blood" in methemoglobinemia. Arterial blood gas measurements are less useful since they measure dissolved O_2 in serum
Acid-base disorders	Any age at particular risk, diabetics, alcoholics	Some diseases (e.g., diabetic ketoacidosis, lactic acidosis) seen more common than others	Patient aware of "deep" breaths, not always "air hunger." Associated disorder (e.g., diabetes, aspirin ingestion, methanol ingestion)	May have findings of underlying disease. Nonspecific for dyspnea	Arterial blood gas, serum bicarbonate, serum potassium, ketone or lactate levels
Hyperventilation syndrome	Most common in adolescent and young adults. Patients frequently have history of anxiety-related disorders	Often provoked by environmental or personal factors, but these are frequently not obvious to the patient and physician	History of previous stress-related attacks. Frequently complaints of circumoral and extremity paresthesias	Normal except for tachypnea and frequent sighing	Blood gas: high P_{O_2}, low P_{CO_2}, high pH

TABLE 37–5. Radiographic Findings in Common Causes of Dyspnea

Condition	Chest Radiograph Findings
Asthma/emphysema	Usually normal, may show hyperinflation, fibrotic changes, peribroncheolar cuffing, or bullous disease
Pneumonia	Lobar or alveolar infiltrates
Pulmonary embolism	Nonspecific, may be normal. Atelectasis, infiltrates, effusion, Hampton's hump
Pneumothorax	Lung collapse, mediastinal shift, subcutaneous emphysema. Inspiratory-expiratory films may benefit the diagnosis.
Noncardiogenic pulmonary edema (acute respiratory distress syndrome)	May be normal early. Later cardiogenic pulmonary edema pattern may be present without cardiomegaly.
Cardiogenic pulmonary edema	Venous engorgement and redistribution, bilateral alveolar edema, Kerley's B lines. May see left ventricular enlargement.

regions of decreased ventilation are noted. The $\dot{V}/\dot{Q}$ scan is high probability for a pulmonary embolus when perfusion defects correspond to areas of normal ventilation. A completely normal $\dot{V}/\dot{Q}$ scan has a sensitivity of 99% and can essentially rule out pulmonary embolus. Interpretation of the $\dot{V}/\dot{Q}$ scan is influenced by the patint's risk for pulmonary embolism after clinical assessment.

Helical Computed Tomography (Spiral CT). Spiral CT images the pulmonary vasculature and other chest cavity structures. CT is most accurate in the diagnosis of large central emboli versus small peripheral emboli. In the emergency department, this test is helpful for patients who have a high likelihood of a nondiagnostic $\dot{V}/\dot{Q}$ scan, such as those with significant underlying pulmonary disorders like COPD, pneumonia, or malignancy. Reported sensitivities for spiral CT are 90% to 100%, with specificities ranging from 78% to 100%.

Pulmonary Angiography. Although $\dot{V}/\dot{Q}$ scanning is the first-line testing for PE, it can be falsely negative or positive. The gold standard diagnostic evaluation for pulmonary embolism is pulmonary arteriography and should be performed within 24 to 48 hours of the embolic episode. It should be completed for patients with doubtful diagnosis, especially patients with risk factors for successful therapeutic anticoagulation.

Electrocardiogram

An electrocardiogram is ordered for all critically ill patients and any patient for whom there is possible primary cardiac disease or dysrhythmia. The electrocardiogram is evaluated for evidence of cardiac ischemia or infarction as the cause of dyspnea. Other subtle findings may reveal pericardial disease, left ventricular hypertrophy, right-sided heart strain, or dysrhythmia.

Special Tests

Pulmonary Function Testing. Simple bedside testing of peak expiratory flow rates can be used to assess the severity of dyspnea and to follow patient response to therapy. There is current controversy about the use of peak flow measurement as a predictor for hospitalization need. Improvement of peak expiratory flow rates after bronchodilator therapy is a good indicator that the dyspnea is a result of reactive airway disease. This measurement is most useful in asthmatics, but it can be used in the assessment of any dyspneic patient. In COPD patient groups, pulmonary function testing is best used for outpatient care and assessment of relapse and is not recommended for acute episodes.

Echocardiography. Emergency department use of echocardiography has become more prevalent in recent years. The rapid assessment for the presence of pericardial effusion and tamponade can be accomplished; however, the presence of wall motion abnormalities, left ventricular function, and valvular disease typically requires a formal assessment.

B-Type Natriuretic Peptide. This peptide is released from the cardiac ventricles as a response to increased tension in the ventricular wall. Recent studies suggest B-type natriuretic peptide levels are more accurate in differentiating congestive heart failure from noncardiac causes of dyspnea than any other noninvasive assessment. Availability of rapid measurements may be a significant diagnostic addition to emergency and subsequent care.

PRINCIPLES OF MANAGEMENT

The key principle for managing patients with dyspnea is the delivery of adequate oxygenation. Other principles include the relief of bronchospasm, elimination of edema, pain management, and treatment of infection. Each is applied, as appropriate, while managing the most common causes of dyspnea, detailed here.

COPD (Chronic Bronchitis, Emphysema) and Asthma

Oxygen. A Venti mask is used with a controlled O_2 flow. If this is not available, O_2 administration is begun with 1 to 2 L/min by nasal cannula, and the patient's response is monitored. Carbon dioxide retention is a concern in COPD. Patients may become lethargic as PCO_2 rises with loss of their hypoxic drive as high-flow O_2 is given. Ensuring adequate oxygenation is of greater importance than suppression of the hypoxic drive. A sufficient concentration of oxygen is provided to maintain oxygenation, and close monitoring of mental status and respiratory status is maintained.

Bilevel Positive Airway Pressure (BiPAP). BiPAP ventilation is a noninvasive ventilatory adjunct used in the care of patients with acute respiratory failure. BiPAP has been shown to decrease the need for intubation and mechanical ventilation and to increase ventilation, improving PO_2 and lowering PCO_2 levels. A decrease in the number of days in an intensive care unit and the overall hospital stay has also been demonstrated. Active airway management is instituted, as necessary.

β_2-Adrenergic Agonist Agents. β_2-agonist medications, preferably in the nebulized and inhaled form, have become the mainstay of therapy for patients with decompensated COPD and acute asthma exacerbations (see Chapter 38, Wheezing). When these agents are inhaled, local bronchodilatation occurs, opening the airways and lowering resistance.

Anticholinergic Agents. Nebulized anticholinergic agents are effective in COPD patients and are used primarily in conjunction with β agonists. Combination therapy has demonstrated superior bronchodilation without added side effects. They have a slower onset of action (5 to 15 minutes) and a longer time to peak effect but are as effective as β_2 agonists for improving pulmonary function.

Theophylline. Theophylline is a methylxanthine, traditionally used in COPD and asthma patients as a bronchodilator. Studies indicate that there is limited benefit when theophylline is added to β_2 agonist and anticholinergic inhaled medications, primarily in patients who are resistant to the first-line therapy. An initial loading dose of aminophylline is given, with a subsequent continuous infusion. Blood levels must be closely followed, because aminophylline has a very narrow therapeutic window and can rapidly reach toxic levels. Adverse effects with theophylline typically occur at higher blood levels and include nausea, vomiting, dysrhythmia, and seizures.

Corticosteroids. The early use of corticosteroids has a clearly demonstrated benefit and may improve responses, by asthmatics and COPD patients, to other medications. A corticosteroid bolus is given to patients who are already corticosteroid dependent, to asthmatic outpatients, and to patients who are not responding to optimal treatment. Corticosteroid burst therapy (5 to 7 days) decreases inflammation and does not cause adrenal suppression. Acute COPD exacerbations may require up to 2 weeks of systemic corticosteroid therapy, with subsequent taper.

Patients receiving corticosteroid therapy should be monitored for hyperglycemia. Most respiratory infections are viral, but a bacterial source should be sought because prophylactic antibiotics have no benefit.

Antimicrobial Therapy. Antibiotics should be administered to patients with signs or symptoms of an associated bacterial respiratory infection, which is a common cause of acute exacerbations. These include increased dyspnea, increased sputum volume, and purulent sputum. When an infection is found, typical antibiotic regimens last for 7 to 14 days.

Pneumonia

Oxygen. Oxygen is provided, and the patient is monitored with pulse oximetry and arterial blood gas analysis. Active airway management is instituted, as necessary.

Antimicrobial Therapy. Antimicrobial therapy is directed by the clinical condition and results of Gram's stain and culture. Macrolides provide the best coverage for the organisms most likely to cause community-acquired pneumonia. Patients with underlying disorders (e.g., diabetes, alcoholism, emphysema, immunosuppression) are admitted to the hospital for intravenous antibiotics (usually a macrolide plus a second- or third-generation cephalosporin).

β_2-Agonist Therapy. Bronchospasm, if present, is treated with inhaled β_2 agonists.

Spontaneous Pneumothorax

Patients with a tension pneumothorax require immediate needle decompression as a temporizing measure, followed by a tube thoracostomy. A

14- or 16-gauge needle is inserted at the ipsilateral second intercostal space in the midclavicular line for temporary pressure release. Patients with a simple pneumothorax are treated differently depending on the severity of collapse. Those patients with less than 15% to 20% collapse may be treated with observation and serial chest radiographs. Those with greater than 15% to 20% collapse are usually treated with tube thoracostomy and suction or water seal.

Needle or Catheter Aspiration. Aspiration of air with a needle or 16-gauge catheter connected to a three-way stopcock has been successfully used in young patients with spontaneous pneumothorax. Patients with no air leak for over 6 hours are discharged from the emergency department, and a follow-up visit along with a chest radiograph is scheduled for the next day.

Tube Thoracostomy. Placement of a chest tube is the standard of care for patients with a large (over 15% collapse) pneumothorax or a tension pneumothorax. A 22- to 28-French tube is placed in the fifth intercostal space at the mid to anterior axillary line, under local anesthesia. This procedure is supplemented with an intravenous sedation, if the clinical condition permits. After the tube is secured, it is connected to suction at 20 cm H_2O and then water-sealed as tolerated. A chest radiograph is obtained to confirm reexpansion and tube placement.

Pulmonary Embolus

Oxygen. Oxygen is provided and adjusted using the results of the arterial blood gas analysis and the patient's clinical condition.

Anticoagulation. Low-molecular-weight heparin is started, if there is no contraindication, with an initial weight-based intravenous bolus followed by an infusion. The rate of the infusion is subsequently adjusted according to the partial thromboplastin time, with a goal of 1.5 to 2.0 times the normal value.

Thrombolytic Therapy. Thrombolytic therapy with recombinant tissue plasminogen activator (rtPA) is considered in patients with massive pulmonary embolus, presenting with hemodynamic instability, severe hypoxia, and progressive shock.

Vena Cava Interruption. Patients with contraindications to anticoagulation and those with recurrent emboli despite adequate anticoagulation are candidates for caval interruption with a Greenfield filter. Patients should be carefully chosen and closely followed, because over time there is an increased risk of recurrent thromboembolism.

Congestive Heart Failure

Oxygen. High-flow oxygen is started on all patients. Active airway management is instituted as necessary.

Nitrates. Preload and afterload reduction, secondary to venodilation (and arteriodilatation) by nitrates will often lead to prompt improvement in the patient's clinical status. No other pharmacologic intervention improves the symptoms of CHF as rapidly as nitrates. Sublingual nitroglycerin, 0.4 mg, has an onset of action of 30 seconds and is usually well tolerated. This dose is repeated every 5 minutes, for a total of three doses. An intravenous infusion is also useful, is easily titrated, and is particularly helpful in hypertensive patients and those with myocardial ischemia. Serial monitoring of blood pressure is essential.

Diuretics. Diuretics have a dual role in patients with congestive heart failure. Within minutes, there is an initial preload reduction owing to increased venous capacitance (dilatation). Second, the renal diuretic effect begins within 20 minutes. A first choice is typically furosemide, a loop diuretic. The usual starting dose is 20 to 80 mg intravenously. Lower dosages are used in patients new to the drug. Patients with renal insufficiency or those on chronic diuretic therapy usually require the higher doses. Other more potent loop diuretics (e.g., bumetanide) may be used if there is a poor response to standard therapy.

Morphine Sulfate. Intravenous low-dose morphine sulfate (2 mg to 4 mg) reduces venous return (preload), dilates pulmonary vasculature, and acts as an analgesic and anxiolytic. Dosing may be repeated every 5 to 10 minutes if necessary, if tolerated by the patient's clinical condition and vital signs. An atropine-like action may cause first- or second-degree heart block in susceptible patients, and patients should remain monitored.

Bronchodilators. Patients with reflex bronchospasm will benefit from inhaled β_2 agonists. Baseline tachycardia is likely caused by hypoxia, and cautious β_2 agonist use may improve oxygenation.

Inotropic Agents. Inotropic agents are required for patients not responding to other medical management. Dobutamine, a β_1 agonist, is considered the drug of choice for treatment of congestive heart failure in normotensive patients (mean arterial blood pressure > 80 mm Hg). Dobutamine has a potent inotropic effect without peripheral vasoconstriction and is usually well tolerated. Dopamine is preferred in the presence of shock (mean arterial blood pressure < 80 mm Hg) because of a constrictive effect on the peripheral vasculature. Amrinone, a phosphodi-esterase inhibitor with inotropic and vasodilatory effects, may improve the hemodynamic status of patients with cardiogenic pulmonary edema. Most of these patients are taking a digitalis preparation before their emergency department visit. On rare occasions, intravenous digitalis may be given in the emergency setting.

Angiotensin-Converting Enzyme (ACE) Inhibitors. Acutely, these medications reduce preload and afterload, improve kidney flow, and decrease sodium retention. They may be administered intravenously or sublingually, with effects in 10 to 60 minutes. The exact role of ACE inhibitors in the emergency department therapy of acutely decompensated left ventricular function is evolving. They are worthy of consideration in patients in whom they are not contraindicated—pregnancy, ACE angioedema history, or hyperkalemia.

Hyperventilation Syndrome

Diagnosis. Although hyperventilation may be readily apparent, other causes of dyspnea, particularly pulmonary embolus and myocardial ischemia, must be ruled out. Arterial blood gas analysis typically confirms a significant respiratory alkalosis with normal oxygenation. This test is ordered on a case-by-case basis.

Rebreather. The use of a paper bag "rebreather" is discouraged because it may lead to significant hypoxia if the patient is not closely observed.

Reassurance. Reassurance is of the utmost importance. Hyperventilation events are common, and patients require sympathetic support.

Medication. The patient may be treated with a mild anxiolytic and discharged. Close follow-up with a primary physician is recommended, particularly in recurrent cases. A discussion of life stressors or trigger events may benefit the patient and lead to coping mechanisms.

UNCERTAIN DIAGNOSIS

If the final diagnosis or the separation of pulmonary versus nonpulmonary causes is unclear, the extent of the emergency department workup depends on the general condition of the patient. The respiratory rate, breath sounds, and presence of underlying medical problems are reviewed a second time. The minimum diagnostic tests include pulse oximetry, arterial blood gas analysis, and a chest radiograph. Other studies are ordered as needed, based on the clinical situation. Discussion with a consultant may be necessary. If

patients remain hypoxic or in distress, hospital admission for observation and further workup becomes necessary. A bedside echocardiogram may reveal an unanticipated pericardial effusion. If the patient appears well, has a normal baseline PO_2, and a normal chest radiograph and does not have significant medical problems (e.g., diabetes, cardiac disease, immunosuppression), then discharge is allowed, with a follow-up appointment scheduled for the next day.

SPECIAL CONSIDERATIONS

Pediatric Patients

A wide variety of disorders cause dyspnea in the pediatric population, including the majority of those affecting adults and some entities unique to children. Common causes of shortness of breath in children include

- Upper airway
  Croup
  Epiglottitis
  Foreign body aspiration
  Retropharyngeal abscess
- Lower airway
  Anaphylaxis
  Asthma
  Bronchiolitis
  Bronchopulmonary dysplasia
  Cystic fibrosis
  Foreign body aspiration
  Pneumonia

Dyspnea in children seldom presents with the same manifestations that occur in adults. Children are usually brought to medical providers because of fever, cough, or generalized illness. An accurate respiratory rate is essential, and normal ranges in children vary with age.

Pregnant Patients

Many physiologic changes occur during pregnancy. Respiratory physiology compensations include increased oxygen consumption and delivery, decreased resistance, decreased functional residual capacity, and increased minute ventilation. Frequently, these changes may produce the complaint of dyspnea in the final trimester of pregnancy. Additionally, the pregnant patient has an increased risk for developing pulmonary complications. The most common problems are venous thrombosis or pulmonary embolism, asthmatic exacerbation with dyspnea, and pulmonary edema.

Pulmonary Embolism. There is an increased incidence of venous thrombosis (up to 3 per 1000 pregnancies) and pulmonary embolism during pregnancy. This may be secondary to compression of the vena cava by the uterus and by hypercoagulation. Anticoagulation therapy is achieved with heparin (unfractionated or low molecular weight) until the time of delivery, because warfarin is contraindicated because of its teratogenic effects. Heparin is started intravenously in the hospital and continued subcutaneously as an outpatient, adjusted for a partial thromboplastin time of two to two and one-half times normal (5,000 to 10,000 units subcutaneously throughout pregnancy). The therapeutic dose of enoxaparin is 1 mg/kg subcutaneously twice a day, and the prophylactic dose is 30 to 40 mg subcutaneously once a day. Complications of heparin therapy include bleeding and heparin-induced thrombocytopenia or osteopenia. The risk of pulmonary embolism continues to the postpartum period. Use of elastic stockings and efforts at early ambulation are recommended for lowering this risk.

Asthma. Asthma worsens in a third of patients during pregnancy, improves for another third, and has no change in the remaining third. Exacerbations of asthma during pregnancy can lead to maternal stress and hypoxia with serious negative impact on the fetus. Treatment is the same as in the nonpregnant patient (see Chapter 38, Wheezing). Assessment of peak expiratory flow baseline values may be an objective measurement to be used for respiratory status throughout pregnancy.

Pulmonary Edema. Pulmonary edema, related to preeclampsia or cardiomyopathy, can occasionally occur in the peripartum period. Peripartum cardiomyopathy may have nonspecific symptoms initially, but has an extremely high morbidity and morality if undetected and untreated.

DISPOSITION AND FOLLOW-UP

The disposition for dyspneic patients will depend on the cause of the dyspnea and the response to therapy in the emergency department. Suggestions for admission and follow-up for patients with common causes of dyspnea are described here.

COPD. Most patients with a primary bronchospastic component to their disease improve with emergency department treatment and can be discharged with close follow-up by their personal physician. General criteria for admission include

- Presence of pneumonia
- Presence of pneumothorax

- Mental status changes
- Failure of hypercarbia or acidosis to resolve with treatment
- No subjective improvement after 4 to 6 hours of treatment

Pneumonia. Nontoxic patients, who are otherwise healthy, may be discharged on oral antibiotics with follow-up in 24 to 48 hours. Patients with risk factors such as age (very young and very old), significant tachypnea, multilobar involvement, preexisting lung disease, PO_2 less than 60 mm Hg, diabetes, alcoholism, chronic renal failure, and sickle cell anemia and those with ongoing emesis are admitted for intravenous therapy (antibiotics and crystalloid).

Pulmonary Embolism. All patients with confirmed or suspected pulmonary embolism are admitted, and most can be placed on the regular ward if they are hemodynamically stable.

Pneumothorax. A select group of patients with pneumothorax may be discharged if there is no reaccumulation of air after catheter aspiration, if there has been a minimum of 6 hours of observation, and if there is no increased collapse on a repeat chest radiograph. A 24-hour follow-up including a repeat radiograph is necessary. If these criteria cannot be met, the patient is admitted.

Pulmonary Edema. Most patients with pulmonary edema are admitted to the intensive care unit. Many will require invasive monitoring, complicated pharmacologic therapy, and a "rule out myocardial infarction" protocol.

Myocardial Infarction. All patients of myocardial infarction are admitted to the intensive care unit for cardiac monitoring, serial electrocardiogram, and cardiac enzyme analysis. These patients are at high risk for dysrhythmias, valvular complications, congestive heart failure, and hypotension.

Hyperventilation Syndrome. Symptoms usually resolve after a short period of observation in the emergency department and after the appropriate reassurance has been provided. These patients are discharged home when other causes of dyspnea have been ruled out. Patients are referred to a primary care physician for a follow-up visit.

FINAL POINTS

- Dyspnea is a common complaint in people presenting to the emergency department.
- Although the sensation of dyspnea is poorly understood, the amount of dyspnea usually correlates with the severity of the causative illness.

- The complaint of dyspnea has high potential for significant morbidity and should never be taken lightly by a physician.
- The respiratory rate is one of the most sensitive indicators of respiratory distress.
- The chest radiograph is an important diagnostic test for evaluating the dyspneic patient.
- The diagnosis of dyspnea is divided into pulmonary and nonpulmonary causes.

Pulmonary causes may be explored anatomically. Nonpulmonary causes include primary cardiac disorders, acid-base disorders, central nervous system problems, and deficiencies in oxygen-carrying capacity of hemoglobin.
- Although the treatment of dyspnea is primarily directed at the specific cause, supplemental O_2 remains the mainstay of therapy in the acute phase.

CASE *Study*

The 19-year-old man who presented after a sudden onset of left-sided chest pain and difficulty breathing while playing basketball had a blood pressure of 125/85 mm Hg, pulse of 105 beats per minute, and respiratory rate of 32 breaths per minute. The physical examination demonstrated decreased breath sounds and hyperresonance at the left chest. An oxygen mask was adjusted to give 4 L/min, and an intravenous line was started with normal saline running at KVO (keep-vein-open, approximately 30 mL/hr).

The history and physical examination suggests a spontaneous pneumothorax. In many patients with a simple spontaneous pneumothorax, the findings are subtle and may be overlooked in the activity and noise of the emergency department. Moving a patient to a quiet room where careful percussion and auscultation can be appreciated is the best course of action, when the patient is stable. The patient's complaint was rapidly localized to a pulmonary disorder occurring anatomically at the left thoracic cage/lung interface: a pneumothorax. Until it was definitively diagnosed, other possibilities were not excluded.

Posteroanterior and lateral chest radiographs were ordered and revealed a 50% pneumothorax on the left side. The mediastinal structures were in their normal position, and no midline shift had occurred.

Occasionally there is a high suspicion of pneumothorax, but the routine inspiratory film does not reveal a collapse. An expiratory view, reducing the chest cavity/lung volume ratio (improving contrast between the lung parenchyma and air) may reveal the presence of a small pneumothorax.

Because this was a moderate to large pneumothorax, the decision was made to place a chest tube. Informed consent was obtained, and the patient was prepped and draped under strict sterile technique. A 28 French chest tube was placed through the fifth intercostal space at the midaxillary line, with blunt dissection. Before the procedure, the patient was given narcotic analgesia and a benzodiazepine for sedation. A portable chest radiograph confirmed tube placement and reexpansion of the lung after the procedure. The patient's vital signs improved and remained stable. Bilateral breath sounds were auscultated on the postprocedure examination.

The patient was admitted, and the chest tube was subsequently placed to water seal. No air leak was noted, and the chest tube was removed within 24 hours. Follow-up radiographs were normal. The patient was discharged with information about recurrent spontaneous pneumothorax and was cautioned that he was at high risk for recurrence.

Bibliography

TEXTS

Baum GL, Wolinsky E (eds): Textbook of Pulmonary Diseases, 6th ed. Philadelphia, Lippincott Williams & Wilkins, 1997.

Fishman AP (ed): Fishman's Pulmonary Diseases and Disorders, 3rd ed. New York, McGraw-Hill, 1998.

JOURNAL ARTICLES

Bach PB, Brown C, Gelfand SE, et al: Management of acute exacerbations of chronic obstructive pulmonary disease: A summary and appraisal of published evidence. Ann Intern Med 2001; 134:600–620.

Barnes D: Chronic obstructive pulmonary disease. N Engl J Med 2000; 343:269–280.

Bosker G: Community-acquired pneumonia (CAP): Antibiotic selection and management update (I and II). Emerg Med Rep 2002; 23:93–108, 109–128.

Emerman CL, Bosker G: Community-acquired pneumonia (CAP) update year 2000 (I and II). Emerg Med Rep 1999; 20:237–248, 248–260.

Goldhaber SZ: Pulmonary embolism. N Engl J Med 1998; 339:93–104.

Hirsh J, Bates S: Clinical trials that have influenced the treatment of venous thromboembolism. Ann Intern Med 2001; 134:407–417.

Hsieh M, Auble TE, Yealy DM: Predicting the future: can this patient with acute congestive heart failure be safely discharged from the emergency department? Ann Emerg Med 2002; 39:181–189.

Kline JA: Dyspnea: Fear, loathing, and physiology. Emerg Med Pract 1999; 1(3):1–22.

Kline JA, Johns KL, Colucciello SA, Israel EG: New diagnostic tests for pulmonary embolism. Ann Emerg Med 2000; 35:168–180.

Kosowsky JM, Kobayashi L: Acutely decompensated heart failure: diagnostic and therapeutic strategies for the new millenium. Emerg Med Pract 2002; 4(2):1–28.

LeConte P, et al: Prognostic factors in acute cardiogenic pulmonary edema. Am J Emerg Med 1999; 17:329–332.

Metlay JP, Kapoor WN, Fine MJ: Does this patient have community acquired pneumonia? JAMA 1997; 278:1440–1445.

Michelson E, Hollrah S: Evaluation of the patient with shortness of breath: An evidence based approach. Emerg Med Clin North Am 1999; 17:221–237.

Niewoehner DE, Erbland ML, Deupree RH, et al: Effect of system glucocorticoids on exacerbations of chronic obstructive pulmonary disease. N Engl J Med 1999; 340:1941–1947.

Peacock WF: Heart failure in the elderly. Geriatr Emerg Med Rep 2000; 1(6):41–52.

Peacock WF, Freda BS: The clinical challenge of heart failure: Comprehensive, evidence-based management of the hospitalized patient with acute myocardial decompensation (I,II). Emerg Med Rep 2002; (23):83–108.

Robinson DJ, Rogers R: The clinical challenge of congestive heart failure (I and II). Emerg Med Rep 1999; 20:121–130, 131–142.

Ryan MT, Radeos MS: Acute exacerbations of COPD: a practical approach to differential diagnosis and management. Emerg Med Pract 2002; 4(4):1–20.

Sahn SA, Heffner JE: Spontaneous pneumothorax. N Engl J Med 2000; 342:868–874.

Snow V, Lascher S, Mottur-Pilson M: Evidence base for management of acute exacerbations of chronic obstructive pulmonary disease. Ann Intern Med 2001; 134:595–599.

Ware LB, Matthay MA: The acute respiratory distress syndrome. N Engl J Med 2000; 342:1334–1349.

Wolfe TR, Hartsell SC: Pulmonary embolism and making sense of the diagnostic evaluation. Ann Emerg Med 2001; 37:504–514.

CHAPTER 38

Wheezing

STEVE SIGRIST
LESLIE WOLF

CASE*Study*

The mother of a 17-year-old young woman called 911 because her daughter was "wheezing and can't catch her breath." The mother was very agitated, begged for immediate help, and could give no more information to the dispatcher.

INTRODUCTION

Definitions

A *wheeze* (sibilant rhonchus) is a continuous, musical sound produced by vibration as air moves past a resistance or partial obstruction in the lower respiratory tract. It is a common finding in patients presenting to the emergency department with shortness of breath or cough.

There are numerous causes of wheezing that are important to consider in patients with no prior history of obstructive airway disease (Table 38–1). Wheezing is most frequently associated with asthma and chronic obstructive pulmonary disease, and these diseases are the primary focus of this chapter.

Asthma is defined by the American Lung Association as a disease characterized by inflammation of the airways and increased responsiveness to various stimuli called "triggers." These trigger factors include inhaled antigens, exercise, cold air, irritant gases (e.g., cigarette smoke), animal dander, dust, drugs (aspirin, β blockers), and emotional stress. The resultant widespread airway narrowing may vary in severity depending on the nature of the "trigger" and the effectiveness of therapy.

There are approximately 14.6 million asthmatics in the United States, and the numbers are increasing. A 61% increase in the number of asthmatics has occurred between 1982 and 1996, and a 20% increase in emergency department visits for asthma was noted between 1992 and 1995. There are more than 2 million emergency department visits, 500,000 hospital admissions, and approximately 5,600 deaths due to asthma in the United States each year. Despite advances in treatment, the mortality rate has continued to climb at an alarming rate (almost 80% increase since 1980), particularly among the young (<19 years) and minority groups.

Chronic obstructive pulmonary disease (COPD) is a term encompassing a spectrum of respiratory diseases. Emphysema and chronic bronchitis are identifiable points on this continuum. The American Thoracic Society defines *emphysema* as an anatomic alteration characterized by an abnormal enlargement of the air spaces distal to the terminal, nonrespiratory bronchioles accompanied by destructive changes of the alveolar walls. *Chronic bronchitis* is a clinical disorder associated with excessive secretion of mucus in the bronchial tree. It is characterized by a chronic or recurrent productive cough during most days of the month for a minimum of 3 months a year for not less than 2 successive years. The major predisposing factor for COPD is cigarette smoking. Other processes can lead to its development, including exposure to industrial or vegetable dusts, cystic fibrosis, and α_1-antitrypsin deficiency. Most patients with COPD have features of both emphysema and chronic bronchitis. COPD has tremendous morbidity and is responsible for almost 87,000 deaths annually in the United States. Patients with decompensated COPD are commonly evaluated in the emergency department.

Pathophysiology

The pathophysiology of asthma involves many body systems that contribute to increased airway reactivity and lung tissue inflammation. The autonomic nervous system is important in determining bronchomuscular tone. The smooth muscle of the airways is innervated by both adrenergic (bronchodilating) and cholinergic (bronchoconstricting) fibers. The cholinergic fibers are carried by the vagus nerve. When stimulated, they cause constriction of small airways and increased glandular secretions. This vagally mediated bronchoconstriction can result from the triggering of

TABLE 38–1. Differential Diagnosis of the Wheezing Patient (ASTHMATIC)

A—Asthma

Asthma (varies by severity, precipitating factors)

S—Stasis

Pulmonary embolism

T—Toxins

Toxic gases
Smoke inhalation
Insecticides
Cholinergic poisonings
Chemical irritants, hydrocarbons

H—Heart

Congestive heart failure, pulmonary edema ("cardiac asthma")
Noncardiogenic pulmonary edema
Acute respiratory distress syndrome (any cause)

M—Mechanical

Foreign body (upper airway, lower airway)
Foreign body embolism (intravenous drug abuse)

A—Allergy, Aspiration

Anaphylaxis
Laryngeal edema
Organic particle exposure
Extrinsic allergic alveolitis
Aspiration of gastric contents, esophageal reflux
Near-drowning

T—Trauma, Tumor

Upper airway trauma
Pneumothorax, tension pneumothorax
Endobronchial tumor

I—Infection

Bronchitis
Pneumonia
Bronchiolitis
Croup, epiglottitis (more often stridor)
Pertussis
Fungal diseases

C—Chronic Lung Disease, Congenital Lung Disease

Chronic obstructive pulmonary disease (emphysema, bronchitis)
α_1-Antitrypsin deficiency
Cystic fibrosis
Congenital abnormalities of the respiratory, cardiovascular, or gastrointestinal systems
Bronchopulmonary dysplasia

irritant receptors in both the large and small airways, as well as by centrally activated chemoreceptors. There is evidence of an exaggerated parasympathetic response in the airways of asthmatic patients.

There are both α- and β_2-adrenergic receptors in airway smooth muscle. Stimulation of α receptors causes bronchoconstriction, however the number of α receptors is small and probably does not significantly contribute to bronchial hyperreactivity. The β_2 receptors are plentiful and are potent bronchodilators.

The systemic release of chemical mediators has a significant role in increasing airway resistance and producing lung tissue inflammation. In "extrinsic" asthma, specific extracorporeal allergens bind with IgE on mast cells lining the tracheobronchial tree, stimulating the release of preformed mediators (e.g., eosinophilic chemotactic factor, neutrophilic chemotactic factor, and histamine) and the synthesis of others (e.g., leukotrienes, platelet-activating factors, and prostaglandins). These mediators stimulate bronchial smooth muscle constriction, secretion of mucus, bronchial wall edema due to vasodilation, and interstitial influx of eosinophils and neutrophils. A similar release of chemical mediators occurs in patients with intrinsic asthma in response to intracorporeal stimuli.

The pathophysiologic changes in asthma result in increased airway resistance, air trapping, and ventilation/perfusion mismatch. Symptoms include dyspnea and cough, and decreased air exchange and wheezing are evident on physical examination.

The pathologic changes characteristic of COPD include hypertrophy and hypersecretion of mucus-secreting glands, bronchial smooth muscle hypertrophy, mucosal inflammation, and destruction and enlargement of alveoli. The end result of these changes is variably reversible airway obstruction and diminished oxygen diffusion capacity. Over time, the COPD patient usually develops carbon dioxide retention and hypoxemia. As chronic carbon dioxide retention progresses, the patient's stimulation to breathe becomes more reliant on hypoxia ("hypoxic drive") and less on hypercarbia. Pulmonary hypertension and cor pulmonale are complications from severe or long-standing COPD.

INITIAL APPROACH AND STABILIZATION

Priority Diagnoses

If the patient is in severe respiratory distress, early intervention precedes or accompanies the rapid assessment. The emergency physician must make a rapid assessment of the patient's airway and determine what early interventions are required. If the patient is in less distress, management can proceed in a more traditional sequence.

The priority list of diagnoses in the patient with wheezing and respiratory distress includes the following:

- Status asthmaticus
- Decompensated COPD
- Congestive heart failure
- Anaphylaxis
- Pneumonia
- Pulmonary embolus
- Pneumothorax

Rapid Assessment

1. Does the patient have known asthma or COPD? Are there any other possible causes for the wheezing?
2. What is the length of the episode?
3. What is the patient's assessment of the current severity?
4. Are there known risk factors for mortality?
   a. Sudden, acute exacerbations that do not respond quickly to treatment
   b. History of intubation or near-fatal episode
   c. History of admission to an intensive care unit (ICU)
   d. Current systemic corticosteroid use
   e. More than two β-agonist inhalers used per month
5. What are the present medications, especially corticosteroids, and the ones most recently taken?
6. What is the patient's position on the stretcher? Sitting up is consistent with higher severity.
7. What is the patient's mental status and ability to cooperate?
8. What is the ability of the patient to speak, and how long are the sentences?
9. Auscultation of the heart and lungs is performed, and the inspiratory-to-expiratory ratio of breathing is noted.
10. The use of accessory muscles is noted.
11. Is there jugular venous distention or peripheral edema?
12. Is there cyanosis or diaphoresis?

Early Intervention

The initial steps in management include

1. If the patient is in severe respiratory distress, *high-flow oxygen* at a rate sufficient to maintain normal saturation is administered. In COPD patients suspected of carbon dioxide retention, there is a theoretical risk of hypoventilation induced by high levels of oxygen. Sufficient oxygen is not withheld in these patients, but the physician must be aware of the possible need for ventilatory support.
2. *Pulse oximetry* is measured. Decreased oxygen saturation may be an early finding in airway obstruction. Levels less than 91% suggest a severe problem.

3. *Cardiac monitoring* is implemented because dysrhythmias are often seen in these patients and can be caused by hypoxia, adrenergic stimulation or therapy, and underlying disease (e.g., myocardial infarction with secondary congestive heart failure).

4. An *intravenous line* is placed and isotonic crystalloid is infused initially at a keep-open rate.

5. If the patient is wheezing significantly or if there is little or no air exchange, *aerosolized bronchodilator therapy* is begun immediately. A β-adrenergic agonist, typically albuterol, is given by nebulizer or metered-dose inhaler (MDI).

6. If the patient is believed to be in severe respiratory distress, but not in immediate need of intubation, *arterial blood gas (ABG) measurements* and a portable *chest radiograph* are obtained. Aerosol therapy is not delayed for either of these assessments.

7. In patients with asthma, intubation and assisted ventilation are required only in less than 1% of patients. Absolute indications for immediate intubation of the wheezing patient are apnea and coma. Intubation (see Chapter 2, Airway Management) is considered if

- PO_2 is less than 50 mm Hg (with supplemental oxygen).
- PCO_2 is greater than 50 mm Hg with acute respiratory acidosis.
- PCO_2 is increasing despite maximal therapy.
- Patient is fatigued.
- Mental status is depressed.

Before intubation every attempt is made to reverse the bronchoconstriction with aerosolized β-adrenergic agonists, corticosteroids, and other medications.

CLINICAL ASSESSMENT

History

A careful history is the key to determining the etiology of wheezing and respiratory distress. Whereas the majority of patient presentations are related to asthma or COPD, a careful history may suggest pursuing a different direction. A full history may be delayed until the patient is stabilized and able to converse.

1. Does the patient have a known history of asthma or COPD?

2. What is the *time of onset* and *duration of symptoms*? The longer the symptoms have lasted, the more likely is the need for admission. Sudden onset may suggest aeroallergens, inhaled foreign body, acute congestive heart failure, or spontaneous pneumothorax.

3. *What events preceded the symptoms*, including *exposure* to known *trigger factors* (e.g., exposure to allergens, preceding respiratory infections, situational stress, exercise, or cold air)?

4. *What elements* of this episode are *atypical relative* to *previous episodes*? Is there chest pain, a productive cough, or fever and chills? Ischemic heart disease, pneumothorax, and pulmonary infection should always be considered in the patient with acute wheezing.

5. *What medications* does the patient take, and what is the *level of compliance*? Data are obtained about the amount and most recent dosage of β-adrenergic agonists, corticosteroids, leukotriene antagonists, and other medications.

6. *What treatment has been tried* by the patient *since* becoming ill? Specifically, inhaler and over-the-counter medication use is discussed. Resistance to β-adrenergics (tachyphylaxis) can occur with overuse.

7. *What is the severity of the patient's underlying COPD or asthma* (mortality risk factors)? Has hospitalization (especially admission to an ICU) or endotracheal intubation occurred in the past? Are corticosteroids given as part of care? When was the patient last treated with corticosteroids? Asthma or COPD tends to follow previous patterns. A patient with a history of frequent admission or previous intubation requires heightened concern.

8. *What is the patient's assessment* of the *severity* of this episode *relative* to *prior episodes*? Patients may be helpful in judging the severity of their attacks and their progress during acute intervention. Still, up to 25% of patients, especially the elderly and men, underestimate the severity of their bronchoconstriction.

9. What is the *past medical history*— cardiopulmonary disease, hypertension, or diabetes? Is there a history of smoking or exposure to a smoker or illicit drug use? Does the patient have allergies?

In a patient without a prior history of asthma or COPD, the history is aimed at ruling out other causes of wheezing. All of the previous points are ascertained, and other questions are asked:

1. Is there *recent-onset dyspnea on exertion, orthopnea, or paroxysmal nocturnal dyspnea*?

2. Is there *recent weight gain* or *peripheral edema*?
3. What *nonpulmonary medications* have been taken (e.g., especially β-adrenergic blocking agents)?
4. Has there been *possible toxic gas exposure*? *What is the patient's occupation*?
5. Is there a possibility of *foreign-body aspiration*, especially in children?

Physical Examination

Ominous findings consistent with severe bronchospasm and pulmonary insufficiency are sought immediately:

1. Excessive use of accessory muscles of respiration, with visible retractions
2. Diaphoresis
3. Altered mental status
4. The need to sit upright to breathe
5. An inability to speak or one- and two-word replies because of dyspnea
6. Presence of central cyanosis
7. Visible fatigue

In the wheezing patient who is less severely ill, the physical examination focuses on the following:

Vital Signs. Vital signs are taken and compared with those obtained by prehospital personnel, if applicable. In adults, a persistent heart rate over 130 beats per minute despite therapy suggests serious disease. Respiratory rates of less than 12 and more than 40 breaths per minute are signs of significant problems. Fever suggests possible infection and warrants a more extensive evaluation. Pulsus paradoxus can be measured, and when elevated above 20 mm Hg it indicates severe airway obstruction. An elevated pulsus is an insensitive parameter and is highly dependent on respiratory effort. It is absent in almost half of asthmatics with severe respiratory obstruction.

Ear, Nose, and Throat. The nose and throat may reflect acute or chronic allergic disease. Increased nasal secretions, mucosal swelling, and findings consistent with sinusitis may be found. Difficulty swallowing may represent a pharyngeal, esophageal, or laryngeal lesion. These may be associated with acute wheezing.

Neck. The neck is examined for jugular venous distention, suprasternal retractions, the use of accessory musculature, and the midline position of the trachea. Neck veins that distend during inspiration represent a significant increase in right-sided pressure (e.g., tension pneumotho-

rax or pericardium). The neck is auscultated to determine if the "wheezing" is actually upper airway stridor.

Thorax. The thorax is assessed for respiratory excursion and prolongation of the expiratory phase and palpated for subcutaneous air. A "barrel chest" with an increased anteroposterior diameter may be seen in the patient with severe chronic airway disease. The thorax is percussed for hyperresonance (air) or dullness (fluid or consolidation). The lungs are auscultated for rales, wheezing, adequate air exchange, signs of consolidation, and symmetry of breath sounds. The experienced examiner can roughly gauge severity based on the lung examination, but there can be significant errors. In the patient with severe respiratory insufficiency, inadequate air exchange may not create sufficient turbulence to produce wheezing. The "silent chest" in a patient working hard to breathe represents a critical situation.

Cardiac. During the cardiac examination the point of maximal cardiac impulse is determined to estimate heart size and position. The heart is auscultated for rate and rhythm, the presence of any gallops, murmurs, or rubs, and the possible presence of mediastinal "crackling" with the heartbeat, indicating pneumomediastinum.

Abdomen. The abdomen is assessed for hepatomegaly, hepatojugular reflux, or ascites.

Extremities. The extremities are examined for adequacy of circulation (cyanosis or prolonged capillary refill), clubbing, and the presence of edema.

Neurologic. The patient's mental status and ability to cooperate remains the final common pathway for assessing the effectiveness of oxygenation, ventilation, and circulation. Fatigue may play a significant role in the patient's ability to respond.

Special Tests

Expiratory Flow Measurements. The peak expiratory flow rate (PEFR) or the forced expiratory volume in 1 second (FEV_1) may be a useful parameter both for assessing the severity of disease and the response to treatment. To properly interpret the results, it is useful to know the patient's baseline. Results are dependent on patient effort and proper technique and should not be relied on as the sole indicator of severity of disease.

CLINICAL REASONING

At this point, three questions are addressed.

If the Patient Does Not Have Known Asthma or COPD, What is the Potential Cause of the Wheezing?

Table 38–1 lists the major diseases in the differential diagnosis of the wheezing patient, using the pneumonic ASTHMATIC. Only a few of these may be difficult to distinguish from bronchospasm caused by asthma or COPD.

Congestive heart failure (CHF) can represent a difficult differential diagnosis in the patient with exacerbated COPD or when asthma-like symptoms appear in an elderly patient. Because management of CHF is quite different from that of asthma or COPD, it is an important differential decision to make early in the course of care. Historical points indicative of left-sided heart failure include nocturnal dyspnea or orthopnea preceding the wheezing and a prior history or symptoms consistent with ischemic heart disease. Physical findings include an S_3 or S_4 extra heart sound, rales, and peripheral right-sided CHF signs: peripheral edema, jugular venous distention, or hepatojugular reflux. A portable chest radiograph may resolve the issue.

Pulmonary embolism—"the great imitator"—occasionally presents as wheezing, but usually there is associated dyspnea and pleuritic chest pain; and in more than 90% of patients an associated predisposing factor will be present. COPD is a known predisposing condition for the development of pulmonary embolism, and therefore it is necessary to consider it in the known COPD patient who presents with acute shortness of breath and chest pain.

Certain life-threatening disorders of the *upper airway* may be mistaken for lower airway disease if care is not taken to differentiate the high-pitched, predominantly inspiratory sound of stridor from true wheezing. These disorders include epiglottitis, croup, and laryngeal foreign body. Failure to diagnose the disorder in such cases can lead to disastrous consequences.

If the Patient Has Known Asthma or COPD, What May Have Exacerbated the Problem?

There are a number of common precipitants of asthma and COPD. They may be short-lived or exist as significant diseases by themselves. The following precipitating causes are listed in order of decreasing relative concern:

- Pulmonary embolism
- Congestive heart failure
- Pneumothorax
- Infection
- Noncompliance with medications
- Irritant/allergic exposure

What is the Estimated Severity of Respiratory Difficulty Associated with the Patient's Wheezing?

Table 38–2 lists the classic physical findings that may discriminate between the three categories of respiratory severity. Although spirometric results are sometimes available (Table 38–3), the physical findings and history are usually enough to categorize the distress as mild, moderate, or severe. This information is most pertinent to decision making in patients with known asthma. COPD patients are optimally evaluated with serial ABG analyses. This initial classification is only a first impression of severity. Reassessment after the first aerosol treatment is often more useful in assessing the patient's true clinical status.

DIAGNOSTIC ADJUNCTS

Each of the following ancillary tests plays a role in the assessment of the patient with asthma or COPD. The usefulness of each measurement varies with the underlying disease.

Laboratory Studies

Arterial Blood Gas Analysis. In asthmatic patients, ABG measurements are not routinely obtained. Indications may include the patient presenting in severe respiratory distress, failure to respond to emergency department therapy, or a history of complex disease. The ABG analysis results do not always correspond to pulmonary function test results. In severe disease, the P_{CO_2} level may rise to normal and even to hypercarbic levels ($P_{CO_2} > 45$ mm Hg). This can be an ominous finding and may indicate impending respiratory failure. The degree of hypoxemia in this setting is usually severe ($P_{O_2} < 50$ mm Hg on room air).

In COPD patients, ABGs are obtained routinely. The physical findings and pulmonary function test results are difficult to interpret in these patients. Optimally, ABG analysis results can be compared with the patient's previous values. If not, one can get some idea of the ventilatory status by evaluating the pH. Patients who chronically retain CO_2 should have a compensatory increase in bicarbonate to maintain a normal pH range.

Complete Blood Cell Count and Differential. If an infectious cause is suspected in the wheezing patient, a white blood cell count

TABLE 38–2. Severity of Asthma as Gauged by Physical Findings

Degree of Severity	Physical Findings
Mild	Tachypnea—30 breaths per minute Patient tolerance good when recumbent Accessory musculature not used Pulsus paradoxus not present Wheezing audible
Moderate	Tachypnea—30–40 breaths per minute Patient tolerance fair with sitting Accessory musculature not used Pulsus paradoxus not present Wheezing diffuse, may be higher pitched
Severe	Tachypnea greater than 40 breaths per minute or inappropriately "normal" or slow Mental status may be confused or depressed Patient tolerance poor with sitting, diaphoresis Accessory muscles active Pulsus paradoxus present, 10–20 mm Hg Wheezing may be high pitched, of low intensity, or absent ("silent chest")
Drawbacks of assessing severity by physical examination	Assessment varies with examiner and patient Provides only late signs Accessory musculature use and pulsus paradoxus related to FEV_1 (latter not always present)

TABLE 38–3. Use and Interpretation of Pulmonary Function Testing in Asthma

PEFR (Ls/min)	% Predicted	FEV_1 (Ls)	% Predicted	Significance
Pretreatment				
<100	<20	<0.7	<20	Severe exacerbation. Early aggressive therapy required. Intubation may be required. ABGs and CXR appropriate. Most patients require admission.
100–200	20–30	0.7–1.0	20–25	Moderate exacerbation. ABGs appropriate in 16- to 40-year-old asthmatics (individualize in other age groups). CXR indicated if improvement is slow.
200–300	30–60	1.0–2.1	25–60	Mild exacerbation
>300	>60–70	>2.1	>60–70	Goal of therapy (but must be individualized).
After Initial Aerosol Therapy				
Improve <60		Improve <0.03		Severe exacerbation. Early aggressive therapy required. Intubation may be required. ABGs and CXR appropriate. Most patients require admission.
Final Value after Maximal Emergency Department Therapy				
<300	<60	<2.1	<60	Admit or schedule early follow-up. If discharged, adequate bronchodilator therapy and, if indicated, corticosteroids are continued.
>300	>60	>2.1	>60	Discharge on appropriate medications and with early follow-up arranged.

ABGs, arterial blood gases; CXR, chest radiograph.

may be helpful. It has limited use in the asthmatic patient because it is increased in about half of these patients, often with a left shift in the differential count owing to endogenous catecholamine release or the administration of adrenergic agonists. The white blood cell count also may be elevated in patients on chronic corticosteroid therapy.

Serum Electrolytes. In the asthmatic or COPD patient, serum electrolytes are generally required only when there is concern about significant dehydration. In the patient with CHF, electrolyte evaluation may be very helpful in those individuals receiving diuretics.

Serum Theophylline. In any patient with exacerbated pulmonary disease who is taking theophylline, a serum level of the drug is measured. The therapeutic range of serum theophylline is 10 to 20μg/mL. Theophylline metabolism is affected by a number of factors. This study is important if theophylline will be added to the patient's medication regimen or if theophylline toxicity is suspected.

Other Studies. Cardiac markers are ordered if there is the potential of an acute coronary syndrome causing the wheezing. B-type natriuretic peptide (BNP) is an endogenous hormone released as part of the response to stretch. It has some correlation with left ventricular overload and may have utility in differentiating CHF from COPD.

Radiologic Imaging

Chest radiographs are indicated if the cause of wheezing is in question. The films should be examined closely for signs of left-sided cardiac failure (cardiomegaly, cephalization of vascular flow, Kerley's lines, alveolar infiltrates), pulmonary infiltrate, pneumothorax, pneumomediastinum, interstitial lung disease, or asymmetric hyperinflation from foreign body or mass.

Chest radiography has limited usefulness in asthmatics. It influences the management in less than 10% of patients. Indications for chest films in asthmatics include fever, change in sputum production, clinical suspicion of other diseases, immunocompromised host, and unexplained chest pain. The radiograph in patients with asthma often shows hyperinflation or atelectasis secondary to plugging with mucus.

In patients with COPD, a chest radiograph is a routine part of the assessment because infection and pneumothorax are common and physical findings may not be accurate. These patients also have limited respiratory reserve and do not tolerate complications superimposed on their disease.

Electrocardiogram/echocardiography

An electrocardiogram generally has limited usefulness in the asthmatic or COPD patient. It is indicated in the wheezing patient if there is a complaint of chest pain or a history of prior cardiac disease or dysrhythmia. The most common abnormal findings include right ventricular strain with right-axis deviation and premature ventricular contractions. These findings are reversible and resolve with therapy and improvement in respiratory status. The electrocardiogram is important in patients suspected of wheezing secondary to left-sided cardiac failure ("cardiac asthma"). Echocardiography may have benefit in assessing

chamber dilatation or left ventricular function, as part of the differential diagnostic assessment of the wheezing patient.

Pulmonary Function Tests

Pulmonary function tests (PFTs) using simple hand-held devices are helpful in determining the initial severity of airway obstruction in the wheezing patient. Repeated measurements aid in following the patient's response to therapy and are valuable in determining appropriate disposition. Parameters most often measured are the FEV_1 and the peak expiratory flow rate (PEFR). Each measures the velocity of air flow and estimates the degree of airway obstruction. Both are effort dependent and can be altered by changes in lung volume. The results are compared with a table of normal values and the patient's historical values. Table 38–3 is a basic guide to interpreting PFT results in asthma. The patient should be asked what his or her baseline peak flow values are. Many patients can provide this valuable information. Values less than 30% of predicted suggest increased severity.

Sputum Analysis

If the wheezing patient has a productive cough, a sputum specimen can be obtained for wet mount examination, Gram's stain, and culture. The wet mount is examined for neutrophils and eosinophils. Eosinophils are cells with shiny green granules and represent an allergic component in the cause of bronchospasm. These studies are particularly important in COPD patients in whom infection is a frequent complication.

PRINCIPLES OF MANAGEMENT

Consistent application of effective clinical guidelines can result in decreased emergency department stay and fewer admissions. Currently, there are no national level evidence-based guidelines in common use.

The basic principles of management in the wheezing patient are protection and patency of the airway, relief of bronchospasm and hypoxia, rehydration, and the treatment of causes or complications (e.g., pneumothorax and pneumonia). Management proceeds following these guidelines:

1. Each patient is unique, and therapy is tailored to the patient's needs and response.
2. Because of differences in age groups and pathophysiology, patients with asthma and

COPD with wheezing are not managed in the same manner. Treatment in asthmatics should emphasize reversal of bronchospasm and hypoxemia. In patients with COPD the highest priority is reversal of hypoxemia. Bronchospasm is treated to the degree it contributes to the patient's underlying respiratory problem.

3. Initial management is based on the category of severity that applies to the patient. This categorization is adjusted according to the patient's response to treatment.

4. A useful time for categorizing the severity of a patient's wheezing is after the first β-adrenergic aerosol treatment. Inhaled aerosol is the first therapy used in patients with essentially all categories of wheezing, except patients needing immediate intubation.

Figure 38–1 is an algorithm for management of reversible obstructive airway disease based on the broad categories of mild, moderate, and severe. It is intended as a guide to therapy and cannot replace attentive assessment, clinical judgment,

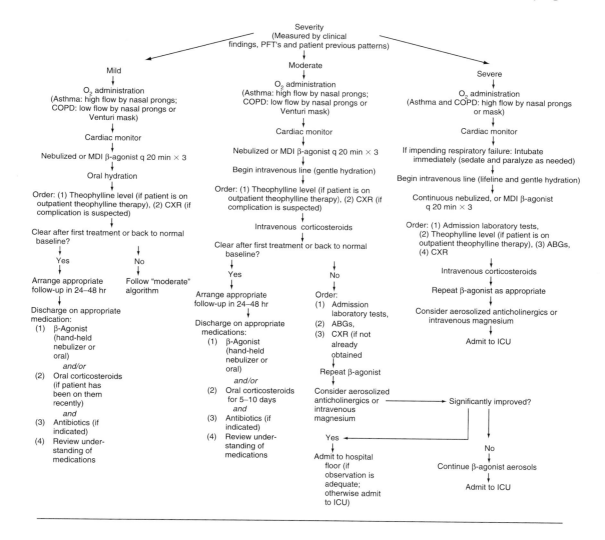

SQ = subcutaneous; ABGs = arterial blood gases; CXR = chest radiograph; MDI = metered dose inhaler, PFTs = pulmonary function tests.
This algorithm is meant only as a management guideline. It cannot replace good clinical judgment, especially in response to changes in patient condition.

FIGURE 38–1 • Management algorithm for reversible obstructive airway disease. This algorithm is meant only as a management guideline. It cannot replace good clinical judgment, especially in response to changes in patient condition. ABGs, arterial blood gases; CXR, chest radiograph; ICU, intensive care unit; MDI, metered-dose inhaler; PFTs, pulmonary function tests.

and appropriate response to changes in the patient's condition. More information on the measures applied within this algorithm is supplied next.

General Measures

Rehydration. Most decompensated asthmatics are mildly dehydrated from increased insensate fluid losses (tachypnea, fever) and decreased oral intake. Mucous viscosity may be increased and clearance decreased by dehydration. Oral fluids may be satisfactory, but intravenous hydration is often necessary. Overhydration is avoided because it may worsen mucosal edema and precipitate pulmonary edema. COPD patients are less likely to have concomitant dehydration than are asthmatics.

Antibiotics. Antibiotics are added to the treatment regimen if there is evidence of bacterial infection (e.g., purulent sputum with a predominance of neutrophils on wet mount). Broad-spectrum antibiotics are selected (i.e., an expanded-spectrum penicillin or a second- or third-generation cephalosporin). Macrolide antibiotics should be administered to any patient at risk for pneumonia from atypical bacteria (e.g., *Mycoplasma, Legionella*). Patients with pneumonia are admitted to the hospital for intravenous antibiotics unless they respond promptly to bronchodilator therapy. The choice of antibiotic is guided by the patient's history and age. Routine administration of antibiotics for exacerbations of COPD without clinical evidence of infection should be discouraged. They may offer modest benefit to patients who suffer from chronic bronchitis.

Sodium Bicarbonate. Significant acidemia of metabolic origin may inhibit the effectiveness of β-adrenergic agonists. Some authors recommend infusing small amounts of sodium bicarbonate if the arterial pH is less than 7.1 and then monitoring the clinical and acid-base response. However, acidemia caused by respiratory acidosis is treated with improved ventilation.

Relief of Bronchospasm

"β₂-Selective" Adrenergic Agonists. Stimulation of β_2 receptors in the tracheobronchial tree results in bronchial smooth muscle relaxation and decreases in mediator release from mast cells, enzyme release from neutrophils, and antibody production in lymphocytes. Avoidance of β_1-receptor stimulation reduces the side effects of tachycardia, tremor, and anxiety. Table 38–4 lists the route, dose, and frequency of administration of the most commonly used agents.

The aerosol produces excellent bronchodilation and reduced adverse systemic side effects. Albuterol or metaproterenol given by hand-held nebulizer or MDI with a spacer are the first line of treatment in patients with exacerbations of asthma or COPD. They are given as often as every 20 to 30 minutes as needed to reverse severe wheezing episodes. They can also be administered as a continuous aerosol in severe or refractory cases. This approach is gaining more acceptance, but close monitoring is advised. Intravenous administration of β agonists in addition to aerosol dosage remains controversial and currently is rarely indicated.

The β_2 agents are the first-line therapeutic choice. Patients who will respond to β agonists usually do so early in their treatment.

Subcutaneous Epinephrine. Epinephrine has a long history of use in patients with asthma. It is a very effective bronchodilator that has significant β_1 and α effects. It is specifically effective in wheezing associated with allergic reactions, including anaphylaxis. However, it can cause unpleasant and sometimes dangerous side effects: muscle tremors, tachycardia, dysrhythmias, and cardiac ischemia. It should be used cautiously or not at all in the elderly or those with known coronary artery disease.

Corticosteroids. Research has shown inflammatory processes play a key role in bronchiolitis, exacerbations of asthma, and COPD. Corticosteroids, once controversial, are now a cornerstone of treatment. The primary mechanisms of action include prevention of activation of inflammatory cells (e.g., eosinophils and T lymphocytes), interference with the synthesis of inflammatory mediators such as leukotrienes and prostaglandins, and upregulation of the β receptor. Although they have minimal effects acutely, they have been shown to reduce recurrences and subsequent hospitalizations. Most studies fail to show any significant difference between oral or intravenous administration. The onset of action of corticosteroids is within typically 4 to 6 hours, but an early effect may be related to β receptor responsiveness to adrenergic aerosols. Therefore, early administration is recommended in moderate and severe asthma. The use of inhaled corticosteroids (budesonide) in acute asthma is promising, and research continues.

Corticosteroids should be given to all but the most mild exacerbations of asthma. Those ultimately discharged to home should be treated with at least a 5- to 7-day course. If patients are treated for longer than 8 to 10 days, they may require a tapering dosage. In general, those patients who use corticosteroids chronically should be given

TABLE 38–4. Medications Commonly Used in Acute Asthma and Chronic Obstructive Pulmonary Disease

Drug	Route	Dose	Frequency	Comment
Adrenergic				
Epinephrine 1:1000	SQ	Adults: 0.3–0.5 mL	q20 min up to three doses	Peak effect: 15–30 min, higher dosage above 70 kg Duration: up to 3 hr Do not use concurrently with terbutaline
		Children: 0.01 mL/kg (0.3 mL max)	q20 min up to three doses	Avoid in first-trimester pregnancy, patients older than 40 yr, hypertension, or coronary artery disease
Sus-Phrine (epinephrine in oil)	SQ	Adults: 0.1–0.3 mL	q6h	Peak effect: 2 hr
		Children: 0.005 mL/kg (0.15 mL/max)	q6h	Duration: up to 6 hr Avoid in first-trimester pregnancy, patients older than 40 yr, hypertension, or coronary artery disease
β-Adrenergic-Continuous nebulization is another evolving administration route for β-adrenergic agents				
Albuterol	MDI	1–2 puffs (90 mEq/spray) Children: 0.10 mg/kg	q20 min tid–qid	Duration: 4–6 hr, optimal with spacer
	Aerosol (0.5% soln)	Adults: 0.5–1.0 mL in 2 mL saline	q20 min up to three doses	Peak effect: 30–60 min
		Children: 0.01 mL/kg (1 mL max) in 2 mL saline	q20 min up to three doses	Duration: 4–6 hr
Metaproterenol	MDI	1–2 puffs Children: 0.3–0.5 mg/kg	q20 min tid–qid	Duration: 4–6 hr, less B₂ specific
	Aerosol (5% soln)	Adults: 0.3 mL in 2 mL saline	q20 min up to three doses	Peak effect: 30–60 min
		Children: 0.01 mL/kg (0.3 mL max) in 2 mL saline	q20 min up to three doses	Duration: 4–6 hr
Terbutaline	MDI	2 puffs	q20 min	Duration: 3–5 hr Not currently recommended in patients <12 yr
	SQ	Adults: 0.25 mL	May repeat once in 30 min (max of 0.5 mL in 4 hr)	Peak effect: 30 min Duration: 4–6 hr Do not use concurrently with epinephrine
Corticosteroids				
Methylprednisolone	IV	Adults: 40–60 mg	q6h	After the first two doses, the dosage can be doubled until a response is noted. Tapering is done rapidly. This is inpatient therapy
Prednisone	Oral	Adults: 40–60 mg Children: 1–2 mg/kg	qd divided bid	If used for only 7–10 days, can stop without tapering. Usually for outpatient therapy

Continued on following page

TABLE 38-4. Medications Commonly Used in Acute Asthma and Chronic Obstructive Pulmonary Disease *Continued*

Drug	Route	Dose	Frequency	Comment
Anticholinergics				
Ipratroprium	MDI Aerosol	1–2 puffs	q20 min	Use with β agonists. Effect variable Caution in glaucoma, urinary obstruction
Other Medications				
Aminophylline	IV	Loading dose adults and children (based on actual body weight): 5.6 mg/kg given over 20 min		This drug is rarely given in acute asthma or COPD exacerbation
		0.9 mg/kg/hr May vary with underlying disease	Continuous infusion	Optimally, the serum level is measured before administering dose. Adjustments can be made when the value returns from the laboratory
Magnesium sulfate	IV	1–2 g over 20 min		Limited benefit, more in severe asthma Does not significantly decrease hospitalizations

MDI, Metered-dose inhaler.

longer, tapering regimens. Corticosteroid inhalers have been shown to be an effective means of preventing relapse. Patient compliance may be limited, because of the cost of the medication. Interestingly, despite more than two decades of demonstrated efficacy, emergency physician use of corticosteroids, defined by, dosage, route of administration, and prescriptions at discharge remains highly variable.

Leukotriene-Modifying Agents. Cysteine leukotrienes are a group of mediators derived from arachidonic acid. They produce changes in lung tissue characteristic of asthma. They increase vascular permeability and facilitate inflammatory cell migration. Cys-leukotriene-1 receptor antagonists block their production and site of actions. Currently available antagonists are zafirlukast (Accolate) and montelukast (Singulair). There are a few studies that measure the effectiveness of these drugs in acute asthma, but a potential benefit of concurrent administration with other treatments has been shown. They have demonstrated benefit in prevention of exercise-induced asthma and in decreasing exacerbations in chronic asthmatics. The effects of leukotriene-modifying agents are thought to be additive to the effects of inhaled corticosteroids.

Anticholinergic Agents. Ipratropium is a derivative of atropine but is less lipid soluble and thus is less systemically absorbed, resulting in fewer adverse effects. Its primary role has been in the treatment of COPD. It is generally given as a combined nebulized treatment with albuterol. Its use in asthma has shown no conclusive evidence to support its use routinely, although pediatric studies do show some trends toward improvement. In adults, its most consistent benefit is demonstrated in patients with pulmonary function tests less than 35% of predicted. It is the treatment of choice in β-blocker–induced asthma.

Magnesium. Magnesium is a well-known smooth muscle relaxant that works by inhibiting cellular calcium uptake and inhibiting calcium release from the sarcoplasmic reticulum. Through this mechanism it also causes bronchodilation. Its primary role is as an adjunct to other treatments in the setting of severe or refractory status asthmaticus. Its potential therapeutic impact is usually noted within 2 to 5 minutes of administration.

General Anesthesia/Heliox. As a last resort in the wheezing asthmatic whose condition continues to deteriorate despite maximal therapy (including intubation and mechanical ventilation), general anesthesia with halothane or derivatives can be used. Halothane has a direct bronchodilating effect on airway smooth muscle. The risks of halothane include myocardial depression, vasodi-lation, and dysrhythmias. It is not readily available in the emergency department. Ketamine, an intravenously administered general anesthetic, is a fairly potent bronchodilator but has the disadvantages of increasing bronchial secretions and causing emergence reactions. For this reason, it is often given with an anticholinergic agent and a benzodiazepine. Helium-oxygen mixtures (heliox) have inconsistently demonstrated decreased airway resistance and less dyspnea in asthmatic patients. This therapy currently has limited application.

Medications to Avoid. A number of medications are not advised in the treatment of acute asthma. These include intravenous aminophylline, sedatives or tranquilizers, most cell mediators (cromolyn), antihistamines, and mucolytics.

Ventilatory Support

BiPAP (Bilevel Positive Airway Pressure) Support. This noninvasive approach has demonstrated utility in hemodynamically stable patients as a means of avoiding intubation and mechanical ventilation. Mild sedation may be required. Noninvasive ventilation with bilevel positive airway pressure may have promise as an alternative to intubation in seriously ill asthmatics.

Endotracheal Intubation and Ventilation. If, in the extreme circumstance (<0.3% of cases), intubation is necessary, assisted ventilation is supplied with a volume-cycled respirator. Initial settings are inspiratory-to-expiratory ratio at 1:3 allowing for a prolonged expiratory phase, tidal volume at 5 to 7 mL/kg with 8 to 12 breaths per minute, and F_{IO_2} set to maintain adequate tissue oxygenation. If the patient is not tolerating assisted ventilation, a long-acting intravenous paralyzing agent (e.g., vecuronium) is used in combination with sedation. Paralytics can be useful to help reduce peak airway pressures. The risk of pneumothorax is significant in these patients. In asthmatic patients, controlled hypoventilation using a slower respiratory rate and lower tidal volumes allows for adequate expiration and helps minimize peak airway pressures and the possibility of barotrauma. Close monitoring with serial examination and ABG measurements is necessary. Initial hypercapnia does not need to be rapidly corrected.

Specific Principles

Whereas asthma and COPD have similar treatment approaches, a number of other causes of wheezing and respiratory distress have specific therapies.

Status Asthmaticus

Primary goals in the patient with status asthmaticus are to reverse bronchospasm, support ventilation and oxygenation as needed, rehydrate, and treat infection if applicable.

1. Supplemental oxygen is given as needed to maintain normal saturation.
2. Intravenous access is established for fluid and medication administration.
3. Bronchodilator therapy is implemented.
4. The need for active airway management is anticipated, and intubation is done if necessary.
5. Corticosteroids may be indicated.
6. ABG analysis and a chest radiograph may be indicated.
7. Antibiotic therapy may be necessary if an infection is suggested.

COPD Exacerbation

Therapy for COPD is generally the same as for asthma. Notable exceptions are that an ABG analysis and chest radiograph should be obtained in most cases and anticholinergics (e.g., ipratropium bromide) are generally given along with the β_2 agonist.

Congestive Heart Failure

Primary goals are to support oxygenation and ventilation as needed, decrease fluid overload, and determine precipitating causes (particularly acute myocardial infarction). A chest radiograph helps confirm pulmonary edema, and an electrocardiogram and cardiac enzymes studies may indicate whether myocardial ischemia or infarction is the precipitating cause. Treatment includes venodilators (e.g., nitroglycerin and morphine) to reduce preload and diuretics (e.g., furosemide) to diurese.

Anaphylaxis

Primary goals are to support oxygenation and blood pressure and block allergic response. Patients are treated with bronchodilators, epinephrine (helps reverse bronchoconstriction and vasodilation), corticosteroids, antihistamines, and fluid (see Chapter 12, Anaphylaxis).

Pulmonary Embolism

A pulmonary embolism is unlikely to present solely as wheezing without chest pain and hypoxemia. Diagnosis is with a ventilation/perfusion scan, spiral CT, and/or pulmonary angiography. Treatment is primarily anticoagulation with heparin. Thrombolytics are sometimes used for massive embolism.

Pneumothorax

A pneumothorax is unlikely to present solely as wheezing but is often seen in COPD and asthmatic patients. Treatment is with tube thoracostomy, preceded by needle decompression if a tension pneumothorax is suggested.

Pneumonia

Hypoxemia and wheezing are frequent signs encountered in patients with pneumonia. Treatment is primarily supplemental oxygen, bronchodilators, and antibiotics. Intubation may be required for severe cases.

UNCERTAIN DIAGNOSIS

Bronchospasm and wheezing are commonly reversed in the emergency setting. Once treated, the focus of assessment must shift to the underlying disease, especially in the patient with the first-time manifestation of wheezing. If a pursuit of the differential diagnosis results in continued uncertainty, and the patient is free of wheezing, a careful review of the history and physical examination is important before discharge. Referral to a primary physician or pulmonologist is recommended. Optimally, this appointment is made at the time of discharge.

Any patient with continued wheezing of unknown etiology after appropriate therapy should be admitted for further testing or, at a minimum, a pulmonologist should be consulted before discharge and close follow-up.

SPECIAL CONSIDERATIONS

Pediatric Patients

Wheezing is common in infants and children younger than 2 years of age. It is most commonly caused by viral infections and is usually diagnosed as *bronchiolitis*. This disorder is characterized by inflammatory obstruction of the small airways, and its incidence peaks at approximately 6 months of age. It occurs most frequently during the winter and early spring and can be either sporadic or epidemic. The question of asthma often arises in the course of treating these children, and there is controversy about the possible relationship of bronchiolitis to later development of asthma. Factors that suggest a diagnosis of asthma include

- A family history of asthma
- Recurrent attacks (less than 5% of recurrent attacks of wheezing are caused by viral infections in this age group)
- Sudden onset without evidence of a preceding viral infection
- Markedly prolonged expiration
- Eosinophilia
- Response to bronchodilators

Once other disorders are ruled out, such as foreign-body aspiration or cardiac disease, children in this age group who present with wheezing should receive a trial of bronchodilator therapy to judge the response. If the patient responds, further bronchodilator therapy can be instituted as outlined for asthma. If there is no response and the child is in any respiratory distress, he or she is treated with humidified oxygen and parenteral fluids and admitted for observation.

Elderly Patients

This fastest-growing segment of the emergency department population has up to a 10% prevalence of asthma. The combination of reactive airway disease with COPD is common in this group. Mortality rates and medication side effects are higher in the elderly. Lengths of stay and complications once admitted are also greater. The therapeutic approach in this group is similar to that for younger individuals. Dosage complications are more common. Ipratropium has shown some specific benefit in this population.

Pregnant Patients

Approximately one third of pregnant asthmatics will experience worsening of the course of their disease during their pregnancy, one third will show improvement in their symptoms, and one third will remain unchanged. Management of wheezing in the pregnant asthmatic can proceed as in the nonpregnant patient with the following cautions:

1. Care must be exercised in using parenteral β agonists in the pregnant patient near term because these drugs may decrease uterine contractility and inhibit labor. When required in this setting, β agonists are given as aerosols to limit systemic absorption.
2. Subcutaneous epinephrine used during the first trimester may be associated with increased fetal malformations and should be avoided.
3. Extra care is necessary to prevent hypoxia in the pregnant asthmatic to prevent fetal anoxia.

The pregnant state is a predisposing factor to the development of deep venous thrombosis and subsequent pulmonary embolism. This possibility must be considered when treating the wheezing, pregnant woman, especially if there is associated chest pain and/or no prior history of asthma.

DISPOSITION AND FOLLOW-UP

More than 80% of patients who present with wheezing are discharged from the emergency department. The emergency physician must use all available parameters in deciding the appropriate disposition for a wheezing patient. This decision usually is made after 2 to 4 hours of therapy, although longer stays or use of an "observation" unit is common.

Admission

Patients who continue to wheeze despite aggressive treatment but are not in sufficient respiratory distress to warrant ICU admission are admitted to a regular hospital bed if the nursing staff is adequate to maintain close observation. This also applies to patients who are not in significant distress but who have complications such as pneumonia, dehydration, or inability to tolerate oral medications.

Admission to Intensive Care Unit

Admission to an ICU is necessary for the following patients:

- Patients requiring intubation
- Patients with severe obstruction and failure to improve after initial bronchodilator therapy (e.g., PFTs < 50% of predicted post treatment)
- Patients with altered mental status
- Patients with acute hypercapnia and respiratory acidosis
- Patients with dysrhythmias other than sinus tachycardia
- Patients with borderline reserve and complications such as pneumothorax, pneumomediastinum, or pneumonia
- Any patient who is believed to have borderline indications for admission to an ICU when close observation is unavailable on a regular hospital unit

It is better to err on the side of ICU admission and transfer the patient to a regular unit after the patient becomes stable than it is to place a potentially unstable patient in a regular hospital bed.

Discharge

Patients are discharged from the emergency department when they are generally asymptomatic. Although not always possible, it is best for them to be free of wheezing. In one study of asthmatics, the FEV_1 was 40% of predicted when the patient subjectively was without wheezes and 60% of predicted when the wheezing was resolved on auscultation. This result implies significant bronchospasm can still be present despite resolution of wheezes on examination. Other guidelines include a peak expiratory flow rate of more than 300 L/min, an FEV_1 of more than 2 L, or PFTs more than 70% of predicted.

Resolution of wheezes does not always correlate well with outcome. Up to 25% of patients may return with a relapse within 10 days. Recent studies have demonstrated prescribing 5 to 10 days of oral corticosteroids as part of the discharge medications decreased the rate and severity of relapse. A practical test before discharge is to ask the patient to walk 30 to 50 feet in the emergency department. If this brief exercise results in wheezing or significant desaturation on retesting, the appropriateness of discharge is reconsidered.

Before discharge the following points are addressed:

1. Patients are prescribed adequate outpatient bronchodilator therapy.
2. If corticosteroid treatment has been initiated in the emergency department, oral prednisone for 5 to 10 days is continued after discharge. A tapering dosage is not necessary in these cases. Addition of inhaled corticosteroids (budesonide) may decrease relapses and subsequent symptoms.
3. The patient's understanding of the dose and use of medication is clarified, particularly with regard to proper technique used with MDIs.
4. An understanding of the patient's environment (home, work, recreation) is necessary. Is an element present that may precipitate bronchospasm?
5. Patients are instructed to return promptly to the emergency department at the earliest sign of relapse.
6. All discharged patients must have appropriate follow-up arranged with their primary physician 24 to 48 hours after their emergency department visit.

FINAL POINTS

- The most common cause of wheezing is reactive airway pulmonary disease (e.g., asthma, emphysema, chronic bronchitis). However, wheezing may be the symptom of other disorders such as congestive heart failure, anaphylaxis, or pulmonary embolism.
- The underlying pathologic process is severe bronchospasm and tissue inflammation resulting in hypoxemia and acidemia.
- The only absolute indications for endotracheal intubation in the wheezing patient are apnea and coma.
- When assessing the patient with asthma and wheezing, the potential complications of pneumothorax and pneumonia are considered.
- The severity of wheezing is gauged by physical findings, PFT results, and ABG measurements. The degree of wheezing on auscultation is a poor indicator of severity. Air flow may not be sufficient to create enough turbulence to generate the sound of wheezing.
- ABG analysis is rarely necessary in patients with asthma and wheezing. It is obtained only in patients with severe attacks or in those who do not respond to therapy.
- PFT results may be useful, but they can be effort dependent and may not be readily available.
- The β_2-selective aerosols are the first-line therapy for acute wheezing from obstructive pulmonary disease.
- Corticosteroids are administered early in the course of moderate or severe attacks or if indicated by history.
- Fluid replacement is important to reduce the viscosity of pulmonary secretions and to promote their clearance from the bronchial tree.
- The decision to discharge a patient after treatment of an acute attack of wheezing is not based on a single clinical or laboratory parameter. Patients must believe they have returned close to their normal state; wheezing must have resolved even with limited exercise; vital signs must be near normal; and bedside PFTs must be significantly improved (more than 70% of predicted).

CASE *Study*

The mother of a 17-year-old young woman called 911 because her daughter was "wheezing and can't catch her breath." The mother was very agitated, begged for immediate help, and could give no more information to the dispatcher.

On arrival, EMS personnel found the patient was tachypneic, had loud expiratory wheezes, and appeared to be in moderate distress. She was given an albuterol aerosol treatment en route, and intravenous access was established. On arrival, the patient was taken to a monitored bed and the emergency physician was notified. She was placed on O_2, 4 L/min, per nasal cannula.

Initial vital signs were temperature, 101.5°F; pulse, 130 beats per minute; respiratory rate, 35 breaths per minute, and blood pressure, 135/82 mm Hg. The patient was noted to be sitting up and having labored breathing. A second albuterol aerosol treatment was given while the physician examined the patient and obtained her history. The cardiac monitor showed a sinus tachycardia.

Although the patient could speak only two to three words at a time because of her distress, the physician was able to ascertain that she had been sick for 2 days, with intermittent episodes of wheezing and shortness of breath. The patient had a history of wheezing in the past and sometimes used an inhaler but did not know if she was asthmatic. She had a productive cough and fever at home. She had self-medicated with over-the-counter cold remedies and a nasal spray mist. Her breathing became abruptly worse 2 hours before arrival. She had never been admitted to the hospital for respiratory problems and had no other medical history.

On examination, she was tachypneic and marked intercostal retractions were noted. Her lung fields revealed diminished breath sounds bilaterally, with harsh inspiratory and expiratory wheezes and a prolonged expiratory phase. Her ear, nose, and throat examination was unremarkable, and her neck revealed no jugular venous distention or lymphadenopathy. Heart sounds were normal but tachycardic. The abdomen was soft and nontender. Extremities showed no clubbing, cyanosis, or edema.

At this point, several principles should be emphasized. Any patient in respiratory distress should be seen as soon as possible. Because of her condition, treatment was initiated concurrently with her clinical assessment. The patient's medical history is somewhat unclear but is consistent with asthma. The fever and productive cough suggest infection as the inciting event for this episode. Her marked tachypnea, difficulty speaking, use of accessory muscles, and inspiratory and expiratory wheezes put her in the severe category. This patient requires aggressive therapy.

The physician ordered another albuterol aerosol treatment and intravenous administration of corticosteroids. He also gave her subcutaneous epinephrine. To evaluate for infection, a chest radiograph was ordered and a sputum specimen was obtained for Gram's stain and culture. The radiograph revealed a left lower lobe infiltrate. A complete blood cell count was ordered as part of routine admission laboratory studies, and the patient was started on a macrolide antibiotic. The patient's initial peak flow was 120 L/min, and repeat testing improved only to 180 L/min. On reevaluation, the patient's respiratory rate had slowed to 24 breaths per minute and she was no longer using accessory muscles. On auscultation, she still had significant respiratory wheezes but demonstrated increased air movement. An additional albuterol aerosol was given, with minimal change in the patient's status. At this point, the physician contacted her family doctor, and the patient was admitted to the ICU for further evaluation and treatment.

Asthma is one of the few medical illnesses that can kill an otherwise healthy young person, and it should be treated aggressively. In this case, the patient is aggressively treated and intubation is avoided. An infectious cause is identified, and antibiotic treatment is promptly initiated. Although the patient showed a marked improvement, she was still significantly symptomatic and thus was admitted to the ICU rather than a regular floor bed.

Bibliography

TEXTS

Clark TJH: Asthma, 4th ed. New York, Oxford University Press, 2000.

Fishman AP (ed): Fishman's Pulmonary Diseases and Disorders. New York, McGraw-Hill, 1998.

George RB, Light RW, Matthay MA, Matthay RA: Chest Medicine—Essentials of Pulmonary and Critical Medicine, 4th ed. Philadelphia, Lippincott Williams & Wilkins, 2000.

JOURNAL ARTICLES

Barnett PL, Caputo GL, Baskin M, Kuppermann N: Intravenous versus oral corticosteroids in the management of acute asthma in children. Ann Emerg Med 1997; 29:212–217.

Bloch H, Silverman R, Mancherje N, et al: Intravenous magnesium sulfate as an adjunct in the treatment of acute asthma. Chest 1995; 107:1576–1581.

Busse WW, Lemanske RF: Asthma: Advances in immunology. N Engl J Med 2001; 344:350–362.

Cullison B, Emerman C: The clinical challenge of acute asthma: Diagnosis, disposition, and outcome-effective management. Emerg Med Rep 2001; 22(11):119–130.

Drugs for Asthma. Med Lett 2000; 41:19–24.

Emond SD, Camargo CA Jr, Nowak RM: 1997 National Asthma Education and Prevention Program guidelines: A practical summary for emergency physicians. Ann Emerg Med 1998; 31:579–589.

Gibbs MA, Camargo CA, Jr, Rowe BH, et al: State of the art: Therapeutic controversies in severe acute asthma. Acad Emerg Med 2000; 7:800–815.

Jagoda A, Shepherd SM, Spevitz A, Joseph MM: Refractory asthma: I. Epidemiology, pathophysiology, pharmacologic interventions. II. Airway interventions and management. Ann Emerg Med 1997; 29:262–274; 29:275–281.

Lin RY, Pesol GR, Bakalchuk L, et al: Superiority of ipratropium plus albuterol over albuterol alone in the emergency department management of adult asthma: A randomized clinical trial. Ann Emerg Med 1998; 31:208–213.

MacIntyre N: Mechanical ventilation in asthma. Respir Care Clin North Am 1995; 1:333–343.

Reilly MK, Kaufmann MA, Cydulka RK: Asthma: An evidence-based management update. Emerg Med Pract 2001; 3(2):1–28.

Rennard SI: COPD: Overview of definitions, epidemiology, and factors influencing its development. Chest 1998; 113:s235–s241.

Rowe BH, Bota GW, Fabris L, et al: Inhaled budesonide in addition to oral corticosteroids to prevent asthma relapse following discharge from the emergency department: A randomized controlled trial. JAMA 1999; 281(22):2119–2126.

Rya MT, Radeos MS: Acute exacerbation of COPD: A practical approach to differential diagnosis and management. Emerg Med Pract 2002; 4(4):1–20.

Senior RM, Anthonisen NR: Chronic obstructive pulmonary disease. Am J Respir Crit Care Med 1998; 157:s139–s147.

Thomas JA, Potter MW, Counselman FL, et al: Emergency physician practice and steroid use in the management of acute exacerbation of asthma. Am J Emerg Med 2001; 19:465–468.

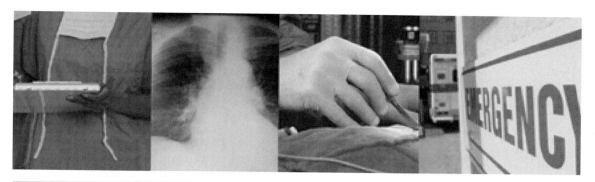

UROGENITAL DISORDERS

CHAPTER 39

Acute Pelvic Pain

JOSEPH J. MOELLMAN
JENNIFER M. BOCOCK

CASE *Study*

A 21-year-old woman presents to the emergency department with the complaint of lower abdominal pain associated with fever, nausea, and vomiting. In the triage area her vital signs include pulse, 100 beats per minute; blood pressure, 110/70 mm Hg; respiratory rate, 12 breaths per minute; and temperature, 100.9°F (38.6°C). The patient states she currently uses no method of birth control.

INTRODUCTION

Acute pelvic pain is one of the most common complaints of women who present to the emergency department. The reported incidence varies greatly among institutions. Those serving patient populations in lower socioeconomic urban areas treat high numbers of women with this complaint. Abdominal pain accounts for up to 5% of all emergency department visits, with pelvic pain occurring in 7% to 20% of those patient encounters. Distinguishing the various causes of pelvic pain remains a diagnostic challenge for numerous reasons. One is the broad differential diagnosis encompassed by the symptoms (Table 39–1).

A primary factor in this wide differential diagnosis is the complex pelvic anatomy and the physiologic principles of pain transmission from the pelvic structures. Somatic and visceral afferent fibers are the two pathways responsible for transmission of pain from the abdomen and pelvis to the central nervous system. Somatic afferent fibers originate from the skin, abdominal wall, and parietal peritoneum and are activated by mechanisms of cutting, burning, and chemical irritation. Somatic pain is usually described as sharp and is readily localized to a specific region. Visceral afferent fibers originate from the walls of the hollow viscus, solid organs, and the visceral peritoneum. Activation of these fibers occurs by mechanisms of stretch, inflammation, and ischemia. Visceral pain is often described as "achy and dull" and is poorly localized.

Visceral afferent fibers in the pelvis follow the autonomic nervous system to plexuses and then join the thoracic, lumbar, and sacral nerve roots at several levels. Pelvic referral patterns are not as constant and predictable as abdominal ones because of these multiple levels. Some general referral patterns have been observed: ovarian—(T10) pain to the infraumbilical region; fallopian and uterine—(T11, T12) pain to the lower abdomen and inguinal regions; inferior uterine, vaginal, and perineal—(sacral roots) pain to the sacral area, buttocks, and suprapubic region.

Incorrectly diagnosing the cause of acute pelvic pain may have devastating sequelae. For example, pelvic inflammatory disease (PID) is an infection of the upper genital tract and may be a complication of chlamydial and gonococcal lower tract (vaginal, cervical, urethral) infections. Chlamydia and gonorrhea are present in one third of PID, with the remainder being polymicrobial. With a *single* episode of PID, the risk of infertility is 11%. The risk rises to 34% with two episodes and to 54% with three or more infections. The equivalent population (females of childbearing age) has an infertility rate of 3% (without salpingitis). The most severe consequence of PID is subsequent ectopic pregnancy. Nearly 5% of total malpractice claims against emergency physicians are because of missed ectopic pregnancy. The emergency physician must approach patients with acute pelvic pain conservatively, with accuracy and efficiency, while recognizing the potential for serious sequelae.

INITIAL APPROACH AND STABILIZATION
Priority Diagnoses

Hemorrhagic shock secondary to ruptured interstitial ectopic pregnancy and septic shock caused by PID or tubo-ovarian abscess are the two most clinically emergent conditions associated with pelvic pain. In *all* female patients of childbearing age, priority diagnoses include ectopic pregnancy (intact or ruptured), infection (appendicitis, PID, and ruptured viscus), adnexal torsion, and intra-abdominal hemorrhage secondary to a ruptured ovarian cyst (corpus luteum cyst), intrauterine

---

TABLE 39–1. Etiologic Classification of Pelvic Pain

I. True Pelvic Etiology

  A. Ovaries, uterus, adnexa
      1. Torsion of ovarian pedicle, cyst or tumor
      2. Polycystic ovaries
      3. Ruptured ovarian cyst
      4. Ruptured ectopic or ovarian pregnancy
      5. Pelvic inflammatory disease, salpingitis, tubo-ovarian abscess
      6. Endometriosis, adenomyosis
      7. Degeneration of uterine myoma, fibroid
      8. Mittelschmerz
      9. Puerperal infections, endometritis
    10. Incomplete septic abortion
    11. Dysmenorrhea
  B. Premenstrual syndrome (PMS)

II. Abdominal Pelvic Pain

  A. Gastrointestinal tract
      1. Appendicitis
      2. Diverticulitis
      3. Femoral hernia
      4. Incarcerated hernia
      5. Small bowel obstruction
      6. Volvulus
      7. Dietary indiscretion, gastroenteritis
      8. Constipation
      9. Parasites
    10. Dysentery, diarrhea
    11. Colitis
    12. Regional enteritis
    13. Carcinoma
    14. Ruptured viscus
    15. Trauma
    16. Mesenteric adenitis
  B. Urinary tract
      1. Cystitis
      2. Pyelonephritis
      3. Ureteral stone
      4. Urethral syndrome
  C. Vascular causes
      1. Aortic or iliac aneurysm
      2. Pelvic thrombophlebitis
      3. Mesenteric vein thrombosis
  D. Liver and gallbladder
      1. Hepatitis
      2. Cholecystitis, cholelithiasis
      3. Fitz-Hugh-Curtis syndrome
  E. Pancreas
      1. Acute pancreatitis
      2. Pancreatic pseudocyst
  F. Primary streptococcal or pneumococcal peritonitis
  G. Leukemia and other lymphomas
  H. Sickle cell crisis
   I. Metabolic causes
      1. Lead poisoning
      2. Diabetic acidosis
      3. Acute porphyria
      4. Hereditary angioedema
   J. Musculoskeletal causes
      1. Ankylosing spondylitis
      2. Degenerative joint disease of symphysis
      3. Osteitis pubis
      4. Prolapsed intervertebral disc
      5. Spondylolisthesis
      6. Muscular strain
  K. Psychogenic causes

---

pregnancy, and spontaneous abortion. In post-menopausal patients, vascular pathology (abdominal aortic aneurysm and mesenteric ischemia), infectious processes (appendicitis, ruptured viscus, and abscesses), and neoplastic processes are the major concerns.

Rapid Assessment

1. The emergency medical services report is reviewed if ambulance transport occurred. Family and friends are asked to remain available for additional history.
2. Key historical features include

   - Description of the onset and duration of pain
   - Last normal menstrual period
   - Pregnancy status
   - Presence or absence of vaginal bleeding and/or discharge
   - Fever
   - Systemic symptoms (vomiting, fatigue, diarrhea, syncope)
   - Past medical history (including gynecologic history)
   - Current medications
   - Drug allergies
   - Last oral intake

3. Early physical examination

   - *General appearance.* Clinical observation of whether the patient is "sick" or "not sick." Pallor, diaphoresis and respiratory pattern are noted, as is the patient's position (writhing, still, or fetal position).
   - *Vital signs.* Temperature, heart rate, respiratory rate, and blood pressure are measured immediately. Orthostatic vital signs may detect significant volume depletion. An increase in pulse of 20 to 30 beats per minute or a decrease in systolic pressure of 20 to 30 mm Hg with position change is suggestive of a 30% or more loss of intravascular volume. Frequent, serial vital sign assessments, including temperature, should occur throughout the patient encounter.
   - *Abdominal examination.* Inspection, auscultation, percussion, and palpation remain the basic examination components. Findings consistent with a surgical acute abdomen are sought (guarding, rebound tenderness, or distention). Caution is used in "ruling out" a life-threatening pathologic process on the presence or absence of findings at this stage, because the process may be evolving (e.g., the lack of a pulsatile mass does not exclude an abdominal aortic aneurysm; the presence

   of bowel sounds does not exclude peritonitis or bowel obstruction).
   - *Pelvic and rectal examination.* If the patient's hemodynamic status is unstable, these assessments are performed concurrently with stabilization to assess potential sources of hemorrhage. A repeat examination may be completed after the patient's condition is stabilized.

Early Intervention

1. The clinician must adhere to the principles of airway, breathing, and circulation (see Chapter 2, Airway Management) when patients present with signs of shock. Oxygen supplementation, intravenous access, and volume resuscitation are among the primary interventions. Early laboratory testing (β-human chorionic gonadotropin [β-hCG], urinalysis, blood type and crossmatch) may help narrow the differential diagnosis.
2. Continuous monitoring of pulse, blood pressure, O_2 saturation, and respiratory rate is maintained in these patients, because clinical instability may rapidly occur.
3. If a patient presents hemodynamically unstable or a surgical intervention is likely, a surgical consultant is notified immediately. The choice of general or gynecologic surgeon remains case specific.
4. All patients with abdominal or pelvic pain remain NPO (nothing by mouth) until the evaluation is complete.
5. Analgesic medication (small doses, with a rapid half-life) may be required for patient comfort and a thorough examination. Studies have shown that small doses of analgesics *do not* mask an intra-abdominal pathologic process or compromise surgical consultation and evaluation.

CLINICAL ASSESSMENT

A well-organized history and a focused physical examination often provide a presumptive diagnosis in the patient with acute pelvic pain. Serial examinations are valuable, because many patients present early in the course of their illness and clinical findings evolve over time.

History

An adequate history and description of pelvic pain may be difficult to obtain. Many women keep poor menstrual histories or have no record at all. Not all patients are comfortable volunteering information regarding sexual behavior and reproductive organs. Patients may be embarrassed or ashamed of their answers, and the physician must maintain a sensitive demeanor to gain patients' confidence.

Characteristics of the Pain

Quality of the Pain. The patient is asked to describe the nature of the pain as being sharp, dull, heavy, or crampy. Inflammatory conditions such as cystitis, PID, or appendicitis often cause "dull" pain initially and, later, after the peritoneum is irritated, evolve into "sharp" pain. Crampy or colicky pain is the result of smooth muscle contraction in a hollow viscus (the result of a ureteral stone) or from the organ itself (uterine contractions).

Onset. The circumstances and pattern of pain onset are both extremely important. Sudden onset of pelvic pain suggests rupture of a structure (i.e., ectopic pregnancy or ovarian cyst). The onset of pain in relation to the patient's menstrual cycle may also provide clues to the diagnosis. Pain associated with salpingitis often occurs shortly after menses, whereas pain in mid cycle can be the result of a follicle cyst rupture (ovulatory pain or Mittelschmerz). Pain occurring consistently with the onset of menses may represent endometriosis. The sudden onset of pain during coitus or exercise often results from a ruptured ovarian cyst.

Severity. The severity of pain is obtained to gauge improvement or worsening of the patient's condition during evaluation. A severity scale of 1 to 10 is often helpful to objectively define the patient's perception of the pain and assess efficacy of treatment interventions.

Site and Radiation. The location of pain may mislead the emergency physician. There are *no* consistent findings on abdominal examination that link the location of pain to a specific source. However, some features of pain location may be helpful in defining a presumptive diagnosis. Unilateral pain often results from adnexal disease (ectopic pregnancy, tubal torsion, cystic rupture or tubo-ovarian abscess), pelvic appendicitis, or ureteral colic. Bilateral pelvic pain is often associated with PID. Central (suprapubic) pain may be the result of PID, endometritis, or cystitis. Pain radiation may suggest a certain pathologic process but is not disease (or organ) specific. Radiation to the flank may occur with ureteral colic, but it also results from localized peritoneal irritation from a ruptured cyst. Shoulder pain should alert the clinician to diaphragmatic irritation, secondary to free fluid or blood in the peritoneum (Kehr's sign).

Duration and Pattern. The duration and pattern of pain associated with either ruptured

ectopic pregnancy or ovarian cyst generally begins abruptly and sharply in a single, focal location and, over hours, evolves into a generalized, constant, diffuse pain. Insidious, bilateral pain is often described with PID; yet as peritonitis evolves, generalized pain also occurs.

Previous History of Pain. Has the same type of pain been previously experienced? How does this pain episode compare? What was the previous diagnosis given to the patient? How was the problem treated?

Previous Treatment. How has this pain been treated? Has the patient recently been seen by another health care provider for this condition? The use of sporadic antibiotics or an analgesic before the visit to the emergency department may alter the presentation. Efforts to remedy the pain at home can offer some insight into the severity.

What is the Patient's Gynecologic, Obstetric, and Sexual History?

1. When was the *last menstrual period* (LMP) and *last normal* menstrual period (LNMP)?
2. Is there a history of any *sexually transmitted diseases*? Was she (and her partner) treated? Was a complete course of medication taken?
3. What is the *gravida, parity, and abortus history*? (Specify number of pregnancies and clarify spontaneous and elective abortion history, because these may be difficult for some women to discuss.)
4. What *method of contraception* is or has been used? If a barrier method, is it *every* encounter? If an oral pill method, is it taken consistently each day?
5. Is the patient *sexually active*? How often and with how many partners? When was the last sexual intercourse?
6. Has the patient had any *obstetric or gynecologic surgical* (or instrumented) *procedures*? Were there any complications?

Associated Symptoms

Fever or Chills. The finding of fever or chills is often associated with PID, appendicitis, or urinary tract infection.

Syncope and Dizziness. These features may suggest hypovolemia or hemorrhagic shock (ruptured ectopic pregnancy or hemorrhagic cyst) or septic shock (perforated appendix or PID). Up to 33% of patients with ruptured ectopic pregnancy will present with these symptoms and the absence of abdominal pain.

Nausea and Vomiting. Classically, nausea and vomiting begin before the pain of appendicitis. Nausea and vomiting that occur simultaneously with onset of pain can be associated with torsion, ectopic pregnancy, ureteral colic, or bowel obstruction. In patients with PID and other infectious processes, nausea and vomiting usually occur late, as a result of the disease progression.

Vaginal Bleeding or Amenorrhea. The presence of vaginal bleeding should always raise the possibility of ectopic pregnancy. Twenty to 50 percent of patients (with ectopic pregnancy) do not have this finding. Amenorrhea raises the suspicion of pregnancy, whether intrauterine, ectopic, or heterotopic. Amenorrhea for greater than 12 weeks can occur in 15% of women with ectopic pregnancy and, conversely, for less than 4 weeks in another 15%. A precise history of the patient's normal menstrual cycle is necessary to determine whether the vaginal bleeding or amenorrhea is related to the pain.

Vaginal Discharge. Vaginal discharge is associated with vaginitis, cervicitis, and PID. It is important to note whether the patient has chronic discharge, because many patients with pelvic pain and chronic discharge are erroneously diagnosed with PID.

Urinary Symptoms. The presence of dysuria, frequency, urgency, and hesitancy may lead to the presumptive diagnosis of urinary tract infection. There have been many reports of such symptoms occurring as the result of bladder irritation secondary to ectopic pregnancy or free peritoneal fluid. The presence of hematuria may point to ureteral pathology, yet concomitant vaginal bleeding may be falsely attributed as the cause.

Risk Factors for Ectopic Pregnancy and PID

Previous Ectopic Pregnancy. Patients with a previous ectopic pregnancy have a greater than 10% chance of repeat ectopic pregnancy with each subsequent pregnancy.

Previous PID. The risk of ectopic pregnancy increases fivefold to sevenfold after an initial episode of PID. Previous PID is associated with recurrent (or chronic) PID, chronic pelvic pain, tubo-ovarian abscess, Fitz-Hugh-Curtis syndrome (perihepatitis), and Reiter's syndrome (urethritis, conjunctivitis, and arthritis—primarily caused by *Chlamydia*).

Presence of Intrauterine Devices. The IUD is placed in the cervical canal and is used to prevent pregnancy. There are two types currently available in the United States, the copper T 380A and a progesterone-releasing IUD. Overall, the IUD reduces the rate of pregnancy. Therefore, the number of ectopic pregnancies in IUD users is also reduced (versus women using *no* contra-

ceptive method). If pregnancy does occur in a patient using an IUD, particularly the progesterone-releasing variety, relative risk of ectopic pregnancy may be as high as 1.5 to 2.8 times the normal population. The use of an IUD increases the risk of both PID and ectopic pregnancy when patients are not screened and selected appropriately. The risk of contracting PID with IUD use is highest at insertion, especially in women with multiple PID risk factors. Recent European and U.S. studies have shown that screening patients for the selection of IUD-appropriate users has decreased the number of PID cases. Uterine perforation occurs in 1/750 to 1/1500 cases of IUD insertion. The most significant risk factor is an inexperienced provider inserting the IUD.

Previous Tubal Surgery/Ligation. There is a post-tubal ligation failure rate that ranges from 7.5 per 1000 patients to 36 per 1000. Thirty to 40 percent of pregnancies occurring after ligation are ectopic. In vitro fertilization, embryo transfer, and gamete intrafallopian transfer all increase the risk of an ectopic pregnancy because the embryos may implant in multiple areas. Ectopic pregnancy, intrauterine pregnancy (IUP), or heterotopic pregnancy (IUP and ectopic together) all occur with increased frequency in this population of patients.

Multiple Partners. A woman with multiple sexual partners has an increased risk of contracting PID. A complete sexual history should be obtained, including the use of contraceptives, history of sexually transmitted disease occurrence, and treatment.

Young Age. The anatomic structure of the cervix and exposure of endocervical cells may allow for an increased susceptibility to *Neisseria gonorrhoeae* and *Chlamydia trachomatis* in the second and third decades. The cervical mucus in the adolescent group is more easily penetrated by these organisms. These facts, combined with increased numbers of partners, late health care seeking, and noncompliance with contraceptive methods, all lead to an increased risk of sexually transmitted diseases and PID.

Additional Risk Factors. Vaginal douching, tobacco use, and bacterial vaginosis are also risk factors for PID. Approximately 50% of patients with ectopic pregnancy have no apparent risk factors.

Past Medical History

Medical Conditions. Medical conditions of importance include diabetes, hypertension, cardiac disease, or immunosuppressive disorders. Susceptibility to infection or complications from anemia may complicate the patient's clinical course.

Past Surgery or Recent Trauma. Any past abdominal or gynecologic surgery (including elective abortion or dilatation and curettage procedures) should be noted.

Medications. Use of chronic corticosteroids or current antibiotics that may mask an intra-abdominal infectious process should be noted.

Allergies. An attempt should always be made to determine specific allergic reactions, especially to medication.

Physical Examination

General Appearance. The presence of pallor, diaphoresis, restlessness, or calm should be noted. Colic tends to cause the patient to be constantly moving (unable to be comfortable), whereas peritonitis causes the patient to remain still, avoiding aggravation of an already inflamed peritoneum.

Vital Signs. Serial assessment of vital signs is essential. The patient's pathologic process may be dynamic and evolve over time. Hypotension and tachycardia are strongly suggestive of ruptured ectopic pregnancy with hemorrhagic volume loss; however, not all patients present with these findings. Several case reports have documented patients with ruptured ectopic pregnancies and normal vital signs. The mechanism of this finding is unclear. However, it is a reminder to use *all* available clinical information and not rely solely on one data point for diagnosis or assessment of severity.

Head and Neck. Pallor of the conjunctiva may suggest underlying chronic anemia. The presence of icteric sclera suggests an elevated bilirubin level, which may be caused by hepatic dysfunction or hemolysis. The status of mucous membranes may reveal hydration status; however, this is not a sensitive or specific sign.

Chest. Breath sounds are evaluated for quality and symmetry. The presence of a heart murmur may lead the clinician to suspect anemia, a hyperdynamic state (pain or fever), or hypovolemia. Breast engorgement and tenderness may suggest menstrual cycle changes or pregnancy.

Abdomen. Inspection should note the presence of distention, because peritoneal irritation may lead to ileus. Specific discoloration on the abdominal wall may be seen in patients (including ruptured ectopic pregnancy) with intraperitoneal or retroperitoneal bleeding. These signs are Cullen's sign (periumbilical) and Grey Turner's sign (flank). These signs represent blood traversing the peritoneal fascia layers where weakened support (periumbilical) or gravity (flanks) assists the spread of the fluid.

Auscultation for bowel sounds is completed, and the presence or absence of these sounds is noted. Palpation is performed in all four quadrants beginning at the site farthest from the primary pain. Voluntary and involuntary guarding should be determined, as well as the presence of rebound tenderness. The exact location of tenderness and the severity are noted. Any palpable masses are identified. Repeat examinations are the cornerstone of diagnosis, unless peritoneal signs are initially detected. Fifty percent of patients with ruptured ectopic pregnancy may have no tenderness on initial abdominal examination.

Pelvic Examination. Visual inspection focuses on the presence or absence of a vesicular rash, which suggests genital herpes. The external genitalia is examined for the presence of a Bartholin's gland abscess, which is commonly associated with gonococcal infections. Trauma such as bruising or tears should raise the question of sexual assault. On speculum examination, the vagina is inspected for the presence of blood, discharge, or tissue. The presence and character of discharge at the cervical os is noted (bloody, purulent, frothy, or mucoid).

A bimanual examination includes lateral movement of the cervix to evaluate for cervical motion tenderness. The presence of cervical motion tenderness is nonspecific and may be produced from fluid or blood in the pelvic cul-de-sac (ruptured cyst or ectopic pregnancy) or from direct irritation caused by an inflamed appendix. Uterine size and tenderness are noted, as well as the presence of masses. The adnexa are palpated and examined for tenderness and fullness. In the obese patient or in a patient with severe pain, adnexal palpation may be difficult, and analgesia may be necessary to allow an adequate examination. An enlarged adnexal mass is palpable in fewer than one third of all patients with diagnosed ectopic pregnancy.

Rectal Examination. A digital examination is performed as part of the pelvic examination to assess fullness in the posterior wall of the cul-de-sac, possibly caused by peritoneal fluid or blood. Stool is tested for blood.

Extremities. Maneuvers that may elicit retroperitoneal irritation are performed. The presence of a psoas sign or obturator sign may indicate this possibility. Lower extremity swelling may represent compression of venous return by a pelvic mass.

Neurologic Examination. The patient's overall awareness and mentation may be affected by hypovolemia, sepsis, or shock. The status and symmetry of lower extremity strength, sensation, and reflexes should be assessed because a pelvic pathologic process (i.e., mass, tumor) may affect these functions.

CLINICAL REASONING

Answering the following key questions will guide future diagnosis and therapy.

Is the Patient Hemodynamically Stable?

The presence of hemodynamic instability prompts early volume resuscitation and surgical consultation. The most common causes of shock in the setting of pelvic pain are hemorrhage and sepsis. Diagnoses include ruptured ectopic pregnancy, rupture of a hemorrhagic cyst, pelvic infection, and, in the postmenopausal patient, abdominal aortic aneurysm and appendicitis with rupture.

Does the Patient Require Surgical Intervention?

Hemodynamically unstable patients will likely need surgical intervention. Hemodynamically stable patients with severe pain and signs of peritoneal irritation (guarding or rebound tenderness) need further evaluation for appendicitis, tubo-ovarian abscess, or ovarian torsion. Ultrasonography or computed tomography (CT) may help discover the cause of the patient's symptoms. It is also important to consult the patient's gynecologist early in the care of these patients.

Is the Patient Pregnant?

All female patients with abdominal pain or pelvic pain, of childbearing age, must have pregnancy testing. In the presence of even benign diagnoses, the presence of a pregnancy must be identified to guide diagnostic or therapeutic choices.

If the Patient is Not Pregnant, is the Pain Pelvic in Origin?

When the presence of pregnancy has been ruled out, the clinician must determine, based on historical and physical examination features, the most likely source of the patient's pain (gynecologic, urologic, neurologic, or gastrointestinal). Serial examinations and diagnostic results may reveal further information and may alter first impressions. Table 39–2 describes conditions that present as true pelvic pain.

Is the Patient's Fertility at Risk?

Salpingitis and other pelvic infections may significantly alter the reproductive capability of affected women. A single infection may result in a 10% to 20% infertility rate. While considering life-threatening illness, the potential for creating future life must be considered.

If the Pain is Not Pelvic in Origin, What Abdominal Causes are Considered?

Table 39–3 lists the common abdominal causes of pelvic pain.

DIAGNOSTIC ADJUNCTS

Several diagnostic adjuncts are useful in narrowing the differential diagnosis and assisting the clinician in the patient's management.

Laboratory Studies

Pregnancy Tests. The most useful test for evaluating the patient with pelvic pain is the serum or urine assay for human chorionic gonadotropin (hCG). The urine assay involves detection of the entire hCG molecule, whereas the serum assay detects the β subunit of the hCG molecule. Urine pregnancy tests can detect hCG levels as low as 25 mIU/mL. Studies have demonstrated an adequate sensitivity of the urine assay for excluding ectopic pregnancy (1 in 2000 false-negative rate). Most serum assays detect a low limit concentration of 10 mIU/mL and are able to detect pregnancy within 7 to 10 days of gestation.

Some laboratories use the same test approach for either urine or blood. The exact test and its values should be assessed at each hospital. Although these assays can detect the presence of the β-hCG or hCG molecule itself, they are qualitative (presence or absence), not quantitative (amount present). When a qualitative test is positive, a quantitative test should be performed to provide a specific level of β-hCG present. The initial β-hCG measurement can guide care in suspected ectopic pregnancy cases by providing a baseline level. Subsequently, levels of the β-hCG hormone will typically double every 48 hours in normal intrauterine pregnancies.

Other serum markers have been investigated for pregnancy detection (creatine kinase, progesterone, amylase, α-fetoprotein, and prolactin) but are of limited value because of lack of sensitivity or lack of availability at hospital sites. The use of progesterone testing appears to be the most promising of this group, when combined with the

TABLE 39–2. Differential Diagnosis of True Pelvic Pain

Illness	Pain History	Precipitating or Relieving Factors	Associated Signs and Symptoms	Key Laboratory or Radiologic Data	Management or Disposition
Pelvic inflammatory disease	Sudden or gradual; colicky pain usually bilateral in lower pelvis, but unilateral salpingitis can occur	Occurs 2–3 days after menstruation due to gonorrhea or *Chlamydia*, after recent D&C or intrauterine device insertion	Fever, chills, malaise, vomiting uncommon; marked tenderness and moderate rigidity of lower abdomen with distention; tenderness or fullness on either adnexa; enlarged uterus with post abortion or puerperal sepsis; cervical motion tenderness; possible rebound tenderness	Leukocytosis, purulent urethral or cervical discharge in gonococcal infection; uterine bleeding with infected abortion; profuse fetid discharge in puerperal sepsis; culdocentesis may reveal pus; ESR often increased	See text
Ruptured corpus luteum cyst, twisted ovarian cyst	Sudden onset; initially severe, intermittent, and localized to one adnexa; becomes continuous with local then general peritonitis	Usually no apparent precipitating factor; may have history of similar episodes lasting from hours to days; corpus luteum cyst usually ruptures 6–8 weeks from LNMP	Normal menses, afebrile or tachycardia out of proportion to fever; abdomen tender; distended, rigid pelvic mass may be palpated in abdomen; pain on cervical motion; adnexal tenderness; discrete cystic adnexal mass palpated independently from uterus	Leukocytosis; culdocentesis may yield serosanguineous fluid; ultrasound may reveal pathologic process causing torsion, but laparoscopy needed to establish diagnosis. Type and crossmatch or type and screen blood	Ruptured cysts usually resolve in 2–4 hr with pain relief. Twisted cysts require further diagnostic and therapeutic interventions (ultrasound, surgery)
Ruptured ectopic pregnancy	Sudden onset, severe, continuous, unilateral pelvic pain; rapidly becomes diffuse across entire lower abdomen and pelvis; may radiate to shoulder	Occurs usually 5–8 wk after LNMP (3–6 wk after ectopic fertilization); with rupture, the sharp localized pain is replaced by generalized hypogastric pain. Timing dependent on location of implantation	Nausea and vomiting are rare but may occur prior to rupture; afebrile; dizziness, pallor, tachycardia, hypotension, breast tenderness, uterus enlarged with cervical motion tenderness; adnexal mass palpated in 50% of cases (+ tender)	ESR normal, possible anemia noted; positive results on serum β-hCG; diagnosis is made by positive culdocentesis, ultrasound, laparoscopy, or diagnostic peritoneal lavage; type and cross match	See text
Endometriosis	Tends to be constant, beginning 2–7 days before onset of menses, increases in intensity until menstrual flow lessens; may radiate to back, thighs, rectum, bladder, vagina, or adnexa, usually history of repeated attacks, associated with menses, and can be very severe (due to chemical causes, i.e., blood peritonitis)	Limited to reproductive years, more frequent in whites and nulliparas; tenderness on examination; more prominent during menses; all sites of endometriosis symptomatic during menses	May palpate tender indurated nodules in cul-de-sac or on rectal examination; dyspareunia more prominent near the menses; 50% have hypermenorrhea; associated with infertility or sterility; dyschezia (painful defecation) is common	Laboratory tests of no immediate value; laparoscopy can confirm the diagnosis, but even laparotomy may fail to identify lesions	Usually can be managed with pain relief at home. Eventually may require surgery.
Degeneration of uterine myonas/fibroids	Sudden onset, severe pain, poorly localized in the pelvis	Older females, especially blacks	Menorrhagia, intermenstrual bleeding, occasionally dysmenorrhea or urinary frequency depending on size of fibroid; bimanual examination demonstrates mobile, usually nontender, firm, smooth masses; degeneration of myonas (ischemic episode) can occur in 30%–35% of women older than age 35 yr	CBC, ESR, β-hCG, ultrasound, laparoscopy, or computed tomography needed to confirm	After diagnostic workup, patients often require admission for volume replacement and pain relief. Surgery is considered
Mittelschmerz	Sudden onset, sharp, continuous, sometimes severe and localized to one adnexa; may radiate to ipsilateral shoulder	History of similar episodes	Afebrile; may have nausea and fever; adnexal tenderness, guarding; may have rigidity and rebound; uterus normal size and no adnexal mass	ESR normal; no leukocytosis; may have positive culdocentesis but no anemia; negative β-hCG results	Managed with pain relief at home

CBC, complete blood cell count; D&C, dilatation and curettage; ESR, erythrocyte sedimentation rate; β-hCG, β human chorionic gonadotropin (pregnancy test); LNMP, last normal menstrual period.

TABLE 39–3. Differential Diagnosis of Abdominal Causes of Pelvic Pain

Illness	Pain History	Precipitating or Relieving Factors	Associated Signs and Symptoms	Key Laboratory or Radiologic Data	Management or Disposition
Ureteral calculus	Intermittent, severe; comes in spasms of several minutes and then generally decreases, but can be constant; maximal in flank or lower abdomen; may radiate to iliac crest	May be precipitated by exercise, motion, or dehydration	Nausea, vomiting, sweating, syncope, even shock; fever and chills if associated with infection; rigidity of abdomen with pain; soreness and tenderness to palpation may persist between attacks of pain	Generally red cells in urine, occasionally WBCs, albumin, and crystals. Radiopaque stones seen often (80%) on abdominal plain film. IVP or CT shows filling defect (in 80%)	Most patients can be managed with pain relief and fluids at home with close follow-up. Continued obstruction requires relief
Acute pyelonephritis	Continuous, aching pain; maximally felt in flank, upper/lower abdomen, or midback	Asymptomatic bacteriuria or partially treated urinary tract infection	Shaking, chills, and fever; skin hot and dry; tachycardia; frequently nausea and vomiting; occasional dysuria; flank tenderness to palpation or percussion	Many WBCs in urine; occasional RBCs and WBC casts; leukocytosis	Can be treated with antibiotics as outpatient if not toxic or vomiting
Acute pelvic appendicitis	Unruptured pelvic appendicitis presents as tense, peristaltic pain felt chiefly in epigastrium or periumbilical area; after rupture, epigastric pain diminishes to give rise to local right-sided pelvic peritonitis that is less severe	Pain worsened with flexion of right thigh with internal rotation	Pain in both left and iliac fossae preceded by anorexia, nausea, or vomiting; may have frequency of urination or dysuria, diarrhea or tenesmus; right pelvic wall tenderness with rectal examination or pelvic mass (abscess) in later stage	Leukocytosis, occasional mild hematuria, low-grade fever; low-lying fecalith present or ileus; ultrasound of abscess present; barium enema sometimes advocated	Requires surgical removal if suspected
Strangulated femoral hernia	Often small fluctuant sac appears suddenly; may become larger and painful; may easily escape notice in thick fat in saphenous region	History of previous unilateral pelvic fullness or pain; occasionally incarceration associated with activities precipitating increasing intra-abdominal pressure	Generalized abdominal pain and vomiting with or without a palpable hernial sac; generally a painful swelling is noted in femoral ring	Late stages may be leukocytosis; may show obstructed pattern on acute abdominal radiologic series	Requires prompt surgical intervention
Leaking or ruptured abdominal aortic (or iliac) aneurysm	Variable; may be no symptoms before rupture; main symptoms may be unbearable pain starting in thorax, gradually extending to abdomen, hip, or thigh, not relieved with narcotics; history of aneurysm	Significant arterial hypertension of long duration is usually a forerunner; with rupture, hypovolemic shock is common	Throbbing pain before rupture; steady pain after rupture; pain possible for 4–5 days before rupture and collapse; nausea and vomiting rare; pulsatile mass anywhere in abdomen but left side most common site; back pain common; occasional unequal femoral pulses	Chest, flat-plate abdomen, or cross-table lateral plain radiograph usually demonstrates calcifications of aortic aneurysms; hematuria and elevated blood urea nitrogen are present if renal artery is involved; type and crossmatch blood. Ultrasound diagnostic	Requires immediate surgical intervention

standard β-hCG. Although an exact level at which a normal IUP is present has not been established (may be > 25 to 30 ng/mL), investigators suggest that at a level below 10 to 15 ng/mL, nonviable IUP versus ectopic pregnancy should be considered.

Complete Blood Cell Count and Differential. A hemoglobin or hematocrit is obtained when hemorrhage (vaginal or suspected intra-abdominal) occurs. *Normal* baseline values may be the result depending on the rate and duration of bleeding. Initial levels establish a baseline to guide management and intervention.

A normal white blood cell count can be insensitive and an elevated count with a left shift in the differential is nonspecific when diagnosing the cause of pelvic pain. An initial white blood cell count can only suggest or add clinical suspicion to the presence or absence of inflammation and infection. It cannot "rule in" or "rule out" PID or appendicitis.

Blood Type and Crossmatch/Screen. A type and screen, or type and crossmatch, should be obtained in patients with findings of, or history suggestive for, blood loss. Pregnant patients with vaginal bleeding require screening of Rh factor, because they may require RhoGAM. Component therapy may be necessary in patients suspected of having hemorrhage and abnormal clotting.

Hemostatic Studies. Platelet counts and coagulation studies (prothrombin time/partial thromboplastin time) should be obtained on patients with a family history of clotting abnormalities, those on anticoagulants, or patients with a history of prolonged bleeding, to detect possible disseminated intravascular coagulation.

Urinalysis. A urinalysis is required in patients with pelvic pain to determine the presence of either pyuria (secondary to peritoneal irritation or pyelonephritis/cystitis) or hematuria (secondary to renal calculi). The specimen should be obtained through straight bladder catheterization because vaginal bleeding or discharge may lead to erroneous diagnoses. The presence of pyuria does not solely diagnose urinary tract infection; adjacent organs (appendix, diverticula, fallopian tubes, uterus) that are inflamed may also inflame the bladder or ureter. It is not uncommon for a clean catch or catheterized urine specimen to have 5 to 10 cells per high-power field without bacteria in this setting (sterile pyuria).

Microbial Studies. Cervical cultures are obtained in patients who have risk factors for PID, vaginal discharge, or fever associated with pelvic pain. Traditional media-based culture methods for *N. gonorrhoeae* and *C. trachomatis* have largely been replaced by enzyme immunoassay and DNA probe assays, which have been shown to have equal sensitivity in the majority of cases.

Radiologic Imaging

Plain Radiographs. The sensitivity and specificity of plain radiographs in the evaluation of pelvic pathology is poor. The acute abdominal series (AAS) is occasionally useful when intestinal obstruction, perforated viscus, and ureteral calculi are suggested clinically. The AAS is composed of upright chest (most sensitive for the detection of free air), upright abdomen, and supine abdomen films, and the series can vary between institutions.

Computed Tomography. The use of helical CT for evaluation of acute abdominal and pelvic pain is increasingly useful owing to availability, high sensitivity and specificity for *certain* diagnoses, and ability to provide the clinician with relatively rapid results. Abdominal and pelvic CT is helpful in cases with an inflammatory process (appendicitis, pelvic abscesses, and diverticulitis). Recent applications for detection of renal calculi are extremely helpful. In elderly patients, the CT is able to provide information to the clinician regarding potential catastrophic illness (e.g., abdominal aortic aneurysm).

Ultrasonography. High-resolution ultrasonography (particularly the transvaginal probe) has become one of the most commonly used diagnostic tools in the assessment of pelvic pain. In the nonpregnant patient, ultrasonography is able to identify tubo-ovarian abscesses, complex ovarian cysts, adnexal torsion (with color Doppler flow application), and free fluid in the cul-de-sac. The most common application in the emergency department is the evaluation of pelvic pain with a positive pregnancy test, looking for the presence of an IUP or ectopic pregnancy (Fig. 39–1).

By the fifth week of conception, transvaginal ultrasound can clearly demonstrate the findings of an IUP, and by the sixth week it is able to identify the IUP.

A critical aspect of ultrasonography in diagnosing ectopic pregnancy is the correlation with the quantitative level of β-hCG. Transabdominal ultrasound is typically able to detect an IUP at 6500 mIU/mL of β-hCG, and transvaginal ultrasound is able to detect an IUP at between 1500 and 2000 mIU/mL of β-hCG. Higher β-hCG levels, coupled with an "empty" uterus, suggest an ectopic pregnancy. Each institution has different discriminatory zones (the level of hCG at which every viable IUP is seen and the absence of the visualization is diagnostic of nonviability) and must be taken into account when interpreting studies. Most patients with ectopic pregnancy

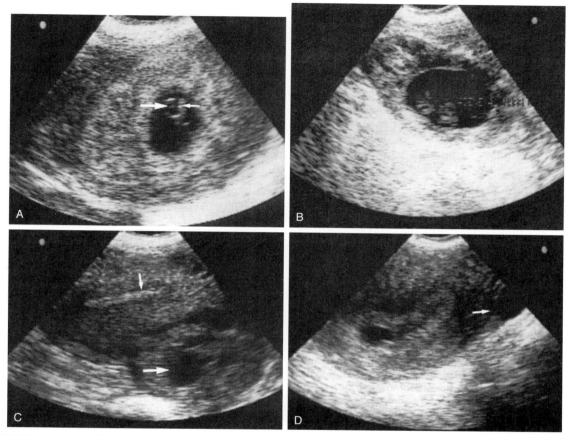

FIGURE 39–1 • *A,* Yolk sac *(large arrow)* visualized within the intrauterine gestational sac. A tiny embryo is beginning to form on the right side of the yolk sac *(small arrow). B,* Definite ectopic pregnancy. A transverse view of the right adnexa reveals an extrauterine gestational sac containing a fetal pole. The gestational sac is surrounded by a thick, brightly echogenic ring. Real-time ultrasonography revealed a fetal heartbeat present within the fetal pole. *C,* Empty gestational sac. This endovaginal longitudinal view demonstrates an empty gestational sac *(large arrow)* surrounded by a thick, brightly echogenic ring found outside the endometrial echo *(small arrow)* in the cul-de-sac. *D,* Pseudogestational sac of ectopic pregnancy. An endovaginal longitudinal view reveals a pseudogestational sac with a thick and prominent decidual reaction surrounding endometrial fluid. Internal debris can be present mimicking embryonic tissue. A complete evaluation of the adnexa revealed an ectopic pregnancy. The gestational sac containing an ectopic pregnancy can be seen adjacent to the uterus *(arrow).* (From Phelan MB, Valley VT, Mateer JR: Pelvic ultrasonography. Emerg Clin North Am 1997; 15:789–824.)

have some abnormality found on ultrasonography, including a complex adnexal mass (60% to 90%), free peritoneal fluid (25% to 35%), or extrauterine fetal heart activity (10% to 15%).

The presence of an IUP by ultrasound will usually rule out the presence of ectopic pregnancy; however, ultrasound images of an intrauterine gestational sac may be seen in up to 20% of ectopic pregnancies (false-positive finding). Also, with the increased incidence of ectopic pregnancy and dizygotic twinning secondary to in vitro fertilization and ovulation agents, the suspicion of heterotopic pregnancy must remain high.

Diagnostic Procedures

Culdocentesis. This procedure is rarely performed, owing to the widespread availability of ultrasonography. The current role of culdocentesis is in cases requiring rapid diagnosis of possible pelvic hemorrhage (patients persistently hypotensive with suspected ectopic pregnancy) or in sites that do not offer ultrasound technology. A hollow needle is inserted through the speculum into the posterior pericervical vaginal wall and into the peritoneal space of the pouch of Douglas. An attempt at fluid withdrawal is made. Historically, the procedure also yielded important culture information in the setting of PID. There are several contraindications, including the presence of a pelvic mass (especially a tubo-ovarian abscess that could rupture), a retroverted uterus, and prepubescent patients.

The interpretation of culdocentesis varies according to the type of fluid withdrawn (or the absence of fluid). In cases where no fluid is obtained, the procedure is of no diagnostic value and does not exclude the presence of ectopic pregnancy. In the normal patient, a few milliliters of clear, yellow fluid can be obtained. A positive tap is the aspiration of nonclotting blood (as little as 0.3 mL), with a spun hematocrit greater than 3%. This finding is indicative of hemoperitoneum but *cannot* delineate the cause. A positive tap does not prove the presence of ectopic pregnancy.

The most serious complication of culdocentesis is the rupture of an unsuspected tubo-ovarian abscess into the peritoneal cavity. Other serious complications include bowel perforation, pelvic kidney perforation, and bleeding from the puncture site.

PRINCIPLES OF MANAGEMENT

General Principles

Anticipation of the most catastrophic possibility should guide the management of patients with acute pelvic pain. Hemorrhagic or septic shock should be anticipated and preparation should be made for rapid treatment. Potential surgical cases must be recognized immediately for early consultation and mobilization of resources.

The three general principles of management focus on the serious complications associated with pelvic pain: volume restoration, early treatment of infection, and pain management.

Volume Restoration. Patients with evidence of volume loss (tachycardia, hypotension, or orthostasis) need two large-bore intravenous lines (14 to 16 gauge) with initial administration of isotonic crystalloid, 1 to 2 L over 20 to 30 minutes. This is followed by vital sign reassessment and another liter of fluid, if necessary.

Heart rate and blood pressure are checked every 5 minutes until stabilized, then every 15 minutes. All patients with signs of hypotension are placed on continuous cardiac monitoring and oximetry. Any patients suspected of being in hemorrhagic shock require aggressive crystalloid replacement, followed by the appropriate packed red cell transfusion, depending on the severity of the patient's condition (typically 2 to 3 L of crystalloid then 1 unit of packed cells).

Early Antibiotic Therapy. When clinical findings suggest sepsis, antibiotic administration must be carried out immediately. In the young patient with acute pelvic pain and sepsis, antibiotic regimens need to cover organisms such as *Neisseria* and *Chlamydia*, as well as anaerobic coverage for potential tubo-ovarian abscess and gut flora.

Pain Management. Multiple studies have demonstrated that analgesic therapy does not mask pelvic pain and can allow the clinician to assess pain more accurately. In patients exhibiting signs of hypotension, analgesic therapy should be reserved or cautiously titrated, because many agents may worsen hypotension.

Preparation for Potential Surgical Therapy. Patients must remain NPO throughout the course in the emergency department.

Specific Management

Selected conditions requiring specific management are listed next. For a more comprehensive list, see Tables 39–1, 39–2, and 39–3.

Ectopic Pregnancy

A diagnostic algorithm for suspected ectopic pregnancy is given in Figure 39–2. It combines hCG levels and ultrasound findings to assist in the diagnosis.

Once the diagnosis of ectopic pregnancy has been made, therapy has traditionally been surgical. Recently, pharmacologic agents have been used for early medical adjunct therapy.

Laparoscopy and laparotomy are typical surgical management. Conservative approaches, such as linear salpingostomy and segmental excision, are usually performed to preserve future fertility. Salpingectomy is preferred in those who are not desiring future pregnancy.

Methotrexate is a folate antagonist (dihydrofolate reductase inhibition) that subsequently interferes with DNA synthesis and stops cell proliferation. It is given at a dose of 1 mg/kg intramuscularly, every other day, for a total of three doses. An alternate single dose therapy is available but has a higher failure rate. Current data seem to support the use of this medical therapy for hemodynamically stable patients with early ectopic pregnancy and a low probability of rupture. Patients are excluded from methotrexate therapy if β-hCG is more than 10,000 mIU/mL, if the gestational sac is greater than 3.5 cm in diameter, or if fetal cardiac activity is noted. In spite of these careful selection criteria this management has a 70% to 85% success rate, but surgical intervention

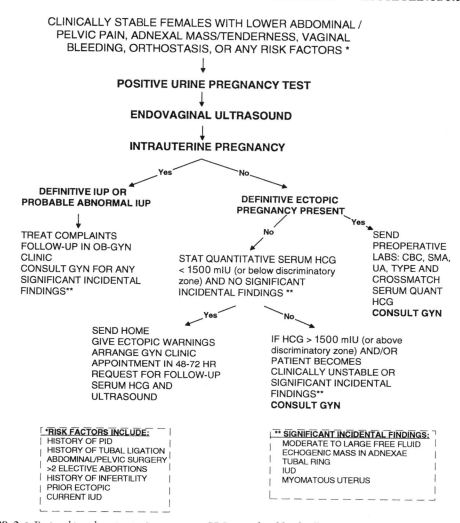

CLINICALLY STABLE FEMALES WITH LOWER ABDOMINAL /
PELVIC PAIN, ADNEXAL MASS/TENDERNESS, VAGINAL
BLEEDING, ORTHOSTASIS, OR ANY RISK FACTORS *

↓

POSITIVE URINE PREGNANCY TEST

↓

ENDOVAGINAL ULTRASOUND

↓

INTRAUTERINE PREGNANCY

Yes / No

**DEFINITIVE IUP OR
PROBABLE ABNORMAL IUP**

**DEFINITIVE ECTOPIC
PREGNANCY PRESENT** — Yes →

TREAT COMPLAINTS
FOLLOW-UP IN OB-GYN
CLINIC
CONSULT GYN FOR ANY
SIGNIFICANT INCIDENTAL
FINDINGS**

No ↓

STAT QUANTITATIVE SERUM HCG
< 1500 mIU (or below discriminatory
zone) AND NO SIGNIFICANT
INCIDENTAL FINDINGS **

SEND
PREOPERATIVE
LABS: CBC, SMA,
UA, TYPE AND
CROSSMATCH
SERUM QUANT
HCG
CONSULT GYN

Yes ← / No →

SEND HOME
GIVE ECTOPIC WARNINGS
ARRANGE GYN CLINIC
APPOINTMENT IN 48-72 HR
REQUEST FOR FOLLOW-UP
SERUM HCG AND
ULTRASOUND

IF HCG > 1500 mIU (or above
discriminatory zone) AND/OR
PATIENT BECOMES
CLINICALLY UNSTABLE OR
SIGNIFICANT INCIDENTAL
FINDINGS**
CONSULT GYN

*RISK FACTORS INCLUDE:
HISTORY OF PID
HISTORY OF TUBAL LIGATION
ABDOMINAL/PELVIC SURGERY
>2 ELECTIVE ABORTIONS
HISTORY OF INFERTILITY
PRIOR ECTOPIC
CURRENT IUD

** SIGNIFICANT INCIDENTAL FINDINGS:
MODERATE TO LARGE FREE FLUID
ECHOGENIC MASS IN ADNEXAE
TUBAL RING
IUD
MYOMATOUS UTERUS

FIGURE 39–2 • Protocol to rule out ectopic pregnancy. CBC, complete blood cell count; SMA, electrolytes, blood urea nitrogen, creatine; UA, urinalysis; IUP, intrauterine pregnancy; HCG, human chorionic gonadotropin; PID, pelvic inflammatory disease; IUD, intrauterine device. (Modified from Phelan MB, Valley VT, Mateer JR: Pelvic ultrasonography. Emerg Clin North Am 1997; 15:789–824.)

is still required in the remaining cases (ongoing ectopic pregnancy or rupture). Administration of the therapy is conducted by a gynecologist. The patient requires close follow-up and receives a repeat β-hCG in 48 hours, on day 4, on day 7, and weekly until the level is zero. If the level does not decline or the patient has pain, surgical intervention is warranted.

Pelvic Inflammatory Disease

Diagnostic criteria for PID include

- Major (all these necessary)
  - Abdominal pain
  - Adnexal pain

- Cervical motion tenderness
- Minor (one necessary)
- Fever greater than 102.2°F (39°C)
- Vaginal discharge
- Leukocytosis
- Positive cervical culture
- White blood cell count increased on vaginal smear
- Gonococcus evident on Gram's stain

Initiation of antibiotic therapy must begin before culture results and must include broad-spectrum coverage to address a wide range of pathogens. Antimicrobial choice should cover *N. gonorrhoeae*, *C. trachomatis*, anaerobes, gram-negative facultative bacteria, and streptococci. All regimens should cover both *Neisseria* and *Chlamydia*, because simultaneous infection is present in 30% to 40% of PID cases. Recent data suggest that even with negative endocervical cultures for *Neisseria* and *Chlamydia*, a significant infection of upper reproductive tract organs may occur, secondary to anaerobic bacteria.

Although there have been no studies comparing efficacy of parenteral versus oral therapy, experts suggest parenteral therapy for 48 hours in those with persistent vomiting, signs of systemic toxicity (septic shock), previous failure of oral regimens within 72 hours of therapy onset, the presence of tubo-ovarian abscess, and in patients who are immunosuppressed or immunocompromised (e.g., human immunodeficiency virus [HIV] infection).

Current parenteral antibiotic therapy, initiated in the emergency department, for inpatients consists of a second-generation cephalosporin (e.g., cefotetan or cefoxitin) combined with doxycycline. An alternative regimen (for penicillin-allergic patients) is clindamycin combined with gentamicin. Once the patient responds clinically (usually within 48 hours), oral agents can be started to complete a 14-day course of antibiotics.

There are several regimens approved by the Centers for Disease Control and Prevention for outpatient management of mild PID. Ceftriaxone intramuscularly (one dose) in the emergency department combined with 14 days of doxycycline is a common regimen. Ofloxacin and metronidazole is another recommended regimen. It is stressed that a positive response should be noted within 72 hours of oral therapy. Failure to respond within this time limit should prompt exploration of an alternative diagnosis or the need for admission and parenteral antibiotics.

Patients are relatively volume depleted in severe cases of PID, secondary to insensible losses from fever or from persistent vomiting. If needed, intravenous fluid should be administered aggressively and is usually well tolerated by these young patients.

Analgesic therapy for PID should not be withheld or delayed. As well as being unethical, the practice of withholding pain medication may prevent the clinician from obtaining an accurate abdominal examination.

Tubo-ovarian Abscess

These occur in 3% to 16% of women with PID. All patients are hospitalized and given parenteral antibiotics. Surgical drainage of the abscess or removal of the tube may be necessary.

Adnexal Torsion

The majority of torsion cases involve a diseased ovary (cystic tumor) or fallopian tube, rotating about an axis, decreasing blood flow. The mainstay of therapy for adnexal torsion is laparoscopy or laparotomy. Conservative management has no place in the management of suspected torsion, even if pain improves in the emergency department (the structure may be spontaneously torsing and de-torsing). Failure to surgically correct this entity may result in ischemia and subsequent necrosis of the involved ovary. Ultrasonographic findings of a single enlarged ovary with follicular (multiple) enlargement or adnexal mass (cystic, solid or complex) are seen. Color flow Doppler studies may be of benefit in this condition; however, because of two blood supplies to the ovary, there may be difficulty with result interpretation (i.e., positive flow on a patient with confirmed torsion or no flow in a normal patient). Further study is warranted.

Ruptured Ovarian Cyst

A ruptured ovarian cyst may cause significant intra-abdominal hemorrhage; and if the rupture transects a large blood vessel, exsanguination may occur. In severe cases, laparoscopy or laparotomy is needed to control the site of hemorrhage. In cases of mild or moderate hemorrhage, close observation with serial hematocrits and abdominal examinations may be sufficient.

UNCERTAIN DIAGNOSIS

The patient with acute pelvic pain often does not receive a specific diagnosis, despite emergency department evaluation and diagnostic testing. Time is a critical aspect in these cases, because many disease entities will become evident during serial examination of the patient. The following steps may assist the emergency physician in cases with an uncertain diagnosis:

1. Reassess the patient history and information. If necessary, speak with family, friends, or prehospital personnel for information that may have been omitted (do not break patient confidentiality—use caution when speaking to spouse or family).
2. Reexamine the patient frequently, reassess clinical status, and recheck vital signs.
3. Evaluate for other potential causes of the pain.
4. Discuss the case with consultants, the patient's primary physician, and other health care providers (another perspective may lead to a different interpretation of the case).

5. Additional observation time can provide information on the evolution of the process.

6. If the case is unclear and the patient's condition is not improved, admit the patient for further observation. Catastrophic illness and a surgically correctable process should not be evident. The physician admitting the patient may not physically evaluate the patient for a significant period of time, depending on the structure of the service. If doubt remains and emergent evaluation is needed, a request can be made that the consultant examine the patient in the emergency department.

SPECIAL CONSIDERATIONS

Prepubertal Patients with Pelvic Pain

In the prepubertal patient, pelvic pain is most likely the result of either a vaginal foreign body, urinary tract infection, or sexual abuse. Malodorous vaginal discharge in the female child is suggestive of a foreign body. Although the patient may be embarrassed giving a thorough gynecologic and sexual history (especially in the presence of parents), such information is critical to patient management. Ectopic pregnancy must be entertained in patients in the perimenarchal age group and a sample should be sent for β-hCG testing regardless of the history. Both adnexal torsion and appendicitis (the most common emergency surgery in childhood) must be considered and ruled out before attributing the pain to a less serious cause. As in adult women, PID may have a disastrous impact on future fertility if missed.

The physical examination in the female prepubescent patient must include inspection of external genitalia to look for signs of sexual abuse or trauma. In young patients, a modified pelvic examination with moistened cotton swab (for cultures) and visual inspection may be adequate to determine the source of pain; however, some specific circumstances may require a full pelvic examination using a pediatric speculum and bimanual examination. Conscious sedation may be needed for the gynecologic examination, and a pediatric gynecology specialist is recommended.

Laboratory testing for prepubertal female patients should include a urinalysis (urinary tract infection is common in this age group), and, in the perimenarchal patient, a β-hCG should be added. Radiographic studies that may be useful include plain radiographs (for potential foreign body) and/or pelvic ultrasound (color Doppler included) to evaluate ovarian vessel blood flow and organ structure.

In cases of pelvic pain in young children, when a sexually transmitted disease, endangerment, or abuse is considered the cause, child protective services and social services are required consultants for the case.

Additional causes of pelvic pain in the prepubertal patient include congenital abnormalities of the genitourinary tract, vulvovaginitis, imperforate hymen, and sickle cell crisis.

Elderly Patients and Patients with Postmenopausal Pelvic Pain

Evaluating the postmenopausal or elderly patient with pelvic pain can be very challenging for the emergency physician. Elderly patients present with atypical features of common pathology, particularly appendicitis, perforated viscus, and mesenteric ischemia. It is a challenge for the emergency physicians to identify catastrophic illnesses, including abdominal aortic aneurysm, perforated viscus, mesenteric ischemia or infarct, bowel obstruction, and inflammatory processes (appendicitis, diverticulitis, and pyelonephritis) in this age group.

Elderly patients may not be able to give a detailed history; therefore, family or skilled nursing facility personnel should be questioned to determine the clinical course before arrival in the emergency department. Particular attention should be given to associated symptoms such as vaginal bleeding (uterine fibroid or carcinoma) or rectal bleeding (diverticulitis, colon cancer, or mesenteric ischemia). The physical examination may not reveal the cause. Elderly patients frequently do not present with classic symptoms (fever, leukocytosis, and right lower quadrant pain) with acute appendicitis. There are multiple reasons why elderly patients with pelvic pain do not present with the classic features of catastrophic illness. The "atypical is typical" in elderly patients with pelvic pain.

There are many relatively benign processes that are also prevalent in the elderly female population with acute pelvic pain, including senile vaginitis secondary to decreased estrogens, uterine prolapse, cystourethrocele, rectocele, cervical polyps, and endometrial hyperplasia.

Patients with Chronic Pelvic Pain

Chronic pelvic pain is defined as pain, in the same location, that lasts longer than 4 to 6 months. One third of cases are due to adhesions secondary to infection, one third are due to endometriosis, and one third are of unknown cause. Despite a negative pelvic examination, the majority of these patients, on subsequent laparoscopic evaluation, have a cause for the pain. A pathologic process is found in over 50% of these cases; however, it may not be causing their pain. In such patients, when evaluated in the emergency department, future gynecologic referral is recommended.

Pelvic congestion syndrome is a specific entity responsible for cases of chronic pelvic pain. This syndrome is thought to be due to dilatation of the veins in the broad ligament and the ovarian plexus, with overfilling of the pelvic venous system. Pelvic ultrasonography may reveal uterine enlargement, thickening of the endometrium, and dilated pelvic veins. Gynecologic follow-up is recommended.

DISPOSITION AND FOLLOW-UP

The decision-making process ends at the final disposition: admission or discharge. In this aspect, the "sixth sense" of clinical judgment can play a critical role. The great challenge for the emergency physician is to predict those patients with the potential to become seriously ill.

Admission

Suspected Ectopic Pregnancy

- Any evidence of hemodynamic instability
- Evidence by ultrasound of ectopic pregnancy
- Combined evidence of no IUP on ultrasound with quantitative hCG greater than discriminatory zone (usually 1500 to 2000 mIU/mL combined with transvaginal ultrasonography) and significant abdominal tenderness
- Severe intractable pain even in the absence of laboratory findings

Pelvic Inflammatory Disease

- Suspected tubo-ovarian abscess or pelvic abscess
- Surgical emergencies such as appendicitis that cannot be excluded
- Intrauterine pregnancy
- Failure of previous oral treatment regimen
- Vomiting, hemodynamic instability, or high fever
- Inability to follow outpatient regimen (poor compliance) or poor follow-up care
- Immunocompromise or immunodeficiency (HIV infection)

Ruptured Ovarian Cyst

- Signs of hemodynamic instability
- Intractable pain

Elderly Patients

Consider admission for any elderly patient, because significant abdominal tenderness with a negative workup has a high likelihood of potential catastrophic medical or surgical illness.

Discharge

Suspected Ectopic Pregnancy

All discharge decisions are optimally made in dialogue with a gynecologic consultant.

- Patients are hemodynamically stable without significant abdominal tenderness.
- Ultrasound evaluation is without signs of masses or clinically significant amounts of free fluid.
- A serum quantitative β-hCG is below the discriminatory zone and is combined with a negative ultrasound (no IUP).
- An IUP is documented by ultrasound and there is minimal abdominal pain and no suspicion of heterotopic pregnancy.
- Consultation with a gynecologist is done, a 48-hour repeat of the quantitative β-hCG is planned, and the patient will be reliable with follow-up care.
- The patient acknowledges a good social environment and support and is able to access care and return if symptoms worsen.

Pelvic Inflammatory Disease

- Admission criteria are not met.
- Close, reliable follow-up is possible.

Ruptured Ovarian Cyst

- Patient is hemodynamically stable.
- Minimal pain is controlled with analgesia.
- Significant anemia is absent.
- Early, reliable follow-up is available.

Uncertain Diagnosis

- Hemodynamic instability is not evident.
- There is no emergent potential for a surgical process (appendicitis).
- Patient exhibits understanding that etiology of pain has not been apparent yet a small potential for illness remains.
- Reliable follow-up is available.

FINAL POINTS

- The emergency physician must rapidly and accurately identify catastrophic illness in patients with acute pelvic pain.
- In patients of childbearing age, diagnoses include ectopic pregnancy, PID, adnexal torsion, ruptured ovarian cyst, and appendicitis.
- In the older patient, diagnoses also include abdominal aortic aneurysm, perforated viscus, appendicitis, mesenteric ischemia, and uterine pathology.
- When evaluating the patient with suspected ectopic pregnancy, the classic presentation of abdominal pain, amenorrhea, and vaginal bleeding is not sensitive or specific.
- Failure to visualize an IUP by transvaginal ultrasonography when the serum β-hCG level is above 1500 to 2000 mIU/mL or by transabdominal ultrasonography with a β-hCG level above 6500 mIU/mL is *highly* suspicious for ectopic pregnancy.

- Empirical therapy should be initiated for suspected PID prior to cultures, because infertility and possible abscess formation are major sequelae.
- Early consultation for potential surgical processes (e.g., appendicitis) should be obtained, because such diagnoses, especially in females, may be missed by attributing the pain to a gynecologic cause.
- Not all pelvic pain is secondary to pelvic pathology. Because of complex innervation of pelvic structures, pain may be referred and can represent another catastrophic illness.
- Repeat examinations are essential and often reveal diagnoses that were not initially apparent.
- Use good clinical judgment and the "sixth sense" in cases of uncertain diagnoses. Reassess frequently, perform additional tests, liberally consult with others, and admit the patient if any doubt remains.

CASE *Study*

A 21-year-old woman presents to the emergency department with the complaint of lower abdominal pain associated with fever, nausea, and vomiting. In the triage area her vital signs include pulse, 100 beats per minute; blood pressure, 110/70 mm Hg; respiratory rate, 12 breaths per minute; and temperature, 100.9°F (38.6°C). The patient states she currently uses no method of birth control.

The patient was hemodynamically stable and was moved to the gynecologic area. She was seen by the emergency physician within 15 minutes. History revealed pain had begun 2 days after the onset of menses, which was heavier than usual. The pain was sharp, was located in the lower abdomen, but was worse in the right lower quadrant. The patient experienced nausea with one episode of vomiting. Past medical history was significant for one episode of trichomonal vaginitis. There are no prior pregnancies. She was on no medication and had no allergies. There were no prior surgeries.

This patient encounter is common. The emergency physician is faced with a wide array of potential catastrophic illness in the differential diagnosis. Possible life-threatening diagnoses in this scenario include ectopic pregnancy, appendicitis, PID, ruptured ovarian cyst, and possibly adnexal torsion. Urinary tract infection, ureteral colic, and early gastroenteritis are also in the

differential diagnosis. Note that the pain began during the patient's reported menses. PID can begin in this manner.

The patient appeared uncomfortable and was lying still on the stretcher with obvious pain on movement. Chest, heart, and flank examinations were unremarkable. Abdominal assessment demonstrated tenderness in the right lower quadrant with involuntary guarding. Bowel sounds were present, and no masses were appreciated. The pelvic examination had minimal blood in the vaginal vault, and the cervix appeared reddened and friable. The os was closed. Both adnexae were tender, with the right more so than the left. Cervical motion tenderness was present. The uterus did not feel enlarged. The rectovaginal examination noted fullness in the cul-de-sac area with tenderness. Cervical studies for *N. gonorrhoeae* and *Chlamydia* were sent.

The examination is consistent with a serious condition. Abdominal tenderness with involuntary guarding indicates peritoneal irritation. The two most common causes of peritoneal irritation in this setting are inflammation and blood. Blood can come from a ruptured cyst or an ectopic pregnancy. The critical piece of information needed at this time is the pregnancy test.

Continued on following page

Laboratory testing revealed a white blood cell count of 12,900/mm^3 with a left shift, a hemoglobin of 12 g, a hematocrit of 36%, and a normal platelet count. A urinalysis was negative, and urine hCG was also negative. A repeat abdominal examination revealed rebound tenderness with decreased bowel sounds. In response to the history of nausea and vomiting, an intravenous line was started for rehydration. Cefotetan was administered intravenously, and doxycycline was given orally. At this point the most likely diagnosis was PID. The history, fever, findings on pelvic examination, and negative pregnancy test all lead to this diagnosis. It is clear this patient will require admission, both for parenteral therapy and to maximize the potential for her future fertility.

A formal ultrasound examination was performed and revealed an inflammatory mass extending from the right fallopian tube to the cul-de-sac. There was a moderate amount of free fluid. A defined abscess was not seen.

A gynecologist was consulted and agreed that the patient required admission for continued intravenous antibiotics, supportive care, and close follow-up until clinical resolution. Aggressive care, with full understanding by the patient, has the ultimate goal of preserving her fertility.

Bibliography

TEXTS

Mishell DR Jr, Brenner PF: Management of Common Problems in Obstetrics and Gynecology. Cambridge, UK, Blackwell Scientific, 2001.

Wolfson AB, Paris PM: Diagnostic Testing in Emergency Medicine. Philadelphia, WB Saunders, 1996.

JOURNAL ARTICLES

Abbott J: Pelvic pain: Lessons from anatomy and physiology. J Emerg Med 1990; 8:441–447.

Baines PA, Allen GM: Pelvic pain and menstrual-related illness. Emerg Med Clin North Am 2001; 19:763–780.

Barnhart K: An update on the medical treatment of ectopic pregnancy. Obstet Gynecol Clin North Am 2001; 27:653–667.

Bent S, Nallamothu BK, Simel DL, et al: Does this woman have an acute uncomplicated urinary tract infection? JAMA 2002; 287:2701–2710.

Braverman PK: Sexually transmitted diseases in adolescents. Med Clin North Am 2000; 84:869–889.

Butler KH, Fidler DK, Grundmann KA: Right lower quadrant abdominal pain in women of reproductive age: an algorithmic approach. Emerg Med Rep 2002; 23(1):1–16.

Centers for Disease Control and Prevention: 1998 Guidelines for Treatment of Sexually Transmitted Diseases. MMWR Morbid Mortal Wkly Rep 1998; 47(No. RR-1):79–85.

Dart RG: Predictive value of history and physical examination in patients with suspected ectopic pregnancy. Ann Emerg Med 1999; 33:283–290.

Nadel E, Talbot-Stern J: Obstetric and gynecologic emergencies. Emerg Med Clin North Am 1997; 15:389–397.

Nelson AZ: The intrauterine contraceptive device. Obstet Gynecol Clin North Am 2000; 27:723–740.

Ness RB, Soper DE, Peipert J, et al: Design of the PID Evaluation and Clinical Health (PEACH) Study. Controlled Clin Trials 1998; 19:499–513.

Newkirk GR: Pelvic inflammatory disease: A contemporary approach. Am Fam Physician 1996; 53:1127–1135.

Phelan MB, Valley VT, Mateer JR: Pelvic ultrasonography. Emerg Med Clin North Am 1997; 15:789–824.

CHAPTER 40

Vaginal Bleeding

COURTNEY HOPKINS

THOMAS KRISANDA

CASEStudy

A 28-year-old woman was in her primary physician's office awaiting an examination for recent irregularity of her menstrual cycle. After calling her to an examining room, the nurse noted that the patient appeared pale and unsteady in her gait. The nurse obtained a pulse of 120 beats per minute and a blood pressure of 90/50 mm Hg in a sitting position. After a brief assessment by the physician, a decision was made to transfer the patient to the emergency department by rescue squad.

INTRODUCTION

Vaginal bleeding is the visible result of hemorrhage occurring anywhere along the female reproductive tract. It is one of the 10 most frequent complaints seen in the emergency department. In premenarchal and postmenopausal patients, vaginal bleeding is almost always the result of a nonhormonal cause. Women of reproductive age may exhibit physiologic vaginal bleeding that reflects cyclic endometrial stimulation orchestrated by the interplay between estrogen and progesterone. These ovarian hormones in turn are controlled by a complex endocrine system mediated by the hypothalamus and pituitary gland and incorporating multiple hormonal feedback loops. This system, although providing the hormonal integration necessary for female reproduction, also produces opportunities for dysfunction.

It is important to distinguish abnormal from the "normal" variations that occur in the menstrual cycle. Most cycles during the first years after the onset of menarche are anovulatory. Menses can be irregular and scant for a short time but usually settle into a regular cycle that varies from 21 to 40 days. The mean duration of menses is 4.7 days with an average blood loss of 35 mL. Recurrent bleeding in excess of 80 mL can lead to anemia. The onset of menopause results in a progressively irregular cycle length, as more cycles become anovulatory.

Abnormal uterine bleeding can be described by using several sometimes confusing terms. *Oligomenorrhea* is bleeding that occurs at intervals of greater than 40 days, and *polymenorrhea* is bleeding at intervals (either regular or irregular) of less than 22 days. Other terms are *menorrhagia* and *metrorrhagia*. To eliminate the uncertainty that can be caused when using these terms, it is best to be descriptive by using nontechnical words and phrases. For example, a patient with polymenorrhea is best recorded as having "heavier than usual bleeding at irregular intervals that are shorter than her regular cycle." This documentation requires greater effort, but decreases confusion.

Vaginal bleeding is caused by one of six basic pathophysiologic mechanisms. These are pregnancy-related, neoplastic, infectious, traumatic, hormonal, and hematologic. The most potentially immediately life-threatening mechanism is pregnancy related. Pregnancy can cause abnormal bleeding in three ways. The ovum can fail to develop properly, in which case its growth will be terminated and it will be expelled from the uterus (spontaneous abortion). Implantation can occur in a site other than the uterus; bleeding will then occur when the site of implantation (ectopic pregnancy) can no longer accommodate the fetus. Later in pregnancy, the placenta can bleed profusely if it is located over the os at the time of cervical dilatation and effacement or if the placenta prematurely separates from the uterine wall (placenta previa or abruptio placentae).

Neoplasms cause bleeding by invading normal pelvic structures or by necrosis of the tumor mass itself. Both benign and malignant processes can cause bleeding. For example, uterine polyps occur in 4% of women and can ulcerate and bleed. Postmenopausal bleeding always raises concern that a malignancy is present, but malignancy is found in only 20% of cases. A neoplasm can invade any anatomic structure from the introitus to the ovary. The goal of routine screening of women with regular pelvic examinations and cervical cytology is to find early signs of cancer.

Infection can cause abnormal bleeding at one or multiple anatomic sites. It may be caused by

677

many organisms, the most important being *Neisseria gonorrhoeae* and *Chlamydia trachomatis.* In one clinical setting, when other causes of bleeding were excluded in sexually active, reproductively capable patients, gonococcal infection (as proved by culture) was the cause of bleeding in 30% of cases. It is routine in many centers to obtain a cervical culture for *N. gonorrhoeae* in all sexually active females with vaginal bleeding. Abnormal bleeding resulting from infection can be very subtle and difficult to diagnose.

Trauma as a cause of bleeding is more common in the pediatric age group. The bleeding is usually the result of lacerations of the perineum, vulva, or vagina. In adults, traumatic bleeding can be caused by sexual intercourse.

Unless prolonged, hormonally related hemorrhage rarely poses a significant risk to the patient. It is often a diagnosis of exclusion, made after other possible mechanisms have been ruled out.

Finally, hematologic causes result from abnormalities of hemostasis. Platelet disorders more commonly present as abnormal vaginal bleeding than coagulopathies. A disorder of the pelvic organs may secondarily "unmask" a defect of the clotting mechanism.

Depending on the time course, rate, and compensatory response to bleeding, the presentation of the patient may range from a "normal" condition to overt shock. The emergency physician must work quickly to identify the patient at high risk from this hemorrhage.

INITIAL APPROACH AND STABILIZATION

Priority Diagnoses

In women of childbearing age, attention is primarily directed toward the pregnancy-related condition: abortion, ectopic pregnancy, placental origin. These cause much of the life-threatening vaginal bleeding seen in the emergency department.

Rapid Assessment

On arrival, patients with a complaint of vaginal bleeding are evaluated and managed according to the following general guidelines. Patients with supine or orthostatic vital signs indicative of hemodynamic compromise secondary to blood loss, with other evidence of hypovolemia (pallor, diaphoresis, apprehension), or with objective evidence of significant vaginal bleeding are triaged to the resuscitation area of the emergency department and seen immediately by the physician. Patients without these findings are placed in a gynecologic examination area and seen in order of their time of appearance in the emergency department.

Initial questions to the patient center on the presence and severity of symptoms such as shortness of breath, orthostatic weakness, abdominal pain, and bleeding. It is critical to establish as early as possible the presence or absence of pregnancy.

On examination, a primary survey of the airway, breathing, and circulation is combined with a rapid assessment of the level of consciousness and an abdominal examination. Supine and orthostatic vital signs are measured.

Early Intervention

The following steps are carried out for the unstable patient:

1. One or more large-bore (16- or 14-gauge) intravenous lines are established, and isotonic crystalloid solution is given.
2. Oxygen therapy at 8 to 10 L/min is begun or continued.
3. Cardiac monitoring is started.
4. A blood sample is sent to the laboratory for initial hematocrit and also for type and screen or for crossmatch for 4 to 6 units.
5. Blood or urine samples are obtained for pregnancy testing by a rapid measurement of β-human chorionic gonadotropin (β-hCG). Blood is saved in anticipation of additional blood tests (e.g., serum quantitative β-hCG, platelet count, coagulation studies).

Patients in labor who are experiencing vaginal bleeding and beyond 20 weeks of pregnancy are handled in a similar manner. It is important to avoid performing a digital or speculum vaginal examination in these patients. Any manipulation of the cervix and os can cause a massive hemorrhage in patients with placenta previa. In any pregnant patient with vaginal bleeding an ultrasound examination is performed as soon as possible.

Patients of reproductive age who are complaining of vaginal bleeding accompanied by abdominal pain but have no evidence of significant distress, obvious bleeding, or hemodynamic instability can be triaged to a gynecology examining room and seen expeditiously by the physician. An intravenous line is established at the discretion of the nursing staff. Serum or urine pregnancy testing is carried out. The possibility of ectopic pregnancy is a foremost concern in these patients.

CLINICAL ASSESSMENT

The goals of the history and physical examination in the patient with vaginal bleeding are to elicit clues to the etiology of the bleeding, discover signs and symptoms of pregnancy, and determine the extent and effect of the blood loss.

History

1. *What is the reproductive status of the patient?* The physician determines whether the patient is reproductively capable or is either prepubertal or postmenopausal. The span of reproductive ability usually ranges from 12 to 55 years of age, but exceptions occur at both extremes. The potential causes of the bleeding are profoundly influenced by this determination.
2. *When did the bleeding begin?* The time of onset of the bleeding is noted. Recent onset of abnormal bleeding is consistent with more immediately threatening problems such as ectopic pregnancy. Abnormal bleeding that has occurred over a prolonged period of time is more consistent with hormonal dysfunction or uterine problems such as malignancy or leiomyomas.
3. *What is the extent of the bleeding?* The amount of bleeding, as reported by the patient, is notoriously unreliable. As a rough gauge, the patient can be asked to measure the blood flow as more or less than her usual menses. Attempts to quantify the bleeding are less important than questioning about easy fatigability or postural dizziness, symptoms that might indicate significant blood loss.
4. *What is the menstrual history of the patient?* A careful menstrual history is essential to evaluate the complaint of vaginal bleeding. If the patient is menstruating, the cycle length, the number of days of menses, and any associated symptoms such as cramping or back pain are determined. The most common cause of cessation of menses is pregnancy. Subtle changes in cycle length or amount of menses may be the only clinical signs of chlamydial or gonorrheal infection of the reproductive organs. Bleeding that occurs outside of the regular menstrual cycle may indicate malignancy or a blood dyscrasia.
5. *Is the passed blood clotted or nonclotted?* Menstrual blood usually does not clot. Clotting occurs with heavy bleeding when the blood does not remain in the uterine cavity long enough to undergo fibrinolysis.
6. *Is the patient sexually active?* Sexually active women are at greater risk for serious bleeding because of possible pregnancy. The method of birth control used is determined.
7. *What is the pregnancy history?* The number of previous pregnancies, live births, and any spontaneous or induced abortions are recorded. It is easiest to record these in annotated form, using the respective terms *gravida, para*, and *abor-*tion (or G–P–Ab). For example, a woman with four previous pregnancies, three live births, and one miscarriage is noted as $G_4P_3Ab_1$.

8. *Are there associated symptoms?* It is important to elicit any history of fever, abdominal or pelvic pain, and vaginal discharge. Pain may be caused by distention of a hollow organ, such as a fallopian tube secondary to an ectopic pregnancy. Sudden vascular occlusion (e.g., torsion of an ovary or uterine fibroid) can cause sudden severe pain. Peritoneal irritation from blood or pus may result in diffuse abdominal pain with rigidity and guarding. Disorders confined to the pelvis may present as pain referred to the back.
9. *Is there a pertinent past medical history?* Inquiries are made about any previous abdominal or pelvic surgeries. Any previous episodes of pelvic inflammatory disease are noted. Both are important risk factors in ectopic pregnancy. Is there endocrine disease? Diabetes mellitus, hyperthyroidism and hypothyroidism, pituitary disease, or adrenal disease can be associated with vaginal bleeding.
10. *Does the patient have a known disorder of hemostasis?* Platelet disorders are more common in women and present primarily as mucosal bleeding. The patient is asked whether other problems with abnormal bleeding have occurred (e.g., nosebleeds, dental extraction, menorrhagia). Use of platelet-inhibiting drugs such as aspirin is explored. A brief family history is obtained.

Physical Examination

Although the physical examination should be complete, inevitably the examiner focuses on vital signs, general appearance, the abdomen, and the reproductive tract.

Vital Signs

Heart Rate. Tachycardia may be secondary to pain, anxiety, or hypovolemia.

Blood Pressure. Hypotension (systolic blood pressure less than 80 to 90 mm Hg) is a serious sign reflecting significant blood loss. All normotensive patients with abnormal bleeding should have their orthostatic vital signs measured. A drop in the systolic pressure of 20 to 30 mm Hg or a rise of 20 to 30 beats in the pulse rate may indicate a significant volume loss. Women in the later stages of pregnancy have a physiologic augmentation of circulating blood volume approaching 40%. Hypotension in this setting indicates major hemorrhage, presenting grave risks to mother and fetus. On the other hand, hypotension in pregnancy may be due to uterine pressure on the inferior vena cava, which can lead to decreased venous return to the heart. Placing the patient on the left side may correct this problem.

Respiratory Rate. Like tachycardia, tachypnea may reflect hypovolemia, pain, or anxiety.

Temperature. The presence of fever points to an underlying infectious etiology for the bleeding.

General Appearance

Patients with significant bleeding or a life-threatening pelvic organ disease often have signs of serious illness. They will look "uncomfortable" and are not inclined to voluntary movement on the stretcher. If hypovolemia is present, pallor, moist skin, and apprehension are observed in spite of a normal blood pressure reading. Conversely, patients with early ectopic pregnancy can appear remarkably well and in no distress. Pursuit of the diagnosis by appropriate testing must be particularly diligent in these cases.

Abdomen

Inspection. The abdomen is inspected for pregnancy or abdominal distention.

Auscultation. Auscultation is carried out to assess bowel sounds or bruits if they are present.

Fetal Heart Tones. If the patient is pregnant, a Doppler stethoscope is used to detect fetal heart tones, but this test may not be detectable at less than 8 to 10 weeks of gestation.

Palpation. All four quadrants of the abdomen are palpated. Any areas of tenderness are noted, especially if there is associated involuntary rigidity or rebound or signs of peritoneal irritation. If the uterus is palpable, the fundal height is determined. Uterine tenderness, rigidity, and contractions are assessed. The location of the uterine fundus may be used as a rough estimate of fetal gestational age as follows: top of symphysis pubis, 12 weeks; level of umbilicus, 20 weeks; and tip of xiphoid, 36 weeks. After the 36th week, the uterine fundus recedes slightly as the fetal head drops into and engages the pelvis.

Pelvic Examination

Reassurance and positioning of the patient are the keys to an adequate pelvic examination. Ideally, the patient is placed in the dorsal lithotomy position; however, if the patient's condition is unstable and the workup needs to proceed more rapidly, the examination can be performed with the patient in a frog-leg position and the buttocks elevated on a bedpan on the stretcher. Because the potential for additional harm is real, pregnant patients with vaginal bleeding after the 20th week should NOT receive a pelvic or rectal examination unless provisions are made for both emergency surgical and vaginal delivery in a delivery suite.

Inspection. The external genitalia are carefully inspected. Bleeding, discharge, inflammation, and infection are noted. Particularly in the elderly, it is important to do a digital vaginal examination before inserting the speculum. This step will serve to detect foreign bodies, atrophic vaginitis with synechiae, and evidence of trauma or masses. It will also allow the position of the cervix to be located in advance of the speculum examination.

Speculum Examination. After insertion of the speculum, bleeding may be observed as originating from the external cervical os or elsewhere. The os is visually inspected, and whether it appears open is noted. An open os is indicative of an ongoing abortion in the pregnant patient. The nonpregnant cervix is firm to the touch, with a uniform pink color. A bluish, soft cervix suggests pregnancy. If indicated, cervical cultures and specimens for microscopic examination are obtained at this time.

Bimanual Examination. A careful bimanual examination is performed. The consistency of the cervix (patulous, firm, nodular) and the presence of any cervical motion tenderness are useful findings. The external cervical os is digitally palpated to reveal any dilatation or cervical effacement. The cul-de-sac is examined. Any fullness could indicate fluid, blood, or pus. The uterus is palpated for size, position, asymmetry, and tenderness. A "nodular" feel is suspicious of fibroids, malignant tumor, or endometriosis. Tenderness or masses (or both) are the important findings in the examination of the adnexae. Two important points to be remembered: the round ligaments are often mistaken for the fallopian tubes, especially in young, thin women, and the ovaries are not palpable in a postmenopausal woman. Because the ovaries are atrophic after menopause, any palpated mass is abnormal.

Rectal Examination. A rectal examination confirms the position of the uterus and the presence or absence of fluid in the cul-de-sac. If the patient has had previous infections, the cul-de-sac may be obliterated.

CLINICAL REASONING

After initial stabilization and data gathering, preliminary diagnostic impressions are organized. The emergency physician seeks to answer four questions.

Does the Patient Have Severe Blood Loss with or without Hemodynamic Instability?

Regardless of the cause of bleeding, the initial resuscitation and stabilization of the patient are directed toward correcting the blood loss and volume depletion. Once appropriate resuscitative measures have been taken, a search for the source of hemorrhage is begun. If the hemorrhage has occurred over an extended time period, compensatory mechanisms may mask a significant loss of red blood cell mass.

Is the Patient Pregnant?

Because the disorders of pregnancy that cause abnormal vaginal bleeding (e.g., ectopic pregnancy, placenta previa, abruptio placentae) tend to be more immediately life threatening than non–pregnancy-related causes, determining the pregnancy status of the patient is paramount.

Is the Source of Bleeding the Reproductive Tract, or is it Related to Other Anatomic Areas?

The woman complaining of abnormal vaginal bleeding is usually accurate in localizing the site. In some cases, particularly in elderly women, the bleeding may be originating from the urinary or gastrointestinal tract. Occasionally, the bleeding originates from other anatomic sites but enters the vagina through a fistula. This finding is usually caused by malignancy.

Is the Bleeding of Systemic Origin?

Systemic disorders of hemostasis, especially platelet disorders, may manifest as mucosal bleeding. Most of these problems are drug related (aspirin inhibition of platelet aggregation or thrombocytopenia due to chemotherapeutic agents) or acquired from immunologic (idiopathic thrombocytopenic purpura), infectious (disseminated intravascular coagulation), or unknown (thrombotic thrombocytopenic purpura) origins.

DIAGNOSTIC ADJUNCTS

The laboratory evaluation of abnormal vaginal bleeding is straightforward. Considerable information can be gained from only a few tests.

Laboratory Studies

Complete Blood Cell Count and Differential. Patients presenting with a complaint of vaginal bleeding require a complete blood cell count if there is evidence of significant blood loss by the history or physical examination (pallor or abnormal orthostatic vital signs). If the hemoglobin and hematocrit are in the normal range, the results will allow comparison at a future time to assess the degree of ongoing blood loss. Low levels represent chronic loss or acute loss of some severity. An elevated white blood cell count and left-shifted differential suggest underlying infection or inflammation as a cause. A platelet count of less than $100,000/mm^3$ is diagnostic of thrombocytopenia. Interpreting the red blood cell indices may provide evidence of iron deficiency or megaloblastosis.

Pregnancy Testing. In general, all women of reproductive capability with a complaint of vaginal bleeding should have an analysis of the β subunit of human chorionic gonadotropin (β-hCG). These tests have a sensitivity as low as 5 to 25 mIU/L and are greater than 96% specific for the β subunit of hCG. A highly sensitive test, able to measure small amounts of hCG, is important because up to 50% of women with ectopic pregnancies have serum hCG levels of less than 100 mIU at the time of discovery. A positive qualitative urinary β-hCG analysis is just as useful as a positive serum assay. However, a negative urine test is not as reassuring as a negative serum test. Urine tests can be falsely negative because of dilution in urine samples with a low specific gravity. When certainty is paramount, then a serum test is obtained.

When an ectopic pregnancy is suspected, a quantitative test for β-hCG is performed in addition to the qualitative test. A low level of hCG can be indicative of an ectopic or failed intrauterine pregnancy. It also provides a baseline against which subsequent levels can be compared. When used in combination with ultrasound, a quantitative β-hCG test can be very accurate in the diagnosis of an ectopic gestational sac (see Chapter 39, Acute Pelvic Pain).

Cervical Cultures. Endocervical gonococcal cultures should be performed in all sexually active women. Cultures or antigen screening for *Chlamydia trachomatis* are strongly suggested when infection is suspected as the cause of the bleeding.

Radiologic Imaging

The cornerstone of radiologic imaging for the evaluation of vaginal bleeding is ultrasonography. The advent of transvaginal ultrasonography has revolutionized the early diagnosis of ectopic pregnancies. A complete evaluation, however, must include both transabdominal and transvaginal approaches. Although transvaginal ultrasound is superior for evaluation of the pelvis and detection of fluid in the cul-de-sac, the transabdominal approach is optimal for the evaluation of free fluid in Morison's pouch and paracolic gutters. Obvious ectopic pregnancies, which were not detected transvaginally, have been identified by transabdominal ultrasound. The two techniques should be considered complementary. Normal and abnormal ultrasound findings are listed in Table 40–1. The gestational sac normally increases by 0.7 mm/day.

Ultrasound is excellent for detecting an intrauterine pregnancy and for evaluating the position of the placenta. It is also good for detecting other adnexal abnormalities and the presence of as little as 5 to 20 mL of blood or fluid in the cul-de-sac. Although it can detect an abruptio placenta, it is less reliable in determining the degree of placental separation.

EXPANDED DIFFERENTIAL DIAGNOSIS

This section is organized with the various causes of vaginal bleeding grouped according to the presence or absence of pregnancy (Table 40–2).

Conditions Causing Vaginal Bleeding when the Pregnancy Test Result is Positive

Ectopic Pregnancy

Ectopic pregnancy is a true emergency and is the most serious cause of vaginal bleeding. It is the leading cause of maternal mortality and occurs in 1:100 to 1:200 pregnancies. Ectopic pregnancy can become manifest in a variety of ways. The presentation of abdominal pain, vaginal bleeding, adnexal mass, and confirmatory laboratory evidence of pregnancy is straightforward. However, the diagnosis can be difficult in many cases. A high index of suspicion is always maintained. The symptoms and signs of ectopic pregnancy, with their approximate incidence, are listed here:

Symptoms
- Abdominal pain (97%)
- Symptoms of pregnancy: amenorrhea, nausea, breast tenderness (75%)
- Vaginal bleeding (55%)
- Syncopal or presyncopal symptoms (34%)

Signs
- Lower abdominal tenderness (83%)
- Adnexal tenderness (72%)
- Clinical evidence of hypovolemia (38%)
- Blood in the cul-de-sac (30%)
- Adnexal mass (25%)
- Uterine enlargement (25%)

In short, any woman capable of reproduction who presents with abdominal pain, abnormal vaginal bleeding, and a positive test for pregnancy is assumed to have an ectopic pregnancy until proved otherwise. Confirming the diagnosis of ectopic pregnancy is by no means easy. The differential diagnosis is extensive and includes conditions of varying severity in both the pregnant and nonpregnant conditions. Table 40–3 categorizes some commonly encountered conditions often confused with ectopic pregnancy. (Also see Chapter 39, Acute Pelvic Pain.) An algorithmic approach to the assessment of suspected ectopic pregnancy is given in Figure 40-1.

Spontaneous Abortion

Spontaneous abortion is commonly seen in the emergency department. Spontaneous abortion, or "miscarriage," is defined as the natural termina-

---

TABLE 40–1. Common Findings in Ultrasonography of the Patient with Potential Pregnancy and Vaginal Bleeding

Normal Findings		
Gestational Age	*Gestational Sac Size*	*Transvaginal Ultrasound Findings*
5.5 weeks	8 mm	Yolk sac present
6.0 weeks	16 mm	Embryo present
6.5 weeks	20 mm	Fetal cardiac activity

Abnormal Findings
6.5 weeks estimated gestational age without cardiac activity
Gestational sac > 1 cm without yolk sac
β-hCG > 10,800 without cardiac activity
Gestational sac > 20 mm without cardiac activity

TABLE 40–2. Differential Diagnosis of Vaginal Bleeding

Pregnancy Status	
Positive	*Negative*
<20 Weeks' Gestation	**Vaginal**
Ectopic pregnancy	Trauma
Threatened abortion	Foreign body
Inevitable abortion	Infection
Incomplete abortion	Neoplasm
Completed abortion	Vascular—arteriovenous malformation
Missed abortion	Atrophic vaginitis
Infection, septic abortion	Endometriosis—cervical/vaginal
Trophoblastic disease	Immunologic—lichen sclerosis et atrophicus or lichen simplex chronicus
>20 Weeks' Gestation	**Uterine**
Placenta previa	***Ovulatory***
Abruptio placentae	Menses
Uterine rupture	Infection
Vasa previa	Neoplasms, benign or malignant
Premature labor	Hematologic
Normal labor	Iatrogenic
	Anovulatory
	Endocrine
	Psychogenic

TABLE 40–3. Differential Findings in Conditions Mimicking Ectopic Pregnancy

Diagnosis	Amenorrhea	β-hCG	Adnexal Mass or Tenderness	Vaginal Bleeding
Ectopic pregnancy	+	+	+	+
Corpus luteum cyst	+	−	+	+/−
Threatened abortion	+	+	−	+
Pelvic inflammatory disease	−	−	Bilateral	+/−
Appendicitis	−	−	RLQ tenderness	−
Degenerating fibroid	−	−	Uterine mass	+/−
Ovarian torsion	−	−	Adnexal mass, tenderness	−

+, present; −, absent; RLQ, right lower quadrant.

tion of a pregnancy before the fetus is capable of extrauterine life, which is approximately 20 weeks' gestation and 500 g fetal weight.

Six subcategories of spontaneous abortion concern the emergency practitioner. *Threatened abortion* is defined as any uterine bleeding that occurs in the first half of a normal pregnancy. This definition is thus met in 20% to 25% of all pregnant women, and in half of these the process will go on to completion. There is no dilatation of the internal cervical os at the time or at presentation to the emergency department. An *inevitable abortion* occurs when the above definition is met and the bleeding increases and pain persists. Dilatation of the internal cervical os is the major differential point. There is no possibility of fetal survival in this circumstance.

An *incomplete abortion* is the natural evolution of an inevitable abortion, but only some of the products of conception from the uterine cavity are passed. A *complete abortion* may be suspected when there is cessation of "pregnancy symptoms" (breast engorgement and tenderness, nausea) after passage of the entire conceptus.

A *missed abortion* occurs when the conceptus dies but is not passed. This condition usually is not accompanied by vaginal bleeding. *Second-trimester abortions* are rare but often are due to identifiable causes such as abruptio placentae, chorioamnionitis, uterine anomalies, cervical

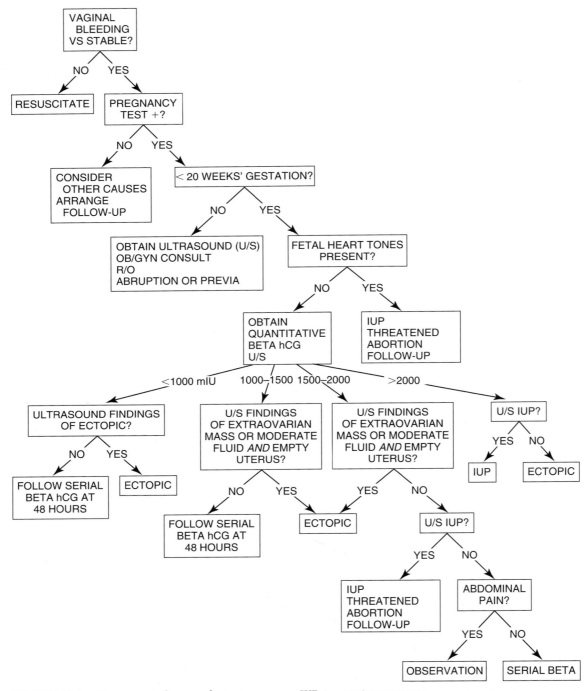

FIGURE 40–1 • Management of suspected ectopic pregnancy. IUP, intrauterine pregnancy.

incompetence, and the lupus anticoagulant syndrome.

Occasionally after the termination of an early pregnancy, infection sets in, leading to septic complications. These cases quickly can become life threatening. Retained products of conception

or injured endometrium and myometrium are susceptible to invasion by facultative and anaerobic bacteria. Septic shock complicates 5% to 15% of these cases. The diagnosis of an infected abortion has to be considered in any febrile, bleeding patient who is pregnant. Aggressive fluid resuscitation and administration of antibiotics is required at the outset of care of these patients.

Bleeding in Late Pregnancy

Third-trimester bleeding is an unusual event, occurring in only 2% to 3% of patients. Although a trivial etiology such as vaginal condylomas, cervical polyps, or minor trauma may be the cause, placental abnormalities and uterine rupture must be considered first. As such, pelvic and rectal examinations are avoided until provision is made for management of severe hemorrhage, including emergent delivery in an operating suite.

Placenta Previa. Placenta previa is the condition in which placental implantation has occurred in the lower uterine segment. Placenta previa is characterized by bright red, painless vaginal bleeding that is initiated by the beginnings of cervical effacement and dilatation. Complications of placenta previa are fetal distress and demise secondary to a reduction or interruption of the fetoplacental circulation. Maternal morbidity or mortality is a direct result of the degree of hemorrhage that occurs before definitive control.

Abruptio Placentae. Abruptio placentae is the complete or incomplete detachment of the normally implanted placenta at any time before the birth of the infant. Placental separation may be complete or partial, and the bleeding is either *revealed* after dissection under the membranes to the outside or *concealed* behind the placenta or membranes. The patient classically presents with a painful, tender uterus that demonstrates variable degrees of uterine contraction with incomplete relaxation. Vaginal bleeding is usually dark red. Fetal distress or demise is usually seen. In the latter instance, fetal heart tones are unobtainable.

Conditions Causing Vaginal Bleeding when the Pregnancy Test is Negative

When the pregnancy test is negative, abnormal vaginal bleeding may be secondary to lower genital tract (vaginal or cervical) pathologic processes or to upper tract (uterus, fallopian tubes, ovaries) disease (see Table 40–2).

Bleeding secondary to a vaginal abnormality is easily evaluated by speculum, digital, and microscopic examinations. All these examinations are easily performed in the emergency department. Many of the conditions resulting in lower genital tract bleeding can be diagnosed and treated primarily in the emergency department. Upper genital tract bleeding usually originates in the uterus. Abnormal uterine bleeding may be either *ovula-*

tory or *anovulatory*. Ovulatory refers to bleeding interspersed with what is otherwise regular, cyclic ovulatory uterine bleeding. Anovulatory bleeding is usually associated with an underlying endocrine disturbance.

Common causes of ovulatory abnormal uterine bleeding include neoplasms (benign and malignant), endometriosis, infections, intrauterine devices, endogenous sex steroid hormones, and blood dyscrasias. Common causes of anovulatory uterine bleeding include endocrine disturbances, most commonly physiologic immaturity of the hypothalamic-pituitary-ovarian axis; psychogenic causes including stress, athletic activity, and eating disorders; and "dysfunctional uterine bleeding."

Dysfunctional uterine bleeding is often construed as a "catch-all" diagnosis. Actually it is defined as abnormal uterine bleeding with no organic cause, and therefore it is a diagnosis of exclusion. This exclusion often cannot be properly made in the emergency department. Causes of dysfunctional uterine bleeding may be grouped according to the age and menstrual status of the patient as follows:

1. *Menarche to age 20.* The usual cause of dysfunctional uterine bleeding in this age range is immaturity of the hypothalamic-pituitary-ovarian axis. Anovulatory cycles with irregular spotting and bleeding are the most common cause of abnormal bleeding in teenagers. Other causes include use of oral contraceptive agents or an intrauterine device.
2. *Ages 20 to 40.* Anovulatory abnormal uterine bleeding is responsible for less than 20% of cases in this age group. In this group, causes are more likely to be psychogenic, (e.g., stress, depression). Rapid weight changes and intense physical activity can also alter menses significantly.
3. *Age older than 40.* As in the young perimenarchal patient, anovulation again becomes the major cause of abnormal bleeding; however, malignancy *must* be assumed until a thorough evaluation excludes it. Endometrial cancer has now superseded invasive cervical carcinoma as the most frequent gynecologic cancer.

PRINCIPLES OF MANAGEMENT

General Principles

The first principle of management of the patient with abnormal vaginal bleeding is to ensure hemodynamic stability. Volume loss must be vigorously treated with fluid or blood component therapy and oxygen and the patient continuously monitored. If the emergency evaluation reveals evidence of surgical disease (e.g., ruptured ectopic pregnancy or a complication of late pregnancy), then provisions for immediate transfer to the operating suite are made. The second major principle is to maintain fetal viability in women with advanced pregnancies but not at the expense of maternal safety. Early consultation with an obstetrician or gynecologist is essential in all cases in which either the mother or the fetus is endangered.

Specific Situations

Ectopic Pregnancy. Once an ectopic pregnancy is diagnosed, preparations for urgent laparotomy are made while the emergency department resuscitation is underway. The definitive surgical procedure of choice is a total salpingectomy. Refined, newer surgical techniques, including use of the operating laparoscope, make it possible to consider tubal salvage rather than removal. Systemic methotrexate therapy has shown promise as a nonsurgical therapy in some cases of unruptured ectopic pregnancy. All therapeutic decisions are made in consideration with a gynecologist. (See Chapter 39, Acute Pelvic Pain.)

Spontaneous Abortion. No specific treatment regimen has proved efficacious in *threatened abortion*. Generally, patients are reassured and sent home with instructions to avoid sexual activity and to remain at bed rest for several days, although the latter has not been conclusively shown to be of benefit. The patient is instructed to return if bleeding persists or becomes worse, if pain increases, or if tissue is passed. Obstetric referral is mandatory and pelvic ultrasonography is performed within a few days to evaluate fetal viability. Doppler ultrasonographic determinations of fetal heart tones provide useful prognostic information, although it may be falsely negative before 8 to 10 weeks' gestation. A pregnancy test that reverts to negative is diagnostic of fetal demise.

The mainstay of treatment for *inevitable, incomplete, completed,* and *missed abortions* is uterine suction curettage. Curettage is necessary even after complete abortion because small tissue products can remain behind, resulting in unnecessary bleeding or infection. When the bleeding is severe, an oxytocin infusion can be initiated in the emergency department until the patient can be transferred for curettage. The final diagnosis of abortion rests on pathologic examination of the products of conception. Any tissue seen on examination is preserved for further evaluation. Finally, all patients should have an Rh determination. Rh-negative patients who are unsensitized following an abortion or ectopic pregnancy need $Rh_0\langle D\rangle$ immune globulin. The consultant obstetrician-gynecologist usually makes this determination, but occasionally it is the responsibility of the emergency physician.

Placenta Previa. Diagnosis and management occur simultaneously in the patient with third-trimester bleeding. When the diagnosis of placenta previa is suspected, diagnosis and management are determined by the amount of ongoing bleeding. If the bleeding is minor and the mother remains hemodynamically stable, a diagnostic ultrasound examination is performed. A blood sample is sent for complete blood cell count and type and cross-match. Fetal heart tones are recorded. When the fetus is immature and the patient has only minimal bleeding, tocolytics and bed rest may suffice. If the bleeding is unremitting or copious, immediate cesarean section is the treatment of choice.

Abruptio Placentae. Again, resuscitation and diagnosis must proceed simultaneously. Placental abruption may release large quantities of thromboplastin into the systemic circulation, placing the patient at risk for a coagulopathy. Therefore, coagulation studies are routinely ordered. Management consists of a vaginal examination and immediate amniotomy. An oxytocin infusion is started if labor does not ensue immediately. Cesarean delivery is performed if there is any evidence of fetal distress or delay in the establishment of effective labor.

Ovulatory Causes of Bleeding. Unless vaginal bleeding has led to hemodynamic instability, severe chronic blood loss, or anemia (hematocrit < 30%), then suspected malignancies, fibroid tumors, and endometriosis are expeditiously referred to a gynecologist for further management. Treatment of infections is initiated in the emergency department, and specific treatment guidelines are discussed in Chapter 39, Acute Pelvic Pain.

Dysfunctional Uterine Bleeding. Patients with anovulatory, or "dysfunctional," uterine bleeding are generally best served by reassurance and referral. Anovulatory bleeding in young women may be treated with birth control pills or other hormone formulations. Hormonal manipulation to arrest bleeding is considered only after consultation with a gynecologist.

UNCERTAIN DIAGNOSIS

In spite of the best efforts of the emergency physician to find the cause of vaginal bleeding, many patients have to be discharged without a specific diagnosis. In the nonpregnant patient, the cause of undiagnosed, abnormal vaginal bleeding is likely to be hormonal. However, the emergency physician cannot confidently make that diagnosis without, for example, cervical culture results. At the follow-up visit, a gynecologist or primary provider can review the case, as well as culture or ultrasound results, and secure the diagnosis of dysfunctional uterine bleeding.

In the pregnant patient, there are few situations in which a patient would be sent home without a clear diagnosis. In stable patients with a suspected ectopic pregnancy that cannot be seen on ultrasound, home management with close follow-up with serial quantitative β-hCG tests can be tried (see "Disposition and Follow-Up").

SPECIAL CONSIDERATIONS

Premenarchal Patients

Abnormal vaginal bleeding in premenarchal girls is an uncommon problem. Seventy percent of

cases are due to vulvovaginitis of either infectious or inflammatory etiology, usually from poor perineal hygiene or nonspecific irritants such as soaps, bubble baths, or clothes. "Sandbox vulvitis" is a well-known clinical entity in this category. Proven cases of sexually transmitted disease require appropriate medical therapy and an evaluation for child sexual abuse.

Traumatic "straddle" injuries and foreign bodies are not uncommon. An uncooperative child may require either examination or treatment while under sedation if this problem is suspected. Table 40–4 lists the common and uncommon causes of vaginal bleeding seen in prepubertal girls.

Postmenopausal Patients

Bleeding in the older, postmenopausal woman immediately raises the suspicion of malignancy.

TABLE 40–4. Causes of Vaginal Bleeding in Prepubertal Girls

Infectious, Inflammatory

Inflammatory processes
Poor hygiene
Chemical irritants (soaps, clothes, cosmetics)
Sexually transmitted diseases
Nonsexually transmitted disease (*Staphylococcus, Streptococcus,* gram-negative enteric organisms, molluscum contagiosum, condylomata acuminata)
Parasitic infections (amebiasis, *Enterobius vermicularis,* fungal)

Traumatic

Physical activity (bicycle riding)
Sexual abuse
Foreign bodies

Hormonal

Neonatal hormone withdrawal
Accidental hormonal ingestions—birth control pills, estrogen creams
Precocious puberty
Sex hormone–producing tumors

Urologic

Urinary tract infections (bacterial, viral, chlamydial)
Urethral prolapse
Hematuria
Neoplasm

Neoplasms

Gonadal stromal tumors (granulosa-theca cell)
Benign tumors (polyps, condylomata acuminata)
Sarcoma botryoides

Dermatologic

Lichen sclerosis et atrophicus
Lichen simplex chronicus
Atopic or irritant dermatitis

Carcinomas of the endometrium and cervix are common; those of the vagina and ovary are less so, but all can result in vaginal bleeding. Invasive colorectal carcinoma is also considered. Fortunately, however, 80% of cases of postmenopausal bleeding ultimately prove to have a nonmalignant cause. Most cases of bleeding originate in the endometrium and are related to estrogenic overstimulation and understimulation.

DISPOSITION AND FOLLOW-UP

The following are guidelines for the disposition and follow-up of patients with vaginal bleeding.

Admission

Patients requiring hospital admission have evidence of hemodynamic instability or unremitting hemorrhage. Also, patients in need of immediate surgery and most pregnant patients with the exception of threatened abortions are admitted. Patients with hemodynamic stability but with severe chronic blood loss anemia (hematocrit of < 30%) are considered for admission.

Discharge

There is a certain subset of patients with suspected early ectopic pregnancy but are otherwise stable and reliable who are candidates for outpatient management. These patients are hemodynamically stable, have minimal abdominal pain and pelvic tenderness, and are less than 6 weeks from their last normal menstrual period. These patients may be observed with serial *quantitative* β-hCG testing and ultrasonography. Women with ectopic and other abnormal pregnancies produce lower serum levels of hCG than those with normal pregnancies of similar gestational age. Serial serum hCG levels drawn 48 hours apart allow quantitation of this level as well as a determination of its rate of rise in the serum. Both quantitation and the rate of rise of hCG are abnormal in the setting of an ectopic pregnancy (see Fig. 40–1).

The patient with a threatened abortion may be safely discharged from the emergency depart-

ment to receive outpatient follow-up. She is asked to return if bleeding, pain, cramping, or the suspected passage of tissue occurs.

Nonpregnant patients without evidence of hemodynamic instability generally do not require hospital admission. Patients with pelvic and vaginal infections, foreign bodies, minor genital trauma, and atrophic vaginitis are usually treated in the emergency department. Patients with suspected neoplastic disease (benign or malignant) and endometriosis are referred to a gynecologist for further evaluation.

FINAL POINTS

- The emergency evaluation of the patient complaining of vaginal bleeding should be geared to detect the few instances in which the correct diagnosis is "not to be missed." These situations include a bleeding complication of pregnancy, sexual abuse in children, and malignant disease.
- Because bleeding in the setting of a pregnancy is a potentially life-threatening problem, a rapid qualitative pregnancy test is performed in *all* women of reproductive capability.
- Ectopic pregnancies are common, can be disastrous, and are often confused with other entities (e.g., threatened abortion).
- The resuscitation of the woman with vaginal bleeding is initially no different from the resuscitation of any hemorrhaging, hemodynamically unstable patient.
- Vaginal bleeding in the premenarchal patient is sexual abuse until proved otherwise.
- Postmenopausal bleeding is caused by malignancy until proved otherwise.
- Infection should not be forgotten as a common cause of vaginal bleeding.
- Dysfunctional uterine bleeding is a diagnosis of exclusion and cannot be made with certainty in the emergency department.
- Always encourage a return emergency department visit for a discharged patient in whom symptoms become worse before a follow-up appointment can be kept.

CASE *Study*

A 28-year-old woman was in her primary physician's office awaiting an examination for recent irregularity of her menstrual cycle. After calling her to an examining room, the nurse noted that the patient appeared pale and unsteady in her gait. The nurse obtained a pulse of 120 beats per minute and a blood pressure of 90/50 mm Hg in a sitting position. After a brief assessment by the physician, a decision was made to transfer the patient to the emergency department by rescue squad.

On arrival in the emergency department, the patient was assigned immediately to the resuscitation area. She was pale and complained of pain in the lower abdomen. There was blood staining on her pants. Her vital signs, taken by the nurse, were blood pressure, 80/40 mm Hg; pulse, 130 beats per minute; and respiratory rate, 24 breaths per minute. She was afebrile but was restless and complaining of thirst. The nurse ensured that the intravenous lines established by the rescue squad were patent and contained isotonic crystalloid. Both lines were increased to a maximum rate. Blood was drawn for an immediately spun hematocrit, type and crossmatch for 6 units of packed red cells, and a rapid serum assay for β-hCG. The physician was asked to see the patient immediately and to speak briefly with the rescue squad. Five hundred milliliters of fluid had been given in the field.

This patient's condition has become worse during transport despite the initial volume resuscitation. Active bleeding is present. The patient needs rapid and aggressive volume resuscitation. Because hypotension is present, blood transfusion is likely in addition to crystalloid. Patients who are actively bleeding and hypotensive on arrival to the emergency department usually have hematocrits that are below 30%. Thirty percent is a guideline cutoff point below which acutely hemorrhaging patients are considered for transfusion.

A brief history revealed that the patient usually had a regular menstrual cycle with routine flow. She was $G_0P_0Ab_0$. Her last regular menstrual period had been shorter than usual, followed now, 2 weeks later, by a heavy flow with accompanying abdominal pain. She had been treated 1 year before for an infection of her "tubes" and used foam for contraception but not consistently. She denied any recent medication use, including aspirin. After 2 L of lactated Ringer's solution had been infused, her pulse had decreased to 110 beats per minute and her blood pressure had increased to 100/60 mm Hg. Her skin was cool, but there was no abnormal bruising. She had mild lower abdominal tenderness on palpation. Her pelvic examination showed blood clots in the vaginal vault and active bleeding from the cervical os. She had right-sided tenderness and a sensation of "fullness" on bimanual examination. The uterus was normal, and movement did not significantly increase the pain.

The patient clearly was in hemodynamic jeopardy and remained so in spite of her improving vital signs. Based on the historical findings, the pain accompanying the bleeding, and the risk factors elicited by the history (prior infection, less than adequate birth control practices), she was likely to be pregnant. Ectopic pregnancy is the most common serious complication of pregnancy and the most likely diagnosis in this patient. The decision was made to continue rapid fluid administration, obtain additional diagnostic data, and consult with a gynecologist.

The pregnancy test result was unequivocally positive. The patient's hematocrit was 28%. After 2000 mL of lactated Ringer's solution had been infused, the patient remained pale with a pulse rate of 110 beats per minute and a blood pressure of 100/60 mm Hg. Packed red blood cell replacement was started. The emergency physician performed bedside abdominal ultrasonography. No gestational sac was visible, and free blood was present in the lower peritoneal and cul-de-sac region. The gynecologist arrived in the emergency department and, after evaluating the patient and other findings, made arrangements for immediate transfer to the operating area.

The use of ultrasound by emergency physicians is a new trend and not uniformly practiced in all emergency departments. Decisions made by this procedure need to be confirmed by the gynecologist. Another test to confirm the presence of blood from an ectopic pregnancy is the culdocentesis. When nonclotting blood is obtained, in the face of a positive pregnancy test, the diagnosis of ectopic pregnancy is virtually ensured.

The patient was admitted to the operating suite from the emergency department. On laparotomy, the gynecologist found 1000 mL of free blood in the peritoneal cavity. The bleeding site was identified as a right-sided tubal pregnancy and controlled. Further volume resuscitation restored the patient to a normal hemodynamic status. Unfortunately, the site and extent of the ectopic mass did not allow tubal salvage and a unilateral salpingectomy was performed. The patient recovered uneventfully.

Bibliography

TEXTS

Hammond CB, Riddick DH: Menstruation and disorders of menstrual function. In Scott JR, et al (eds): Danforth's Obstetrics and Gynecology, 8th ed. Philadelphia, Lippincott Williams & Wilkins, 1999.

Stovall TG, McCord ML: Early pregnancy loss and ectopic pregnancy. In Berek JS, et al (eds): Novak's Gynecology, 12th ed. Baltimore, William & Wilkins, 1996.

JOURNAL ARTICLES

Alexander JD, Schneider FD: Vaginal bleeding associated with pregnancy. Prim Care 2000; 27:137–151.

American College of Emergency Physicians Clinical Policies Committee: Clinical policy for the initial approach to patients presenting with a chief complaint of vaginal bleeding. Ann Emerg Med 1997; 29:435–458.

Barnhart K, Mennuti MT, Benjamin I, et al: Prompt diagnosis of ectopic pregnancy in an emergency department setting. Obstet Gynecol 1994; 84:1010–1015.

Baron F, Hill WC: Placenta previa, placenta abruptio. Clin Obstet Gynecol 1998; 41:527–532.

Buckley RG, King KJ, Disney JD, et al: Derivation of a clinical prediction model for the emergency department diagnosis of ectopic pregnancy. Acad Emerg Med 1998; 5:951–960.

Carson SA, Buster JE: Ectopic pregnancy. N Engl J Med 1993; 329:1174–1181.

Frates MC, Laing FC: Sonographic evaluation of ectopic pregnancy: An update. AJR Am J Roentgenol 1995; 165:251–259.

Luciano AA, Roy G, Solima E: Ectopic pregnancy from surgical emergency to medical management. Ann NY Acad Sci 2001; 943:235–254.

Munro MG: Dysfunctional uterine bleeding: advances in diagnosis and treatment. Curr Opin Obstet Gynecol 2001; 13:475–489.

Phelan MB, Valley VT, Mateer JR: Pelvic ultrasonography. Med Clin North Am 1997; 15:789–824.

Pisarska MD, Carson SA, Buster JE: Ectopic pregnancy. Lancet 1998; 351:1115–1120.

Zinn HL, Cohen HL, Zinn DL: Ultrasonographic diagnosis of ectopic pregnancy: Importance of transabdominal imaging. J Ultrasound Med 1997; 16:603–607.

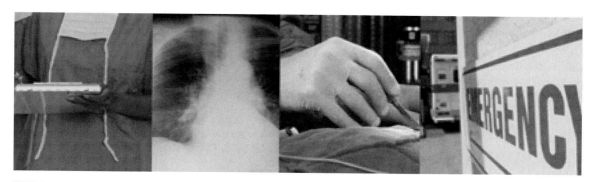

TRAUMA

CHAPTER 41

Multiple Blunt Trauma

JOHN M. WIGHTMAN

CASE *Study*

Emergency medical services (EMS) personnel notified the emergency department they were en route with a 19-year-old man who was the unrestrained driver of a car that struck a tree. His female passenger was dead at the scene.

INTRODUCTION

Trauma is the leading cause of death for people 1 to 44 years of age, and it is common in all age groups. Almost 200,000 people die each year and many more become permanently disabled as a result of a traumatic injury. These injuries commonly occur at ages when times lost from societal productivity are the greatest. The cost of traumatic injury in the United States has been estimated at almost $400 billion annually.

Trauma can be divided into blunt and penetrating types. There are also a number of special cases such as environmental injury, burns, blast overpressure, and others. Blunt injury often results in simultaneous damage to multiple organ systems. The management principles for multiple blunt trauma (MBT) can be used as the general approach to clinical problem-solving in all trauma patients. A discussion of penetrating trauma is presented in Chapter 42, Penetrating Trauma.

Injury Prevention

Another method of classifying trauma is intentional *versus* unintentional. Over 60% of deaths from trauma are considered unintentional (i.e., accidental) and are thus potentially preventable. Up to half of these deaths occur out of the hospital, most before arrival of medical assistance. It is estimated that up to a third of all deaths from injury can be prevented.

Haddon's 3 × 3 matrix provides a useful approach for injury prevention strategies. The matrix examines three general categories of factors that contribute to injury: (1) factors intrinsic to humans; (2) factors intrinsic to the injurious object; and (3) environmental factors that affect the interaction. These factors are then examined relative to (1) the pre-event phase; (2) the event itself; and (3) the post-event phase. This matrix may be applied to any cause of injury. The most common is a motor vehicular crash. Preventable pre-event human factors include driver experience, visual acuity, reaction time, and sobriety. Vehicle operating capabilities such as exterior visibility and tire traction are pre-event factors affecting the vector of injury. Vehicle safety features may mitigate the effects of the event itself. Highway design may affect injury rates in both pre- and intra-event phases.

Strategies to control injuries can be classified as passive or active measures. Passive measures require no thought or effort on the part of the persons being protected. Air bags are an example of a passive vehicle factor protecting individuals in the event phase. Seat belts require active placement by a human to confer protection. They are an active human factor affecting injury during the event. Health care workers can improve both passive and active prevention measures by lobbying for safer roads and vehicles and by providing patient and parent education.

Trauma Mechanisms

The term *mechanism of injury* is used to describe the traumatic forces applied to a given patient. These forces can be subdivided into the amount of force and its direction as applied to the victim. Specific mechanisms can lead clinicians to suspect higher likelihoods of certain injuries but do not preclude the need for a complete evaluation. Table 41–1 matches some of the more frequent causes of MBT seen in the United States to their most common injury patterns.

The pathophysiology of MBT is complex. Dividing trauma into primary and secondary effects is a useful approach for emergency physicians. Primary traumatic injury results from the direct and indirect effects of the damaging forces themselves. When an object strikes the body or the body impacts an object (direct primary

---

TABLE 41–1. Common Injuries Resulting from Blunt Mechanisms

Motor Vehicle Crash (unrestrained)

Frontal impact	Scalp lacerations, intracranial injuries
	Facial lacerations and fractures
	Sternal and costal fractures, pulmonary and cardiac contusions
	Traumatic aortic disruption
	Laceration of the spleen and liver
	Pelvic ring disruption, posterior hip dislocation
	Extremity fractures
Lateral impact	Intracranial injuries
	Costal fractures, pulmonary contusion
	Laceration of spleen or liver (depending on side impacted)
	Pelvic ring disruption
Ejection	Intracranial injuries
	Spinal injuries
	Thoracic and abdominal trauma
	Pelvic ring disruption, extremity fractures

Injuries Specific to Restraints (though overall injuries reduced)

Lap belt only	Small bowel rupture, mesenteric tears
	Transverse (Chance) fractures of lumbar spine
Shoulder belt under arm	Pulmonary and cardiac contusions
	Laceration of liver
Airbags	Eye injuries
	Upper-extremity fractures

Motorcycle Crashes

Thrown forward	Same as ejection above
Lateral impact	Abdominal trauma
	Pelvic ring disruption, lower extremity fractures

Pedestrians/Bicyclists Struck by Vehicles

Initial impact	Lower extremity fractures
Roll over vehicle	Intracranial injuries
	Spinal injuries
	Costal fractures, pulmonary contusion
	Laceration of spleen
Roll under vehicle	Abdominal trauma
	Pelvic ring disruption

Fall from Height

Landing on feet	Spinal injuries
	Pelvic ring disruption
	Foot and ankle fractures
	Other lower extremity fractures
Landing otherwise	Intracranial injuries
	Costal fractures, pulmonary and cardiac contusions
	Traumatic aortic disruption
	Abdominal trauma
	Pelvic ring disruption
	Extremity fractures

Thermal Exposure

Flame/heat	Burns with fluid loss
	Eschar restriction of ventilation or distal circulation
Smoke	Smoke inhalation
	Toxic inhalation (particularly carbon monoxide)

Blast Overpressure

Primary injury	Perforation of tympanic membranes
	Pulmonary contusion
	Ruptured bowel
Structural collapse	Crushing injury of any location

---

injury), two important vectors of energy transmission occur in biologic structures. The first type comprise *stress waves*, which are propagated deep into tissues in the direction of the applied external force and are proportional to the rate of acceleration of the body surface. Intraparenchymal hemorrhage is the typical result when the energy is sufficiently great. The second type are *shearing forces*, which are dependent on the total amount of body surface deformation. Shearing forces occur perpendicular to the impact, producing tearing motions tangential to the surfaces of underlying organs; hence, lacerations and ruptures are common results. Because of their relatively lower elasticity, solid organs such as the liver and spleen seem to be more susceptible to the effects of shear forces.

Tissue damage can occur when the whole body experiences rapid deceleration (indirect primary injury). Organs with relative mobility can continue to move when the body stops or is rapidly slowed. These organs can either tear their attachments or less-compliant components or impact the inside of their bony protection. The brain can disrupt its bridging veins to cause a subdural hematoma or impact the skull with resulting contusion or intraparenchymal hematoma. The aortic arch may move forward, tearing its least-compliant layer, the intima, allowing blood to dissect into the media or rupture through the adventitia. The heart may strike the sternum with subsequent contusion.

Secondary injury results from the effects of hypoxia, hypoperfusion, hypothermia, and dysfunction of other homeostatic functions on critical organ systems. A severe pulmonary contusion with hypoxia may lead to secondary encephalopathy without primary brain injury. Prolonged hypovolemic shock from external extremity hemorrhage may cause acute renal failure and intestinal ischemia without direct abdominal damage. A patient with preexisting coronary artery disease could sustain a myocardial infarction as the result of either hypoxia or hypoperfusion without thoracic trauma.

Trauma Centers

The American College of Surgeons Committee on Trauma has developed criteria for categorizing medical facilities as trauma centers. Level I trauma centers are usually regional tertiary medical centers with clinical and academic dedication to management of all types of traumatic conditions, immediate access to multiple subspecialties, and active research and education programs. They should be leaders in injury prevention and treatment for the communities and regions they serve. Level II trauma centers maintain a clinical commitment to trauma care but cannot meet the same requirements for subspecialty availability and academic pursuits. Nonetheless, they must have the capability for initial definitive care, although some patients may have to be transferred for additional services. Level III hospitals participate in regional trauma systems but serve communities where trauma centers are not in the immediate vicinity. They will generally have 24-hour-a-day emergency department availability with laboratory and radiologic support. Surgeons are capable of providing initial definitive care but are often not in the hospital. Level IV facilities are usually those in remote areas where they are the only medical care available. They could even be clinics without physicians as long as they have personnel trained in the initial management of trauma and predefined methods of rapid evacuation to higher levels of care. An additional category called an acute care facility recognizes that other hospitals may receive victims of trauma on occasion. They should be part of an organized trauma system but are not designated for receipt of patients by emergency medical services. Other facilities may offer specialty care for pediatric cases, burn victims, neurosurgical intervention, or rehabilitation. It is clear from the literature that trauma patients treated at trauma centers with coordinated, multidisciplinary teams who manage major trauma on a regular basis have better outcomes.

INITIAL APPROACH AND STABILIZATION

Knowing the mechanism of injury helps anticipate possible problems (see Table 41–1). If emergency department personnel are notified prior to the patient's arrival, the initial approach always includes consideration of potential injuries and preparation for receipt of the patient.

Priority Diagnoses

Priority diagnoses in MBT represent the most common life-threatening injuries to be addressed during the rapid assessment. They are listed in the middle column of Table 41–2.

Rapid Assessment

The *primary survey* is the first phase of trauma management. The letters *ABCDE* correspond to assessment and intervention for the *airway, breathing,* and *circulation,* as well as determining gross intracranial neurologic *disability* and fully *exposing* the patient to identify all emergent

TABLE 41–2. Identification and Management of Life-Threatening Problems after Multiple Blunt Trauma

Assessment	Problem	Intervention
Global assessment	Shock	100% oxygen
		Intravenous access
		Volume resuscitation
Airway status	Airway compromise	Definitive airway (tube w/ cuff)
		Endotracheal intubation
		Cricothyroidotomy
Ventilatory function	Tension pneumothorax	Needle thoracentesis
		Tube thoracostomy
	Massive hemothorax	?Needle thoracentesis (if unsure)
		Tube thoracostomy
		Autotransfusion
		Surgery
	Open pneumothorax	Temporary defect closure
		Tube thoracostomy
		Surgery
	Flail chest	100% oxygen
		? Positive-pressure ventilation
Cardiovascular hemodynamics	External hemorrhage	Direct pressure on wounds
	Shock	Volume resuscitation
		Prepare for blood administration
	Cardiac tamponade	Pericardiocentesis
		?Resuscitative thoracotomy
		Surgery
Neurologic parameters	Brain herniation	Airway management
		Intracranial pressure control maneuvers
		?Skull trephination
		Surgery
Patient exposure	External hemorrhage	Direct pressure on wounds
Cardiac monitor	Dysrhythmias	Medical management
Pulse oximetry	Hypoxia	Improve oxygenation
Serum glucose	Hypoglycemia	Dextrose administration
Gastric intubation	Gross hemorrhage	Surgery
Chest radiograph	Pneumothorax	Tube thoracostomy
	Hemothorax	Tube thoracostomy
		?Surgery
	Aortic disruption	?Computed tomography and/or aortography
		Surgery
	Pulmonary contusion	Improve oxygenation and ventilation
	Pneumomediastinum	Determine source
		Surgery
	Diaphragmatic rupture	Surgery
	Pneumoperitoneum	Surgery
	Thoracic spine disruption	Spinal immobilization
		?Fluids and/or vasopressors
Pelvic radiograph	Pelvic ring disruption	External fixation
		Arteriographic embolization
		?Surgery
Hematocrit	Anemia	Packed red blood cells
Electrocardiogram	Myocardial ischemia or infarction	Medical management
		Caution with vasodilators, aspirin,
		anticoagulants, and thrombolytics
Ultrasonography	Intrapericardial fluid	Pericardiocentesis (if compromised)
		Surgery
	Intraperitoneal fluid	Surgery (if compromised)
Diagnostic peritoneal tap and lavage	Gross hemoperitoneum	Surgery
	Minor hemoperitoneum	?Surgery
	Other criteria	Surgery
Cervical spine series	?Cervical spine instability	Spinal immobilization
		?Fluids and/or vasopressors

injuries. These are the priorities in the initial approach. As soon as a life-threatening problem is identified, immediate intervention is accomplished. Table 41–2 matches the most common life-threatening injuries identified in the different phases of management with their immediate interventions. Although presented in a sequential manner here, much of the evaluation and treatment during a coordinated trauma resuscitation occurs as a multitasking event.

Global Status. The initial patient evaluation in a dynamic situation starts with a global assessment of general status. Asking patients their name is a quick method of accomplishing this. Not only does it begin to establish a rapport with the conscious patient, it may provide useful physiologic information. If patients answer with an appropriate reply, they can be assumed to have sufficient cerebral oxygenation and perfusion to hear the question and formulate an answer. If their voice is reasonably normal, they must have a patent airway and adequate ventilatory exchange to phonate their answer. Patients who do not respond appropriately may have one or more problems that require early intervention.

Patients must be undressed or their clothing cut away while the physician conducts the initial assessment. A rapid search for obvious life-threatening injuries is conducted over all body surfaces. Pallor, skin mottling, diaphoresis, or cyanosis can be quickly noticed and may represent severe oxygenation or perfusion abnormalities.

Any verbal history required from the patient is obtained concurrently with the resuscitation. If the patient cannot provide information, an effort to question paramedics, police officers, bystanders, or family is made. A detailed physical examination will follow later; but once any identified problems are addressed, the patient should be covered, and dried as necessary, to prevent hypothermia.

Airway Status. Ensuring a patent and protected airway are top priorities in trauma management. Victims of MBT are at significant risks for both airway problems and trauma to the cervical spine. Cervical immobilization or actual spinal cord injury complicates airway management, and the possibility of an unstable cervical spine cannot be excluded at the time the airway is first evaluated. The clinician makes an immediate assessment of the need for performing an airway procedure versus the risk of damage to the spinal cord (see Chapter 2, Airway Management).

Breathing Status. Once airway adequacy (patency and protection) is assessed and any required intervention accomplished, ventilatory function is evaluated. The chest is observed for symmetric rise and fall with spontaneous respirations or artificial ventilations. Lack of expansion on one side may indicate a pneumothorax or hemothorax. Paradoxical motion (i.e., a portion of the chest wall moves inward with the negative pressure generated by the majority of the chest moving outward on spontaneous inspiration) indicates a flail chest with the high probability of significant underlying pulmonary contusion. An open pneumothorax may result in air entering the pleural space through a defect in the chest wall during negative-pressure inspiration (i.e., sucking chest wound). Chest wall defects are covered with an occlusive dressing.

Diminished or absent breath sounds on one or both sides indicate poor ventilation. If the patient is intubated, the tube may have been placed in the right mainstem bronchus instead of the trachea. Most commonly, asymmetric breath sounds indicate a pneumothorax or hemothorax. If the patient appears to be in shock with unilaterally decreased breath sounds, the emergency physician must assume that a tension pneumothorax or massive hemothorax exists. A needle thoracentesis is performed to emergently relieve excessive air pressure before placing a chest tube for more definitive management.

The highest possible concentration of oxygen is delivered to all patients in this phase of management to maximally saturate circulating hemoglobin. This is accomplished through a nonrebreather mask connected to oxygen at 10 L/min or a self-inflating resuscitation bag at 15 L/min.

Circulation Status. After auscultation of breath sounds, cardiac sounds may be evaluated. "Distant" tones may result from blood in the pericardial sac. Holosystolic murmurs or diastolic blows may indicate traumatic valvular incompetence. Patients are assessed for rate, rhythm, and strength of their carotid pulses. A weak pulse usually is caused by a diminished pulse pressure. Patients who are frankly hypotensive or bradycardic, unless these problems are caused by medications or drugs, have passed the point where their homeostatic mechanisms can compensate. This state must be rapidly reversed and adequate perfusion restored.

Blood loss usually follows a predictable continuum from minimal findings to irreversible shock and death. Table 41–3 shows the compensatory factors associated with this progression. Although divided into four main categories, evolving shock is most often a progression of findings and any assessment only represents a patient's state at a given time. In all cases, shock occurs when there is inadequate delivery of oxygen and other metabolic substrates to tissues (see Chapter 4, Shock).

TABLE 41–3. Continuum of Pathophysiologic Changes Associated with Hemorrhage

Phase of Hemorrhage	Phase 1: Sympathoexcitatory Phase				Phase 2: Sympathoinhibitory Phase	
Blood Loss						
Blood loss out of cardiovascular system (% of total blood volume)	0–10%	10–20%	20–30%	30–40%	40–50%	>50%
Volume of blood loss from a 25-lb (12.5-kg) child	0–100 mL	100–200 mL	200–300 mL	300–400 mL	400–500 mL	>500 mL
Volume of blood loss from a 160-lb (72-kg) adult	0–500 mL	500–1000 mL	1000–1500 mL	1500–2000 mL	2000–2500 mL	>2500 mL
Neurohumoral Processes	Venous capacitance allows passive constriction of vascular circuit	Compensation primarily through increased heart rate to maintain DO_2	Added compensation through increased vasoconstriction of arterioles	Sudden withdrawal of vasoconstriction initiated by unknown trigger in humans	Humoral mechanisms unable to overcome withdrawal of neural vasoconstriction	Lack of atrial pressure leads to arrest with pulseless electrical activity until heart dies
Central parasympathetic nerves	Baseline	Decreased when upright to increase HR	Decreased at all times to keep HR increased	Negligible activity to maximize HR	Unknown whether cardiopulmonary afferents increase parasympathetic activity at this point	Unknown level of activity in humans during traumatic cardiac arrest
Peripheral sympathetic nerves	Baseline	Vasoconstriction in skin, skeletal muscle, and gut	Vasoconstriction in kidney (in addition to previous vessels)	Moderate withdrawal of vasoconstriction in noncritical vessels	Major diffuse withdrawal of vasoconstriction	Intravascular volume loss exceeds system's limits
Renin activity and angiotensin II	Baseline	Baseline	Mild increase	Moderate increase	Major increase	Major increase
Adrenal medulla catecholamines	Baseline	Baseline	Mild preferential release of norepinephrine	Moderate release of both norepinephrine and epinephrine	Major preferential release of epinephrine	Major preferential release of epinephrine until exhausted
Clinical Manifestations	None	Orthostatic light-headedness	Apprehension and light-headedness	Anxiety to confusion	Confusion to coma	Coma to complete unresponsiveness
Vital signs (for adults)	Normal	HR incr but < 100; SBP normal supine; DBP increased; RR normal	HR 100–120; SBP nrml – slight incr; DBP further increase; RR 20–30	HR 120–140; SBP moderate decr; DBP major decrease; RR 30–40	HR > 140; SBP major decrease; DBP major decrease; RR > 40	HR < 80; SBP not measurable; DBP not measurable; RR 0 or agonal
Electrocardiographic changes	None	None	Tachycardia	Tachycardia	Tachycardia with ventricular ectopy	Pulseless electrical activity to bradycardia to asystole
Urine output	>0.50 mL/kg/hr	>0.50 mL/kg/hr	0.25–0.50 mL/kg/hr	0.10–0.25 mL/kg/hr	<0.10 mL/kg/hr	<0.10 mL/kg/hr, if any
Fluid Management						
Crystalloid fluid replacement	None required	Up to one 20-mL/kg bolus before reassess	Up to two 20-mL/kg boluses before blood	Up to three 20-mL/kg boluses but second two with blood	Normal saline in conjunction with blood	Normal saline in conjunction with blood
Red blood cell replacement	None required	Unlikely without preexisting anemia	Yes, if no response to first fluid bolus or only get transient response	Initiate blood therapy in all cases unless hemorrhage ruled out	Initiate blood therapy in all cases unless hemorrhage ruled out	Initiate blood therapy in all cases unless hemorrhage ruled out

HR, heart rate; SBP, systolic blood pressure; DBP, diastolic blood pressure; RR, respiratory rate; DO_2, Oxygen delivery.

The first priority for intervention in the bleeding patient is to stop active hemorrhage and loss of oxygen-carrying hemoglobin. If the bleeding is external, direct pressure is applied to the wound(s). If other injuries allow for elevation of the wound site, this is accomplished. Application of pressure to superficial proximal arteries or use of an arterial tourniquet is almost never necessary in the emergency department. Bleeding vessels should not be clamped unless they are going to be tied off later. The evaluation for internal hemorrhage is discussed later in this chapter.

In the absence of invasive hemodynamic monitoring, other therapeutic interventions for hemorrhage should be guided by responses of end-organ functions (e.g., mental status improvement, elimination of cardiac ectopy or dysrhythmias, adequate urine output). Not all therapy is beneficial; attempts to bring a mildly hypotensive patient's systolic blood pressure from 90 to 120 mm Hg may actually be detrimental by artificially circumventing natural defenses. Rapid reestablishment of normal oxygen delivery may also result in permanent reperfusion injury to cells. Current controversies involve the rate and amount of volume resuscitation.

Isotonic crystalloid fluids such as lactated Ringer's solution or normal saline are administered in repeated boluses of 20 mL/kg in an attempt to restore intravascular volume when MBT victims are hemodynamically compromised. Whenever possible, these fluids are warmed to 39°C to 40°C. Patients without ongoing hemorrhage often respond to one or two boluses with improved mental status, change of vital signs toward normal, and adequate urine output. Transient responses suggest continuing blood loss or other abnormality affecting hemodynamics. Lack of response, especially after 2 L of fluid, in the compromised patient is an ominous sign and should prompt more aggressive assessment and resuscitative effort.

Depending on the urgency, there are three choices by which packed red blood cells (RBCs) may be administered. Blood products must be warmed and diluted with normal saline, not lactated Ringer's solution.

- Type O blood can be running within 5 to 10 minutes in many trauma centers but has some risk of minor transfusion reactions. In general, O-positive packed RBCs are administered to males and O-negative packed RBCs are administered to premenopausal females, the latter because of the potential Rh factor risk to any current or future fetus.
- Type-specific packed RBCs may be released and administered within 20 to 30 minutes.
- Crossmatched packed RBCs may take up to 60 minutes but offer the lowest risk of a minor transfusion reaction. If the patient possesses antibodies to any blood antigens, crossmatching may take even longer.

Resuscitative thoracotomy is a highly invasive procedure used to emergently open the left anterolateral chest of moribund patients to relieve cardiac tamponade, stop major intrathoracic hemorrhage, cross-clamp the descending thoracic aorta to preserve blood flow to the heart and brain, and provide direct cardiac compressions. It has a limited role in the management of MBT, because of its success rate of less than 1%.

Neurologic Disability Status. Initially, only gross information related to function of the central nervous system is necessary. The patient's mental status and pupillary responses make up the initial assessment. Alterations of consciousness must first be assumed to be the result of direct or indirect brain injury (e.g., inadequate oxygen delivery), but they can also be secondary to many nontraumatic causes (e.g., hypoglycemia, alcohol or drug use, stroke). An often-used mnemonic is **AVPUP**: Is the patient **alert** and moves spontaneously, does the patient respond only to **verbal** or **painful** stimuli, or is the patient **unresponsive**? The **pupils** are then checked for symmetry and reactivity to light.

The Glasgow Coma Scale (GCS) (Table 41–4) is an accepted measure of brain function at any given moment, but it is more useful when monitoring a patient for changes in level of consciousness over time. The best patient responses to stimuli for eye opening, verbal ability, and motor function are assessed, scored, and summed for a total of 3 to 15. Although there are no absolute levels for any individual, patients with a score of 13 or less are considered impaired and those with a score of 8 or less are considered comatose. Decorticate and decerebrate posturing indicates severe disruption of brain function.

Slowly reactive pupils may result from central hypoperfusion or drug use. The most important causes of equal but nonreactive pupils are brain injuries. A unilaterally dilated pupil may be caused by stretching of the ipsilateral oculomotor nerve, if an intracranial hematoma causes herniation of the temporal lobe over the tentorium cerebelli. MBT victims who exhibit progressive neurologic deterioration, accompanied by a dilated pupil, are candidates for emergent neurosurgical intervention. If a neurosurgeon is not available within a short period, the emergency physician may elect to perform skull trephination (burr hole) through the temporal bone on the side of the dilated pupil. The likelihood of making contact with an offending hematoma is reasonably good and the procedure can be lifesaving.

TABLE 41–4. Glasgow Coma Scales for Adult and Pediatric Patients

	Adults / Children	Infants
Eye-Opening Response		
4	Spontaneous	Spontaneous
3	To verbal stimuli	To verbal stimuli
2	To painful stimuli	To painful stimuli
1	No eye opening	No eye opening
Verbal Response		
5	Answers questions appropriately	Coos and babbles
4	Confused replies	Irritable cries
3	Inappropriate words	Cries to pain
2	Nonspecific sounds	Moans to pain
1	No sounds	No sounds
Motor Response		
6	Follows commands	Appropriate for age
5	Localizes toward painful stimulus	Withdraws from touch
4	Only withdraws from pain	Only withdraws from pain
3	Flexion (decorticate) posturing	Flexion (decorticate) posturing
2	Extension (decerebrate) posturing	Extension (decerebrate) posturing
1	No movement with painful stimulus	No movement with painful stimulus

Revised Trauma Score (RTS). The GCS generally predicts the outcome of patients with isolated head injuries, but it does not take into account other physiologic derangements that may cause or contribute to mortality in MBT patients. The originally proposed Trauma Score for Adults and the Pediatric Trauma Score tended to underestimate the life-threatening nature of isolated system trauma, especially head injuries. More recently, the RTS (Table 41–5) has been developed as a tool to predict the likelihood of survival in both adults and children.

The approximate probabilities of survival based on the GCS and RTS are shown in Table 41–6. Although these scores are mostly used as quality tools to identify potentially preventable deaths and improve processes, they also demonstrate the importance of head injury in MBT patients. Furthermore, trauma patients with a GCS motor response less than 5 (inability to localize to a painful stimulus) or any one of the three RTS component scores less than 4 should be considered for management in a trauma center. These scores only help predict survival, not functional recovery or quality of life.

Early Intervention/Monitoring

All victims of MBT must be constantly monitored and frequently reassessed for any change in condition. The possibility of deterioration always exists until each potentially serious injury has been treated or excluded. The entire primary survey may need to be repeated when any life-threatening problems are identified later in a patient's course. A deterioration in mental status (disability) may be from poor perfusion (circulation) caused by a new tension pneumothorax (breathing). To aid the team in monitoring for changes, a variety of electronic and clinical tools have been developed.

Vital Signs. Pulse and respiratory rates, blood pressure, and temperature must all be accurately measured, and all abnormal vital signs obtained by EMS and emergency department personnel must be explained. However, even "normal" vital signs may be abnormal for certain patients.

Heart rate has a direct effect on cardiac output. It increases to meet oxygen delivery demands, if not inhibited by drugs or other factors. Patients with pacemakers or those taking β-adrenergic blocking medications may not be able to respond with tachycardia when needed. Many individuals, especially children, only manifest tachycardia before the sudden onset of life-threatening hypotension when preload can no longer be maintained.

Respiratory rate and depth are evaluated to estimate any distress resulting from inadequate oxygen delivery; aberrations in ventilatory mechanics, caused by thoracic or neurologic injuries; and the need to blow off CO_2 secondary

TABLE 41–5. Revised Trauma Score (RTS)

Respiratory Rate (RR; breaths per minute)	Systolic Blood Pressure (SBP; mm Hg)	Glasgow Coma Scale (GCS)	RTS Component Coded Value
10–29	90+	13–15	4
29+	76–89	9–12	3
6–9	50–75	6–8	2
1–5	1–49	4–5	1
0	0	3	0

Formula: $RTS = 0.2908 (RR_{code}) + 0.7362 (SBP_{code}) + 0.9368 (GCS_{code})$
Maximums: $7.8552 = 1.1632 + 2.9448 + 3.7472$
Percentage: $100.0\% = 14.8\% + 37.5\% + 47.7\%$

TABLE 41–6. Probabilities of Survival using Two Scoring Systems

Glasgow Coma Scale (GCS)	Percent Probability of Survival
15	99
14	97
13	88
12	83
11	83
10	83
9	79
8	77
7	77
6	75
5	50
4	50
3	16

Revised Trauma Score (RTS)	Percent Probability of Survival
max	99
7	96
6	92
5	81
4	61
3	36
2	18
1	7
0	2

to the metabolic acidosis, which can develop during shock or after certain poisonings.

Blood pressure is auscultated whenever possible, so values may be obtained for systolic and diastolic blood pressures. The difference between the two is the pulse pressure. The pulse pressure decreases as the diastolic pressure increases secondary to increasing systemic vascular resistance during hemorrhage. Serial measurements are accomplished with automatic sphygmomanometers, but pulse pressure is not commonly displayed. When Korotkoff sounds cannot be heard, the systolic pressure is palpated at a distal pulse site or a Doppler device is used.

Core body temperature is an important, but frequently overlooked, parameter. Hypothermia can occur with exposure in the emergency department and administration of cold resuscitation fluids. Fever can signal an established infection, if there is a delay between injury and patient presentation.

Cardiac Monitoring. Standard cardiac monitors, whether fixed or portable, usually provide a continuous tracing of cardiac electrical activity. In the setting of trauma, these allow early recognition of problems with cardiac rate or rhythm, as well as the appearance of ectopic complexes indicative of cardiac irritability. It is important to correlate electrical activity with the presence of palpable pulses.

Continuous Pulse Oximetry. Early identification of hypoxia by clinical findings is particularly problematic in the emergency department. Tachycardia and tachypnea have a host of other causes, and central cyanosis is a late finding. Pulse oximeters provide continuous averaging of hemoglobin oxygen saturation (SpO_2) readings over the previous several seconds. Any decrease in a trauma patient may represent a decrease in oxygen delivery heralding a slide toward irreversible shock. Pulse oximetry may be inaccurate during low-flow states or when saturation is less than 70%.

Glasgow Coma Scale. The GCS is a clinical tool used to follow alterations in mental status (see Table 41–4). Improvement or deterioration over time will affect management decisions more than a single value assessed on admission.

Urine Output. When measurable, urine output indicates the state of renal perfusion. Only changes over each 15 minutes are calculated and extrapolated to a volume per hour (see Table 41–3). Initial collections immediately after insertion of a catheter only measure how much urine is in the bladder. Large returns may give false impressions of adequate active urine formation.

Newer Modalities. Monitoring end-tidal CO_2 from an endotracheal tube may help determine the adequacy of perfusion. Additionally, utilization of transcutaneous measurements of thoracic bioimpedance and arterial and venous oximetry may help guide trauma resuscitations in the future by indirectly measuring all parameters necessary to calculate oxygen delivery and tissue oxygen extraction. These devices may be able to monitor moment-to-moment changes and alert the trauma team to subclinical deterioration in a patient's condition.

CLINICAL ASSESSMENT

Once the interventional resuscitation has been completed (i.e., all known life-threatening injuries have been identified and corrected), a directed history and physical examination is accomplished. This is considered the *secondary survey*.

History

As much information as possible is obtained early in the course of management in case the patient's condition deteriorates to the point where questions cannot be answered. A useful mnemonic to remember the most important questions is: *Take an AMPLE history.*

1. Do you have any *Allergies* to medications?
2. Are you taking any prescription or over-the-counter *Medications*?
3. Do you have any *Past or present* medical problems? Have you had any *Past* surgeries? Could you be *Pregnant*?
4. When was your *Last tetanus shot*? When did you *Last eat or drink*? When did you *Last use alcohol or drugs*? When did your *Last normal menstrual period* begin?
5. What were the *Events surrounding the injury,* especially the mechanism by which it occurred?
6. If time allows, a brief *review of systems* should include any history of loss of consciousness; amnesia regarding events before, during, or after the incident; the location and nature of any pain; the presence or absence of dyspnea, visual disturbances, or nausea; or neurovascular symptoms such as paresthesias, numbness, or weakness.

If EMS personnel transported the patient, they can provide an immediate verbal report to the emergency physician receiving the patient. They may be the only source of critical information early in the course of management. Police may be used to question bystanders at the scene or contact family members. On site photography can be especially helpful in vehicular crashes in estimating the mechanisms of injury. Images of the vehicle's interior and exterior, as well as damaged items in the area, usually enhance the emergency physician's awareness and concern. Nonetheless, trauma teams are often faced with the need to make rapid decisions with little historical data.

Physical Examination

Victims of MBT frequently have several injuries to be discovered only through a careful examination in a systematic manner. This is often called the *head-to-toe assessment* or "fingers and tubes in every orifice."

Head and Face. The scalp is examined for swelling, ecchymosis, and open wounds. Deformity of the skull may signify a depressed fracture. The facial and nasal bones are palpated for tenderness, movement, and crepitus. Extraocular muscle movements are checked in cooperative patients. The pupils are reexamined, and attempts to measure gross visual acuity and visualize the fundus are made. The ears are examined for damage to the pinna and any blood or cerebrospinal fluid behind the tympanic membrane. The interior of the nose is visually inspected. Dental trauma is noted. Malocclusion is assessed by alignment of the patient's bite. Fractures of the mandible or maxilla may lacerate the oral mucosa. The pharynx is examined for potential airway compromise from swelling, blood, emesis, or secretions.

Neck. If the patient is immobilized in a cervical collar, an assistant is necessary to stabilize the patient's head before examination of the neck. A hematoma or other swelling in the neck may compromise the airway. The trachea is palpated for midline position and crepitus indicative of a fracture. Jugular venous distention and carotid bruits are noted, if present. Careful palpation of the cervical spine involves assessment for tenderness, deformity, "step-off," and crepitus. Any suspected injury of the cervical spine is correlated with a rapid motor and sensory assessment of the upper extremities.

Chest. All thoracic evaluations performed in the primary survey are repeated during the secondary survey. The chest wall is inspected for ecchymosis and palpated for bony tenderness, deformity, and subcutaneous emphysema. Percussion may reveal asymmetric hyperresonance, indicating the possibility of pneumothorax, or dullness, caused by hemothorax. The lung fields are auscultated more thoroughly in the secondary survey. The heart is auscultated for murmurs and extracardiac sounds.

Abdomen and Flanks. Inspection should seek to identify distention and ecchymosis. Seat belts may leave characteristic marks and place patients at risk for certain injuries (see Table 41–1). Ecchymosis of the flank or umbilicus may indicate significant extraperitoneal hemorrhage. Auscultation may reveal a bruit, but the presence or absence of bowel sounds is not helpful in the acute phase after MBT. The abdomen is palpated to determine areas of tenderness and assess for peritoneal irritation. Unfortunately, abdominal tenderness alone is an unreliable indicator of injury severity, but unequivocal signs of peritonitis are indications for exploratory laparotomy.

Pelvis. Gentle pressure on the pelvis and iliac crests is usually done. Because pressing on the pelvic ring can increase hemorrhage in patients with unstable fractures and dislocations, clinical assessment is usually accompanied by an anteroposterior pelvis radiograph. The combination usually yields all information necessary in the emergency department for decision making.

Perineum and Rectum. Perineal ecchymosis and scrotal hematoma are noted if present. Blood at the urethral meatus may indicate lower urinary tract injury. Males should receive a testicular examination. Females may undergo visual inspection of the vagina and cervix. A digital rectal examination is performed on all patients, unless there is a perianal laceration that could become contaminated. A hematoma in the vicinity of the male prostate or displacement of the gland itself are indicators of urethral injury and preclude early insertion of a urinary catheter. Perianal sensation and sphincter tone are assessed to add to the neurologic examination.

Extremities. Inspection and palpation may reveal ecchymosis, swelling, deformity, abnormal position, crepitus, and open wounds. Skin tension from displaced fractures or dislocations is corrected as soon as possible. Paresthesias or tense muscle groups may indicate a compartment syndrome. Distal neural, vascular, and muscular functions are assessed in all injured extremities to the extent possible in individual patients.

Back. Patients are carefully "log-rolled," maintaining spinal alignment, to examine their backs. Tenderness, deformity, and crepitus of the spine are sought. Components of the chest and flank examinations are repeated for those areas not seen with patients supine.

Neurologic Examination. An assessment of the patient's GCS and pupils is repeated. Awake and cooperative patients are evaluated for sensory and motor levels, if spinal cord injury is suspected. Bilateral normality is the optimal outcome of this examination. Impaired patients can be assessed for lateralizing responses to painful stimuli or lack of response below a certain dermatomal level.

Special Tests

Bedside tests are directed toward identifying potentially life-threatening problems, which are often clinically occult. Although many tests may be accomplished at the bedside, particularly portable radiographs, only a few are necessary early in the course of a resuscitation.

Serum Glucose. Test-strip measurement of serum glucose is indicated in all patients with altered mental status. Although glucose is one of the most common laboratory abnormalities found when screening all trauma patients, it is rarely in the hypoglycemic range.

Hematocrit. A low hematocrit in the emergency department represents previous anemia, or significant hemorrhage with compensatory fluid shifts. It represents impaired oxygen delivery capability in the patient. Determination of hematocrit has limited value in the acute emergency department management of trauma patients not taken to the operating theater. It is reasonable to obtain a baseline value with bedside testing before induction of anesthesia.

Gastric Intubation. Placement of a tube in the upper gastrointestinal system allows the clinician to identify gross hemorrhage. However, the absence of blood does not exclude significant injury to the esophagus, stomach, or duodenum. Gastric intubation likely decreases the risk of aspiration and may lessen the effects of an ileus or obstruction. Ideally, it should be performed before chest radiography so that the esophageal lumen can be identified on a plain film.

CLINICAL REASONING

The clinical appraisal for trauma patients focuses on determining the presence or absence of injuries requiring treatment, as well as identifying any issues that may complicate management. The priorities for subsequent decisions are based on the answers to the following questions:

Does the Patient Require Emergent Procedural Intervention?

If this is the case, what type of procedure or surgery must be performed and where are the necessary personnel and equipment resources located? Life-threatening hemorrhage may occur from any combination of external, intrathoracic, intraperitoneal, extraperitoneal, or perifemoral bone bleeding. External hemorrhage can be at least temporarily corrected in the emergency department. Temporary or definitive surgical or radiologic intervention may be necessary for internal bleeding sites and other conditions in which, if the proposed procedure was delayed, death or disability may result. The following are the most common examples seen in emergency department patients:

- Inability to obtain a definitive airway, when necessary
- Persistent tension pneumothorax, despite appropriately placed chest tube(s)
- Exsanguinating arterial hemorrhage of the neck or extremity
- Diagnostically positive pericardiocentesis, regardless of therapeutic results
- Initial chest tube drainage of more than 20 mL/kg of blood
- Successful stabilization after resuscitative thoracotomy
- Persistent aspiration of blood from a gastric or duodenal tube
- Unequivocal evidence of traumatic aortic dissection
- Evidence of abdominal viscera in the chest, secondary to diaphragmatic rupture
- Unequivocal signs of peritonitis
- Gross blood from a diagnostic peritoneal tap in a hemodynamically compromised patient
- Pelvic ring disruption with mechanical instability or persistent transfusion requirements after mechanical stabilization
- Space-occupying lesion within the cranium

If the necessary resources are not available or cannot be coordinated in a timely manner at the receiving facility, immediate arrangements for patient transfer to a trauma center must be made. Having prearranged protocols for these transfers will greatly facilitate the process.

Does a Known Mechanism of Injury Indicate an Occult Injury for which the Patient Has Not Yet Been Evaluated?

In addition to the relationships outlined in Table 41–1, details of the traumatic event combined with physical examination help prioritize further assessment. Human vulnerabilities, contact location and vector, potential amount of energy transfer, and a myriad of other factors determine the likelihood of subsequent injuries, and hence the priority of their evaluation.

Which Diagnostic Modalities Should Be Used to Detect or Exclude Common Occult Injuries or Those Suggested by the Mechanism of Injury?

Are tests necessary to separate possible causes of observed abnormalities? Because blunt trauma may result in serious injuries to multiple body regions and physiologic systems, additional studies may need to be employed to thoroughly exclude all potential life threats. Diagnostic testing may also differentiate possible causes of certain problems (e.g., computed tomography [CT] of the head to rule out intracranial hemorrhage as a cause of altered mental status). Any deterioration noted on the requisite reevaluations should prompt a new interventional resuscitation and clinical assessment.

Are There Coexistent Medical Problems to Manage or Consider in the Assessment?

Chronic medical problems, medications, and toxicologic problems may complicate a patient's perception of pain, awareness of surroundings, or physiologic compensation for systemic insults such as shock. These must be considered during the evaluation and before consideration of any procedure requiring conscious sedation or general anesthesia. They also may address the corollary question, *What happened to cause this traumatic event?*

Does the Patient Require Antimicrobial Prophylaxis?

Antimicrobial prophylaxis can be divided into two types: postexposure immunization (e.g., tetanus shot) and bacterial growth prevention. All MBT victims with open wounds need to have their tetanus-immunization status documented or a booster immunization injected intramuscularly. Patients who have not completed their primary series should also receive tetanus immune globulin, 4 U/kg (up to 250 U), intramuscularly. Antibiotic prophylaxis, on the other hand, is not routinely required for MBT patients unless there is an external wound in communication with the cranial or peritoneal cavities; a fracture, its hematoma, or a joint capsule; or suspicion of gastrointestinal perforation.

Are There Minor Injuries to Treat when Time Allows?

All open wounds should be thoroughly explored under local, regional, or general anesthesia when time allows. Foreign bodies are removed when the entire extent of them can be visualized and it is deemed safe to do so. Meticulous inspection and palpation may reveal damage to underlying structures (e.g., tendons, joint capsules). Whenever possible, fractures should be splinted before patients are moved.

The emergency physician must constantly assess and reassess whether a specific diagnostic or therapeutic course of action will alter management decisions and potential outcome.

DIAGNOSTIC ADJUNCTS

Many trauma centers obtain a standard battery of tests on all victims of MBT at the time of arrival. Proponents of these protocols cite the advantages of the following:

- Efficiency by not forgetting to order needed tests during the potential chaos of a trauma resuscitation
- Receiving the results as early as possible, so they will be available when decisions must be made
- Not missing potentially occult injuries when comprehensive testing panels are ordered

Depending on the tests considered, the disadvantages of this approach include

- Potential risks of the test itself to the patient
- Risks of delaying treatment for diagnostic testing
- False results leading to erroneous decision making
- Exposure of emergency department personnel to ionizing radiation and body substances
- Costs of tests that may not contribute to the patient's care

Hundreds of thousands of dollars per facility are spent on "routine" testing in many level I trauma centers every year. This practice has been questioned because the usual battery of tests (arterial blood gas analysis, complete blood cell count, type and crossmatch, seven-chemistry profile, amylase, liver function tests, ethanol level, coagulation studies, urinalysis, and toxicologic screen) uncommonly produce results that aid in medical decision making or change management plans.

Laboratory Studies

Arterial Blood Gas (ABG) Analysis. ABG analysis may not be necessary in many trauma patients. If an accurate reading can be obtained, pulse oximetry may be used to assess for hypoxemia, because it is the SaO_2 not the P_aO_2 that is the important parameter in oxygen delivery. ABG analysis is obtained in all MBT victims with significant chest injuries. Respiratory acidosis from occult hypoventilation can result from ineffective breathing from neurogenic causes, deformity of the chest wall, decreased compliance of injured lungs, or even painful respirations. Blood pH levels may be useful in monitoring systemic perfusion. Venous blood can also be used for this measurement.

Complete Blood Cell Count. Hemoglobin concentration and hematocrit are poor guides to the quantity of acute blood loss. Sudden hemorrhage of whole blood will not change these proportional values until the red blood cells are diluted by fluid drawn from the interstitium, retained by the kidneys, or exogenously administered. Abnormal results, which would mandate administration of packed RBCs, are often returned after the clinical decision to transfuse has been made and blood products already given. The white blood cell and platelet counts are not generally the focus of concern, unless preexisting disease is involved.

Electrolytes and Glucose. Abnormalities of sodium and chloride are rare in patients with acute trauma. Low bicarbonate levels and an increased anion gap are relatively common during the acidosis that accompanies hypovolemic shock but are not required to make the diagnosis or begin treatment. Severe MBT can cause hypokalemia, but urgent potassium replacement is rarely necessary in the emergency department. Glucose level is seldom significantly elevated in patients who are not otherwise known to have diabetes mellitus.

Organ Function Tests. Renal function abnormalities may be more common in elderly patients but not at a level requiring dialysis. Although abnormal hepatic function tests may be associated with liver damage, it is unlikely that they will be elevated in MBT victims who will not have their intraperitoneal contents evaluated by other means. Elevated serum amylase does not correlate with the likelihood of pancreatic injury. These are often ordered as "baseline" levels to assess the impact of the injury and treatment over time.

Coagulation Studies. Prothrombin time, activated partial thromboplastin time, and platelet counts are indicated for patients who are found to have clinically abnormal bleeding, especially those receiving large quantities of packed RBCs. In contrast to whole blood, packed RBCs have small amounts of coagulation factors and platelets, thus further diluting the patient's circulating levels already being lost through bleeding or consumed in an effort to abate active hemorrhage. Platelet counts do not accurately reflect platelet function, which may be impaired by aspirin or nonsteroidal anti-inflammatory drugs and contribute to bleeding.

Urinalysis. Although currently routine, obtaining a urinalysis on all MBT trauma patients is controversial, because the clinical significance of microscopic hematuria is unclear. Although it may represent trauma anywhere along the urinary tract, it cannot be correlated to injuries requiring surgical repair or other interventions. Most useful information can be gained from urine dipstick testing in the emergency department. Gross hematuria should be investigated with CT (usually with contrast) in stable patients. Patients whose condition is unstable may require urgent laparotomy. Intravenous pyelography can be performed during surgery before retroperitoneal exploration. Myoglobinuria secondary to rhabdomyolysis may present as measured hemoglobinuria without associated red blood cells on microscopic analysis.

Toxicologic Screens. Routine screening for ethanol and other drugs should be discontinued. Blood ethanol level may be useful in patients with altered mental status, but its presence probably has less effect on hemodynamics and temperature regulation than is commonly assumed, and no specific reversal agent is available. Other drugs with potentially adverse pathophysiologic effects on trauma patients must be considered and may be recognized by their toxidromes (see Chapter 15, The Poisoned Patient). By the time most toxicologic screens are returned from the laboratory, the information will be of little clinical use. The counter argument is that identification of alcohol and drug abusers creates opportunities for rehabilitation, education, and subsequent injury prevention. Postsurvival interviews can probably be used just as effectively to identify those individuals at risk for recurrent trauma.

Pregnancy Testing. A screening urine or serum pregnancy test is ordered on every female patient of childbearing age, unless she is known to be pregnant or has a reliable history of prior hysterectomy. If positive, the mother's Rh status is also determined.

Radiologic Imaging

A "standard" radiographic series for all MBT victims has been recommended in the past. The usual portable views ordered (*cross-table lateral film of the cervical spine and anteroposterior films*

of the chest and pelvis) are designed to screen for occult injuries, which if missed may lead to catastrophic outcomes. Failure to discover an unstable cervical spine, aortic disruption, or pelvic ring disruption may lead to improper patient handling or delays in treatment resulting in permanent disability or death. Still, indiscriminate application of routine testing can lead to enormous costs with very little impact on patient outcomes.

Radiographs in the emergency department are divided into those used for screening purposes and those ordered for diagnostic confirmation. The three films just mentioned are examples of screening radiographs. When the likelihood of abnormality detection is high or the consequences of missing a problem are severe, screening tests are appropriate. Diagnostic radiographs are used to refine or better delineate diagnoses suspected by clinical examination or other diagnostic tests. For example, determination of fracture displacement or angulation can be suspected by swelling and deformity, but its exact geometry may directly impact management decisions.

Chest. A portable anteroposterior chest radiograph may reveal a number of initially occult problems after MBT. Life-threatening injuries such as simple pneumothorax or hemothorax, traumatic aortic disruption (TAD), pulmonary contusion, and rupture of the large airways, esophagus, or diaphragm may require chest radiography for early detection. Although other studies may be selected to confirm the diagnosis or decide on a procedural intervention, a portable anteroposterior chest film is obtained for virtually all MBT victims as soon after the primary survey as practical. A more selective approach may be applied to isolated chest injuries. If the patient can tolerate it, an upright film is beneficial. Small pneumothoraces may be missed without an upright or expiratory film. Findings for small hemothoraces may be extremely subtle.

Pelvis. Pelvic ring disruptions may be identified rapidly with a portable anteroposterior pelvis film. They may be defined as symphyseal diastasis greater than 20 mm or fracture or joint displacement greater than 5 mm. Pelvic ring disruptions can cause severe extraperitoneal hemorrhage owing to tearing of the sacral plexus of veins, disruption of named arteries, and bleeding from sheared bone edges. The presence of a pelvic ring disruption indicates that life-threatening hemorrhage not amenable to easy surgical control is possible. The clinician must be prepared for large fluid and blood requirements early in the resuscitation, so the film is obtained immediately after the chest radiograph. When discovered, pelvic ring disruptions further mandate a thorough evaluation of the pelvic contents to include vascular, intestinal, neurologic, musculoskeletal, gynecologic, and, in particular, genitourinary systems. Vascular and rectal trauma can be life threatening, whereas other injuries, especially to the male urethra, can lead to significant morbidity. On the other hand, recent data indicate that patients who are alert, respond appropriately, are not obviously impaired by alcohol, drugs, or head injury, and are not hemodynamically compromised or unstable may not need a pelvis film if they also have no pelvic tenderness or instability, gross hematuria, or clinical evidence of lumbar or femur fractures. Clinically occult pelvis fractures rarely cause significant hemorrhage or require emergent orthopedic stabilization.

Cervical Spine. Almost all MBT victims are brought to the emergency department by EMS personnel who have immobilized the patient's spine with a cervical collar and backboard. Past recommendations have been to obtain cervical spine radiographs on every patient with a mechanism of injury that could produce damage to bony or ligamentous structures. Proponents of this approach have been willing to accept that 98% of all studies will be negative so as not to miss any fractures. The consequences of missing an occult cervical spine fracture and subsequent high cord damage could be devastating. Cross-table lateral, anteroposterior, and open-mouth odontoid views are considered the minimum set of films.

Despite these concerns, it is now acceptable to "clinically clear" the cervical spine in the emergency department. Patients who are alert and oriented, not intoxicated by alcohol or other drugs, and not distracted by significant pain in another location should be able to relate cervical discomfort or tenderness and allow an accurate neurologic examination. Many of these patients do not require cervical spine radiography if they have no anterior or posterior midline neck pain or tenderness and no neurologic deficits. Pain or tenderness in the posterior paraspinal muscles is common after violent movement of the head but is not independently associated with the likelihood of detecting a fracture radiographically. Even with negative readings on the films, the emergency physician must consider the following:

- Radiolucent ligamentous injuries may result in an unstable spine without fracture.
- Cord damage may occur without bony fracture or ligamentous instability.

Therefore, when cervical cord injury cannot be excluded or is suspected by neurologic exam, the patient's spine must remain immobilized. Early CT or MRI of the vertebral column or spinal cord is becoming available as necessary diagnostic adjuncts. (See Ch. 48, Head and neck Trauma.)

Thoracic and Lumbar Spines. Any patient with a neurologic deficit or radiographic evidence of one spinal fracture or dislocation should receive a complete evaluation of the entire spinal column from the occiput to the sacrum. Falls from heights causing axial loads on the spine are common. Concomitant injuries such as calcaneal and ankle fractures should usually prompt thoracic and lumbar spine films. Patients wearing only lap-belt restraints when injured in a vehicle with a decelerating mechanism have a relatively higher incidence of thoracic and lumbar spine fractures, too. Unfortunately, few studies have reported the clinical manifestations of thoracic and lumbar fractures in MBT patients. There are no known criteria that may be used to avoid unnecessary radiographic evaluation.

Extremities. Fractures and dislocations occur in the extremities of MBT patients. Plain films including the joint above and below the injured bone are routine. Patients who require an emergent surgical procedure to save their lives and who may also have vascular compromise of an extremity owing to local injury may have a one-shot arteriogram performed in the emergency department or operating theater via proximal intra-arterial injection of contrast medium.

Skull. Plain skull radiographs offer few advantages over cranial CT in MBT victims, although there may be some specific indications in pediatric patients with isolated head trauma and normal results on neurologic examination. Any patient with MBT and a moderate risk of having an intracranial pathologic process requires CT evaluation and neurosurgical consultation.

Abdomen. Although some signs of abdominal trauma may be identified on a plain radiograph (e.g., pneumoperitoneum), most are nonspecific and do not impact emergency department or surgical management. A normal abdominal radiograph does not exclude intraperitoneal or extraperitoneal injury requiring procedural intervention. Nonetheless, if films of the chest, pelvis, or lumbar spine are obtained for other reasons, they should also be scrutinized for evidence of abdominal trauma. Ultrasound and CT of the abdomen are important for a thorough evaluation. They are discussed under "Diagnostic Procedures."

Intravenous Pyelography. Gross hematuria, advanced age, multiple rib fractures, and extrarenal trauma place patients at higher risk for upper urinary tract injuries requiring surgical repair. Lack of a nephrogram on a one-shot intravenous pyelogram in a hemodynamically compromised patient who cannot be taken to the radiology suite for CT could indicate a renal-pedicle disruption as one potential cause of hypovolemia. A pyelogram is also preferred over CT for ruling out ureteral injury, although extravasation, hematoma, or urinoma can be seen when CT is performed for other reasons.

Retrograde Urethrography. Tearing of the urethra usually occurs from either direct impact (e.g., straddle injury), shearing forces on the urogenital diaphragm by displaced fractures of the anterior pelvic ring, or indirectly from deceleration forces on a full bladder. Absence of the classic signs of urethral injury (blood at the meatus, perineal or scrotal ecchymosis, and abnormal prostate examination) cannot be relied on to exclude either partial or complete disruption. A urinary catheter should never be placed through or removed from a potentially damaged urethra by a nonurologist, because of the risk of converting common partial tears into complete discontinuities. Conversely, the presence of any one clinical sign or identification of pelvic ring disruption by plain radiography mandates dynamic retrograde urethrography in males. This involves active injection of 0.25 mL/kg (up to 25 mL) of contrast medium from the fossa navicularis of the penis retrograde into the bladder. A slightly oblique pelvis radiograph is taken near the end of the contrast medium administration. The column of contrast medium on the film is then examined for narrowing, extravasation, and inability to reach the bladder. If the injection is paused, sphincter closure may not allow visualization of a continuous line of contrast medium. A normal study allows for cautious insertion of a transurethral urinary catheter. Retrograde urethrography is not necessary in females unless a catheter meets resistance during an attempt to insert it or urine is not recovered after placement.

Retrograde Cystography. Once urine has been drained from the bladder, retrograde cystography may be performed by infusing contrast under gravity. The volume of contrast is calculated by (years old + 2) × 30 mL (up to 400 mL). It is important to adequately distend the bladder to avoid false-negative results. The catheter is then clamped, and an anteroposterior radiograph of the pelvis is obtained. A postdrainage anteroposterior film is also taken to detect small extravasations obscured by a bladder full of contrast medium. Large extravasations can complicate other contrast studies to be performed later, so retrograde cystography is delayed until CT or angiography has been accomplished or is deemed no longer necessary.

Computed Tomography. CT has revolutionized trauma care by enabling clinicians to image the location, character, and extent of internal injuries without exploratory surgery. For acute decision making in the emergency department, CT has its greatest applicability to the head, cervical spine, chest, abdomen, and pelvis.

CT of the head is the diagnostic modality of choice for patients with moderate or high risk for an acute intracranial pathologic process after head trauma. Any abnormal mental status, focal neurologic finding, or depressed skull fracture mandates CT, unless the patient must first be taken to the operating theater for emergent hemorrhage control. Some patients with a normal and stable examination, no history of loss of consciousness or post-traumatic seizure, no associated symptoms such as severe headache, visual changes, or vomiting, and no history of a bleeding disorder might be admitted for observation in lieu of CT in some centers. CT is obtained if any deterioration is noted.

One life-threatening thoracic problem only hinted at by plain radiographic findings is disruption of the thoracic aorta. Most of these patients die before reaching the hospital, but some have defects in the intima or media of their thoracic aorta before frank rupture and rapid exsanguination. Early discovery and proper treatment can save at least three of every four initial survivors. Although there are numerous findings that may suggest thoracic aorta disruption, most are only helpful if present. Widening of the mediastinum (8 cm measured at T4), a mediastinum-to-chest ratio greater than 1:3 (also at T4 level), and loss of aortic contour seem to be the best predictors. Stable patients with chest radiographic findings suggestive of thoracic aortic disruption may have thoracic CT as a screening test before invasive aortography in some centers. Absence of positive findings in technically good studies read by radiologists experienced in management of trauma can reliably exclude thoracic aortic disruption. Aortography is usually required in other circumstances. Some trauma surgeons will operate on patients based on a positive CT alone, but aortography is usually obtained to better plan the vascular repair.

CT studies of the abdomen and pelvis are performed together on the majority of MBT patients, except patients who may be pregnant. Evaluation of the pelvic contents are important components of a complete examination. During this process, the bony pelvis will also be imaged, which may yield useful information for orthopedic consultants if fractures are present. Retrograde CT cystography may be performed, but CT cannot reliable exclude urethral injury.

CT scans are usually read by radiologists in most trauma centers. Nonetheless, emergency physicians and surgeons should be able to identify gross, life-threatening problems on the studies they order when no radiologist is immediately available. Importantly, CT is notoriously insensitive for excluding injuries of the diaphragm and bowel. If the mechanism of injury suggests that these are a concern (see Table 41–1), additional studies may be required.

Electrocardiogram

A 12-lead ECG is ordered for patients who have an abnormal heart rhythm, for those who manifest persistent shock without another obvious cause, and when there is medical suspicion of a pre- or post-traumatic cardiac event (e.g., myocardial infarction). In the absence of hemodynamic compromise or rhythm disturbances, screening for myocardial contusion with serial 12-lead ECGs, cardiac enzymes, and echocardiography does not significantly affect management decisions.

Diagnostic Procedures

The modalities discussed in this section relate to determination and characterization of internal injuries, for which standard laboratory and radiologic examinations are inadequate or only suggestive. Most are performed, and all are interpreted, by physicians and surgeons.

Exploratory Surgery. The ultimate diagnostic procedure is exploratory surgery. Damaged organs may be visualized directly and repair undertaken if indicated. However, not every injured patient can or should receive an operation. Victims of MBT have two or more organ systems involved by definition. It has been shown that the risks of an exploratory laparotomy with no repairable injury carries a much higher morbidity and mortality in the presence of associated trauma such as closed-head injury, pneumothorax or hemothorax, mediastinal trauma, or fractures of the pelvis or long bones than it does in their absence. Therefore, unless mandated by clinical findings, early exploratory surgery is being replaced by more extensive radiologic assessment.

Transabdominal Ultrasonography. Although it is possible, most clinicians do not use ultrasonography in the emergency department to characterize the actual damage to solid organs for surgical decision making. This is mostly because of the length of time required to complete these additional studies in potentially unstable MBT patients and the technical difficulty in making sure that all injuries are identified to avoid false-

negative results. It may be accomplished by ultrasonographers and radiologists, but some important types of injuries can still be missed. Hollow viscus injuries, in particular, are not well detected by transabdominal ultrasonography, which has its greatest use in pregnant MBT patients.

Focused Abdominal Sonography for Trauma (FAST). One of the newer modalities employed in the emergency department is FAST performed by emergency physicians or trauma surgeons. The four ultrasonic views most commonly employed are listed here:

- Subxiphoid view of the pericardial space
- Right upper quadrant view of the hepatorenal space (Morison's pouch)
- Left posterolateral view of the perisplenic space
- Suprapubic view of the rectovesicular gutter (pouch of Douglas)

In less urgent circumstances, additional views of the chest (bilateral costophrenic angles for intrapleural fluid) and abdomen (bilateral pericolic gutters) may be added. After acute injury and in the likely absence of preexisting effusion or ascites, anechoic fluid can be assumed to be blood. In the abdomen, 70 to 100 mL of intraperitoneal fluid is required for detection by experienced ultrasonographers, but 150 to 200 mL can be found by most trained emergency physicians and surgeons. This test can be performed very rapidly, depending on the number of views obtained and the experience of the operator. In many centers, the identification of free intraperitoneal fluid in a hemodynamically compromised patient is a sufficient criterion for surgeons to perform exploratory laparotomy to identify and repair any life-threatening intra-abdominal injuries.

Diagnostic Peritoneal Tap and Lavage (DPTL). DPTL shares many of the advantages of FAST when searching for fluid representing hemoperitoneum. Regardless of which DPTL technique is employed (closed, semi-closed, semi-open, or open), it can be performed safely and rapidly in experienced hands. It has been a sensitive test to determine the presence or absence of intraperitoneal hemorrhage or hollow-organ rupture since it was introduced in 1965. Access to the peritoneal cavity is gained either through a needle or through incisions in the skin, linea alba, and peritoneum. Any free intraperitoneal fluid or other intraperitoneal contents near the anterior abdominal wall in a supine patient are then aspirated. Withdrawal of 10 mL of gross blood is considered a positive tap result, so the remainder of the procedure becomes unnecessary. If the tap is negative, a dialysis catheter is placed into the lowest part of the peritoneal cavity and the tap

TABLE 41–7. Diagnostic Peritoneal Lavage: Criteria for Positive Results in Multiple Blunt Trauma

Cell Counts

Red blood cells: $\geq 100,000$ RBCs/μL (1.0×10^{11} RBCs/L)
White blood cells: ≥ 500 WBCs/μL (5.0×10^{8} WBCs/L)

Enzymatic Assays

Amylase: ≥ 200 U/L (some authors use $\geq$ upper limit of normal for serum)
Alkaline phosphatase: ≥ 10 U/L (no longer used in most centers)

Abnormal Intraperitoneal Contents

Bacteria
Bile
Feces
Food
Urine

Abnormal Fluid Effluent Location

Gastric tube
Rectum
Thoracostomy tube
Urinary bladder catheter

repeated. If this second tap is also negative, a peritoneal lavage is performed by instilling 15 mL/kg (up to 1 L) of warmed normal saline through the catheter. Once the fluid has filled the intraperitoneal space, gravity drainage is used to collect the effluent.

Criteria for a positive lavage in MBT are listed in Table 41–7. DPTL is sensitive for detecting intraperitoneal injuries requiring surgical repair. Less than 25 mL of whole blood from a previously healthy person in 1 L of lavage fluid will cause the test to be positive. False-negative results are rare. Therefore, a negative DPTL in a hemodynamically compromised patient should provide evidence that ongoing, intraperitoneal hemorrhage is extremely unlikely, and additional bleeding sites or other cause(s) of cardiovascular abnormalities should be sought.

Recently, use of DPTL has been criticized for being overly sensitive or too nonspecific. It has been argued that positive DPTL results have led to laparotomies being performed for abdominal injuries that did not require surgical repair. Because DPTL cannot identify the type of injury causing the hemorrhage, it may not have a role in stable patients with blunt trauma who are likely to have isolated, mild-to-moderate spleen or liver damage. Victims of MBT with actual or potential instability, however, may have severe solid organ injury, as well as trauma to organs not normally at risk from localized, relatively low-energy mecha-

nisms. Therefore, DPTL still plays an important role in the evaluation of occult intracavitary hemorrhage in the hemodynamically compromised MBT patient.

Tests for Evaluation of Abdominopelvic Contents. Immediate laparotomy is generally reserved only for MBT victims who will likely die without emergent intervention. Patients are usually severely compromised hemodynamically and demonstrate minimal, if any, response to resuscitative measures. Data gathering, beyond enough history and physical examination to determine which operation(s) to attempt, is unwarranted in these cases.

Emergency physicians must remember that both FAST and DPTL address only one test question: *Does the patient require emergent surgical intervention?* The result is either *yes or no.* If this is not the question being asked or decision making will not be based on one of these dichotomous answers, these are not the tests to employ. Because it takes more blood for a positive FAST than DPTL, FAST can be applied first. If FAST is positive for free intraperitoneal fluid, invasive DPTL would be unnecessary. If FAST is negative, the more sensitive DPTL could then be performed. FAST cannot be used once normal saline is instilled into the peritoneal cavity during DPTL.

Abdominopelvic CT has been directly compared with both transabdominal ultrasonography

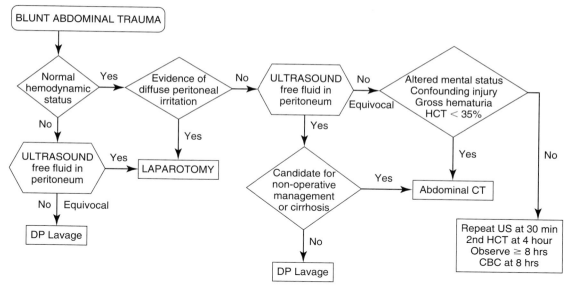

FIGURE 41–1 • Algorithm for diagnosis of intra-abdominal injuries used at the Denver Health Medical Center. CBC, complete blood count; CT, computed tomography; HCT, hematocrit; US, ultrasound. (From Branney SW, Moore EE, Cantrill SV, et al: Ultrasound-based key clinical pathway reduces the use of hospital resources for the evaluation of blunt abdominal trauma. J Trauma 1997; 42:1087; with permission.)

and DPTL for determination of the need for exploratory laparotomy. However, its role is actually more complementary, because it provides different information. CT can visualize free fluid at about the same volume as FAST. However, unlike the usual applications of FAST or DPTL to detect a hemoperitoneum, CT can characterize the nature and extent of damage to most intraperitoneal and extraperitoneal structures. Radiographic grading systems for various injury patterns often facilitate surgical decision making.

CT is noninvasive like transabdominal ultrasonography and FAST, but it cannot be accomplished in the emergency department. If examining for organ injury and not free intraperitoneal fluid only, it can be performed after DPTL. DPTL is still used in hemodynamically compromised patients when FAST does not demonstrate free intraperitoneal fluid. One algorithmic approach is shown in Figure 41–1. However, because the patient should not be moved to the radiology suite in an unstable condition, its applicability is limited to patients who are not hemodynamically compromised. In selected cases, the potential information gained from CT clearly outweighs the risk of possibly conducting a resuscitation outside the emergency department, and a well-equipped team transports the patient.

Angiography. Performed by an interventional radiologist, angiography seeks to identify the location and quantity of active hemorrhage in

trauma patients. Like exploratory surgery, angiography can be both diagnostic and therapeutic.

Arteriography of the thoracic aorta is the gold standard for identification of thoracic aortic disruption. Strong suspicion of thoracic aortic disruption based on clinical and plain radiographic findings mandates aortography. However, thoracic CT may be used to screen patients with only one or two radiographic abnormalities consistent with thoracic aortic disruption. Aortography is not required when the CT is negative in these questionable cases. Inconclusive CT results and most positive studies will still be followed by aortography for definitive diagnosis.

If the patient would not suffer undue morbidity without blood flow distal to any location of arterial hemorrhage, the radiologist may inject an autologous clot or other substance through the intraluminal catheter proximal to the site. If the bleeding stops with arteriographic embolization, surgical repair may not be necessary. Perhaps this technique's greatest role lies in managing the often severe extraperitoneal hemorrhage associated with pelvic ring disruptions. Surgically opening a pelvic hematoma, which may contain up to 3 L of blood, frequently results in immediate, uncontrollable hemorrhage and is associated with a high mortality. When employed appropriately, angiography can be added to the list of diagnostic modalities that can be used in a complementary manner in the treatment of MBT.

PRINCIPLES OF MANAGEMENT

General Principles

Optimal management of the MBT victim demands a team effort, but a single individual must be in charge who can coordinate simultaneous evaluation and therapeutic intervention in a synergistic manner. *As with any emergency department patient, the guiding principle is always to assume that the patient has one or more life-threatening problems.* Conducting a rapid assessment, directed toward potential problems consistent with the mechanism of injury, and intervening when necessary are the key skills that emergency physicians bring to their teams.

1. *Preparation,* based on any information obtained before patient arrival, involves anticipating likely scenarios and readying sufficient personnel and equipment necessary for those contingencies. The interventional resuscitation comprises the first steps in evaluation and management. Treatment is planned and accomplished in accordance with the findings.
2. *Maintaining adequate oxygenation, ventilation, and tissue perfusion* are the general goals of trauma management. Oxygen administration is always maximized in the emergency department, but correction of fluid and blood losses is not. Crystalloid fluids should be given in 20 mL/kg (up to 2 L) boluses. Packed RBCs may be given at 10 mL/kg (up to 1 to 2 U) at a time. Each of these should be followed by an assessment of their hemodynamic and end-organ effects. Absent or transient responses often signify ongoing hemorrhage. Titration is especially important in preventing secondary brain and lung injuries.
3. *The clinical assessment is based on knowledge of the mechanisms of injury;* history, physical examination, and adjunctive modalities prioritized by likelihood and life-threatening potential; and understanding of literature evidence regarding the utility of tests and outcomes of treatment options.
4. *Pain control* may be provided by repeating small doses of intravenous narcotics, once an evaluation and management plan for any abnormality in mental or hemodynamic status has been established. Aspirin and other non-steroidal anti-inflammatory agents are not given acutely to avoid any potential adverse affects on platelet function.

Specific Principles

The general principles of trauma management focus on maintaining oxygen delivery and preventing or reversing increased intracranial pressure (ICP). Other principles must also be considered when injuries to specific organs or body regions are discovered.

Head. No victim of MBT is assumed to be at low risk for significant brain damage. CT evaluation of moderate- and high-risk patients has already been discussed. Careful wound exploration may be the only method of identifying an open skull fracture, particularly near the vertex of the cranium where CT may miss those that are not displaced. Neurosurgical consultation is mandatory for all open fractures. It remains controversial whether prophylactic antibiotics are of additional benefit for basilar skull fractures, despite their potential open communication with the sinuses or middle ear.

Increased ICP can result from a hemorrhagic mass lesion (e.g., subdural or epidural hematoma), contusion, or diffuse swelling. The emergency physician's first duty is to prevent further ICP elevations. Patient movement and testing responses to painful stimuli are kept to a minimum. Pretreatment with lidocaine (1.5 mg/kg intravenously) and rapid sequence intubation should be accomplished during airway intervention (see Chapter 2, Airway Management). Delivery of oxygenated blood and sufficient metabolic substrates is critical. If increased ICP is suggested, efforts to decrease it are undertaken. All patients should receive high-flow oxygen. Intubated patients may be mildly hyperventilated to a P_aCO_2 no lower than 32 to 34 mm Hg (4.25 to 4.50 kPa). In the absence of significant hypovolemia, mannitol (0.25–0.50 g/kg intravenously) may be given as a bolus to stimulate an osmotic diuresis. Each of these methods is used to decrease the vascular volume within the head to reduce increased ICP. Corticosteroids do not appear to help decrease cerebral swelling after acute injury. Lipid antioxidants may be helpful in the future once clinical trials are completed (see Chapter 48, Head and Neck Trauma).

Eyes. Eye trauma can frequently present with dramatic appearances, but there are no immediately life-threatening ocular injuries. Emergency physicians must not allow these and other distractions to interrupt their initial interventional resuscitation or preoccupy their attention to more important tasks. The details of an eye evaluation are discussed in Chapter 25, The Red Painful Eye.

Face. Disfiguring facial trauma should not distract the clinician from focusing on more serious problems. The major goal of managing facial injuries in the MBT patient is protection of the airway from anatomic derangement, swelling, bleeding, and the inability to handle secretions. Head injuries are relatively common with significant facial fractures, although cervical spine injuries are not. In the emergency department, identification of facial injuries in the MBT victim mostly involves inspection, palpation, and determination of mobility of the facial bones, hard palate, and mandible.

Neck. For purposes of evaluation and management, the neck is divided into anterior and posterior components. Anterior injuries usually result from direct trauma to the anterior neck. Laryngeal and tracheal disruptions are infrequent but life-threatening sequelae requiring aggressive surgical airway control. Subcutaneous or retropharyngeal emphysema may indicate injuries to the larynx or trachea, the pharynx or esophagus, or other gas-containing structures in the thorax. Once the airway is secure, further evaluation of these structures is left to specialists.

Posterior (cervical spine) injuries are much more common, and indeed must be a consideration in every MBT patient. Because spinal cord damage at the cervical level can directly lead to death (e.g., C4 and above causing diaphragmatic paralysis) and permanent disability (e.g., quadriplegia), spinal immobilization must be maintained until an unstable injury can be excluded. A detailed neurologic examination is performed to document any deficits and subsequent changes over time. Specifically, the clinician must seek evidence for abnormal sensory or motor examinations below a certain spinal cord level, keeping in mind that not all injuries are complete transections. Additionally, complete transverse myelopathies can ascend from the original point of injury as cord edema increases. For these reasons, methylprednisolone is administered as a bolus (30 mg/kg intravenously) followed by a drip (5.4 mg/kg/hr) to help decrease swelling. Unstable injury of the spinal column or any transient or persistent neurologic deficit demands consultation with a neurosurgeon (see Chapter 48, Head and Neck Trauma).

Chest. Thoracic trauma has the potential to compromise the airway with blood or fluid in the lumina of the tracheobronchial tree, breathing via alterations in ventilatory mechanics and alveolar-capillary interfaces, and circulation through vascular or cardiac injury. Many of these will be identified and initially managed in the interventional resuscitation. Others will be discovered during physical examination or diagnostic tests. If a properly functioning large-bore chest tube cannot evacuate a pneumothorax, a bronchopleural communication should be suspected (see Chapter 44, Chest Trauma).

Abdomen. MBT victims can rapidly exsanguinate from clinically occult abdominal trauma. The primary focus of the evaluation of abdominal trauma is the determination of whether surgery may be indicated, because the initial operative procedure (i.e., laparotomy) is the same for all intraperitoneal injuries. Maintenance of oxygen delivery and hemodynamic stability are the principal *therapeutic* objectives in the emergency department (see Chapter 43, Abdominal Trauma).

Pelvis. Minimally displaced (≤5 mm) fractures of the pelvis rarely bleed sufficiently to cause hemodynamic compromise. Wider displacement or distraction associated with pelvic ring disruption signify tearing of the strong ligamentous structures that bind and traverse the pelvic ring. When the symphysis pubis of cadavers is experimentally divided but other ligaments are left intact, the pelvis will spring open but symphyseal diastasis will always be less than 25 mm. Further opening of the ring requires disruption of the sacrospinous, sacrotuberous, and anterior sacroiliac ligaments on at least one side. The ring may also be crushed closed by compression from the side. Vertical displacement of one hemipelvis may also occur. Stabilization of the pelvic ring disruption will often decrease pain, bleeding, and the likelihood of causing additional vascular or visceral damage during patient movement. External fixation may be applied by an orthopedic surgeon if the posterior sacroiliac ligaments are intact. If the ligaments are not intact, open reduction and internal fixation is often required. A relatively new device that resembles a large C-clamp can be used for "open book" injuries. If the patient requires transfer to another facility and no orthopedic surgeon is available, a pneumatic antishock garment may be used as a temporary stabilization adjunct, if other injuries allow inflation of all three of the garment's compartments. A full-length vacuum splint can also be used.

External Genitalia. Blunt testicular and penile trauma occurs from any one of several mechanisms, ranging from crushing damage to degloving injuries. Doppler ultrasonography may provide information regarding the testes. Any abnormality, even if nonspecific for rupture, should be evaluated by a urologist for possible scrotal exploration. Direct trauma to the penis or perineum may result in disruption of the anterior urethra. Retrograde urethrography may be used for evaluation of all but the most distal portion. Simple lacerations of the penis or scrotum may be closed in the emergency department. Any wound penetrating fascia must be managed by a urologist. A gynecologist should be consulted for significant wounds to the external genitalia of females.

Back. Injuries to the thoracic, lumbar, and sacral spines may cause similar neurologic deficits as they do in the neck. Examination and management are identical, remembering that the whole spine requires imaging if one fracture or dislocation is found. Methylprednisolone is used for cord injuries. Other back injuries are managed as thoracic, abdominal, or pelvic trauma.

Extremities. Splinting fractures and dislocations reduces bleeding, swelling, and pain. Realignment in the emergency department may be required if the skin is stretched taut or there is evidence of distal vascular compromise. "Hard" signs of arterial injury include continuous external bleeding, expanding or pulsatile hematoma, bruit or thrill, diminished distal pulses, or evidence of distal ischemia. "Soft" signs include a history of pulsatile bleeding or large blood loss before application of direct pressure, unexplained hemodynamic compromise, a large hematoma that is not expanding, or a neurologic deficit related to a nerve in proximity to an artery. Loss of two-point discrimination and paresthesias may also be early signs of rising pressure within the fascial investments of muscular compartments. Compartment pressure can be measured directly with any number of needle-and-manometer devices. Pressure that exceeds 15 mm Hg (2.0 kPa) is considered elevated. Intervention, in the form of an emergent fasciotomy, is entertained for any pressure greater than 30 mm Hg (4.0 kPa). Identification of compartment syndrome can be elusive in patients who cannot communicate pain or other abnormal sensations, but failure to make the diagnosis may result in neuromuscular ischemia and subsequent loss of the limb (See Ch. 47, Lower Extremity Injury).

UNCERTAIN DIAGNOSIS

The central guideline of trauma management is to reevaluate the patient frequently, because any assessment is only a snapshot in time. Dynamic situations call for anticipation of problems, rapid analysis of options, and timely intervention. The major life-threatening problems, which can be subtle at first and then progress rapidly to a moribund state, are increasing ICP and decreasing oxygen delivery. Causes for either may be direct or indirect.

Most of the uncertainty in the primary survey is in decision making, not diagnosis. Noisy resuscitation areas may make auscultation of the lungs or heart difficult, but most parameters in this phase are objectively observed or measured. Inexperience with trauma management or lack of confidence in skills may lead to inaction when lifesaving intervention is required. Indecision regarding the symmetry of breath sounds, for example, may lead to missing a tension pneumothorax, which can kill a patient in less than 5 minutes.

Some of the more common uncertainties leading to preventable mortality are listed here:

1. *Uncertainty regarding the order of interventions.* Altering a rehearsed, step-wise approach to address obvious or dramatic injuries, which may not be life threatening, is common in inexperienced clinicians. However, the converse is not altering a dogmatic approach to address an obvious life threat just to stay in the proscribed order (e.g., seeking a potential airway problem when severe external hemorrhage is readily apparent).

2. *Uncertainty regarding the etiology of altered mental status.* Ascribing altered mental status to ethanol intoxication based on a patient's appearance, social situation, or even actual detection of ethanol in the blood can lead to missing important physiologic derangements. Hypoglycemia, increased ICP, and decreased oxygen delivery are the threats to life that require management.

3. *Uncertainty regarding reported untoward effects of interventions.* Concern over the effects of high-dose oxygen therapy on lung tissue or on the ventilatory drive of some patients with chronic obstructive pulmonary disease may lead to failure to deliver maximal amounts and undertake interventions for relative hypoxemia. Subsequent brain swelling or poor tissue perfusion may result. Isotonic crystalloid fluid should not be curtailed when needed acutely, because of concern about its pH or chloride ions causing a metabolic acidosis.

4. *Uncertainty regarding the contribution of quality indicators to numerical vital signs.* Failure to appreciate hypoventilation leading to hypercarbia and acidemia can markedly increase brain edema. Diffusely weak or "thready" pulses indicate decreased pulse pressure, which may be an indication of hypovolemia before systolic blood pressure crashes (see Table 41–3).

5. *Uncertainty regarding assessment of shock in the absence of invasive monitoring.* Not providing sufficient volume resuscitation to maintain preload leads to inadequate cardiac stroke volume, hypoperfusion, and decreased oxygen delivery. However, overzealous crystalloid fluid administration dilutes the hemoglobin concentration, which also decreases oxygen delivery. It may also increase ICP. MBT patients should be resuscitated to adequate end-organ function and then serially reassessed to assure the clinical gains are maintained.

6. *Uncertainty regarding the reliability of history and physical examination.* Clinicians may be placed in the dilemma of not believing patients who are telling the truth and believing patients who are telling lies. The result is misinterpretation of essential information. If a patient says his abdomen hurts, but the examiner does not acknowledge the complaint because the abdomen is soft to palpation, subtle injuries causing morbidity and mortality may be missed. Patients not wanting to reveal information may conceal the true mechanism of injury, leading to failure to anticipate organ damage.

DIAGNOSTIC ADJUNCT UNCERTAINTY

Time constraints may be imposed by more serious problems or standard methods may have to be altered. Some studies, particularly radiographic evaluations, may also yield equivocal results. Because many patients cannot relate symptoms or respond to tenderness during physical examination, the importance of subtle radiographic findings can be difficult to interpret on occasion. These equivocal findings can contribute to uncertain diagnoses.

Incomplete or Equivocal Cervical Spine Evaluation. Obtaining complete plain radiographic views of the cervical spine in a supine patient secured to a backboard is often difficult. The patient's shoulders commonly obscure adequate visualization of lower portions of the spine on the lateral view. Overlapping lines and pseudo-subluxations may be overinterpreted. Facial bones, teeth, tubes, and slight head rotation can make reading the open-mouth odontoid view confusing. Repeated attempts may delay further care with a relatively low chance of better films. CT is a viable alternative in these patients once hemodynamic stability is achieved.

Equivocal Chest Radiography. CT of the thorax detects smaller pneumothoraces and hemothoraces, pulmonary contusions, and diaphragmatic rupture with herniation much better than plain chest radiographs. However, plain radiographs identify most of those that are immediately compromising, particularly if upright and expiratory exposures can be obtained. In the presence of a decreased P_aO_2/F_IO_2 ratio caused by pulmonary contusion, CT delineation of the extent of lung involvement may possess some predictive value, which may impact the decision to transfer a patient from a smaller facility to more specialized care.

- If mediastinal widening is close to the numerical criteria but thoracic aortic disruption is not sus-

pected clinically, additional chest radiographs may help, if the patient can tolerate being placed upright. A sitting anteroposterior film in the emergency department or a standing posteroanterior film in the radiology suite may correct positional and projectional aberrancies.

Equivocal FAST or DPTL. Some of the emergency medicine and surgical literature separate FAST and DPTL results into positive, equivocal, and negative. Emergency physicians should not use the equivocal category. For the FAST examination, free intraperitoneal fluid is either seen or not seen. If the operator is unsure, DPTL or CT should follow. DPTL lavage results of 50,000 to 100,000 RBCs/μL only affect surgical decision making, and then more for penetrating trauma. In the setting of MBT, this "equivocal" result still indicates that active intraperitoneal hemorrhage is unlikely, just as a negative result does.

Equivocal Pelvic Fracture Displacement. A single, anteroposterior radiograph may not demonstrate significant bony displacement, especially in injuries where one hemipelvis is driven toward the midline. Some of these are listed here:

- The pubic rami may fracture in the coronal plain en face to the x-ray beam.
- The sacrum may manifest only buckle fractures of the sacral arcuate lines.
- The ilium may have a crescentic fracture at an angle difficult to detect.
- Nondisplaced acetabular fractures are not pelvic ring disruptions but still warrant admission.

Mild diastasis of one sacroiliac joint may also be subtle in open-book injuries with borderline symphyseal diastasis. An inlet view is used to image the anterior ring in another plane. An outlet view may show sacral fractures and vertical displacement better. Oblique views are used to better image the iliac wing or detect acetabular fractures.

SPECIAL CONSIDERATIONS
Patients with Hypothermia

Humans conserve heat primarily by alterations in their behavior. They remove themselves from cold, wet, and windy environments; position themselves to minimize exposed body surfaces; increase protective clothing; and seek external warmth when possible. Not only are these compensatory mechanisms impossible for many MBT victims who may be unable (e.g., head injury) or unwilling (e.g., intoxication) to modify their circumstances, but EMS personnel and hospital workers often limit patients' capabilities by confining them to backboards, restraining extremities, cutting away all their clothes, and administering large volumes of room-temperature fluids. Injury in a cold environment or prolonged exposure before rescue may initiate loss of body heat, which may be exacerbated by hemorrhaging warm blood. Head injury may ablate the shivering reflex, and disruption of the sympathetic nervous system in spinal injury may cause vasodilation instead of heat-conserving vasoconstriction.

If normal core body temperature is 98.6°F (37.0°C), signs of mild hypothermia most commonly occur in the range of 90°F to 95°F (32°C to 35°C). These include slow decision making, mild confusion or amnesia, and difficulty with fine motor skills or ataxia. More severe hypothermia can cause frank alterations in mental status progressing to coma, impaired ventilatory capabilities, and atrial and ventricular dysrhythmias leading to fibrillation or asystole. Although mild hypothermia may actually have a beneficial effect by decreasing the oxygen demand of tissues, loss of body heat is not good for seriously injured MBT patients. Emergency physicians must prevent further cooling by removing wet or constricting clothing, drying and then covering patients, and keeping the resuscitation area as warm as possible. Patients must be shielded from drafts, and cold backboards and splints should be removed as soon as practical. Fluids should be warmed to 102°F to 104°F (39°C to 40°C). Blood products are also warmed adequately (see Chapter 18, Hypothermia).

Pediatric Patients

Management of critically injured children is a difficult and demanding task. Although priorities are generally the same as in adults, pediatric MBT victims require different methods for many aspects of their care.

1. During the interventional resuscitation, anatomic differences in airway anatomy require alteration of intubation techniques (see Chapter 2, Airway Management), ventilation parameters have to be adjusted, and total blood volume (approximately 80 mL/kg) is deceptively small. Loss of 500 mL of blood does not cause significant hemodynamic changes in the adult (see Table 41–3). Loss of the same amount from a 20-kg child would be almost a third of his or her blood volume and represents life-threatening hemorrhage. Unlike adults, infants can lose enough blood volume into their cranial vault to cause hypovolemic shock.

2. Pediatric patients represent a heterogeneous group by virtue of the changes that occur from birth to adolescence. Knowing what is an appropriate mental status and the normal ranges for vital signs are important considerations during management of MBT in this population. Use of the GCS must be modified for infants and children who do not understand verbal communication (see Table 41–4). Upper limits of heart rate are 160 beats per minute in the newborn, 140 beats per minute in the toddler, and 120 beats per minute in the preadolescent child. The lower limit of systolic blood pressure can be calculated as 70 + (age[in years] × 2) mm Hg. Moreover, many laboratory parameters have different reference ranges.

3. Use of length-based tapes or weight-based tables greatly speeds decisions regarding appropriately sized equipment and medication doses.

4. Vascular access can be problematic in infants and small children, especially if they are also significantly hypovolemic. The general rule of thumb is that if two attempts at peripheral access are unsuccessful, intraosseous infusion through the proximal tibia or distal femur of an uninjured lower extremity is indicated. If this is not possible or is deemed inadequate, a cutdown should be performed on a peripheral vein. High flow can be achieved with any of these methods if short, maximum-caliber devices are used.

5. Isotonic crystalloid fluids should be administered in repeated boluses of 20 mL/kg. The need for more than two boluses may signify active hemorrhage requiring blood replacement. Packed RBCs may be administered in repeated boluses of 10 mL/kg. The acute replacement of more than half of a child's blood volume (four boluses) is an indication for exploratory surgery in some institutions.

6. Abdominal trauma may be evaluated in a manner similar to adults with the caveat that solid-organ injury is often managed conservatively. If nonoperative treatment is considered, DPTL RBC counts should not be used to determine necessary laparotomy, although a positive tap and other abnormalities on lavage (see Table 41–7) are still indications for exploration.

7. It is also important to relate the reported mechanism of injury to what is likely for a given child's age. MBT may be the result of abuse.

Space precludes a detailed discussion of the variations in injury patterns specific to children of different ages, but the one general point that needs to be made is that pediatric bones are more pliable than adult bones. This affects decision making in two ways:

1. Serious organ injury can occur without obvious external signs or evidence of overlying bony fracture.
2. When fractures are identified, major forces must have been applied to them and underlying structures.

For example, significant pulmonary contusions may not have associated rib fractures, but the presence of rib fractures makes pulmonary contusion much more likely, even if it is not yet manifested radiographically. Interpreting plain films of the spine can be made difficult by children's relatively increased column flexibility and the frequent occurrence of pseudosubluxation. Spinal cord injury can also occur in the absence of fracture or dislocation.

Finally, it should be remembered that injured children have age-specific psychological needs, which must be provided to responsive patients in verbal and nonverbal ways. Even the care received in the emergency department can be as traumatic to an intellectually or emotionally immature child as the original injury was. Pediatric patients who cannot effectively communicate their needs are at additional risk. Emergency department personnel must make every effort to display a calm and reassuring demeanor, to constantly communicate with the child in an honest and caring manner, and to involve emotionally supportive parents or other caregivers as soon as practical.

Pregnant Patients

Early pregnancy does not directly affect the physiologic state of the mother to any significant degree, nor is the fetus able to survive on its own. As pregnancy progresses, however, increased total blood volume may mask serious hypovolemia, and fetal viability becomes an important consideration. Nonetheless, the way to save the fetus is to save the mother. Overall, the management of MBT differs little between patients who are pregnant and women of similar ages, except on a few points:

1. Mild hyperventilation, tachycardia, and hypotension are normal in the third trimester, but these may also be indicators of hypovolemia and impending shock. It is usually best to assume the worst and act early than to fall behind resuscitation requirements and develop an oxygen debt.
2. Up to 20% of a patient's blood volume may be lost acutely before there are noticeable changes in her vital signs, so correction of fluid and blood loss must be started early to prevent a precipitous change. Patients with fundal heights above their umbilicus are also at risk for uterine compression of their inferior vena cava. If a wedge is not placed under the patient's right hip and back or the backboard is not angled to the left, venous return to the heart may be diminished and cardiac output decreased up to 25%. Lactated Ringer's solution is the crystalloid fluid of choice for pregnant patients, except as a diluent for packed RBCs.
3. Acquisition of a directed history should include questions to determine the estimated gestational age of the fetus, complications with the present or any previous pregnancy, and the presence or absence of abdominal pain, contractions, fetal movement, and vaginal bleeding or discharge.
4. In addition to the standard examination of the abdomen of any MBT victim, pregnant patients should also receive fundal-height measurement; palpation for uterine tenderness, with firmness indicating distention from blood or a coincident contraction, and exposed fetal parts; and auscultation of the fetal heart rate. Doppler devices or transabdominal ultrasonography can be very useful adjuncts for determination of fetal heart rate, which should be 120 to 160 beats per minute. These portions of the physical examination should be repeated every 5 to 10 minutes. Vaginal examinations beyond Nitrazine testing for amniotic fluid at the introitus are generally not necessary before arrival of an obstetrician.
5. Rh-negative mothers should receive Rh_0 (D) immune globulin (300 μg intramuscularly) empirically.
6. Pregnancy should not deter clinicians from ordering necessary radiographic examinations. If the number of plain films are kept to a minimum and the abdomen is shielded, fetal exposure will be insignificant. If CT is used to evaluate intraperitoneal and retroperitoneal organs, most information can be gained by scanning only the upper abdomen. If transabdominal ultrasonography did not identify free intraperitoneal fluid, there will not likely be much additional information gained by scanning the lower abdomen and pelvis. Pelvic CT and angiography result in the greatest exposure of the fetus to ionizing radiation. If they are

truly needed for decision-making purposes, however, they should be performed. CT has the additional advantage of being able to image the intrauterine cavity, and angiography has the potential for therapeutic intervention.

7. If the reported mechanism of injury seems inconsistent with examination findings, the patient should be questioned about the possibility of domestic violence or other battery.

Pregnant victims of MBT, who are beyond 20 weeks' gestation, should be placed on a tococardiographic monitor as soon as possible and then for at least 4 hours more. Any abnormality demands 24 hours of additional monitoring. This protocol is much more sensitive than transabdominal ultrasonography for identifying placental abruption and fetal distress, evidence of which may indicate the need for emergency cesarean section. Although a relatively rare occurrence, uterine rupture requires an immediate laparotomy.

Elderly Patients

Preexisting medical conditions such as atherosclerosis, congestive heart failure, chronic obstructive pulmonary disease, and osteoporosis are some of the many factors that complicate the management of MBT in elderly patients.

1. Even mild brain atrophy may stretch bridging veins attached to the fixed dural sinuses. Movement of the brain during trauma may shear these small vessels, making a subdural hematoma three times more frequent in older than younger patients. This leads to a lower tolerance for ordering CT of the head.
2. Elderly patients may have reduced pulmonary reserve. ABG analysis is obtained on all elderly patients with chest injuries. Even those found to have only simple chest wall contusions or rib fractures may require admission for pain control and observation for the sequelae of hypoventilation such as atelectasis and pneumonia.
3. Preexisting anemia may have lowered the patient's baseline oxygen delivery. This can be rapidly worsened when the patient is losing blood and receiving crystalloid fluids.
4. Overaggressive fluid resuscitation can exacerbate poor cardiac function, lead to congestive heart failure with pulmonary edema, and make oxygenation difficult. On the other hand, elderly victims of MBT have poor tolerance for even brief periods of shock. The trauma team must carefully balance fluid and blood requirements by adequately but not overly resuscitat-

ing these patients. Invasive hemodynamic monitoring is always considered.
5. Elder abuse may present as MBT.

The elderly are also more likely to be malnourished and have subtle immunologic deficiencies. Reduced body fat in many individuals makes hypothermia even more of a concern, especially when early signs such as slow decision making, confusion, and poor motor coordination may be interpreted as the expected effects of aging.

DISPOSITION AND FOLLOW-UP

No patients are discharged if it is determined they have multiple injuries. Patients brought to the emergency department for evaluation of MBT but found to have relatively minor, isolated injuries may be discharged with next-day follow-up arranged.

Consultation

Although covered late in the chapter, the simple truth, "the earlier, the better" always operates in determining the timing of communication between the emergency physician and the surgeon. Trauma care is a time for aggressive cooperation using mutually accepted principles of assessment and intervention.

Admission

Admission to the hospital may occur from the emergency department to an operating theater, intensive care unit, "step-down" unit, or ward. In all cases, it is the emergency physician's responsibility to ensure each patient is appropriately evaluated and safely taken to the indicated level of care.

Transfer

Any patient requiring surgery or admission is transferred to an accepting trauma center if all needed resources are not available at the initial hospital. Preestablished transfer agreements and protocols greatly facilitate this process. The transferring physician must call the receiving trauma center to present the case and obtain permission for the transfer. As much of the evaluation and management as is appropriate should be accomplished before patient transportation. Anticipation of potential deterioration in the patient's condition en route is essential. The airway is secured if there is any possibility of compromise during transfer. Chest tubes are placed for even small pneumothoraces, especially if the patient is being transported by aeromedical services. Sufficient supplies such as procedural equipment, fluids, blood, and medications should accompany the patient. The transfer crew must have adequate interventional skills for all potential problems.

Death and Organ Donation

Patients who die of MBT in the emergency department often do so from one of two principal causes: severe head injury or prolonged irreversible shock. Patients with the latter usually arrest after severe metabolic derangements have occurred. Organ explantation is generally not undertaken in these circumstances, although postmortem recovery of corneal tissue and bone is possible. Those with brain death but relatively preserved homeostatic functions may be candidates for organ donation. Protocols vary with each facility, but all patients and their families deserve a respectful approach to the process. The emotional needs of survivors must be constantly kept in mind. The local coroner must be informed of all deaths and any desires for transplantation. The need for an investigative autopsy might preclude organ donation.

FINAL POINTS

- The emergency department management of MBT requires a multidisciplinary team approach directed by a single individual experienced and confident in his or her decision-making abilities for critical patients.
- Personal protective equipment is essential to reduce the exposure of health care workers to blood, other body substances, and ionizing radiation.
- Priorities are established early to assess the most likely life-threatening problems first.

- Intervention is accomplished as soon after identification as is possible with available personnel, equipment, and other resources.
- Repeated determination of vital signs, monitoring data, and physical examinations are conducted throughout the patient's course until care is explicitly transferred to a surgeon.
- Ancillary studies are ordered as needed for screening or diagnostic purposes, each with a specific purpose based on knowledge of the literature.
- Inattention to existing hypothermia or failure to prevent additional heat loss during the resuscitation and evaluation may result in unrecoverable physiologic derangements.
- Findings inconsistent with the reported mechanism of injury should raise suspicion for the possibility of a criminal act.
- Consultants are requested when the emergency physician requires assistance from others with specialized knowledge or skills; definitive care often demands specialty intervention; some or all of the consultants may not be at the same facility as the emergency department initially receiving the patient.
- If interhospital transfer is considered, the benefits should always outweigh any potential risks and these decisions should be discussed in a transfer note.
- Careful documentation of both positive and pertinent negative findings are critical for both medical and legal reasons.
- Not every MBT victim can be saved, but unnecessary deaths still occur. Some causes include the clinician's failure to implement proven emergency systems, take leadership for a team, anticipate individual problems before they occur, adequately resuscitate critically ill patients, and fully evaluate each person for potentially life-threatening injuries.

CASE *Study*

Emergency medical services (EMS) personnel notified the emergency department that they were en route with a 19-year-old man who was the unrestrained driver of a car that struck a tree. His female passenger was dead at the scene.

EMS personnel reported significant damage to the front of the vehicle. The windshield was shattered and the steering wheel was bent. It took 25 minutes to extricate the driver from the wreckage. The patient's vital signs were pulse rate, 120 beats per minute; blood

pressure, 110/80 mm Hg; and respiratory rate, 20 breaths per minute. According to bystanders, he was unconscious earlier but was reported responsive to verbal stimuli from EMS personnel. They immobilized the patient on a backboard with a rigid cervical collar, administered high-flow oxygen by non-rebreather mask, started an intravenous line of normal saline running wide open, and applied a splint to an open left tibial fracture.

Continued on following page

The patient did not respond to questions in the emergency department. He did open his eyes, moan, and withdraw from pain. His skin was cool and moist, but there was no obvious pallor or cyanosis. His teeth were clenched, so his airway could not be inspected directly, but he was moving air and there was no stridor or gurgling. Breath sounds were believed to be equal, although his chest excursions were somewhat shallow. It was decided that no emergent intervention was required for the patient's airway or ventilation for the next minute. Cardiac auscultation revealed normal sounds and no murmurs. Carotid pulses were fast and weak. There was no jugular venous distention. A full-thickness laceration of the left frontoparietal scalp required direct pressure to control bleeding. Lacerations of the left forearm and leg were only slowly oozing. No other sources of external hemorrhage could be immediately identified.

The patient was diagnosed to be in shock, although a significant head injury had not yet been excluded. Thus, the clinical decisions to endotracheally intubate the patient for future airway protection and to assist his ventilations were made. While preparations for rapid sequence intubation were being made, monitoring equipment was applied.

Vital signs in the emergency department were pulse rate, 132 beats per minute; blood pressure, 76/58 mm Hg; respiratory rate, 36 shallow breaths per minute. The cardiac monitor showed sinus tachycardia with occasional premature ventricular complexes (PVCs). The pulse oximeter did not detect a pulse from the patient's finger, but a probe placed on his earlobe registered an S_pO_2 of 88%. The patient received a GCS of 8 (eyes, 2; verbal, 2; motor, 4). His pupils were 5 mm in diameter and sluggishly reactive bilaterally.

An assistant provided in-line stabilization of the patient's cervical spine before the cervical collar was loosened in the front for cricoid pressure applied by another assistant. Based on the patient's estimated body weight of 80 kg; lidocaine, 120 mg, etomidate, 25 mg, and succinylcholine, 150 mg, were pushed intravenously in rapid succession. Suction was required to clear some mild secretions; then the patient was successfully orally intubated with an 8.0-mm endotracheal tube. Placement was confirmed by auscultation of bilateral and equal breath sounds. The cervical collar was replaced, and an orogastric tube was then inserted without difficulty.

Frequent reevaluation of seriously injured patients, especially after each intervention, is a critical component of any resuscitation.

The liter of normal saline given by EMS personnel was completed. An additional large-bore intravenous line was started, tubes of venous blood were obtained for laboratory tests, and 2 L of lactated Ringer's was started. After the 3 L of IV crystalloid fluid, the patient's vital signs were pulse rate, 120 beats per minute, and blood pressure, 102/66 mm Hg. The patient was being ventilated with a self-inflating resuscitation bag connected to high-flow oxygen at a rate of 16 ventilations per minute.S_pO_2 was 94%. The cardiac monitor still showed sinus tachycardia but no more PVCs. His pupils and GCS could not be reassessed, because he was pharmacologically paralyzed.

No immediate history could be obtained from the patient. There was no additional useful information from EMS or law enforcement personnel. The police began attempts to find family or friends of the two victims.

When little history is available and patients cannot relate their symptoms, clinicians must perform a detailed physical examination to identify all important injuries.

Documentation of the physical examination in the medical record was as follows:

The initial physical examination was conducted while the patient was sedated and paralyzed.

General A 19-year-old man in apparently good previous health who is slightly pale. His skin is cool and moist.

HEENT There is no gross deformity or Battle's sign. A 7-cm curvilinear laceration of the left frontoparietal scalp extends to the periosteum. No foreign body or skull fracture could be identified. Pupils are equal at 7 mm but not reactive to light at this time. There is no obvious ocular trauma. The left ear canal is filled with blood, most likely from the scalp wound, but the tympanic membrane could not be visualized. There is no evidence of cerebrospinal fluid leak. The right canal and tympanic membrane are normal. There is no deformity or crepitus of the nasal or facial bones. The nose is clear without septal hematoma. There are no obvious dental injuries, and the maxilla is stable. There is a small laceration at the tip of the tongue that does not require repair. The oropharynx is clear.

Neck The trachea is midline. There are no carotid bruits or jugular venous distention. There is no deformity or stepoff of the cervical spine.

Chest There is no deformity of the chest wall or flail segment, but subcutaneous emphysema is palpable in the left midaxillary line. There is also posterolateral bony crepitus of several ribs. No open wounds or ecchymoses are seen. There is good air entry in both lungs with bag ventilation. Crackles are heard in the left hemithorax. Heart sounds are not distant, and there are no murmurs or extracardiac sounds.

Abdomen There is a semicircular ecchymosis (convex caudad) between the umbilicus and symphysis pubis. Ecchymosis is also present above the posterior portion of the left iliac crest. There are rare bowel sounds. The abdomen is nondistended and soft without hepatosplenomegaly. There are no masses or bruits. There is no blood at the urethral meatus and no perineal or scrotal hematoma. The testes appear normal. Rectal examination reveals no masses or blood. Sphincter tone could not be assessed. The prostate is in normal position.

Pelvis and Lower Extremities Stability testing of the pelvis was deferred until after an anteroposterior radiograph could be obtained. A ladder splint is present on the left leg. There is a 5-cm laceration of the anterior leg with exposed bone. It is not grossly dirty. Despite some lateral angulation, distal pulses are 1 over 4, symmetric with the right, and similar to the upper extremities. The compartments are not tense. There is no obvious deformity of the left knee, thigh, or hip. The right lower extremity is normal with full passive range of motion at all joints.

Upper Extremities The upper extremities are normal, with the exception of a 3-cm laceration over the ulnar surface of the distal left forearm. This was explored to its base and was noted to extend into subcutaneous fat without exposure of underlying structures. No foreign body was present. Both distal pulses were 1 over 4 and symmetric.

Back The patient was log-rolled maintaining in-line cervical stabilization. No wounds are noted. The left flank ecchymosis extends over most of the region of the costovertebral angle. The spine is straight without obvious deformity or stepoff.

Neurologic A detailed neurologic examination could not be performed at this time. The patient had been noted to have symmetric pupillary reactivity and to withdraw from pain in all four extremities before paralyzation.

Vital signs taken after the examination revealed pulse rate, 128 beats per minutes; blood pressure, 88/60 mm Hg; respiratory rate, 16 ventilations per minute; and rectal temperature, 97.7°F (36.5°C).

Given the patient's transient responses to fluid resuscitation, 2 U of O-positive packed RBCs were administered with 2 L of NS. Priorities at this time included determination of whether surgical intervention was indicated for any sources of active hemorrhage or intracranial pathology. Several sets of vital signs after blood-component therapy demonstrated a period of hemodynamic stability: pulse rates, 104 to 112 beats per minute, and blood pressures around 110/70 mm Hg.

The patient received the "standard" diagnostic protocol for MBT victims in effect at the receiving trauma center.

Cross-table lateral, anteroposterior, and open-mouth odontoid radiographs of the cervical spine were normal. The supine chest radiograph demonstrated posterolateral fractures of the left sixth through tenth ribs, clear lung fields, and a normal heart size and shape. There was no hemothorax or pneumothorax. The mediastinal width was 7 cm. Its ratio to the thoracic diameter was 0.29. There were no other radiographic findings suggestive of thoracic aortic disruption, and the patient's blood pressures were equal in both arms. The tip of the endotracheal tube was 2 cm above the carina, and the orogastric tube was in the stomach. The pelvis radiograph was normal. There was a tripartite fracture of the left tibia and fibula with 12-mm posterior displacement of the central fragment and 30 degrees of lateral angulation of the distal extremity.

A 12-lead ECG showed sinus tachycardia without ectopy and no ST-segment or T-wave changes. ABG analysis during assisted ventilations at 16 breaths per minute and F_IO_2 of 1.00 revealed pH, 7.36; $Paco_2$, 32 mm Hg (4.3 kPa); P_aO_2, 62 mm Hg (8.3 kPa); S_aO_2, 92%; HCO_3^-, 17 mEq/L; and base deficit of 8 mEq/L (8 mmol/L). Pulmonary contusion, not yet manifested radiographically, was believed to be the most likely cause of the hypoxemia.

Because the chest and pelvis radiographs indicated no suggestion of significant hemorrhage, the patient's previous hemodynamic compromise was believed to be caused by a combination of

Continued on following page

blood loss from the three lacerations or intraperitoneal bleeding. Rapid decisions needed to be made to determine the most appropriate diagnostic tests. An abdominopelvic CT would have shown detail of any injuries, but the patient had potential for hemodynamic deterioration in the radiology suite, so it was decided to perform FAST to screen the peritoneal cavity for blood. Free intraperitoneal fluid was easily identified, so DPTL was not required.

The large battery of laboratory tests returned at this point had no impact on patient management, except for the type and crossmatch of blood. The patient's ethanol level was 229 mg/dL (50 mmol/L).

With the patient at least temporarily stabilized, it was believed that the potential benefits of a 2-minute head CT outweighed the risks of inability to intervene. Therefore, the patient was transported to the radiology suite with sufficient personnel, equipment, and supplies to manage any eventualities.

No intracranial hemorrhages, midline shift, effacement of the ventricles, bony fractures, or fluid in the air spaces were noted on the cranial CT.

After administration of a tetanus booster and cefamandole nafate for combined coverage of bowel flora and the open tibia fracture, the patient was taken to the operating theater for laparotomy. On abdominal exploration, a mixture of intraperitoneal blood and gastric contents were evident. Additional instillation of 3 U of blood was required. Lacerations of the liver and stomach were repaired. An external fixator was used to immobilize the patient's tibia.

The patient had a complicated hospital course with increased ICP and pulmonary fat embolism. Supportive medical care during 12 days in the ICU eventually resulted in complete recovery. Although he wished to return to college, he was tried and convicted of vehicular manslaughter in the death of his girlfriend and was sentenced to prison for 3 years.

Bibliography

TEXTS

American College of Surgeons Committee on Trauma: Advanced Trauma Life Support For Doctors. Chicago, American College of Surgeons, 1997.

Ferrera PC, Coluciello SA, Marx JA, et al: Trauma Management. St. Louis, Mosby, 2001.

Mattox KL, Feliciano DV, Moore EE (eds): Trauma, 4th ed. New York, McGraw-Hill, 2000.

Scaletta TA, Schaider JJ: Emergent Management of Trauma. New York, McGraw-Hill, 1996.

JOURNAL ARTICLES

Baron BJ, Scalea TM, Sclafani SJA, et al: Nonoperative management of blunt abdominal trauma: The role of sequential diagnostic peritoneal lavage, computed tomography, and angiography. Ann Emerg Med 1993; 22:1556–1562.

Boulanger BR, Brenneman FD, McLellan BA, et al: A prospective study of emergent abdominal sonography after blunt trauma. J Trauma 1995; 39:325–330.

Branney SW, Moore EE, Cantrill SV, et al: Ultrasound-based key clinical pathway reduces the use of hospital resources for the evaluation of blunt abdominal trauma. J Trauma 1997; 42:1086–1090.

Chu UB, Clevenger FW, Imami ER, et al: The impact of selective laboratory evaluation on utilization of laboratory resources and patient care in a level I trauma center. Am J Surg 1996; 172:558–563.

Esposito TJ: Trauma during pregnancy. Emerg Med Clin North Am 1994; 12:167–199.

Feliciano DV: Diagnostic modalities in abdominal trauma: Peritoneal lavage, ultrasonography, computed tomography scanning, and arteriography. Surg Clin North Am 1991; 71:241–256.

Hoffman JR, Schriger DL, Mower W, et al: Low-risk criteria for cervical spine radiography in alert victims of blunt trauma. Ann Emerg Med 1992; 21:1454–1460.

Koury HI, Peschiera JL, Welling RE: Selective use of pelvic roentgenograms in blunt trauma patients. J Trauma 1993; 34:236–237.

Lee CC, Marill KA, Carter WA, et al: A current concept of trauma-induced multiorgan failure. Ann Emerg Med 2001; 38:170–176.

Livingston DH, Lavery RF, Passannante MR, et al: Admission or observation is not necessary after a negative abdominal computed tomographic scan in patients with suspected blunt abdominal trauma: Results of a prospective, multi-institutional trial. J Trauma 1998; 44:273–280; discussion 280–282.

McCabe C, Warren R: Trauma: An annotated bibliography of the Literature—2001. Am J Emerg Med 2002; 20:352–366.

Namias N, McKenney MG, Martin LC: Utility of admission chemistry and coagulation profiles in trauma patients: A reappraisal of traditional practice. J Trauma 1996; 41:21–25.

Nordenholtz KE, Rubin MA, Gularte GG, Liang HK: Ultrasound in the evaluation and management of blunt abdominal trauma. Ann Emerg Med 1997; 29:357–366.

Pryor JP, Pryor RJ, Stafford PW: Initial phase of trauma management and fluid resuscitation. Trauma Rep 2002; 3(3):1–12.

Silka PA, Roth MM, Geiderman JM: Patterns of analgesic use in trauma patients in the ED. Am J Emerg Med 2002; 20:298–302.

Sternbach G: Trauma in older patients. Trauma Rep 2002; 3(1):1–11.

Thomason M, Messick J, Rutledge R, et al: Head CT scanning versus urgent exploration in the hypotensive blunt trauma patient. J Trauma 1993; 34:40–45.

Wightman JM, Manuel TS, Hamilton GC: Objectives to direct the training of emergency medicine residents on off-service rotations: Traumatology, parts 1, 2, & 3. J Emerg Med 1995; 13:99–104; 247–252; 407–414.

CHAPTER 42

Penetrating Trauma

KEVIN W. KULOW

JOHN M. WIGHTMAN

CASE *Study*

A radio call from emergency medical services (EMS) personnel advises the emergency department they are 5 minutes away and bringing a 17-year-old boy with multiple stab wounds to the chest and abdomen. There was a "moderate" amount of blood at the scene, but the patient is conscious. Vital signs are blood pressure, 100/60 mm Hg; heart rate, 100 beats per minute; and respiratory rate, 26 breaths per minute. The patient is on oxygen by mask, and an intravenous line was established with isotonic crystalloid running wide open.

INTRODUCTION

The management of penetrating trauma is an enormous problem in the United States. Each year during the 1990s there were nearly 100,000 injuries from firearms and many more cases of penetrating injuries by other means. The patient population is generally concentrated in urban areas, especially regarding cases involving violent crime. Penetrating trauma in age-matched cohorts from rural areas is distinctly uncommon.

The approach to the patient with penetrating trauma parallels that of multiple blunt trauma (MBT) (see Chapter 41, Multiple Blunt Trauma). The sequence of preparation, evaluation, intervention, diagnosis, and definitive care is identical. However, many of the specifics differ, particularly because the mechanism of injury usually allows the emergency physician to focus on a limited body region.

Mechanisms of Injury

Mechanism of injury refers to physical forces and other interactions between the human body and a damaging object. Elucidating the mechanism(s) by which injuries may have been produced is essential during the assessment of the patient with penetrating trauma. Knowledge of the physical properties of wounding instruments (e.g., knives,

bullets, bomb fragments) establishes appropriate indices of suspicion for certain types of injuries. Although the mechanisms of primary injury are markedly different than those of MBT, secondary effects occur in much the same manner. Therefore, categorizing penetrating trauma into primary and secondary effects has value.

Stab wounds and impalements are the simplest forms of penetrating trauma. Each represents an injury produced by an implement or object with relatively low energy. A *stab wound* occurs when only a wound site is visible. The term *impalement* is reserved for when the injuring object is retained in the body and extends out of the skin. Both mechanisms cause direct trauma to the tissues they penetrate. The wound usually tracks in a relatively straight line, but it can traverse multiple tissue planes, including bone.

The nature of the instrument may affect its injury profile. A dull implement may occasionally push structures aside rather than lacerate them. During the assessment it is assumed that any structure close to the wound tract has been injured. Depth of penetration is an important consideration, and physical examination assists in revealing this information. For example, the presence of a surface contusion caused by the hilt of a knife implies the entire length of blade penetrated the body and considerable force was applied. Knives may also be twisted or levered, resulting in additional trauma.

The wounding mechanisms of projectiles with higher energy represent more complex penetrating trauma. A bullet may take a circuitous path through tissue planes and make sharp turns if deflected by bone. Bones shattered by high-energy missiles may themselves break up and result in secondary injuries from fragments.

Terminal Ballistics

A basic understanding of terminal ballistics (i.e., projectile behavior inside the body) is necessary to predict possible structures at risk and avoid some of the problems inherent in managing gunshot wounds. The most important principle is recognizing the energy transfer from the bullet or other object to body tissues. Although most lower-mass, higher-velocity objects possess more kinetic energy than higher-mass, lower-velocity objects, this does not mean that they always have a higher wounding potential. It is not as simple as multiplying the mass of the projectile (m) by the square of its velocity (v) to obtain the familiar equation for kinetic energy (E_K):

$$E_K = \frac{1}{2} \cdot m \cdot v^2.$$

Given that a projectile will continuously decelerate after entering the body, the amount of energy it transmits to the tissues is due to its kinetic energy at any instant in time and the degree to which its progress through those tissues is retarded by various factors. Thus, the concept of transmitted energy (E'_{tr}) is defined as

$$E'_{tr} = -2 \cdot \Re \cdot E_{K'}$$

where $\Re$ is the retardation coefficient. This concept has direct applicability to wounding potential. The retardation coefficient is dependent on the density of the tissue, its drag coefficient, the area of the moving object that is in actual contact with the tissue, and the inverse of the mass of the projectile. These factors are more critical in predicting extent of injury than the velocity of the missile in air at the time of body contact.

Projectiles of all types produce injury by direct tissue destruction along the missile track in a manner analogous to stab wounds. The primary wound track is typically one and one-half to two times the actual diameter of the intact projectile. Lead "hollow-point" ammunition, used by law-enforcement personnel in an effort to decrease overpenetration and subsequent bystander casualties, may double its original caliber as the nose of the bullet peels back in a "mushroom" manner. This type of handgun round often stays within the body, because the increase in projectile retardation associated with the deformation may lead to complete transfer of energy before exiting the victim. In contrast, military "full metal jacket" ammunition possesses a hard, copper coating inhibiting it from deforming or fragmenting, thus making it possible for these rifle rounds to completely pass through one person with sufficient residual energy to penetrate another.

When a missile traveling through air strikes denser body structures, it creates an instantaneous *superpressure* on the liquid tissues at its point of entry. This produces a shock wave, which travels away from the tip of the bullet at the speed of sound. These high-frequency stress waves travel rapidly through tissues of homogenous density to potentially cause disruption at tissue interfaces and attachments. They may shatter bone remote from the actual wound track cut by the bullet. Within a closed space such as the skull, a hydraulic burst effect may fracture the cranium from the inside out.

Higher-velocity missiles further injure tissue by an additional mechanism termed *cavitation*. Release of a projectile's kinetic energy leads to shear waves that radiate perpendicularly away from the leading edge of the moving object. Shear waves possess a lower frequency than shock waves but are capable of significant displacements of tissue mass. This produces a *temporary cavity* within a few milliseconds, the greatest extent of which peaks after passage of the projectile through the body part. Although the velocity with which this cavity forms around the path of the bullet is about 10% of the speed of that bullet, it is often sufficient to cause extensive damage. The temporary cavity also pulsates, so it collapses in on itself with a pressure of up to 200 kPa (about 70 psi), causing additional injury. The damage from this cavitation is most apparent in less-compliant "solid" organs such as the liver and spleen, in contrast to more compliant tissues such as lung and bowel.

INITIAL APPROACH AND STABILIZATION

Whenever possible, personnel in the resuscitation area should be gowned, gloved, and wearing head, eye, and foot protection before the arrival of the patient. The importance of these measures cannot be overstated when the possibility of pulsatile arterial bleeding or invasive procedures is considered.

Rapid Assessment/Early Intervention

A rapid assessment is done to find and correct any life-threatening injuries. Problems with a patient's airway, difficulty with ventilation, and shock are usually identified and managed in the initial phase of the resuscitation. Gross deficits in neurologic function should also be assessed.

Global Assessment. This "first glance" serves as a rapid overview of a patient's condition. It commonly influences the urgency of the initial phases of management. An awake, talking patient with normal color, who appropriately does not appear anxious, allows time for a more extensive assessment. Changes in mental status and cool, clammy, or pale skin are indicators of shock, which are essential to note quickly.

Airway Status. A definitive airway may be defined as one that both protects from nasal, oropharyngeal, and esophageal foreign material (e.g., blood, vomit) and facilitates positive-pressure ventilation. Cuffed endotracheal or tracheostomy tubes placed inside the tracheal lumen fulfill these criteria. Victims of penetrating trauma may require a definitive airway for one of several indications, which can be categorized as therapeutic, prophylactic, or diagnostic.

Therapeutic airways may be established for problems such as laxity of the tongue due to coma; pharyngeal secretions, vomit, or blood; or positive-pressure ventilation for open pneumothoraces. Prophylactic protection usually occurs after neck wounds with the potential for significant anatomic distortion of airway anatomy or in conjunction with rapid sequence intubation to protect incompetent or combative patients from injuring themselves. Diagnostic airway protection is part of a procedure such as laryngotracheobronchoscopy.

Ventilatory Function. High-flow oxygen is administered to all trauma patients, either by mask or through a definitive airway. Oxygen toxicity is not an issue in the brief time frame of a trauma resuscitation.

Tension pneumothorax is an acutely life-threatening condition requiring immediate intervention to prevent death. Asymmetrically decreased breath sounds after penetrating trauma, with or without concurrent shock, are indicators for needle thoracentesis or tube thoracostomy. A 14-gauge or larger catheter-over-needle device should be immediately placed through the chest wall over the top of the third rib through the second intercostal space in the midclavicular line, even if tension pneumothorax is only suspected. Obtaining a confirmatory chest radiograph or waiting for a thoracostomy tray is inappropriate. Improvement in the patient's hemodynamic status will allow placement of a chest tube after other immediately life-threatening injuries are addressed. Lack of immediate improvement requires a tube thoracostomy to be performed sooner.

Once placed, the tube is connected to a water-sealed collection device with the capability for autotransfusion. An initial hemothorax output of 20 mL/kg is an indication for expeditiously moving the patient to an operating theater for a thoracotomy.

Cardiovascular Hemodynamics. Acute presentations of shock are assumed to represent life-threatening hypovolemia. Cardiac tamponade is also considered after penetrating chest trauma. If suspected, pericardiocentesis may be both diagnostic and therapeutic. Resuscitative thoracotomy may be lifesaving in some victims of penetrating torso trauma who have sustained cardiac arrest but still have signs of life.

Any external bleeding must be controlled by direct pressure. This aspect of the interventional resuscitation is often overlooked by inexperienced clinicians. It is the emergency physician's duty to restore cardiovascular homeostasis to whatever degree possible, and to facilitate the patient's survival until operative intervention, as necessary. Isotonic crystalloid fluids and blood are administered appropriately to restore tissue perfusion, as evidenced by improvement in mental status and vital signs (see Chapter 4, Shock).

Neurologic Parameters. The rapid neurologic assessment is performed in much the same manner as in the MBT setting (see Chapter 41, Multiple Blunt Trauma). The Glasgow Coma Scale is a useful clinical tool to follow neurologic functions over time (see Table 41–4).

Patient Exposure. It is necessary to completely undress and expose the patient with penetrating trauma. This allows careful scrutiny for entrance and exit wounds. Most patients are not aware of all their wounds, even if they are awake and alert. Similarly, many wounds may be concealed in places such as areas covered by dark hair; in the axillae, gluteal cleft, and perineum; and in areas of skin apposition, such as folds of fat or beneath breast tissue. Once all surfaces of the body have been evaluated, the patient should be covered to prevent the potential complications of hypothermia.

Monitoring

All critical patients and those with potential for deterioration require constant monitoring. Several parameters require monitoring for clinical improvement, maintained stability, or deterioration after each intervention or after predetermined intervals of time.

Vital Signs. Vital signs are continuously monitored during the initial resuscitation. An overhead monitor that displays visual and audible information, which can be seen and heard by all personnel involved, is preferred. Alarm features protect the patient and should not be disabled.

Cardiac Monitoring. In the setting of penetrating trauma, a cardiac monitor is useful to identify dysrhythmias caused by myocardial hypoperfusion. Electrical activity on the screen does not guarantee adequate mechanical contractions are occurring or that the patient has sufficient volume to generate a pulse.

Continuous Pulse Oximetry. Pulse oximeters are standard tools in most emergency departments across the country. Their primary function is to display the oxygen saturation of hemoglobin. They measure the differential absorptions of certain wavelengths of light by oxygenated and deoxygenated hemoglobin, but the results must be clinically correlated to the patient. Patients with poor peripheral perfusion may not have sufficient flow for the device to adequately function.

Central Venous Pressure (CVP). Monitoring CVP to identify changes after resuscitative interventions is more useful than obtaining a single, initial value in the emergency department. Emergency physicians rarely require a low CVP to assist them in determining a patient's hypovolemic condition after penetrating trauma. Persistently elevated CVP readings may be a useful early sign of impending cardiac tamponade.

Urine Output. Urinary output is measured for prolonged resuscitations or during transportation. It is interpreted in the same manner as for victims of MBT. Adequate renal perfusion is suggested by a urine output of 0.5 mL/kg/hr.

Newer Modalities. Additional monitoring devices include bedside electroencephalographic machines and end-tidal CO_2 monitors. A bedside electroencephalogram may be used as an early determinator of brain death after transcranial gunshot wounds in patients who may be candidates for organ donation. Measurement of end-tidal CO_2 reliably detects esophageal intubation and may be useful when tissue perfusion changes during shock and subsequent resuscitation.

CLINICAL ASSESSMENT

The clinical assessment of victims of penetrating trauma is necessarily brief and targeted. Prediction of likely injuries is usually easier than for MBT. Discovery of potentially confounding factors such as chronic medical problems, concurrent medications, or prior surgeries may affect decision making, but identifying all wounds and possible trajectories has a greater impact on evaluation and treatment in most instances.

History

Time constraints commonly prohibit a detailed history, but complaints of pain or shortness of breath should be elicited. Additionally, take an AMPLE history by asking the following questions:

1. Do you have any *Allergies* to medications?
2. Are you taking any prescription or over-the-counter *Medications*?
3. Do you have any *Past* or *present* medical problems? Have you had any *Past* surgeries? Could you be *Pregnant*?
4. When was your *Last tetanus shot*? When did you *Last eat or drink*? When did you *Last use*

alcohol or *drugs*? When did your *Last normal menstrual period* begin?
5. What were the *Events surrounding the injury,* and how much *time* has *Elapsed* since wounding? Details of the injury and wounding weapon should be obtained from the patient as well as available bystanders, EMS, and police. EMS personnel are frequently the only people who can provide the most complete picture of the mechanism of injury.
6. If time allows, a brief *review of systems* should include a preoperative assessment and neurovascular symptoms such as paresthesias, numbness, or weakness.
7. *Additional trauma* may occur before or after the penetrating trauma.

Physical Examination

The physical examination is a complete head-to-toe assessment focused on three areas important for further management. The first is a more detailed evaluation of respiratory, cardiovascular, and neurologic parameters. This is essentially an expansion of items first assessed in the primary survey, with the addition of abdominal and rectal examinations. The second involves a careful search for all entrance and exit wounds. The third documents the neurovascular status distal to any wounds. Table 42–1 highlights the essential components of the physical examination in the patient with penetrating trauma.

Local Wound Exploration

Local wound exploration (LWE) may be an adjunct to the physical examination. LWE can be performed in most regions under most circumstances.

- LWE is not performed deeper than soft tissue fascia in the neck (platysma muscle), owing to the risk to underlying structures and to creating a communication from outside to inside.
- LWE over the rib cage and in the supraclavicular areas involves searches for underlying injury, not to determine if the thoracic cavity has been penetrated.
- LWE of anterior abdominal stab wounds has use in separating superficial lacerations from those with potential to have penetrated the peritoneal cavity.
- LWE is an essential component of the evaluation of extremity wounds, if more serious injuries do not take precedence.

TABLE 42–1. Important Aspects of Physical Examination of Penetrating Trauma

General

Complete exposure is mandatory.
Perform stepwise head-to-toe examination, including perineum and axilla.
Find all entrance and exit wounds.

Head and Neck

Confirm or exclude penetration of the platysma.
Exact location of wound is important; treatment is based on zone of injury.
Early neurologic examination if spinal cord injury is suspected.

Chest

Wounds or missile tracks medial to the nipples or scapular tips require mediastinal assessment.
Beware of unilateral absent breath sounds or muffled heart sounds.
Consider diaphragmatic injury.

Abdomen

Local wound exploration is indicated in questionable stab wounds.
Any penetration of the fascia mandates surgery.
Abdominal gunshot wound mandates surgery.
Consider diaphragmatic and extraperitoneal injury.

Extremities

Bilateral extremity blood pressures may expose occult vascular injury.
Even without direct injury, vessels can be injured by cavitation from nearby missile tracks.

Forensic Considerations

Preserve clothing in paper bags, and gather all potential evidence (e.g., shell casings) carefully.
Do not cut through bullet holes in clothing during patient exposure.
Maintain chain of custody with all evidence. Keep evidence in your possession until given directly to a police officer.

Bedside Tests

Because active hemorrhage is the most common cause of early mortality after penetrating trauma to all regions except the head, bedside testing should be considered adjuncts to the interventional resuscitation to determine the location of any bleeding. Additional tests include:

Serum Glucose. Test-strip measurement of serum glucose is indicated in all patients with altered mental status. Although glucose is one of the most common laboratory abnormalities found when screening all trauma patients, it is rarely so low as to necessitate exogenous dextrose administration.

Gastric Intubation. Nasogastric or orogastric intubation is accomplished as soon as possible to sample upper gastrointestinal contents for blood indicative of esophageal, gastric, or duodenal perforation, as indicated by the penetrating injury. Lack of gross blood from the tube or on a digital rectal examination does not exclude hemorrhage in these areas. Gastric intubation with continuous suction may also decrease the risk of aspiration of gastric contents in patients without a definitive airway in their trachea.

CLINICAL REASONING

There are several questions to address before, during, and after the initial assessment and data-gathering phase of the encounter.

Does the Patient Require Emergent Procedural Intervention?

If this is the case, what type of procedure or surgery must be performed, where are the necessary personnel and equipment resources located, and when will they be available?

Excluding penetrating injuries to the brain, which are often not amenable to surgical intervention, the most common cause of early death after gunshot and stab wounds is exsanguination. External hemorrhage must be controlled in the emergency department. Exploratory surgery is often safer than observation for internal hemorrhage, because patients commonly do not have associated injuries as in MBT. On the other hand, tube thoracostomy may be emergently required for some chest injuries, but it is frequently the only intervention required.

Indication for thoracotomy in the emergency department varies with the source. One study lists the following situations caused by penetrating trauma in which emergency department thoracotomy is recommended for moribund patients:

- In patients with penetrating cardiac injuries, emergency department thoracotomy is indicated for those who present with signs of life.
- In patients with penetrating thoracic (noncardiac) injuries, the procedure should be performed despite the low survival rate.
- In patients with penetrating, exsanguinating, abdominal vascular injuries, emergency department thoracotomy should be used judiciously in conjunction with definitive surgical repair.

Are Life-Threatening Problems Present That Are Not Initially Obvious?

If this is true, which diagnostic modalities should be employed to detect or exclude them?

Many immediately life-threatening injuries can be identified during the interventional resuscitation. However, penetrating trauma to the torso may result in serious internal bleeding into the thoracic, intraperitoneal, or extraperitoneal cavities. A neck wound without immediate evidence of swelling may suddenly manifest as an expanding hematoma, a small leak in the myocardium may slowly develop into cardiac tamponade, or a benign abdominal examination may change to that of peritonitis. Thigh wounds can also result in significant internal hemorrhage. Frequent reassessment is a critical component of any evaluation of penetrating trauma.

What Is the Potential of a Residual Foreign Body?

A careful search for retained foreign body from a penetrating injury is essential. Impaled objects may break off, and bullets or pellets may embolize to other areas of the body. Any entrance wound should be matched to an exit wound or retained object. Secondary "foreign bodies" such as bone fragments are actively sought.

Are There Coexistent Medical Problems That Must Be Managed?

Chronic medical problems, medications, and toxicologic considerations may complicate a patient's perception of pain, awareness of surroundings, or physiologic compensation for systemic insults such as shock. These must be considered during the evaluation and before consideration of operative intervention.

Does the Patient Require Antimicrobial Prophylaxis?

Preoperative antibiotics are usually recommended before exploratory laparotomy for unknown injuries. They are definitely indicated when hollow viscera are known to be penetrated (e.g., gross blood discovered after gastric intubation or rectal examination) or diagnostic peritoneal tap and lavage (DPTL) reveals food or fecal material. Open fractures of the skull, pelvis, and extremities also warrant antibiotic prophylaxis. Chest wounds not obviously involving the esophagus or abdominal viscera do not necessarily require early prophylactic antibiotics. Passive immunization against tetanus may be necessary and should not be overlooked.

Are There Minor Injuries That Should Be Treated Before Disposition?

Simple lacerations are not generally repaired in the emergency department, unless the patient is being considered for discharge to home. Gunshot wounds crush tissue at their edges, so they are not closed primarily. Grossly contaminated wounds are also left open in most circumstances. Fractures may need to be splinted before patients are moved.

DIAGNOSTIC ADJUNCTS

Many therapeutic decisions can be made on information gained from the initial resuscitation and clinical assessment. Young, healthy individuals may be taken for emergent exploration without a single laboratory test or radiographic study being performed.

Laboratory Studies

Just as in many cases of MBT, "routine" trauma panels have a low benefit-to-cost ratio. Early determination of the hemoglobin and hematocrit will not affect many emergency department decisions. Whether a patient receives transfusions of packed red blood cells (RBCs) is based on clinical parameters. However, having a baseline before fluid resuscitation may be helpful to surgeons and anesthesiologists before any planned operative intervention. Hematuria indicates the possibility of injury to the kidney, ureter, bladder, or urethra only if present but is not helpful if blood is not found on urinalysis. It could be argued that the only laboratory test indicated in many cases of penetrating trauma would be a pregnancy test on females of childbearing age who are not obviously gravid by clinical examination. However, the result only impacts some decisions regarding medications and elective radiographs, not decisions regarding lifesaving interventions.

Radiologic Imaging

Radiographs are most commonly used to screen for intrathoracic complications of penetrating trauma, confirm suspected fractures, localize projectiles, and determine the attitudes and depth of impaled objects. Regardless of the body region being studied, the last two are evaluated by simple biplanar radiography, where anteroposterior and lateral views are taken to provide a three-dimensional estimation of trajectory and determine structures at risk for injury. The use of radiopaque markers under tape to indicate the position of external wounds is very helpful in this regard.

Plain Films

Chest. The anteroposterior chest radiograph, when used as an adjunct to interventional resuscitation, is often taken with the patient in a supine position. An upright film may be helpful in better delineating mediastinal width, identifying a hemothorax if it layers in the costophrenic angles, and detecting free air under the diaphragm from pneumoperitoneum. Standard chest films are also exposed at the peak of inspiration to maximally inflate the lungs. If a pneumothorax is suspected based on the mechanism of injury, symptoms, and signs but not seen on an inspiratory chest film, an expiratory chest radiograph may be added. A simple, closed pneumothorax represents a constant volume of air outside the lung but inside one hemithorax. Therefore, reduction of the intrathoracic volume by exhalation will make this fixed amount of air a larger percentage of the total volume and make it easier to detect a small pneumothorax, if present.

Skull. Plain radiographs of the skull are used to localize a projectile or impaled object to confirm penetration of the cranium. Anteroposterior and lateral views do not offer much information regarding brain injury. Bullets that cross the midline or traverse more than one cranial fossae on the same side have a worse prognosis. Gunshot wounds to the head do not mandate radiographic examination of the cervical spine. An unstable

fracture or ligamentous injury rarely occurs simply from the force of the projectile striking the skull.

Cervical, Thoracic, and Lumbar Spines. In the absence of neurologic deficits, patients with penetrating trauma to the neck do not routinely require spinal immobilization. They do require radiographic examination of the cervical spine to rule out an open fracture. Stab wounds generally do not cause unstable fractures, if they cause fractures at all. Gunshot wounds rarely result in fractures without a neurologic deficit. No studies have been undertaken to answer the same question for the thoracic, lumbar, and sacral spines. If biplanar radiographs are used to localize a retained projectile anywhere near the spine, the clinician should take the time to fully evaluate the films for fractures and disruption of ligamentous lines.

Pelvis and Extremities. In addition to simple localization of retained foreign bodies, identification of any bony abnormality confirms the diagnosis of an open fracture after penetrating trauma.

Contrast Studies

Urologic Studies. One-shot intravenous pyelography may be accomplished in the emergency department to demonstrate kidney function before surgical exploration and potential renal resection. Formal intravenous pyelography is the study of choice to identify ureteral disruption. Dynamic retrograde urethrography is indicated in all patients with a stab or gunshot wound in the vicinity of the urethra and in male patients found to have penetrating trauma with a trajectory across the pelvic midline. Retrograde cystography may demonstrate bladder perforation. None of these specifically identify immediately life-threatening injuries.

Wound Tract Sinography. Injection of radiographic contrast material directly into a penetrating wound to determine its tract is usually a waste of time. Negative results cannot completely rule out penetration of deeper cavities (e.g., peritoneal). Positive results frequently only confirm what could have been determined quicker and easier by other methods.

Arteriography. Arteriography may be employed whenever a major arterial injury is suspected, providing that the general location of the disruption is not clear on physical examination and the delay in procedure performance will not jeopardize a bleeding patient. Hard signs of injury to an extremity's arterial supply may warrant exploration without preoperative studies, except determination of the presence or absence of fracture. Damage to arteries within the neck, chest, abdomen, and pelvis is more difficult to detect. Arteriography in these locations may be accomplished preoperatively by an interventional radiologist or intraoperatively by surgeons. Active hemorrhage may often be arrested by embolization of the bleeding vessels with an autologous clot, gelatin foam, or other suitable substance.

Ultrasonography

Focused abdominal sonography for trauma (FAST) can be used as a screening test before DPTL. If the surgeon takes a patient to the operating theater when free intraperitoneal fluid is noted on FAST, then DPTL would be unnecessary. If a negative FAST result is obtained because of blood or other fluid in insufficient amounts to be detected, then DPTL could be used for its greater sensitivity.

Computed Tomography

Although computed tomography (CT) is an excellent modality for imaging the abdomen, it is used less frequently after penetrating injury than after MBT. There are no advantages to using CT to identify internal injuries from penetrating trauma that outweigh the risks involved in taking a hemodynamically compromised or unstable patient to the radiology suite for scanning. On the other hand, it may be useful for imaging structures in the head, chest, and extraperitoneal abdominopelvic regions, where plain films and DPTL have limited specificity regarding structures that may require surgical repair. Hemodynamically normal patients with flank and back wounds are often evaluated with spiral or triple-contrast CT using water- soluble intravenous, intragastric, and intracolorectal contrast material. Some centers with experienced trauma teams use CT for selected intraperitoneal gunshot wounds as well.

Electrocardiogram

The electrocardiogram usually does not play a significant diagnostic role in penetrating trauma, except in the elderly patient whose myocardium may be having "bystander ischemia" from global hypoperfusion secondary to a shock state and poor systemic oxygen delivery.

Diagnostic Procedures

Consultants are often required for definitive diagnosis and management of injuries sustained through penetrating mechanisms. Cavity exploration by surgeons and arteriography by radiologists can be both diagnostic and therapeutic during the same procedure.

Exploratory Surgery. In the setting of penetrating trauma, exploration without extensive diagnostic studies may be indicated for the neck, chest, abdomen (intraperitoneal and extraperitoneal spaces), or extremities. The rationale behind each of these is discussed in "Specific Principles." Active bleeding may be identified and controlled during the same procedure. Ideally, a surgeon experienced in trauma management will have been present for most of the interventional resuscitation and clinical assessment, so that early decisions and preparations for operative exploration can be made quickly, if indicated. In many situations, surgeons must come from another location (e.g., home, office, operating room) to the emergency department or the patient must be transferred from the receiving emergency department to a facility where a trained surgeon is available.

Diagnostic Peritoneal Tap and Lavage. DPTL is a highly sensitive method of detecting intraperitoneal blood or the contents of hollow viscera in victims of penetrating trauma, although it cannot determine the sight or extent of specific damage. In the setting of penetrating abdominal trauma, DPTL is useful to answer one of two questions:

1. Did the object enter the peritoneal cavity?
2. Did the object cause an injury potentially requiring surgical repair?

One of these questions is addressed each time DPTL is used, depending on the location of the entry wound and the mechanism of injury. Exploratory laparotomy must be considered after any positive DPTL result in the setting of penetrating trauma. A negative DPTL result should assure the trauma team that active intraperitoneal hemorrhage is highly unlikely. If such a patient is hemodynamically compromised, an alternative location of external or internal bleeding must be sought.

When DPTL is used to determine solely whether the peritoneum has been violated, the RBC criterion is lowered to 5,000 RBCs/μL. Thus, 100,000 RBCs/μL is applied for "injury requiring repair" and 5,000 RBCs/μL is applied for "peritoneal penetration." All other criteria outlined in Table 41–7 remain unchanged (see Chapter 41, Multiple Blunt Trauma). Because 5,000 RBCs/μL may represent as little as 1 mL of whole blood in 1 L of lavage fluid, meticulous hemostasis must be achieved during performance of the procedure. A local anesthetic containing epinephrine should be used, even if the patient is unconscious.

The mechanisms of injury must be considered before DPTL employment. Broad categories are stab wounds, gunshot wounds, and wounds caused by other projectiles. Because impaled objects are almost universally taken to the operating theater for removal under direct visualization, DPTL is not commonly used under these circumstances. There are much fewer data on the specifics of DPTL in cases of non–bullet-penetrating projectiles such as may occur after an explosion. Until studies are published to the contrary, it is probably best to evaluate them as gunshot wounds.

PRINCIPLES OF MANAGEMENT

General Principles

The trauma resuscitation should proceed in a well-orchestrated and systematic fashion. The important components of the resuscitation are performed in order of importance. Knowledge of the mechanism of injury and the circumstances surrounding the trauma are essential in assembling the "big picture" and not missing important diagnostic possibilities.

Open Wounds. The first assessment of all open wounds is their degree of hemorrhage. Although any single wound may be bleeding only to a relatively minor degree, the summation of blood lost from multiple wounds can be significant. All external bleeding should be controlled with direct pressure. Clamping of bleeding vessels is not advised. If the external bleeding stems from a noncompressible site, a surgeon should be contacted immediately.

Stab Wounds. LWE, following the guidelines discussed earlier, is used for lacerations and puncture wounds caused by objects other than missiles. In addition to determination of wound depth and injury to underlying structures, LWE also involves a search for foreign bodies and devitalized tissue, just as it does for other lacerations seen in the emergency department. Depending on wound characteristics (see Chapter 49, Wound Care), some stab wounds can be closed primarily in the emergency department after débridement and high-pressure irrigation. Deep puncture wounds may require surgical referral.

Missile Wounds. The edges of wounds created by projectiles are often crushed by the tearing and energy transfer of the missile. The sudden creation of a temporary cavity inside the body produces a vacuum, which may draw skin debris and clothing fibers into the body through the surface wound. Because gunshot wounds are different from puncture wounds, LWE can be difficult and hazardous. Even if no deep or vital structures are injured, personal or telephone consultation with a surgeon is warranted in most cases. Retrieval of the projectile is rarely necessary and generally not emergent in any case. Long-term sequelae from retained lead or depleted uranium is possible, but it only requires follow-up referral from the emergency department.

Shotgun Wounds. Wounds caused by shotguns deserve special consideration. Penetrating trauma caused by rifle slugs can be managed similar to gunshot wounds of smaller caliber. However, wounds caused by multiple shot pellets must be viewed differently. Shotgun blasts at close range, where the shot is still concentrated after it leaves the barrel, tend to cause massive tissue destruction, gaping open wounds, and heavy bleeding. A large number of pellets, and the wadding that separates the shot from the powder, are frequently imbedded in the wound. Surgical consultation is required.

The farther away the victim is from the muzzle of the shotgun, the wider the roughly circular pattern with more distance between individual pellets. Instead of a concentrated impact on the tissues, multiple individual penetrating wounds are found. Because of lower energy at longer range, many pellets may not penetrate beyond skin. The goal of assessment is to determine if any pellets have injured underlying structures. This normally involves the use of biplanar radiography and careful accounting of where each radiopaque foreign body is located in the body. This can be extremely time consuming, with sometimes over a hundred pellets to examine. A careful physical examination with neurovascular injury emphasis is made on all sites distal to pellet wounds. Disposition of the patient depends on the characteristics of the individual penetrating wounds and final resting places of the projectiles.

Specific Principles

The approach to penetrating trauma greatly depends on the mechanism of injury and the region of the body affected.

Head. Penetrating trauma to the head carries a high mortality. Although these devastating injuries will often require the attention of a neurosurgeon, emergency physicians must consider the patient's prognosis during the interventional resuscitation. Pressures caused by stress waves within the confines of the bony cranium can create a hydraulic effect that may burst the skull open from inside to outside or push cranial contents out the foramen magnum and compress the brain stem. These patients, especially those with brain tissue external to the skull, are frequently moribund on arrival in the emergency department and have limited hope of salvage.

The damaged brain is susceptible to the effects of hypoxia, shock, and increases in intracranial pressure secondary to tissue edema and bleeding. Therefore, the patient must be resuscitated adequately to maintain perfusion pressure to the brain, but excessive fluid administration may lead to additional brain injury. Neurosurgical consultation can help guide treatment modalities such as forced hyperventilation, osmotic diuresis, and intracranial pressure monitoring.

Neck. The airway is of prime concern in neck injuries. Any actual or potential compromise of the patient's airway warrants early definitive intervention. Expanding hematomas are particularly problematic, because blind nasotracheal intubation is contraindicated, anatomic landmarks may be distorted for orotracheal intubation, and cricothyroidostomy may release a partially contained hematoma. Orotracheal intubation by an experienced emergency physician is usually best. Once the patient's airway is secured, definitive intervention for penetrating neck trauma with vascular injury involves transferring the patient to an operating theater for neck exploration, sternotomy, or thoracotomy.

The evaluation of other penetrating neck wounds without obvious damage to important internal structures can be controversial. The initial assessment is based on the location of any entrance or exit wounds (Fig. 42–1). Zone I extends from the thoracic outlet to the level of the cricoid cartilage, where gaining proximal control of major vessels is more complex. Zone II includes the structures from the cricoid cartilage to the angle of the mandible, where surgical exploration is the easiest and least risky. Zone III represents the portions of the neck distal to the angle of the mandible, where distal vascular control below the base of the skull is difficult.

Each of these three zones is approached differently. Zone I requires an extensive evaluation before surgery is normally undertaken. This commonly includes the following tests:

- Four-vessel arteriography (both carotid and both vertebral arteries)
- Fiberoptic laryngotracheobronchoscopy
- Fiberoptic esophagoscopy (some centers prefer rigid esophagoscopy)
- Fluorocine-esophagography with water-soluble contrast

The evaluation of zone II may be accomplished through a similar approach as in zone I, or the surgeon may elect to simply explore the neck

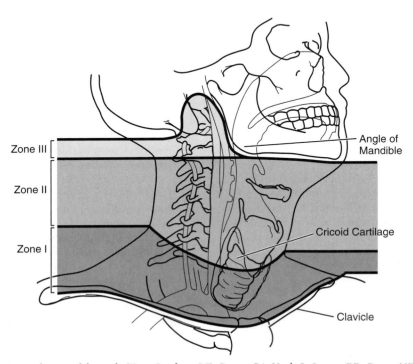

FIGURE 42–1 • Surgical zones of the neck. (From Jacobson LE, Gomez GA: Neck. In Ivatury RR, Cayten NR [eds]: Textbook of Penetrating Trauma. Baltimore, Williams & Wilkins, 1996; with permission.)

without extensive preoperative testing. Both approaches have similar sensitivities and specificities for injuries requiring surgical repair, morbidity and mortality rates, and total monetary costs. Zone III requires only a direct pharyngeal examination for blood and four-vessel arteriography.

Depending on trajectory of the penetrating object, injury to the cervical spine may be a concern. Patients without neurologic deficits are unlikely to have an unstable bony or ligamentous injury. Victims who are neurologically compromised are unlikely to improve significantly, although methylprednisolone may be administered. Neurosurgical decompression of the spinal canal may be warranted in some patients with a deficit that progresses over time.

Central Chest. "The box" refers to the central area of the chest containing the heart, great vessels, tracheobronchial tree, esophagus, thoracic spine, and adjacent structures in the chest and abdomen. It is bounded by the sternal notch superiorly, the midclavicular lines on each side, and the intersection of these lines with the inferior costal margins inferiorly. The evaluation of these structures incorporates similar procedures to those of zone I of the neck. The additional tests required for cardiac evaluation include an electrocardiogram and either FAST examination or CVP manometry. The former may identify cardiac irritability, ischemia, and infarction. The latter two facilitate early detection of free intrapericardial fluid before development of cardiac tamponade.

Lateral Chest. Wounds that have clearly entered or traversed one hemithorax, without involvement of the mediastinal box, often cause simple pneumothoraces and hemothoraces. Appropriate placement of chest tubes may be the only intervention required. Persistent air leaks should raise the suspicion of bronchial disruption. Active hemorrhage from pulmonary or intercostal vessels with persistent drainage of gross blood may necessitate a thoracotomy in the operating theater.

Thorax and Abdomen. A thoracoabdominal wound is one in which the penetrating tract could travel through the chest and into the peritoneal cavity. These are most commonly located between the nipple lines and the inferior costal margins, but the entrance wound could be located anywhere on the chest, neck, or upper extremities. By definition, a wound that enters the thorax and crosses into the abdomen must penetrate the diaphragm. Most diaphragmatic injuries should be surgically repaired acutely. Therefore, the key diagnostic determination to be made in the emergency department is whether the peritoneal cavity is violated, thus implying that the diaphragm is penetrated. This can be done by identifying abdominal contents in the chest on plain radiography, using DPTL with its normal non-RBC criteria and an RBC criterion of 5000 RBCs/μL for peritoneal penetration, or obtaining thoracic and abdominal CT in less urgent stab wound cases.

Anterior Abdomen. Approximately one half to two thirds of anterior abdominal stab wounds enter the peritoneal cavity. However, only about half of those that enter this cavity cause an injury requiring surgical repair. Performing laparotomies on all hemodynamically stable patients with these common injuries is unnecessary. The combination of LWE, FAST, DPTL, or CT can be helpful in sorting out which patients should be referred for surgery. In this setting the question being asked is: Does the patient have an injury requiring operative repair? Figure 42–2 represents an algorithmic approach to addressing this question.

In contrast to low-energy stab wounds, abdominal gunshot wounds commonly cause injuries requiring surgical repair. Therefore, in most settings, the only diagnostic question that must be asked for a hemodynamically stable patient is: Did the bullet enter the peritoneal cavity? As soon as this can be determined by physical examination, radiography, or DPTL, patients are normally taken to the operating theater expeditiously. There are no tests sufficiently specific to directly identify some injuries that are more common after gunshot wounds compared with stab wounds (e.g., bowel perforation). In some high-volume trauma centers with efficient systems and experienced personnel, there are data that support nonoperative management in selected patients. Accurate pre-selection, CT, and serial assessments are central to this evolving approach.

Flanks and Back. The flanks are the areas below the costal margins, above the iliac crests, and between the anterior and posterior axillary lines. The back lies between the posterior axillary lines below the eighth intercostal space. The organs at greatest risk are the ascending and descending colon, major arteries and veins, the kidneys and adrenal glands, the pancreas, and the spinal cord. Intraperitoneal injury is less common than after anterior abdominal wounds.

Unstable or hemodynamically compromised patients are usually taken directly to the operating theater. A one-shot intravenous pyelogram to demonstrate two functioning kidneys before any potential nephrectomy can be accomplished in the operating theater, as appropriate. FAST or DPTL can be employed for evaluation of peritoneal penetration or intraperitoneal injury

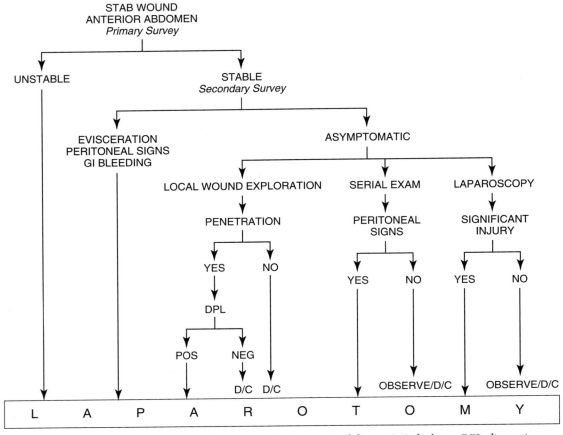

FIGURE 42–2 • Evaluation of the patient with a stab wound to the anterior abdomen. D/C, discharge; DPL, diagnostic peritoneal lavage; NEG, negative; POS, positive. (From Cayten CG, Nassoura ZE: Abdomen. In Ivatury RR, Cayten NR [eds]: Textbook of Penetrating Trauma. Baltimore, Williams & Wilkins, 1996; with permission.)

requiring repair, depending on circumstances. Triple-contrast CT may be ordered for hemodynamically normal and stable patients.

Pelvis. Transpelvic gunshot wounds have a high mortality rate. The most common causes of death are exsanguination from vascular injuries in the early phases and sepsis from colorectal penetration or open fractures in the late phases. The victim should be managed by a multidisciplinary trauma team when any missile fractures bone or enters the abdominopelvic spaces. If coronal and transverse planes are drawn through the greater trochanters, anterior wounds cause significant injury over 90% of the time, whereas posterior wounds cause injury in about one third of cases. Of those that enter posteriorly, superior wounds cause injury requiring surgical repair much more frequently than inferior wounds. Up to two thirds of gunshot wounds and three fourths of stab wounds that enter the buttocks may not violate the pelvis proper, but they can still cause vascular and neurologic injuries.

Extremities. Identifying fractures and neurovascular injuries are the most important aspects of extremity evaluations. "Hard" signs of arterial injury include continuous external bleeding despite direct pressure, expanding or pulsatile hematoma, bruit or thrill, absent distal pulses, or evidence of distal ischemia such as pallor or cyanosis. "Soft" signs include weak distal pulses, a history of pulsatile bleeding or large blood loss before application of direct pressure, unexplained hemodynamic compromise, a large hematoma that is not expanding, an estimated wound trajectory in proximity to an artery, or a neurologic deficit related to a nerve in proximity to an artery.

In the absence of hard signs that mandate surgical exploration, adjunctive testing should involve measurement of an arterial pulse index (API). An API between injured and uninjured extremities of less than 0.9 should prompt additional testing with color-duplex Doppler ultrasonography. Arteriography is commonly reserved for proximal wounds, multiple wounds in the same extremity (especially shotgun injuries), and evaluation of patients in shock where baseline blood flow makes other tests difficult to interpret. Embolized projectiles are also considered.

A compartment syndrome may occur after penetrating trauma and is more likely after high-velocity gunshot wounds and injuries associated with a fracture. Consultation with an orthopedic surgeon is required for any wounds violating joint spaces or bony structures.

UNCERTAIN DIAGNOSIS

Intracranial injury and exsanguination from cardiovascular wounds are the leading causes of death in victims of penetrating trauma who reach the emergency department alive. The former is usually obvious, and little can be accomplished to improve the patient's chances of survival. The latter, on the other hand, can be occult and demands a thorough approach to evaluation and management. Just as in victims of MBT, rapid decisions must be made and positive actions undertaken during the interventional resuscitation. Patients must be repeatedly questioned for new or changing symptoms and frequently reassessed by physical examination or other tests. In addition to those discussed in the previous chapter, some of the more common uncertainties leading to preventable mortality are discussed here.

Uncertainty About Whether a Stab Wound Entered the Pleural Space. Traditional LWE is not used for thoracic stab wounds. Instruments can open a tract from the outside air into the chest, creating a pneumothorax where none existed. However, carefully peeling back the wound edges in patients with normal chest radiographs can establish the superficial nature of many wounds, thus avoiding hospital admission or emergency department observation. When uncertain of the risk of pleural penetration, there is good evidence that patients who remain asymptomatic and have a normal chest radiograph at the end of a 6-hour observation period in the emergency department can be discharged home with simple wound care and rapid access to EMS or follow-up evaluation.

Uncertainty About Route or Extent of Damage of a Gunshot Wound. Gunshot wounds that enter and exit with a trajectory that might not result in penetration of a body cavity are called tangential gunshot wounds. The cranium can be evaluated with plain skull radiographs or CT. Penetration of the platysma in the neck is usually straightforward. The chest is evaluated in the same manner as are stab wounds. An abdominopelvic trajectory is evaluated by employing DPTL for peritoneal penetration with a RBC count of 5000/μL or surgically opening the wound tract in the operating theater. The literature also contains documented cases of intraperitoneal injury with gunshot wounds where the missile did not enter the peritoneal cavity. Given the poor sensitivity of FAST and CT for bowel injuries, DPTL is extremely useful in these situations.

Uncertainty About the Number of Entrance Wounds Relative to the Number of Exit Wounds Plus Retained Projectiles. Although entrance and exit gunshot wounds are not reliably distinct in many cases, there should be just as many entrance wounds as exit wounds, unless one or more missiles are retained in the body, an exit wound is missed, a projectile is radiolucent, or a radiopaque object is not within the regions covered by the films. Bullets do not always travel parallel to the transverse plane. For instance, they may enter the lumbar area and stop in the chest or neck in a victim bending over to run away from an assailant. Bullets falling from the sky during celebratory activities have entered the supraclavicular fossae and ended their tract in the abdomen. Projectiles can embolize in arteries and veins to be carried to the brain or distal extremities, or the heart or lungs, respectively.

Uncertainty Regarding the Utility of a Negative Study. Normal Doppler ultrasonographic and arteriographic studies reasonably exclude vascular injury. However, a negative chest radiograph will not exclude cardiac injury. It can only rule out immediately significant pneumothoraces and hemothoraces. A negative FAST examination only excludes larger amounts of fluid in the pericardial or peritoneal cavities, whereas a negative DPTL result should indicate absence of intraperitoneal hemorrhage significant enough to cause hemodynamic compromise. These last two statements may be less true in patients with prior abdominal surgery leading to adhesions that create exclusionary pockets within the peritoneal cavity. Negative FAST, DPTL, and CT results never fully exclude diaphragmatic or bowel injury. Normal laboratory tests have limited utility in emergency decision making for penetrating trauma. Any single study only provides a snapshot of conditions at that moment and may change later. Serial assessments and studies are often necessary in these patients.

SPECIAL CONSIDERATIONS
Pediatric Patients

Normal vital signs vary at different stages of development of children. Length-based tapes

(Broselow tapes) with specific data may be helpful in this regard. They also provide rapid reference for equipment sizing and medication dosing.

Pediatric trauma victims tolerate hypoxia very poorly. Because of their higher metabolic rates, special attention should be placed on early airway and breathing interventions. Maximizing oxygen saturation of hemoglobin is just as important in improving oxygen delivery to a child's tissues as it is for adults. Respiratory compromise is the most common cause of cardiac arrest in the pediatric population.

Volume-depleted children can often maintain a normal blood pressure for their age with only mild tachycardia until sudden decompensation and cardiovascular collapse. If this is allowed to occur, resuscitation can be difficult. If intravenous access cannot be obtained after two attempts at peripheral cannulation, an intraosseous needle may be inserted into the marrow cavity of the proximal tibia or distal femur. Fluid resuscitation and medication administration may then proceed through this route.

The body surface areas of pediatric patients are larger than adults when compared with their body volumes. This makes maintaining body temperature more problematic in children, so careful attention must be given to keeping them warm during and after resuscitation.

Pregnant Patients

In addition to the physiologic changes induced by pregnancy, the gravid uterus alters the approach to penetrating abdominopelvic trauma. Gunshot wounds that clearly enter the peritoneal cavity or the uterus are normally explored surgically. However, if DPTL is being used to make decisions, two major adjustments must be made. First, the technique must be an open supraumbilical technique to avoid injuring the uterus. Second, because of the compaction of intraperitoneal contents displaced superiorly by the enlarging uterus and increased likelihood of injury for any given peritoneal penetration, the RBC criterion should be $5000/\mu L$ in all stab and gunshot wound cases.

Simultaneous resuscitative thoracotomy with aortic cross-clamping immediately after fetal delivery has resulted in maternal improvement in some cases.

Elderly Patients

Although not statistically likely to be victims of penetrating trauma, elderly patients present a number of additional challenges to the managing physician. The elderly population has a higher incidence of chronic medical conditions, as well as a lower physiologic reserve, than younger trauma victims.

Diabetes, coronary artery disease, and hypertension may complicate management of these patients. The diabetic trauma victim may exhibit wide swings in blood glucose concentration, will have poorer capacity for wound healing, and is likely to have more problems with infection. Elderly patients may suffer watershed cerebral infarctions from untreated hypotension. Because of the autoregulation phenomenon, restoring the blood pressure to "normal" levels may, in fact, be a relative hypotension for chronically hypertensive patients and may be inadequate to perfuse the entire brain. Also, a relative hypotension may insufficiently perfuse stenotic coronary arteries, resulting in myocardial ischemia or infarction. Elderly patients have longer lengths of stay, more complications, and often poorer outcome after penetrating injuries.

DISPOSITION AND FOLLOW-UP

Although some patients may be discharged from the emergency department, this is the exception rather than the rule. Disposition of most victims of penetrating trauma means referring them to the appropriate inpatient services.

Immediate Consultation

The need for immediate consultation is usually obvious early in the resuscitation of the unstable patient. Any serious bleeding or internal injuries require interventional or definitive treatment by the appropriate surgeon. Orthopedic surgeons should be involved in cases with open fractures and joint spaces. Despite the poor prognosis of penetrating cranial and spinal trauma, a neurosurgeon should be consulted early in the management of these patients.

Observation

An observation period in the emergency department is appropriate for some patients. Questionably superficial chest wounds may be observed for development of hemothorax or pneumothorax and discharged from the emergency department. Observation units attached to emergency departments may be ideal for such patients. Patients with stab wounds with negative findings on physical examination and an internal study (i.e., FAST, DPTL, or CT) may take some time to manifest occult bowel injury. If discharge from the emergency department is considered after performance of a DPTL, a period of observation is warranted to be sure there are no complications from the procedure. Any victim of penetrating trauma who would not have rapid access to EMS care may best be observed in the hospital for longer periods.

Admission or Transfer

Admission to the hospital is the appropriate action for most penetrating trauma patients. If observational, ancillary, surgical, or blood-banking services are not sufficient, then transfer to a referral center is appropriate.

Discharge with Follow-up

Patients who may be potentially discharged include those with superficial stab wounds, uncomplicated extremity wounds, and some tangential gunshot wounds of the neck or torso. As always, it is important to ensure that the patient is sufficiently reliable, has understood the discharge instructions, has been appropriately referred for follow-up care, and has rapid access to EMS or other unscheduled care for any problems listed on discharge instructions or any additional concerns.

Death and Organ Donation

Morbidity and mortality from penetrating trauma are commonly preventable once the victim arrives in the emergency department, but there are those patients who will succumb to their injuries despite the best resuscitative efforts. Organ donation may be an option, provided the family is approached with sensitivity and empathy. A transcranial gunshot wound may leave an individual brain dead, but with otherwise intact organs, which might save or improve the quality of multiple other lives. Discussing the possibility of organ donation with family members and notifying the transplantation team is an important responsibility of the emergency physician.

FINAL POINTS

A stepwise process of evaluation and treatment, beginning with the primary survey and continuing through the final disposition of the patient, will ensure that few life-threatening injuries are missed.

- Intervene rapidly for life threats discovered during the primary survey.
- Stop any external or internal bleeding.
- Perform a targeted secondary survey to identify possible occult injuries within any time constraints imposed by the victim's physiologic status.
- Reassess periodically and any time the patient's condition deteriorates.
- Perform or order appropriate ancillary studies to facilitate decision making.
- Consider the potential of embolic or fragment-based secondary injury.
- Arrange an appropriate disposition, taking into account the mechanism of injury, the injuries themselves, and the patient's social situation.

CASE *Study*

A radio call from emergency medical services (EMS) personnel informed the emergency department they were 5 minutes away and bringing a 17-year-old boy with multiple stab wounds to the chest and abdomen. A "moderate" amount of blood was evident at the scene, but the patient was conscious. Vital signs were blood pressure, 100/60 mm Hg; heart rate, 100 beats per minute; and respiratory rate, 26 breaths per minute. The patient was placed on oxygen by mask, and an intravenous line was established with isotonic crystalloid running wide open.

The patient remained conscious during transport. His vital signs en route were pulse, 100 beats per minute; blood pressure, 104/70 mm Hg; and respiratory rate, 20 breaths per minute. EMS personnel started him on oxygen at 4 L/min by nasal cannula but were unable to establish an intravenous line. The victim had one stab wound inferolateral to the left nipple, several in the left anterolateral abdomen and flank, and one in the lateral aspect of his left arm. His left torso had been exposed by EMS personnel and was covered in blood.

The patient appeared drowsy on arrival in the emergency department. He seemed slow to answer questions but did so appropriately without abnormal airway sounds. His skin had no obvious pallor or cyanosis, but he was diaphoretic. When asked to take deep breaths, little air movement could be heard on the left. Breath sounds were normal on the right. Cardiac auscultation revealed normal sounds and no murmurs. Carotid pulses

Continued on following page

were fast and weak. There was no jugular venous distention. Capillary refill over the sternum was 3 seconds. None of the four wounds were actively bleeding. Initial vital signs in the emergency department were pulse, 112 beats per minute; blood pressure, 84/62 mm Hg; and respiratory rate, 28 breaths per minute. The cardiac monitor showed sinus tachycardia without ectopy. The pulse oximeter registered an S_pO_2 of 91%.

Changes in the patient's mental status and vital signs compared with those in the field made the diagnosis of early shock probable. The degree of external blood loss before arrival in the emergency department could not be accurately assessed, but hemorrhage into the pleural, intraperitoneal, and extraperitoneal spaces was possible. Tension pneumothorax was also a consideration. There were no wounds in the mediastinal "box."

While one assistant changed the patient to high-flow oxygen by non-rebreather mask and another obtained intravenous access with a 14-gauge catheter in the patient's right antecubital fossa, the emergency physician performed a needle thoracentesis through the anterior left chest. No rush of air was heard, but air could be withdrawn using a 60-mL syringe.

Reassessment is required after any intervention. Although the S_pO_2 increased to 94%, the patient's mental status did not improve significantly. Either the thoracentesis did not relieve any increased intrathoracic pressure or there was another cause of the hemodynamic compromise. A tube thoracostomy was indicated for the possibilities of a persistent tension pneumothorax or a hemothorax. Volume expansion to restore adequate end-organ perfusion was also indicated.

The emergency physician performed a left lateral tube thoracostomy with a 40-Fr chest tube. An initial rush of air was noted, but then the tube began to return gross blood. A second intravenous line was simultaneously established. A 500-mL bolus of warmed lactated Ringer's solution was infused through one line and a saline lock established on the other. There was little change in the patient's mental status and his vital signs were pulse, 124 beats per minute; blood pressure, 80/60 mm Hg; and respiratory rate, 22 breaths per minute. Another 500-mL bolus of lactated Ringer's was infused and O-positive blood was ordered from the blood bank. The chest tube yielded an immediate return of 650 mL of blood into an autotransfuser. This was administered with warmed

normal saline (NS) solution through the second intravenous line. After this, the patient began responding more appropriately to questions and his vital signs improved to pulse, 108 beats per minute; blood pressure, 96/60 mm Hg; and respiratory rate, 22 breaths per minute.

The victim's only complaint was pain at the site of the thoracostomy. He denied central chest pain, shortness of breath, lightheadedness, nausea, and abdominal pain. He had no known allergies to medications, had no significant medical or surgical history, and was up to date on his tetanus immunization. He admitted to having had two beers, but he denied use of illicit drugs. He had eaten about 1 hour previously. He stated he did not know who stabbed him. His parents' telephone number was obtained so that the police could contact them.

The patient's clothes were removed and saved for investigators. Once additional injuries were excluded, he was covered with a blanket to prevent hypothermia. The physical examination was documented as follows:

General: 17-year-old boy stabbed in chest and abdomen. He is awake, alert, and oriented.

Neck: The trachea is midline. There is no jugular venous distention.

Chest: There is a 2-cm wound in the left fifth intercostal space in the left anterior axillary line. There is another 2-cm wound in the ninth intercostal space in left posterior axillary line. Breath sounds are decreased on the left but improved after chest tube placement. Lungs are clear to auscultation. The heart has a regular rate and rhythm, and sounds are not distant.

Abdomen: There is a 2-cm wound 6 cm below the costal margin just lateral to the left midclavicular line. There is another 2-cm wound just below the costal margin in the left posterior axillary line. The abdomen is nondistended with normal and active bowel sounds. There is some mild left upper-quadrant tenderness but no guarding or rebound tenderness. Rectal examination reveals normal sphincter tone and no gross blood.

Back: No additional injuries were found beyond those noted above.

Extremities: There is a 2-cm wound between the biceps and triceps on the lateral aspect of the left arm near its midpoint. All distal pulses are normal.

A simple drawing can be very effective. Photographs are even better. The emergency physician must always keep in mind that penetrating trauma may necessitate the collection of forensic evidence. Only facts should be documented. Forensic interpretations of those facts have no place in the medical record.

Bloody output from the chest tube had slowed to a trickle. After 1 L of total isotonic crystalloid fluid, as well as the patient's autologous blood, his vital signs were pulse, 88 beats per minute; blood pressure, 122/78 mm Hg; and respiratory rate, 20 breaths per minute. A plain anteroposterior chest radiograph in the sitting position showed a well-positioned chest tube and a slight residual hemopneumothorax. The cardiac and mediastinal shadows appeared normal. There was no free air under the diaphragm. A nasogastric tube returned stomach contents without blood. A transurethral catheter of the bladder returned 220 mL of clear urine.

Because the patient was now hemodynamically normal and there was no immediate evidence of an ongoing transfusion requirement, attention was focused on determining if any of the stab wounds caused an injury requiring surgical repair. Penetrating trauma to the lateral chest can often be managed solely with chest tube drainage. The heart was believed to be at some risk, owing to the proximity of one of the wounds. Other organs at most risk were the diaphragm, stomach, spleen, and colon. No surgeon was immediately available to come to the receiving emergency department, so the emergency physician sought to determine if early surgery might be indicated. LWE of the anterior abdominal stab wound was considered but would take time to perform and would only provide information on one of the wounds. FAST examination would be helpful only if positively identifying free intraperitoneal fluid. It is not designed to detect diaphragmatic violation. DPTL would be difficult to interpret in the context of multiple wounds, unless it was positive for intraluminal contents or blood at the 100,000 RBCs/μL level. CT might show specific injuries, but the scanner was in the basement of the receiving hospital and it was believed to be too risky until the patient was known to be stable for a longer period of time. Thus, sequential use of studies was deemed appropriate.

During the subsequent evaluation, the patient was monitored and frequently reassessed.

FAST examination with good visualization revealed no free fluid in the pericardial sac or peritoneal cavity. Because the FAST examination is less sensitive for free intraperitoneal fluid than is DPTL, the latter was performed using a closed, infraumbilical technique. The tap was negative. The lavage returned a minimally pink fluid, which was sent to the laboratory for analysis. The DPTL cell counts were 14,000 RBCs/μL and 160 WBCs/μL. There were no other abnormalities in the lavage fluid.

The lack of gross blood on the tap from a patient without previous abdominal surgery meant that life-threatening intraperitoneal hemorrhage was highly unlikely. The lavage cell count met the threshold for peritoneal penetration but not for injury requiring surgical repair. If caused by either thoracoabdominal wound, then there would be an indication for surgery. If caused by the anterior abdominal wound, then there would not be. If caused by the flank wound, penetration of the descending colon would be more likely.

Because the patient was hemodynamically normal and currently stable, the decision was made to transfer him to a trauma center where an experienced trauma team was immediately available. The patient's parents were instructed to meet him there. Because of distance and the level of care that could be provided by local EMS and transfer services, a regional rotary-wing ambulance service was used for transportation and continuous monitoring. Four units of type-specific blood and supplies to manage any complications with the chest tube were sent with the patient.

The patient remained stable during transfer to the trauma center, where he was met by the trauma team. After their initial evaluation, the patient received a triple-contrast CT by an experienced trauma radiologist. Contrast medium was noted to leak from the descending colon, so the patient was taken to the operating theater for exploration. In addition to the colonic penetration, the left hemidiaphragm and one loop of small bowel were also violated. The patient had an uneventful postoperative course and was discharged on the fifth hospital day. His left arm wound was débrided and closed before discharge. There was no evidence of bony injury of the humerus on plain radiographs.

Bibliography

TEXTS

American College of Surgeons Committee on Trauma: Advanced Trauma Life Support Program for Physicians. Chicago, American College of Surgeons, 1997.

Cooper GJ, Dudley HAF, Gann DS, et al (eds): Scientific Foundations of Trauma. Oxford, Butterworth-Heinemann, 1997.

Ivatury RR, Cayten CG: Textbook of Penetrating Trauma. Baltimore, Williams & Williams, 1996.

Scaletta TA, Schaider JJ: Emergent Management of Trauma. New York, McGraw-Hill, 1996.

JOURNAL ARTICLES

Bickell WH, Wall MJ, Pepe PE, et al: Immediate versus delayed fluid resuscitation for hypotensive patients with penetrating torso injuries. N Engl J Med 1994; 331:1105–1109.

Boyle EM, Maier RV, Salazar JD, et al: Diagnosis of injuries after stab wounds to the flank and back. J Trauma 1997; 42:260–265.

Branney SW, Moore EE, Feldhaus KM, et al: Critical analysis of two decades of experience with post injury emergency department thoracotomy in a regional trauma center. J Trauma 1998; 45:87–95.

Chan D: Echocardiography in thoracic trauma. Emerg Med Clin North Am 1998; 16:191–207.

Dennis JW, Frykberg ER, Veldenz HC, et al: Validation of nonoperative management of occult vascular injuries and accuracy of physical examination alone in penetrating extremity trauma: 5- and 10-year follow-up. J Trauma 1998; 44:243–253.

Fackler ML: Gunshot wound review. Ann Emerg Med 1996; 28:194–203.

Grossman MD, May AK, Schwab CW, et al: Determining anatomic injury with computed tomography in selected torso gunshot wounds. J Trauma 1998; 45:446–456.

Klyachkin ML, Rohmiller M, Charesh WE, et al: Penetrating injuries of the neck: Selective management evolving. Am Surg 1997; 63:189–194.

Leibner EC, Jackimczyk K: Penetrating extremity trauma: The problem of occult vascular injury, Trauma Rep 2001; 2:1–12.

Mendelson JA: The relationship between mechanisms of wounding and principles of treatment of missile wounds. J Trauma 1991; 31:1181–1202.

Ordog GJ, Wasserberger J, Balasubramanium S, Shoemaker W: Civilian gunshot wounds: Outpatient management. J Trauma 1994; 36:106–111.

Rosemurgy AS, Albrink MH, Olson SM, et al: Abdominal stab wound protocol: Prospective study documents applicability for widespread use. Am Surg 1995; 61:112–116.

Velmahos GC, Demetrious D, Toutouzas KG, et al: Selective nonoperative management in 1,856 patients with abdominal gunshot wounds: Should routine laparotomy still be the standard of care? Ann Surg 2001: 234:395–403.

Working Group, Ad Hoc Subcommittee on Outcomes, American College of Surgeons—Committee on Trauma: Practice management guidelines for emergency department thoracotomy. J Am Coll Surg 2001:193:303–309.

CHAPTER 43

Abdominal Trauma

GREGORY J. FERMANN

CASE *Study*

A rescue squad was called to the scene of a motor vehicle accident involving a 33-year-old male driver whose car collided head on with a truck.

INTRODUCTION

Abdominal trauma is defined as an injury occurring anteriorly from the nipple line to the inguinal creases and posteriorly from the tips of the scapula to the gluteal creases (Fig. 43–1). Respiratory movement of the diaphragm exposes the intra-abdominal contents to injuries that, at first glance, appear to be isolated to the thorax. Traumatic abdominal injuries are further classified as intraperitoneal or retroperitoneal. Intraperitoneal injuries are more amenable to diagnosis by physical examination. In these injuries, both parietal and visceral pain systems are affected. Parietal pain receptors lead to localized pain, such as in hepatic or splenic injuries. Visceral pain receptors classically cause dull, poorly localized pain commonly associated with hemoperitoneum or hollow viscus injuries. Intraperitoneal injuries may present as referred pain to the shoulders, scapula, flank, chest, and back. Retroperitoneal injuries are often less amenable to physical diagnosis. Large amounts of blood can accumulate in the retroperitoneal spaces without causing clear physical findings. Simultaneous injuries to intraperitoneal and retroperitoneal structures are not uncommon and can complicate the physical

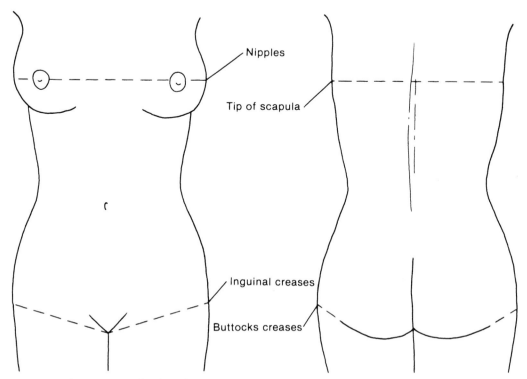

Nipples

Tip of scapula

Inguinal creases

Buttocks creases

FIGURE 43–1 • The anatomic surface boundaries of the abdomen. Anteriorly, the abdomen extends from the nipple line to the inguinal creases. Posteriorly, it extends from the tips of the scapula to the gluteal creases of the buttocks.

examination. Intoxicants, such as alcohol, and other central nervous system depressants, stimulants, and hallucinogens may make the clinical examination unreliable. The presence of underlying medical problems and psychiatric disease may further confuse the trauma evaluation.

Multiple injuries are common in the patient with abdominal trauma. Management of the head-injured patient with an abdominal injury can be particularly challenging because of difficulties with communication that influence the interpretation of the physical examination. Major traumatic injuries to the pelvis, long bones, neck, and thorax may distract the patient from perceiving, and thereby reporting, any initial abdominal discomfort. Providers may focus on more graphic injuries, such as a fractured femur, and fail to identify the presence of abdominal trauma until later in the evaluation. A high index of suspicion is particularly necessary in trauma patients with an altered level of consciousness or with multiple injuries.

Abdominal trauma is categorized as penetrating or blunt in origin, with the spleen, small bowel, and liver being the most commonly involved organs (Table 43–1). Blunt abdominal trauma is five times more common than penetrating injury, with an overall mortality of 10% to 30%. Motor vehicle crashes, motorcycle crashes, and vehicle-pedestrian collisions account for 50% to 75% of blunt abdominal trauma. Direct blows to the abdomen and falls are responsible for the majority of the remaining injuries.

Penetrating trauma is the result of high- or low-velocity firearms, stab injury, and foreign-body penetration into the body (i.e., impaling injuries). Firearms cause a high incidence (90%) of serious peritoneal/solid organ injury, with a 10% to 30% mortality rate. Two thirds of stab wounds penetrate the peritoneum, with 50% to 75% of these patients having significant vascular or solid organ injury. Mortality has been reported at 5% from serious stab injuries.

Stab wounds are more frequent on the left (right-hand dominant assailant) and in the upper quadrants. In 30% of abdominal stab wounds there is 30% concomitant thoracic cavity penetration. Diaphragmatic injury is of particular concern in these cases.

The damage resulting from firearm injury is primarily caused by the impact velocity of the projectile. Weapons with muzzle velocities greater than 2000 ft/sec are considered high velocity (assault), cause devastating injuries, and have a 50% mortality. Most handguns have a muzzle velocity less than 1000 ft/sec and are low velocity. Two thirds of low-velocity (civilian) firearm injuries have a bullet that remains in the body. Organs are injured by direct impact of the projectile and by the concussive effect of dissipating kinetic energy. Primary projectiles may strike bone, produce secondary projectiles, and inflict tissue damage without direct organ penetration. The wound path of a projectile is not a reliable indicator of organ injury.

Emergency trauma management focuses around the "golden hour," the first 60 minutes after any injury, when the greatest impact on morbidity and mortality may be realized. This is particularly true in abdominal trauma. Early death is often the result of uncontrolled hemorrhage from solid organ or vascular injury; therefore, early stabilization, diagnosis, and operative intervention can be lifesaving. Causes of late mortality include sepsis, unrecognized hemorrhage, occult injury (e.g., diaphragmatic rupture with herniation of abdominal contents), hollow organ injury (bowel, gallbladder, and urinary bladder), and pancreatic or renal injury.

INITIAL APPROACH AND STABILIZATION

The initial approach to the trauma patient centers around stabilizing the patient's condition and determining the need for operative intervention. The initial contact must be focused on the most immediately life-threatening conditions.

Priority Diagnoses

Whatever the mechanism of injury, the priority diagnoses in abdominal trauma include violation of the peritoneal cavity or retroperitoneal space, rupture of a hollow viscus, solid organ disruption, and intraperitoneal hemorrhage or bacterial contamination from any source.

TABLE 43–1. Incidence of Organ Injury at Laparotomy Based on Mechanism of Injury at the Presley Regional Trauma Center, 1990–1993

	Penetrating (n = 1272)	Blunt (n = 539)
Liver	357 (28)*	275 (51)*
Spleen	94 (7)	251 (47)
Colon	296 (23)	29 (5)
Small bowel	369 (29)	37 (7)
Stomach	168 (13)	10 (2)
Duodenum	69 (5)	20 (4)
Pancreas	79 (6)	31 (6)

*Figures in parentheses are percentage of laparotomies in which that organ was found to be injured.

From Mattox KL, Feliciano DV, Moore EM: Trauma, 4th ed. New York, McGraw-Hill, 2000, p 585; with permission.

Rapid Assessment

- A brief description of the event and transport care by prehospital personnel is obtained.
- A description of events is obtained from patient. Specific mechanisms of injury are sought.
- Brief symptom review is obtained from the patient with a focus on any dyspnea and pain.
- A primary survey, with assessment of airway and ventilatory status, is followed closely by evaluation of circulation and perfusion. Vital signs are obtained, including pulse oximetry. Signs of advanced hemorrhagic shock are poor capillary refill, cold diaphoretic skin, and confusion.
- After airway, breathing, and circulation are assessed, inspection and palpation of the abdomen is done. Findings consistent with a "surgical abdomen" are sought (i.e., muscle rigidity or guarding, rebound tenderness, or gross distention). A brief neurologic assessment should follow.
- Any trauma patient must be completely disrobed to adequately assess all injuries.
- Particular focus on the most immediate life threats, such as uncontrolled thoracoabdominal hemorrhage, is paramount in the initial trauma physical examination.
- A common mistake in the initial trauma evaluation is extended focus on distracting injuries, such as open fractures, leading to delayed recognition and treatment of intra-abdominal injury.
- Neck, back, axillae, and buttocks are frequently neglected in examinations and need to be assessed for injury.

Early Intervention

1. Airway management is performed as necessary. Cervical stabilization must accompany any attempt at airway manipulation in the patient who has sustained blunt trauma.
2. Two large-bore, 14- to 16-gauge, peripheral intravenous lines are established, depending on field care and the patient's condition. Blood administration sets are included in any potentially serious injury.
3. Spinal immobilization, including thoracolumbar immobilization, is maintained in patients with blunt trauma with any neurologic abnormalities or pain along the spinal column. Patients unable to be evaluated because of altered mental status from head trauma or intoxicants are immobilized until radiographs of the axial skeleton are obtained.
4. Continuous cardiac monitoring and pulse oximetry are maintained on each trauma patient. Complete vital signs are measured every 5 to 10 minutes and after each therapeutic intervention.
5. A laboratory panel, including a complete blood cell count, electrolytes, glucose, coagulation studies, ethanol level, urinalysis, and pregnancy test (if appropriate) is generally ordered.
6. A blood sample for type and screen is sent to the laboratory from hemodynamically stable patients. More seriously injured patients are crossmatched for 6 units of packed blood cells. Uncrossmatched (O negative or O positive in males) blood is used in patients with any immediately life-threatening hemorrhage. As a rule, in patients with hypotension not responding rapidly to crystalloid infusion, rapid transfusion of uncrossmatched blood may be lifesaving.
7. In addition to cervical spine radiographs, anteroposterior portable chest radiographs are done to screen for life-threatening thoracic injury, such as pneumothorax, thoracic aorta transection, and diaphragmatic herniation. Anteroposterior pelvis radiographs are done to evaluate the bony pelvis structure for fracture or distraction, when indicated by patient case (pain, external injury, instability).
8. In the absence of massive facial trauma, a nasogastric tube should be placed for gastric decompression. The presence of blood or bile in the aspirate may suggest significant injury. Enteral contrast agents can easily be administered through a nasogastric tube for later studies if needed.
9. In males, examination for urethral or scrotal injury, and a prostate and rectal examination, must precede any urethral catheterization. The presence of an abnormally placed prostate, blood at the meatus, or pelvic instability suggests urethral injury. If urethral injury is possible, catheter placement is delayed until further evaluation is completed. In the male patient without obvious urethral injury (and in the majority of female patients), the catheter is placed, the urine is tested for the presence of blood, and fluid status is monitored by urinary output volumes (average, >0.50 mL/kg/hr).

CLINICAL ASSESSMENT

For patients who do not require immediate surgery (see Clinical Reasoning), a more complete clinical assessment, often referred to as the secondary survey, takes place. A directed history followed by a head-to-toe physical examination is carried out on all victims of major trauma. The goals of the clinical assessment are to establish the patient's clinical status before the injury, the nature and degree of forces involved, injury extent, and the patient's physiologic response to injury and to monitor evolving signs and symptoms.

History

1. *Patient symptoms.* The location, character, and severity of abdominal pain, as well as symptoms related to other organ systems, should be determined.
2. *Time of incident.* The treatment of life-threatening hemorrhage and irreversible shock is time dependent. Also, delays in treatment may allow for peritoneal signs to evolve or infection to be established.
3. *Mechanism of injury.*
   a. *Motor vehicle:* information on speed, size of vehicles, presence of passive restraints (airbag) or active restraints (seat belt), ejection from auto, and damage to passenger compartment is obtained. Prehospital providers are often equipped with photographic equipment to aid in this process.
   b. *Motorcycle:* whether there was separation of the rider from the bike and the presence of helmet and protective clothing should be ascertained.
   c. *Fall:* distance, secondary impacts, patient position at landing, and surface of landing should be evaluated.
   d. *Gunshot wound:* type of gun and distance from gun are documented, including the number of shots.
   e. *Penetrating injury:* length of weapon and direction of weapon are recorded.
4. *Causation.* Specific questions regarding the injury can elucidate the mechanism. Self-inflicted injury is often noted in the presence of alcohol or drug ingestion. The question, "What caused this injury to happen?" may reveal underlying medical illness or drug/toxin exposure.
5. *Allergy.* Particular attention should be paid to antibiotics, analgesics, anesthetics, and contrast agents.
6. *Medications.* Medications the patient may be taking may provide insight to other illnesses that may complicate care.
7. *Past medical history.* Particular attention is paid to previous heart and lung disease.
8. *Past surgical history.* Previous abdominal surgery may dictate the choice of diagnostic testing. Past abdominal surgery may preclude the use of diagnostic peritoneal lavage (DPL).
9. *Tetanus immunization history.* Immunization history is assessed, and the toxoid or immune globulin is given according to established guidelines.
10. *Most recent food or drink.* Knowing this information is pertinent for those in need of an anesthetic for procedures.

Physical Examination

After the initial evaluation of the ABCs (airway, breathing, and circulation), an evaluation for neurologic disability and a complete head-to-toe examination is performed. Aspects of the physical examination pertinent to abdominal injury are discussed here. Serial examination is essential for these patients, because any underlying pathologic processes may be evolving.

General Appearance. Skin temperature and color, capillary refill, and presence of diaphoresis are clues to the adequacy of perfusion and oxygenation. Hypoperfusion may be present with "normal" blood pressure. In an effort to maintain central circulation, blood pressure is maintained through profound peripheral vasoconstriction. Therefore, the patient with pallor, tachycardia, peripheral cooling, and poor capillary refill must be treated as a shock victim despite a "normal" blood pressure. The cause of blood loss can be intra-abdominal, thoracic, retroperitoneal, pelvic, and extremity hemorrhage.

Neck. Any evidence of spinal cord injury makes abdominal physical examination findings unreliable. Any spinal tenderness or neurologic deficits should lead to aggressive evaluation for occult intra-abdominal injury.

Chest. Concomitant thoracoabdominal injuries are not uncommon. Chest wall tenderness or crepitus from lower rib fractures suggest hepatic, splenic, or renal injuries. Decreased breath sounds at lung bases suggest the presence of hemothorax or diaphragmatic rupture. Bowel sounds heard in the chest also suggest diaphragmatic rupture. Abnormal heart tones, murmurs, and subxiphoid or sternal tenderness should lead the clinician to evaluate for pericardial blood or cardiac contusion.

Abdomen. The solitary abdominal examination is known to be insensitive, with a 69% accuracy, for the presence (or severity) of an underlying injury. Repeated examinations result in a higher rate of significant findings as the patient's clinical condition evolves.

Inspection. Findings of blunt trauma include abrasions or ecchymoses of the abdomen and flank. Linear abrasions consistent with seat belt use are of concern because one third of these patients have bowel or mesentery injury and may have a burst fracture of the lumbar spine (Chance fracture). Abdominal distention is indicative of free intraperitoneal air and a distended viscus.

Meticulous inspection for penetrating abdominal injury includes inspection of the genitourinary structures, gluteal cleft, and axillae.

Auscultation. Presence or absence of bowel sounds or abdominal bruits is rarely helpful in the evaluation of the traumatized patient.

Percussion. Tenderness elicited on percussion is a sign of true peritoneal irritation.

Palpation. Localized tenderness suggests injury to proximate structures. Guarding and rebound are signs of peritoneal irritation but can be unreliable predictors. Thirty percent of patients with intra-abdominal hemorrhage show no evidence of peritoneal irritation on initial examination. In stable patients, the decision regarding surgery or final disposition cannot be made with only one examination of the abdomen. Repeat palpation is necessary, because over time the abdomen will become tender when an injured organ is present. Intoxication, analgesics, and head and spinal cord injuries make the physical examination less reliable.

Rectal. The rectal examination value in the patient with blunt or penetrating abdominal trauma is unclear. Rectal tone evaluation for head-injured patients or those with spinal cord injuries may be useful. Assessment of the bulbocavernosus reflex may be of significance in the patient with sacral fractures, when sensory deficits (S2 to S4) are noted. Abnormal prostate findings (floating, change in location or shape) in males with pelvic fractures indicates the need for urologic evaluation. Acute rectal bleeding solely from abdominal trauma (blunt or penetrating) is a rare phenomenon.

Genitourinary. Trauma patients must receive a complete genitourinary examination. In males, this includes inspection of the urethral meatus, scrotum, and prostate. Blood at the urethral meatus suggests a urethral disruption, which in turn suggests significant abdominal or pelvic trauma. Before placing an indwelling catheter, further studies (e.g., urethrogram) may be necessary. In females, urethral injuries are less common but may occur. Vaginal bleeding may represent a vaginal laceration. Labial ecchymoses or lacerations may be present. Bimanual examination is an important part of the evaluation of injury in the female trauma patient.

Pelvis. Instability to gentle anterior and lateral compression of the pelvis suggests fracture or ligament disruption. Ecchymosis and soft tissue swelling of the pelvis with pain on passive movement suggests direct trauma. Four to six units of blood can be lost through the pelvic venous plexus, representing a significant cause of hemorrhagic shock.

Extremities. Penetrating injuries from gunshot wounds may result in a bullet embolism to a distal extremity. A femur or hip fracture indicates significant mechanical force and can represent an increased potential for abdominal injury.

Neurologic. The initial neurologic examination for trauma patients is relatively limited. The key determinations are the Glasgow Coma Scale score, pupillary function, and the presence of posturing or lateralizing signs. Spinal injury is reflected by a loss of sensation and muscular tone (flaccid paralysis), absent peripheral reflexes, absent rectal tone, and the presence of priapism. Spinal shock occurs after a high spinal cord injury, with loss of sympathetic response and vasomotor tone. Vascular dilation leads to hypotension without tachycardia and warm extremities with good refill. Hypotensive patients usually respond to 1 to 2 L of crystalloid infusion. Abdominal tenderness is a poor indicator of injury in patients with a spinal cord injury, owing to the interruption of visceral and peritoneal nerve pathways.

CLINICAL REASONING

During the initial assessment and stabilization, the decision-making process begins. Almost all traumatic abdominal injuries have the potential to be or become life threatening. Primary decision making is most often determined by the patient's hemodynamic status and the role of the abdominal injury in the context of the patient's total body trauma (Fig. 43–2). Patients can generally be placed into three categories of severity: (1) those in need of emergent operative intervention, (2) those requiring urgent evaluation and possible operative intervention, and (3) those who can be observed and discharged either after a short hospital or observation bed stay or directly from the emergency department.

Does the Patient Require Immediate Operation?

Hemodynamically unstable trauma patients are evaluated and resuscitated simultaneously. Patients who present unstable or become unstable in the emergency department, who develop diffuse tenderness suggestive of peritoneal irritation, or who develop abdominal distention require immediate surgical intervention (Table 43–2). Hemoperitoneum is most often caused by uncontrolled hemorrhage from liver, spleen, renal, or mesentery injury. Aggressive volume replacement with crystalloid and blood products is carried out concomitantly with efforts to immediately transfer the patient to the operating suite.

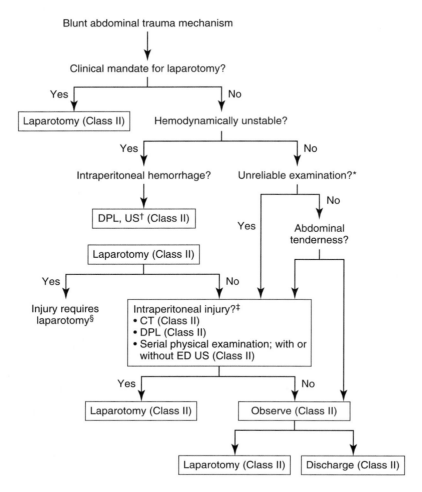

Blunt abdominal trauma mechanism

Clinical mandate for laparotomy?

Yes → Laparotomy (Class II)

No → Hemodynamically unstable?

Yes → Intraperitoneal hemorrhage?

DPL, US† (Class II)

Laparotomy (Class II)

Yes → Injury requires laparotomy§

No → Intraperitoneal injury?‡
• CT (Class II)
• DPL (Class II)
• Serial physical examination; with or without ED US (Class II)

No → Unreliable examination?*

No → Abdominal tenderness?

Yes / No

Yes → Laparotomy (Class II)

No → Observe (Class II)

Laparotomy (Class II)   Discharge (Class II)

*Can be unreliable because of closed-head injury, intoxicants, distracting injury, or spinal cord injury.
†Determined by unequivocal free intraperitoneal fluid on ultrasound or positive peritoneal aspiration on DPL.
‡One or more studies may be indicated.
§Need for laparotomy is based on clinical scenario, diagnostic studies, and institutional resources.

The **evidence for recommendations** is graded using the following scale:
Class I: Definitely recommended. Definitive, excellent evidence provides support. **Class II:** Acceptable and useful. Good evidence provides support. **Class III:** May be acceptable, possibly useful. Fair-to-good evidence provides support. **Indeterminate:** Continuing area of research.

FIGURE 43–2 • Clinical pathway: management of blunt abdominal trauma. CT, computed tomography; DPL, deep peritoneal lavage; ED, emergency department; US, ultrasound.

Penetrating injuries with evisceration of omentum or visible peritoneal contents are an indication for emergent surgery. The contents are not to be reduced into the peritoneal cavity. Sterile, moistened gauze is used to protect the contents en route to the operating suite.

Diaphragmatic rupture with impairment of adequate ventilation is an indication for immediate intervention. The airway and respiratory status must be serially evaluated, because distress occurs rapidly.

An object penetrating into the peritoneal cavity is left in place. Removal of any impaled object or weapon is avoided in the emergency department and accomplished in the operating suite.

Emergency department thoracotomy in the setting of blunt abdominal trauma is rarely advantageous. In a sudden, witnessed hemodynamic collapse, unresponsive to other resuscitative efforts, a thoracotomy with compression of the descending aorta may be considered. The outcome of this procedure is uniformly dis-

TABLE 43–2. Indications for Laparotomy

Blunt	Penetrating
Absolute	
Anterior abdominal injury and hypotension	Injury to abdomen, back, and flank with hypotension
Abdominal wall disruption	Abdominal tenderness
Peritonitis	Gastrointestinal evisceration
Free air on chest radiograph	Positive DPL
CT diagnosed injury requiring surgery (i.e., pancreatic transection, duodenal rupture)	High suspicion for transabdominal trajectory (gunshot wound)
	CT diagnosed injury requiring surgery (i.e., ureter or pancreas)
Relative	
Positive DPL or FAST in stable patient	Positive local wound exploration (stab wound)
Solid visceral injury in stable patient	
Hemoperitoneum on CT without clear source	

CT, computed tomography; DPL, diagnostic peritoneal lavage; FAST, focused assessment with sonography in trauma.
From Tintinalli JE, Kelen GD, Stapczynski JS: ACEP: Emergency Medicine: A Comprehensive Study Guide, 5th ed. New York, McGraw-Hill, 2000, p. 1706; with permission.

mal. In penetrating abdominal trauma with witnessed cardiovascular collapse, thoracotomy may be more successful. The chances are greater that a single vessel injury exists and may be controlled.

Does the Patient Require Urgent Evaluation and Possible Operation?

Hemodynamically stable patients with localized tenderness, ecchymoses, and abrasions over the abdomen, flank, and pelvis are candidates for further diagnostic evaluation. Repeat examinations may reveal progression of worrisome findings such as increased tenderness or distention. Patients with altered mental status or intoxication have unreliable physical findings. For patients undergoing urgent evaluation, the diagnostic tests discussed later may reveal the extent of injury and dictate the course of action.

Is Only Observation Required?

Patients with normal vital signs and minimal physical findings and with normal mentation not altered by drugs, alcohol, or head injury may be observed for a period of time. During this observation period, serial vital sign and abdominal evaluation occurs. A change in vital signs or development of tenderness requires further evaluation. The decision to observe or study a stable patient is often a matter of individual preference. Some physicians will obtain imaging studies for mechanism of injury alone, such as motor vehicle rollover or fall from a motorcycle.

Is the Injury Intra-abdominal, Retroperitoneal, or Both?

The retroperitoneal space can contain 1500 to 2500 mL of blood. It is poorly identified by the neurosensory system, and serious injuries in this location may manifest few localizing signs. Injury to the retroperitoneal organs, such as sections of duodenum, the pancreas, and kidneys, are of great concern in evaluating patients with abdominal trauma. When patients develop unexplained hemodynamic instability, retroperitoneal hemorrhage is high on the list of possible causes.

DIAGNOSTIC ADJUNCTS

The benefits from diagnostic testing in patients with abdominal trauma have steadily increased. More tests are providing definitive results, such as computed tomography, but they must always be placed in the context of the patient's injury and clinical condition. In most cases, a complete blood cell count and urinalysis are the minimum tests ordered. In patients with severe injury, the majority of the tests listed are ordered and additional, case-specific testing may be requested.

Laboratory Studies

Complete Blood Cell Count. A complete blood cell count is obtained for all patients with abdominal injuries. In unstable patients, a spun hematocrit is done in the emergency department, if available. This establishes a baseline hemoglobin and hematocrit reflecting oxygen-carrying capacity.

A normal result does not indicate blood loss or recent hemorrhage. A low value may represent premorbid anemia. White blood cell counts may be elevated as a result of the sympathetic discharge accompanying trauma. This is very common and renders the white blood cell count nondiagnostic initially. Platelet estimates may vary greatly and are useful only if they are under 100,000/mm^3. All such measurements represent "baseline values" and may be repeated during the continuing care of the patient to evaluate trends.

Urinalysis. Injury to the urinary tract is frequently associated with abdominal trauma. Gross blood found in the urine is considered significant and indicative of serious renal or genitourinary trauma. Improvements in the sensitivity of urine dipstick testing have made it a suitable screening test for microscopic hematuria. If there is gross blood or microscopic (dipstick) blood present in a patient with shock, radiographic testing is needed and may include intravenous pyelography, cystourethrography, or computed tomography (CT). Urinalysis should always be done in pediatric trauma patients, because renal injury may be present when 50 cells per high-powered field are present.

Amylase/Lipase. Pancreatic injury occurs in patients with either penetrating or blunt trauma. Initial amylase levels are not a sensitive or specific indicator of this injury. Lipase levels may be evaluated, but sensitivity and specificity for pancreatic trauma are not clear.

Other Laboratory Tests. Other laboratory tests are indicated as necessary: glucose, blood urea nitrogen, and creatinine determinations, coagulation studies, electrolytes, ethanol level, and toxicology screening. Blood type and screen or crossmatching is ordered if hemorrhage is suspected. The number of units crossmatched depends on the estimated severity of injury; 4 to 6 units is a reasonable first estimate. Blood lactate levels and base deficit testing may be used to follow the resuscitation status of patients in shock.

Radiologic Imaging

Most patients with major trauma and suspected abdominal injury will get a chest radiograph, cervical spine films, and pelvis radiograph. Additional imaging studies of the abdomen are ordered as necessary.

Plain Radiograph. In blunt abdominal trauma, plain abdominal radiographs are not often useful and may be omitted in lieu of more definitive studies. In penetrating trauma, anteroposterior and lateral views are used to locate projectiles, foreign bodies, or free air. The location of the skin wound with respect to the projectile may aid in identifying the injured structure and is accomplished by a radiopaque skin marker placed over injury site.

Computed Tomography. CT has been used routinely since the early 1980s for evaluation of suspected intra-abdominal injuries. The patient must be hemodynamically stable to leave the emergency department and undergo CT. Patients who are unstable should be evaluated with ultrasound and/or DPL during the resuscitation or taken directly to the operating suite.

Advantages of CT include specificity, sensitivity, and accuracy equal to DPL without its invasive nature in severely injured patients. Hemoperitoneum of as little as 100 mL can be detected during scanning from diaphragm to symphysis pubis so as to evaluate the entire abdomen. Specific intraperitoneal and retroperitoneal organ injuries are reliably imaged. CT can direct the need for exploratory laparotomy versus conservative management, when combined with the clinical examination. In the setting of significant retroperitoneal hemorrhage and pelvic fracture, CT detects injury where DPL cannot.

Disadvantages of CT include the need to move the patient from the resuscitation area to an imaging suite, the potential of recurrent hemodynamic instability, and the use of ionizing radiation. Uncooperative patients are difficult to evaluate with this test modality and may require sedation. To optimize this test, both oral and intravenous contrast media may be used; however, an oral contrast agent does not necessarily provide a significant benefit in the trauma CT evaluation and may lead to emesis. Injuries to small bowel, mesentery, ureter, pancreas, and the diaphragm are difficult to diagnose with CT, and early findings can be missed. DPL may be considered after CT if there is a high suspicion for a bowel injury and a negative CT or if the CT shows fluid that may not be blood (e.g., ascites). If DPL is done before CT, the radiologist must be made aware of the procedure (remaining fluid).

Ultrasonography. Emergency department ultrasound scanning in the setting of blunt abdominal trauma has demonstrated value, but acceptance into emergency practice in the United States has been slow. Concerns about operator-dependent results and less accuracy in specific organ injury, with comparison to CT, have been raised.

Advantages include portable equipment allowing the patient to remain in the resuscitation suite for imaging, a noninvasive evaluation tool, a completion time of 5 to 15 minutes, and easy serial examination of the patient. The cost of ultrasound evaluation is significantly less than that of CT and DPL.

The indications for emergent ultrasonography are broad, including any significant mechanism with signs of abdominal injury such as pain, tenderness, or skin abrasions. For instance, a driver's-side impact would increase suspicion for splenic or renal injury and a patient with altered mental status would be considered for abdominal imaging because of unreliable examination.

Ultrasonography is noninvasive when compared with diagnostic peritoneal lavage and contrast medium–enhanced CT. Free intraperitoneal fluid of 500 mL or more can be detected. Pericardial, pleural, and retroperitoneal fluid may also be assessed. Ultrasonography has been reported to have a sensitivity of 88% and a specificity of 98% in diagnosing traumatic intra-abdominal injuries (accuracy, 97%). Limiting factors in accuracy of ultrasonography include the presence of subcutaneous emphysema, morbid obesity, and significant bowel gas.

The specific ultrasound technique for abdominal trauma, FAST (*focused assessment with sonography in trauma*), relies heavily on the presence of free fluid (i.e., hemoperitoneum) to identify injury. The FAST examination is used to answer the question "Is free fluid present in the peritoneal cavity?" There are views of Morison's pouch (hepatorenal), splenorenal recess, and the pelvis (pouch of Douglas) to answer this question. A fourth view, subxiphoid, is used to determine fluid in the pericardial space (Fig. 43–3). Subcapsular injury to the spleen, liver, and kidney can be missed because free fluid is not present. Pancreatic, diaphragmatic, and hollow viscus injuries are difficult to assess with this technique. This technique cannot be used to completely rule out a significant intra-abdominal injury, but that is not what the FAST examination is intended to do. Positive identification of free fluid (likely blood) increases the confidence of the surgeon that surgery is necessary and decreases the need for additional testing (with CT or DPL).

Although ultrasonography is dependent on operator experience and training, many studies show that emergency medicine and surgical residents alike can acquire competence and expertise with didactic and practical teaching. The number of studies and didactic sessions to acquire credentialing remains a topic of controversy among emergency physicians, surgeons, and radiologists.

Intravenous Pyelography. If renal injury is suggested, a one-shot intravenous pyelogram can be used to identify the presence of, and function

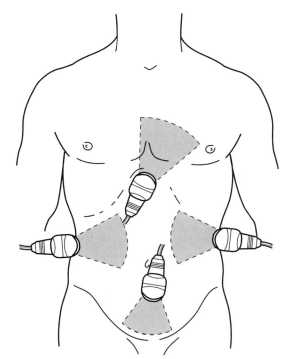

FIGURE 43–3 • Transducer positions for the FAST examination. The transducer positions are pericardial, right and upper left quadrants, and the pouch of Douglas. (Redrawn from Sisley AC, Rozycki GS, Ballard RB, et al: Rapid detection of traumatic effusion using surgeon-performed ultrasonography. J Trauma 1998; 44:292; with permission.)

of, both kidneys. Extravasation of contrast material from the kidney or ureter suggests injury and the need for operative intervention.

Retrograde Cystourethrography. Blood at the urethral meatus, gross hematuria, pelvic fracture, straddle injury, and high-riding prostrate are indicative of urethral or bladder injury. Retrograde cystourethrography is carried out before catheter placement. Extravasation of dye from the urethra or bladder signifies serious injury and requires urologic consultation.

Angiography. Angiography has been the gold standard for evaluating vascular injury. It is not commonly used for initial assessment of abdominal trauma because most patients with major vascular injury require rapid surgical exploration. It may be used to evaluate aortic, inguinal, pelvic, or renal vasculature. It is the method of choice for assessment of patients with uncontrolled retroperitoneal bleeding from pelvic fractures or intraparenchymal (spleen, liver) bleeding from laceration; embolization may be done in the angiography suite.

Diagnostic Peritoneal Lavage

DPL has historically been the procedure of choice in the evaluation of traumatic abdominal injuries. The advent of ultrasonography and CT has led to more selective use of DPL. The primary indication for DPL is in the patient with multiple traumatic injuries and hemodynamic instability. The procedure is performed in a resuscitation suite where continued evaluation and treatment is ongoing. The only absolute contraindication to the DPL is the existence of an indication for immediate exploratory laparotomy, such as a gunshot wound to the abdomen or evisceration. Relative contraindications include pediatric patients, prior abdominal surgery, or advanced pregnancy. Both the stomach and bladder should be decompressed by nasogastric tube and catheter placement before beginning DPL to prevent organ puncture or injury.

The techniques for DPL have been extensively evaluated. The choice of approach depends on patient body habitus, pregnancy, clinical situation (i.e., presence of a pelvic fracture), and operator/institutional preference. The techniques are classified as opened, semi-closed, and closed percutaneous. They can be performed above or below the umbilicus.

Previous abdominal surgeries, coagulopathy, and pregnancy are some common indications for the open technique. Direct visualization is essential to avoid complications and false-positive results. Suspected pelvic fracture with a large retroperitoneal hematoma is better evaluated with the supraumbilical approach because the hematoma often spreads along the linea alba, producing false-positive results. Morbid obesity is often an indication for a closed/percutaneous technique because extensive dissection and local anesthetic infiltration can escalate procedure morbidity. CT may be indicated after DPL if the results are indeterminate and the suspicion of injury is high for retroperitoneal bleeding (i.e., renal injury or duodenal injury). If the DPL is positive, the patient is stable, and more information is desired before surgery, CT may also be done.

As the established standard for the determination of intra-abdominal bleeding, DPL is highly sensitive (indicating bleeding in 97% of cases) and 97% accurate, with as little as 30 mL of blood present, but is nonspecific (not able to identify the bleeding site). Criteria for interpreting the DPL include evaluation of red blood cells, white blood cells, and effluent (Table 43–3). The major advantages of this test are its speed, cost-effectiveness, reliability, and complication rate of 1%. It does not delineate the location or severity of injury and may miss significant retroperitoneal injuries, diaphragmatic injury, and bowel or bladder injuries that do not result in significant bleeding. A false-negative result may occur if previous surgery or infection has resulted in significant abdominal adhesions, preventing blood from freely entering the peritoneal cavity.

EXPANDED DIFFERENTIAL DIAGNOSIS

Evaluation of suspected abdominal trauma requires a thorough understanding of the possible

---

TABLE 43–3. Interpretive Criteria for Diagnostic Peritoneal Lavage

Test Results are Considered Positive If:

1. Immediate return of 10 mL of gross blood or intestinal contents with initial aspiration
2. RBC count >100,000 cells/mL in blunt trauma
3. RBC count >10,000 cells/mL in abdominal stab wound*
4. RBC count >5000 cells/mL in penetrating chest trauma
5. WBC count >500 cells/mL
6. If lavage fluid exits urinary, nasogastric, or tube thoracostomy tubes
7. Urine, feces, bile, or particulate matter is found in the lavage fluid

Test Results are Considered Indeterminate If:

1. RBCs total >50,000 cells/mL and <100,000 cells/mL (blunt trauma)
2. WBCs total >100 cells/mL and <500 cells/mL
3. Less than 600 mL of lavage fluid return

Test Results are Considered Negative If:

1. RBCs total <50,000 cells/mL (blunt trauma)
2. WBCs total <100 cells/mL

RBCs, red blood cells; WBCs, white blood cells.
*If gunshot wounds of the abdomen are assessed using diagnostic peritoneal lavage, the RBC count considered positive falls to 5000 cells/mL.

anatomic structures involved. The findings on physical examination may differ depending on the site of injury and which pain pathways are stimulated. Solid organs may be injured, yet bleeding may be contained within the fibrous capsule, leading to more localized findings. Hollow viscus injuries are classically difficult to diagnose. Perforation caused by concussive effect, sheer effect, or penetrating injury leads to spillage of bowel contents and subsequent peritoneal irritation and may take hours or days to present. The mechanism of initial trauma is vital to formulating a differential diagnosis. Table 43–4 lists signs and symptoms of selected major organ injuries and guidelines for diagnosis and management.

PRINCIPLES OF MANAGEMENT

The approach to any traumatically injured patient begins with the ABCs of airway management, breathing (ventilatory control), and evaluation of circulation (volume status and perfusion). In any unstable patient, evaluation and resuscitation occur simultaneously. In patients with intra-abdominal injury, the decision for immediate surgical intervention is of primary concern. Many institutions have general algorithms for evaluation of the patient with abdominal trauma. The following guidelines are useful when tempered with the experience.

Blunt Abdominal Trauma

Figure 43–2 presents an algorithm for the management of blunt abdominal trauma. Emphasis is increasing on ultrasonography to become the modality of first choice in the trauma patient evaluation. Ultrasonography can be used at the bedside, and resuscitation of the unstable patient continues while the study is completed. In the patient with a distended, tense, rigid abdomen, preparations for exploratory laparotomy accompany the resuscitation. In stable patients, selected liver and spleen injuries, as diagnosed by CT, can be conservatively managed without operative intervention.

Penetrating Abdominal Trauma

Surgical exploration is the rule in virtually all gunshots wounds to the abdomen, because of the high frequency of organ damage. Occasionally, a penetrating wound to the chest extends to the peritoneum; however, abdominal findings may be absent. After management of the chest wound, DPL can be performed. The red blood cell count criteria for a positive DPL is 5000 cells/mm^3 (penetrating injury of the diaphragm).

Stab wounds are evaluated differently than gunshot wounds. Indications for exploratory laparotomy are signs of hemodynamic instability, peritoneal irritation, evisceration, diaphragmatic injury, gastrointestinal bleeding, and implement in situ. Local wound exploration to visualize potential penetration of posterior fascia and peritoneum is used to evaluate the stable patient. If the peritoneum is breached, surgeons may proceed with exploratory laparotomy or use DPL or CT to further evaluate the injuries. A grossly positive DPL or red blood cell count of more than 100,000 cells/mm^3 indicates serious intra-abdominal injury. These patients undergo immediate surgery. If the red blood cell count is indeterminate, close observation with serial abdominal examinations can be considered. Hollow viscus injuries are likely to yield red blood cell counts of less than 100,000/mm^3. There is no substitute for close observation and clinical judgment.

Stab wounds to the flank and back are evaluated differently because retroperitoneal injuries occur. DPL is less sensitive in these cases, and CT with oral, intravenous, and rectal contrast medium enhancement evaluates genitourinary and colonic structures for injury.

Other Measures in Management

Abdominal traumatic injuries with skin abrasions or penetrating injury are treated with tetanus prophylaxis. Patients with penetrating injuries and those requiring emergent surgery are also treated with appropriate antibiotics. Prophylactic antibiotics (e.g., clindamycin plus gentamicin, or second-generation cephalosporin plus anaerobic coverage), with capability of combating bowel organisms, have been shown to reduce the morbidity of penetrating wounds. These medications are important because they may be overlooked after the patient leaves the emergency department. The skin wounds may be closed primarily with sutures if they are clean, sharp, and not devitalized. If so, they can be left to heal by secondary intention or closed over drains. Occasionally, the skin wound from a gunshot can be excised and closed primarily in the operating room.

UNCERTAIN DIAGNOSIS

Uncertain diagnosis is common in abdominal trauma. Aggressive stabilization and thorough clinical and radiologic assessment are often insufficient to determine underlying conditions that may take hours or days to evolve. Repeated clinical assessment, monitored observation, and admission for further evaluation are the mainstays

TABLE 43–4. Differential Diagnosis of Abdominal Injury by Major Organs

Injury	Clinical Signs and Symptoms	Possible Associated Injuries	Diagnosis and Management
Liver injury	Pain or tenderness in right upper quadrant Signs of hypovolemic shock Referred pain to right shoulder from diaphragmatic irritation	Lacerated bowel Right lower rib fractures Hepatic vascular injury Renal injury	Liver injury can range from minor parenchymal injury with confined subcapsular bleeding to massive organ injury with uncontrolled hemorrhage. Significant injury or hemorrhage may be determined in hemodynamically stable patients by peritoneal lavage or CT. CT may delineate extent of injury, but the management of minor injuries with minimal bleeding remains controversial. Significant injury or bleeding requires surgery; in children, conservative expectant management is favored whenever possible. Surgical consultation is indicated for all suspected liver injuries. Patients with subcapsular hematomas are protected from further trauma that might result in rupture of the capsule.
Splenic injury	Tenderness and pain in left upper quadrant Kehr's sign: referred pain to left shoulder from diaphragmatic irritation Muscle spasm, guarding, rigidity Signs of hypoperfusion	Stomach, bowel, and pancreatic injury Renal injury Diaphragmatic injury Left lower rib fractures 20% of fractures of 9th to 10th ribs have associated splenic injury	Splenic injury may range from relatively minor parenchymal injury with confined bleeding within a subcapsular hematoma to complete parenchymal or vascular disruption with uncontrolled hemorrhage. Splenic injuries are the most common cause of intraperitoneal bleeding from blunt abdominal trauma. Enlarged spleen may cause medial displacement of the gastric bubble on plain film. CT can delineate the extent of injury and bleeding and is a useful adjunct in hemodynamically stable patients. A splenectomy is required for unstable patients or those with massive injury. A splenorrhaphy may be attempted in less damaged spleens, and minor injuries (particularly in children) may be treated conservatively by close observation and expectant management.
Pancreatic injury	Mild epigastric pain and tenderness that may decrease initially and then worsen after several hours Guarding and muscle spasm (relatively rare) Signs of hypovolemic shock (may be delayed) Ileus Severe back pain	Seat belt–associated injuries Duodenal injury	Lack of significant acute physical findings from this retroperitoneal structure often make initial diagnosis difficult. A high amylase level in lavage fluid or evidence on CT coupled with a high degree of suspicion may result in early diagnosis. Undiagnosed injury may result in necrosis with subsequent pancreatitis, delayed bleeding, peritonitis, or cyst formation. No definitive diagnostic test exists for early and accurate diagnoses of these injuries following injury. Requires surgical intervention when suspected. High mortality rate (15%–20%) due to other injuries.
Ruptured or perforated gastrointestinal tract (hollow viscus)	Epigastric pain, tenderness, gastrointestinal pain, or guarding; blood in nasogastric fluid or bowels Ileus and distention Free air in peritoneum	Mesenteric vascular injury Solid organ injury (liver and spleen) Most often due to penetrating injury	Free intraperitoneal rupture or air on plain film is presumed to be a perforation of the gastrointestinal tract. These patients require exploratory laparotomy. Immediate symptoms and physical findings may be unremarkable, but over 48–72 hours gradually increasing pain and tenderness may indicate peritonitis from occult injury. Significant injury from blunt trauma may be difficult to diagnose initially when the injury involves the retroperitoneal portion of the duodenum. Contrast duodenography, CT, or exploratory laparotomy may aid in the diagnosis. Perforation in blunt trauma occurs at the points of fixed attachment, particularly the duodenum. Patients with suspected bowel perforation are given antibiotics in anticipation of surgery and a nasogastric tube to remove gastrointestinal contents. Bile or urine in peritoneal lavage fluid suggests biliary perforation or genitourinary disruption; both require surgical consultation and management.
Inferior vena cava	More often due to penetrating trauma Signs of hypoperfusion Signs of retroperitoneal hematoma Abdominal distention, tenderness, and rigidity	Bowel perforation Spinal cord injury Retroperitoneal hematoma	In suspected inferior vena cava injury, intravenous access for fluid resuscitation is placed above the diaphragm. Vascular injury may cause significant hemorrhage and needs both aggressive resuscitation and immediate surgery. This injury is frequently catastrophic; DPL and CT may show hemorrhage while angiography and exploratory laparotomy define the extent of injury. Aggressive fluid resuscitation with acute surgical repair is necessary.

Injury	Clinical Findings	Associated Injuries	Management
Perforation of aorta or vascular rupture	Abdominal distention, tenderness, and rigidity Bruits and lost or decreased distal pulses Signs of hypoperfusion	Bowel perforation Spinal fractures	Emergency department thoracotomy to access the aorta and control bleeding may be required in catastrophic bleeding. The use of PASG to minimize bleeding is controversial.
Genitourinary (kidneys, ureters, urethra, and bladder)	Flank or abdominal pain and tenderness Flank swelling or ecchymosis Blood at urethral orifice Hematuria (95%) Suprapubic tenderness or ecchymosis Displaced prostate Retroperitoneal hemorrhage Distended bladder Suprapubic mass from blood or urine	Pelvic fracture (e.g., 90% of bladder injuries are associated with a pelvic fracture) Vascular injuries Spinal fractures Liver and spleen injuries	Gross hematuria, anuria, and intraperitoneal injury. Suspected renal injury can be evaluated by IVP, angiography, and contrast CT. Suspected urethral injury should be evaluated by urethrogram before placement of an indwelling urinary catheter. Suspected bladder injury or disruption can be evaluated by cystogram, cystoscopy, and CT. In renal injury due to blunt trauma the bleeding is usually confined by Gerota's fascia and the capsule. Therefore, if bleeding is limited, patients may be managed conservatively with supportive care and observation. Penetrating renal injury with uncontrolled bleeding or renal vascular injury usually requires surgical management. Transected or damaged ureters require surgical repair or external drainage; intraperitoneal bladder disruption will require surgical repair; retroperitoneal rupture needs urinary diversion with suprapubic cystostomy. Urethral injury is frequently managed conservatively; however, urinary diversion must be provided by a carefully placed indwelling urinary catheter or suprapubic cystostomy. Urologic consultation is obtained before any procedure.
Fractured pelvis	Pain and tenderness in pelvis Referred pain to abdomen or back Palpable fractures, crepitus, or instability Signs of hypoperfusion or retroperitoneal bleeding	Urethral, bladder, and rectal injury Vascular injury and retroperitoneal bleeding Spinal fractures Uterine and vaginal injury	Patients with significant blunt abdominal injury and the possibility of a pelvic fracture require pelvic radiographs. The pelvis is a ring structure and usually fractures in more than one place. Pelvic fractures may result in uncontrolled life-threatening retroperitoneal hemorrhage and may require aggressive fluid resuscitation and early consultation. Pelvic stabilization with PASG or external fixation may minimize pain and bleeding. Uncontrolled bleeding may require angiography and selective embolization.
Diaphragmatic injury	Ventilation compromise from herniation of intra-abdominal contents Bowel sounds in thorax Hypovolemic shock Stomach, bowel, or nasogastric tube in thorax on chest radiograph Thoracic aspiration of bile, gastric contents, or feces or drainage from chest tube; 95% of lesions are on left side	Liver and spleen injury Renal injury Lung and thoracic injury Stomach and bowel injury	No single diagnostic test will identify all diaphragmatic injuries. Plain chest radiographs with stomach, bowel, or nasogastric tube in the thorax, or CT with thoracic windows, and enhanced upper gastrointestinal radiographs may help diagnose these injuries. Thoracic aspiration of bowel contents or drainage from a chest tube indicates diaphragmatic or esophageal rupture. Surgical exploration may be required to diagnose these injuries, and, when identified, these injuries need surgical repair. Stabilization focuses on maintaining adequate ventilation.
Abdominal wall injury	Pain or tenderness localized to traumatized area Hematoma or localized swelling Increased pain with stress of rectus muscles	Any intra-abdominal injury Liver or spleen injury	Abdominal wall injury is often difficult to differentiate from underlying or concomitant intra-abdominal injury and, therefore, is regarded as a diagnosis of exclusion. Conservative management is appropriate. Significant hematomas of the abdominal wall and along the rectus sheath can complicate DPL or lead to false-positive results. CT can determine the presence of a significant soft tissue hematoma, which may result from direct injury or dissection from retroperitoneal bleeding.
Uterine and ovarian injury	Vaginal bleeding or lacerations Lower abdominal pain, tenderness, and guarding Tender or enlarged uterus or ovaries on bimanual examination Hypovolemic shock, particularly from uterine trauma when pregnant (abruptio placentae or uterine rupture)	Other intra-abdominal injury Pelvic fractures Pelvic vascular injuries Bladder and urethral injury	Uterine disruption or injury may result in significant bleeding and may require hysterectomy. During pregnancy, blunt abdominal trauma may cause a placental abruption, and patients with abdominal pain or vaginal bleeding require obstetric consultation and fetal monitoring. Vaginal lacerations are identified by direct examination with a speculum. They frequently require surgical repair.

CT, computed tomography; DPL, diagnostic peritoneal lavage; IVP, intravenous pyelography; PASG, pneumatic antishock garment.

of unraveling the uncertainty of abdominal trauma.

SPECIAL CONSIDERATIONS

Pediatric Patients

Children with abdominal trauma are diagnostic and therapeutic challenges. Trauma care providers must be familiar with the challenges of intravenous access techniques, nasogastric and urinary catheterization, and airway management in the pediatric population. Psychological stressors of caring for injured children and their families should be anticipated.

Injury patterns in the pediatric patient differ from those in the adult. Head injuries are far more common. Cervical injuries tend to be located higher in the cervical spine. Chest injuries are frequently pulmonary contusions without rib fracture, secondary to the elasticity of the chest wall. Abdominal contents are less well protected by the rib cage in pediatric patients, and splenic and hepatic injuries are more common. The majority of blunt abdominal trauma is caused by motor vehicle and vehicle-pedestrian crashes. Handle-bar bicycle injuries, lap belt injuries, and nonaccidental trauma injuries are situations more unique to the pediatric population. Pediatric abdominal injuries are more frequently managed by noninvasive techniques, such as abdominal serial examinations, ultrasonography and CT, and fluid resuscitation. CT is used for solid organ, retroperitoneal, and peritoneal evaluation. Ultrasonography is used for evaluation of the hemoperitoneum, as in adults. Laboratory testing continues to have a significant role in identifying intraabdominal injuries. Volume resuscitation must be carefully monitored. DPL has a primary role in the unstable patient with multiple injuries when ultrasonography is nondiagnostic. Early pediatric surgical consultation is recommended.

Pregnant Patients

The emergency physician must attend to the needs of both the mother and the fetus. As a rule, the best care for the mother will ultimately be the best for the fetus. Trauma to the fetus and uterus is unusual in the first trimester, and patients in the third trimester are at the highest risk for complications. Vaginal bleeding, abdominal pain or cramping, decreased fetal movement, or changes in fetal heart rate are signs of uterine injury and fetal distress. Aggressive volume resuscitation is indicated, even when minimal instability is noted. The intravascular space is expanded in the preg-

nant patient (35%), and hemodynamic decompensation can occur rapidly in these patients. Motor vehicle crashes, falls, and domestic violence are among the causes of trauma in the pregnant patient. The pregnant patient should be placed in the left lateral decubitus position, or the uterus should be tipped left to relieve pressure on the inferior vena cava. Radiographs are used as indicated and should not be withheld because of concerns regarding ionizing radiation. Indications for emergency laparotomy are the same as in the nonpregnant patient (see Table 43–2).

Even apparently minor trauma, such as a fall, can result in significant issues in the third trimester of pregnancy. Ultrasonography and 6 hours of fetal monitoring are recommended as a standard of care when uterine trauma cannot be ruled out by other means. Psychological concerns of the expectant parents should be addressed freely and as needed in the emergency department. Most pregnant patients with suspected trauma require the insight and guidance of an obstetric consultant. Fetal viability is recognized at 23 to 26 weeks' gestation.

Elderly Patients

Elderly patients with abdominal trauma are more difficult to diagnose, require more diagnostic adjuncts, and have a higher morbidity and mortality than younger patients. Underlying chronic medical problems and medication use can complicate presentation and resuscitation and alter the physiologic response to injury. The elderly often do not develop peritoneal findings even with spillage of blood or bowel contents. The elderly are more likely to suffer complications during hospitalization, such as pulmonary compromise and changes in mental status. The emergency physician should take a conservative approach when determining the need to admit these patients for observation and to request surgical consultation.

DISPOSITION AND FOLLOW-UP

Disposition of patients with abdominal trauma falls into three categories:

1. Direct transfer from the emergency department to the operating suite
2. Hospital admission to an inpatient setting for observation and nonoperative management of selected hepatic, renal, and splenic injuries
3. Emergency department or observation bed placement

Direct Transfer to the Operating Room

Immediate surgical consultation is required for patients with obvious lesions, hemodynamic instability refractory to resuscitation efforts, and/or findings consistent with a surgical abdomen (see Table 43–2). The timing of transfer is made in consultation with the surgeon. Patients with injuries needing care not available at the receiving hospital require transfer to another facility for higher-level services.

Hospital Admission

- Patients requiring peritoneal lavage
- Patients with unexplained pain, tenderness, or vomiting not resolved by a period of observation
- Patients with intra-abdominal injuries amenable to nonoperative approach (e.g., subcapsular splenic injuries, minor liver lacerations)
- Significant mental status changes precluding a reliable examination
- Patients with associated head injury
- Patients with stab wounds or gunshot wounds (rarely) with suspected peritoneal violation but not requiring immediate operation

Observation

Many emergency departments are developing units to rapidly evaluate and treat patients who meet certain low-risk criteria. Minor trauma protocols are becoming more common. Although these protocols are specific to their institutions, common points include the following:

- A negative abdominal radiographic study (e.g., ultrasound, CT)

- Normal mental status
- Normal vital signs
- Absence of major comorbidities, such as coagulopathy or severe heart, kidney, or lung disease
- Reliable social/home situation and adequate follow-up medical care
- Superficial stab wounds in which the peritoneum is clearly intact after local exploration

These patients may be discharged after a period of observation and repeated assessment. Patients need to be advised to return if their clinical condition worsens or they have any concerns.

FINAL POINTS

- The boundaries of the abdomen extend from the nipple line to the inguinal creases.
- The liver, spleen, and small bowel are the most commonly injured abdominal organs.
- Blunt traumatic injuries with retroperitoneal hemorrhage can be difficult to diagnose.
- The management of abdominal trauma still begins with the ABCs: airway, breathing, and circulation.
- Gunshot wounds almost always require operative intervention.
- Failure to adequately and rapidly restore lost blood volume is the most common resuscitation error in management of abdominal trauma patients.
- Injuries to the small bowel and pancreas are difficult to diagnose and are causes of late mortality in abdominal trauma patients of all age groups.
- Ultrasonography and CT have superseded DPL for initial diagnosis of intra-abdominal injury except in selected cases.

CASE *Study*

A rescue squad was called to the scene of a motor vehicle accident involving a 33-year-old male driver whose car collided head on with a truck.

On arrival at the scene and after initial assessment, the rescue squad radioed the base station and reported the patient was awake and alert but intoxicated and was complaining of abdominal pain. He was the driver of a medium-size car that collided head on with a tractor trailer 15 minutes earlier. Each was traveling at approximately 35 miles per hour. The windshield and steering wheel were intact, and the patient was wearing a seat belt. Vital signs were a pulse of 130 beats per minute, respirations of 18 breaths

per minute, and blood pressure of 100/55 mm Hg. The lifesquad medic placed the patient on nasal O_2 at 6 L/min and started a 16-gauge intravenous line with a rapid infusion of isotonic crystalloid. A cardiac monitor was placed, and the patient was transported to the emergency department.

Although the patient appeared alert and "stable," the severity of the accident, the complaint of abdominal pain associated with an increased pulse rate, and the presence of intoxication raise the suspicion of a severe intra-abdominal injury with significant hemorrhage. Any changes during transport indicate further instability and must be reported.

Continued on following page

In the emergency department, the patient is alert. He complains of abdominal pain but no chest pain, shortness of breath, or neurologic symptoms. The rescue squad indicates the patient has had no change in his symptoms or vital signs during transport. The patient is undressed, and vital signs are taken. His pulse rate is 130 beats per minute and blood pressure is 100/60 mm Hg. A cardiac monitor is placed. A primary trauma examination is carried out, revealing no upper airway or chest injury. The pulse volume is diminished, and capillary refill is slowed. The abdomen is tender, but no peritoneal signs are present. All four extremities are intact, and there are no neurologic findings. A second intravenous line is started with a 16-gauge catheter followed by a rapid infusion of 2000 mL of saline. Blood samples are sent to the laboratory, including a type and crossmatch request for 6 units of blood. A nasogastric tube is placed. A portable chest film shows no hemothorax or pneumothorax, and the mediastinum is of normal width and configuration. After an unremarkable rectal examination, a Foley catheter is placed. A urine sample tested for blood is negative. A call goes out for the trauma surgeon.

The emergency department approach to the trauma patient is systematic and thorough. The initial evaluation and stabilization are carried out concurrently. In spite of the obvious abdominal injury, in all cases of trauma the airway examination begins the resuscitation phase of care. Mistakes are made when the sequence is broken and inordinate attention is paid to the clearly evident, but not life-threatening, injuries, such as a bleeding extremity. The change in vital signs (fall in blood pressure) in a short time period is typical of young patients with potential hemorrhagic shock. Aggressive stabilization efforts, in this case primarily volume resuscitation and anticipating the need for a surgeon and blood product replacement, are necessary to prevent further hypoperfusion and complications.

After the rapid, primary evaluation and initial resuscitation, a secondary, more detailed survey is performed. No other injuries are found. The patient continues to have diffuse upper abdominal tenderness with some guarding. After the infusion of 2 L of saline, the pulse rate falls from 130 to 110 beats per minute and the blood pressure rises to 110/70 mm Hg. The extremities remain warm, and the patient continues to be alert. Laboratory results include a hematocrit of 38% and an ethanol level of 0.8 mg/mL; renal function is normal. Because the patient has shown some improvement, clinically, the decision is made to obtain a CT of the abdomen in consultation with the surgeon.

Even though the patient showed some signs of hemodynamic instability, the improvement in his vital signs does not force an immediate operation. Because a CT will reveal occult retroperitoneal blood and accurately delineate the type and extent of most intra-abdominal injuries, it is a good test to perform at this time. The greatest risk is sending the patient to an imaging suite. The patient must be monitored at all times and accompanied by an emergency department or critical care nurse or physician.

The CT of the abdomen shows a small laceration of the left lobe of the liver with free blood in the peritoneum. The spleen, retroperitoneal space, and other organs appear normal. On return from the imaging suite, the patient remains stable but has a persistent tachycardia of 110 beats per minute. A repeat hematocrit is ordered and returns as 27%, and 2 units of crossmatched packed red blood cells are administered. The patient is transferred to the intensive care unit for observation and care by the surgeon.

The early response of the patient to fluids and the CT has allowed the surgeon to determine that the patient can be managed conservatively without operation. Blood is usually administered when a trauma victim's hematocrit acutely falls below 30% in the presence of persistent tachycardia after crystalloid infusion. Type-specific blood may be given to avoid the delay of a full crossmatch. That was not necessary in this case. The risk of administering type-specific blood is very low, and, because of its almost immediate availability in large medical centers, there is no need to give O negative, the universal donor type.

The patient continued to improve. He did well and was discharged after 7 days of hospitalization.

Bibliography

TEXTS

Ferrera PC, Colucciello SA, Marx JA, et al: Trauma Management: An Emergency Medicine Approach. St. Louis, CV Mosby, 2001.

Mattox KL, Feliciano DV, Moore EE: Trauma, 4th ed. New York, McGraw-Hill, 2000.

JOURNAL ARTICLES

Brown CK, Dunn KA, Wilson K: Diagnostic evaluation of patients with blunt abdominal trauma: A decision analysis. Acad Emerg Med 2000; 7:385–396.

Ferrada R, Birolini D: New concepts in the management of patients with penetrating abdominal wounds. Surg Clin North Am 1999; 79:1331–1356.

Holmes JF, Sokolove PE, Brant WE, et al: Identification of children with intra-abdominal injuries after blunt trauma. Ann Emerg Med 2002; 39:500–509.

Ingleman JE, Plewa MC, Okasinski R, et al: Emergency physician use of ultrasonography in blunt trauma. Acad Emerg Med 1996; 3:931–937.

Jones R: Clinical use of ultrasound in thoracoabdominal trauma. Trauma Rep 2000; 1 (Suppl): 1–16.

Knudson MM, Maull KL: Nonoperative management of solid organ injuries: Past, present, and future. Surg Clin North Am 1999; 79:1357–1371.

Livingston DH, Lavery RF, Passannate MT, et al: Admission or observation is not necessary after a negative abdominal computed tomographic scan in patients with suspected blunt abdominal trauma: Results of a prospective, multi-institutional trial. J Trauma 1998; 44:273–280.

Kendall JL: Emergency imaging for the 21st century: where does ultrasound fit in? Emerg Med Pract 2001; 3:1–24.

Marx JA: Blunt abdominal trauma: Priorities, procedures, and pragmatic thinking. Emerg Med Pract 2001; 3(5): 1–28.

Malhotra AK, Fabian TC, Katsis SB, et al: Blunt bowel and mesenteric injuries: The role of screening computed tomography. J Trauma 2000; 48:991–1000.

Pohlgeers A, Ruddy RM: An update on pediatric trauma. Emerg Clin North Am 1995; 13:267–289.

Shah R, Sabanathan S, Mearns AJ, et al: Traumatic rupture of the diaphragm. Ann Thorac Surg 1995; 60:1444–1449.

Udobi KF, Rodriguez A, Chiu WC, et al: Role of ultrasonography in penetrating abdominal trauma: A prospective clinical study. J Trauma 2001; 50:475–479.

CHAPTER 44

Chest Trauma

ALEXANDER T. TROTT

CASE *Study*

A 44-year-old woman is the unrestrained driver in a high-speed motor vehicle accident. She was driving alone. Another car crossed the center line, resulting in a head-on collision with the patient's car. Speeds exceeding 50 mph for both cars are estimated. There is extensive damage to the car, including a crushed steering wheel. The police arrive and find the victim still in the car. She is awake but obviously injured, in respiratory distress, and complaining of anterior chest pain. An immediate call is made to dispatch the rescue squad. Victims in the other car are being transported elsewhere. One person is dead at the scene.

INTRODUCTION

Thoracic injuries contribute to morbidity and mortality in more than 60% of patients with multiple injuries. Blunt thoracic injuries rank second only to head injury as a cause of death and disability in trauma patients. In spite of these statistics, operative thoracotomy is necessary in only 10% to 15% of patients with thoracic trauma. Most are managed with advanced airway care, needle and tube thoracostomy, ventilatory support, or volume resuscitation.

Trauma to the thorax occurs by means of four basic forces: *shearing, compression, torsion*, and *acceleration/deceleration*. The simplest example of shearing is a knife wound. Tissue is divided with little force imparted and the actual damage is small. The critical factor in shearing injuries is the potential involvement of a major vessel, leading to exsanguination, or loss of negative intrapleural pressure that causes lung collapse and ventilatory compromise. An example of compression is the mechanism by which ribs are broken, as the force delivered exceeds the elastic capacity of the bone. The bone fragment can then "shear" lung tissue, leading to a pneumothorax or hemothorax. Significant compression to the thoracic cage can cause a segment of ribs to break in at least two places. This may create a "flail" segment of the chest wall. This segment of chest wall is no longer a stable portion of the thoracic cage and can collapse into the chest cavity with the negative intrathoracic pressure of inspiration. This instability of the thoracic cage may contribute to ventilatory compromise. Significant compressive forces are also imparted to the underlying lung, with resultant pulmonary contusion. Pulmonary contusions beneath the flail segment are the major contributors to ventilation-perfusion abnormalities. Both shearing and compression occur with gunshot wounds. The bullet divides tissue, and the area around the path is directly compressed by the shock wave. In wounds resulting from high-velocity missiles, the area of injury is expanded into tissue by the energy released from the bullet as it decelerates in the body.

Shearing or compression injuries can result in a rapidly fatal outcome. Shearing penetration of the heart usually results from a knife or bullet. Compression against a blood-filled chamber can cause myocardial rupture. Hemorrhage from the myocardial wound ensues, but the pericardial injury often remains closed. The accumulation of blood in the pericardium results in cardiac tamponade. As intrapericardial pressure rises, the return blood flow to the heart decreases until the right ventricular diastolic filling pressure is exceeded. In this setting, as little as 50 mL of blood may cause a pericardial tamponade, resulting in hypotension and shock.

Shearing, compression, and torsion may contribute to creating a tension pneumothorax (Fig. 44–1). When the pleural space or lung is penetrated, a tissue flap is created that can create a one-way valve, allowing air to escape into the pleural cavity but preventing its exit. Because of the one-way valve effect, positive intrapleural pressure quickly builds and begins to compress the lung. As intrapleural (and intrathoracic) pressure increases, it begins to exceed the right ventricular filling pressure and decreases blood return to the heart. The expanding pneumothorax on the affected side compresses the mediastinum and unaffected hemithorax, depending on the mobility of the mediastinum. This pressure and torsion of the mediastinal vessels may contribute to impaired cardiac venous return.

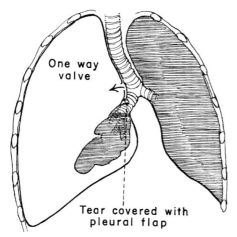

FIGURE 44–1 • Tension pneumothorax. (From Zuidema GD, Rutherford RB, Ballinger WF [eds]: The Management of Trauma, 4th ed. Philadelphia, WB Saunders, 1985.)

The most lethal result of an acceleration-deceleration thoracic injury is transection of the aorta. The aorta is relatively fixed in the mediastinum at a point just distal to the left subclavian artery, the ligamentum arteriosum. Distally, it is more mobile until it reaches the diaphragm. In a rapid deceleration injury, such as occurs with blunt impact of the chest against a steering wheel, the aorta accelerates forward as the thorax decelerates. At the point of fixation, shearing and torsion cause tearing in the aortic intima and media. If the force is sufficient, the adventitia may tear as well, and rapid exsanguination will follow. This mechanism is the underlying cause of immediate death in most fatal motor vehicle accidents. In 10% to 20% of patients with this injury, the adventitia remains intact and the patient has a chance of survival depending on the recognition and treatment of the lesion. As many as 50% of remaining survivors will die within 24 hours if they are not diagnosed and treated expeditiously.

Although the spectrum of injuries occurring in thoracic trauma vary with the mechanism of injury, the underlying result is generally similar: impairments in cardiac output, ventilatory efficiency, and gas exchange may occur with injury to the chest wall, pleura, heart, aorta, tracheobronchial tree, or pulmonary parenchyma whether caused by an ice pick or by impact with a steering wheel.

INITIAL APPROACH AND STABILIZATION

Priority Diagnoses

Early considerations specific to chest trauma include the following immediately life-threatening injuries: airway obstruction, bronchial/tracheal rupture, tension pneumothorax, massive hemothorax, pericardial tamponade, and aortic rupture.

The potential for a rapidly fatal outcome mandates that patients with thoracic injuries be rapidly triaged to the critical care area of the emergency department and seen immediately by the emergency physician.

Rapid Assessment

The prehospital care history is repeated and confirmed while EMS personnel are present.

Airway. The upper airway is assessed for patency and protection. Any obvious sources of obstruction, such as dentures or broken teeth, are removed. The anterior neck is palpated for signs of laryngeal trauma, including tenderness and subcutaneous air (palpable crepitance) in the area of the thyroid cartilage. If shortness of breath is present, the patient is asked about its severity, response to oxygen supplementation, and, if available, any positioning that offers relief. Patients who cannot speak, who are not handling secretions, or who have a depressed/absent gag reflex require immediate airway management.

Respiratory Status. Respiratory rate, ventilatory effort, and skin color are assessed to evaluate respiratory status. Interventions for injury to the chest wall that impair ventilation are discussed later.

Circulation. Blood pressure, pulse rate, mental status, and skin appearance (pallor, diaphoresis) are quickly assessed. Hypovolemia is the most common cause of circulatory compromise in chest trauma, but cardiac tamponade and tension pneumothorax are reversible "obstructive" causes that should be considered and immediately treated.

Chest Wall. The chest wall is compressed anteroposteriorly and laterally to find sites of pain or instability. Areas of pain are palpated for bony or subcutaneous crepitus. The chest is observed for asymmetry during respiration or open pneumothorax. Auscultation and percussion are completed, searching for signs of tension pneumothorax or hemothorax.

Other Injuries. The cervical spine is examined and immobilized as necessary. Significant C-spine injury should be suspected in the injured patient with an altered level of consciousness or evidence of blunt injury above the clavicle. A rapid secondary survey is performed after the primary survey and stabilization is begun. Intraabdominal injuries, head trauma, and fractures of long bones are frequently associated with thoracic injuries.

Early Intervention

Airway Management. Patients in extreme respiratory distress require definitive airway management and ventilatory support (see Chapter 2, Airway Management). Endotracheal intubation is the preferred technique. Nasotracheal and orotracheal intubation should be determined by the skill level and experience of the physician. Nasal intubation is restricted to patients older than 12 years of age when they are breathing and are without midfacial fractures or basilar skull fractures. Cricothyrotomy is the procedure of choice if there are severe injuries to the face or upper airway. In children younger than 12 years of age needle cricothyroidotomy is preferred over surgical cricothyroidotomy. Supplemental oxygen is given to all patients. Pulse oximetry is measured as a screen for hypoxemia and to continuously monitor oxygen levels.

Intravenous Access and Volume Resuscitation. All patients with significant thoracic trauma require two large-bore peripheral intravenous catheters. Unstable patients may need placement of additional intravenous lines. If central venous access is necessary, the internal jugular or subclavian vein on the injured side of the chest is preferred to avoid complications in the functioning hemithorax. Femoral access can also be attempted. Isotonic crystalloid is the fluid of choice; the rate depends on the initial vital signs and estimated blood loss. In patients who do not respond to crystalloid or who arrive with persistent hypotension, uncrossmatched type O or type-specific blood is given.

Needle Thoracostomy. Any patient who has clinical evidence of a tension pneumothorax is decompressed by needle thoracostomy. Clinical features of a tension pneumothorax include respiratory distress, hypotension, tachycardia, contralateral tracheal deviation, distended neck veins, decreased breath sounds, and hyperresonance on percussion. Needle decompression is performed by inserting a 14- to 16-gauge catheter-covered intravenous needle into the second intercostal space at the midclavicular line. The needle is inserted just over the superior edge of the second rib to avoid possible injury to the intercostal artery. On entering the pleural space, there will be an expulsion of air with a characteristic hissing sound. The steel needle portion of the catheter is removed, and the plastic catheter is left in place. Needle thoracostomy is a temporizing measure and is followed as soon as possible by tube thoracostomy.

Tube Thoracostomy. Tube thoracostomy is used for continuous evacuation of air and fluid from the pleural space. In the patient with thoracic trauma, the indications for early tube thoracostomy include pneumothorax (simple, tension, open), hemothorax, hemopneumothorax, and conditions requiring anesthesia or positive-pressure ventilation in patients with penetrating chest trauma. Tube thoracostomy is done in a sterile field. A large-bore (36 to 40 French) chest tube is inserted over the superior edge of the rib in the fourth or fifth intercostal space in the midaxillary line, connected to a closed drainage system with a water seal, and secured in place (Fig. 44–2). Initially, suction is set at –15 to –20 cm H_2O. A chest radiograph to assess the degree of lung reexpansion, tube placement, and presence of associated injuries is mandatory after decompression has been accomplished.

Pericardiocentesis. In the deteriorating or hypotensive patient with clinical findings and a mechanism of injury consistent with cardiac tamponade (e.g., penetrating trauma in the central chest area), subxiphoid pericardiocentesis is a potentially lifesaving procedure (Fig. 44–3). Late clinical signs of cardiac tamponade include Beck's triad of hypotension, jugular venous distention, and muffled heart tones. This combination is seen in only 30% of patients. Other signs include decreased pulse pressure, Kussmaul's sign (distended neck veins with inspiration), and pulseless electrical activity. One early finding is an elevated central venous pressure. Bedside ultrasonography may be diagnostic, but in severe compromise the procedure is initiated based on clinical suspicion. An 18-gauge spinal needle is inserted at the intersection of the xiphoid process and the left costal margin and then directed toward the sternal notch or left shoulder. The only test of its success is restoration of a measurable blood pressure after withdrawal of blood from the pericardial space. If there is time, placement may be aided by attaching the needle to the chest lead of an electrocardiographic machine with the limb leads in place. The needle is advanced with intermittent attempts to aspirate blood. Contact with the myocardium is demonstrated by acute ST-segment elevation. If this distant limit is reached, the needle is withdrawn slightly and an attempt is made to aspirate blood in the pericardial space.

Pericardiocentesis is a hazardous procedure with a high potential for misdiagnosis. For example, in up to 60% of patients with acute traumatic pericardial tamponade the blood is all or partly clotted. At best, the procedure is a high-risk temporizing measure while preparations for surgery are made. Emergency thoracotomy is performed if deterioration continues and suspicion of tamponade remains.

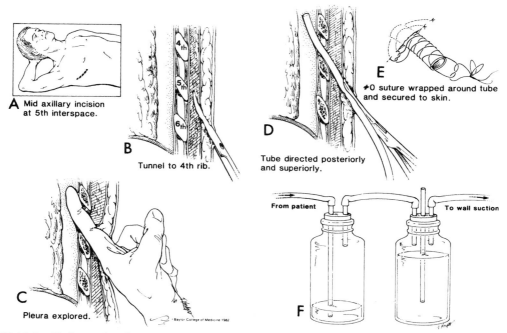

FIGURE 44–2 • Technique for tube thoracostomy. Note that the pleural space is entered with the gloved finger, not a trocar or a sharp instrument. (From Emergency department treatment of chest injuries. Emerg Clin North Am 1984; 2[4]:786.)

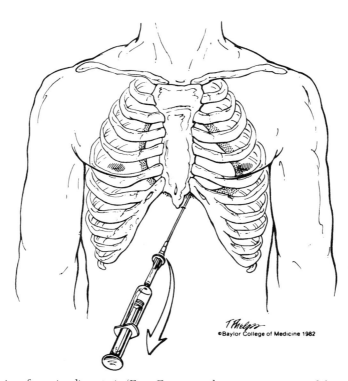

FIGURE 44–3 • Technique for pericardiocentesis. (From Emergency department treatment of chest injuries. Emerg Clin North Am 1984; 2[4]:787.)

Emergency Thoracotomy. Emergency thoracotomy is indicated in the patient with the following:

- Penetrating thoracic or abdominal injuries with vital signs during the prehospital phase of care and who arrives at the emergency department in agonal condition or cardiac arrest.
- Penetrating thoracic or abdominal trauma whose condition deteriorates rapidly in spite of maximal therapy.

Emergency thoracotomy, with few exceptions, has little clinical utility in victims of blunt traumatic cardiac arrest or nontraumatic cardiac arrest. The outcome of thoracotomy in penetrating wound patients varies considerably by type. Patients with stab wounds have a much better outcome than those with gunshot wounds. Resuscitative thoracotomy (Fig. 44–4) is performed by the most experienced physician in the emergency department.

Chest Radiography. Plain chest films are important to order early in the care of any injured patient with thoracic trauma. They are *not* indicated before treatment in the unstable patient suspected of a tension pneumothorax, open pneumothorax, or cardiac tamponade. Treatment in these cases is based on clinical judgment. *Portable* chest radiographs are obtained as soon as possible after stabilization. Upright portable radiographs may be taken in clinically stable patients who are at no risk for spinal injury. Chest radiographs increase the chances of finding small pneumothoraces, hemothoraces, aortic rupture, or pulmonary contusions. A clinically unstable or partially evaluated patient should not leave the emergency department for radiography.

CLINICAL ASSESSMENT

After the initial assessment and necessary interventions have been performed, a more complete history is taken and a physical examination is performed.

History

1. *Mechanism and timing of the trauma.* The time of injury and onset of symptoms (if not simultaneous), mechanism of injury, and amount of force involved are documented. The latter information is particularly important in patients with blunt trauma. It is often available only from EMS personnel. Specific mechanisms of injury should lead the examiner to obtain certain information. For example, in motor vehicle accidents the following information is helpful:

- Type of vehicle and estimated speed at the time of the accident

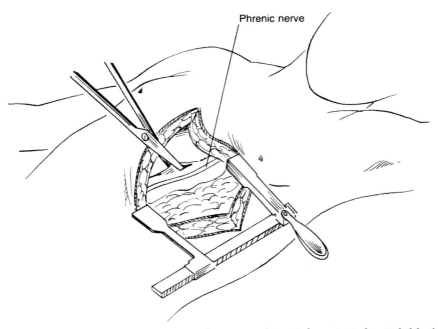

FIGURE 44–4 • Left anterolateral location of resuscitative thoracotomy. (From Roberts JR, Hedges JR [eds]: Clinical Procedures in Emergency Medicine, 2nd ed. Philadelphia, WB Saunders, 1990.)

- Victim's position in vehicle (driver or passenger)
- Amount of damage occurring to the vehicle, particularly to the internal structures (e.g., steering wheel, windshield), and whether airbags were present and deployed
- Where victim was found
- Use and type of restraints (e.g., seat belts)

Most victims of penetrating trauma have either gunshot wounds or stab wounds. For patients with gunshot wounds it is helpful to know the type and caliber of weapon used, victim's distance from assailant, and number of shots fired. For patients with stab wounds, useful information includes the type of weapon used, length of weapon, and direction of stabbing.

2. *Respiratory symptoms*. The sensation of "shortness of breath" is the most common subjective complaint in patients with thoracic trauma. The sensation of dyspnea may result from a number of processes involving the airway, chest wall, lungs, other deep thoracic structures, or hemorrhage (see Chapter 37, Acute Dyspnea).
3. *Presence of chest pain*. Pain is a common symptom after injury to the musculoskeletal chest wall. The pain is usually described as sharp or stabbing and is made worse by deep inspiration or movement of the thorax. Aching or pressure-like pain may be related to injury to the thoracic visceral structures or referred pain from associated injuries. Myocardial contusion or myocardial ischemia may be associated with chest trauma.
4. *Associated symptoms*. Are there other areas of pain and discomfort? Were there symptoms before the accident? Chest pain, dizziness, or syncope from myocardial or cerebrovascular disease may have contributed to the accident.
5. *Past medical history*. Is there a past history of cardiorespiratory disease or previous surgical procedures? When was the patient's last tetanus immunization? A history of other medical problems should be obtained either from the patient or the patient's family.
6. *Current use of medications or other substances*. All medications are noted. Alcohol or drug use is questioned. Use of herbal medications should be noted.
7. *History of allergies*. Allergies to medications, contrast materials, or anesthetics are discussed.
8. *Most recent meal*. This information helps to anticipate the potential for aspiration and is useful for the anesthesiologist and trauma surgeon.

Physical Examination

Table 44–1 summarizes the physical assessment of the patient with chest trauma. Because of the potential for clinical instability of patients with chest trauma, the examination may initially be limited. The importance of repeated evaluation cannot be overstressed. The findings and evolution of response to trauma often change.

CLINICAL REASONING

Throughout the early management of thoracic trauma, the clinician must constantly reevaluate the condition of the patient as well as the differential diagnoses of potentially life-threatening problems. The following questions provide a framework for action.

Do the Mechanisms of Injury Explain the Patient's Findings?

It is important in all traumatic injuries to understand the mechanisms of injury and attempt to explain the patient's injuries through those mechanisms. Inconsistencies between the history and the findings should raise questions about

- Exactly what mechanisms were involved. Could secondary trauma have occurred?
- What clinical events may have occurred before the trauma.
- What clinical events may have occurred after the trauma (e.g., prolonged extrication).
- Whether the clinical examination is complicated by drugs, alcohol, or endogenous/exogenous toxins (e.g., Are β blockers causing the patient's bradycardia?).

The most difficult aspect of caring for the trauma patient is focusing on the entire patient, not just the injuries, and considering pathophysiologic events before and after the actual trauma.

Is the Patient Currently Unstable in Spite of Resuscitative Effort?

Circulatory impairment, massive hemorrhage, and ventilatory insufficiency are the three primary causes of continued instability. Priority diagnoses to be entertained in this setting include those listed in Table 44–2. Although they are considered during the initial stabilization efforts, because of the potential for rapid changes in chest trauma, each is reconsidered at this point. For example, a hemothorax may be missed because 200 to 400 mL of blood must be lost into the chest cavity

TABLE 44–1. Physical Examination in Patients with Chest Trauma

Examination	Observation	Comments
Vital Signs		
Pulse	Pulse deficit	Suspect hypovolemia, tamponade, tension pneumothorax, arterial injury
	Tachycardia	Associated with hypovolemia, hypoxemia, increased sympathetic tone
	Bradycardia	A critical sign; may be a *preterminal event* in patients with airway or ventilatory compromise
Blood pressure	Narrow pulse pressure	Early sign of hypovolemia
	Hypertension	Secondary to increased sympathetic tone
	Hypotension	A critical sign; may be secondary to hypovolemia, tension pneumothorax, or cardiac tamponade
Respiratory rate and effort	Tachypnea	Common, insensitive for serious injury; has multiple causes
	Bradypnea	A critical sign; may be a preterminal event
	Labored	Effort required is indicative of level of respiratory distress.
Temperature	Abnormal	Hypothermia is common in trauma victims.
General		
Appearance	Skin abnormal	Observe for diaphoresis, pallor, cyanosis.
	Wounds	Suspect pneumothorax, cardiac tamponade, or opening to pleural space.
HEENT	Upper airway obstruction	Observe for patency and protection of airway, presence of secretions, fractured larynx.
	Cervical spine	Palpate for tenderness, deformity. Immobilize until cleared.
Neck	Discolored, swollen	Swelling, hematoma. Check position of trachea, carotid pulsations, presence of subcutaneous emphysema, crepitance over fractured larynx.
	Distended neck veins	Suspect tamponade, tension pneumothorax.
Chest	Contusions, tenderness	Compress thorax gently in the anteroposterior and lateral directions to localize fractured ribs. A flail chest may not be readily apparent.
	Asymmetry, hyperresponance, decreased breath sounds	Tension pneumothorax
	Hyporesonance	Hemothorax or other density in chest cavity (e.g., bowel from diaphragmatic rupture)
Cardiac	Decreased heart sounds	Usually indicative of shock. Not sensitive for tamponade
	Regurgitant murmurs	Valvular damage, most often mitral or aortic
Abdomen	Tenderness, decreased bowel sounds	Associated intra-abdominal injuries
Neurologic	Decreased consciousness, neurologic deficits	Intracranial trauma and possible peripheral nerve injuries

before it is detectable on upright chest radiographs. It is often difficult to detect if the patient remains supine during radiography. If the patient continues to bleed, false security in interpreting the first film may hinder discovery of the problem. Even without changes in the patient's condition, equipment failures can complicate the diagnosis (e.g., a treated tension pneumothorax can recur if there is a malfunction of the chest tube apparatus).

What Potential Life-Threatening Problems May Exist in a Currently Stable Patient?

The injuries listed in Table 44–2 are also considered in this setting. Most patients present in a temporarily stable condition at best, which is followed by rapid deterioration.

Patients with thoracic trauma can become unstable at any time. Because changes can be subtle, constant monitoring of vital signs is mandatory.

Are There Associated Injuries or Underlying Conditions? Is the Secondary Survey Complete?

Because of the high association of other injuries with thoracic trauma, a complete assessment is always necessary. One injury with great potential for occult morbidity is the penetrating wound at or below the nipple line. The diaphragm rises up to the fourth intercostal space, and a penetrating injury of the peritoneal cavity may be clinically evident on examination. Other inquiries are related to the mechanism and focus of injury. The most common associated injuries are abdominal (lac-

TABLE 44–2. Immediately Life-Threatening Injuries in Chest Trauma

Condition	Mechanism of Injury	Vital Signs	Physical Findings	Useful Diagnostic Tests	Initial Management	Comments
Tension pneumothorax	Blunt or penetrating trauma	Hypotension Tachycardia Tachypnea	Respiratory distress Decreased breath sounds and hyperresonance on the affected side Tracheal deviation Subcutaneous emphysema	*None* in the unstable patient *Portable anteroposterior* CXR—collapsed lung with deviation of mediastinal structure to the opposite side	Needle thoracostomy followed by tube thoracostomy	CXR is still most common source of diagnosis. Late formation is anticipated in all patients having positive-pressure ventilation.
Open pneumothorax	Blunt or penetrating trauma	Tachycardia Tachypnea	Respiratory distress Open "sucking" chest wound Decreased breath sounds Subcutaneous emphysema	None for initial diagnosis and treatment	Immediate closure of wound with an air-tight or ball-valve type of dressing (e.g. Vaseline gauze) Tube thoracostomy as soon as appropriate Endotracheal intubation and positive-pressure ventilation as necessary	Physiologic mechanism is that of a large functional dead space. Function of both lungs is affected.
Cardiac tamponade	More common in penetrating trauma; in blunt trauma associated with cardiac rupture	Hypotension Tachycardia Tachypnea Narrow pulse pressure	Muffled heart sounds Distended neck veins Cyanosis of head, neck, upper extremities Triad of muffled heart sounds, elevated venous pressure, and hypotension seen in only 30% of patients	Elevated central venous pressure may be earliest finding None in unstable patients with penetrating trauma in the precordial region	Volume repletion Needle pericardiocentesis Emergency thoracotomy for patients who rapidly deteriorate	Occurs in <2% of chest trauma. Rare after blunt injury. Echocardiography may be useful if patient is stable and there is sufficient blood in pericardial space. Patients can deteriorate rapidly.
Large hemo- or hemopneumothorax (>500 mL or continuous hemorrhage)	Blunt or penetrating trauma	Hypotension Tachycardia Tachypnea	Respiratory distress Decreased or absent breath sounds on the affected side May be dullness to percussion	*Portable anteroposterior* CXR—fluid density air-fluid level involving entire hemithorax	Tube thoracostomy	Both chest wall vessels and lung parenchyma are sources of bleeding. More often bleeding results from penetrating injury. These patients are autotransfusion candidates. Chest cavity can hold 2000–3000 mL.
Aortic disruption	Blunt trauma; usually rapid deceleration injury	May be normal Hypotension Tachycardia Tachypnea	Patients may have *no* signs of major trauma Mechanism of injury more important than clinically obvious chest trauma Upper extremity hypertension, attenuation of femoral pulse may be seen	*Portable anteroposterior* CXR—highest yield: widened superior mediastinum (>8 cm) or loss of contour of aortic knob	High index of suspicion required Patients with appropriate mechanism of injury and associated clinical or radiographic findings receive emergency aortic angiography or computed tomography	Only 10%–20% of patients arrive alive. In one third of these exsanguination will occur in 6 hours.
Tracheobronchial disruption	Blunt trauma; usually rapid deceleration injury, less often penetrating injury	Tachypnea Tachycardia	Massive subcutaneous emphysema Pneumothorax Pneumomediastinum	*Portable anteroposterior* CXR; massive SQ and mediastinal air	Airway management Initial tube thoracostomy may be inadequate Bronchoscopy	Rare injury (<3% of chest trauma patients) with high mortality (>30%).
Flail chest and pulmonary contusion	Blunt trauma	Tachypnea Tachycardia	Paradoxically moving segment of chest wall Respiratory distress Tenderness or crepitation of chest wall Chest wall bruising	*Portable or standard CXR;* multiple fracture of adjacent ribs. Infiltrates usually seen within 1–2 hours and always by 4–6 hours after injury *Arterial blood gas measurements:* hypocarbia and hypercarbia, hypoxemia	Observation Supplemental O_2 Ventilatory support Pain control Anticipation and treatment of pulmonary contusion	Majority occur within 3 cm of carina. Usually three or more ribs fractured at two points. Derangement of chest wall expansion contributes to ventilatory compromise. Contusion characterized by edema and hemorrhage without laceration.

CXR = chest radiograph; SQ=subcutaneous.

erated spleen and liver, perforated bowel), craniospinal (subdural and epidural hematomas, cervical spine), and fractures (pelvis, femur).

Patients often have complicating medical illnesses and need to be evaluated for these conditions. The question of "what caused this accident?" cannot be lost in the urgency of management. Myocardial infarction, cerebrovascular accident, hypoglycemia, or a suicide attempt may have precipitated the traumatic event.

Chest trauma often results in a combination of potentially life-threatening injuries. The emergency physician assesses and treats the physiologic derangements while anticipating the underlying pathologic conditions. A reasonable rule is always to search for more than one cause of the patient's condition. At a minimum, this rule encourages repeated examination.

DIAGNOSTIC ADJUNCTS

The use of diagnostic adjuncts is always tempered by the condition of the patient. With the exception of portable chest films, it is common for chest trauma patients to receive definitive care before diagnostic testing.

Laboratory Studies

Trauma Panel. Standard laboratory profiles are often obtained for all seriously injured patients. These include complete blood cell count and differential; determination of levels of serum electrolytes, serum glucose, blood urea nitrogen, and creatinine; blood for type and crossmatch; and urinalysis. Modifications in the "panel" approach are made in context of the patient's determined injuries. These panels are currently considered excessive in terms of efficient laboratory usage, but the practice continues.

Arterial Blood Gas Measurements. Arterial blood gas samples are obtained early in the care of chest trauma patients who have signs of airway or ventilatory compromise, low pulse oximetry values, hemodynamic instability, altered mental status, or a history of significant trauma to the chest. Hypoxemia (PO_2 less than 60 mm Hg on room air) is indicative of a serious derangement of oxygenation. It is often an early finding in patients with pulmonary contusion and a variety of other conditions. Hypercarbia (PCO_2 more than 40 mm Hg) reflects ventilatory insufficiency, which may have a variety of causes (e.g., major hemothorax or pneumothorax or airway obstruction). Acidemia (pH less than 7.35) may be primarily respiratory or secondary to hypoperfusion and shock.

Cardiac Enzyme Levels. The myocardial fraction of creatine kinase (CK-MB) is often measured in patients suspected of having sustained a myocardial contusion. The levels usually peak by 24 hours. A level greater than 5% is considered diagnostic. Unfortunately, patients with normal or minimally elevated CK-MB (less than 2%) have shown significant myocardial wall motion abnormalities consistent with a diagnosis of cardiac contusion. It remains a relatively insensitive test.

Radiologic Imaging

Chest Radiograph. A portable or standard view chest radiograph is obtained as early as possible in the evaluation of all patients with significant thoracic trauma. An upright study is preferable in patients who are not at risk for spinal injury. A pneumothorax and hemothorax may be obscured in the supine position, and the mediastinum may appear falsely widened. The need for chest radiographs should not delay the treatment of a patient with a clinically evident tension or open pneumothorax. Serial radiographs may be useful in evaluating the development or evolution of clinically unapparent pneumothorax or hemothorax. A chest film is also obtained after therapeutic interventions, such as tube thoracostomy or endotracheal intubation, to assess tube position. Chest film findings localized to the site of injury, including patchy alveolar infiltrates or frank consolidation, that are present immediately on arrival or develop within 6 hours are highly suggestive of pulmonary contusion.

A particularly insidious injury is traumatic disruption of the aorta. Suspicion for this injury is raised if the patient has sustained a blunt deceleration injury to the chest, particularly as an unrestrained driver. The most important first study is the chest radiograph, which is preferably taken in the anteroposterior upright position at a distance of 100 cm. An upper mediastinal width of 8 cm or greater (the approximate width of a standard pager), deviation of the nasogastric tube or trachea to the right of the midline, and loss of the shadow of the aortic knob are three key radiographic signs that require further immediate investigation through computed tomography (CT) or angiography.

Aortography. The selection of patients for contrast aortography to evaluate for traumatic aortic disruption is based on the mechanism of injury, primarily rapid deceleration (falls, motor vehicle accidents), and an abnormal chest radiograph.

Computed Tomography of the Chest. Contrast medium–enhanced CT of the chest has been increasingly useful in diagnosing aortic injury. It can detect the extraluminal hematoma but cannot localize the site of the internal tear. In many centers it is performed before aortography.

Echocardiography. Two-dimensional and Doppler pulsed echocardiography may assist in the diagnosis of pericardial tamponade and myocardial contusion and with valvular function abnormalities. In myocardial contusions, findings include right ventricular dilatation and segmental wall motion abnormalities. These studies are obtained relatively easily in patients with chest trauma.

Gated Radionuclide Angiogram (Multiple Gated Acquisition [MUGA] Scan). The MUGA scan is not routinely obtained from the emergency department. It is an excellent diagnostic tool for the patient with suspected cardiac contusion. The scan has a high degree of sensitivity in detecting the segmental wall motion abnormalities characteristic of the condition.

Electrocardiogram

A standard 12-lead electrocardiogram is obtained in all patients with significant thoracic trauma. Cardiac dysrhythmias often occur as a direct result of myocardial contusion or penetrating cardiac injury. They may also be secondary to metabolic derangements such as hypoxemia or acidosis. Rarely, myocardial infarction may result from coronary vascular damage. Electrocardiographic changes compatible with myocardial contusion include ST-T segment elevation or depression, conduction disturbances, and rhythm disturbances. If positive, electrocardiographic findings can support the suspicion of myocardial contusion. A normal electrocardiogram does not rule it out. Additionally, a primary myocardial event may have caused the accident and hypotension or hypoperfusion from any cause may precipitate myocardial ischemia or infarction.

EXPANDED DIFFERENTIAL DIAGNOSIS

After the immediately life-threatening disorders are managed or ruled out, a number of potentially serious injuries are considered. The diagnoses of diaphragmatic rupture, myocardial contusion, simple pneumothorax, hemothorax, sternal fracture, and rib fracture are outlined in Table 44–3. These entities can cause morbidity and even mortality for the patient if appropriate therapeutic modalities are not instituted.

PRINCIPLES OF MANAGEMENT

General Principles

Airway Management. Early, aggressive airway control and constant airway monitoring are essential to patient survival. Supplemental oxygen therapy is initially administered to all patients with thoracic injuries. Continued therapy is guided by arterial blood gas analysis results. Indications for intubation and ventilatory support include (1) PaO_2 of less than 55 mm Hg on room air; (2) $PaCO_2$ greater than 50 mm Hg in previously eucapneic patients; (3) respiratory rate of greater than 40 breaths per minute; (4) inability to protect airway; and (5) need for intubation to provide anesthesia for operative procedures. For further discussion, see Chapter 2, Airway Management.

Volume Resuscitation. Volume resuscitation follows the same guidelines given in Chapter 4, Shock. Close monitoring of the volume is important in lung injuries because of potential complications of acute respiratory distress syndrome.

Monitoring and Recognition of Immediately Life-Threatening Disorders. Rapid recognition and management of respiratory and cardiovascular insufficiency from any cause are essential for patient survival. Constant vigilance is mandatory throughout the course of the patient's management.

Specific Thoracic Injuries

Tension Pneumothorax. Most of the information pertaining to tension pneumothorax is listed in Table 44–2. The absence of near-complete reexpansion of the lung on chest radiograph or a massive air leak as manifested by increasing subcutaneous emphysema and continuous air collection in the chest tube drainage system is an indicator of possible tracheal or bronchial injury. Further evaluation by flexible bronchoscopy and treatment with an additional chest tube are necessary.

Open Pneumothorax. If a tension pneumothorax develops after occlusion of the chest wall defect, immediate decompression by briefly opening the occlusive dressing is required. A chest tube is inserted at a remote site as soon as clinically feasible to ensure continued lung expansion.

Cardiac Tamponade. Patients with penetrating thoracic trauma and suspected cardiac tamponade who respond initially to pericardiocentesis and then whose condition deteriorates or who do not respond at all are candidates for emergency thoracotomy.

TABLE 44–3. Less Potentially Serious Injuries in Chest Trauma

Condition	Mechanism of Injury	Vital Signs	Physical Findings	Useful Diagnostic Tests	Initial Management	Comment
Diaphragmatic rupture	Blunt trauma	If severe, tachypnea Tachycardia	May be respiratory distress, dullness to percussion, bowel sounds in affected hemithorax Most often no specific symptoms	Portable or standard chest radiograph—signs may vary from gastrointestinal gas pattern in hemithorax to blurred diaphragmatic margins. Diagnosis may be aided by contrast studies Arterial blood gas measurements show hypoxemia, hypercarbia	Supplemental O_2 Ventilatory support Operative repair	Usually results from abdominal compression into chest. 95% occur on the left side. Can be very subtle and is often discovered later. Complications are bowel obstruction or strangulation.
Myocardial contusion	Blunt trauma, usually deceleration injuries	Dysrhythmias including sinus tachycardia (70% of cases), premature atrial or ventricular beats. Rarely, ventricular tachycardia or fibrillation, otherwise dependent on associated injuries	Dependent on associated injury. About 75% of patients with same finding: rib fracture, pulmonary contusion, sternal fracture	ECG—Initial and serial 12-lead ECG needed to document dysrhythmias, conduction disturbance (RBBB most common), or ST–T wave changes. Often appear after 24 hr. Changes may be due to other diseases CPK-MB—Initial and serial determination. Usually peaks in 24 hours. Level >5% significant Two-dimensional echocardiogram—excellent sensitivity	Observation Continuous cardiac monitoring Standard pharmacologic therapy for dysrhythmias	Occurs in about 10% of patients with chest trauma. Difficult clinical diagnosis. Major concerns are complications—dysrhythmias, cardiac and valve rupture, coronary vessel injury. May evolve into traumatic myocardial infarction. Most contusions do not result in clinically significant myocardial impairment.
Simple pneumothorax	Blunt or penetrating trauma	Tachypnea Tachycardia	May be respiratory distress (>50% have dyspnea and chest pain) Absent or decreased breath sounds on the affected side Hyperresonance to percussion Trachea in midline (no mediastinal shift)	Portable or standard chest radiograph—shows presence of extrapleural air shadow. Note size as percentage of lung volume	Observation if less than 5% Catheter aspiration or tube thoracostomy if less than 15% Tube thoracostomy if greater than 20% or if patient in distress or requires surgery or mechanical ventilation	Occurs in 10%–30% of patients with blunt chest trauma and almost 100% (to some degree) of those with penetrating trauma
Hemothorax	Blunt or penetrating trauma	Tachycardia Tachypnea	"Effusion" line of dullness to percussion Decreased breath sounds at base	Portable or standard chest radiograph—200 mL of blood necessary to be seen. Supine view may make diagnosis difficult. Costophrenic angle blunting is earliest finding. Repeated chest views may be useful	Volume resuscitation as necessary Tube thoracostomy in most cases	Often seen with pneumothorax, usually self-limited. Tube thoracostomy suitable for almost all cases
Sternal fracture	Significant blunt trauma, usually anterior (e.g., steering wheel)	Tachypnea	Tenderness and pain over sternum	Lateral radiograph of sternum ECG—changes characteristic of myocardial contusion	Search for associated injury Analgesia as allowable	Seen in <5% of chest trauma patients, usually due to severe trauma. Because of this, there may be mortality of up to 30% from associated injuries. High association with myocardial contusion or rupture, pulmonary contusion

| Rib fracture | Blunt trauma | Tachypnea Tachycardia | Tenderness, crepitation of chest wall May be respiratory distress | *Standard chest radiographs*—More than 50% of simple fractures missed on initial standard view. Ordered to evaluate for complications: hemothorax, pneumothorax, pulmonary contusion. Rib views rarely necessary
Arterial blood gas measurements—Ordered to check for evidence of respiratory compromise or underlying pulmonary disease (e.g., COPD) | Observation Analgesia Elderly patients and patients with significant cardiopulmonary disease are admitted and observed. | Accounts for 50% of injuries in cases of blunt chest trauma. Increased morbidity associated with increasing age, number of fractures, and location of fractures. More common in adults. Fractures of the first and second ribs require significant trauma and mandate careful evaluation for associated injuries. Great vessels, lung, and bronchial plexus are at risk. High morbidity if associated with other injuries, including other rib fractures. Fractures of ribs 9–11 can cause intra-abdominal injuries (e.g., splenic puncture). |

COPD, chronic obstructive pulmonary disease; CPK-MB, the myocardial fraction of creatine phosphokinase; ECG, electrocardiogram; RBBB, right bundle branch block.

Massive Hemothorax or Hemopneumothorax. Initial chest tube drainage of 1500 mL of blood or continued drainage of 200 mL of blood per hour for the first 2 to 4 hours indicates significant injury and warrants operative thoracotomy.

Pulmonary Contusion or Flail Chest. Partial ventilatory support using intermittent mandatory ventilation and positive end-expiratory pressure is the most effective means of treatment for these patients.

Myocardial Contusion. There is no evidence that prophylactic antidysrhythmic therapy is beneficial. Commodio cordis is an acute dysrhythmia event potentially causing sudden cardiac death, precipitated by a blow to the chest (e.g., baseball bat). Most occur in teen-aged men who are struck inadvertently. A recent study reported only a 16% survival rate, directly related to the immediate availability of CPR and defibrillation. Ventricular fibrillation was the most commonly found rhythm.

Rib Fracture. Narcotic analgesia improves ventilatory effort and is the only intervention required in the majority of patients. The use of external stabilization devices such as rib belts and tape is discouraged. They may provide some measure of pain relief, but they significantly limit the expansion of the chest and may predispose the patient to atelectasis and pneumonia. If used at all, their use should be limited to young, otherwise healthy patients with isolated rib fractures.

UNCERTAIN DIAGNOSIS

The complications of trauma often evolve over several days. Repeated rib fracture examination may reveal aspiration pneumonia, ligament tears or bone fractures masked by the initial findings, and problems such as drug withdrawal, which may suggest reasons for the traumatic event. Both in the emergency department and after admission or discharge, the potential for a missed or uncertain diagnosis must always be considered. Repeated examinations, careful monitoring, and close follow-up will keep these inevitable complications to a minimum.

SPECIAL CONSIDERATIONS

Pediatric Patients

The management of thoracic injuries is the same in the child as in the adult. The increased elasticity of the chest wall in the child makes injuries to the bony thorax less common, but abdominal injuries occur more often. Patients considered to be at higher risk for thoracic injury in blunt trauma include abnormal chest wall contour on back examination, hypotension, tachypnea, abnormal auscultations, and a Glasgow Coma Scale score of less than 13.

Elderly Patients

As in children, the pathophysiology of thoracic injuries in the elderly patient is not unique. The older patient has less physiologic reserve and is more likely to have significant underlying disease. Elderly patients with thoracic trauma require aggressive monitoring and are frequently admitted for further observation.

DISPOSITION AND FOLLOW-UP

Because operative intervention may be required, consultation with the appropriate surgical specialist is obtained early in the evaluation and management of the thoracic trauma patient in unstable condition. Disposition of the critically injured patient may depend on the facilities available at a particular institution. Patients requiring operative thoracotomy, cardiopulmonary bypass, or specialized critical care support are best treated at a regional trauma center.

Admission to Critical Care Facilities

Critically ill patients require skilled continuous care for an optimal outcome. Patients with the following conditions initially receive close hemodynamic and cardiorespiratory monitoring:

- Tension pneumothorax
- Open pneumothorax (postoperative as necessary)
- Cardiac tamponade
- Postoperative thoracotomy
- Flail chest or pulmonary contusion
- Myocardial contusion, sternal fracture
- First or second rib fracture
- Hemothorax (initially more than 500 mL of blood or with continued hemorrhage)

Patients with simple pneumothoraces or small hemothoraces (500 mL or less without continued hemorrhage) who are hemodynamically stable may be safely observed in a "step-down" unit or other monitored bed.

Admission

Some patients with rib fractures may require admission. Most are treated in a noncritical care setting. Patients in this category include (1) elderly or cardiorespiratory disease patients with isolated fractures, (2) those with inward displacement of jagged fragments, and (3) those with multiple (more than three) rib fractures.

Discharge

Patients with minor blunt trauma, such as isolated rib fractures in an otherwise healthy patient, who remain clinically stable after emergency department observation are discharged with follow-up arranged in 24 to 48 hours. Sufficient analgesia and an awareness of the patient's support system are important concerns when considering discharge.

FINAL POINTS

- Only 10% to 15% of patients with thoracic trauma require operative thoracotomy. The remainder can be appropriately managed in the emergency department.
- Tension pneumothorax, open pneumothorax, and cardiac tamponade are the three rapidly reversible, life-threatening disorders that every emergency physician must strive to recognize and treat appropriately.

- Needle thoracostomy can be lifesaving for patients with tension pneumothorax. It is followed by tube thoracostomy.
- The only measure of success for pericardiocentesis in cardiac tamponade is the restoration of blood pressure. This procedure is frequently unsuccessful, and emergency thoracotomy is often necessary.
- A chest radiograph is obtained early in combination with initial efforts to stabilize the patient with thoracic trauma. Tension pneumothorax, open pneumothorax, and cardiac tamponade are usually diagnosed by clinical assessment.
- Myocardial contusion is common in patients with blunt thoracic trauma. It is rarely associated with significant morbidity or mortality.
- Most patients with thoracic trauma—penetrating or blunt—are admitted to the hospital. Exceptions include single rib fractures in otherwise healthy patients or minor chest wall contusions.

CASE *Study*

A 44-year-old woman is an unrestrained driver involved in a high-speed motor vehicle accident. She was driving alone. Another car crossed the center line and collided with the patient's car head on. Speeds exceeding 50 mph for both cars are estimated. There is extensive damage to the car, including a crushed steering wheel. When the police arrive, the victim is still in the car. She is awake but obviously injured, in respiratory distress, and complaining of anterior chest pain. The rescue squad is called. Victims in the other car are being transported elsewhere. One person is dead at the scene.

The patient is awake and alert but pinned by the collapsed steering wheel. As the rescue squad assesses her, other fire and rescue personnel work to dislodge the steering wheel. She complains of chest pain, difficulty in breathing, and pain from an obviously fractured left femur. A hard cervical collar and short spine board are applied, and the patient is extricated from the vehicle. Spinal immobilization with a cervical collar and a long backboard is secured. The patient's vital signs are blood pressure, 130/70 mm Hg; pulse, 130 beats per minute; and respiratory rate, 24 breaths per minute. A 16-gauge intravenous line is started with isotonic crystalloid, and the patient is placed on 8 L of oxygen

and a cardiac monitor. A traction splint is applied to the left leg.

At this point, the appropriate interventions have been accomplished. Because the patient is alert and able to protect her airway and maintain her perfusion, the rescue squad is able to complete the standard field stabilization procedures at the scene. If the patient were in shock or otherwise unstable, these actions would be performed during transport. The mechanism of injury and the forces involved are significant, and continued observation and monitoring of the patient for deterioration of status is necessary. Focusing on chest trauma, the type of injury sustained raises concerns about aortic tear, myocardial contusion, and pulmonary contusion.

The patient is brought directly to the trauma area in the emergency department. Nursing personnel undress her, take repeat vital signs, obtain additional intravenous access, and continue cardiac monitoring and supplemental oxygen. On the primary survey the patient is found to be alert, diaphoretic, and in moderate respiratory distress. Her upper airway is clear. Her vital signs are blood pressure, 80 mm Hg systolic by palpation; pulse, 150 beats per minute; and respiratory rate, 36 breaths per minute. On

Continued on following page

palpation, tenderness is found in the left lateral chest wall with obvious subcutaneous emphysema. Decreased breath sounds are heard in the left chest. The left hemithorax is hyperresonant to percussion. A needle thoracostomy is performed, and a rush of air is heard. Her respiratory distress improves dramatically. Repeat vital signs are blood pressure, 110/70 mm Hg; pulse, 110 beats per minute; and respiratory rate, 20 breaths per minute. A tube thoracostomy is performed, and a portable chest radiograph is ordered. Surgical consultation is obtained (or may have been contacted upon notification of transport by the rescue squad).

The patient's status changed from that in the field. She became hemodynamically unstable with respiratory distress and manifested clinical evidence of a tension pneumothorax. Immediate decompression was indicated. Lifesaving actions and procedures are straightforward and uncomplicated to perform. Placing a needle into the chest takes less than a minute yet means the difference between life and death. The decision to perform this maneuver, however, is not always easily made. Inexperience of the physician or fear of second guessing by later caregivers can cause hesitation. It is important to remember that the consequences of not proceeding rapidly to treat a tension pneumothorax are far greater than placing a needle into chest without one.

After tube thoracostomy, the patient remains stable. A more thorough examination is completed. Palpation of the chest wall reveals bony crepitance over the left eighth and ninth ribs at the posterior axillary line. Breath sounds are equal bilaterally. There is minimal tenderness in the left upper quadrant of the abdomen. The left femur is obviously fractured, but there are good distal pulses. The traction splint remains in place. The chest tube is actively draining blood, and a total of 250 mL is measured.

In spite of the current stability of the patient's condition, there are several causes for concern. The active bleeding of the left hemithorax, although not yet sufficient to warrant surgical intervention, raises the possibility of an operative thoracotomy if it continues or increases. Fractures of the lower left ribs with their accompanying abdominal tenderness, no matter how mild at present, raise the suspicion of an intra-abdominal process such as a splenic injury. The femoral fracture is often associated with significant blood loss and complications and also represents the significant force involved in the accident.

The patient continues to bleed actively from the chest tube, and 700 mL have accumulated in approximately 30 minutes. She looks less well and now pale. Her pulse is 130 beats per minute, and her blood pressure is 110/90 mm Hg. A chest radiograph shows a well-placed chest tube, an expanded lung, and a poorly defined left hemidiaphragm.

The patient is becoming hemodynamically unstable secondary to continued hemorrhage. She is likely an exception to the 85% of patients with hemothorax who are definitively treated with tube thoracostomy.

The emergency physician continues vigorous fluid resuscitation and considers the use of blood products. A decision is then made with the surgical consultant against further diagnostic efforts in favor of surgical intervention. In spite of infusion of 2 L of isotonic crystalloid and 2 units of type-specific blood, the patient's pulse rises to 140 beats per minute and her blood pressure is 100/80 mm Hg. Her original hematocrit was 32%. Arterial blood gas results were Po_2, 130 mm Hg on 8 L of oxygen; Pco_2, 38 mm Hg; and pH, 7.31. She is increasingly restless, and the chest tube has drained 900 mL of blood. She begins to complain of abdominal pain, and the abdomen is significantly more tender.

At this point, the patient requires surgical intervention for hemorrhage control and clearer delineation of the extent of her injuries. Although diagnostic peritoneal lavage and computed tomography of the abdomen are considered, both the emergency physician and the surgeon agree that little information is to be gained from these studies. She is rapidly prepared for transport to the operating suite.

At surgery, a single lacerated intercostal artery is found to be the source of the continued bleeding. The fractured ribs are the only thoracic injuries found. Abdominal laparotomy reveals a small splenic laceration that is repaired without sacrificing the spleen. Because the chest and spleen injuries are easily managed, open repair and fixation of the femur fracture is performed under the same anesthesia. The patient is transferred to the critical care unit for continued evaluation and monitoring. She remains in the hospital and is transferred to rehabilitation on the sixth postoperative day.

Bibliography

TEXTS

Mattox KL, Feliciano DV, Moore EE (eds): Trauma, 4th ed. New York, McGraw-Hill, 2000.

Westaby S, et al (eds): Cardiothoracic Trauma. New York, Oxford University Press, 1999.

JOURNAL ARTICLES

Demetriades D: Penetrating injuries to the thoracic great vessels. J Card Surg 1997; 12(2 Suppl):173–179.

Dubrow TJ: Myocardial contusion in the stable patient: What level of care is appropriate? Surgery 1989; 106:267–273.

Haenel JB, Moore FA, Moore EE: Pulmonary consequences of severe chest trauma. Respir Care North Am 1996; 2:401–424.

Holmes JF, Sokolove PE, Brant WE: A clinical decision rule for identifying children with thoracic injuries after blunt torso trauma. Ann Emerg Med 2002; 39: 492–499.

Jones EB, Chambers K, Haro L: Thoracic trauma: Principles and practice of emergency stabilization, evaluation and management: I, II, III. Emerg Med Rep 2001; 22:201–210, 211–222, 223–234.

Lindstaedt M, Germing A, Lawo T, et al: Acute and long-term clinical significance of myocardial contusion following blunt thoracic trauma: Results of a prospective study. J Trauma 2002; 52:479–485.

Mansour KA: Trauma to the diaphragm. Chest Surg Clin North Am 1997; 7:373–383.

Maron BJ, Gohman TE, Kyle SB, et al: Clinical spectrum of commotio cordis. JAMA 2002; 287:1142–1146.

Mayberry JC, Trunkey DD: The fractured rib in chest wall trauma. Chest Surg Clin N Am 1997; 7:239–261.

Morgan PB, Buechter KJ: Blunt thoracic aortic injuries: Initial evaluation and management. South Med J 2000; 93:173–175.

Van Hise ML, Primack SL, Israel RS, Muller NL: CT in blunt chest trauma: Indications and limitations. Radiographics 1998; 18:1071–1084.

CHAPTER 45

Open Injuries to the Hand

MELISSA GILLESPIE
DENNIS T. UEHARA

CASE *Study*

A 55-year-old man injured his hand while attempting to manually declog the snow chute of his snow blower. The ambulance was delayed because of heavy snowfall. Neighbors wrapped his gloved hand in a scarf and brought him to the emergency department.

INTRODUCTION

Open hand, wrist, and forearm injuries can result in substantial deformity and functional disability. Initial management of these injuries is often the responsibility of the emergency physician. Many of these injuries will require close follow-up or extended evaluation and definitive treatment by a hand specialist. Because initial management often determines functional recovery, it is essential that all physicians managing injuries of the hand understand the intricacies of its evaluation and treatment. A thorough knowledge of the structural and functional anatomy of the hand is the basis for the proper care of hand injuries. The goal of treatment is to assess the extent of injury rapidly yet thoroughly, prevent infection, achieve early healing, and provide optimal function as quickly as possible.

Acute injuries to the hand constitute 5% to 10% of all patient complaints evaluated in the emergency department. These injuries range from the simple laceration to the complex crush or mutilating injury. Lacerations are the most common injuries, accounting for over 50% of all hand-related complaints. The male-to-female ratio is approximately 2:1. Sixty percent of patients are between the ages of 16 and 32. An emergency physician working in a busy department will see approximately 400 hand injuries per year. Although most physicians will recognize that the grossly traumatized hand needs care urgently, a seemingly innocuous-appearing laceration, puncture, or bite wound can lead to extensive and devastating deep structure damage. Therefore, it is imperative that all wounds be evaluated thoroughly for injuries to nerves, tendons, arteries, and bone.

INITIAL APPROACH AND STABILIZATION

Although patients presenting with a complicated wound, high-energy injury, or severe pain require urgent management, most open injuries to the hand can be managed in the minor treatment area. The notable exceptions are major amputations, rapidly exsanguinating wounds, or those associated with life-threatening injuries.

Priority Diagnoses

The priority diagnoses on initial evaluation include the following:

- Exsanguinating injury to the radial, ulnar, or brachial artery
- Major amputations
- Mutilating or crush injuries
- Open fracture
- Gunshot or stab wounds
- High-pressure injection injuries
- Human bite wounds
- Compartment syndrome
- Flexor tenosynovitis

Rapid Assessment

History

1. What was the mechanism of injury? ("How did it happen?")
2. What was the kind and amount of contamination at the scene?

Physical Examination

1. The hand is completely exposed and examined to assess the type and severity of injury.
2. Is the hand grossly intact? Are there amputated parts?
3. Is the basic grasp function intact?

Early Intervention

Hemostasis. Bleeding is controlled by applying direct pressure. Because arteries are in close proximity to nerves, tendons, and muscle, blind clamping can lead to further injury and is therefore contraindicated.

Intravenous Access. In the patient with a complicated injury, intravenous access may be needed for pain management, fluid or blood replacement, or antibiotic delivery.

Reduction of Edema. The hand is elevated, and ice is applied when significant soft tissue swelling is anticipated. All jewelry should be removed.

Antibiotics. Open fractures are treated prophylactically for infection with intravenous broad-spectrum antibiotics and require early consultation with an orthopedist or hand specialist.

Analgesia. It may be impossible for a patient to cooperate with an adequate examination because of pain. After assessing sensation, pain may be relieved by local or regional anesthesia. Both nonsteroidal anti-inflammatory drugs and either oral or parenteral narcotics are useful for temporary pain relief.

CLINICAL ASSESSMENT

History

An organized and carefully performed history is essential in assessing the hand and wrist. The history can suggest possible diagnoses and help the examiner anticipate specific complications. Important components of the history include the following:

1. *Nature of the injuring force*: Tidy injuries are clean, sharp, and recent and do not involve extensive tissue destruction. Untidy injuries are contaminated, caused by blunt trauma, and associated with significant tissue destruction and have a high risk for infection. Knowledge of the mechanism of injury will determine how the wound should be managed, the likelihood of surgical consultation, and the need for radiography.
2. *Time since the injury*: All traumatic wounds are contaminated. As the time elapsed since injury increases, the bacterial count increases until a point is reached when no amount of wound cleansing is sufficient to allow the laceration to be closed primarily. In general, hand wounds more than 6 hours old are subject to impaired healing and a greater incidence of infection.
3. *Contamination of the injuring force*: Grossly contaminated wounds cannot undergo primary closure regardless of appropriate wound care or time since injury. These wounds are best irrigated and left open. The patient should be started on antibiotics and referred for follow-up care.
4. *Associated medical illnesses*: Certain medical illnesses such as diabetes mellitus, peripheral vascular disease, and malnutrition will alter the healing process. Also, patients who are immunosuppressed or are taking medications such as corticosteroids may have impaired wound healing.
5. *Tetanus status*.
6. *Handedness of the patient and level of use*: Individuals with injury to the dominant hand and those whose livelihood depends on meticulous use of the hands will experience far greater disability from permanent injuries.
7. *Industrial injuries*: Because it is not practical for physicians to have a working knowledge of all industrial equipment, it is essential for the patient to describe carefully the mechanism of injury. The following questions are helpful:
   a. What type of machine caused the injury?
   b. Were rollers used? How wide is the space between the rollers?
   c. What normally passes through the machine?
   d. Was heat generated in the process?
   e. Is there a release mechanism? If not, how was the hand released?
   f. How long was the hand trapped?

Physical Examination and Functional Anatomy

The physical examination is the most important step in evaluating open injuries of the hand. A thorough examination will reveal the majority of injuries. To perform this assessment and interpret the findings, one must be familiar with the functional anatomy of the hand. The following discussion will review the physical examination in the context of functional hand anatomy. Of special significance is the concept of *topographic anticipation*. This refers to the process of anticipating a deep structural injury based on knowledge of the surface anatomy.

Three lines on the palm accurately establish the position of the underlying structures (Fig. 45–1):

1. The cardinal line of Kaplan extends from the apex of the thumb-index interdigital fold across the palm parallel to the midpalmar crease.
2. The radial border line is an extension of the radial border of the long finger. The point of

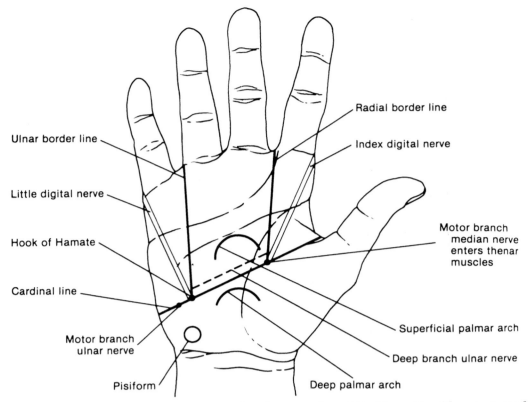

FIGURE 45–1 • Emmanual Kaplan described reference lines that accurately established the position of deep structures of the hand. (Adapted from Spinner M: Kaplan's Functional and Surgical Anatomy of the Hand, 3rd ed. Philadelphia, JB Lippincott, 1984; with permission.)

intersection with the cardinal line represents the point where the motor branch of the median nerve enters the thenar muscles. A line drawn from this radial reference point to the radial border of the base of the index finger overlies the course of the radial digital nerve to that finger.

3. The ulnar border line is an extension of the ulnar border of the ring finger. The place where it intersects the cardinal line closely approximates the location of the hook of the hamate. A line drawn from this point to the base of the ulnar border of the small finger overlies the course of the ulnar digital nerve to that finger. The pisiform is easily palpated at the base of the hypothenar eminence at the wrist crease.

The ulnar nerve and artery enter the palm radial to the pisiform and ulnar to the hook of the hamate (Guyon's canal). The nerve then divides, sending a deep motor branch across the palm. The course of this nerve is just distal to the cardinal line. The ulnar and radial arteries form the superficial palmar arch, which is 2 to 3 cm distal to the cardinal line, and the deep palmar arch, which is just proximal.

With these surface landmarks in mind, the examination proceeds as follows:

Observation. Lacerations, puncture wounds, soft tissue swelling, deformity, and color are noted. The normal posture of the resting hand reveals increasing flexion from the index to the small finger. Deviation from this resting posture may indicate a laceration of an extensor or flexor tendon (Figs. 45–2 and 45–3).

Palpation. Gently performed palpation of the injured hand may yield valuable information. The examination is performed with the patient's hand resting comfortably on the table. The finger or an instrument such as the eraser end of a pencil or a cotton-tipped applicator can be used to find the exact location of maximal tenderness.

Circulation. The radial and ulnar arteries provide the major blood supply to the hand. These arteries terminate by branching into deep and superficial branches, which anastomose to form the superficial and deep palmar arches

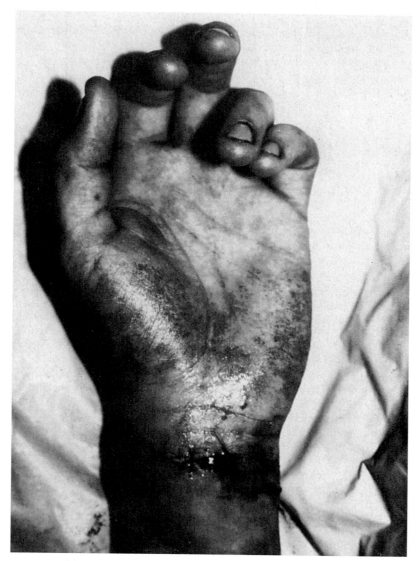

FIGURE 45–2 • Laceration of the wrist with flexor tendon injuries to the middle finger. Notice the middle finger falling outside the normal resting patterns of increasing flexion from index finger to little finger.

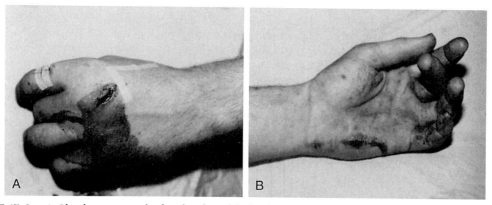

FIGURE 45–3 • *A,* Glass laceration on the dorsal surface of the hand. *B,* Complete transection of the extensor tendon to the middle finger demonstrated by altered normal alignment at rest.

(Fig. 45–4). Blood to the superficial arch is primarily supplied by the ulnar artery, and it is usually larger and more important than the deep arch.

Circulation is evaluated by observing the color, capillary filling time, and temperature of the skin. A hand that is edematous and cyanotic has venous insufficiency. A pale cool hand with poor capillary filling has arterial insufficiency.

Neurologic Examination

Sensation. Sensation to the hand is mediated by three nerves: the ulnar, median, and radial nerves (Fig. 45–5). The ulnar nerve supplies sensation to the small finger and the ulnar half of the ring finger. The median nerve supplies sensation to the thumb, index, long, and radial half of the ring finger, the central palmar area, and the distal portions of the dorsum of the ring, long, and index fingers. The radial nerve supplies sensation to that portion of the dorsum of the hand not supplied by the ulnar and median nerves. Although there is sensory overlap among adjacent nerves, autonomous areas do exist. These are the tip of the small finger for the ulnar nerve, the tip of the index finger for the median nerve, and the dorsal thumb-index web space for the radial nerve. The best assessment of sensory function is obtained by checking two-point discrimination, the normal range of which is 2 to 5 mm.

Motor. The median and ulnar nerves innervate all the intrinsic muscles of the hand, and the radial nerve innervates all of the extrinsic extensors (Table 45–1). Injuries to their main trunk can be diagnosed by testing one muscle only for each nerve. The ulnar nerve is tested by placing the patient's hand on a table on its ulnar side and having the patient elevate the index finger against resistance. The muscle belly of the first dorsal interosseus is palpated in the thumb-index web space. This muscle is reliably innervated by the ulnar nerve.

The median nerve can be tested by placing the patient's hand on a flat surface palm up and then asking the patient to raise the thumb toward the ceiling against resistance (palmar abduction). The belly of the abductor pollicis brevis, which is reliably innervated by the median nerve, can be palpated on the radial border of the thenar eminence.

The radial nerve is tested by placing the patient's forearm on a table and asking the patient to extend the wrist against resistance. The thumb is then extended and abducted, followed by extension of the other fingers. A laceration of the main trunk results in paralysis of the wrist and finger extensors and reveals an obvious "wristdrop."

Distal forearm lacerations, however, may result only in weak thumb and index finger extension. This is because of the more proximal innervation of the muscles to the wrist and finger extensors.

Tendon Examination

Either flexor or extensor tendons may be involved in hand or wrist lacerations. Extensor tendons are more superficial, easier to visualize, and easier to repair and generally heal without difficulty. Flexor tendons run through deep structures and are encased in a tendon sheath. They can be very difficult to visualize and repair, and complications are common.

Volar lacerations and potential flexor tendon injuries require a meticulous examination. The complex anatomy and the patient's resistance to examination because of pain can make this difficult. An appropriate nerve block or local infiltration with an anesthetic agent will facilitate this part of the examination. *Sensation is documented before instillation of anesthetic agents.*

Additionally, direct observation of the tendon through the lacerated skin may not reveal an injury. With potential tendon injuries, an additional historical factor to consider is the position of the hand at the time of injury. Flexor tendon lacerations that occur with the fingers in flexion will not be seen through the wound when the hand is examined with the fingers in the extended position. To evaluate the tendon directly, the fingers must be flexed to reproduce its position at the time of injury. This maneuver usually brings the tendon laceration into view. If a tendon laceration is not seen but the sheath is cut, it should be assumed that the tendon is also lacerated.

The anatomy of the flexor tendons is complex (Fig. 45–6). All these tendons enter the hand through the carpal tunnel. In the palm, the flexor digitorum profundus (FDP) and the flexor digitorum superficialis (FDS) travel together to all the fingers except the thumb. At the level of the metacarpophalangeal (MCP) joints, a fibrous canal, the flexor tendon sheath, surrounds them. Condensations of these sheaths form the pulley system of the fingers, which, along with the transverse carpal ligament, prevents bow-stringing of the tendons and allows the flexor tendons to flex the joints fully with little dissipation of energy. At the proximal phalanx, the FDP passes through the superficialis tendon and continues distally to insert on the proximal portion of the distal phalanges of the index, middle, ring, and small fingers. The FDP mainly flexes the distal interphalangeal (DIP) joint. Testing for injury to the FDP is done by immobilizing the MCP joint

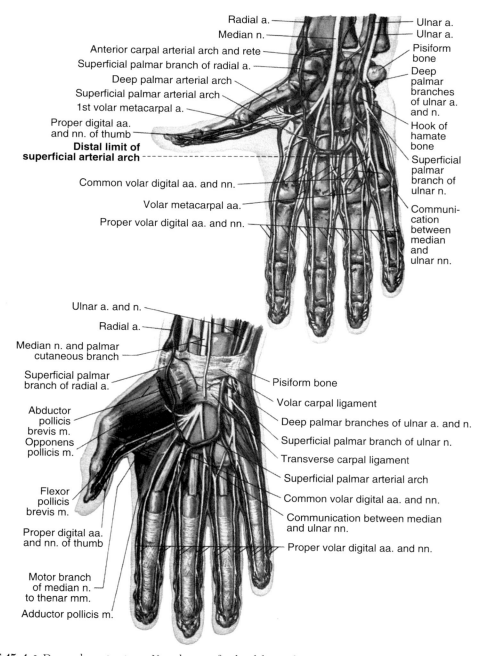

FIGURE 45–4 • Deep palmar structures. Note the superficial and deep palmar arterial arches. (Copyright ©1988 CIBA-GEIGY Corporation. Reproduced with permission from the CLINICAL SYMPOSIA by Frank H. Netter, MD.)

and the proximal interphalongeal (PIP) joint while the patient flexes the DIP joint against resistance.

The FDS splits around the FDP to insert on the middle phalanx of the index, middle, ring, and small fingers. Inactivating the profundus by extending the fingers not tested and having the patient flex the PIP joint against resistance tests it. This test is not reliable for the index finger because this finger has an independent profundus muscle belly and cannot be inactivated in this manner. Having the patient flex the PIP joint while the physician feels for laxity of the distal phalanx tests the index finger. Another maneuver is to have the patient pinch the thumb forcefully against the index finger with the DIP joint hyperextended. Patients with superficialis tendon

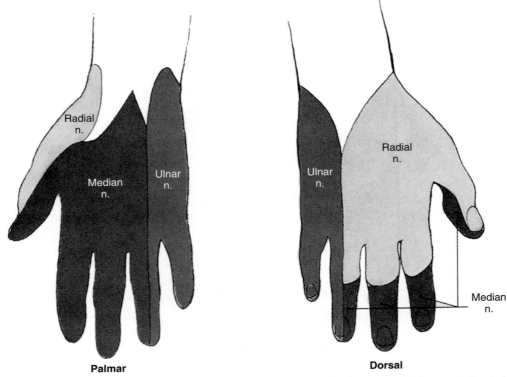

FIGURE 45–5 • Sensory distribution in the hand. (From Carter PR: Common Hand Injuries and Infections: A Practical Approach to Early Treatment. Philadelphia, WB Saunders, 1983; with permission.)

TABLE 45–1. Motor Innervation and Testing

Nerve	Innervation	Test
Ulnar	Muscles of the hypothenar eminence, two ulnar lumbricals, interossei, adductor pollicis, flexor carpi ulnaris, deep head of the flexor pollicis brevis, and flexor digitorum profundus of the ring and little fingers	Index finger abduction (first dorsal interosseus)
Median	Muscles of the thenar eminence, two radial lumbricals, palmaris longus, flexor carpi radialis, flexor pollicis longus, flexor digitorum superficialis, and flexor digitorum profundus of the index and long fingers	Thumb palmar abduction (abductor pollicis brevis)
Radial	All extrinsic muscle extensors	Wrist and finger extension

injuries tend to flex the DIP joint during this maneuver.

The flexor pollicis longus (FPL) inserts on the thumb's distal phalanx and is tested by immobilizing the MCP joint and having the patient flex the interphalangeal joint against resistance.

Extensor tendons travel through six osseofibrous canals on the dorsal surface of the wrist (Fig. 45–7). Cross-linking of these tendons can make testing difficult. The testing of these extensor tendons is outlined in Table 45–2.

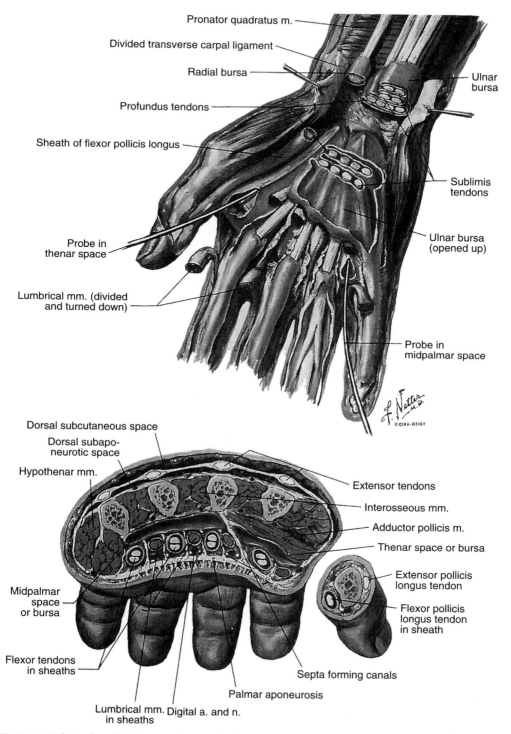

FIGURE 45–6 • Relationship of the flexor tendons to other deep structures of the hand. (Copyright ©1988 CIBA-GEIGY Corporation. Reproduced with permission from the CLINICAL SYMPOSIA by Frank H. Netter, MD.)

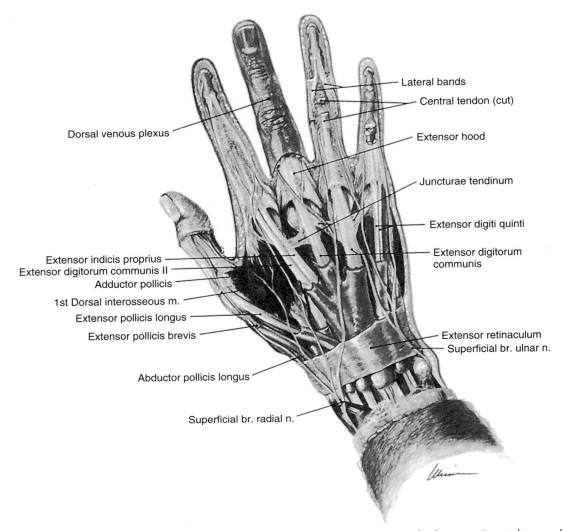

FIGURE 45–7 • Extensor surface of the hand. (From Carter PR: Common Hand Injuries and Infections: A Practical Approach to Early Treatment. Philadelphia, WB Saunders, 1983; with permission.)

Examination in a Bloodless Field

With uncooperative patients or when occult injuries such as partial flexor tendon lacerations, open joint injuries, or retained foreign bodies are suspected, examination in a bloodless field is performed. This is accomplished by applying a layer of Webril around the patient's arm and elevating it for 2 minutes. A blood pressure cuff or a pneumatic tourniquet is inflated to 250 mm Hg. Patients can generally tolerate this procedure for 15 minutes.

CLINICAL REASONING

As covered under "Clinical Assessment," the key questions in approaching hand injuries are as follows:

1. What was the *mechanism of injury* and what is the *extent of soft tissue injury* and/or *injury to deeper structures* such as nerves, tendons, or vessels?

TABLE 45–2. The Extensor Tendons of the Hand

Compartment	Tendons	Insertion	Test of Function
First	Abductor pollicis longus	Dorsum of the base of the thumb metacarpal	Extension and abduction of the thumb
	Extensor pollicis brevis	Dorsum of the base of the thumb proximal phalanx	Extension and abduction of the thumb
Second	Extensor carpi radialis longus	Dorsum of the base of the index metacarpal	Making fist while extending the wrist
	Extensor carpi radialis brevis	Dorsum of the base of the long metacarpal	Making fist while extending the wrist
Third	Extensor pollicis longus	Dorsum of the base of the thumb distal phalanx	Lifting the thumb off the surface of a table while the palm is flat against the table
Fourth	Extensor digitorum communis	Dorsum of the base of the proximal phalanges	Extension of the fingers at the MCP joints
	Extensor indicis proprius	Dorsum of the base of the proximal phalanx of the index finger	Extension of the index finger at the MCP joint with the other fingers in a fist
Fifth	Extensor digiti minimi	Dorsum of the extensor hood of the small finger	Extension of the small finger while making a fist
Sixth	Extensor carpi ulnaris	Dorsum of the base of the small finger metacarpal	Extension and ulnar deviation of the wrist

MCP, metacarpophalangeal.

2. Do the *physical examination findings* fit with the *reported mechanism*? If not, should an *uncertain diagnosis* be *considered*?
3. What is the *potential* for *infection*? What is the degree and kind of contamination and what is the degree of soft tissue injury?
4. What *impact* will this *injury* have on the *patient's occupation* or *recreational activities*?

DIAGNOSTIC ADJUNCTS

Laboratory Studies

Laboratory work is rarely indicated in the care of open injuries to the upper extremity. A few exceptions are listed here:

* Complete blood cell count in exsanguinating injuries
* Type and screen (for potential crossmatch) in exsanguinating injuries
* Coagulation studies with excessive ecchymoses or poorly controlled bleeding
* Blood glucose in the nonhealing wound or severe infection
* Wound cultures when indicated. Cultures are often used with open fractures, but this use is controversial.

Radiologic Imaging

Radiographs are commonly used in evaluating hand injuries. The decision to use radiography depends on several factors, including medical indications, patient expectations, time management, medicolegal considerations, and physician uncertainty. The medical indications for obtaining radiographs of the hand are listed below:

* To determine the extent of injury
* To diagnose an occult injury
* To detect a foreign body
* To document results of therapy (postreduction alignment, foreign body removal)

Routine plain radiographs include the anteroposterior, oblique, and lateral views. It is important that a true lateral view be obtained because any degree of obliquity may obscure a subtle but functionally significant injury.

PRINCIPLES OF MANAGEMENT

General Principles

Management of patients with an open injury to the hand requires attention to four factors.

Hemorrhage Control. This has been discussed earlier in "Initial Approach and Stabilization."

Wound Care. Detailed discussion of wound care is found in Chapter 49, Wound Care. The following elements are basic to wound care:

1. Moderate-pressure irrigation with a 19-gauge needle, 35-mL syringe, and at least 250 mL of normal saline. (Do not irrigate the pure puncture wound, because debris can be forced farther into the wound.)

2. Skin cleansing with an agent such as povidone-iodine solution, Hibiclens, or Shur-Clens.
3. Judicious débridement of wound edges and devitalized tissue, especially in animal and human bites.
4. Sutures of the skin with a nonreactive monofilament material such as 5-0 nylon. Generally, a single-layer closure is sufficient. (Do not close bite wounds to the hand.)
5. Routine antibiotics for uncomplicated lacerations of the hand have not been found to be effective in preventing infections. Instead, early treatment and meticulous wound care are the more important factors.

Dressing. The dressing serves several functions:

- Absorption of drainage
- Support and protection
- Prevention or reduction of edema
- Provision of a framework for the application of topical antibiotics

The dressing consists of three parts:

1. The first layer is a nonadherent, fine-mesh layer that is applied directly over the wound. This layer allows seepage to occur without allowing the layer above to adhere to the wound.
2. The second layer is the absorbent and protective layer and consists of several fluffed gauze pads.
3. The final layer is stretchable and conforming and serves to provide even pressure without constriction.

Immobilization and Elevation. It is important to immobilize the hand in a position that will not result in functional impairment once the acute event has resolved. For most injuries this consists of placing the hand in the "safe position," with the wrist in 30 degrees of extension, the MCP joints in 60 to 90 degrees of flexion, the interphalangeal joints in 10 to 20 degrees of flexion, and the thumb in palmar abduction (Fig. 45–8). This position maximally stretches the collateral ligaments of the MCP and interphalangeal joints and reduces the danger of joint stiffness from collateral ligament shortening (Fig. 45–9). Other splinting techniques include the radial and ulnar gutter splints, the thumb spica, and the mallet finger splint. Aluminum splints as well as preformed splints may be used.

Elevation is important when one is attempting to prevent or reduce edema. When combined with pressure and splinting, elevation markedly reduces edema and improves functional outcome.

Management of Specific Injuries

Flexor Tendon Lacerations. The anatomy of the flexor tendons is quite complex. These tendons travel through a dense osseofibrous canal and are in close proximity to bones, nerves, arteries, and other tendons. Surgery is difficult, and functional recovery is often disappointing. Consequently, repair in the emergency department is not indicated. Instead, the wound is cleansed and the skin is loosely sutured. Prophylactic antibiotics, usually cephalosporins,

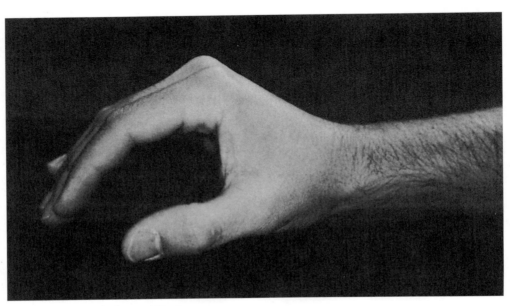

FIGURE 45–8 • Position of safe immobilization.

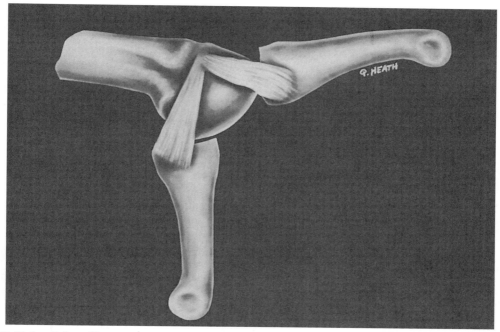

FIGURE 45–9 • Collateral ligaments at the metacarpophalangeal and interphalangeal joints are taut in flexion and lax in extension. (Adapted from Eaton RG: Joint Injuries of the Hand. Springfield, IL, Charles C Thomas, 1971; with permission)

are started and the hand is splinted in flexion. The patients are promptly referred to a specialist in hand surgery.

Extensor Tendon Lacerations. The superficial location of extensor tendons makes them susceptible to injury and accessible to repair. So, some extensor tendon lacerations, unlike flexor tendons, may be repaired in the emergency department by an experienced physician. Although repair may take place from the distal insertion to a level proximal to the wrist, the tendons most easily repaired are those in the area of the metacarpals. If one is unfamiliar with the repair of extensor tendons, the wound is treated as a flexor tendon laceration except that the hand is splinted in extension.

Nerve Injury. The diagnosis of a nerve injury is made on physical examination. Emergency treatment consists of wound care, suturing the skin, prophylactic antibiotics, and splinting. Referral to a specialist for consideration of repair is essential and should be arranged before the patient is discharged from the emergency department.

Vascular Injury. Vascular injuries are referred to a vascular or hand surgeon.

UNCERTAIN DIAGNOSIS

Uncertainty frequently surrounds hand injuries regarding the degree of soft tissue injury or specific structures injured. This is caused by local swelling, patient apprehension, other distracting injuries, and the inability to achieve visualization of deeper structures that may be injured. If the clinician suspects injury to underlying nerves, vessels, tendons, or possibly joints, then the patient should be referred to a hand specialist after the wound is cleaned, examined, sutured, and dressed as outlined earlier.

SPECIAL CONSIDERATIONS

Infections

Infections of the hand may result from a break in the skin or, rarely, from hematogenous spread. The infections reviewed here are primary infections rather than complications of existing wounds.

Paronychia. A paronychia, or "run-around abscess," is an infection of the soft tissue surrounding the base and sides of the nail, usually caused by *Staphylococcus aureus* or *Streptococcus pyogenes* (Fig. 45–10). Drainage is accomplished by entering it just above the nail with a No. 11 blade. After drainage, treatment consists of trimming of the nail, warm soaks, and oral antibiotics.

Felon. A felon is a distal pulp space infection characterized by swelling, erythema, and pain. The causative organisms are the same as those

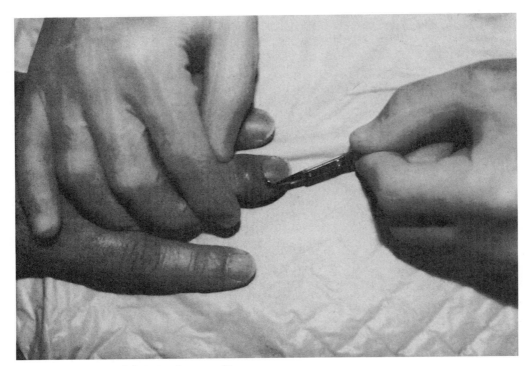

FIGURE 45–10 • Incision and drainage of a paronychia.

causing paronychias. Treatment is surgical decompression. Although there are several methods of treatment, the preferred method is a longitudinal incision over the area of "pointing," which is usually over the central pad. The wound is loosely packed, and the patient is started on antibiotics such as a penicillinase-resistant penicillin or a cephalosporin. This procedure is preferably done in consultation with a hand surgeon.

Deep Space Infections. There are many spaces in the hand that can harbor infection. These spaces include the web space, palmar space, thenar space, hypothenar space, ulnar bursae, radial bursae, and Parona's space. The patient presents with pain, swelling, tenderness to palpation, erythema, localized warmth, and, sometimes, systemic symptoms such as fever and chills. Treatment is emergent operative débridement.

Suppurative Flexor Tenosynovitis. This infection is an acute inflammation of the flexor tendon sheath characterized by Knavel's four cardinal signs of flexor tenosynovitis:

- Finger in slight flexion
- Uniform swelling of the finger
- Tenderness along the course of the tendon sheath
- Pain on passive extension

Pus forms in the closed flexor tendon sheath, which causes an increase in pressure, leading to tissue ischemia, tendon necrosis, and finally tendon adhesions (Fig. 45–11). The infection may remain localized or may extend into the thenar or midpalmar bursa (Fig. 45–12). Treatment is prompt surgical decompression in the operating room.

Human Bites

Human bite injuries to the hand often occur during an altercation. A direct bite to the hand or a clenched fist bite injury are both common. The direct bites to the hand tend to have more soft tissue injury and can be dorsal or volar in location. The clenched fist injury, the "fight bite," will have a small puncture/laceration overlying the metacarpophalangeal joint. Puncture wounds caused by a human bite are far more prone to infection than a similar injury caused by an animal.

These infections are often caused by a mixture of oral and skin flora. In addition, risk of exposure to fungi and viruses must be considered. The physician treating patients with puncture or lacerations over the dorsal MCP joint must have a high index of suspicion for a bite injury because the patient will often not volunteer this information. Initial

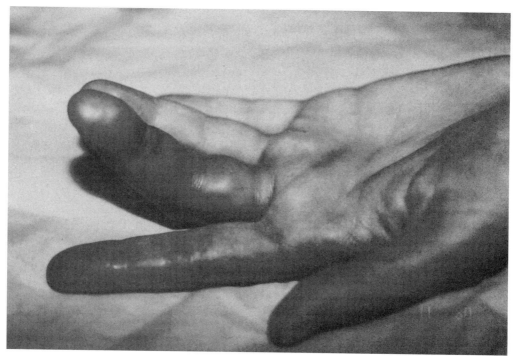

FIGURE 45–11 • Suppurative tenosynovitis of the long finger. This was caused by an untreated seemingly minor laceration at the distal interphalangeal crease. Note Knavel's signs of suppurative tenosynovitis.

inspection of the wound may appear benign. Discovery of a tract or deeper injury may be dependent on mimicking hand position at the time of the injury. Surgical exploration of the wound with thorough irrigation and débridement is required. Intravenous antibiotics are begun immediately. Despite aggressive therapy these injuries may progress to extensive soft tissue infection, joint sepsis, and osteomyelitis. Some cases may require repeat débridement and rarely amputation.

Nail Bed Injuries

The role of the fingernail is cosmetic, protective, and functional. The nail, by stabilizing the finger pad, allows greater sensitivity and precise touch and grasp and is therefore vitally important to the function of the hand (Fig. 45–13).

Injuries to the hand often involve the nail bed. A neglected injury may cause pain as well as splitting, ridging, and clawing of the nail. These problems are extremely troublesome for the patient, so efforts directed at diagnosis and precise repair at the time of injury will ensure the best functional and cosmetic results.

Subungual hematomas are common injuries that often occur when a door is closed on a fingertip. The patient complains of pain, and physical examination reveals a swollen, tender distal phalanx with a nail discolored owing to hematoma. Radiographs should be taken to rule out a distal phalanx fracture. Treatment consists of nail trephination, which may be done with an 18-gauge needle or electrocautery. This releases the blood and results in immediate relief from pain.

Traditional literature states that a subungual hematoma is more extensive, covering more than 25% of the visible nail; or if there is an obvious nail bed injury, the nail should be removed. Newer data suggest that even larger hematomas of more than 25% of the visible nail can be treated with trephination and splinting if associated with a stable distal phalanx fracture. Nail removal should be performed in cases involving open nail plate/nail bed injuries or with unstable or comminuted distal phalanx fractures to permit better fracture reduction and alignment and nail bed repair. This can be accomplished by using a mosquito hemostat while sharply dissecting the nail from the nail bed and eponychium. The nail should be thoroughly cleansed and saved. The nail bed is irrigated and minimally débrided, and lacerations are repaired using 6-0 absorbable sutures on a fine needle. The principles of repair include preservation and accurate apposition of tissue.

After the nail bed has been repaired, the nail plate is placed beneath the nail fold (eponychium).

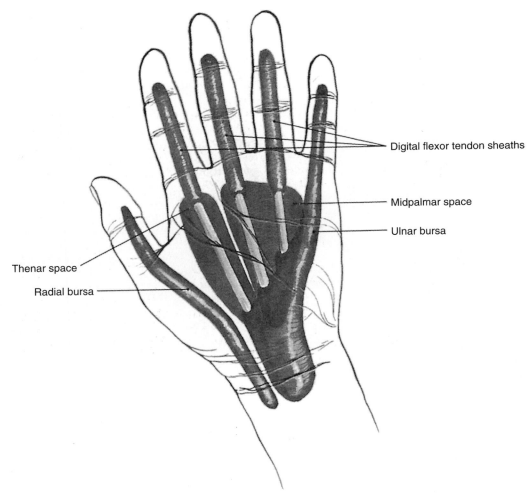

FIGURE 45–12 • Relationship of flexor tendon sheaths and palmar spaces. Tendon sheath infection can spread into these spaces. (From Carter PR: Common Hand Injuries and Infections: A Practical Approach to Early Treatment. Philadelphia, WB Saunders, 1983; with permission.)

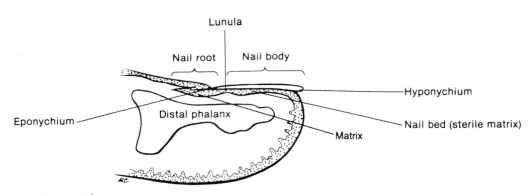

FIGURE 45–13 • Nail anatomy.

This will prevent adhesions between the nail fold and the repaired bed. If the nail plate is not available, a trimmed nonadherent material such as the aluminum wrapper of the suture may be used.

Extensive injuries such as unstable distal phalanx fractures, severe crush injuries, and nail bed avulsions are best referred to a specialist.

Open Fractures

An open fracture is defined as an interruption in the integument communicating with an underlying fracture. These are often associated with lacerations or puncture wounds. Sometimes they will have visible protruding bone or bony fragments in the wound. There are many classification schemes described in the literature. The Gustilo-Anderson classification separates open fractures into three types:

1. Type 1 fractures are clean and have less than 1 cm openings.
2. Type 2 open fractures have extensive soft tissue damage, with openings greater than 1 cm.
3. Type 3 open fractures involve high-energy trauma, severe soft tissue injury associated with segmental or comminuted fractures, and occasional vascular injury.
   a. Type 3A fractures are defined as injuries with comminution or segmental fracture, regardless of the size of the soft tissue injury.
   b. Type 3B injuries are more severe and are associated with massive contamination, severe periosteal stripping and soft tissue loss, and significant fracture and bone exposure.
   c. Type 3C fractures are those with vascular injury that require repair to restore perfusion.

All open fractures require orthopedic consultation. The very simple open fracture with a small perforating injury is débrided and left open and the fracture stabilized as in a closed injury. For all other open fracture injuries (Gustilo types 2, 3A, 3B, and 3C) meticulous débridement, irrigation, and fracture stabilization are required. Tetanus prophylaxis and intravenous antibiotics (usually a cephalosporin) are started. An aminoglycoside should be added to antibiotic coverage in type 3 injuries, and triple antibiotics should be considered for the patient with a severely contaminated wound.

Gunshot wounds may be a common source of open fracture in the upper extremity in the urban emergency department. There are many variables that determine severity. In general, low-velocity handguns cause less severe injury than the high-velocity rifle or shotgun. Additional consideration should be the caliber of the weapon used and whether the missiles used were soft or hollow point bullets designed to expand on impact. All missile wounds must be considered contaminated because the heat of firing does not sterilize the gunshot wound or the bullet. Bacteria and foreign material can be drawn into the wound from both the entrance and the exit by formation of a temporary cavity, and surrounding soft tissue injury further increases the risk of infection.

Basic management is similar to that of the open fracture. All damaged skin margins, devitalized fascia, and muscle are débrided. Copious irrigation is necessary for removal of gross contaminants. The wound is then immobilized and placed in a bulky compressive dressing for absorption of drainage and to prevent hematoma formation. Low-velocity wounds may often be managed on an outpatient basis with oral antibiotics and close follow-up, whereas high-velocity wounds will require admission and management as that described for open fracture.

Amputations and Replantations

Replantation is a commonly accepted medical practice, as evidenced by the number of centers specializing in this procedure and by its popularity in the lay press. In fact, "educated consumers" expect that all amputated parts will be replanted with subsequent return to full function. Physicians responsible for the initial care of patients with amputations need to be aware of the indications and contraindications for replantation and of the proper handling and transport of the amputated part.

Replantation is considered in the following situations:

- Thumb amputations
- Multiple digit amputations
- Wrist and forearm amputations
- Amputations in children
- Single-digit amputations proximal to the MCP joint or distal to the FDS insertion

Contraindications to replantation are generally considered to include

- Severe crush injuries, severe degloving injuries
- Multiple levels of amputation
- Single-digit amputations between the MCP joint and the FDS insertion
- Mental instability of the patient (those with severe psychiatric illness or self mutilators)

- Severe medical illness
- Injuries that are more than 8 hours old
- Other life-threatening injuries that take priority

Transporting the amputated part appropriately is important if replantation is to be considered. It is best to wrap the part in saline-moistened sterile gauze, seal it in a plastic bag, and place it on crushed ice.

Physicians involved in the care of patients with amputations should understand that functional recovery is never assured, prolonged morbidity is common, and multiple surgeries over years may be required. The decision to attempt replantation depends on many factors, including the age and occupation of the patient, level of amputation, condition of the amputated part, patient motivation, and the absence of medical illness.

High-Pressure Injection Injuries

The use of high-pressure compression equipment for the application of grease, paint, paint solvents, and hydraulic fluid is common. These devices can generate emission pressures of 1500 to 12,000 pounds per square inch (psi). Associated with the proliferation of this equipment is an increase in the number of patients who sustain high-pressure injection injuries. These injuries usually occur at work, with the index finger of the left hand the most common site.

The pathophysiology is related to two major factors. First, the amount of material injected influences the mechanical distention and subsequently the pressure in the tissue. More injected material results in greater pressures, which decrease arterial inflow and reduce venous outflow. Additionally, a local physical effect results in edema, which further increases tissue pressure and ischemia. Second, the type of material injected is important. Agents such as paint, solvents, and fuels produce an intense inflammatory reaction and are extremely damaging to tissue. These substances cause edema by direct chemical irritation, further increasing tissue ischemia. Other factors include the compression pressure generated by the device, which influences the spread through tissue, the anatomic areas involved, and any delay in diagnosis and treatment.

The diagnosis is made by the history and by observing the site of entry, which may be only 2 to 3 mm. Although the initial physical findings may be scant and the patient's complaints minimal, the injury is significant, and the likelihood of a poor outcome is great. Radiographs of the fingers and hand may demonstrate the presence of the foreign substance (Fig. 45–14). The patient should be prepared for surgery, which consists of decompression, débridement, and thorough irrigation. Consultants should be contacted early because a delay of surgery beyond 6 hours post injury increases the incidence of amputation, which may be as high as 60% to 80% with injectants such as paint and solvent.

Farm Injuries

Significant injury to the upper extremity by farm machinery can be devastating. The power take off (PTO), augers, balers, corn pickers, moving chains, belts, and rollers are examples of potentially dangerous yet common farm machinery. Most farm equipment causes injury by a combination of compressive, shearing, and thermal forces. Injuries vary from the simple distal fingertip amputation to the mangled extremity. Hydraulic lines account for high-pressure injection injuries. Most farm injuries are significantly contaminated and will require extensive débridement and irrigation. After fracture stabilization, wound closure with a drain or delayed wound closure are options to consider. Wound closure may be a delayed primary closure 48 to 72 hours after the initial examination and irrigation. Therapy with broad-spectrum antibiotics is recommended.

DISPOSITION AND FOLLOW-UP

The great majority of patients with open hand injuries and infections are managed as outpatients. A few injuries, however, demand special attention and require hospitalization:

1. Mutilating hand injuries
2. Injection injuries
3. Highly contaminated lacerations requiring operative débridement
4. Open fractures and dislocations requiring operative intervention
5. Complex infections such as suppurative flexor tenosynovitis, deep space infections, and septic arthritis
6. Nerve trunk lacerations
7. Multiple tendon or nerve lacerations

Patients who have isolated digital nerve or tendon lacerations may have prompt surgical follow-up rather than immediate surgery. Because the type and timing of surgery are operator dependent, each surgeon will have his or her own preference. For tidy wounds, it is appropriate to irrigate copiously, suture the skin, splint, and treat with prophylactic antibiotics. Untidy wounds are dressed and left open.

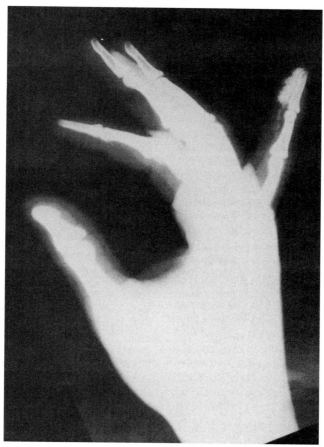

FIGURE 45–14 • High-pressure paint injection to little finger. Note paint visible in soft tissue and along the course of the tendon sheath. (From Rudzinski J, Uehara D: Radiology of the hand. Trauma Q 1986; 2(4):61, with permission of Aspen Publishers, Inc. Copyright © 1986.)

FINAL POINTS

- Open injuries often harbor an injury to bone, nerves, tendons, and arteries. A high index of suspicion and "topographic anticipation" based on the cardinal line of Kaplan are the keys to diagnosis.
- An abnormal position of the hand at rest may indicate a tendon laceration.
- When evaluating a hand laceration, it is more important to test for the function of the structures at risk than to attempt to visualize damaged structures in the depth of the wound.
- Sensory examination using two-point discrimination is accurate and reliable. The normal range is 2 to 5 mm.
- Examination in a bloodless field is often rewarding and is essential if the diagnosis is in doubt.
- Ice, elevation, and splinting reduce edema and shorten recovery time.

- Radiographs are used frequently to determine the extent of injury, diagnose occult injuries, detect foreign bodies, and document results of therapy.
- Principles of management of hand injuries include hemorrhage control, irrigation and débridement, dressing, immobilization in the proper position, and elevation.
- Suppurative tenosynovitis is a surgical emergency. Diagnosis is by observing flexion of the finger, uniform swelling of the finger, tenderness along the course of the tendon sheath, and pain on passive extension.
- The paucity of physical findings in patients with high-pressure injection injuries belies the catastrophic nature of this injury.
- Patients with single nerve or tendon injuries are generally referred to a hand surgeon for delayed repair.

CASE *Study*

A 55-year-old man injured his hand while attempting to manually declog the snow chute of his snow blower. The ambulance was delayed because of heavy snowfall. Neighbors wrapped his gloved hand in a scarf and brought him to the emergency department.

On arrival the patient's blood pressure was 120/90 mm Hg, pulse rate was 110 beats per minute, and respiratory rate was 20 breaths per minute. Initial examination revealed no evidence of injury except to the right hand, which on inspection was found to have multiple severe lacerations involving the volar aspect of the wrist and the radial half of the palm. There was diffuse bleeding.

This patient is hemodynamically stable. He is somewhat tachycardic and tachypneic, most likely from pain and anxiety. While the injury to the hand is significant, the first priority is always to evaluate for life-threatening injuries or impairment of vital functions. Finding none, attention can be redirected to the hand injury. Control of bleeding in the hand is best accomplished with direct pressure. When the hand is not being examined or treated, it can be wrapped in a tight dressing using sterile gauze. This patient should receive pain medication early in the course of care.

An intravenous line is established and a normal saline infusion is started. Analgesia is provided intravenously using small doses of morphine as needed. Serial monitoring of the patient's blood pressure and respiration is ordered.

Meticulous examination of the wrist and hand is needed but is impaired by the bleeding. The patient's arm is elevated for 2 minutes, followed by placement of a blood pressure cuff on the upper arm. The cuff is inflated to 250 mm Hg and maintained at that pressure during the examination.

Use of a blood pressure cuff or a pneumatic tourniquet in the manner described is essential for most severe hand injuries. A thorough examination cannot be accomplished when there is continued, active bleeding from the site being examined.

Using an inflated cuff to provide a bloodless field for examination is essential, but examination and treatment must proceed promptly. Typically, the patient will begin to complain of ischemic pain after about 15 minutes of use.

Examination reveals a 4-cm laceration of the radial aspect of the volar surface of the wrist. Exploration reveals severing of the radial artery and of two major tendons at the wrist, the flexor carpi radialis and the flexor pollicis longus.

Although the bleeding from this patient's injuries was significant, there was no arterial pulsation observed, in spite of the fact that the radial artery was found to be severed. With complete transection, arteries retract and go into spasm, therefore reducing the amount of bleeding. It is the incompletely severed artery that cannot retract and close down that creates pulsatile bleeding.

On observation of the hand at rest, the index and long fingers are abnormally straightened. The ring and little fingers have a normal degree of flexion at rest. On specific testing, flexion of the ring and little fingers is found to be intact.

The flexor digitorum sublimis tendon to the long finger is not functioning (this finger cannot be flexed when the neighboring fingers are fixed in position), but the flexor digitorum profundus is intact (the distal interphalangeal joint can be flexed when the MCP and PIP joints are fixed in position). In the index finger, neither of these tendons is functional. The interphalangeal joint of the thumb also cannot be flexed when the MCP joint is fixed in position.

Sensation, tested with two-point discrimination, is intact throughout. The patient begins to complain of severe aching in the entire arm distal to the blood pressure cuff after about 15 minutes of examination and cleaning of the wounds. The cuff is deflated, and the aching resolves.

Examination of the tendons indicates severing of the flexor pollicis longus (this injury was also detected by exploration at the wrist), both flexor tendons to the index finger, and the flexor digitorum sublimis to the long finger. These tendon injuries may also be demonstrated by exploration of the palmar lacerations. The injury itself may be difficult to detect, however, because severed tendons usually retract out of the field of view. Even partially severed tendons may be difficult to visualize, because the cut may have occurred at a point when the tendon was significantly flexed or extended. At rest, the point of injury may not be visible. Therefore, efforts to visualize tendon injuries should include examination throughout the entire range of movement of the tendon.

Sensation to the hand was found to be intact. Palmar sensation is provided via the ulnar and median nerves that were not involved in this injury.

Plain films of the hand revealed no fractures. The patient was taken to the operating room where the following injuries were found:

- Radial artery transection
- Flexor pollicis longus laceration
- Flexor carpi radialis laceration
- Flexor digitorum profundus and sublimis laceration of the index finger
- Flexor digitorum sublimis laceration of the long finger

All injuries were repaired. One year after the incident the patient is working at his previous job with nearly complete functional recovery.

Even without the arterial injury, this patient's tendon injuries would have required repair in the operating room. Flexor tendon repairs are difficult, and recovery of full function may not always occur. Even single flexor tendon injuries require repair in the operating room and should not be attempted in the emergency department.

Bibliography

TEXTS

Brinker M, Miller M: Fundamentals of Orthopaedics. Philadelphia, WB Saunders, 1999.

Hart RG, Uehara DT, Wagner MJ: Emergency and Primary Care of the Hand. Dallas, American College of Emergency Physicians, 2001.

Martin DS, Collins ED: Manual of Acute Hand Injuries. St. Louis, Mosby–Year Book, 1998.

Reider B: The Orthopaedic Physical Examination. Philadelphia, WB Saunders, 1999.

JOURNAL ARTICLES

American College of Emergency Physicians: Clinical policy for the initial approach to patients presenting with penetrating extremity trauma. Acad Emerg Med 1999; 33:612–636.

Bhende MS, Dandrea LA, Davis HW: Hand injuries in children presenting to a pediatric emergency department. Ann Emerg Med 1993; 22:1519–1523.

Harrison BP, Hilliard MW: Emergency department evaluation and treatment of hand injuries. Emerg Med Clin North Am 1999; 17:793–822.

Hausman MR, Lisser SP: Hand infections. Orthop Clin North Am 1992; 23:171–185.

Kieban M, Kanes D, Buckman RF: Gunshot wounds of the hand: Anatomic patterns of injury. Ann Emerg Med 2000; 36:523–524.

Lampe E: Surgical anatomy of the hand: With special reference to infections and trauma. CIBA Symp 1988; 40(3):1–36.

Perron AD, Miller MD, Brady WJ: Orthopedic pitfalls in the ED: Fight bite. Am J Emerg Med 2002; 20:114–117.

Steinberg DR: Acute flexor tendon injuries. Orthop Clin North Am 1992; 23:125–140.

Vasilenski D, Noorbergen M, Dipiertem M, Lafontraine M: High pressure injection injuries to the hand. Am J Emerg Med 2000; 18:820–824.

CHAPTER 46

Closed Injuries of the Upper Extremity

VALERIE NEYLAN

CASE *Study*

A 27-year-old man presents to the emergency department after sustaining trauma to the right upper extremity while playing racquetball. He says he ran into the wall with his extended right arm and now complains of severe pain to the right shoulder.

INTRODUCTION

The diagnosis and treatment of acute injuries of the extremities is facilitated by taking a thorough history of the mechanism of injury, noting specific physical findings, and maintaining an awareness of associated injuries. Twenty-five percent of all emergency department visits are for orthopedic complaints. Approximately half of these involve acute injuries of the upper extremity.

Although these injuries are seldom life threatening, they may have a major impact on an individual's lifestyle and livelihood. The hand and the upper extremity are important in almost every activity of daily living, including routine personal care, occupational activities, and recreational activities. This active role predisposes the hand and arm to injury. The protective response of the body, using the arm to ward off a blow or to brace the body during a fall, increases the risk of injury.

Failure to adequately diagnose and appropriately treat an upper extremity injury may result in major functional impairment or deformity. Because the majority of patients incurring upper extremity injury are young, healthy individuals, the functional, financial, and potential medicolegal impact is even greater. A thorough knowledge of the anatomy of the upper extremity, the potential injuries that can occur, and the mechanisms that are likely to result in specific injuries forms the basis for the clinical evaluation and management of these injuries in the emergency department.

INITIAL APPROACH AND STABILIZATION

Priority is given to resuscitation of vital functions and to injuries that are potentially life threatening. Once life threats have been treated or ruled out, attention can be focused on injuries of the extremities.

Rapid Assessment

The necessary history is brief and focused, but the details of the events are important in assessing the likelihood of various specific injuries.

1. A vascular examination is performed to rule out deficits requiring immediate reduction. The morbidity of limb ischemia is directly proportional to time without blood flow. A cold, pale, pulseless distal extremity is an indication for immediate reduction before radiography.
2. What kind of *activity* was the patient involved in at the *time of injury*? This information helps to determine a logical sequence between the activity and the injury. It is important to consider the possibility that a different disease process caused the injury (e.g., a "fall" may turn out to be syncope on more specific questioning).
3. *Exactly what happened* to the injured extremity? The mechanism of injury is very helpful in identifying the specific injury. A fall on an outstretched arm predisposes to certain injuries, such as wrist fractures, supracondylar fractures, elbow dislocations, and proximal humeral shaft fractures.
4. What *symptoms* has the patient noticed since the injury? Increasing pain suggests a compartment syndrome. Numbness, weakness, or tingling suggests nerve injury or compression. Limitation of movement suggests a fracture or joint injury. The course of the symptoms can help to differentiate acute injury from chronic conditions, such as arthritis or overuse syndromes.
5. What sort of *occupational and leisure activities* does the patient engage in, and which is the patient's *dominant hand*? The significance of an upper extremity injury may be magnified many times depending on the patient's livelihood. An injury to the dominant hand of a professional

violinist or sculptor may be treated more aggressively than that of a debilitated person.

Early Intervention

1. Jewelry and constricting clothing are removed to avoid a tourniquet effect as local swelling occurs.
2. Ice and elevation of the extremity will help to minimize edema. A carefully interposed barrier, such as a hand towel, is necessary to protect against thermal injury.
3. Padded, preformed aluminum splints, inflatable air splints, arm slings, or other "universal" devices are used to increase patient comfort initially. These devices are suitable for temporary use only and will usually be replaced with a molded splint.
4. Open wounds are covered with sterile, saline-soaked gauze to minimize contamination and tissue loss through drying. Tetanus status should be addressed.
5. Application of splints, fracture or dislocation manipulation, and movement needed for radiographic assessment all cause discomfort for the patient. Providing early adequate analgesia will result in a grateful, more comfortable, and more cooperative patient. Patients requiring conscious sedation should be monitored appropriately.

CLINICAL ASSESSMENT

History

Additional history taking is directed toward the patient's past medical history, including significant underlying illness, allergies, and medications.

Physical Examination

Exposure. The entire extremity must be uncovered to allow adequate examination. The joints above and below the suspected site of injury are included in the examination. This allows the physician to examine the impact of forces transmitted along the bone to the joint.

Inspection. *Deformity* may be caused by displaced or angulated fractures, dislocations, or edema. *Ecchymosis* requires time to develop, but with major disruptions it may be present initially. *Skin integrity* is important because any open wound over or adjacent to a fracture site is considered to communicate with the fracture (open fracture) and should be considered an orthopedic emergency.

Palpation. *Neurovascular status* is determined by checking for the presence and strength of the brachial and radial pulses, as well as for capillary refill time and skin temperature. Motor and sensory integrity of the radial, median, and ulnar nerves, which supply the hand, is evaluated as described in Chapter 45, Open Injuries to the Hand. The axillary nerve innervates the skin over the lateral shoulder, and the musculocutaneous nerve innervates the dorsum of the forearm.

Tenderness is the observation of a painful response to palpation. Although pain may be perceived over a wide area, the point of maximal tenderness is an objective sign that correlates well with the location of pathology. Careful palpation, working from uninvolved to involved areas, is required.

Swelling is also time dependent but is likely to be present to some degree at the time of initial evaluation.

Bony crepitus is perceived when bone fragments move against one another. If noted during palpation, crepitus is significant, but it is not necessary for diagnosis. Because it is associated with significant pain, it is not routinely sought in the examination.

Range of Motion. *Active and passive range of motion* is determined. Active range of motion implies patient-originated movement. Diminished active range of motion is evidence of either loss of joint integrity or injury to the musculotendinous elements that produce the movement. Passive range of motion, in which the examiner initiates the movement, is a means of evaluating joint integrity alone. An abnormally large passive range of motion implies complete rupture of the joint capsules and supporting ligaments. Testing of range of motion may lead to severe pain, complicating interpretation of these tests.

CLINICAL REASONING

After completion of the history and physical examination, the following questions are asked:

Is a Fracture or Dislocation Likely?

If a fracture or dislocation is suspected, appropriate radiographic assessment is ordered to confirm this suspicion and to delineate the exact pathologic process.

Does the Fracture or Dislocation Require Immediate Reduction?

Although rare, neurovascular complications must always be considered. If they are present, they can usually be relieved by bony realignment. Some injuries have a high incidence of neurovascular complications (e.g., supracondylar fracture is associated with ischemia and distal radioulnar ligament disruption is associated with median nerve injury).

If Bone or Joint Disruption Is Not Suggested, What Other Soft Tissue Injuries Need to Be Considered?

Contusions are usually caused by direct blows. They are associated with tenderness, swelling, and, with time, ecchymosis. There is no deformity, and any reduction in range of motion of the adjacent joints is minimal and caused by the discomfort of the contusion.

Sprains are injuries to the ligamentous structures surrounding the joint and result from abnormal or excessive joint movement that is less than that necessary to result in dislocation. This amount of ligament tear is clinically divided into three classes according to severity:

- *First-degree* (minimal) *sprains* result in tenderness on stressing the joint but do not result in joint instability.
- *Second-degree* (partial) *sprains* are significant enough tears to allow abnormal joint motion. Signs of swelling, tenderness, and ecchymosis make fracture a distinct possibility.
- *Third-degree sprains* result in complete ligamentous disruption and a grossly unstable joint. Signs of swelling, tenderness, and ecchymosis are invariably present, and a joint effusion is frequently palpable. Associated fractures are common. These injuries may heal slowly and incompletely.

Strains are injuries to musculotendinous units secondary to a violent contraction or overstretching. Mild strains are diagnosed by finding local tenderness and pain in the muscle or tendon with contraction. Severe or complete disruptions result in severe pain, loss of function, and often a palpable defect in the muscle. Avulsion of bone where the tendon inserts may be seen.

DIAGNOSTIC ADJUNCTS

Laboratory Studies

There are no laboratory tests to assist in the diagnosis of acute upper extremity injury, but they may be of use in investigating syncope or associated injuries.

Radiologic Imaging

Plain Films

Radiographs are crucial to the proper diagnosis and treatment of extremity injuries. They do not,

however, replace the history or examination. Differentiating the point of maximal tenderness from the subjective location of pain is necessary for proper selection of radiographs.

A *standard radiographic series* of any anatomic location consists of anteroposterior, lateral, and occasionally oblique views. Special views may be required for some unusual cases. Stress views, in which the integrity of one or more ligamentous structures is indirectly evaluated, may be of benefit in some cases. If suspicion of significant bony pathology is not confirmed by the standard views, one may request a magnified "coned-down" view to enhance the image of a well-localized injury site. Frequent communication with the radiology technician will enhance the usefulness of the films obtained.

Trauma to long bones seldom creates an isolated injury. The joints at either end are often affected and, therefore, must be included in the radiographs obtained.

At the extremes of age or in the presence of degenerative bone disease, injury to bone is more difficult to detect. Familiarity with the characteristics of age-dependent normal bone radiographs is helpful. "Mirror image symmetry" can be used in questionable cases by obtaining comparison views of the presumed normal extremity. This technique is used in evaluating epiphyseal regions, such as the pediatric elbow, where considerable variation exists among patients.

Certain orthopedic injuries defy standard radiographic diagnosis because the classic radiolucent fracture line is lacking. Secondary radiographic evidence may be useful. The "fat pad" sign about the elbow, described later under "Specific Injuries," is a good example. Ultimately, clinically suspected fractures should be treated with immobilization regardless of the presence or absence of radiographic signs. After a sufficient period of time, bone resorption and callus formation make radiographic diagnosis possible. Initial immobilization of any injured extremity is indicated until fracture is definitely ruled out.

Other Imaging

Tomography and *computed tomography*, in which selective "slices" of a given bone or joint are visualized, are used less commonly. These studies are used when plain radiographs are inconclusive and a definitive diagnosis is needed. *Bone scans* detect the increased bone metabolism found at a fracture site and are used to identify occult fractures. These are most helpful in chronic overuse injuries such as stress fractures. *Magnetic resonance imaging* may play a useful role in assessing soft tissue injury and determining the presence of intramuscular or ligamentous injury or hemorrhage.

Although there are "grading systems" to aid physicians in deciding what types of injuries are to be assessed radiographically, most injuries of the upper extremity are imaged. It is important not to overestimate the diagnostic powers of radiography. Some subtle fractures and most soft tissue injuries are not visualized with present techniques.

PRINCIPLES OF MANAGEMENT

General Principles

The major principles of management for all orthopedic injuries include the following:

- Analgesia and sedation, as appropriate
- Reduction to anatomic alignment
- Immobilization to allow healing
- Rehabilitation

Long-term pain control and measures to limit inflammation are useful adjuncts.

Analgesia/Anesthesia. Early administration of analgesics is indicated for patients who are stable and have purely orthopedic injuries. Major fractures and dislocations are extremely painful, and narcotic analgesics, such as meperidine or morphine, are needed. For minor reductions, such as interphalangeal dislocations, local anesthesia such as a digital block is adequate. For major reductions, such as shoulder dislocations, conscious sedation using intravenous analgesics, such as etomidate or fentanyl, and muscle relaxants such as diazepam or midazolam, may be used. Conscious sedation should be used in conjunction with proper cardiovascular and vital sign monitoring. Reversal agents for these medications as well as airway equipment, such as a bag-valve-mask and oral or nasal airway, should be available at the bedside. Anesthetic techniques that are also useful include hematoma blocks, nerve blocks, and intravenous regional anesthesia.

Reduction. Closed reduction of fractures and dislocations can, in most cases, be performed in the emergency department. Fractures and dislocations are invariably associated with spasm of the surrounding musculature. The resultant deformities can be explained based on the pertinent anatomy. Reduction is much easier after spasm has been alleviated with analgesia and/or anesthesia. Overriding or shortening at the site of a fracture or dislocation is overcome by applying steady longitudinal traction to fatigue the contracting musculature. In most cases, this can be followed by appropriate manipulation of the distal bone to

produce anatomic alignment. Periarticular fractures are often not amenable to closed reduction because the lever arm is too short to be manipulated. In cases of distal ischemia, reduction is attempted immediately to improve circulatory status. In less urgent circumstances, orthopedic consultation is obtained, after which the emergency physician or the orthopedist may perform the indicated reduction.

Immobilization. Short-term immobilization is the appropriate treatment for the majority of extremity injuries. When there is a questionable fracture, immobilization and referral are standard procedures. Invariably, if there is significant suspicion of fracture, there is sufficient soft tissue injury alone to justify a period of rest.

Because most extremity injuries seen in the emergency department are acute and tissue edema has not yet reached maximum levels, circumferential rigid casting carries the real possibility of vascular compromise. For this reason, injuries are immobilized almost exclusively with noncircumferential plaster splints. This allows the elastic bandage to be loosened as the edema increases and the neurovascular status to be easily monitored.

Therapeutic splinting decreases pain by limiting fragment movement, inflammation, and bleeding, as well as by lessening the risk of neurovascular compromise. As a general principle, immobilization of the joints above and below the site of the pathology is indicated. Joints not involved in the fracture are not splinted, and, unless contraindicated, joints are immobilized in a neutral position of function.

Commercially available, prefabricated plaster and fiberglass splints are available. They have the advantage of speed and ease of use but are not custom-made for the injury or the patient. Customized (as opposed to preformed) plaster splints provide individualized immobilization and can be designed to fit specific patients and injuries or combinations of injuries. Custom-made plaster splints, however, are time consuming and messy to apply.

Techniques of Splint Making

The standard technique of splinting is making a plaster of Paris splint specifically for the patient. Before splinting, the extremity is padded with the joints in the desired positions. The padding is applied at least two layers thick in a circumferential manner, proceeding in a distal to proximal direction. Bony prominences and taut tendons receive a minimum of two additional layers. Padding is carried well beyond the limits of the plaster both distally and proximally. Trimming excessive padding can be done easily, but plaster must not be allowed to come into direct contact with the skin. Using a roll of padding with a small diameter and applying it with tension will avoid wrinkling. Rolls of plaster are measured on the patient; a general guideline is 8 to 10 layers on the upper extremity. Vigorous young people may require additional layers. The splint is molded to fit the body contours while an assistant supports the limb in the exact position desired. Any movement at this stage creates hinging and renders the splint useless. An elastic bandage is applied from distal to proximal, and the splint is allowed to dry for approximately 30 minutes.

Some of the more commonly applied upper extremity splints and indications for their use are presented in Table 46–1. Splinting is designed to provide proper fit, durability, comfort, and immobilization.

Increased pain in the extremity after a splint is applied necessitates removal of the splint to evaluate for compartment syndrome or pressure sores.

Long Arm Posterior Splint. Fractures and dislocations near the elbow are best treated with a long-arm posterior splint. This splint is applied beginning at the ulnar aspect of the metacarpal heads, proceeding over the olecranon and up the posterior border of the arm to as proximal a position as is comfortable. Standard flexion is 90 degrees at the elbow. Usually, neutral pronation-supination is appropriate and is achieved by placing the patient's arm with the thumb up.

Sugar Tong Splint. This splint is used for radial head and Colles' fractures. It is a long splint extending dorsally from the metacarpal heads around the elbow and then volarly back to the metacarpal heads. The advantage of this splint is that it gives both volar and dorsal fixation without the disadvantages of circumferential casting. Supination-pronation is eliminated at the elbow, but a moderate degree of elbow flexion and extension will remain.

Short Arm Splint. More stable wrist injuries, such as extensor strains and impacted distal radius fractures, may be treated with either dorsal or volar short-arm posterior molds. The elbow is left free, and iatrogenic stiffness is avoided. Volar-applied splints severely limit any functional use of the hand.

Ulnar Gutter Splint. Ulnar gutter splints are applied in the same way as the simple wrist splint. They are used for fractures of the fourth and fifth metacarpals and proximal phalanges of the ring and little fingers. The splint is extended nearly to the end of the little finger and includes the ring and little fingers.

Radial Gutter Splint. The radial gutter splint is indicated for fractures of the second and third metacarpals and proximal phalanges of index and long fingers. Application necessitates a wide hole cutout for the thumb and thenar musculature.

Thumb Spica Splint. An effective thumb spica splint can be made by applying a dorsal wrist splint along with a 2- to 3-inch strip of plaster applied to the dorsum of the thumb. The thumb should be placed in opposition to the fingers as if a beverage can were being held in the hand.

Padded Aluminum Splint. Fractures of the middle and distal phalanges and post-reduction

TABLE 46–1. Immobilization of Specific Injuries

Injury	Usual Treatment
Shoulder dislocation	Reduction, sling and swathe
Rotator cuff tear	Sling and swath
Acromioclavicular joint sprains	Sling (pulled tight)
Clavicular fracture	Sling or "figure of eight"
Elbow dislocation	Reduction, long arm posterior splint
Supracondylar fracture	Long arm posterior splint
Radial head fracture	Sugar tong splint
Olecranon fracture	Long arm posterior splint
Subluxation of radial head (nursemaid's elbow)	Reduction only
Midshaft ulnar (nightstick) fracture	Long arm posterior splint
Both-bone forearm fracture	Long arm posterior splint
Wrist fractures	Sugar tong splint or long arm posterior splint
Navicular fracture, thumb metacarpal fracture	Short arm thumb spica splint
Metacarpal fracture (e.g., fifth metacarpal head, boxer's fracture)	Ulnar gutter or radial gutter splint
Metacarpophalangeal joint dislocation	Short arm posterior splint
Ulnar collateral ligament tear (gamekeeper's thumb)	Short arm thumb spica splint
Phalangeal tuft fracture	Aluminum splint
Proximal phalanx fracture	Short arm posterior splint
Middle phalanx fracture	Aluminum splint
Interphalangeal joint injuries	Reduction, aluminum splint

dislocations of the interphalangeal joints are treated with padded aluminum splints applied to the involved digit from the fingertip to the distal wrist crease. In general, all hand joints are placed in moderate flexion (the "Position of function") to avoid shortening of collateral ligaments and resultant stiffness. If there is rotatory deformity, as in spiral or long oblique fractures, an adjacent digit is "buddy splinted" to the involved one.

Slings. Simple slings are useful in a number of situations to immobilize the upper extremity. For hand or wrist injuries, they should be applied so that the hand lies higher than the heart rather than with the traditional 90-degree flexion at the elbow. Slings may be used in combination with a swathe, which is a circumferential bandage holding the arm adducted to the trunk to limit motion at the shoulder.

Specific Injuries

Shoulder Injuries

The shoulder has an extensive range of motion that predisposes it to instability. The shallow glenohumeral joint allows for extremes in movement. Joint stability is provided primarily by muscular and ligamentous attachments.

ANTERIOR SHOULDER DISLOCATION

The shoulder is the most commonly dislocated major joint. Dislocations can be anterior, posterior, inferior, and superior. Ninety-five percent are anterior dislocations, in which the humeral head lies anterior to the glenoid fossa.

Mechanism. The usual mechanism of injury is the application of leverage forces to the arm when it is in abduction and external rotation. Occasionally, direct force from behind, applied to the humeral head, can result in the same injury.

Presentation. Patients present in extreme pain, slumped forward supporting the injured arm with the well arm. Extreme pain occurs with internal rotation. There is a characteristic squared-off contour of the lateral deltoid and a prominence of the acromion. The humeral head may be palpated anteriorly. Neurapraxia of the axillary nerve, producing hypesthesia over the deltoid, may be associated and is usually transient. Avulsion fractures of the head of the humerus and inferior lip of the glenoid may also be associated. Uncommonly there are associated vascular injuries to the axillary artery and veins, especially in elderly patients.

Radiologic Diagnosis. The standard antero-posterior and scapular lateral view or "Y" views of the shoulder are adequate to make the diagnosis. If these views are inconclusive or a fracture is sug-gested, an axillary view should be obtained. Axillary views are excellent for diagnosis of dislocations and fractures but are difficult to obtain because there is the requirement for painful abduction of the injured extremity.

Management. The dislocation can be reduced by several methods. A common theme for all methods is to use adequate analgesia, muscle relaxation, and gentle and steady force. *Scapular manipulation* is highly effective and is done by an assistant applying steady traction to the involved arm or using weights suspended from the forearm while the physician rotates the tip of the scapula medially. This can be done in the prone or sitting position. The *external rotation method* has the patient supine with the elbow flexed 90 degrees at the side while the arm is slowly externally rotated with longitudinal traction. The *Milch technique* places the patient in a supine position. The patient is then guided to slowly extend and externally rotate the affected arm over the head while the physician applies gentle traction. If reduction is incomplete, the physician may manipulate the humeral head into the glenoid fossa using the thumb or fingers. *Traction-countertraction methods* can also be used involving two people and several sheets. One sheet is wrapped under the axilla of the affected shoulder and directed toward the opposite shoulder. The second sheet is applied to the flexed elbow of the injured arm. Steady gentle traction is applied in opposite directions. Successful reduction is usually appreciated palpably and visually and is confirmed by the patient's ability to internally rotate the shoulder, as evidenced by the ability to touch the uninvolved shoulder with the index finger of the injured side.

After reduction, the shoulder is held in adduction and internal rotation with a sling and swathe or shoulder immobilizer and confirmatory radiographs are done. In general, a period of 3 weeks of immobilization is necessary to reduce the incidence of repeat dislocations. Patients are informed that there is a 25% chance of recurrence after one episode and a 50% chance after two, and nearly all patients who have had three dislocations require a surgical procedure to prevent chronic recurrent dislocation.

ROTATOR CUFF TEAR

The rotator cuff tear is an injury of a group of muscles that cross the shoulder and give stability to it. The rotator cuff muscles are often mnemonically referred to as the **SITS** muscles (Fig. 46–1A):

Supraspinatus
Infraspinatus

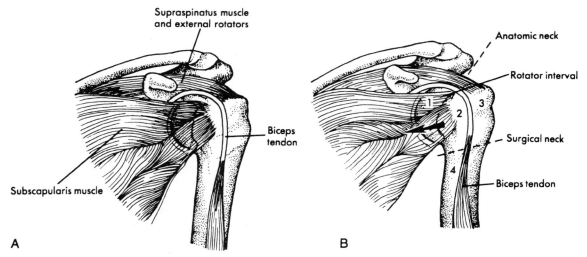

FIGURE 46–1 • Anatomy of the shoulder: *1,* head; *2,* lesser tuberosity; *3,* greater tuberosity; *4,* shaft. (From Orban DJ: Shoulder. In Rosen P, et al [eds]: Emergency Medicine: Concepts and Clinical Practice, 2nd ed, vol 1. St. Louis, CV Mosby, 1988.)

Teres minor
Subscapularis

The supraspinatus is the most frequently torn muscle/tendon.

Mechanism. A fall on the outstretched arm may tear any of these muscles without producing a fracture or dislocation.

Presentation. There is *relatively* painless passive range of motion. Active range of motion, notably initiation of external rotation and abduction, is very painful because the patient is asked to forcefully contract a muscle that has been partially torn.

Radiologic Diagnosis. The shoulder joint is intact and has a normal radiographic appearance. Magnetic resonance imaging or intra-articular contrast injection may be necessary for diagnosis. These tests are done outside of the emergency care setting.

Management. Emergency treatment consists of short-term (usually only 2 to 3 days) therapy with sling and swathe and analgesics. When consultant referral may be delayed, the physician should instruct the patient in passive range of motion exercises. Pendulum motion with the olecranon describing larger and larger diameter circles is used to avoid the development of adhesive capsulitis, which can result in decreased range of motion.

ACROMIOCLAVICULAR SEPARATIONS

The clavicle is bound to the scapula by two sets of strong ligaments (the coracoclavicular and acromioclavicular ligaments) and an acromioclavicular joint capsule.

Mechanism. When a strong force displaces the scapula inferiorly, these ligaments may tear. Commonly, this injury occurs when a football player, carrying the ball with adducted arm, is tackled and falls on the lateral shoulder.

Presentation. A complete tear (class 3) results in a "free floating" clavicle. Physical examination displays a superiorly displaced, easily visualized lateral end of the clavicle, which is ballotable. Lesser tears may produce partial separations that result in displacement only with stress (class 2) or that result only in point tenderness at the sites of attachment, anterior and inferior to the lateral aspect of the clavicle (class 1).

Radiographic Diagnosis. Comparison films of the normal side may be made, looking for relative widening. Weights can be held in the hands to confirm a suspected class 2 injury.

Management. Most partial separations are treated with a sling to elevate the scapula indirectly into apposition with the clavicle, along with analgesics. Complete separations are sometimes corrected surgically, especially in very active individuals such as athletes.

Clavicular Fractures

The clavicle functions as a strut that fixes the arm to the thorax.

Mechanism. A fall on the lateral aspect of the proximal arm is the usual mechanism of injury, and the middle third of the clavicle is the usual site of fracture.

Presentation. The clavicle is a subcutaneous structure. Therefore, an injury will present with well-localized pain, swelling, and tenderness over the site of fracture. The arm is usually held against the chest to minimize movement.

Radiologic Diagnosis. Standard clavicular views demonstrate the fracture without difficulty.

Management. Realignment of fragments is difficult because the clavicle is the site of attachment of so many strong muscles, both superiorly and inferiorly. Unless cosmesis is a strong concern, symptomatic treatment consists of a sling (to remove the weight of the arm from the lateral fragment) and possibly the "figure-of-eight" bandage for more anatomic alignment. No great effort need be made for anatomic alignment because it is said that, "two pieces of clavicle in the same area code will heal fine." The patient is informed that a visible and palpable subcutaneous callus will form as the clavicle remodels.

Humeral Fractures

PROXIMAL HUMERUS

The proximal humerus is anatomically divided into four functional parts: anatomic neck, greater and lesser tuberosities, and surgical neck (see Fig. 46–1B). The surgical neck is the site of most fractures.

Mechanism. Most proximal humeral fractures result from distal forces transmitted from a fall on the outstretched arm. A direct blow to the lateral shoulder may also be responsible.

Presentation. There are usually no findings except for pain and tenderness in the proximal upper arm and shoulder.

Radiologic Diagnosis. Standard shoulder views (anteroposterior and lateral) demonstrate the fracture in most cases.

Management. Rather impressive angular deformities may be tolerated in the interest of early movement. The inherent range of motion of the shoulder joint is far greater than that used by most individuals, so the shoulder is able to compensate for deformities that in other locations could not be tolerated. The issue of early motion of the shoulder joint is paramount. Even an uninjured shoulder that is immobilized for as little as 1 to 2 weeks may form an extremely debilitating adhesive capsulitis or "frozen shoulder." For this reason, proximal humerus fractures are immobilized acutely with sling and swathe and definite orthopedic referral is arranged within 48 hours.

HUMERAL SHAFT FRACTURES

Mechanism. A blow to the lateral aspect of the arm or a fall is the typical mechanism of injury.

Presentation. The patient complains of well-localized upper arm pain, and the extremity may be shortened or rotated. A wristdrop may be present, owing to radial nerve injury. The radial nerve is the most common complication associated with this injury, especially with midshaft and distal humeral fractures, because it travels in the spiral groove along much of the humeral shaft.

Radiologic Diagnosis. These fractures are readily appreciated on plain radiographs of the humerus. The shoulder and elbow joints should also be visualized.

Management. Early management consists of sling and swathe or sugar tong splint with the elbow held in 90 degrees of flexion. Plaster or fiberglass is placed high in the axilla and extends down and under the elbow and back up the lateral arm to the top of the shoulder. Close follow-up with outpatient orthopedic referral is adequate. Surgical management may be elected later. Return to early motion is of paramount importance.

SUPRACONDYLAR FRACTURES

Mechanism. A fall on the outstretched arm with the elbow in flexion is the usual mechanism of injury.

Presentation. Supracondylar fractures are more common in children. The child usually presents while holding the arm as still as possible at 90 degrees of flexion at the elbow. There is usually marked swelling and tenderness about the elbow, and this injury can be clinically indistinguishable from an elbow dislocation.

Radiologic Diagnosis. The intra-articular hemorrhage produced by the fracture displaces the fat occupying the coronoid fossa anteriorly and the olecranon fossa posteriorly. These displacements are seen radiographically as a triangle-shaped radiolucency anterior to the distal humeral shaft (sail sign) and a more linear lucency posterior to the distal humeral shaft (Fig. 46–2). These signify joint effusion, which is always presumed to be blood in the context of acute trauma. To evaluate the degree of posterior angulation that is present a straight line is traced down the anterior border of the humerus and should bisect the capitellum (Fig. 46–3).

Management. Supracondylar fractures are potentially limb threatening, since they may compromise the blood supply from shearing forces or pressure from developing hematoma and edema. Ischemia of the forearm is devastating. Close monitoring of vascular status is necessary. Long-arm splinting, maintaining accessibility to both the antecubital fossa and the distal neurovascular examination sites, is recommended. Hospitalization or close follow-up to monitor neurovascular status is indicated.

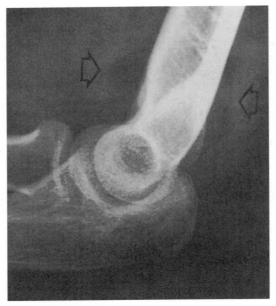

FIGURE 46–2 • The typical roentgen configuration and appearance of the anterior and posterior olecranon fat pad signs *(open arrows)* in the lateral radiograph. (From Harris JH Jr, Harris WH [eds]: The Radiology of Emergency Medicine, 2nd ed. Baltimore, Williams & Wilkins, 1981. Copyright © 1981, The Williams & Wilkins Co.)

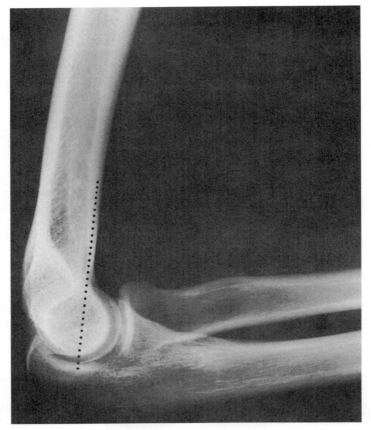

FIGURE 46–3 • Supracondylar fracture: line traced down anterior border of capitellum to evaluate degree of posterior angulation.

Elbow Injury

ELBOW DISLOCATION

Mechanism. Falls on the outstretched arm, usually with the elbow in some degree of flexion, are responsible for this injury.

Presentation. The patient presents with shortening of the forearm and with the olecranon tenting the skin posteriorly. This injury can be confused with a supracondylar fracture.

Radiologic Diagnosis. Anteroposterior and lateral views of the elbow reveal the coronoid process below the trochlea and displaced posterior to the humerus (Fig. 46–4). The coronoid and medial epicondyles are commonly fractured in conjunction with the dislocation.

Management. Reduction should be prompt. It is performed by reproducing the mechanism of injury with inferior traction on the proximal forearm, followed by longitudinal traction on the forearm and then flexion. Reduction of the radius may not occur simultaneously with that of the ulna and is confirmed with smooth supination-pronation.

RADIAL HEAD SUBLUXATION (NURSEMAID'S ELBOW)

Mechanism. An unsuspected longitudinal traction applied to the hand is the cause of the injury. This usually occurs when a toddler is rescued from falling or possibly "encouraged" to hurry up. This injury happens commonly in children younger than age 5 years and is usually caused by a well-meaning adult. It should not be construed as evidence of child abuse.

Presentation. Children display a phenomenon called "pseudoparalysis" when a limb is injured anywhere along its length. A child's apprehension over any manipulation of the injured arm can make the examination challenging at times. Careful palpation, observation, and ingenuity in examining the extremity will elucidate the site of injury and avoid unnecessary entire limb radiographs. On careful examination, the hand will be found to function normally if objects are brought to it. Similarly, shoulder motion is unlimited and is not associated with tenderness. The specific motion of supinating the pronated elbow elicits exquisite pain.

Management. The same motion, supination, followed by flexion at the elbow, reduces the injury. Within a short time (usually about 15 minutes), most children will have forgotten that their elbow was painful and will be using the limb normally (a near miracle in the eyes of a grateful parent). This is a very satisfying reduction. No immobilization is necessary.

RADIAL HEAD FRACTURE

Radial head fractures are the most common elbow injuries in adults.

Mechanism. A fall on an outstretched hand is the typical mechanism of injury. This forces the radial head into the capitellum. Although the

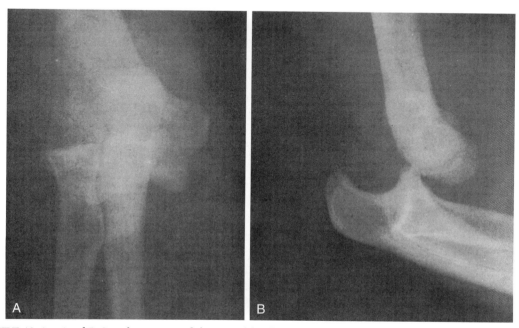

FIGURE 46–4 • *A* and *B*, Complete posterior dislocation of the elbow. (From Harris JH Jr, Harris WH [eds]: The Radiology of Emergency Medicine, 2nd ed. Baltimore, Williams & Wilkins, 1981. Copyright © 1981, The Williams & Wilkins Co.)

capitellum of the humerus may be fractured, the radial head is fractured far more commonly.

Presentation. The usual presentation is point tenderness of the radial head deep in the proximal extensor forearm muscles that is exacerbated by supination of the forearm, which the patient holds in pronation. Examination of the wrist for tenderness is important to identify an Essex-Lopresti injury, a radial head fracture with disruption of the distal radioulnar ligaments.

Radiologic Diagnosis. Often, no fracture line is visible on radiologic examination. The pathologic fat pad signs discussed earlier under "Supracondylar Fractures" may be seen, leading to the diagnosis.

Management. Minimal fractures, with essentially no depression of the articular surface, require only brief immobilization with a sling or posterior splint and early range of motion exercises. More extensive fractures in which a large percentage of the articular surface is depressed may require removal and prosthetic replacement of the radial head. Aspiration of the hemarthrosis and injection of an anesthetic such as bupivacaine into the joint space may be indicated for pain relief and early mobilization.

OLECRANON PROCESS FRACTURES

Mechanism. Falls directly on the elbow and forceful contraction of the triceps muscle resulting in avulsion are the mechanisms of injury.

Presentation. There is well-localized swelling. Tenderness over the olecranon and separation at the fracture site is sometimes palpable because the olecranon is covered by minimal tissue. Elbow extension will be weak or absent. Sensory and motor deficits in the hand caused by ulnar nerve dysfunction are possible.

Radiologic Diagnosis. The lateral view of the elbow will demonstrate the fracture nicely. The distractive forces created by the triceps muscle frequently cause proximal migration of the fragment.

Management. Long-arm splinting with the elbow held at 90 degrees is adequate emergency department management. Most of these injuries will require open reduction and internal fixation.

Forearm Fractures

The forearm, with its vulnerable position and protective function, is commonly injured. Direct blows aimed for the head are commonly absorbed or deflected by the ulnar aspect of the forearm. Falls on the outstretched arm continue to be the most common mechanism for the great majority

of upper extremity injuries and account for countless forearm fractures.

An important orthopedic principle, illustrated in the forearm, is that injury to one of two bones running parallel to each other by necessity affects the other bone. This second injury may be another fracture or a joint dislocation at the proximal or distal end.

ULNAR SHAFT FRACTURE (NIGHTSTICK FRACTURE)

Mechanism. A direct blow to the elevated ulnar shaft in a maneuver to defend the face or head is the usual scenario.

Presentation. Well-localized swelling and tenderness on the ulnar aspect of the forearm is usually the only finding.

Radiologic Diagnosis. Anteroposterior and lateral forearm views will demonstrate the fracture. This is the one exception to the previously stated principle of both-bone involvement in an injury. With neither tenderness nor radiographic evidence of radial injury at the elbow or wrist, one may presume the ulna alone to be injured.

Management. The intact radius and significant surrounding muscle bellies provide a splint. A long-arm plaster or fiberglass splint adds to the immobilization and provides protection against further injury.

COMBINED RADIAL AND ULNAR SHAFT FRACTURE

Mechanism. A very forceful direct blow is necessary to fracture both bones. Sometimes the bones of the forearm will fracture if too much force is applied to either end.

Presentation. These patients frequently present with marked swelling and tenderness, involving a large portion of the forearm. The elbow or the wrist may be involved.

Radiologic Diagnosis. With the splinting action of the intact radius lost, these fractures tend to be displaced or badly angulated. Commonly, subluxations at the wrist or elbow are associated.

Management. These injuries generally require urgent orthopedic referral for reduction under general anesthesia.

Wrist Fractures

The wrist in its role of supporting and moving the hand is prone to many injuries. By far the most common mechanism of injury is a fall on the outstretched hand. Depending on the exact vector of forces applied, distal radial and ulnar fractures, carpal fractures, or intercarpal dislocations (lunate and perilunate dislocations) can occur. The dorsally displaced radial and ulnar fracture (Colles' fracture) is by far the most common type.

Forced volar flexion of the wrist is an unusual mechanism of injury, but it can occur during falls or fights. A dorsal sprain of the wrist joint is possible, but if there is significant ligamentous injury, instability will again lead to intercarpal dislocation.

Smith's fracture may result from severe volarly directed forces on the distal forearm. The result is a distal radial and ulnar fracture with volar displacement.

COLLES' FRACTURE

Mechanism. The common mechanism is a fall on the outstretched arm with the wrist in dorsiflexion.

Presentation. Swelling and tenderness at the wrist are present, and, depending on the degree of displacement, there may be significant deformity with the distal radial fragment angulating dorsally to form the "dinner fork" deformity. Median nerve dysfunction may result in numbness in the hand.

Radiologic Diagnosis. Fracture of the distal radius with dorsal displacement is obvious on standard anteroposterior and lateral views of the wrist. Sixty percent of patients have an associated ulnar styloid fracture.

Management. A dorsal-volar splint such as a "sugar tong" is the preferred treatment. Orthopedic follow-up within 24 hours is recommended.

NAVICULAR FRACTURES

Mechanism. A fall on the outstretched arm is the cause.

Presentation. These fractures are suspected when the maximal point of tenderness is in the anatomic snuffbox with ulnar wrist deviation. The anatomic snuffbox is the depression formed at the radial aspect of the wrist when the thumb is abducted and extended, as in a hitch-hiking sign. The tendons forming the anatomic snuffbox are the abductor pollicis longus and the extensor pollicis brevis on the volar boundary and the extensor pollicis on the dorsal boundary.

Radiologic Diagnosis. The absence of radiographic visualization of an acute fracture must not dissuade the clinician from treating this injury. These fractures are notoriously difficult to visualize and may require a repeat radiograph in 2 weeks when resorption of bone along the fracture line allows visualization.

Management. Immobilization must include the forearm, wrist, and thumb to minimize an impressive 30% rate of nonunion or avascular necrosis. A tenuous blood supply, distal to proximal, combined with the absence of any muscular attachments contributing perforating arteries, predisposes this bone to poor healing. A period of immobilization followed by repeat radiographs is often necessary. Even with optimal care these fractures have high complication rates. Patients with these injuries should have early orthopedic referrals (Fig. 46–5).

Hand Fractures and Joint Injuries

The hand is subject to a great array of trauma given its vulnerable position and its relationship to labor. Associated disability can be economically devastating.

METACARPAL FRACTURES

Mechanism. The fifth metacarpal is by far the most commonly fractured bone in the hand, usually when its owner strikes a mandible, wall, or other nonforgiving structure with a closed fist (boxer's fracture).

Presentation. The patient may be reluctant to give an honest history. Any abrasion, laceration, or puncture wound in the area should arouse the suspicion of a human bite. Even an apparently trivial skin disruption over a metacarpophalangeal joint may be an injury from a tooth, with joint penetration and subsequent bacterial seeding.

Radiologic Diagnosis. Anteroposterior, lateral, and oblique views of the hand are standard. Metacarpal shaft fractures are usually obvious but a minimally displaced fracture of the head of a metacarpal can be quite subtle.

Management. Immediate exploration or at least admission for elevation, intravenous antibiotics, and observation is indicated when joint penetration is a possibility. It is indeed fortunate that this most commonly fractured metacarpal is also the most mobile. This mobility allows compensation for the volar angulation of the distal fragment without loss of function.

An identical fracture of the index or long finger metacarpal needs anatomic reduction through operative means to avoid functional loss. Percutaneous Kirschner wires are usually placed to hold the reduction in place. Fractures of the fourth metacarpal fall somewhere between these two extremes. Twenty-four-hour orthopedic referrals are recommended because many of these fractures will start to heal quickly, in whatever position the bones are in.

Fractures of the first metacarpal result in the thumb becoming unstable relative to the rest of the hand. The proximal fragment invariably carries with it the only strong ligamentous

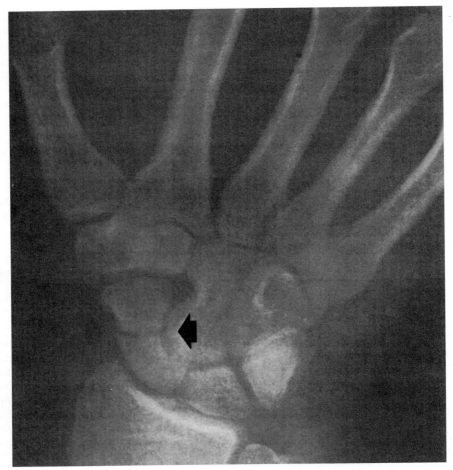

FIGURE 46–5 • Navicular fracture. (From Harris JH Jr, Harris WH [eds]: The Radiology of Emergency Medicine, 2nd ed. Baltimore, Williams & Wilkins, 1981. Copyright © 1981, The Williams & Wilkins Co.)

attachments to the carpals. Repair requires operative management, but in the acute situation the joint can be splinted with a thumb spica pending further treatment.

METACARPOPHALANGEAL DISLOCATIONS

The fifth and index metacarpophalangeal (MCP) joints are most likely to be involved in dislocations. These injuries are termed *dorsal dislocations* because of the dorsal position of the proximal phalanx relative to the metacarpal.

Mechanism. The mechanism is a volar depression of the head of the metacarpal through the volar plate (Fig. 46–6). The metacarpal head comes to lie in a bayonet apposition with the proximal phalanx, and the finger flexors come to lie in a noose-like fashion around the neck of the metacarpal.

Presentation. There is well-localized tenderness and swelling at the base of the involved finger.

Radiologic Diagnosis. Standard hand films reveal dorsal dislocation of the MCP joint, with the proximal phalanx lying dorsal to the metacarpal head. The fifth and index MCP joints are most likely to be involved, because of their greater mobility.

Management. Longitudinal traction on the digit to effect a reduction results in tightening of these tendons and the inability to reduce the metacarpal head through the rent in the volar plate. Operative reduction is necessary.

THUMB METACARPOPHALANGEAL ULNAR COLLATERAL LIGAMENT SPRAIN (GAMEKEEPER'S THUMB)

Mechanism. The mechanism of this injury is transient lateral dislocation of the thumb at the MCP joint that has spontaneously reduced. Strong acute or repeated lateral stresses act to deviate the mobile thumb away from the fixed elements of the hand, with subsequent rupture of the

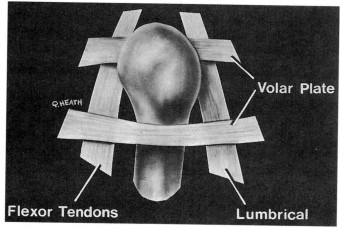

FIGURE 46–6 • Irreducible dislocation of the digital metacarpophalangeal joint, with metacarpal head rupturing through the volar plate. Arranged in a tight, sphincter-like fashion are the split-volar plate, lumbricals, and long flexor tendons. Attempts at reduction with longitudinal traction further tighten the ring by tightening the lumbricals and flexors against the thin metacarpal neck. (From Hossfeld GE: Joint injuries of the hand. Trauma Q 1985; 1:80. Reprinted with permission of Aspen Publishers, Inc., © February 1985.)

ulnar collateral ligament. Today it is seen most commonly with ski pole injuries.

Presentation. Stress testing of the ulnar collateral ligament will display more than 40 degrees angulation with the MCP in extension if there is complete rupture.

Radiologic Diagnosis. Radiographic assessment of the joint will be normal.

Management. Surgical repair is necessary because in two thirds of cases the abductor pollicis lies interposed between the two ends of the torn ligament and no amount of immobilization will allow healing. Repair can be done electively at a later date.

MIDDLE AND PROXIMAL PHALANGEAL FRACTURES

Mechanism. Hyperextension, torsion, and direct blows to the digit are common mechanisms.

Presentation. Deforming forces of the musculotendinous attachments may result in angulation or rotational deformity. Both abnormalities must be sought and corrected.

Radiologic Diagnosis. Standard hand or single finger views adequately demonstrate the disruption of the shaft.

Management. Many of these injuries are unstable to closed reduction and require internal wire fixation. This is true even of avulsion fractures. The insertions of the extensor and flexor tendons as well as the volar plate and collateral ligaments all may avulse their bony attachments given a strong enough deforming force. These injuries are often best treated with open wire fixation. Emergently, splinting in the position of

relaxation of the involved avulsed structure with timely (within 48 hours) referral to an orthopedist is indicated to ensure rapid return to functional stability without unnecessary stiffness, after prolonged immobilization. Fractures entering the articular surfaces are also generally unstable and are best treated by prompt referral. Anatomic reopposition of the articular cartilage is mandatory to minimize joint stiffness.

DISTAL PHALANGEAL TUFT FRACTURES

Mechanism. These injuries usually result from a crush mechanism.

Presentation. These fractures may be open or may be associated with subungual hematoma. The patient complains of marked throbbing of the fingertip.

Radiologic Diagnosis. The specific finger in question can be visualized separately if the injury is isolated. Comminution of the tuft is common.

Management. These fractures heal satisfactorily if they are protected with a padded aluminum splint. Prophylactic antibiotics may be given if the fracture is open. In addition, nail plate removal and nail bed repair may be indicated as discussed in Chapter 45, Open Injuries to the Hand.

DISLOCATIONS OF THE PROXIMAL INTERPHALANGEAL JOINTS

Mechanism. These injuries occur with or without concomitant fracture, but all involve rupture of the ligamentous structures. Hyperextension and a lateral force with the joint extended are common mechanisms.

Presentation. Because of minimal surrounding soft tissue, the dorsal displacement of the middle phalanx relative to the proximal phalanx is obvious.

Radiologic Diagnosis. A radiograph is useful in identifying concomitant fractures. It is repeated after reduction.

Management. Reduction is easily accomplished with longitudinal traction to reduce the bayonet apposition, followed by appropriate manipulation of the middle phalanx to alignment. Reduction is best done after a digital block, both for patient comfort and to enable the physician to assess the stability of the joint after reduction. If the reduced joint can be passively or actively put through a range of motion without recurrent dislocation, management is conservative. Avoidance of open repair obviates foreign body reaction with resultant stiffness.

DISLOCATIONS OF THE DISTAL INTERPHALANGEAL JOINTS

Mechanism. Strong hyperextension or a lateral deforming force with the joint in extension is necessary to produce these injuries. Multiple strong osteocutaneous fibers stabilize these joints.

Presentation. These injuries usually present as open dislocations. The same osteocutaneous fibers that provide stability result in shearing injuries to the overlying skin.

Radiologic Diagnosis. These dislocations are obvious. Radiographs may reveal concomitant fracture.

Management. Irrigation, débridement, reduction by longitudinal traction, and prophylactic antibiotics are indicated.

SPRAINS OF THE FINGER JOINTS

Mechanism. Hyperextension and abduction forces applied across the proximal interphalangeal (PIP) joint are the most common mechanisms. These injuries occur most frequently in contact sports.

Presentation. The patient complains of tenderness about the PIP joint. Stress testing of the lateral collateral ligaments and joint capsule, after adequate anesthesia, may demonstrate incomplete ligamentous tears.

Radiologic Diagnosis. Standard films will be normal. Stress views will demonstrate the instability, but these are rarely done in the emergency department.

Management. Although the ligamentous disruption may be nearly complete, surgical repair is seldom indicated because the remaining intact fibers align the torn segments anatomically, where they will heal nicely with minimal fibrosis.

Stiffness rather than instability is a more likely complication.

Whenever possible, immobilization should be accomplished with the joint in the flexed position and should be of brief duration. Referral is helpful to ensure proper rehabilitation.

BOUTONNIERE DEFORMITY

Rupture of the central slip of the extensor tendon occurs where it inserts at the base of the middle phalanx. The lateral extensor tendons slip down to act as partial flexors. The result is flexion of the PIP and hypertension of the DIP.

Mechanism. Usually a sharp force is applied to the end of a partially extended finger.

Presentation. Patients may present with the deformity just described and will be unable to fully extend the PIP and will have difficulty flexing the DIP. However, patient presentation may be delayed and the diagnosis is often missed initially. Initial findings may be minimal and include weak and painful extension of the PIP against resistance and point tenderness at the base of the middle phalanx.

Radiologic Diagnosis. Standard films will be normal.

Management. Isolated splinting of the PIP in extension is done for 4 weeks along with outpatient referral to an orthopedist.

MALLET FINGER

Hyperflexion and loss of extensor tendon attachment to the distal phalanx occurs by disruption of the tendon or avulsion of a chip from the base of the distal phalanx. This results in flexion or volar displacement of the distal phalanx with an inability to actively extend it.

Mechanism. Forceful flexion of the distal interphalangeal (DIP) joint, such as occurs from jamming the fingertip, is the mechanism of injury.

Presentation. Patients may present acutely with a tender DIP joint and flexion deformity. Others may present with a history of trauma that occurred days to weeks before and with a persistent deformity.

Radiologic Diagnosis. Plain films may be normal or may reveal an avulsed fragment at the base of the distal phalanx.

Management. Dorsal splinting of the DIP joint only, in slight hyperextension, is usually effective if it is maintained for 6 to 12 weeks. If there is an avulsed fragment or if splinting is ineffective, open reduction and internal fixation are indicated.

UNCERTAIN DIAGNOSIS

As with any acute orthopedic injury, initial examination is usually limited by acute swelling and

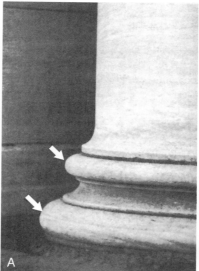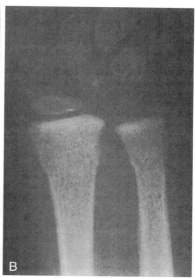

FIGURE 46–7 • *A,* The convex moldings at the base of a column are the origin of the term *torus fracture.* The tori are indicated by arrows. *B,* The pronounced bulging of the cortex *(arrows)* represents buckling bone, a so-called torus fracture. (From Kirschner SG, et al [eds]: Advanced Exercises in Diagnostic Radiology. Philadelphia, WB Saunders, 1981.)

pain. It is critical that the emergency physician understand the mechanisms associated with certain injuries and that physical or radiographic findings will be minimal in such injuries as navicular fracture, Salter-Harris fractures (especially types I and V), gamekeeper's thumb, boutonniere deformity, and other sprains of the hand and digits. In addition, any suspected or questionable fracture should be referred to an orthopedist. Usually it is appropriate to do this on an outpatient basis.

SPECIAL CONSIDERATIONS

Pediatric Patients

Although many of the principles of adult orthopedics can be applied to the pediatric population, there are many special considerations. Accurate historical information is often unavailable, and an adequate physical examination may be difficult. Moreover, radiographic diagnosis is difficult, owing to the radiolucency of developing bone and the variable appearance of secondary centers of ossification. Comparison radiographic views of the contralateral "normal" extremity are often essential in diagnosing abnormalities. In general, children's fractures heal more rapidly and are more likely to undergo extensive remodeling with age compared with adults, but epiphyseal (growth plate) injuries may lead to growth arrest or progressive deformity of the extremity. The pediatric patient with an extremity injury cannot be treated merely as a "little adult."

Torus and Greenstick Fractures. Torus and greenstick fractures are common and unique to children. These fractures occur when the relatively resilient bone of children allows only a localized break in the cortex. As the analogy implies, a

greenstick fracture occurs when bowing of a long bone results in an incomplete fracture. A part of the cortex breaks while the cortex opposite it undergoes only a plastic deformity. The torus fracture is similar but involves a localized buckling of the cortex, secondary to an axial load rather than bending (Fig. 46–7). The torus fracture may be quite subtle and is often missed on initial review of the radiographs.

Epiphyseal Injuries. The presence of epiphyseal plates in the growing bones of children creates a whole class of injuries that are unknown in adulthood. Because their ligaments are strong relative to the areas of calcifying cartilage in the growth plate, stress near a joint is likely to cause a fracture or fracture-separation in the zone of the epiphysis. With this in mind, one cannot dismiss stress-induced pain and swelling near a joint in a child as a "sprain." Several classifications of these fractures have been proposed, but the Salter-Harris classification (Fig. 46–8) has provided the basis for discussion of these injuries for the past 30 years. Not only does classifying a pediatric fracture according to Salter-Harris criteria provide a clear picture of the fracture to the consulting orthopedist on the phone, but it also provides some prognostic value.

Salter-Harris type I fractures involve only the epiphyseal plate. No fracture line is seen because the epiphyseal plate is radiolucent. Displacement of the epiphysis makes diagnosis obvious, but a nondisplaced type I fracture may appear radiographically normal. It is of paramount importance that any injury in a child with tenderness over an epiphyseal plate be treated as a nondisplaced type I injury despite the normal appearance of the appropriate radiographs. *This is a clinical diagnosis.* Failure to immobilize and protect this injury

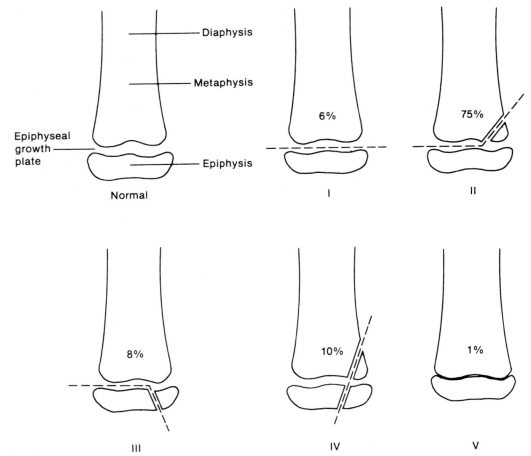

FIGURE 46–8 • Salter-Harris classification of epiphyseal injury. Percentages shown represent the relative incidences. *Dotted lines* represent the path of fracture.

adequately may lead to subsequent subluxation of the epiphysis, thereby causing additional injury to the growth plate and necessitating a reduction. The epiphyseal area of growing bone is delicate. Failure to treat these injuries may increase the incidence of growth disturbance and subsequent dysfunction.

Type II Salter-Harris fractures account for up to 80% of all Salter-Harris injuries. They are similar to type I injuries in that the translucent epiphyseal plate remains contiguous and attached to the epiphyseal fragment. Type II injuries differ only in that the fracture line exits from the metaphyseal bone, creating a small radiologically visible fragment. Because the epiphyseal plate remains intact, type I and type II injuries have a lower incidence of growth disturbance and later deformity. The most common epiphyseal injury is a type II fracture-separation of the distal radius.

The type III Salter-Harris fracture is an injury in which the fracture line exits through epiphyseal bone, revealing an epiphyseal fragment on the

radiograph. The fracture is not only intra-articular but also causes injury to the epiphyseal plate. The epiphyseal plate, although radiographically invisible, always remains with the visualized epiphysis.

Salter-Harris type IV fractures have a fracture line vertical to the epiphyseal plate, which results in epiphyseal *and* metaphyseal fragments. As in type III fractures, they are intra-articular and injurious to the epiphyseal plate. Types III and IV injuries may require open reduction to restore articular and epiphyseal anatomy. Both have a poorer prognosis than types I and II.

Type V injuries are potentially devastating injuries that may appear radiographically benign. An axial loading force may crush the epiphyseal plate, but only a subtle decrease in the height of the radiographically lucent space represents the area of calcifying cartilage. As in nondisplaced type I injuries, this injury must be suspected and diagnosed clinically.

All epiphyseal injuries (except presumptively diagnosed nondisplaced Salter-Harris I fractures) require prompt orthopedic consultation. The injury is immobilized in a plaster splint. Rapid follow-up is important because children undergo rapid bone repair, and extensive bony bridging may hinder reduction if it is performed late. Hospitalization may be indicated for Salter-Harris fractures types III, IV, and V. Parents are made aware immediately that epiphyseal injuries may give rise to deformity or growth arrest in the involved limb in spite of appropriate and timely care.

Elderly Patients

The important principle in treating fractures or postreduction dislocations in the elderly is to limit the time of joint immobilization. This may be difficult because healing times may be longer, but recovery from a "frozen" joint is slow and painful.

Wrist or other bony fractures in the elderly may be an opportunity to discover and discuss the potential of osteoporosis. This serious and significant disease of aging, especially in women, may be initially identified or suspected by the astute emergency physician.

DISPOSITION AND FOLLOW-UP

Admission or Immediate Orthopedic Consultation

Certain orthopedic injuries will require urgent operative intervention, and others are associated with complications frequent enough to warrant immediate telephone or on-site consultation. These include the following:

1. Open fractures or dislocations
2. Injuries associated with actual or potential neurovascular compromise
3. Injuries known to be unstable to closed management
4. Salter-Harris types III, IV, and V epiphyseal injuries in pediatric patients
5. Irreducible fractures and dislocations
6. Any injury with which the emergency physician feels uncomfortable

Discharge and Follow-up

Most orthopedic injuries can be effectively treated with emergency department management and timely orthopedic follow-up. Follow-up is essential, and the patient's compliance with the recommended referral is improved markedly if the patient is given explicit instructions as to who to see, the location of the doctor's office, and the specific time of the appointment.

Patient education includes instructions for the following:

1. Keeping splints dry
2. Elevating the limb and using ice packs liberally for the first 24 hours
3. Loosening the Ace wrap if tingling or coolness of the fingers develops or if there is increased pain
4. Returning to the emergency department if these problems do not promptly resolve or if any difficulty with treatment or follow-up is encountered

Adequate pain medication is supplied. The type and severity of injury will dictate the need for oral narcotics, nonsteroidal anti-inflammatory drugs, or acetaminophen.

FINAL POINTS

- Upper extremity injuries are rarely life threatening, and they must never take priority over life-threatening illness or injury.
- Injuries to the hands and arms may have significant impact on a patient's ability to hold gainful employment and enjoy leisure activities.
- The mechanism of injury is delineated when possible because it will assist in determining potential injuries.
- Knowledge of the involved anatomy is important in the diagnosis of associated injuries.
- Physical findings on careful examination will reveal the specific site of injury in most patients and will guide the ordering of diagnostic radiographs.
- Emergency department reduction and immobilization followed by orthopedic referral are appropriate for most fractures and dislocations.
- Reduction of fractures and dislocations should be done using a steady and gentle technique. Patients should receive adequate anesthesia and analgesia and be monitored appropriately.
- Immediate orthopedic consultation and consideration for admission are indicated for open fractures or dislocations, neurovascular compromise, fractures that are not amenable to closed management, irreducible fractures or dislocations, and high-grade epiphyseal fractures.

CASE*Study*

A 27-year-old man presents to the emergency department after sustaining trauma to the right upper extremity while playing racquetball. He says he ran into the wall with his extended right arm and now complains of severe pain to the right shoulder.

The patient states he was running backward with his right arm extended, abducted, and externally rotated when he ran into the wall with his right arm. On arrival, he is in moderate pain and holds his right arm splinted to his side. The right arm is slightly externally rotated and abducted. The vital signs are normal in triage. He reports no other injuries and has no medical problems. He denies previous injury to the shoulder.

A deformity to the right shoulder with a squared-off appearance to the deltoid is noted. The humerus and elbow are noted to be nontender without deformity.

It is important to evaluate the contiguous structures to evaluate for associated injuries that may be missed.

With all extremity injuries, it is important to do an appropriate neurovascular examination tailored to the anatomic area. With shoulder injuries and proximal humeral injuries, it is important to examine for brachial plexus injuries, in particular the axillary and musculocutaneous nerves and the axillary artery and vein. These should be documented on initial presentation and after any reduction or manipulation.

The patient is noted to have decreased sensation over the insertion of the deltoid. The patient is medicated with intramuscular ketorolac and is referred to radiology for a shoulder series, which is to include a standard anteroposterior film as well as a scapular "Y" view.

The diminished sensation over the deltoid indicates axillary nerve injury. This finding usually is caused by a neuropraxia, which is temporary and requires no intervention. No vascular injuries are noted. The scapular "Y" view is added because this presentation is consistent with a shoulder dislocation.

It is important to consider pain management in all patients with orthopedic injuries. Because the patient is leaving the emergency department to go to radiology, a nonnarcotic analgesic was selected. It would be dangerous to give narcotics and not observe the patient properly while he was away from the emergency department.

The radiographs demonstrated a subcoracoid anterior dislocation. There was a Hill-Sachs impaction fracture.

Radiographs are done to confirm the diagnosis and also to look for associated fractures that would make the reduction difficult. Large fractures through the glenoid rim or humerus should be considered unstable and referred for operative intervention. This fracture, however, is very stable and should not preclude the examiner from reducing the dislocation. It occurs when the posterolateral aspect of the humeral head becomes impacted on the glenoid rim. This may occur acutely, but most often it occurs with recurrent shoulder dislocations.

The patient needs to have the shoulder reduced promptly. The longer the patient waits, the worse the muscle spasm and pain becomes, making the reduction more difficult. Several methods can be used. If anxiolytics or analgesics are used, the patient must be monitored appropriately.

A preferred method is the scapular manipulation or the Milch technique. The key is to use a steady gentle reduction technique with adequate analgesics. The reduction is complete when the patient or physician appreciates a normal contour to the shoulder with good range of motion.

It is important to know several techniques to use when a difficult reduction is encountered, but it is also important to know when to stop if you are unsuccessful. If multiple attempts have been made using appropriate techniques and adequate medications but the reduction has not occurred, then the physician should stop and refer the patient for possible operative intervention. Failed attempts may indicate soft tissue entrapment or loose foreign bodies in the joint space.

The patient is placed in a shoulder immobilizer. A repeat neurovascular examination is done to document any injury that may have occurred during the reduction. Repeat radiographs are done to document the reduction and to reassess for any associated fractures. He is discharged with analgesics, such as a nonsteroidal antiinflammatory agent, and instructed about the use of ice and the shoulder immobilizer. He is sent to an orthopedic surgeon for follow-up.

Injuries in young patients are typically immobilized for several weeks. Those in elderly patients are immobilized for shorter periods of time, with early passive range of motion exercises beginning within 2 to 3 days, to prevent adhesive capsulitis.

Bibliography

TEXTS

Della-Giustina D, Coppola M (eds): Orthopedic Emergencies: I and II. Emerg Med Clin North Am 1999; 17(4) and 2000; 18(1).

Hart RG, Uehara DR, Wagner MJ: Emergency and Primary Care of the Hand. Dallas, American College of Emergency Physicians, 2001.

Magee DJ: Orthopedic Physical Assessment, 3rd ed. Philadelphia, WB Saunders, 1997.

Neylan VD, Wols M: Principles of orthopedic reductions. In Hart RG, Rittenberry TJ, Uehara DT (eds): Handbook of Orthopedic Emergencies. Philadelphia, Lippincott-Raven, 1999.

JOURNAL ARTICLES

Brady WJ: Challenging and elusive orthopedic injuries: Diagnostic and treatment strategies for optimizing clinical outcomes: I. Upper extremity fractures and dislocations. Emerg Med Rep 1999; 20(9):87–97.

Freiberg A, Pollard BA, Macdonald MR, Duncan MJ: Management of proximal interphalangeal joint injuries. J Trauma 1999; 46(3):523–528.

Hendy GW: Necessity of radiographs in the emergency department management of shoulder dislocation. Ann Emerg Med 1999; 36:87–97.

Hill S, Wasserman E: Wrist injuries: Emergency imaging and management. Emerg Med Pract 2001; 3(11):1–24.

Kothari RU: Prospective evaluation of the scapular manipulation technique in reducing anterior shoulder dislocations. Ann Emerg Med 1991; 21:1349–1352, 1992.

Johnson G: The Milch technique for reduction of anterior shoulder dislocations in an accident and emergency department. Arch Emerg Med 1992; 9:40–43.

Perron AD, Brady WJ, Keats TE, et al: Orthopedic pitfalls in the emergency department: Closed tendon injuries of the hand. Am J Emerg Med 2001; 19:76–80.

Perron AD, Miller MD, Brady WJ: Orthopedic pitfalls in the ED: Pediatric growth plate injuries. Am J Emerg Med 2002: 20:50–54.

Riebel GD: Anterior shoulder dislocation: A review of reduction techniques. Am J Emerg Med 1991; 9:180–188.

Stewart C: Hand injuries: A step-by-step approach for clinical evaluation and definitive management. Emerg Med Rep 1997; 18:223–233.

CHAPTER 47

Lower Extremity Injury

T. J. RITTENBERRY
EDWARD P. SLOAN
STEPHEN W. DAILEY

CASE *Study*

A 28-year-old man was transported to the emergency department after a motorcycle accident. The accident occurred at low speed, and the rider was wearing a helmet. The patient complained of left hip and lower leg pain and inability to bear weight. He was evaluated by the rescue squad and was transported on a backboard with his left leg carefully splinted to the right.

INTRODUCTION

Orthopedic injuries account for 10% of all emergency department visits. Although most of these injuries are not life threatening, orthopedic injuries to the lower extremities account for the majority of true orthopedic emergencies. For example, while pelvic fractures represent only 3% of all fractures, they are second only to head injuries as the leading cause of morbidity and mortality in patients with major trauma.

The lower extremity includes the structures from the forefoot to the pelvis. Injuries can be the result of direct forces applied to a specific structure or by indirect forces transmitted along the chain of structures resulting in injuries that are more complex and less apparent. For this reason, patients with trauma to the lower extremities must be examined for potential injury along the entire limb, direct or remote from the apparent site of applied force. The joints above and below the site of injury must be examined even if no injury is apparent to those adjacent structures.

Lower extremity injuries do not usually represent a threat to life, yet limb-threatening injuries do occur, mandating rapid diagnosis and management to maximize salvage. In the more likely event of injuries that are not limb threatening, an aggressive approach aimed at pain relief, anatomic reduction, and immobilization is necessary for prompt reestablishment of lower extremity function. Failure to diagnose and treat an injury adequately may lead to cosmetic deformity, impaired function, and chronic pain. An aberration in long bone or joint architecture that results in a gait disturbance may have a "domino" effect that over time causes dysfunction and pain in other joints of the legs and back.

INITIAL APPROACH AND STABILIZATION

Priority Diagnoses

Many injuries are commonly associated with vascular injury or compromise. These "true" emergencies include anterior hip dislocations, knee dislocations (especially posterior), proximal tibial fractures, fracture-dislocations of the ankle (bimalleolar and trimalleolar fractures), and Lisfranc fracture-dislocations of the midfoot.

Rapid Assessment/Early Intervention

Patients often present to the emergency department with isolated orthopedic injuries. The physician, however, must always suspect the presence of associated and potentially life-threatening injuries. The patient with multiple trauma who has suffered an assault, a significant fall, or a motor vehicle accident is assessed with the dictum, "life before limb" in mind. Three major problems should be looked for and addressed early: hemorrhage (internal or external), vascular compromise, and open fractures.

Hemorrhage

Victims of trauma are addressed according to the ABCs. Obvious and often impressive injuries of the extremities must not distract the physician from immediately assessing and managing the patient's airway, breathing, and circulatory status. Any site of external bleeding is controlled with pressure. Internal bleeding is considered, and aggressive intravenous hydration is instituted. The patient with a deformed or swollen thigh may lose 1 to 2 L of blood at the site of a femoral fracture and may present in a hypotensive state. A fractured pelvis may sequester up to 3 to 4 L. As with all trauma victims, concealed bleeding in the thoracic or peritoneal cavity is a major consideration.

Neurovascular Injury

All lower extremity injuries are assessed immediately for vascular compromise by palpating the femoral, popliteal, dorsalis pedis, and posterior tibial pulses. If pulses are not felt in the presence of adequate systemic blood pressure, flow can be assessed using a Doppler unit. Evaluating color, warmth, and capillary refill time in the feet and toes is also informative. Because major vessels are usually accompanied by nerves, associated neurologic, motor, and sensory deficits are sought on examination as well. The complete neurovascular examination is an integral part of the evaluation of the patient with *any* extremity injury.

Closed fracture-dislocations with vascular compromise are immediately reduced in an attempt to reestablish blood flow to the distal extremity. In the absence of vascular compromise, deformities usually require splinting and prompt radiologic evaluation before manipulation to obtain information for use in reduction as well as for medicolegal documentation.

Open Fractures

Emergency department care of open injuries differs from that of closed injuries in that manipulation is not performed unless there is vascular compromise. The wound is not explored digitally, and exposed bone is not reduced back into the wound. Instead, the site is first cleansed with a povidone-iodine solution and copiously irrigated before covering it with a saline or povidone-iodine–soaked dressing. This step is followed by placing a noncompressive sterile wrap and splinting. The patient is given intravenous antibiotics as soon as possible, most commonly a second- or third-generation cephalosporin. Fractures or dislocations with vascular compromise and all open injuries require immediate orthopedic consultation for aggressive débridement, irrigation, and reduction in the operating room.

CLINICAL ASSESSMENT

History

The history is an essential part of assessment in lower extremity injuries. It provides clues useful for identification of *all* the patient's injuries and may prevent iatrogenic morbidity.

1. *When did the injury occur?* Knowing the amount of time that has elapsed since an injury is most helpful in treating open injuries or those with vascular compromise and potential vascular injury. The longer an injury is open, the greater the degree of contamination and the greater the risk of wound infection or osteomyelitis. If vascular compromise has occurred, blood flow must be reestablished in 4 to 6 hours or tissue necrosis distal to the obstruction will occur.
2. *How did the injury occur?* Knowledge of the mechanism of injury helps the physician diagnose the primary as well as associated injuries. For example, a patient who has jumped two stories to avoid a fire is a likely candidate for any combination of lower extremity injuries but is at especially high risk for calcaneal fractures. Consideration of this mechanism of injury also leads one to seek out associated injuries such as compression fractures of the lumbar spine. The mechanism of injury is also important in determining the method of repair or reduction.
3. *Has the patient had a previous injury to the same extremity?* Knowledge of previous injury of the extremity in question will not only influence the physician's expectations during the examination but also help in interpreting radiographs.
4. *Is there a significant past medical history?* Eliciting a history of past illness, current medications, or allergies is important in all cases to anticipate complications and prevent unnecessary drug interactions or reactions. All patients in need of surgery are also asked about previous surgeries, transfusions, and the time elapsed since the last meal.

Physical Examination

The physical examination includes inspection, palpation, and a quantitative functional analysis: testing the range of motion in degrees. Auscultation is rarely used, although a Doppler blood flow detector may be necessary to confirm the distal pulses. Attention to surface structures is important and emphasizes the need to know the associated underlying bony anatomy. The uninjured opposite extremity provides the best source of what should be considered "normal" for that patient.

The Hip

The femur is the strongest bone in the human body as well as the longest. It can be divided into the head, neck, and shaft (Fig. 47–1). The hip articulation is composed of the spherical head of the femur and the acetabulum of the pelvis, forming a ball-and-socket joint. The capsule of this joint extends from the rim of the acetabulum to the junction of the femoral neck and the trochanters of the femoral shaft. A significant but somewhat tenuous

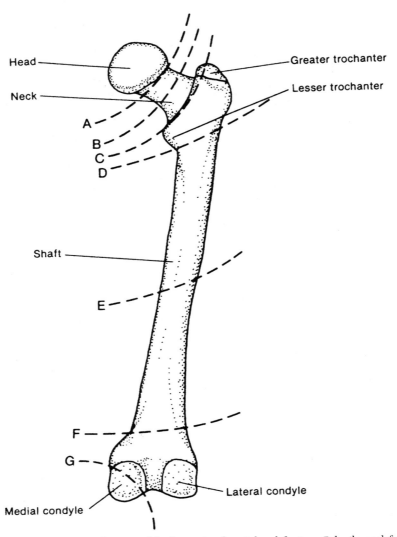

FIGURE 47–1 • Anatomy and common fractures of the femur: *A*, subcapital neck fracture; *B*, basilar neck fracture; *C*, intertrochanteric fracture; *D*, subtrochanteric fracture; *E*, shaft fracture; *F*, supracondylar fracture; *G*, condylar fracture.

portion of the blood supply to the head and proximal neck of the femur arises from the central acetabulum through the artery of the ligamentum teres. This relationship is important in the development of nonunion or avascular necrosis after femoral neck fractures or hip dislocations.

Careful observation of the position of the lower extremity can often lead to a strong presumptive diagnosis before radiographic evaluation of a hip injury. The examiner should note the presence of hip flexion as well as abduction or adduction compared with that in the uninjured leg. Comparison of the relative positions of the knees and malleoli or heels may reveal shortening of the extremity. Rotational deformity is best observed with regard to the position of the great toe and knee relative to the superior iliac crest. Range of motion of the hip in flexion, extension, abduction, adduction, and internal and external rotation is performed and quantified in terms of degrees while noting associated pain.

The Thigh

The femoral shaft and its attendant muscle groups comprise the musculoskeletal thigh. Physical examination of the thigh is as straightforward as its anatomy. Observation is often all that is necessary to make a presumptive diagnosis of a femoral shaft fracture. A swollen or deformed thigh that is tender to palpation after trauma is assumed to be a femoral shaft fracture until proven otherwise. Further evaluation and care must be undertaken on the assumption that an unstable fracture of the femur exists.

The Knee

The knee is actually a combination of three joints: the medial condylar joint, the lateral condylar joint, and the patellofemoral articulation. The articular capsule is intimately associated with the ligaments and aponeuroses of several muscle insertions as well as the knee's intrinsic ligamentous structures (Fig. 47–2). The medial and lateral collateral ligaments are separate structures that provide support, especially on knee extension.

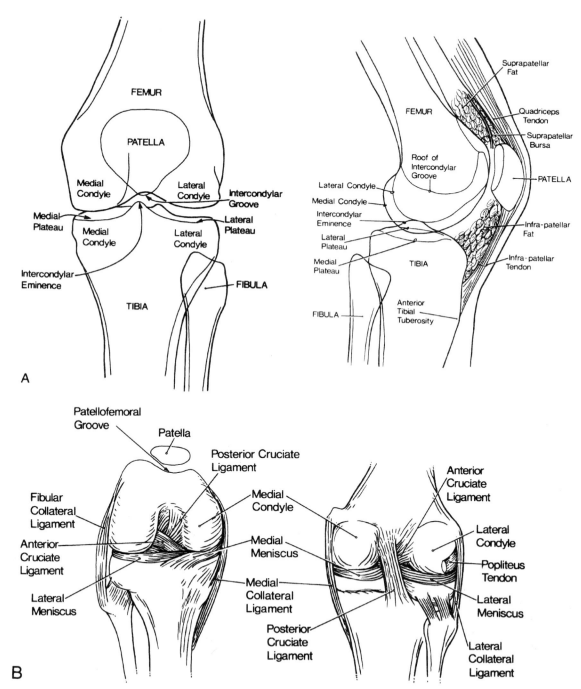

FIGURE 47–2 • *A* and *B*, Principal anatomic structures of the knee. (*A*, From Rogers LF: Radiology of Skeletal Trauma, vol 2. London, Churchill Livingstone, 1982. Used by permission of the Churchill-Livingstone Co.; *B*, adapted from Schultz RJ: The Language of Fractures. Huntington, NY, Robert E. Krieger, 1972. Copyright © 1972 by the Williams & Wilkins Co., Baltimore.)

Within the capsule lie the menisci and the cruciate ligaments. The anterior and posterior cruciate ligaments are strong, rounded cords arising from the anterior and posterior aspects of the tibial surface, respectively. The anterior cruciate extends posteriorly to connect to the femoral joint surface, whereas the posterior cruciate attaches to the anterior aspect of the femur. The menisci are crescent-shaped pads of fibrocartilage that extend to the outer borders of the tibial condyles; they have concave surfaces superiorly that correspond to the femoral condyles. This complex arrangement of cartilage and connective tissue gives remarkable stability to an intrinsically unstable arrangement of vertically apposed bones while simultaneously allowing weight bearing as well as free movement in the vertical plane.

During the physical examination of the knee the integrity of the supporting cartilage and ligaments must be evaluated because injuries to these structures are more common than fractures of bones. The examination and documentation should include the following essential components: neuromuscular evaluation, patellar and joint line palpation, valgus and varus stress test, and anterior and posterior cruciate ligament and extensor mechanism function.

Gross Examination. Apparent swelling of the knee is often caused by joint effusion rather than the result of local soft tissue swelling. Careful ballottement will usually help to differentiate between the two. A "patellar tap" may be noted when the patella, separated from the femoral condyles by the effusion, "taps" the femur as it is ballotted. If an effusion occurs rapidly or has been present for less than 24 hours, it is presumed to be bloody; in 70% to 90% of cases it is associated with an internal injury of a cruciate ligament or meniscus. The extensor mechanism is tested by observing straight-leg raising against gravity. If the patient cannot do this, then quadriceps rupture, patellar tendon rupture, patellar fracture, and tibial tubercle fractures are all possibilities.

Joint Line Palpation. If the joint line is tender, injury of the meniscus or collateral ligaments is suspected because it is here that they are attached to the bone.

Collateral Ligament Palpation. The attachments of the medial and lateral collateral ligaments to the femur, tibia, and fibula extend beyond the joint line. These attachments must be fully palpated to diagnose sprains about the knee. Tenderness without laxity indicates largely intact ligaments and a first-degree sprain.

Ligamentous Laxity Examination. Valgus and varus stresses of the extended knee are used to evaluate the laxity of the medial and lateral col-lateral ligaments. With the lower leg stabilized in extension, 20 degrees of flexion force applied to the lateral knee will provide a valgus stress, whereas varus stress will result from force applied to the medial knee. Anterior and posterior drawer tests of the knee in flexion are used to evaluate laxity in the anterior and posterior cruciate ligaments, respectively. For the drawer test, the patient is placed in the supine position with the hip in 45 degrees of flexion and the knee flexed to 90 degrees. While the patient's foot and pelvis are stabilized, two hands are used to push the proximal tibia posteriorly (posterior drawer test) or pull it anteriorly (anterior drawer test). There should be no movement in either of these tests in the healthy knee. A more appropriate test in the acutely injured knee is the Lachman test. The knee is flexed 15 degrees and while the femur is stabilized with one hand the proximal tibia is first pulled anteriorly and then pushed posteriorly. The presence of laxity with stress indicates at least a second-degree ligamentous sprain. Unrestricted joint movement with stress indicates a complete ligamentous disruption or a third-degree sprain.

Range of Motion. The knee joint should be evaluated for its ability to extend and flex, both actively and passively. If the injured knee cannot be fully extended, disruption of the quadriceps or patellar tendon may be present as well as a transverse patellar fracture. A "locked knee" that does not allow full range of motion suggests a meniscal cartilage tear with a loose foreign body within the joint, thus blocking movement.

Meniscal Cartilage Evaluation. In McMurray's test the knee is extended from the fully flexed position with the foot externally rotated. The presence of palpable crepitance, locking, or pain with full extension of the knee suggests injury to the medial meniscus. Identifying meniscal lesions by physical examination has a low accuracy, especially after an acute injury. Follow-up examinations are recommended.

The Leg

The anatomy of the leg is relatively simple and consists of the parallel arrangement of the tibia and fibula, which are joined by a fibrous interosseous membrane (Fig. 47–3). On this structure are layered the various flexor and extensor muscles of the ankle divided into well-circumscribed compartments. The tibia and fibula are poorly protected by soft tissue anteriorly, increasing their vulnerability. The common peroneal nerve winds around the proximal neck of the fibula, and the anterior tibial artery penetrates the interosseous membrane, posteriorly, in the

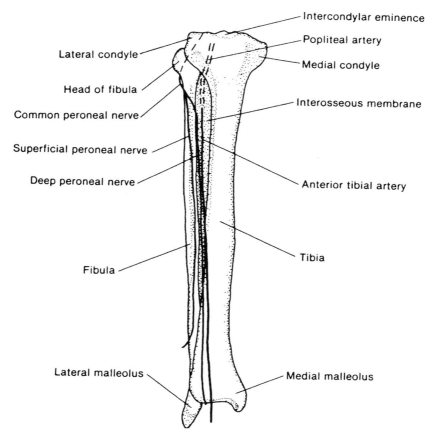

Intercondylar eminence

Popliteal artery

Medial condyle

Lateral condyle

Head of fibula

Common peroneal nerve

Superficial peroneal nerve

Deep peroneal nerve

Interosseous membrane

Anterior tibial artery

Fibula

Tibia

Lateral malleolus

Medial malleolus

FIGURE 47–3 • Basic anatomy of the leg.

proximal leg. Benign-appearing fractures in these two areas may be associated with unsuspected nerve or vascular injury.

The physical examination of the leg is easier than that of the knee. Fractures of the tibial and fibular shafts are often obvious, as they often have angular or rotational deformity and localized soft tissue injury. Palpation may elicit point tenderness. The skin is carefully examined for small wounds that can occur when bone fragments puncture the surface from within, indicating an open fracture. The compartments of the leg are also examined (as described later under "Compartment Syndromes").

The Ankle and Foot

The ankle and foot consist of an intricate complex of tendons, ligaments, and bones with innumerable interdependent articulations and relationships (Fig. 47–4). The ankle is a hinge joint that

has 13 tendons but no muscles that cross the joint. The weight-bearing tibia forms the plafond, or ankle ceiling, in the talocrural joint (the joint between the tibia and the talus). The support of the ankle exists circumferentially about it, with strong ligaments securing the fibula, talus, and tibia. Injuries occur either because of pulling forces along these ligaments (which cause sprains or transverse avulsion fractures) or abnormal movement of the talus within the ankle joint (which causes oblique fractures). Injuries that cause two or more disruptions in this ligament and bone ring render the ankle unstable. Fractures that occur through the malleoli above the tibial-talar interface are assumed to have rendered the ankle unstable.

The foot may be divided anatomically into the hindfoot, midfoot, and forefoot. The hindfoot is made up of the calcaneus and talus. It receives the majority of the weight-bearing load transferred from the tibia. The rigid midfoot is composed of

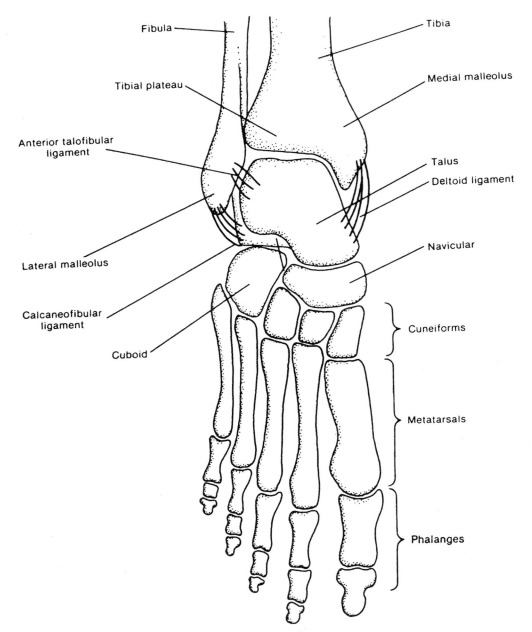

FIGURE 47–4 • Basic anatomy of the ankle and foot.

the tarsal navicular, the cuboid, and the three cuneiform bones, tightly joined by multiple ligamentous structures. The forefoot is made up of the five metatarsals and phalanges. Ligamentous connections in the forefoot decrease with increasing distance from the tarsometatarsal articulations, allowing more flexibility distally in the foot. The complex articulations and ligamentous connections in the foot help to equally distribute the loads incurred with normal gait.

Foot and ankle injuries are common and can alter this elaborate architecture, leading to dysfunctional use if they are unrecognized or untreated. A thorough examination will identify likely injuries. The examination should include the three following aspects:

Gross Examination. The presence of moderate to severe soft tissue swelling is typical in the presence of ligamentous sprains of the ankle. This is especially true of lateral ankle sprains because the lateral ankle ligaments form part of the lateral joint capsule. Ecchymosis usually occurs late after injury. Fracture-dislocations of the ankle are common and can be readily recognized by the gross deformity and extensive soft tissue swelling that accompany them. Dislocations of the tarsals, metatarsals, and phalanges are less easily diagnosed without radiographs. The diffuse pain and foot swelling that occur acutely often obscure bony landmarks and prevent the use of aggressive palpation to pinpoint the problem.

Palpation. Point tenderness of the ankle or midfoot ligaments suggests a common sprain. Point tenderness of the malleoli, proximal fibula, calcaneus, or base of the fifth metatarsal suggests that a fracture is more likely. All of these locations are examined in the patient with a chief complaint of an ankle "sprain."

Examination of Ligamentous Laxity. Laxity about the ankle is diagnosed using anterior drawer and talar tilt stress testing. The anterior drawer examination of the ankle is similar to that of the knee. It is performed by pulling the heel anteriorly while flexing the knee 45 degrees and keeping the lower leg stabilized. Movement of the foot relative to the lower leg suggests anterior talofibular ligament disruption. The talar tilt examination is performed by forcing the heel into inversion while the lower leg is stabilized. Abnormal movement of the foot reflects injury to both the anterior talofibular and calcaneofibular ligaments. These laxity tests should be performed whenever the ankle is significantly tender both medially and laterally, suggesting extensive ligamentous disruption. They are not necessary in the presence of severe ankle joint deformity, because in such cases the diagnosis of ankle instability is already made. Furthermore, the presence of severe swelling and pain may prevent adequate stressing or interpretation.

CLINICAL REASONING

When the data gathering is complete, the emergency physician answers three questions before moving on to diagnostic adjuncts.

Is There a Persistent Life-Threatening Problem?

As previously mentioned, the presentation of lower extremity injury can be dramatic and can distract the physician from focusing on potentially catastrophic problems. These problems can also evolve over time. Therefore, before ordering diagnostic studies and moving on, the physician may find a brief review of the secondary survey

very rewarding. This is also an appropriate time to check the volume of fluid given and the patient's level of pain.

Is There a Persistent Limb-Threatening Problem?

Limb-threatening problems from vascular, nerve, or other pressure-related damage can also evolve over time. A rapid reassessment of warmth, capillary refill time, and gross neurologic status relative to the initial examination provides valuable information.

Is There a Need for Any Further Testing?

This is a question that applies to the more benign patient problems. Radiographs are never "routine"; it is important that there be reasonable indications for ordering them. For example, several studies have found that a careful ankle examination using specific criteria, known as the *Ottawa Ankle Rules,* can decrease the number of ankle films ordered by almost 40% without missing significant problems. These rules state that an ankle radiograph is indicated only if (1) there is tenderness over the distal 6 cm of the tibia and fibula (near the malleoli); (2) there is an inability to bear weight for four steps both immediately and in the emergency department; or (3) there is bone tenderness at the posterior edge or tip of either malleolus. The *Ottawa Knee Rules* have also been shown to decrease the number of knee radiographs ordered by 2% and are both highly sensitive and specific. These Knee Rules state that radiographs are not indicated if the patient is younger than 55 years of age, is without isolated bone tenderness, and can actively flex the knee to 90 degrees and walk four steps. Although these guidelines are well accepted, many films are ordered by rote rather than by reason. Each test should be thoughtfully justified before it is requested. For equivocal clinical findings or inexperience, the threshold for ordering radiographs should be lowered.

DIAGNOSTIC ADJUNCTS
Radiologic Imaging

Plain film radiographs are the standard measure of bone injury. As in all cases of trauma to an extremity, anteroposterior and lateral views are mandatory. A view of the full length of the long bone including both joints is necessary for optimal interpretation.

Indications

Several considerations influence the need for radiographs when evaluating lower extremity trauma. Radiographic examination is appropriate in the following situations:

- *High likelihood of fracture.* Any bone that is likely, based on the history or physical examination, to have been fractured or dislocated is radiologically examined.
- *High incidence of associated injury.* If an injury is frequently associated with a certain fracture, both areas are viewed. One example is injury to the contralateral calcaneus when a calcaneal fracture has resulted from a fall.
- *High morbidity of a missed fracture.* If the suspected fracture is known to lead to long-term complications, radiographs are used liberally. For example, failure to radiograph and diagnose a slipped capital femoral epiphysis will lead to further irreversible slippage, gait aberration, degenerative changes, and potential avascular necrosis. Therefore, any child with hip pain or a limp should undergo radiographic evaluation.
- *Significant soft tissue injury.* If there is significant soft tissue disruption of an extremity after trauma, an open fracture must be ruled out with radiographs.
- *High patient expectations.* Patients or family members may be adamant in requesting radiographic evaluation of a bone that is judged clinically by the physician to be at low risk of fracture. Radiographs are strongly considered if the request is reasonable.
- *High litigation potential.* Injuries that result from accidents in which one party is alleged to be at fault require radiographs to document the true extent of injury. Occupational injuries fall into this category.
- *Poor patient follow-up.* If patients are thought to be poorly compliant, radiographs are obtained to document the exact injury that is present, because conservative treatment with later radiographs as appropriate is not a treatment option.
- *Potential foreign body risk.* If there is a possibility that a foreign body is present in an injured extremity, radiographs are indicated for localization and documentation.

Specific Radiographic Evaluation

Hip. Anteroposterior and lateral views of the femoral head and neck as well as an anteroposterior view of the pelvis are usually adequate for delineating hip fractures. An additional frog-leg lateral view is often obtained in children in whom a slipped capital femoral epiphysis is suspected.

Femur. Anteroposterior and lateral views will reveal fractures as well as their angulation. The *entire* length of the femur should be visible in both views.

Knee. The routine knee examination includes anteroposterior and lateral views as a minimum. Most radiology departments also include an intercondylar view, which gives better visibility of the joint space and femoral condyles, as well as a patellar (or sunrise) view, which assists in identifying fractures of the patella. When an occult tibial plateau fracture is suspected, oblique views or tomograms may be indicated.

Tibia and Fibula. As with the femur, anteroposterior and lateral views reveal fractures. Again, the entire length of the tibia and fibula must be visible.

Ankle. Anteroposterior, lateral, and mortise views will provide information about fractures and ankle stability. The anteroposterior film will show the medial and lateral malleoli, and the lateral view reveals the talus, posterior malleolus, calcaneus, and base of the fifth metatarsal. The mortise view (an anteroposterior view with 10 degrees of internal rotation) shows the mortise en face. This view will reveal osteochondral fractures on the superior surface of the talus and will show the superior, medial, and lateral clear spaces of the talar articulation. Any variance from a constant width of 3 to 4 mm in these spaces is considered evidence of an unstable disruption of the ankle mortise.

Foot. Anteroposterior, lateral, and oblique views are needed because the many bones of the foot overlap. Anteroposterior and oblique views are useful in the examination of the tarsals, metatarsals, and phalanges. The lateral view reveals the calcaneus, talus, and superior portion of the tarsals.

Calcaneus. If abnormalities of the calcaneus are suggested on foot radiographs, or if tenderness and swelling are restricted to the heel, specific calcaneus films including lateral and axial views should be obtained.

Specialized Techniques

Computed Tomography (CT). CT is useful in evaluating fracture-dislocations of the hip. It reveals both the fractures of the acetabulum and the location of the femoral head. This information is particularly useful in defining central hip dislocations.

Magnetic Resonance Imaging. Magnetic resonance imaging (MRI), like CT, is useful for evaluating the femoral head and acetabulum. It also has been used for evaluating intra-articular pathology, such as meniscal tears in the knee and ligament status in knee and ankle sprains.

Radioisotope Scanning. Although bone scans are rarely indicated in the ED, nuclear scans that reveal "hot spots" in areas of increased metabolic activity may be useful in the evaluation of systemic bone disease (Paget's disease, rheumatoid arthritis) or metastatic lesions. Bone scans may help in the diagnosis of occult fractures, stress fractures, or osteomyelitis in a patient with persistent symptoms of bone pain with unremarkable radiographs. They may also be used to evaluate local vascularity and occasionally to help define avascular necrosis of bone, as in Legg-Calvé-Perthes disease.

Arteriography. Although not useful in defining bony injury per se, arteriography may be indicated when vascular compromise is not readily corrected by reduction of an angulated deformity. It may also be indicated when there is a high likelihood of arterial injury, as in posterior knee dislocations.

Laboratory Studies

Although laboratory values have little bearing on the specifics of lower extremity injuries, certain assays are important.

Pregnancy Test. In females of childbearing age, especially those with abnormal menstrual histories, who are about to undergo pelvic irradiation or surgery, a pregnancy test should be ordered.

Hemoglobin and Hematocrit. These hematologic values are needed in patients with external or potential internal bleeding.

Type and Crossmatch. In patients with significant or potentially significant blood loss, blood type and crossmatch are ordered. They may also be ordered in consultation with an orthopedist, in preparation for surgery.

Presurgical Testing. Presurgical testing is initiated in the emergency department for all patients whose injury will require immediate treatment in the operating room. Specific tests ordered will vary with the institution and the consultant.

Special Tests

Arthrocentesis

Arthrocentesis, the needle aspiration of intra-articular fluid, is commonly used for diagnostic and therapeutic reasons in the emergency department. It is sometimes used in conjunction with local instillation of bupivacaine (Marcaine) or lidocaine (Xylocaine) after acute knee or elbow trauma to relieve a painful hemarthrosis. It is of diagnostic value when gross blood or fat globules are aspirated from a radiographically normal joint, suggesting such intra-articular injury as a torn cruciate ligament or occult osseocartilaginous injury. In the setting of trauma, any analgesic or diagnostic value of arthrocentesis must be weighed against the risk of providing entry to the joint space for pathogenic bacteria, creating an iatrogenic septic joint. Oral analgesics and a compressive wrap may be entirely adequate treatment for a traumatic joint effusion if pain is not severe. Traumatic effusions causing more significant pain, however, require therapeutic arthrocentesis (see Chapter 30, The Swollen and Painful Joint).

PRINCIPLES OF MANAGEMENT

In the emergency department management of lower extremity injuries, the physician considers all aspects of the injury: the integrity of the skin, the neurovascular status, and the severity and stability of a fracture or dislocation. Appropriate timing for surgery, if indicated, is important, as is the patient's ability to undergo and participate in the proposed treatment plan. Throughout, attention is paid to patient comfort.

Analgesia. The methods used for pain control are the same as those used with upper extremity injury. No patient should have to suffer without some form of analgesia. Dislocations and long-bone fractures can be very painful and use of intravenous morphine, meperidine, or fentanyl is usually indicated.

Closed Reduction of Dislocations. Prompt closed reduction is completed if vascular compromise is confirmed. If the dislocation occurs with an open fracture in which bone is protruding from the wound, reduction should occur as soon as possible in the operating room after wound culture and irrigation. If immediate reduction is delayed and vascular compromise threatens the viability of the lower extremity, wound culture and copious irrigation are followed by reduction and immobilization in the emergency department.

Immobilization. Immobilization of lower extremity injuries minimizes pain and further soft tissue injury in prehospital as well as in hospital and outpatient settings. Emergency department splinting is a temporizing procedure until definitive casting can occur, but it can provide the long-term immobilization necessary for minor injuries. Splinting should be used *liberally* because complications of short-term immobilization are negligible, whereas failure to immobilize may indeed complicate an injury. *When in doubt, splint!*

Hare Traction Splint. The Hare traction splint (Fig. 47–5) provides an excellent first response for suspected closed fractures below the femoral neck and above the ankle. It is especially appropriate for patients with suspected femoral fractures to reduce pain and, more importantly, to limit additional soft tissue injury and bleeding at the fracture site.

Long-Leg Splint. Long-leg splinting is useful for fractures of the distal femur (involving the knee joint), tibia/fibula, and those that severely disrupt the ankle mortise. The knee should be splinted in 10 to 15 degrees of flexion and the ankle in 90 degrees of dorsiflexion.

Knee Immobilizer. A knee immobilizer limits flexion and extension at the knee. Several types are available. It is used most often to immobilize a knee that has suspected cartilaginous or ligamentous injuries. It is ideal in this setting because it is adjustable and removable and can be placed over a bandage or clothing. Because it is adjustable, it can be used comfortably as knee swelling varies. A knee immobilizer does not, however, provide the same degree of rigidity as a plaster splint and can be easily removed by a noncompliant patient. Therefore, patients with injuries that must remain absolutely immobile, such as fractures about the knee, should receive a long-leg plaster splint.

Short-Leg Splint. Posterior short-leg splinting, which extends from the plantar aspect of the forefoot to the proximal leg, restricts plantarflexion and dorsiflexion of the ankle. This protects the ankle from further injury and pain in patients with ankle fractures that await definitive casting or repair. These splints also promote healing in patients with severe ankle sprains and foot fractures who are sent home. Placement of a short-leg splint increases not only the likelihood that the patient will avoid weight bearing on the affected extremity but also that the patient will seek appropriate follow-up.

Sugartong (Stirrup) Splint. Although posterior short-leg splinting restricts plantarflexion and dorsiflexion, some inversion and eversion can still occur, especially as swelling subsides and the splint loosens. Applying a strip of plaster that runs along the lateral and medial sides of the leg, around the posterior plantar surface of the foot, will provide stability against eversion and inversion. Combining this stirrup splint with a posterior short-leg splint provides the best ankle immobilization short of circumferential casting.

Ankle Splint Alternatives. Many minor ankle sprains can be managed without a plaster splint. Bandaging alternatives include circumferential cast padding followed by an Ace wrap, a gel or air splint, or an Ace wrap alone. These bandages minimize swelling and limit motion, so that healing occurs more quickly and less painfully. As with all dressings or splints, the patient should be instructed to loosen the bandage if signs of vascular compromise occur, especially when the bandage is placed soon after the injury occurs, before maximal swelling.

Management of Specific Injuries

Injuries of the Hip and Thigh

The patient who complains of groin, hip, or knee pain may have one of a variety of hip injuries. In a young person who has suffered major trauma, a

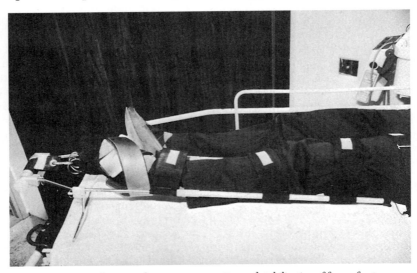

FIGURE 47–5 • The Hare traction splint provides temporary traction and stabilization of femur fractures.

pelvic fracture near or at the acetabulum, an anterior or posterior dislocation of the femoral head, or a proximal femoral fracture is most likely. In an adolescent with no trauma, the diagnosis of a slipped capital femoral epiphysis should be considered, whereas Legg-Calvé-Perthes disease is a possibility in preadolescent children. When the patient is elderly, a femoral neck fracture or an intertrochanteric fracture is a likely diagnosis even when a history of trauma is seemingly trivial or absent. Patients of any age who are subjected to major deforming forces may sustain any of a variety of femoral fractures (see Fig. 47–1).

Femoral Neck Fractures

Mechanism. The mechanism of injury is often a trivial force applied to the greater trochanter or is forced rotation of the extremity such as might occur in a simple fall. These shear forces coupled with the decreased bone density of osteoporosis may result in a fracture.

Presentation. A femoral neck fracture typically presents in an elderly patient who complains of hip pain and inability to walk. Some patients give no history of trauma. Impacted femoral neck fractures or those that are nondisplaced may result in minimal symptoms and findings, with pain elicited only at the extremes of range of motion. Displaced fractures cause more pain and an inability to walk. The hip is typically found in abduction and external rotation with associated shortening of the leg.

Radiologic Diagnosis. Routine anteroposterior and lateral views of the hip are usually adequate for diagnosis. With the exception of minimally displaced impacted fractures, these fractures are usually obvious. Oblique films are used when suspicion is high but routine views are nondiagnostic.

Management. All patients with femoral neck fractures (except possibly those with nondisplaced, impacted fractures that are weeks old and allow ambulation) require hospitalization to prevent further displacement until open reduction and internal fixation (ORIF) or prosthetic replacement can be performed. Because of the tenuous blood supply to the proximal femoral neck and head, failure to provide such care will increase the risk of aseptic necrosis or ultimate nonunion of the fragments.

Intertrochanteric Fractures

Whereas fractures of the femoral neck occur within the joint capsule, intertrochanteric fractures occur along a line between the greater and lesser trochanters and are extracapsular. Both fractures occur in older, osteoporotic patients, with a higher frequency in females.

Mechanism. The mechanism of injury is almost always a fall involving both direct and indirect forces.

Presentation. The classic presentation is severe hip pain in an older patient, in whom the leg appears markedly shortened and is held in as much as 90 degrees of external rotation. Any movement of the lower limb is painful and can potentially cause further soft tissue injury or bony comminution.

Radiologic Diagnosis. These fractures are readily demonstrated on routine hip films as a lucent fracture line extending from the greater to the lesser trochanter.

Management. Patients with a possible hip fracture should have the affected limb stabilized with sandbags before radiographic examination. In general, more comminuted fractures are more unstable and more difficult to reduce. Immediate hospitalization and orthopedic consultation should be sought. Aseptic necrosis and nonunion are uncommon complications of intertrochanteric fractures, because there is a generous extracapsular blood supply in this area.

Hip Dislocations

Another cause of hip pain and dysfunction is dislocation or fracture-dislocation of the hip. This was once a rare injury but has become more frequent, related to the intense forces generated in motor vehicle accidents. Less severe forces may be adequate to cause luxation of a prosthetic femoral head. Dislocations are described according to the positional relationships of the femoral head and acetabulum and may be categorized as anterior, posterior, or central.

POSTERIOR HIP DISLOCATIONS

Posterior hip dislocations are much more common than anterior or central dislocations.

Mechanism. The mechanism of injury is a force applied axially along the femur with the knee and hip in flexion, such as may occur when a seated passenger's knee strikes the dashboard during a head-on car accident.

Presentation. The patient generally has multiple injuries. The affected hip is typically held in adduction, internal rotation, and flexion, and the leg is shortened. Ten to 15 percent of patients with posterior hip dislocations have various degrees of sciatic nerve dysfunction because the dislocated femoral head approaches the sciatic notch, stretching or compressing the nerve.

Because of the intense force necessary to produce a hip dislocation, associated damage to the femoral shaft and knee must be ruled out. As many as one third of patients will have an associated knee injury.

Radiologic Diagnosis. Radiography will reveal the femoral head lying posterior to a coronal plane dividing the acetabulum. Additional views as well as CT may be necessary to fully assess the femoral head's position and the integrity of the acetabulum, because an axial load applied to an abducted femur is likely to fracture the posterior acetabular lip.

ANTERIOR HIP DISLOCATIONS

Anterior dislocations comprise less than 15% of hip dislocations.

Mechanism. The mechanism responsible for injury is similar to that causing a posterior dislocation except that the femur undergoes axial loading while in a more abducted position. An anterior dislocation may also occur if a patient is struck from behind while squatting. The femoral head may assume a superior (iliac or pubic) or inferior (obturator) position.

Presentation. A patient with an anterosuperior dislocation will present with a palpable mass in the inguinal area, with the leg held in abduction and external rotation. Because of the close proximity of this region to the femoral neurovascular bundle, direct injury to the femoral nerve, artery, or vein may result. A patient with an anteroinferior dislocation will present with more hip flexion.

Radiologic Diagnosis. Anteroposterior, lateral, and oblique hip views will reveal the nature of the dislocation, showing the femoral head anterior to the acetabulum. In an anteroinferior dislocation, radiographs will show the femoral head overlying the obturator canal, inferior to the acetabulum.

CENTRAL HIP DISLOCATIONS

Central dislocations are always associated with acetabular fracture.

Mechanism. These injuries occur when an extreme axial force is transmitted to the femoral neck, shattering the acetabulum as the femoral head is driven centrally into the pelvis. The femoral head remains in contact with the comminuted acetabulum.

Presentation. The presentation is that of a pelvic fracture—severe hip and pelvic pain with movement. Hypotension from blood loss as well as associated intra-abdominal and genitourinary injuries are frequent accompaniments.

Radiologic Diagnosis. Plain films or CT scans will demonstrate the acetabular injury with the femoral head lying within the confines of the pelvis.

MANAGEMENT

All hip dislocations are true orthopedic emergencies, and immediate orthopedic consultation is necessary. Prompt reduction will increase limb viability, decrease pressure-induced nerve ischemia, and reduce the incidence of subsequent avascular necrosis of the femoral head. Further long-term complications include myositis ossificans, post-traumatic arthritis, recurrent dislocation, and thrombosis of the femoral artery or vein. Multiple manipulations are used to reduce anterior or posterior hip dislocations, and some authors advocate the immediate use of open reduction. If no fracture is present, closed reduction may be attempted in the emergency department with intravenous sedation and analgesia. The exception is the central dislocation, which mandates immediate surgical treatment. In the likely event that reduction is unsuccessful or cannot be maintained, general anesthesia is required for closed or open reduction in the operating room.

Fractures of the Femoral Shaft

Mechanism. Femoral shaft fractures occur commonly as a result of a direct force, torsional stress, or a high-velocity missile injury. Unless a pathologic fracture has occurred, the injury is usually the result of significant trauma.

Presentation. The patient will complain of pain exacerbated by movement or palpation of the thigh. Findings may include angulation, shortening, and rotational deformity of the lower limb. Because of the generous blood supply to the femoral diaphysis, the thigh is routinely swollen by local hemorrhage. The bleeding is significant and is often an ignored source of vascular volume loss. Up to 1.5 L of blood may be lost from a femoral shaft fracture, leading to hypotension and tachycardia.

Radiologic Diagnosis. Anteroposterior and lateral views of the entire femur are obtained to demonstrate the nature of the fracture. Depending on the mechanism of injury, the fracture may be transverse, oblique, spiral, or comminuted, with varying degrees of angulation and shortening.

Management. Use of a Hare traction device is ideal for these fractures because it corrects angulation and shortening while preventing further soft tissue injury at the fracture site. Nerve involvement and vascular injury are rare occurrences. Patients require aggressive fluid resuscitation with large-bore intravenous catheters, admission to the hospital, and orthopedic consultation. Comminuted fractures are often treated initially with traction, whereas internal fixation with medullary nailing is often advocated in patients with simple fractures to facilitate early mobilization. The prognosis for repair of a femoral shaft fracture is generally excellent.

Injuries of the Knee and Leg

PATELLAR FRACTURES

Mechanism. Patellar fractures occur with either direct trauma or forced flexion of the knee.

Presentation. Localized soft tissue swelling, point tenderness over the patella, and joint effusion are common. In patients with displaced transverse patellar fractures, the horizontally aligned bone defect is often palpable. The patient is usually unable to extend the knee.

Radiologic Diagnosis. Radiographs of the knee (including a "sunrise" view of the patella) facilitate diagnosis of these fractures. Because the anteroposterior view shows the patella superimposed over the knee joint, careful scrutiny is needed to discover any pathologic process.

Management. Nondisplaced or minimally displaced (by less than 2 mm) horizontal fractures are treated with immobilization and a compressive bandage, whereas displaced patellar fractures will require eventual surgical repair. Most patients may be discharged from the emergency department with knee immobilization and crutches after orthopedic consultation.

DISTAL FEMORAL FRACTURES

Fractures of the femur in or about the knee joint are infrequent. The femoral shaft is the more likely site of fracture. Fractures involving the supracondylar or intercondylar femur with intra-articular involvement are complex problems requiring immediate orthopedic referral. Patients with such injuries are likely to require hospitalization for traction or open reduction.

TIBIAL PLATEAU FRACTURES

Mechanism. Patients with a history of direct knee trauma, sudden axial loading, or a violent twisting force may fracture one of the tibial condyles, disrupting the tibial plateau, which provides an articulating surface for the femur (Fig. 47–6).

Presentation. Patients are unable to bear weight without pain, and a knee effusion is typically present.

Radiologic Diagnosis. Anteroposterior, lateral, and oblique views of the knee are usually adequate to define the fracture, although CT may be necessary.

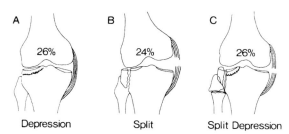

FIGURE 47–6 • Classification and incidence of fractures of the tibial plateau. (Adapted from Hohl M: Tibial condylar fractures. J Bone Joint Surg [Am] 1967; 49:1455.)

Management. Nondisplaced fractures are often treated solely with immobilization, whereas displaced fractures (with greater than 5 mm of depression or widening) may require open reduction. Immediate orthopedic consultation is required in deciding the disposition of the patient.

COLLATERAL AND CRUCIATE LIGAMENT INJURIES

Mechanism. Direct or indirect ("twisted knee") trauma to the knee can result in forced hyperextension, forced hyperflexion, valgus stress, or varus stress, any of which may be superimposed on rotational forces. These may lead to an isolated collateral ligament injury or may cause complete disruption of the collateral ligaments with injury to the cruciate ligaments.

Presentation. Swelling and effusion that develop immediately, or within 6 hours, of the injury often indicate a serious ligamentous injury, specifically a tear of the anterior cruciate ligament. Swelling that develops more slowly can be caused by less severe, but still significant ligamentous or cartilaginous injuries.

Radiologic Diagnosis. Knee radiographs will show knee effusion only.

Management. A severe traumatic effusion may require arthrocentesis. A compressive wrap, knee immobilizer, and crutches used in coordination with ice, elevation, and analgesics are prescribed until follow-up with an orthopedist can be arranged.

KNEE DISLOCATION

Perhaps the most serious diagnostic consideration in acute injury of the knee is that of knee dislocation.

Mechanism. The most common type is the anterior dislocation, which is usually due to forced hyperextension. Posterior dislocation may occur when a severe force strikes the proximal tibia anteriorly (e.g., when the leg strikes the dashboard in an auto accident). This type of dislocation should be considered whenever the mechanism of injury suggests high-energy transfer to the knee.

Presentation. Massive knee swelling with deformity or complete joint instability occurs. Lack of deformity does not rule out the possibility of dislocation, because "spontaneous" reduction or reduction by trainers or emergency medical services personnel may occur in the prehospital setting. Consequently, obtaining a thorough history of mechanism, prior deformity, and any prehospital intervention is critical in making this diagnosis, guiding the physical examination, and obtaining the appropriate studies.

Radiologic Diagnosis. If reduction has not already occurred, the lateral view of the knee reveals abnormal juxtaposition of the tibia and femur.

Management. Because of the high incidence of popliteal artery injury associated with knee dislocation, this injury requires immediate reduction. Placing the hip in flexion and applying longitudinal traction to the leg will facilitate the realignment of the tibia and femur. Angiography *after reduction* is indicated to rule out arterial injury. This is a true orthopedic emergency.

PATELLAR DISLOCATIONS

Mechanism. Patellar dislocations typically occur when there is an underlying abnormality of the patellofemoral anatomy. Direct trauma to a flexed knee may result in dislocation, but more commonly the injury occurs when the quadriceps forcibly contracts when the knee is flexed and the tibia is externally rotated, dislocating the patella laterally.

Presentation. The patient presents with a painful swollen knee, stating that the knee "went out." There is often a history of previous patellar dislocations. The knee is found to be swollen and warm, often because of an associated hemarthrosis. The patella is palpated lateral to its normal position. If reduction has occurred before presentation, there will be positive results on the patellar apprehension test (Fairbands test): on pushing the patella laterally, the patient will grasp the physician's hand because of the sensation of impending dislocation.

Radiologic Diagnosis. Anteroposterior, lateral, and oblique views of the knee are required to rule out associated fracture, which occurs in 28% to 50% of these dislocations. Prereduction and postreduction films should be obtained. The patella typically appears in a lateral position, although superior, horizontal, and intercondylar patellar dislocations do occur.

Management. Lateral patellar dislocations are reduced by placing the patient in a posture of hip flexion and knee extension to achieve maximum relaxation of the knee's extensor mechanism. The patella is then gently moved medially to its normal position. After postreduction films show the patella in its normal position, orthopedic consultation is needed. Although some orthopedists elect to repair first-time dislocations surgically, others treat these injuries with a long-leg cast for 6 weeks. The patient may be discharged for follow-up care with a posterior long-leg splint or a knee immobilizer.

FIBULAR FRACTURES

Mechanisms. Fibular shaft fractures result from direct trauma. Isolated proximal fibular fractures are suspected in patients who are struck by a car's bumper while walking. Fibular shaft fractures tend to occur in association with tibial shaft fractures, because of their parallel positions and tight interosseous membrane connection. Ankle stress is likely to cause a distal fibular fracture but can produce a fracture throughout the length of the fibula if it is forceful enough.

Presentation. Patients with isolated fibular fractures present with local pain and swelling. Pain may not be exacerbated by weight bearing. If associated peroneal nerve injury occurs, there is weakness in ankle dorsiflexion.

Radiologic Diagnosis. Anteroposterior and lateral tibia-fibula views will delineate a fracture.

Management. Because the fibula has no role in weight bearing, the rare isolated fracture of the fibular shaft usually is not problematic; it can be treated without casting when pain is minimal. Fractures of the lateral malleolus or distal fibula are more serious because the lateral support of the ankle joint is jeopardized. Depending on the severity of injury, surgical repair may be required.

TIBIAL SHAFT FRACTURES

Mechanism. Tibial fractures occur secondary to direct trauma or torsional stress.

Presentation. Because the anterior aspect of the tibia lies immediately below the skin, fractures of this bone are often readily apparent. Examination may reveal laxity and crepitance at the site associated with pain. Nerve or vascular damage is rare except in instances of comminuted and displaced fractures of the proximal third of the tibia, near the anterior tibial artery's passage through the interosseous membrane.

Radiologic Diagnosis. Anteroposterior and lateral views of the entire tibia and fibula will reveal the fracture.

Management. Emergency department treatment involves reduction of gross deformities through longitudinal traction and immobilization in a long-leg posterior mold until definitive reduction and casting can be performed. Fractures of the proximal tibia may require angiographic evaluation of the popliteal and tibial arteries.

Injuries of the Ankle and Foot

MECHANISMS OF ANKLE INJURY

The ankle is a complex structure of interdependent articulations and ligamentous supports (Fig. 47–7). The mechanism of injury will indicate the type of pathologic process to be expected. The three common mechanisms of injury can be correlated with distinct constellations of findings:

1. Inversion injury
   • Lateral ligamentous sprain or avulsion fracture of the lateral malleolus from local distractive forces

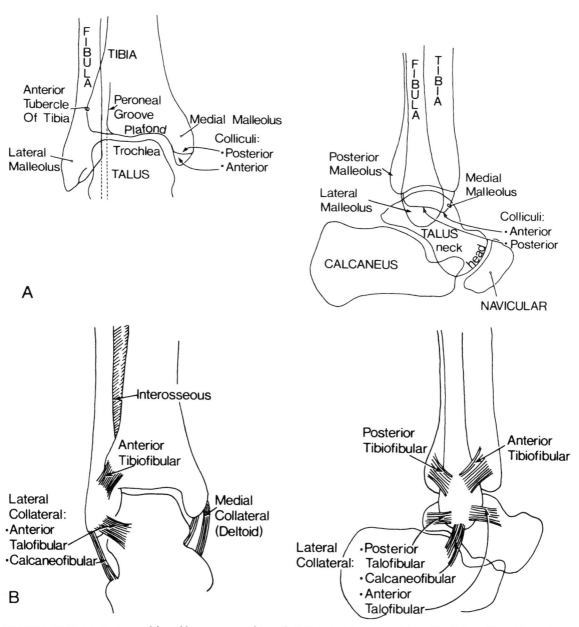

FIGURE 47–7 • *A,* Anatomy of the ankle as seen on radiograph. *B,* Principal ligaments of the ankle. (Adapted from Rogers LF: Radiology of Skeletal Trauma, vol 2. London, Churchill Livingstone, 1982. Used by permission of the Churchill-Livingstone Co.)

- Oblique fracture of the medial malleolus as the talus is driven into the inferolateral tibia from below (Fig. 47–8)
2. Eversion injury
   - Deltoid ligament sprain or avulsion fracture of the medial malleolus from local distractive force
   - Oblique fracture of the fibula as the talus is driven into the lateral malleolus from below (Fig. 47–9)
3. External rotation injury (occurs as the foot and talus rotate externally relative to the leg)
   - Disruption of the syndesmosis between the tibia and fibula or a fibular fracture above the plafond as the talus moves laterally
   - Anterior or posterior tibial fracture with separation of the distal tibia and fibula
   - Deltoid ligament sprain or tibial avulsion fracture

These findings may occur singly, in combination, or not at all, depending on the forces

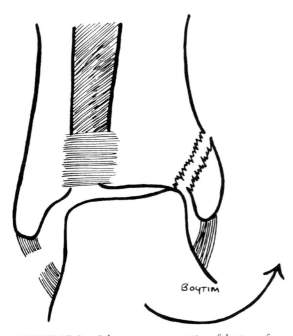

FIGURE 47–8 • Schematic representation of the type of injury caused by forced inversion of the ankle with medial displacement and rotation of the talus. The effect of the impaction force on the medial malleolus resulting from the displacement of the talus is the vertical fracture through the base of the medial malleolus. The avulsion force may either disrupt the lateral collateral ligament (as depicted here) or, if the lateral collateral ligament remains intact, produce an avulsion fracture of the styloid process of the lateral malleolus. Note that the distal tibiofibular ligaments and the interosseous membrane remain intact. (From Harris JH, Harris WH: The Radiology of Emergency Medicine, 2nd ed. Baltimore, Williams & Wilkins, 1981. Used by permission of the Williams & Wilkins Co.)

involved. Keeping these patterns in mind is helpful when interpreting radiographs.

ANKLE SPRAIN

Sprain is the most common diagnosis in ankle injury. An injury that appears to be a simple ankle sprain to the naive examiner is often more complex when it is fully evaluated. The common injuries about the ankle that may simulate the pain found in simple ankle sprains are listed in Table 47–1. These must be considered and ruled out before the diagnosis of ankle sprain can be comfortably made.

Mechanism. Inversion, eversion, or rotation about the ankle lead to variable degrees of stretching and tearing of the medial deltoid ligament or lateral ligamentous complex.

Presentation. The patient presents with local swelling and pain. Lateral sprains are more common than medial sprains, because the deltoid ligament has greater strength and the lateral malleolus is slightly longer than the medial malleolus. These anatomic differences result in more inversion injuries.

Radiologic Diagnosis. All but the most minor ankle injuries require radiographic evaluation to rule out the presence of a fracture (note Ottawa Ankle Rules presented earlier). Anteroposterior, lateral, and mortise views are appropriate. MRI is of significant use in the diagnosis of ligament injuries but is currently not routinely ordered for emergency department patients.

Management. Pain control, elevation, and immobilization (ranging from a bulky Ace wrap to splinting with a posterior plaster mold) are appropriate treatment regimens. Patients with all injuries are given crutches to keep them from bearing weight until they can do so without pain.

MALLEOLAR FRACTURES

Mechanism. Transverse avulsion fractures of the medial and lateral malleoli imply pulling forces along the supporting ligaments. Oblique malleoli fractures imply injury caused by the moving talus.

Presentation. Significant ankle swelling, tenderness, and occasionally gross deformity are found in patients with malleolar fractures. Distal vascular compromise may occur with the deformity caused by a severe fracture-dislocation.

Radiologic Diagnosis. Anteroposterior, lateral, and mortise views show fractures of the involved malleolus, which may appear as small avulsion injuries. The mortise view is carefully evaluated for any evidence of joint instability. A bimalleolar fracture involves the lateral and

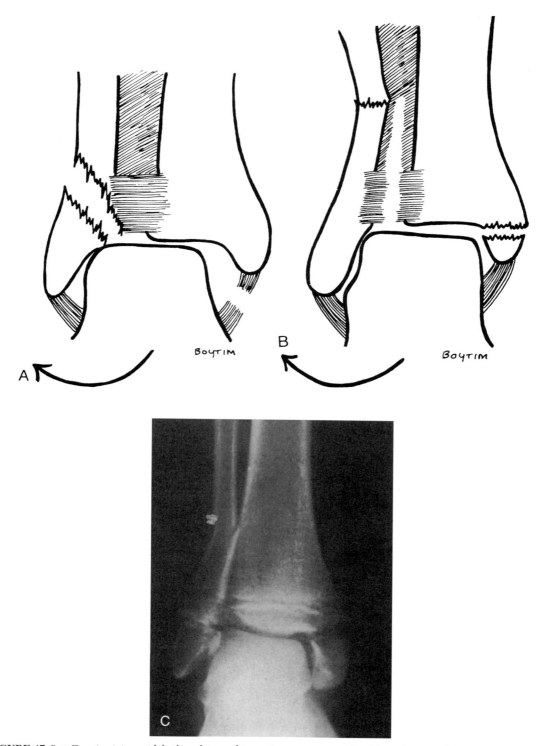

FIGURE 47–9 • Eversion injury with both avulsion and impaction components. The oblique fracture of the distal fibula represents the impaction force of the talus against the lateral malleolus, as the deltoid ligament is torn or an avulsion fracture of the medial malleolus occurs. (Adapted from Harris JH, Harris WH: The Radiology of Emergency Medicine, 2nd ed. Baltimore, Williams & Wilkins, 1981. Used by permission of the Williams & Wilkins Co.)

TABLE 47–1. Injuries Mimicking Ankle Sprain

Injury	History	Physical Findings
Calcaneal fracture	Axial load to ankle	Severe pain, swelling of heel
Proximal fibular fracture	Ankle eversion or rotation	Point tenderness along the fibula, especially near the knee
Fifth metatarsal fracture	Ankle inversion	Point tenderness at the proximal fifth metatarsal with pain on ankle inversion
Tarsal fracture midfoot	Severe foot twisting or direct trauma	Diffuse midfoot tenderness

medial malleoli, whereas a trimalleolar fracture also includes the posterior malleolus (the infero-posterior lip of the distal tibia).

Management. Isolated transverse lateral malleolus fractures often can be treated much like sprains. Bimalleolar and trimalleolar fractures, however, render the ankle unstable. Gross deformity is corrected before immobilization in a posterior mold, and patients are usually hospitalized for ORIF. It is imperative that a description of bimalleolar and trimalleolar fractures and disruption of the ankle mortise be made to the orthopedist so hospitalization or 1- to 2-day follow-up is achieved.

MAISONNEUVE FRACTURES

Mechanism. Isolated sprains of the strong deltoid ligament are not common. Medial tenderness should raise one's index of suspicion for an associated lateral injury. This lateral injury could be a Maisonneuve fracture, in which the proximal fibula is fractured as forces are transferred axially and proximally along the length of the bone and interosseous membrane. This injury should be considered as an isolated fracture of either the medial or the posterior malleolus.

Presentation. In addition to pain and swelling of the medial ankle, tenderness is noted along the proximal fibula. The patient may deny any direct trauma to the area. Including palpation of the proximal fibula as a standard part of the ankle examination ensures that a Maisonneuve fracture will not be missed.

Radiologic Diagnosis. The key to this diagnosis is a high index of suspicion. Clinical examination of the area is followed by anteroposterior and lateral radiologic views of the entire tibia and fibula as well as an ankle mortise view (Fig. 47–10).

Management. Treatment principles for this injury are the same as those for ankle fractures in general. The unstable ankle, as evidenced by a disrupted mortise, is likely to require ORIF if closed reduction cannot achieve a stable, anatomic alignment. After orthopedic consultation, placement of a long-leg posterior mold is appropriate, whether inpatient or outpatient treatment is chosen.

FRACTURE-DISLOCATIONS OF THE ANKLE

Mechanism. The three mechanisms of ankle injury described earlier may lead to a fracture-dislocation. Forces strong enough to cause bimalleolar or trimalleolar fractures may force the talus out of the ankle mortise.

Presentation. The deformity of an ankle dislocation is readily apparent in the form of swelling and angulation. If the injury is severe, a distally cyanotic foot with an absent dorsalis pedis pulse may be noted.

Radiologic Diagnosis. The three views of the ankle will show a bimalleolar or trimalleolar fracture with disruption of the mortise.

Management. It is necessary to check immediately for the integrity of the overlying skin and distal neurovascular function. Early reduction is completed after the initial radiographs. Reduction is achieved simply by returning the talus to its position in the ankle mortise using in-line traction. Documentation of the neurovascular status after reduction and splinting is mandatory. As with other bimalleolar or trimalleolar fractures, hospitalization for ORIF is usually indicated.

CALCANEAL FRACTURES

Mechanism. Injuries of the calcaneus result from axial loading, usually derived from a fall or jump from a significant height. Although the calcaneus is not easily fractured, it is the most commonly fractured tarsal bone. Posterior avulsion fractures due to forceful contraction of the Achilles mechanism may also occur.

Presentation. A patient may present with any constellation of lower extremity injuries after a fall. Avulsion fractures are characterized by pain, swelling, and an inability to walk caused by the impaired plantarflexion mechanism. Plantarflexion is weak or absent on examination, and the area of the avulsion is tender. Fractures of the body of the calcaneus result in severe pain and tenderness, extensive swelling and ecchymosis, and inability to bear weight.

Radiologic Diagnosis. Calcaneal fractures are often apparent on lateral views of the foot or ankle. More subtle compression fractures are

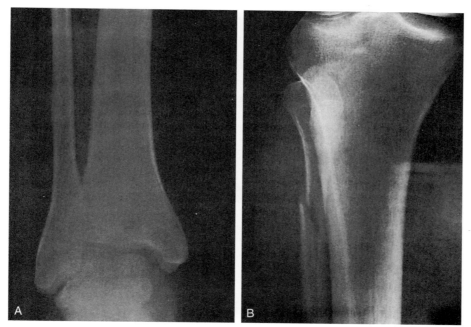

FIGURE 47–10 • The Maisonneuve fracture. Note that the talus is displaced laterally, indicating disruption of the distal tibiofibular ligaments, while the propagation of forces proximally has caused a proximal fibular fracture. (Adapted from Harris JH, Harris WH: The Radiology of Emergency Medicine, 2nd ed. Baltimore, Williams & Wilkins, 1981. Used by permission of the Williams & Wilkins Co.)

diagnosed by evaluating Boehler's angle on the lateral radiograph. A decrease in the described angle (which is usually 30 to 40 degrees) usually indicates a fracture (Fig. 47–11). Axial views of the calcaneus are also useful.

Management. Because 10% of patients have associated vertebral or contralateral calcaneal fractures, emergency department treatment is incomplete until these injuries are ruled out. It is important to institute ice, elevation, and a compressive dressing as soon as possible to prevent the extensive soft tissue swelling that follows these injuries. Depending on the severity of the calcaneal pathology or the associated injuries, hospitalization may be indicated.

TALAR FRACTURES

Mechanism. The talus has an anterior head, posterior body, and intermediate neck. The neck is highly vulnerable to fracture, because of its lesser diameter, relative position in bearing stress, minimal supporting cartilage, and numerous vascular foramina. These transcervical fractures are caused by forced dorsiflexion of the foot (e.g., when violently forcing the foot against a car's brake pedal). The body of the talus may move posteriorly after a transcervical fracture. This results in impairment of its blood supply because the

majority of the vessels of the talus enter at the neck. Avascular necrosis is a possible complication. Up to 20% of talar fractures are associated with a medial malleolar fracture. The most common fracture of the talus is an osteochondral fracture of the talar dome due to compression.

Presentation. Fracture of the talar dome has presenting signs similar to those seen with ankle sprains and is often overlooked. A clue to its presence is a click felt on ankle movement. More severe talar fractures present as intense pain and swelling and often a loss of the normal contour of the anterior ankle.

Radiologic Diagnosis. Anteroposterior, lateral, and oblique views of the ankle, often with comparison views of the uninjured ankle, are needed. Small irregularities of the superior surface of the talus are seen best on the mortise view of the ankle and indicate an osteochondral fracture of the talar dome. Fractures of the head, body, or neck of the talus will cause a fracture line or an abnormal talar profile.

Management. Fracture of the neck of the talus must be reduced as soon as possible, and prompt orthopedic consultation is important. Nondisplaced linear fractures of the body are less urgently addressed, needing short-leg casting for 6 to 8 weeks. Displaced fractures of the talar body

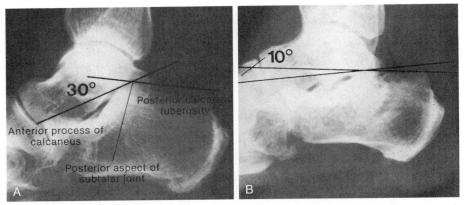

FIGURE 47–11 • Boehler's angle is described by drawing a line from the posterior aspect of the subtalar joint to the anterior process of the calcaneus and another from the posterior aspect of the subtalar joint to the posterior calcaneal tuberosity. *A*, Normal Boehler's angle of 30 to 40 degrees. *B*, Abnormal Boehler's angle of 10 degrees indicates flattening of the calcaneus consistent with a fracture. (From Nance EP, et al [eds]: Advanced Exercises in Diagnostic Radiology. Philadelphia, WB Saunders, 1983, pp 88 and 92.)

require prompt reduction. As with neck fractures, hospitalization for immediate surgical intervention is the rule. Osteochondral dome fractures may also require surgery to remove any fragments that may lead to locking of the ankle.

TALAR DISLOCATIONS

Most ankle dislocations are examples of single talar dislocations in which only the tibiotalar joint is disrupted. More complex dislocations also involve luxation at the subtalar joint and talonavicular joint.

Mechanism. Total dislocation of the talus is rare. In this entity, the talus moves forward and laterally, losing its anatomic proximity to the tibia *and* tarsals.

Presentation. Patients have severe pain and swelling, often with severe tenting of the skin overlying the deformity.

Radiologic Diagnosis. Plain films of the ankle show complete loss of the normal position of the talus.

Management. Immediate orthopedic consultation is necessary for reduction. This injury invariably leads to avascular necrosis of the talus and a poor outcome. Failure to reduce the talus in a timely fashion can also lead to necrosis of the overlying skin.

TARSAL FRACTURES

Mechanism. The rigid midfoot has multiple articulations but limited joint movement. Therefore, twisting foot injuries cause only small avulsion fractures of the tarsals. Other tarsal fractures are caused by direct trauma, as when an object falls onto the foot or when violent forces twist the midfoot.

Presentation. A tarsal fracture may simulate a simple ankle sprain. However, palpation about the ankle will be unremarkable. Palpation of the painful midfoot may reveal point tenderness. A combination of tarsal fractures and dislocations may occur, causing severe soft tissue swelling and pain. Any movement of the midfoot causes discomfort.

Radiologic Diagnosis. Anteroposterior, lateral, and oblique views of the foot are necessary to locate an abnormality. Because of the many articulations, multiple oblique views may be necessary to evaluate an injury fully.

Management. Orthopedic consultation is obtained. Minor injuries in inactive patients may be adequately treated with a compressive dressing, elevation, ice, and crutches. More severe injuries may necessitate a short-leg walking cast once swelling subsides. Severe and complicated injuries will require ORIF and immediate hospitalization.

TARSOMETATARSAL FRACTURE-DISLOCATIONS

Mechanism. Lisfranc's joint (the tarsometatarsal joint) separates the midfoot from the forefoot. It is injured when there is severe forefoot twisting or a direct axial load on the foot with the toes hyperextended. This can occur when an equestrian falls off a horse with the foot caught in the stirrup or when a heavy object falls on the heel while the subject is kneeling.

Presentation. Severe pain and swelling of the midfoot-forefoot complex are present, sometimes with distal vascular compromise from involvement of the dorsalis pedis artery.

Radiologic Diagnosis. Anteroposterior, lateral, and oblique views of the foot are needed. Any fracture of the base of the second metatarsal or of the cuboid is pathognomonic for disruption of the tarsometatarsal joint. The metatarsal complex is usually translocated laterally, and the dislocation is obvious on radiographs.

Management. Hospitalization for surgical reduction and stabilization is indicated. Immediate orthopedic consultation is obtained.

METATARSAL FRACTURES

Mechanism. Direct trauma or twisting of the forefoot is the usual cause of metatarsal fractures.

Presentation. Patients have pain on ambulation and palpable tenderness. As in other injuries of the foot, swelling and ecchymosis may be impressive if the foot has remained dependent for any length of time.

Radiologic Diagnosis. Anteroposterior, lateral, and oblique views of the foot are necessary to evaluate the metatarsals fully.

Management. The soft tissue injury may become the most important focus of treatment. Patients with little or no fracture angulation and mild to moderate swelling may be managed with immobilization in a short-leg splint and discharged with instructions to elevate the foot, apply ice as needed, refrain from bearing weight, and secure prompt orthopedic follow-up. Severely injured patients with poor fracture alignment and extensive swelling may require hospitalization for fracture reduction followed by frequent skin and neurovascular checks.

STRESS (MARCH) FRACTURES

Mechanism. Stress fractures, which occur commonly in the second and third metatarsals, result from repetitive and seemingly trivial trauma. They are so named because of their occurrence in recruits to the armed services who develop forefoot pain after extended periods of marching.

Presentation. Patients complain of foot pain that is worse with weight bearing. Localized tenderness and swelling occur at the fracture site.

Radiologic Diagnosis. These nondisplaced shaft fractures often cannot be seen on initial films. If symptoms persist, repeated radiographs or bone scans may be required to delineate the fracture.

Management. The diagnosis is presumptive when initial radiologic evaluation is unremarkable. Treatment is conservative, with splint immobilization and crutches to prevent weight bearing. Definitive treatment will require short-leg casting for 3 to 4 weeks.

FRACTURE OF THE PROXIMAL FIFTH METATARSAL

Mechanism. This fracture can occur through one of three mechanisms: inversion injury with bony avulsion caused by the pull of the peroneus brevis tendon, direct trauma, or indirect stress.

Presentation. Patients with this type of fracture (Jones fracture) have a history and physical findings consistent with those characteristic of an ankle sprain.

Radiologic Diagnosis. The proximal fifth metatarsal can be evaluated on either a lateral ankle or foot radiograph (Fig. 47–12).

Management. In patients with avulsion injuries in which displacement is small, a dressing that supplies some local compression followed by a posterior plaster mold is usually adequate. Patients with transverse fractures through the base of the metatarsal are treated similarly but receive a short-leg cast at orthopedic follow-up.

METATARSOPHALANGEAL DISLOCATIONS

Mechanism. Patients who "stub" their toes may dislocate the metatarsophalangeal (MTP) joint.

Presentation. The area of the MTP joint is swollen, painful, and obviously deformed.

Radiologic Diagnosis. Even though these injuries usually are not associated with phalangeal fractures, plain films are obtained before reduction.

Management. Reduction requires accentuation of the mechanism of injury followed by axial traction. Difficulty in reduction can be caused by entrapment of the plantar joint capsule (similar to entrapment of the volar plate in phalangeal dislocations) or entrapment of a sesamoid bone. Either taping the involved toe to its neighbor, using a metallic splint, or using a cast shoe is appropriate treatment.

PHALANGEAL FRACTURES

Mechanism. Stubbed toes that do not dislocate may fracture instead.

Presentation. Any tender, swollen foot phalanx is potentially a fractured phalanx.

Radiologic Diagnosis. A limited survey of the toes or a complete view of the foot will demonstrate a fracture.

Management. Any marked angulation can be reduced with axial traction, and the injured toe can be "buddy taped" to a neighboring toe. In the case of a fracture of the great toe, buddy taping is inadequate stabilization; plaster splinting is needed.

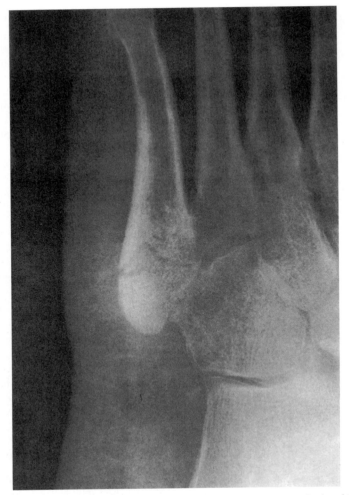

FIGURE 47–12 • The transverse lucency at the base of the fifth metatarsal represents a nondisplaced Jones fracture. (From Nance EP, et al [eds]: Advanced Exercises in Diagnostic Radiology. Philadelphia, WB Saunders, 1983, p 64.)

INTERPHALANGEAL DISLOCATIONS

Mechanism. Direct trauma is usually involved in phalangeal dislocations.

Presentation. The patient with a history consistent with this mechanism of injury presents with a tender, deformed phalanx.

Radiologic Diagnosis. Views of the toes or entire foot will show loss of the normal alignment at the interphalangeal joint.

Management. Interphalangeal joint dislocations are evaluated in the same way as MTP dislocations. Similar problems with reduction occur. Great toe phalangeal dislocations are most often dorsal and are significant because of their tendency to redislocate with weight bearing. Buddy taping is usually adequate. The great toe will need stabilization with a plaster splint, however.

SPECIAL CONSIDERATIONS

Legg-Calvé-Perthes Disease

Legg-Calvé-Perthes disease, also known as *coxa plana* or *osteochondrosis of the femoral head*, results from transient ischemia and consequent avascular necrosis of the femoral head. The exact etiology of the condition is controversial, but it is presumed to be directly related to the particularly tenuous blood supply of the capital femoral epiphysis in children between the ages of 3 and 11. The typical presentation is a preadolescent boy complaining of hip or knee pain with an antalgic gait. Males are affected four times as often as females. Range of motion at the hip may be limited in abduction and external rotation. Clinical suspicion is confirmed by hip radiographs, including one with the patient in a frog-leg position. Early abnormalities include flattening (coxa plana) or increased bone density of the femoral capital epiphysis. Radiolucent areas below the cortical margin of the epiphysis consistent with subchondral fractures may also be seen. Radiologically, the disease progresses over 4 to 6 years, resulting in further fragmentation and flattening of the epiphysis, shortening and widening of the femoral neck, and femoral head subluxation. Later in life this residual joint incongruity will lead to degenerative joint disease. Once the diagnosis has been made, the child should have prompt orthopedic referral. A variety of treatment regimens exist, all of which incorporate containment of the femoral head well within the acetabulum by long-term splinting of the hip in abduction and flexion. This "protects" the femoral head and minimizes further flattening of the epiphysis.

Slipped Capital Femoral Epiphysis

Another cause of hip pain and limp in children is a slipped capital femoral epiphysis. This entity is most common in older children and adolescents from 9 to 16 years of age. It occurs predominantly in obese males and is a bilateral disease in 30% of cases. Chronic shear stress encountered by the obliquely situated upper femoral epiphyseal plate coupled with other possible predisposing factors (previous radiation or chemotherapy, hypothyroidism, renal osteodystrophy) leads to separation of the growth plate and progressive posterior and medial slippage of the femoral head. The history is typically significant for an absence of direct trauma. The development of hip or knee pain and limp is generally insidious. Range of motion at the hip is painful and is limited in adduction and internal rotation. Diagnosis is made by often subtle radiographic findings (Fig. 47–13).

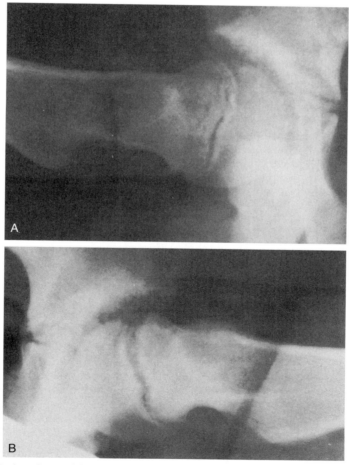

FIGURE 47–13 • *A,* This lateral view of the femoral head is normal. *B,* This lateral view of a slipped capital femoral epiphysis shows a loss of continuity along its superior edge where the metaphysis has moved cephalad with respect to the epiphysis. One might imagine this pathology to be similar to "the ice cream sliding off the cone." (From Nance EP, et al [eds]: Advanced Exercises in Diagnostic Radiology. Philadelphia, WB Saunders, 1983, p 15.)

Radiographs may show widening and irregularity of the proximal epiphyseal plate. Anteroposterior and frog-leg views of the hip will show the epiphysis projecting beyond the inferior border of the femoral neck while remaining flush or caudad to the superior edge of the neck. This abnormality is more easily seen when comparison views of the healthy hip are obtained. The overall picture is one of ice cream (the femoral head) sliding off an ice cream cone (the femoral neck). The slipping capital femoral epiphysis that remains undiscovered is likely to progress until bone maturity and fusion of the epiphyseal plate occur, decreasing hip mobility and increasing the risk of avascular necrosis or early osteoarthritis. Patients must refrain from weight bearing, usually in the hospital, until surgical pinning can be performed.

Osgood-Schlatter Disease

Another entity to be considered in the differential diagnosis of adolescent knee pain is Osgood-Schlatter disease. Repeated forceful contraction of the quadriceps mechanism causes serial partial avulsions of the tibial tubercle at the site of insertion of the patellar tendon. This apophysis is particularly prone to injury in active males between ages of 10 and 15. Repeated injuries of this growing tubercle, with subsequent avascular necrosis of the proximally avulsed portion, lead to local swelling and pain, which is exacerbated by palpation as well as extension of the knee against resistance. Radiographically, the tubercle appears elevated, irregular, and fragmented compared with the normal tibia. Treatment is usually conservative. Avoidance of kneeling, jumping, and excessive running will allow healing to occur. Some authors recommend a more aggressive approach: keeping the knee immobilized with no weight bearing for 4 to 6 weeks and resuming normal activities after 3 months. Fusion of the apophysis with increasing bone maturity at 16 to 18 years of age makes Osgood-Schlatter disease a self-limiting problem.

Compartment Syndromes

A compartment syndrome is a condition in which the vascular supply and function of tissues within a closed space are compromised by increased pressure within that space. The fascia, skin, and bones of the lower leg form the anterior, lateral, deep posterior, and superficial posterior compartments, any of which may be involved in an acute compartment syndrome. Compartment syndromes in the thigh and gluteal regions may occur but are rare. Failure to recognize an impending compartment syndrome will lead to progressive ischemic necrosis of nerve and muscle, with subsequent loss of function of the extremity.

Because the development of a compartment syndrome depends on the relationship between the available enclosed space and the tissue contents within it, any decrease in compartmental size or increase in compartmental content can initiate this entity. Decreased compartmental size may result from inordinately tight dressings or casts. Compartment volume may increase secondary to intercompartmental edema resulting from direct trauma such as crush injuries or from postischemic swelling, as in cases of proximal vascular occlusion. Less common causes include burns, vigorous exercise, intracompartmental bleeding (as may occur in patients with coagulopathies), venous obstruction, muscle hypertrophy, and nephrotic syndrome.

Clinically, the most important symptom that arouses a physician's suspicion of an impending compartment syndrome is pain that is out of proportion to that expected for the degree of soft tissue or bony injury present. This ischemic pain will not be relieved by immobilization or elevation. Patients may also complain of distal paresthesias. Early findings include swelling and palpable tenseness of an entire muscular compartment, which is often hard to appreciate in the presence of extensive but more superficial soft tissue swelling. Pain with passive stretch of the muscles within the compartment is common. Paresis is difficult to appreciate because motor testing may be biased by pain. The most reliable physical finding is a deficit in soft touch and pinprick sensation in an area supplied exclusively by a nerve that travels through the compartment in question. In all compartment syndromes, a pulse deficit is an uncommon early finding. Dependence on a diminished pulse to make the diagnosis is a grave error. Among the five "Ps" characteristic of compartment syndrome—*pallor, paralysis, pulselessness, paresthesias, and pain (out of proportion to injury as well as with passive muscle stretching)*—the latter two are the most important early findings in making a prompt diagnosis.

Of the specific syndromes, the *anterior compartment syndrome* is encountered most commonly (Fig. 47–14). As intercompartmental pressure increases, passive stretching of the tibialis anterior, extensor hallucis longus, and extensor digitorum longus muscles (as in plantarflexion of the ankle or toes) will be painful. Weakening of these muscle groups may be detected on forced extension of the toes or dorsiflexion of the ankle

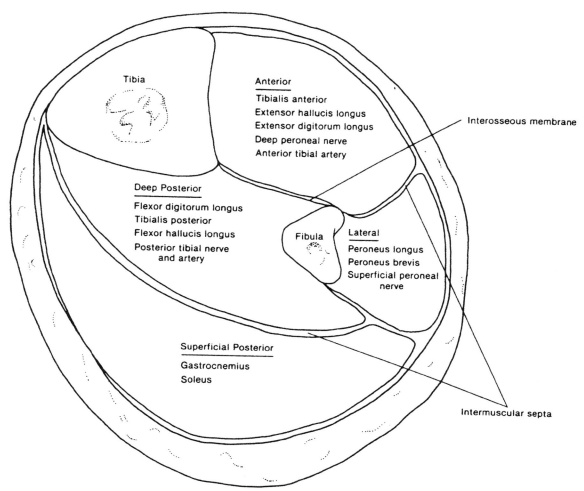

FIGURE 47–14 • Cross-sectional anatomy of the leg showing the contents of the anterior, lateral, posterior, and deep posterior compartments.

against resistance. Impairment of anterior tibial nerve function will lead to hypesthesia in the distribution of its sensory branch, the deep peroneal nerve, which supplies the dorsum of the foot and, most exclusively, the dorsum of the web space between the great and second toes.

In *deep posterior compartment syndrome*, hypesthesia develops on the sole of the foot with weakness noted in the toe flexors. Passive extension of the toes will elicit pain in the calf.

The *lateral compartment syndrome* results in sensory loss on the lateral dorsum of the foot, weakness in foot eversion, and pain with passive inversion of the foot.

The key to diagnosing all compartment syndromes is a high index of suspicion and frequent, careful examinations of the extremity to elicit these findings. If compartment syndrome is sus-

pected, testing of compartment pressures may be performed in the emergency department, depending on the institution. Normal compartment pressure ranges from 0 to 10 mm Hg. Pressures of 10 to 20 mm Hg should prompt consideration of admission for observation or repeat evaluation. A compartment pressure of 30 to 40 mm Hg is markedly elevated and requires admission and fasciotomy.

DISPOSITION AND FOLLOW-UP

Indications for Immediate Operative Intervention

The following lower extremity injuries usually require immediate orthopedic consultation and operative intervention:

1. Open fracture with gross bone or joint contamination
2. Irreducible fracture-dislocation associated with neurovascular compromise
3. Partial or complete amputation in which the limb can be salvaged or that is associated with uncontrolled hemorrhage
4. Compartment syndrome

Indications for Admission

The following lower extremity injuries usually require orthopedic consultation and admission of the patient to the hospital:

1. Hip fracture
2. Femoral fracture, because of the severity of the trauma that caused the fracture, the potential for local hemorrhage, and the need for operative management or traction
3. Knee fracture or dislocation, because of the likelihood of increased displacement of fracture fragments with even partial weight bearing and the high probability of operative management
4. Fracture of the tibia and fibula, because of gross instability and the potential for development of vascular compromise or compartment syndrome
5. Unstable ankle fracture (bimalleolar or trimalleolar fracture)
6. Calcaneal fracture, because of the significant associated pain and swelling
7. Open fractures that require operative irrigation or intravenous antibiotics

Outpatient Management

Minor sprains, strains, and contusions are best treated with (1) RICE therapy (rest, ice, compression, elevation) for 24 to 48 hours, (2) weight bearing only when it is painless, (3) nonsteroidal anti-inflammatory therapy for 5 to 7 days, and (4) follow-up if pain persists beyond 3 to 5 days.

Minor fractures or suspected cartilaginous or ligamentous injury of the knee may be treated with (1) RICE therapy for 24 to 48 hours with plaster immobilization or a knee immobilizer, (2) absolute absence of weight bearing, (3) narcotic analgesics for 24 to 72 hours as needed, (4) nonsteroidal anti-inflammatory therapy for 5 to 7 days, and (5) follow-up with an orthopedic consultant in 2 to 3 days for splint removal, reexamination, and casting as appropriate.

Crutches

Lower extremity injuries that are initially managed with the RICE method can be expected to heal more quickly and less painfully. To improve outcome and to limit liability, patients are told to refrain from bearing weight on the extremity during the first 24 to 48 hours after the injury. This can be best achieved with crutches, but a cane can be used if the patient cannot tolerate or handle crutches.

FINAL POINTS

- Injuries to the lower extremity can be life threatening through blood loss or late sepsis.
- The most important immediate examination priority is directed toward assessing the presence of pulses and vascular integrity.
- Because of the anatomic complexity of the lower extremity and the nature of injury forces, the joint above and below the site of injury must be examined.
- A negative radiograph is rarely reassuring in lower extremity injuries. Soft tissue injuries can be more problematic to diagnose and treat than fractures.
- Not all fractures are seen on initial radiographs. When in doubt, splint the extremity and arrange for close follow-up. Educate the patient about this possibility.
- Elevation and immobilization are the foundation of any treatment of lower extremity injuries.

CASE *Study*

A 28-year-old man was transported to the emergency department after a motorcycle accident. The accident occurred at low speed, and the rider was wearing a helmet. The patient complained of left hip and lower leg pain and inability to bear weight. He was evaluated by the rescue squad and transported on a backboard with his left leg carefully splinted to the right.

On arrival at the emergency department, the patient was placed in the resuscitation bay. The emergency physician and nursing personnel initiated the trauma protocol on arrival. The airway was checked for patency and the lungs auscultated. The chest wall was palpated for obvious rib or sternal tenderness. Simultaneously, the nurse obtained vital signs, placed the patient on a cardiac monitor, and established a second intravenous line with normal saline. The cervical spine was palpated for point tenderness, and the abdomen was surveyed for visible contusions, distention, and tenderness. An initial neurologic assessment revealed a Glasgow Coma Scale score of 15 (normal).

In spite of the obvious left lower extremity injury, the resuscitation proceeded in an orderly and step-wise fashion that addressed the life-threatening priorities first. Anticipation of airway compromise or hemorrhage always takes precedence over extremity trauma even if there is a vascular threat. A limb-threatening extremity injury has up to 4 to 6 hours within which to reverse it, whereas an airway disorder can cause irreversible organ damage within minutes.

The initial survey did not reveal any immediate life-threatening injuries. The vital signs are a blood pressure of 130/80 mm Hg, pulse of 90 beats per minute, and a respiratory rate of 16 breaths per minute. The chest and cervical spine radiographs are negative. A spun hematocrit is 40%, and the urine has no measurable blood. Femoral, dorsalis pedis, and posterior tibial pulses are equal bilaterally. On inspection, the left leg appears shortened and externally rotated. There is marked tenderness of the proximal femur. There is also a laceration over the mid anterior tibia and bony crepitance. Additional plain films are ordered.

Clinically, there appears to be a closed fracture of the femur and an open one of the tibia. A Hare traction splint is the recommended splint for the femur; however, the tibial fracture precludes its application. The extremity can be managed by placing the leg in a long-leg aluminum splint and by keeping the patient on a backboard. Every precaution is taken to minimize the manipulation of the leg.

Before being moved to the radiology suite, a short-acting narcotic, fentanyl, is administered for pain. In addition, a second-generation cephalosporin is given to treat the open fracture. The open wound is gently cleansed and irrigated. A moist povidone-iodine dressing is placed. Radiographs reveal a comminuted proximal shaft fracture of the femur. The tibia is also comminuted in the midshaft. An orthopedic surgeon is consulted.

At this point the responsibility for the patient is transferred to the orthopedic surgeon. The trauma is localized to the extremity and all subsequent care is directed toward those injuries. In this case, the next step in the management is likely to be operative. Most closed femur fractures can be repaired primarily. The tibia will need open exploration, irrigation, and débridement before repair. Both open and closed techniques can be used to reduce tibia fractures. The first priority, however, is to prevent infection of the bone or soft tissues.

In the operating room, the femur is repaired primarily. The tibia is débrided, and an external fixator is placed. In a subsequent operation, plates and screws are used to complete the tibia repair. Over the next several months, the patient undergoes intense physical therapy to restore function of the left leg. A year later, he has returned to his normal life but no longer rides motorcycles.

Bibliography

TEXTS

Della-Ginstina D, Coppola M (eds): Orthopedic Emergencies: I. Emerg Med Clin North Am 1999; 17(4).

Della-Ginstina D, Coppola M (eds): Orthopedic Emergencies: II. Emerg Med Clin North Am 2000; 18(1).

Rockwood CA, Green DP, Bucholz RW (eds): Fractures in Adults, 4th ed. Philadelphia, Lippincott-Raven, 1996.

Ruiz EE, Cicero JJ (eds): Emergency Management of Skeletal Injuries. St. Louis, Mosby–Year Book, 1995.

JOURNAL ARTICLES

Birrer RB, Fani-Salek MH, Totten VY: Managing ankle injuries in the emergency department. J Emerg Med 1999; 17:651–660.

Brady WJ, Degnan GG, Buchanon LP, et al: Challenging and elusive orthopedic injuries: Diagnostic and treatment strategies for optimizing clinical outcomes. Emerg Med Rep 1999; 20:99–108.

Dougall TW, Duthie R, Maffulli N, Hutchinson JD: Antibiotic prophylaxis: Theory and reality in orthopedics. J R Coll Surg Edinb 1996; 41:321–322.

Harrington KD: Orthopedic management of extremity and pelvic injuries. Clin Orthop 1995; 26:136–147.

Kaufman D, Leung J: Evaluation of the patient with extremity trauma: An evidence-based approach. Emerg Med Clin North Am 1999; 17:77–95.

Markert RJ, Walley ME, Guttman TG, Mehta R: A pooled analysis of the Ottawa ankle rules used in the ED. Am J Emerg Med 1998; 16:564–567.

Perron AD, Brady WJ, Keats TE: Orthopedic pitfalls in the ED: Lisfranc fracture-dislocation. Am J Emerg Med 2001; 19:71–75.

Pijnenburg ACM, Glas AS, De Roos MAJ, et al: Radiography in acute ankle injuries: The Ottawa Ankle Rules versus local diagnostic decision rules. Ann Emerg Med 2002; 39:599–604.

Prokuski LJ, Saltzman CL: Challenging fractures of the foot and ankle. Radiol Clin North Am 1997; 35:655–670.

Reddy PK, Posteraro RH, et al: The role of MRI in evaluation of the cruciate ligaments in knee dislocations. Orthopedics 1996; 19:166–170.

Reisdorff ES, Coroling KM, Gavin L: The injured ankle: New twists to a familiar problem. Emerg Med Rep 1995; 16(5):39–48.

Seybold EA, Buscon BD: Traumatic popliteal artery thrombosis and compartment syndrome of the leg following blunt trauma to the knee: A discussion of treatment and complications. J Orthop Trauma 1996; 10:138–141.

Solomon DH, Simel DL, Bates DW, et al: Does the patient have a torn meniscus or ligament of the knee? JAMA 2001; 286:1610–1620.

Stewart C: Knee injuries: Diagnosis and repair. Emerg Med Rep 1997; 18:1–12.

Stiell IG, Wells GA, Hoog RH, et al: Implementation of the Ottawa Knee Rule for the use of radiography in acute knee injuries. JAMA 1997; 278:2075–2079.

Wasserman E, Hill S: Ankle injuries in the ED: How to provide rapid and cost-effective assessment and treatment. Emerg Med Pract 2002; 4(5):1–28.

CHAPTER 48

Head and Neck Trauma

RAY LEGENZA

JAMES BROWN

CASE *Study*

A 67-year-old woman is involved in a major motor vehicle accident. The driver, her husband, is dead at the scene. She is extricated from the car and is noted to be confused. A cervical collar is placed. Her vital signs are blood pressure, 150/95 mm Hg; heart rate, 105 beats per minute; and respiratory rate, 22 breaths per minute on 10 L of oxygen by face mask. Estimated time of arrival is 5 minutes.

INTRODUCTION

Trauma to the head and neck is a frequent presenting complaint in the emergency department. Each year, nearly 500,000 Americans incur a head injury requiring medical evaluation. Of these approximately 50,000 suffer severe brain injury and between 50,000 and 100,000 people die. Of the 500,000 patients with head injuries, most (80%) can be classified as having only mild injuries. Ten percent have moderate injuries, whereas the remaining 10% have severe brain trauma. Almost 10,000 new cases of spinal cord injury occur annually in the United States. A clear, concise, and practical approach to evaluate head and neck trauma in the emergency department is necessary to minimize further injury, avoid delays in management, prevent errors in diagnosis, and optimize resources. Prompt, effective care reduces patient mortality and morbidity.

Head and neck trauma is usually classified as either blunt or penetrating. Most blunt head and neck trauma has no intrusion through the dura of the skull or the platysma muscle of the neck. Each usually occurs as a result of motor vehicle accidents, falls, assaults, or recreational and sporting events. Penetrating trauma is usually caused by gunshot or knife wounds and occasionally by impalement and blast injury.

Management of head and neck trauma is focused on the potential damage to the nervous system, which is protected by bone. The damage can be divided into primary and secondary injury. Primary injury is the immediate mechanical disruption of brain or spinal cord tissue. It occurs at the time of impact. Its treatment is anticipatory through prevention and protection. A cascade of neurochemical and cellular mediators causes secondary injury. These excitatory amino acids, eicosanoids (from lipid hydrolysis), and inflammatory mediators alter normal neural functioning, change local cerebral blood flow, and may damage the cellular metabolic environment. The first goals of emergency care are preventing further direct insult to the central nervous system (CNS) with stabilization of the patient's head and spine and medically modifying the secondary injury cascade to minimize indirect injury.

Anatomy and Pathophysiology

Knowledge of the normal anatomy of the head and neck is necessary to understand the significance of abnormal findings on physical examination or radiographic studies.

Head

The scalp consists of five layers, the most important of which are the galea aponeurotica and dermis. The galea is a fibrous nonelastic covering that lies adjacent to the skull. The cranial vault encloses the brain and its three meningeal layers: dura mater, arachnoid, and pia mater. The dura mater, or dura, is the dense, fibrous, nonelastic outermost component of the three layers and is part of the protective structure for the brain. The arachnoid is the thin, vascular middle layer. The innermost layer, the pia, closely envelops the brain matter throughout its sulci and gyri. The meningeal arteries course between the innermost layer of the skull and the dura mater. Injury to these vessels may result in arterial epidural bleeding in the potential epidural space between the dura and the cranial vault.

The skull is composed of a base and the cranial vault. The inferior portion of the cranial vault is further divided into an anterior cranial fossa, a middle cranial fossa, and a posterior cranial fossa. Anatomically important structures in the anterior fossa include the cribriform plates and the frontal lobes of the brain. In the middle fossa are multiple cranial nerve and vascular foramina and the temporal lobes of the brain. The cerebellum and brain stem are found in the posterior fossa. The cerebrospinal fluid (CSF) is conveyed in a system of ventricles and foramina: the large, paired lateral ventricles, the two interventricular foramen (of Monro), the singular third ventricle, the cerebral aqueduct (of Sylvius), and the fourth ventricle near the cerebellum.

Skull injuries include (1) fractures of the cerebral vault, in which location and depth of the fracture are clinically important, and (2) fractures of the skull base, which may be difficult to demonstrate radiographically but may be clinically inferred (e.g., CSF rhinorrhea [anterior fossa fracture], hemotympanum or CSF otorrhea [middle fossa fracture], cerebellar hematoma [posterior fossa fracture]).

Brain tissue injury may be divided into focal injury and diffuse brain injury. *Focal injuries* include

1. *Cerebral contusion,* demonstrated by multiple small isolated hemorrhages in the brain parenchyma.
2. *Epidural hematoma,* caused by arterial bleeding that produces a hematoma external to the dura. It often results from a skull fracture lying adjacent to the middle meningeal artery.
3. *Subdural hematoma,* caused by venous bleeding between the dura and subarachnoid membrane after blunt trauma.
4. *Intracerebral hematoma,* resulting from intracerebral bleeding after severe brain parenchymal disruption or subsequent tissue ischemia and necrosis.

Diffuse brain injuries include:

1. *Mild concussion,* manifested as rapidly resolving temporary neurologic dysfunction, typically memory loss or short-term loss of consciousness (less than 5 minutes).
2. *Classic cerebral concussion,* manifested as slowly resolving temporary neurologic dysfunction often accompanied by a significant loss of consciousness (from 5 minutes to hours).
3. *Diffuse axonal injury,* resulting in a prolonged comatose state. Mild and moderate forms of diffuse axonal injury rarely result in coma lasting more than 24 hours. The severe form of diffuse axonal injury is associated with brain stem dysfunction and is caused by the involvement of the reticular activating system; the coma may last for months.

Brain injury can be devastating because the cranial vault acts as a closed box. Its normal contents are brain tissue, CSF, and blood. Because fluids are nearly incompressible, any swelling or mass will tend to displace brain tissue, CSF, or venous volume in an attempt to maintain near-normal intracranial pressure (ICP). When these compensating mechanisms are exhausted, further mass effect will increase ICP and result in a decrease in cerebral perfusion pressure (CPP). The CPP is the difference in mean arterial blood pressure (MAP) minus ICP. As ICP increases, CPP decreases and relative brain hypoxia ensues. An ICP greater than 20 mm Hg is considered abnormal, and CPP less than 70 mm Hg is associated with worse outcomes in severe brain injury. As ICP increases, swelling or mass effect results in physical compression and shifting of brain tissue.

Neck

The neck extends from the floor of the mandible to the manubrium of the sternum and along the clavicles to the acromion process of the shoulder. It encompasses the trachea, esophagus, and the cervical spine, along with a complex array of major vessels and nerves. The bones of the neck consist of the hyoid bone and the seven cervical vertebrae.

The components of a cervical vertebrae allow rotation, flexion, extension, and lateral movement of the head while protecting the spinal cord, the roots of the brachial plexus, and the vertebrobasilar vascular network supplying the brain. The first cervical vertebra (C1), the atlas, has a ring-like structure with an absent vertebral body. The second cervical vertebra (C2), the axis, has a vertically enlarged vertebral body called the dens axis or odontoid process protruding just posterior to the anterior aspect of the atlas (Fig. 48–1). All subsequent cervical vertebrae have a similar appearance albeit with a cannular vertebral body (Fig. 48–2).

Causes of cervical spine injuries may be categorized into four major mechanisms of injury, linked to the direction of force involved. These are (1) flexion injuries, (2) extension injuries, (3) rotational injuries, and (4) vertical compression injuries. The results of these four mechanisms (or combinations) are the potential disruption of three distinct anatomic "columns": the anterior, middle, and posterior. Violating any two of the three columns implies an unstable cervical spine and increased risk for causing or exacerbating an existing spinal cord injury. The anterior column consists of the anterior longitudinal ligament and anterior two thirds of the vertebral body and disc. The middle column consists of the posterior third of the vertebral body and disc and posterior longitudinal liga-

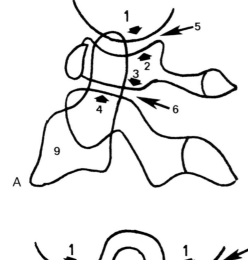

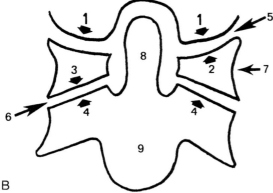

FIGURE 48–1 • Lateral and odontoid views of the occipitoatlantoaxial joints. *A,* Lateral view. *B,* Dens or odontoid view. (1) Articular surface of occipital condyles, (2) superior articular facet of C1, (3) inferior articular facet of C1, (4) superior articular facet of C2, (5) occipitoatlantal joint, (6) atlantoaxial joint, (7) lateral mass of C1, (8) odontoid process, (9) body of C2. (From Gerlock AJ: Advanced Exercises in Diagnostic Radiology: The Cervical Spine in Trauma. Philadelphia, WB Saunders, 1978.)

ment. The pedicles, lateral masses, intertransverse ligaments, lamina, ligamentum flavum, and spinous processes and supraspinous ligaments are found in the posterior column (Fig. 48–3).

The spinal cord is enclosed by the vertebral bodies anteriorly and the paired laminae posterolaterally. The major descending motor pathway in the cord is the lateral corticospinal tract which is anteriorly placed in the cord. The ascending sensory pathways are the posterior columns, conveying position sense, light touch, and vibration, and the spinothalamic tracts, conveying pain and temperature sensation. A spinal cord injury can result from a bony injury such as a fracture, dislocation, or both. It can also be caused by soft tissue injuries, such as a ruptured or buckled ligament, disc extrusion, or vascular compromise. The cervical plain film series examines only the bony structures and cannot rule out significant, acute cord or soft tissue damage. The acronym SCIWORA stands for "spinal cord injury without radiologic abnormality." In a recent study, less than 1% of patients with identified cervical spine injury—all adults—had this type of injury.

INITIAL APPROACH AND STABILIZATION

Priority Diagnoses

Patients with significant head or neck trauma are brought immediately into a major resuscitation room. Priorities of initial management include the following:

- A primary and secondary trauma survey
- Respiratory and hemodynamic stabilization
- Assessment and monitoring of consciousness
- Protecting the patient from further injury

Rapid Assessment

In any trauma, a *brief* initial history is necessary. The ABCDEs of trauma, also known as the primary survey, are uniformly applied (see Chapter 41, Blunt Trauma). They specifically address life-threatening injuries. Universal safety precautions including eye protection, mask, gloves, and protective garments are required. Important information to obtain either from the prehospital personnel, patient, or witnesses includes mechanism of injury; time elapsed since the injury; change in consciousness; major medical problems, including allergies; medications; and possible use of drugs or alcohol.

The initial physical examination must include the following:

- Airway status: patency and protection of the airway. Can the patient swallow, talk, and answer questions?
- Breathing status: spontaneous breathing, respiratory effort required (use of accessory muscles)
- Cardiovascular status: blood pressure, pulse rate, and peripheral circulation
- Level of consciousness: the Glasgow Coma Scale (GCS) is used to measure the level of consciousness, including eye opening, verbal response, and motor response (Table 48–1). A score of less than 8 is defined as coma.
- Presence of neck pain
- Location and extent of other injuries
- A screening neurologic examination to include pupillary size, symmetry, and reactivity, symmetry of motor movement, motor and verbal response to

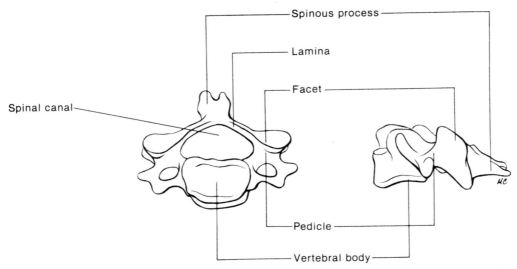

FIGURE 48–2 • Cervical vertebrae C3 through C7, superior and lateral aspects. (Redrawn from Gerlock AJ: Advanced Exercises in Diagnostic Radiology: The Cervical Spine in Trauma. Philadelphia, WB Saunders, 1978.)

noxious stimulus (if necessary), reflexes of extremities, and gross respiratory pattern

Early Intervention

An immediate assessment is done to correct problems in airway, breathing, and circulation. Large-bore intravenous access is established, vital signs (to include pulse oximetry) are taken, and cardiac monitoring is begun. Proper spine immobilization is ensured.

Airway Management and Cervical Spine Immobilization

Cervical spine immobilization is initiated simultaneously with airway management. Proper spinal immobilization includes a properly sized and applied firm cervical collar (e.g., Philadelphia-type collar), foam bolsters or towels (to minimize lateral and rotational head displacement), and a long spine board with the patient securely attached. Until the spine has been completely cleared of injury, an unstable vertebral fracture is assumed and the patient should always be moved with in-line spinal integrity. A patient who vomits while immobilized requires prompt recognition and rotation of the entire long spine board to the patient's side while manually maintaining cervical alignment. The vomitus should be suctioned and serious consideration given to airway protection.

Because hypoxia has such a profoundly detrimental effect on neuronal injury, airway maintenance with cervical spine immobilization and ensurance of ventilation and oxygenation takes priority. Indications for an early definitive airway (oral or nasal endotracheal intubation or surgical cricothyroidotomy) in the head and neck trauma patient are as follows:

- Unconscious head injury
  - Airway protection
  - Oxygenation and ventilation
  - Potential need for hyperventilation
- Maxillofacial injury
  - Airway protection
  - Obstruction cannot be cleared
- Neck injury
  - Risk for obstruction from expanding hematoma
  - Laryngeal or tracheal injury

Orotracheal intubation, with in-line cervical immobilization, has been found to be safe and effective with minimal risk of aggravating occult spinal cord injury. Rapid sequence intubation in a nonobstructed airway minimizes ICP elevation and allows safe, rapid airway management in the comatose head-injured patient (see Chapter 2, Airway Management). Blind nasotracheal intubation is contraindicated in patients with severe maxillofacial trauma, frontal sinus or cribriform plate fractures, or evidence of potential laryngeal or tracheal trauma.

Breathing and Oxygenation

Breathing or ventilation may be impaired in the trauma victim with multiple injuries. Respiratory effort may be hindered from CNS injury, mechanical

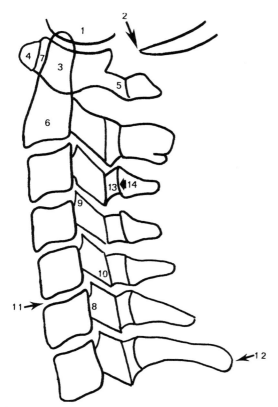

FIGURE 48–3 • Cervical vertebrae C1 through C7, lateral aspects. (1) Occipital condyle of skull, (2) posterior margin of foramen magnum, (3) odontoid process or dens of C2, (4) anterior arch of C1, (5) posterior arch of C1, (6) C2 vertebral body, (7) space between the posterior surface of the anterior arch of C1 and the anterior surface of the odontoid process, (8) pedicle of C6, (9) superior articular process of C4, (10) inferior articular process of C5, (11) intervertebral disc space between C5 and C6, (12) tip of spinous process of C7, (13) lamina of C3, and (14) spinolaminar junction of C3. (From Gerlock AJ: Advanced Exercises in Diagnostic Radiology: The Cervical Spine in Trauma. Philadelphia, WB Saunders, 1978.)

trauma to the chest, or concomitant respiratory suppression from narcotics or other drugs. All patients receive supplemental oxygen. Hypoxia has been documented in up to 40% of patients with significant head injury. Head-injured patients with even one episode of hypoxia (defined as an $Sao_2 < 90\%$) have a marked increase in morbidity and mortality.

Intravenous Access

Patients in shock with associated head or neck trauma are assumed to be hypovolemic until proven otherwise. Neurogenic shock rarely presents in patients with isolated head or thoracolumbar spinal injuries because it is usually seen in severe high cervical cord injuries. At least one large-bore intravenous catheter ($\geq$16-gauge) is placed. Isotonic fluid replacement is the appropriate initial treatment. The goal is correction of hemodynamic instability and perfusion deficits without excessive fluid replacement. Maintenance of an adequate MAP is essential to provide an adequate CPP. Hypotension (mean arterial blood pressure measurement of < 90 mm Hg) has also been associated with poor outcome in head-injured patients. If spinal shock has been identified as the cause of hypotension, Neo-Synephrine for vasoconstriction, dopamine for increasing cardiac output, and atropine to counteract bradycardia may be given.

Metabolic Substrate Replacement

Patients with a depressed consciousness (GCS < 13) on initial examination are given 100 mg of thiamine, bedside glucose measurement or 50 g of dextrose (1 ampule of $D_{50}W$), and 0.4 to 2 mg of naloxone. A bedside blood glucose test strip may substitute for glucose administration because elevated glucose levels have a potential to worsen secondary brain injury. The patient is observed for improvement, and response to treatment is noted.

CLINICAL ASSESSMENT

The history and physical examination are important means of determining signs or symptoms of neurologic dysfunction after head or neck trauma. Serial examinations are necessary to demonstrate an evolving neurologic injury.

History

1. *Trauma event.* Two important goals are identifying mechanisms of injury and assessing the patient's ability to reconstruct the events. The initial history should be obtained from prehospital personnel, police, or possibly witnesses. When possible, additional information is sought directly from the patient. The patient is asked: What *events preceded* the *trauma*? What is *remembered* of the trauma? Was there *loss of consciousness*? Were any *drugs* or *alcohol* involved? When was the patient's *last meal*?
   a. If a *motor vehicle accident:* Was the seat belt worn? Was the patient a passenger or the driver? Where was the site of impact to the vehicle? Was the airbag deployed? Was the steering wheel crushed? Was the windshield shattered? Damage to the steering wheel or windshield has an increased association with chest, maxillofacial, and neck injuries.

TABLE 48–1. Glasgow Coma Scale

Eyes Open

Never	1
To pain	2
To verbal stimuli	3
Spontaneously	4

Best Verbal Response

No response	1
Incomprehensible sounds	2
Inappropriate words	3
Disoriented and converses	4
Oriented and converses	5

Best Motor Response

No response	1
Extension (decerebrate rigidity)	2
Flexion abnormal (decorticate rigidity)	3
Flexion withdrawal	4
Localizes pain	5
Obeys	6

Total	**3–15**

From Jennett B, Teasdale G: Aspects of coma after severe head injury. Lancet 1977; 1:878–881.

  b. If a *penetrating injury:* What was the size, shape, speed, and direction of the penetrating object?
2. *Systemic symptoms*
  a. *Pain.* Is pain or discomfort present? If so, where is it located? What is its character and intensity? Where did it begin? Does it radiate?
  b. *Nausea, vomiting.* Is nausea or vomiting present? Nausea and vomiting may be indicative of increased ICP. Vomiting may predispose the patient to aspiration. If the patient is actively vomiting, log-rolling the patient onto his or her side, keeping the neck aligned, may protect the airway. Consideration is given to performing endotracheal intubation for airway protection.
  c. *Numbness or weakness.* Does the patient have any area of unusual sensation or perceive any decreased strength?
  d. *Bowel and bladder function.* Is the patient incontinent of bowel or bladder?
3. *Medications.* What medication is the patient taking? When was the last dose taken? These medications may indicate significant underlying medical disorders or may have contributed to decreased consciousness. The patient may have this information on a Medic-Alert bracelet or in pockets, purse, or wallet. All should be examined.

4. *Past medical history.* The patient is asked about conditions that could predispose to syncope, such as prior cardiac dysrhythmia or infarction, known seizure disorder, diabetes mellitus, bleeding, hypovolemia, or dehydration. The background medical/surgical history, including pregnancy, is obtained.

Information about the patient's usual mental status is sought from old charts, wallet or purse, family, and primary physician. What appears to be altered mental status may actually be the patient's baseline condition.

Physical Examination

The patient with head and neck trauma receives a full primary and secondary survey (see Chapter 41, Blunt Trauma). The survey's emphasis is on gauging the patient's level of consciousness, discovering neurologic deficits, and monitoring the changing nature of the findings.

Vital Signs. Blood pressure, pulse, and respirations are evaluated. Bradycardia and hypotension are a late finding of increased ICP and impending herniation. Hypotension is usually caused by bleeding elsewhere in the body, although scalp wounds may result in significant blood loss. Hypertension may be seen with intracranial hemorrhage, especially in children. The pulse has no characteristic pattern in the patient with head trauma, although the rate is usually increased secondary to pain in the conscious patient. Respirations have different patterns reflecting the level of cortex and brain stem that is involved. These patterns are often not established in the emergency department and are of little value in predicting the patient's course. The diagnosis of "central hyperventilation" is reserved until the patency of the airway (particularly endotracheal tube patency), acid-base status, toxicologic status, and circulatory condition are evaluated.

Head. The head is carefully palpated for pain and tenderness. Special attention is given to possible entrance or exit wounds and to the presence of foreign bodies or lacerations. A sterile glove is used to examine open wounds, enabling the examiner to palpate the skull carefully for fractures. Raccoon's eye (periorbital bruising) and Battle's sign (mastoid ecchymosis) are late signs of a possible basilar skull fracture.

Ears. The ears are examined for blood behind the tympanic membrane (hemotympanum), which indicates a basilar skull fracture. Serous fluid draining from the ear is presumed to be CSF, and this is best confirmed by laboratory analysis. Analysis of the glucose level in the fluid to identify CSF is unreliable.

Eyes. Pupillary size, equality, and reflexes are noted. Most structural lesions influencing the pupil will affect both size and reflex reactivity: "the dilated and fixed" pupil. Extraocular movements and reflexes are important and are discussed in Chapter 25, The Red Painful Eye. Examination of the fundus may reveal papilledema with absence of venous pulsations or may show retinal hemorrhage. A subhyoid or preretinal hemorrhage may be seen, especially in children with head trauma; this indicates an underlying intracerebral hemorrhage.

Nose. The presence of a clear discharge may indicate a CSF leak. Bedside testing for glucose levels in suspected CSF is no longer recommended, and laboratory testing is necessary. Tenderness of the nose may indicate an underlying nasal fracture.

Face. The face is palpated for tenderness, deformity, or instability with gentle movement of the maxilla. The mandible is examined for loss of teeth, bite occlusion, tenderness of the jaw, and soundness of the temporomandibular joint. Maxillofacial fractures are described by three Le Fort classifications. Clinically, malocclusion will be evident in all Le Fort fractures. A *Le Fort I fracture* is horizontal fracture across the lower maxilla and nasal opening. Therefore, the roof of the mouth is separated from the cranial base and zygoma. The roof of the mouth will move with distraction while the midface remains stable. A *Le Fort II fracture* is triangular and occurs along the zygomaticomaxillary region and extends into the frontal bone. On examination, the nasal bones and midface move with the maxilla. Cribriform plate fracture can occur. A *Le Fort III fracture* implies complete craniofacial disruption. The maxilla, zygoma, nasal bones, ethmoid, and inferior orbit are separated from the skull. The airway is often obstructed, and the face appears flattened. With trauma involving the zygomatic arch, a fracture may cause trismus as the coronoid process of the mandible becomes obstructed (Fig. 48–4).

Mouth and Throat. The mouth and throat are examined for lacerations, bleeding, foreign bodies, patency of the upper airway, and ability to swallow or presence of a gag reflex.

Neck. In the alert and cooperative patient, the cervical spine collar may be removed while in-line immobilization is maintained. If the patient is free of pain and without deformity on palpation, he or she is asked to lift the head slightly. If there is no pain on limited movement, the patient is asked to raise the head more and turn it slowly from side to side. If the patient remains free of pain, the posterior section of the collar is removed. If neck pain or limited movement occurs at any time, the collar is replaced. In the uncooperative or unconscious patient, the collar is not removed. The examination is postponed until the condition of the cervical spine is clearer radiologically and optimally when the patient is alert, calm, and cooperative. It is important to complete a brief examination of strength and symmetry of the upper extremity and shoulder muscles innervated by the cervical nerve roots to document function. All patients are examined for subcutaneous emphysema, lacerations, deformity, or tracheal deviation of the anterior neck. In patients with penetrating trauma, attention is given to whether the platysma muscle is violated. If so, surgical consultation is necessary. Patients with a local hematoma are closely observed for signs of expansion, indicating the need for protection by endotracheal intubation.

The neck in penetrating trauma is divided into three zones: zone I is inferior to the sternal notch, zone II extends from the sternal notch to the angle of the mandible, and zone III extends superior to the angle of the mandible (Fig. 48–5). The platysma, a thin muscle layer within the superficial fascia of the neck, extends from the deltoid and pectoralis region and overlies the anterior triangle and inferior third of the posterior triangle to insert on the inferior border of the mandible. In the emergency department, possible penetrating head and neck wounds are examined using sterile gloves and superficially probed to determine only if they reach the skull or penetrate the platysma. Vascular beds are auscultated for bruits.

Neurologic Examination. The level of consciousness is the single most important indication of an underlying pathologic process. Level of consciousness can be most objectively categorized by use of the Glasgow Coma Scale (see Table 48–1). This scale is useful to (1) standardize the degree of brain stem and cerebral function, (2) document objectively changes in the level of consciousness, and (3) predict on a preliminary basis the morbidity associated with head trauma. Patients with a score of 8 or less usually have significant morbidity. Hypothermia, ethanol, or drugs of abuse (e.g., benzodiazepines) can complicate the interpretation of the Glasgow Coma Scale.

The remainder of the initial examination includes examination of the sensory, motor, and cranial nerves. In cooperative patients, simple observations of extremity movements, symmetry of reflexes, smile, and grimace along with response to pain or touch are sufficient. Any abnormal finding prompts a detailed examination. In patients with suspected cervical spine injury,

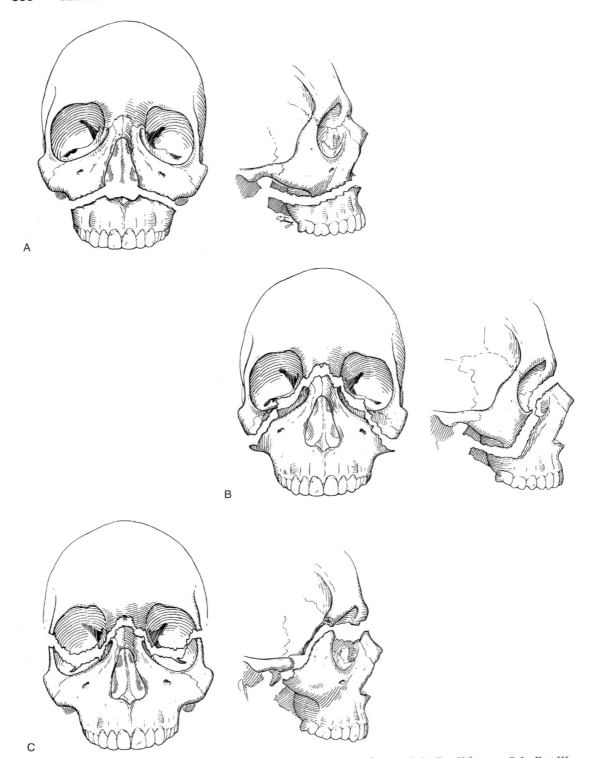

FIGURE 48–4 • The Le Fort classification of maxillary fractures. *A*, Le Fort I fracture. *B*, Le Fort II fracture. *C*, Le Fort III fracture. (*A* to *C* from Fonseca RJ, Walker RV [eds]: Oral and Maxillofacial Trauma, 2nd ed. Philadelphia, WB Saunders, 1997, pp 654–655.)

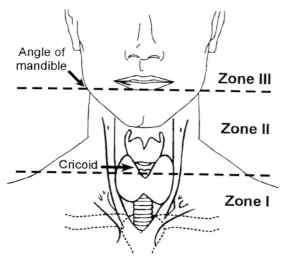

FIGURE 48–5 • Zones of the anterior neck. (From Rosen P, Barkin R [eds]: Emergency Medicine: Concepts and Clinical Practice, 4th ed. St. Louis, CV Mosby, 1998, p 506.)

TABLE 48–2. Motor Deficits and Corresponding Cervical Cord Segments

Motor Deficit	Cervical Cord Segment Injured
Respiratory failure	C4 and above
Quadriparesis with preservation of shoulder elevation and diaphragmatic breathing	C5
Wrist extension and elbow flexion. Biceps reflex may be absent	C6
Elbow extension, partial paralysis of finger and wrist flexions: result in preacher's hand	C7
Complete paralysis of finger flexors	C8
Partial paralysis of hand muscles (interossei and lymbricals) and abductor pollicis	T1

each segment of the cervical cord is examined, as are the anterior and posterior columns (Fig. 48–6). Motor deficit findings for each segment are listed in Table 48–2. An illustration of the sensory dermatomes is often useful in localizing findings to a particular level (Fig. 48–7).

Certain cerebral herniation syndromes may be determined by physical examination. These syndromes represent a rise in ICP, creating pressure gradients. Brain tissue may shift along these gradients and result in a brain herniation syndrome. There are at least four clinical patterns, discussed later under "Special Considerations."

CLINICAL REASONING

Clinical reasoning guides the physician in ordering diagnostic studies and implementing therapy. Most traumatic injuries are assessed by initially interpreting the historical and clinical findings as a means of understanding the nature and extent of the underlying pathological processes. These are addressed by answering three essential questions.

Are There Obvious or Evolving Life-threatening Injuries Discovered After Data Gathering?

If critical problems are discovered, they will require immediate or additional management

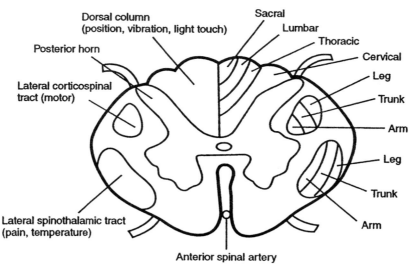

FIGURE 48–6 • Anatomic/clinical relationships in the spinal cord. The anterior columns (lateral corticospinal and spinothalamic tracts) and posterior (dorsal) columns are assessed separately for a full examination.

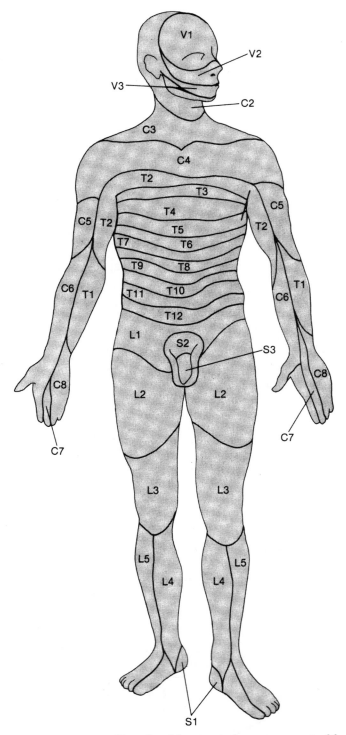

FIGURE 48–7 • Distribution of spinal nerves and branches of the trigeminal nerve to segments of the body surfaces. Each segment is named for the principal spinal nerve that serves it. C, cervical segments; T, thoracic segments; L, lumbar segments; S, sacral segments; V, trigeminal segments. (From Solomon EP, Davis PW [eds]: Human Anatomy and Physiology. Philadelphia, WB Saunders, 1983.)

beyond the initial stabilization measures. Most of these immediately life-threatening injuries are addressed in the initial assessment and stabilization. Some, such as evolving uncal herniation, may require additional aggressive therapy (skull trephination) and early consultative assistance. In neurologic injuries, much of the effort in emergency care is focused on thorough assessment and protection from further injury. The two most common causes of death with associated neuronal injury are hypotension and respiratory failure. Death from massive injury or uncontrolled cerebral edema is less common in patients who survive to undergo emergency care.

Are There Treatable Pathologic Processes That Could Worsen the Original Injury?

The major concern in regard to head and neck trauma is its effect on the brain and spinal cord. Primary injuries comprise actual structural damage to neuronal tissue inflicted by the traumatic forces. These injuries heal with scar tissue, and recovery from them is very limited. A common set of "secondary" processes exists that can worsen the degree and extent of injury to neuronal tissue. Some of these processes are initiated as the tissue responds to injury, some may result from trauma to other organs, and others may exist at the time of the injury and contribute to its cause. To prevent the damaging effects of these secondary processes, they must always be considered early in the care of any brain-injured patient.

Metabolic Substrate Replacement. Oxygen, glucose, and thiamine are important metabolic substrates in brain and spinal cord tissue. Low levels or absence of these substrates can have a damaging effect on neurons. Oxygen and thiamine are usually supplied before they are measured. Glucose is optimally measured and then supplied in the amount deemed necessary. Hyperglycemia in injured tissues is a potentially harmful effect of superfluous glucose administration.

Toxins. The presence of endogenous (renal, hepatic) or exogenous (poisons, intoxicants) toxins is assessed in head-injured patients. Such toxins may cause or result from the injury. But in either case they can complicate the patient's presentation and clinical course, further injuring damaged cells. Appropriate laboratory testing and administration of a narcotic antagonist, naloxone, are part of the management protocol.

Mass Lesions. Mass lesions result from either intracranial or intraspinal hemorrhage or edema. In the skull, they can cause pressure shifts, resulting in herniation, and may increase ischemia to tissues at and near the area of primary damage. Computed tomography (CT) has dramatically changed the diagnosis and management of mass lesions. Skull trephination (bur holes) in the emergency department is reserved for only the most extreme situations.

Metabolic Rate. The metabolic rate of the brain determines its oxygen demand. Increased rates increase oxygen demand when there may not be sufficient supply; therefore, at a minimum a "normal" rate is desirable. Two controllable factors that have the potential to increase this rate are fever and seizure activity.

Ischemia. Neuronal tissue does not tolerate vascular ischemia well. Cerebral vessels have the ability to autoregulate their resistance to maintain a relatively constant flow in the presence of a fluctuating blood pressure. Their lower effective operating range is 60 to 70 mm Hg MAP. This self-regulating ability may also be lost in severe injury. It is recommended that the MAP be maintained between 90 and 110 mm Hg. Isotonic crystalloid and blood are the fluids of choice *up to* this level. Above this level the fluid is changed to 0.25% to 0.50% normal saline and flow is reduced to decrease cerebral edema. It is important to remember that an adequate MAP does not guarantee blood flow to the brain. CPP is equal to the MAP minus the ICP. Therefore, the ICP is a major determinant of flow.

Tissue Edema. Both primary injury and secondary processes can promote tissue swelling. This can cause direct intracellular injury and ischemic injury from increased ICP. In the emergency department, tissue edema is treated, although not always successfully, with judicious use of blood pressure control and mannitol. Mannitol, an osmotic diuretic, is thought to temporarily reduce water content in normal and injured brain tissue. Mild hyperventilation to Pco$_2$ levels of 25 to 30 mm Hg is reserved for acute neurologic deterioration suggesting herniation.

What is the Mechanism and Nature of Injury?

Is the head or neck, or both, injured? Are the injuries blunt or penetrating or a combination? Answers to these questions help divide the injuries into major categories. Each of these five groups has key questions guiding management.

Blunt Head Trauma

The key question in blunt head trauma is not is there a bony injury but is there CNS injury?

Suspicion of such injury is based on risk stratification after the clinical assessment (Table 48–3). The best method to structurally identify suspected CNS injuries is with CT.

Penetrating Head Trauma

Has the object (e.g., bullet, shrapnel) penetrated the cranium and, if so, has it traversed the midline? Anteroposterior and lateral plain radiographs can usually provide this information. Skull penetration connotes CNS injury. Traversing the midline by a penetrating object means both cerebral hemispheres have been damaged, and this type of trauma is linked to a significantly worse outcome. Given the force of missile injury, CT should be performed on all patients with gunshot wounds to the head, regardless of penetration of the cranium.

Maxillofacial Blunt Trauma

What is the status of the airway and need for acute airway management? Can the injury be classified using the Le Fort system? Is there associated CNS or neck injury? Airway management takes top priority over concerns for spine movement. Intracranial injuries are common with facial

injuries, and identification and management of these injuries take priority. The incidence of cervical spine injury is less than 10%, even in severe facial trauma.

Blunt Neck Trauma

Is there bony, soft tissue, or cord injury, or a combination? Can the patient's cervical spine be cleared without radiographs? Cervical spine (C-spine) radiographs cannot replace a careful physical examination. The most common error in the assessment of blunt neck trauma is considering a normal C-spine series the equivalent of an intact cervical spinal cord. Table 48–2 lists motion deficits with corresponding injured cord levels.

Generally, a low threshold to obtain C-spine plain films is necessary. Recent evidence has shown that when the risk of occult spine injury is low, the patient can be cleared from spine immobilization clinically. One set of criteria is listed in Table 48–4.

The cervical spine is palpated throughout its course in the neck. Then the patient is asked to actively move the head laterally and then flex and extend it first without resistance and then against resistance provided by the examiner. Finally, axial loading is performed. Any pain with motion requires cessation of that activity, reimmobilization, and a C-spine imaging series. If no hesitation or pain is present, the cervical spine is believed to be clear from fracture.

The prevalence of spinal fractures with craniocerebral injury is controversial. It is prudent to assume fractures of the cervical spine in any patient with a head injury who has altered mental status.

Blunt trauma, especially force applied directed to the neck in a small area (e.g., strangulation, clothesline injury, impact on steering wheel) may cause laryngotracheal and neurovascular injury. Laryngeal edema or fracture should be suspected and the airway protected. Stridor, hoarseness, and

---

TABLE 48–3. Risk Stratification for Intracranial Injury

Low Risk

GCS = 14–15 (mild head injury)
Mild headache
Minor scalp wound
Mild dizziness
Scalp contusion or abrasion
Asymptomatic

Moderate to High Risk

GCS = 9–13 (moderate head injury)
GCS < 8 (severe head injury)
Focal neurologic signs
Loss of consciousness
Amnestic to the events
Decreasing level of consciousness
Depressed skull fracture
Penetrating skull trauma
Suspected open skull fracture or cerebrospinal fluid leak
Suspected basilar skull fracture
Post-traumatic seizures
Persistent vomiting
Anticoagulated or with coagulopathies
Severe or worsening headache
Unreliable or inadequate history
Multiple trauma
Suspected physical child abuse

TABLE 48–4. NEXUS Criteria for Clinical Cervical Spine Clearance

1. No cervical pain or posterior midline tenderness
2. Normal mental status
3. No evidence of intoxication (drug or alcohol)
4. No focal neurologic deficits
5. No distracting injury or conditions (pain, emotional stress)

From Hoffman JR, Mower WR, Wolfson AB, et al: The National Emergency X-Radiography Utilization Study Group: Validity of a set of clinical criteria to rule out injury to the cervical spine in patients with blunt trauma. N Engl J Med 2000; 343: 94–99.

dysphasia are ominous signs. Direct or fiberoptic laryngoscopy to evaluate the laryngotracheal area is performed. In addition, there may be damage to the carotid and jugular vasculature with development of thrombus or intimal tears. Evidence of stroke-like symptoms suggests vascular injury.

Penetrating Neck Trauma

What is the status of the airway? What are the soft tissues that may be injured? What zones of the neck may be involved in the penetrating injury (see Fig. 48–5)? The neck is especially vulnerable to penetrating injury. Multiple important structures are closely confined in the neck, making even small injuries potentially devastating. Loss of airway integrity from direct injury or expanding hematoma warrants early and aggressive airway management.

Penetrating neck wounds usually result in four types of injuries:

1. *Vascular* (carotid artery, jugular and subclavian veins)
2. *Neurologic* (spinal cord, recurrent laryngeal nerve, sympathetic chain); the presence of Horner's syndrome (miosis, ptosis, and anhidrosis) should raise suspicion of an ipsilateral vascular injury because the stellate ganglion is closely approximated to the carotid artery.
3. *Laryngotracheal* (larynx, vocal cords, trachea)
4. *Visceral* (pharynx and esophagus)

Because of the difficulty in proximal and distal surgical control of vascular structures, injuries in zones I and III are evaluated nonsurgically. Zone I injuries may cause damage to the thoracic outlet, whereas zone III injuries can damage multiple structures in the jaw, mouth, and sphenopalatine area. Initial diagnostic evaluation on hemodynamically stable patiens with zone III injuries consists of angiography to identify injury to the internal and external carotid and cerebral arteries. Zone I injuries may need a chest radiograph to evaluate for pneumothorax, pleural effusion, or mediastinal widening; angiography to evaluate the integrity of the thoracic outlet vessels; an esophageal contrast study (Gastrografin or barium) with or without esophagoscopy to identify perforation; and direct laryngoscopy or bronchoscopy to identify laryngotracheal injuries. Zone II injuries that penetrate the platysma can cause primarily airway and circulatory injuries. Most require operative evaluation, although some authors prefer diagnostic evaluation and a selective approach to surgery.

DIAGNOSTIC ADJUNCTS

After the history and physical examination, radiographic studies are helpful in making a definitive diagnosis. However, serious head and neck injury can exist in the presence of apparently normal radiologic studies.

Laboratory Studies

With the exception of low blood glucose and electrolyte abnormalities, most head and neck trauma is managed clinically. A few basic laboratory tests can assist with the management of head and neck trauma and may provide an initial reference during the reparative or recovery phase of an injury.

Arterial Blood Gas (ABG) Analysis. An ABG analysis assists with the oxygenation and management of ventilated patients. It is critical to avoid inadvertent hypoxia and excessive hypocarbia in the patient with a severe head injury. Hyperventilation is no longer recommended to control elevated ICP, unless there are associated signs of herniation. ABG analysis is used in conjunction with pulse oximetry and end-tidal CO_2 monitoring. Base deficit has been used to predict outcome and guide resuscitation.

Hematology. A hemogram with initial hemoglobin, hematocrit, and platelet count should be performed and will establish a baseline to evaluate the extent of hemorrhage.

Chemistry. Electrolytes, blood urea nitrogen, creatinine, and blood glucose are obtained to evaluate metabolic derangements. Serum osmolality measurements will help guide diuresis from mannitol for severe head injury.

Toxicology. An ethanol level may assist with determination of altered mental status in a patient. It is most useful when a low or nondetectable value can rule out intoxication as a cause for altered mental status. Ethanol is a common complicating factor in the head and neck, but rarely is the only problem.

Brain Injury Serum Markers. Identifying serum markers is part of the continued search for both sensitive and specific tests capable of identifying traumatic brain injury and predicting outcome. Both neuronal and axial cell proteins have been studied. Creatine kinase BB, serum S-100B, and cleaved tau protein have all shown promise, but research continues. These markers have potential value in identifying brain injury in patients with normal CT scans, localizing the tissue site of injury, monitoring efficacy of treatment, and predicting short-term and long-term prognosis of the brain-injured patient.

Radiologic Imaging

Computed Tomography. Nonenhanced CT of the head should be obtained in all hemodynamically stable patients who have sustained recent severe head trauma. In addition, patients who possess high-risk criteria for intracranial injury should undergo a head CT. In patients with minor head injury (witnessed loss of consciousness, amnesia, or disorientation in patients with GCS 13 to 15) the Canadian CT rule is helpful (Table 48–5). Although a normal head CT does not rule out the possibility of intracranial bleeding, it is 90% to 95% sensitive for fresh bleeding. If the trauma occurred 5 to 14 days earlier, blood may have similar density to brain tissue. A normal nonenhanced CT can be followed with intravenous injection of contrast medium to help intensify the isodense old blood. Low-risk patients for intracranial injury can be briefly observed and discharged from the emergency department after a thorough history and neurologic examination without a head CT.

In patients with a significant brain injury or mechanism of injury, spiral CT of the cervical spine is performed at the same time as the cranial CT. The extent of CT of the cervical spine is controversial, but most authorities agree that imaging from the base of the skull through C2 is appropriate. Others would advocate that CT of the entire cervical spine is an appropriate and cost-effective screening tool in high-risk patients.

Skull Radiographs. Except in the infant population (age 2 years), skull films should not routinely be obtained for blunt head trauma. Skull radiographs cannot identify intracranial bleeding and mass effect and merely identify depressed or nondepressed fractures. If a plain film of the skull is obtained and a fracture is identified, CT of the head should be considered, because the risk for intracranial injury is more likely.

Cervical Spine Series. A complete C-spine series includes the lateral, anteroposterior, and odontoid (open mouth) views. These studies can be completed with a cervical collar in place.

Indications for C-spine radiographs are liberal. They include (1) a mechanism compatible with C-spine injury (e.g., trauma to the head or neck, or flexion, extension, or axial loading of the head); (2) altered mental status with suspected head or neck trauma; (3) cervical spine pain after trauma; and (4) focal or bilateral neurologic deficits that may be consistent with cervical spine injury.

In obtaining and interpreting these films, several aspects must be clear to the emergency physician.

1. There is *no* urgency to remove the cervical collar. The patient's head must remain fixed relative to the body until the C-spine films *and* repeat neurologic screening examination are normal. This priority is communicated to the radiology staff. In high-risk situations, a portable lateral film is obtained first or a physician accompanies the patient to the radiology department.
2. The lateral C-spine film is taken first, and absence of a pathologic process is confirmed before the anteroposterior and odontoid views are completed. These subsequent views require some movement of the patient and may be avoided if an unstable fracture is seen on the lateral radiograph.
3. All seven cervical vertebrae should be seen on the lateral C-spine film, including the C7-T1 interspace. This may require the use of traction on the arms or special radiographic techniques such as the transthoracic view.
4. Significant injuries to the spine and cord may be present despite "normal" radiographs.
5. Patients who continue to have severe neck pain or neurologic findings despite normal C-spine radiographs are studied more definitively by CT or magnetic resonance imaging (MRI) of the cervical spine.

A critical skill of the emergency physician is the ability to differentiate abnormal from normal C-spine radiographs. The lateral view is most important in this regard, although the other views contribute valuable information. In the normal lateral view, four contour lines must be aligned (Fig. 48–8): (1) the anterior vertebral line, (2) the posterior vertebral line, (3) the spinolaminar line, and (4) the line connecting the tips of the spinous processes. These four lines delineate the normal lordotic curve of the cervical spine and establish

---

TABLE 48–5. Canadian CT Head Rule

High risk (for Neurologic Intervention)

GCS < 15 at 2 hours after injury
Suspected open or depressed skull fracture
Any sign of basal skull fracture
Vomiting > two times
Age > 65 years

Medium risk (for CT abnormality)

Amnesia before impact > 30 minutes
Dangerous mechanism (pedestrian struck by car, occupant ejected from vehicle, fall from > 3 feet or five stairs)

From Stiell I, Wells GA, Vandemheen K, et al: The Canadian CT head rule for patients with minor head injury. Lancet 2001; 357:1391–1396.

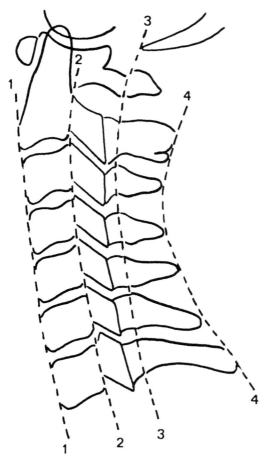

FIGURE 48–8 • The four contour lines of the cervical spine, normal anatomy: (1) anterior vertebral line, (2) posterior vertebral line, (3) spinolaminar line, and (4) line connecting the tips of the spinous processes. (From Gerlock AJ: Advanced Exercises in Diagnostic Radiology: The Cervical Spine in Trauma. Philadelphia, WB Saunders, 1978.)

the relationship between the "anterior" vertebral body and the "posterior" structures around the spinal cord, the pedicle, lamina, facets, and spinous process.

Interpreting this view requires experience, and a few points may be helpful:

1. The absence of the normal lordotic curve may indicate a ligamentous injury or may be the result of severe cervical muscle strain.
2. Each vertebral body is identified on the lateral radiograph. If one vertebral body is "out of alignment," it is said to be "subluxed" with respect to its next lower vertebral segment. Such a subluxation is considered a serious injury until proved otherwise.
3. The "parallel" alignment of lines 3 and 4 to lines 1 and 2 on Figure 48–8 establishes the relationship of the "anterior" and "posterior" elements.

4. The soft tissue areas ventral to the spinal column (along line 1) are important. The prevertebral soft tissue width at C3 should be less than half the width of the adjacent vertebral body (or less than 7 mm), and the width at C6 should be less than 22 mm. Any increased size of the prevertebral soft tissue may indicate a bony fracture or ligamentous disruption.
5. The normal anatomy of the spinal vertebrae and the "posterior" anatomy are recognizable and are duplicated for each cervical vertebra from C2 through C7.
6. The next most important view is the odontoid (open mouth) view. This may be difficult to obtain in an uncooperative patient. The normal odontoid relationships are illustrated in Figure 48–1A; the odontoid view most closely resembles the schematic depicted in Figure 48–1B. The key elements are (a) absence of a fracture of the dens itself and (b) alignment of the inferior articular facet of C1 directly over the superior articular facet of C2. Additionally, the gap between the anterior ring of C1 and the dens (pre-dens space) should be less than 3 mm in adult patients.

Any observations inconsistent with these guidelines are brought to the attention of an experienced emergency physician and, optimally, a radiologist. Cautious interpretation is in the best interest of the patient.

A ligamentous injury may be present in a patient with significant neck pain but normal C-spine films. Flexion and extension views may demonstrate subluxation, but their use recently has been questioned. Flexion and extension films may also be useful in the evaluation of the elderly patient with severe degenerative changes. Flexion and extension films are contraindicated in the patient with focal neurologic deficit. They should only be taken in the alert, nondistracted patient. A neck CT may identify occult fractures, but for ligamentous injury MRI offers better imaging.

For inadequate C-spine films, fractures visualized on plain radiographs, or evidence of focal neurologic signs, thin-cut CT (2- or 3-mm slices) of affected area plus one vertebrae above and below the area in question should be obtained. CT is best at evaluating the bony architecture and involvement of the spinal canal.

Magnetic Resonance Imaging. MRI currently has a limited role in acute brain trauma. However, its role is expanding in the management of acute spinal trauma. It is the study of choice to image the spinal cord. In addition, it can reveal ligamentous injuries not found in other imaging modalities.

Arteriography. Carotid arteriography is considered for neck wounds that penetrate the platysma muscle and may cause occult vascular injury. Arteriography is also indicated in patients with signs of or mechanism consistent with blunt vascular injury.

EXPANDED DIFFERENTIAL DIAGNOSIS

Initial data gathering and serial observations combined with proper use and interpretation of laboratory values, radiographs, and CT often allow the differential diagnosis to be further refined.

Blunt Head Trauma

Blunt head trauma can result in epidural, intracerebral, or subarachnoid hemorrhage. An *epidural hematoma* is classically described as transient loss of consciousness immediately after injury, followed by a lucid period. However, this clinical picture is seen in only 20% of cases. This period of consciousness may deteriorate rapidly and is often associated with signs of uncal herniation. The patient may exhibit an ipsilateral dilated pupil and contralateral hemiparesis relative to the side of the hematoma. Epidural hemorrhage is usually caused by arterial bleeding and may be associated with a skull fracture over the middle meningeal artery. The hemorrhage is distinctly seen as a biconvex density on the CT scan (Fig. 48–9A).

Subdural hematoma is the result of venous bleeding beneath the dura. Elderly patients, alcoholics, patients with cerebral atrophy, and those with hemostatic disorders are susceptible to subdural hemorrhage. Symptoms result from direct pressure to the cortex under the hemorrhage. Subdural hemorrhage may be classified as acute, subacute, or chronic based on the time course of the development of symptoms. Acute symptoms develop within 24 hours, subacute symptoms take 1 day to 2 weeks to develop, and chronic hematomas become symptomatic after 2 weeks. A chronic subdural hemorrhage is often difficult to diagnose because a history of head trauma days or weeks ago may not be available, and the appear-

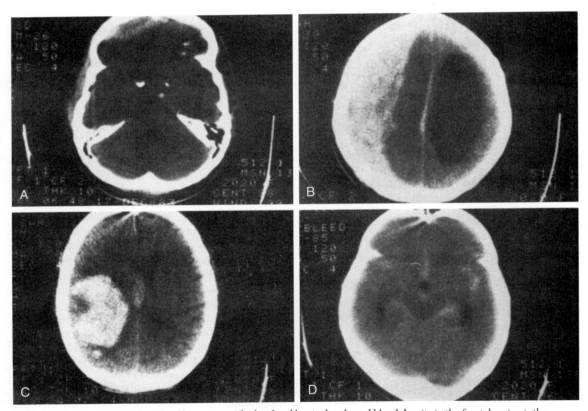

FIGURE 48–9 • *A,* Frontal epidural hematoma. The localized lenticular-shaped blood density in the frontal region is the common configuration of an epidural hematoma. *B,* Subdural hematoma. This massive, panhemispheric collection of blood assumes a typical shape as it outlines the cortex. There is also ventricular enlargement. *C,* Intracerebral hematoma. The localized blood density mass in the parietal region has associated edema surrounding it, seen as a darker band. *D,* Subarachnoid hemorrhage. Blood in the subarachnoid spaces appears as faint white lines in the major fissures. (From Tintinalli JE: Emergency Medicine: A Comprehensive Study Guide. New York, McGraw-Hill, 1985.)

ance of symptoms can be insidious (e.g., slightly increased irritability, unstable gait, or a chronic headache without focal neurologic findings). CT of the head often shows a crescent-shaped deficit (see Fig. 48–9*B*).

Intracerebral hemorrhage is bleeding within the parenchyma of the cerebral hemispheres. It may occur at the time of trauma or may appear a few days later. Symptoms are usually dramatic and include acutely depressed level of consciousness and signs of increased ICP (see Fig. 48–9*C*). Subarachnoid hemorrhage may occur spontaneously as a result of an aneurysmal hemorrhage, or it may be caused by head trauma (see Fig. 48–9*D*).

Skull fractures are considered in all patients with head trauma and may be classified as linear, depressed, or basilar. Linear fractures are important because they may be the precursor of subsequent intracranial events such as epidural hemorrhage. Depressed skull fractures are indications of severe traumatic force and are often associated with cerebral contusion, a bruising of the cerebral cortex. If the fracture is depressed more than 5 mm, it requires neurosurgical elevation (Fig. 48–10). *Basilar skull fractures* are usually *inferred* from the characteristic clinical signs, including Battle's sign, raccoon eyes (periorbital ecchymoses), and CSF rhinorrhea or otorrhea. They are not usually well identified by plain films, but CT and MRI may be diagnostic.

Temporary loss of consciousness (longer than 5 minutes) or temporary neurologic deficits that resolve in less than 24 hours may be categorized as *cerebral concussion* or *cerebral contusion*. In the patient with cerebral concussion, the CT scan is normal, whereas in the patient with cerebral contusion CT shows microhemorrhages of the cerebral cortex. Patients with cerebral contusion are at high risk for subsequent intracranial bleeding.

In both cerebral contusion and concussion, the most common deficit is memory loss. Memory loss may be retrograde (loss of memory a time period before the injury) or antegrade (loss of current memory). In the latter situation the patient may ask the same question repeatedly, because he or she does not remember asking it. This can be very annoying to staff and family, and the underlying problem must be explained to them.

Neck Injuries

Common Fractures

A *"hangman's" fracture* is suspected when the spinolaminar line reveals that the spinous process of C2 is posteriorly subluxed. The anterior and posterior vertebral lines often remain in alignment. Thus, a hangman's fracture is a fracture through the pedicle of C2 (Fig. 48–11). This is a highly unstable fracture involving the posterior elements.

Another fracture best seen on lateral C-spine radiographs is the *teardrop fracture*, a small anteroinferior chip fracture of the vertebral body. This is a flexion-type injury and has a high incidence of ligamentous disruption and cord compression (Fig. 48–12).

The *clay shoveler's fracture* is a fracture of the spinous process of C6 or C7. It is generally considered a stable fracture but may be unstable if the nuchal ligament is fully avulsed.

The dens or odontoid view may reveal a fracture in one or more areas of the atlas, the ring comprising C1. This is called *Jefferson's fracture*. The odontoid view shows one or both lateral masses of C1 located lateral to their usual positions (Fig. 48–13). This very unstable fracture is usually the result of axial loading. It can result from falling from a significant height, diving into shallow water, or being thrown against the car roof in an abrupt deceleration.

Ligament and Muscle Strain

Abrupt deceleration in a motor vehicle accident causes a flexion-extension injury ("whiplash"). It often damages, to varying degrees, the muscular and ligamentous supporting tissue of the cervical spine. The extent of injury depends on the prior condition of the cervical spine, the degree and direction of the force, and the patient's opportunity and ability to protect himself or herself. Although pain usually appears during the first few hours, the full intensity and range of symptoms may be delayed for 2 to 3 days. These symptoms include stiffness, radicular pain, paresthesias, paresis, headache, and dizziness or a sense of instability. These symptoms can occur in the presence of normal alignment on the C-spine series. All patients who have neck pain or have sustained a mechanism of injury with the potential to produce this injury are warned of these possible complications. Under controlled situations, lateral view radiographs of the neck in flexion and extension may identify instability in the cervical spine. CT or MRI is recommended in suggested cases.

Cord Syndromes

Injury to the spinal cord can occur with or without bony injury. Spinal cord deficits are divided into complete and incomplete syndromes. The *complete cord syndrome* is a loss of motor and sensory

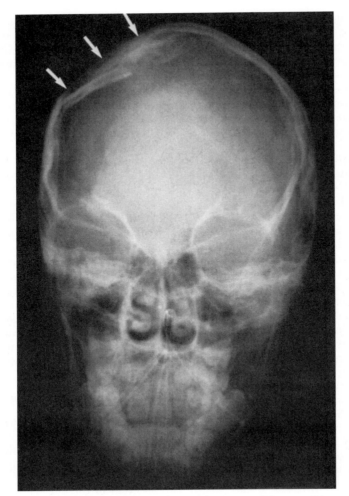

FIGURE 48–10 • Anteroposterior view of the skull shows a depressed comminuted fracture of the parietal bone *(arrows)*. Injury occurred after a blow with a blunt object. (From Rosen P: Diagnostic Radiology in Emergency Medicine. St. Louis, CV Mosby, 1992, p 35.)

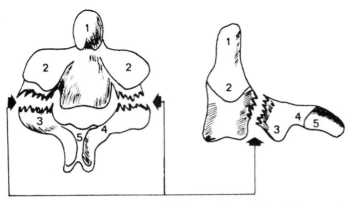

FIGURE 48–11 • Hangman's fracture. The *arrows* point to the fractures through the pedicles anterior to the inferior articular facets and posterior to the superior articular facets: (1) odontoid process, (2) superior articular facets, (3) inferior articular facets, (4) laminae, and (5) spinous process. (From Gerlock AJ: Advanced Exercises in Diagnostic Radiology: The Cervical Spine in Trauma. Philadelphia, WB Saunders, 1978.)

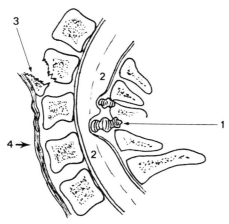

FIGURE 48–12 • Teardrop fracture and contusion of the spinal cord: (1) buckled ligamenta flava compressing the spinal cord, (2) spinal cord, (3) the teardrop—an avulsed fracture fragment from the anterior margin of a vertebral body, and (4) anterior longitudinal ligament. (From Gerlock AJ: Advanced Exercises in Diagnostic Radiology: The Cervical Spine in Trauma. Philadelphia, WB Saunders, 1978.)

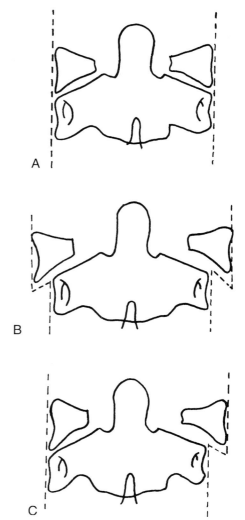

FIGURE 48–13 • Jefferson's fracture, showing relationship of C1 to C2. *A,* Normal atlantoaxial anatomy as seen from the odontoid view. *B,* Bilateral displacement of the lateral masses of C1. *C,* Unilateral displacement of the lateral masses of C1. (From Gerlock AJ: Advanced Exercises in Diagnostic Radiology: The Cervical Spine in Trauma. Philadelphia, WB Saunders, 1978.)

function below the level of injury. It is often accompanied by neurogenic or "spinal" shock. Loss of sympathetic tone results in hypotension. Differentiating between hypovolemia and neurogenic shock can be problematic. Findings consistent with spinal shock include warm, dry skin (from vasodilation) accompanying complete paralysis below the site of injury. Blood pressure is rarely lower than 80 mm Hg systolic in neurogenic shock, although 20% to 30% of patients will require vasopressors. Hemorrhagic shock, however, is usually accompanied by cool, clammy skin. Careful testing may reveal sacral sparing on the sensory examination and an intact bulbocavernous reflex or perceptible rectal tone. These findings point to an incomplete cord lesion.

The three common incomplete cord syndromes are central, anterior, and Brown-Séquard. The *central cord syndrome* is most commonly caused by hyperextension of the neck that contuses the central area of the spinal column. This injures the central fibers of the corticospinal tract. It is characterized by a disproportionately greater weakness in the upper extremity. Sensory deficits are variable. Resolution of the neurologic deficits is unpredictable, although a speedy recovery and preservation of bowel and bladder function are positive prognostic signs.

The *anterior cord syndrome* is usually caused by hyperflexion injuries. The anterior spinal artery is injured or the anterior cord contused by vertebral fragments or a herniated intervertebral disc. The syndrome is characterized by complete paralysis and loss of sensation to pain and temper-

ature bilaterally below the lesion. Dorsal column function such as light touch, proprioception, and vibratory sensation are usually spared. Most patients show some neurologic improvement but do not completely recover.

The *Brown-Séquard syndrome,* a hemisection of the cord, is most commonly seen with a penetrating injury. This syndrome evolves to ipsilateral motor and contralateral sensory dysfunction. Bowel and bladder function is retained.

Spinal cord contusion presents as transient neurologic signs following a traumatic injury that resolves in minutes to 72 hours. Symptoms vary in severity and duration from mild paresthesias or weakness of the upper extremities to complete flaccid paralysis. Sacral sparing with or without an intact bulbocavernosus reflex leads the physician to suspect contusion versus complete cord syndromes. The symptoms may completely resolve during the emergency department visit. The prognosis for full recovery is excellent.

PRINCIPLES OF MANAGEMENT

General Principles

The general principles of head and neck trauma management are to support the patient's cardiovascular status and to prevent further injury. Most of this information was given earlier in the section on "Clinical Reasoning." A few additional points are provided here.

Immobilization. All patients who exhibit a decreased level of consciousness after trauma are presumed to have injured the cervical spine until proved otherwise. Spinal immobilization is continued until a fracture of the cervical spine is ruled out. Patients with simple neck muscle strain may be treated with analgesics and muscle relaxants.

Measures to Decrease Intracranial Pressure. The initial response to evidence of increased ICP is elevation of the head. Second, mannitol may be given as a 20% solution, 0.25 to 1 g/kg intravenously, as a bolus. Prolonged hyperventilation and prophylactic hyperventilation have been shown to worsen outcome and are currently recommended only for signs of neurologic deterioration suggesting herniation. Furosemide (20 to 40 mg) is given as an adjunct to mannitol in some patients, usually after admission to the intensive care unit. ICP monitoring is useful to help guide treatment. Neither induced hypothermia nor the use of corticosteroids in patients with head trauma has been demonstrated to be effective.

High-Dose Corticosteroids. Patients with acute spinal cord injuries should be treated with large doses of corticosteroids within 8 hours. In those treated within 3 hours of injury, an initial loading dose of 30 mg/kg of methylprednisolone is followed by an infusion of 5.4 mg/kg/hr for 24 hours. In those treated between 3 and 8 hours, the infusion should be continued for 48 hours.

Scalp Lacerations. Significant bleeding from scalp lacerations is treated initially with direct pressure. Local anesthesia with lidocaine and epinephrine will decrease pain and bleeding, often resulting in hemostasis. Depending on other priorities, Ramey clips or immediate rapid closure with staples or running suture will result in control of the hemorrhage. Scalp wounds involving the galea are closed in two layers, the galea separately, with absorbable suture, to avoid subgaleal hematoma formation. A single-layer nonabsorbable suture closure is used for most scalp wounds.

Nasogastric Tube. Because of the likelihood of vomiting and subsequent aspiration, nasogastric tube placement is considered in all patients with head injuries. If a cribriform plate fracture or nasal fracture is a possibility, the nasogastric tube is inserted orally.

Foley Catheter. A Foley catheter is placed if (1) a pelvic examination reveals no instability, (2) a rectal examination shows absence of a high-riding prostate, and (3) the external meatus has no blood on examination. The Foley catheter will help in monitoring the patient's fluid status and response to resuscitative efforts.

Specific Treatments

Blunt Head Trauma

For severe head trauma (GCS score of 11 or signs of herniation/focal neurologic deficit), airway management with rapid sequence intubation, controlled ventilation with oxygenation, and protection of cervical spine alignment are the mainstays of initial therapy. Blood pressure should be maintained above 90 mm Hg systolic.

Mannitol (0.25 to 1 g/kg) is an osmotic diuretic indicated for focal neurologic signs (posturing, altered pupillary function, worsening coma) in severe blunt head trauma. It is used to decrease suspected increases in ICP. Early neurosurgical consultation can assist in decisions about administering mannitol.

The head of the bed can be elevated slightly (15 degrees) to help reduce ICP if the thoracolumbar spine is clear. Corticosteroids have not been shown to be beneficial in closed-head injury. If uncal herniation is suspected, and head CT is not practical, the patient's condition deteriorates, and there is no immediate neurosurgical assistance, then emergent cranial burr holes may be performed on the ipsilateral side of the dilated pupil. If this procedure is not effective, another burr hole may be performed on the contralateral side. Skull trephination is a rare procedure in the ED but potentially life-saving.

Neurosurgical consultation is obtained for any intracranial injury, focal neurologic finding, or moderate to severe brain injury (GCS score of 13). Prompt neurosurgical evaluation is required for potential evacuation of epidural and subdural hematomas and elevation of depressed skull fractures. Operative evacuation of subdural hematomas within 4 hours of injury has been shown to improve outcome.

In the trauma patient with multiple injuries in whom laparotomy or thoracotomy is immediately required, CT of the head can be delayed. If signs or symptoms of intracranial injury exist, either an ICP monitor or decompressive craniotomy can be performed in the operating suite by the neurosurgeon. The risk of concomitant operative neurosurgical and thoracoabdominal injuries has been shown to be low in several studies.

Penetrating Head Trauma

CT may be difficult to interpret in the patient with penetrating trauma, owing to interference from metal (bullets, shrapnel). Penetrating and open skull fractures are not routinely treated with prophylactic antibiotics. Early neurosurgical consultation is mandatory. In patients in whom the projectile has traversed the midline, extensive injury has usually occurred and death is almost always inevitable. Airway management and hemodynamic stabilization are combined with consideration of organ donation. The emergency physician may have a substantial role in this discussion.

Maxillofacial Trauma

Bleeding can be difficult to control after severe facial trauma. Isolated hemorrhage can be managed with direct pressure but surgical control of bleeding vessels is difficult in the maxilla and anterior face. Angiography with embolization of an arterially bleeding vessel may be required. Severe hemorrhage often presents as airway obstruction, and orotracheal intubation or surgical cricothyroidotomy is necessary. The oropharynx can be packed in an attempt to control hemorrhage while awaiting surgical or angiographic intervention.

The nose may require anterior packing for persistent nosebleeds. The patient is given appropriate antibiotic coverage and referred to the facial surgeon. Facial surgeons may apply intermaxillary (arch bars) fixation for Le Fort I fractures, whereas Le Fort II and III fractures may need open reduction and internal fixation.

Cervical Vertebrae Fracture with and without Spinal Cord Injury

Fractures of the spine with or without neurologic involvement consist of continued spinal immobilization, immediate neurosurgical consultation, and surveillance for other associated injuries. If there is evidence of acute spinal cord injury (within 8 hours of presentation), intravenous methylprednisolone is started immediately.

Penetrating Neck Trauma

After securing the airway, management depends on the zones of injury, as previously discussed. A nasogastric tube should not be placed. General supportive care, including tetanus immunization and broad-spectrum antibiotic coverage is indicated. The specific management (whether mandatory or selective surgical exploration) is determined by the surgical consultant.

UNCERTAIN DIAGNOSIS

There are some uncertain diagnoses in patients with head and neck trauma. Most of the concern is which diagnostic study is appropriate. Examples include whether the patient's hypotension is related to "spinal shock," a post–closed-head injury patient with a complaint of a focal neurologic injury but a nondiagnostic head CT and a normal neurologic examination, or the intoxicated patient with an altered sensorium but normal diagnostic studies (except for ethanol level). Prudent management in essentially all uncertain cases is early consultation, observation, regular neurologic checks, and often a repeat or more sophisticated diagnostic study (e.g., MRI) later in the course of care.

SPECIAL CONSIDERATIONS

Pediatric Patients

Blunt head trauma is common in children. Its occurrence should always raise the question of child abuse. An expanded history may identify events and an environment associated with child abuse. Skull or other radiographs may be taken in children younger than 2 years of age to help identify findings consistent with child abuse (e.g., post-traumatic leptomeningeal cysts).

The GCS was not originally developed for infants. A revised GCS that addresses the verbal abilities of young children is given in Table 48–6.

Children who have one to three episodes of vomiting or slight sleepiness without neurologic deficit are observed in the emergency department for several hours. Should their vomiting persist or symptoms increase, emergency CT is done and they are admitted. If the child has reliable, competent parents and the vomiting ceases, he or she may be safely sent home, providing the parents can comply with strict "head" instructions.

Children rarely suffer cervical spine injury. The age group that is younger than 15 years represents only 1% to 2% of all patients with spinal injuries. Those children who are at increased risk for suffering cervical spine injury usually have preexisting conditions that allow less latitude in the upper cervical region and may have serious neurologic loss (e.g., quadriplegics). When they do suffer cervical spine injury, it is seen higher on the spinal column (their relatively larger head causes a higher fulcrum), with devastating consequences. Radiographic findings also differ for the pediatric population. The pre-dens space may measure up to 5 mm in children and still be considered normal. Also, *pseudosubluxation*, a normal finding, may be found in up to 40% of children younger than 8 years. This is a subluxation of the C2 vertebral body on C3 (Fig. 48–14). A disruption or subluxation at the spinolaminal line of C2, however, is abnormal. Often, prevertebral soft tissue swelling accompanies a true subluxation.

Elderly Patients

The cerebral atrophy and diminished vascular resiliency found in elderly patients places them at higher risk for intracranial hemorrhage after head trauma, particularly subdural hematoma. Mechanisms of injury that might usually be considered minor can create significant hemorrhage in this population. Some individuals may have underlying functional brain impairment, making reliability of signs and symptoms difficult. Osteoporosis and osteosclerosis may have a significant impact on the radiographic interpretation and clinical outcome of head and neck trauma. There is a low threshold for ordering diagnostic studies in the elderly population. This population generally has higher morbidity and mortality after head or neck trauma.

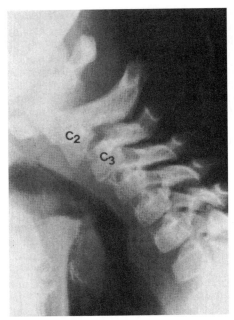

FIGURE 48–14 • Pseudosubluxation of C2-C3 in a 7-year-old girl. (From Wilberger JE [ed]: Spinal Cord Injuries in Children. Mt. Kisco, NY, Futura, 1986.)

Patients With Herniation Syndromes

Figure 48–15A illustrates the normal intracranial relationships and the three herniation syndromes.

Uncal Herniation. Unilateral cerebral swelling or mass lesions force the ipsilateral medial portion of the temporal lobe into the tentorial hiatus, compressing the parasympathetic fibers of oculomotor nerve (CN III) (see Fig. 48–15B). This parasympathetic compression results in unopposed sympathetic dilation of the involved pupil. The result is a fixed, dilated pupil. This dilated pupil is ipsilateral to the mass lesion 85% of the time. The cerebral peduncle is also compressed, causing a contralateral hemiparesis and

TABLE 48–6. Glasgow Coma Scale for Infants

Assessment	Score					
	6	5	4	3	2	1
Eye opening	—	—	Spontaneous	To speech	To pain	None
Verbal response	—	Smiles, babbles	Irritable	Cries with pain	Moans with pain	None
Motor response	Appropriate for age	Withdraws to touch	Withdraws from pain	Decorticate posturing	Decerebrate posturing	None

Scale scores range from 3 to 15, <13 is considered altered mental status, <8 is consistent with coma.

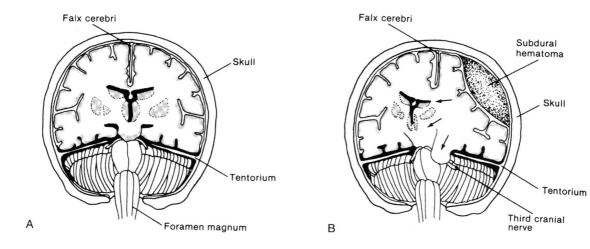

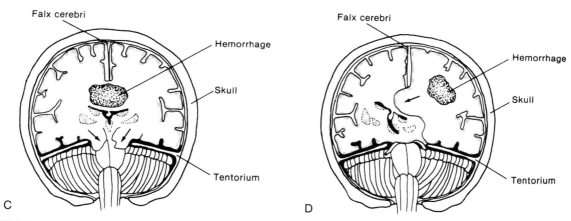

FIGURE 48–15 • Herniation syndromes. *A,* Normal relationship of intracranial structures. *B,* Uncal transtentorial herniation syndrome. *C,* Central herniation syndrome. *D,* Cingulate herniation. (From Rosen P: Emergency Medicine: Concepts and Clinical Practice. St. Louis. CV Mosby, 1988.)

a depressed level of consciousness. Roughly 15% of the time, the patient may have contralateral pupillary dilatation and paralysis.

Central Herniation. Bilateral uncal herniation occurs secondary to downward displacement of both hemispheres from diffuse swelling or bilateral lesions (see Fig. 48–15*C*). This leads to coma, Cheyne-Stokes respirations, decorticate posturing, and, eventually, death.

Cingulate Herniation. The cingulate gyrus shifts laterally underneath the falx cerebri, leading to cerebral ischemia. It is difficult to diagnose clinically (see Fig. 48–15*D*).

Cerebellar Tonsil Herniation. Medullary compression may occur from a posterior cranial fossa mass lesion. Respiratory arrest and

death often result. It is rarely seen with blunt head trauma, but it may be a common cause of death in high velocity penetrating injuries to the brain.

Patients With Mild Traumatic Brain Injury (MTBI)

Evaluation and management of the patient with mild head injury are controversial. Some would advocate CT for all patients with a loss of consciousness. Others advocate a more selective approach. The Canadian CT Head Rule appears to be a valid, reasonable approach. Patients with GCS of 13 or more who meet none of the seven criteria in Table 48–5 are observed for 2 hours. If their GCS does not return to 15, they undergo CT. Otherwise, they may be discharged.

DISPOSITION AND FOLLOW-UP

"Mild" to Moderate Closed-Head Trauma without Evidence of Intracranial Injury or Focal Neurologic Deficit. Patients who present in the mild risk category who have a normal neurologic examination can be discharged home. CT of the head is rarely appropriate in this group and is guided by clinical findings.

The following factors are addressed before the patient is sent home:

1. The patient must be supervised by a responsible person. The role of this person is to wake the patient every few hours through the night and monitor the patient's responsiveness and behavior during a full 24-hour period.
2. The supervising person understands that he or she is observing the patient for lethargy, confusion, vomiting, ataxia, or increasing pain. The patient needs to return immediately to the emergency department if any of these conditions become evident.
3. Studies show that patients with mild head injuries may indeed suffer from subsequent deficiencies in learning, memory, or visual motor speed. Up to 15% of these patients demonstrate some degree of disability 1 year after injury. Therefore, careful physician follow-up of the patient is necessary.

Intracranial Brain Hemorrhage, Severe Brain Injury, or Penetrating Head Injuries. The patient is admitted to an intensive care bed with neurosurgical consultation. Transfer to a trauma or brain injury center may be required.

Maxillofacial Injuries. The patient is referred to a facial surgeon.

Neck Pain without Evidence of Fracture/ Instability (Cervical Strain, Muscular Sprain, Contusion). Analgesics with or without a muscle

relaxant are provided for several days. Early follow-up with a primary physician is important for reevaluation and establishing the need for further evaluation (e.g., MRI) and treatment (e.g., physical therapy).

Spinal Column Fracture or Ligamentous Injuries. Patients with unstable fractures are admitted to the neurologic or spine service. Stable fractures may be discharged after review with orthopedic or neurosurgical consultants.

Spinal Cord Injury. After initial management, including spinal immobilization, care is decided in consultation with the neurosurgeon. Transfer to a trauma or spinal cord injury center is often considered.

Penetrating Neck Trauma. These patients are admitted for surgical exploration, repair, or observation for airway status.

FINAL POINTS

- Head and neck trauma is common and has a wide range of presentations and outcomes.
- The primary goals of emergency care are assessing the extent of the injury, protecting the patient from further injury, and stabilizing the airway and cardiovascular status.
- Normal initial C-spine films do not rule out a cervical spine fracture or cervical cord injury.
- A normal nonenhanced CT of the head does not rule out a CNS hemorrhage.
- Part of the assessment is searching for the cause of the trauma. Underlying metabolic, neurologic, or cardiovascular disorders may be the inciting event, especially in the elderly patient.
- All patients with head and/or neck trauma with associated neurologic deficits are admitted for further management.
- Early transfer of patients is done in those whose injuries exceed the capability of the hospital.

CASE*Study*

A 67-year-old woman is involved in a major motor vehicle accident. The driver, her husband, is dead at the scene. She is extricated from the car and is noted to be confused. A cervical collar is placed. Her vital signs are blood pressure, 150/95 mm Hg; heart rate, 105 beats per

minute; and respiratory rate, 22 breaths per minute on 10 L of oxygen by face mask. Estimated time of arrival is 5 minutes.

The patient arrives at the emergency department in C-spine immobilization and on a long board. She is on oxygen, and an intravenous line is in her left antecubital fossa. The paramedics report that she was initially awake with mild confusion but is now less responsive. She has a history of coronary artery disease and hypertension. Her medications are diltiazem, aspirin, and an unknown water pill. She is allergic to penicillin and cephalosporins. Previous surgery was for a hysterectomy with a bilateral salpingo-oophorectomy.

Her husband was killed at the scene. The car was smashed and rolled twice with the passenger side caved in. She was a front seat passenger and was wearing her seat belt. There were no airbags deployed in the car.

On examination in the emergency department, her airway is patent and the gag reflex is present but weak. Her vital signs are a heart rate of 92 beats per minute, blood pressure of 110/65 mm Hg, a respiratory rate of 8 breaths per minute, and rectal temperature of 36.1°C (97°F). Her breathing is very shallow and periodically irregular, and breath sounds are slightly diminished on the right. Pulse oximetry reads 92% on 4 L of oxygen by nasal cannula. A cardiac monitor shows a normal sinus rhythm with periodic unifocal premature atrial contractions. There are no obvious signs of bleeding. She responds only to a painful sternal rub with a moan and does not open her eyes spontaneously. Her pupils are 4 mm, round, and sluggish but reactive. She withdraws all extremities to noxious stimulus, but she will not move her extremities to command. The patient is undressed and covered with a warm blanket.

The primary survey is completed in this trauma patient, and initial findings indicate potential for loss of airway protection, discordant breathing, hypoventilation, and relative hypotension in this patient who normally has hypertension for a disease state. She needs urgent airway management with endotracheal intubation for a number of reasons: (1) airway protection from a risk of aspiration, (2) dysfunctional respiratory state, (3) suggestion of severe head injury with a GCS of E = 1, V = 2, M = 4, totaling 7 (consistent with coma). While preparations for intubation are made, the primary survey can be continued. Rapid sequence intubation with premedication can best avert increased ICP as long as her oxygen saturation and her blood pressure are stable. Her asymmetric breath sounds can be further evaluated by a chest radiograph because there is no impending respiratory or circulatory collapse. Of great concern is her diminishing neurologic condition. She has deteriorated from awake and confused at the scene to comatose in the emergency department. Whatever processes are causing these changes

must be found and reversed, if possible. Volume resuscitation in this patient would initially consist of two to three 250- to 500-cc isotonic crystalloid boluses to determine her response and fluid needs. An initially conservative approach is taken to lessen cerebral edema.

She is placed on 10 L of oxygen via face mask, which improves her oxygenation to 97%, and arrangements for rapid sequence intubation and endotracheal intubation are initiated. A second intravenous line is started and blood is drawn (for bedside glucose, complete blood cell count, electrolytes, blood urea nitrogen, creatine, and serum glucose). Blood is also drawn and held for a type and screen, coagulation panel, and cardiac markers. The patient responds well to the initial fluid challenge with a blood pressure of 130/100 mm Hg. The secondary survey is completed, and her only injury appears to be neurologic. The bedside glucose value is 122 mg /dL. She responds to painful stimulation globally and withdraws all four extremities to pain; there are no pathologic reflexes and no evidence of vascular impairment.

With a normal bedside glucose value and a low suspicion for narcotic overdose, there is no current need for thiamine, dextrose, or naloxone. In this patient, appropriate radiographic studies include chest, pelvis, and lateral C-spine films. This patient is at high risk for an intracranial pathologic process, and a CT of the head and C-spine radiograph should be performed urgently. Furthermore, with her hypotension that responded to crystalloid fluids, an appropriate diagnostic survey to identify occult intra-abdominal hemorrhage is necessary. The patient is unable to provide clinical examination assistance because of her altered mental status. With her history of coronary disease, an electrocardiogram is helpful to identify potential coronary ischemia.

The chest radiograph revealed three rib fractures on the right with evidence of early pulmonary contusion but no pneumothorax. A pelvic series was unremarkable. The lateral C-spine radiograph showed degenerative changes but no obvious fractures, although C1 and C2 vertebrae were not well visualized. The odontoid image was suboptimal and nondiagnostic. The electrocardiogram was read as normal.

A nasogastric tube and Foley catheter were placed. After rapid sequence intubation, the patient was placed on a ventilator with a goal of oxygen saturation above 97% and a CO_2 of 35 to 40 mm Hg. An ABG analysis was requested in 15 to 20 minutes. The CT of the head demonstrated a large subdural hematoma on the right

Continued on following page

with evidence of intraparenchymal hemorrhage and subarachnoid bleeding. There was evidence of early mass effect and cerebral hemispheric shift. A neurosurgeon was consulted, and 0.25 mg/kg of mannitol was administered. The CT of the abdomen revealed a small (grade 1) splenic laceration without evidence of intra-abdominal hemorrhage.

This patient has evidence of severe focal brain injury with evidence of mass effect. Management included protecting the airway, ventilation control, preventing hypotension, and osmotic diuretics to relieve ICP. Emergent neurosurgical intervention is planned.

The patient's bony spine is still not cleared from fracture. With the poor visualization of C1 and C2, the chronic degenerative changes, and the evidence of severe brain injury, a CT of C1 and C2 was obtained and indicated a small fracture through the pedicle of C2.

This is a highly unstable fracture and the neurosurgeon was notified. Careful and complete immobilization is necessary. CT of the entire spine eventually may be required. A detailed neurologic examination is impossible in this patient. There is no evidence of focal spinal cord injury. If there were such indication, methylprednisolone, 30 mg/kg intravenously, would be given and a 5.4 mg/kg intravenous drip started over the next 24 hours. The neuromuscular paralyzing agent from the rapid sequence intubation would have worn off by now. If the patient is spontaneously moving, a short-acting paralytic agent may be necessary to prevent the patient from inadvertent movement (protective pain mechanisms are lost) and resultant spinal cord injury. The splenic injury can be observed for the time being.

The patient was transferred to the operating room for decompression of her subdural hemorrhage and fixation of her C2 pedicle fracture. Her prognosis is uncertain.

Bibliography

TEXTS

American College of Surgeons. Committee on Trauma: Advanced Trauma Life Support Program for Doctors, 6th ed. Chicago, American College of Surgeons, 1997.

Bullock M, Chestnut R, Clifton G, et al: Guidelines for the Management of Severe Traumatic Brain Injury. New York, Brain Trauma Foundation, 2000.

Ferrera PC: Trauma Management: An Emergency Medicine Approach. St. Louis, CV Mosby, 2001.

Scaletta T, Schaider J: Emergent Management of Trauma, 2nd ed. Boston, McGraw-Hill, 2001.

JOURNAL ARTICLES

Atkinson PP, Atkinson JL: Spinal shock. Mayo Clin Proc 1996; 71:384–389.

Barron DN, Levitt MA, Clements RC: Head trauma and subdural hematoma: I and II. Emerg Med Rep 2001; 22:299–314.

Bracken MB: Pharmacological interventions for acute spinal cord injury. Cochrane Database Syst Rev 2000; (2): CD001046.

Bracken MB, Shepard MJ, Holford TR, et al: Administration of methylprednisolone for 24 or 48 hours or tirilazad mesylate for 48 hours in the treatment of acute spinal cord injury: Results of the Third National Acute Spinal Cord Injury Randomized Controlled Trial. National Acute Spinal Cord Injury Study. JAMA 1997; 277:1597–1604.

Brooks RA, Willett KM: Evaluation of the Oxford protocol for total spinal clearance in the unconscious trauma patient. J Trauma 2001; 50:862–867.

Chesnut RM, Marshall LF, Klauber MR, et al: The role of secondary brain injury in determining outcome from severe head injury. J Trauma 1993; 34:216–222.

Clifton GL, Miller ER, Choi SC, et al: Lack of effect of induction of hypothermia after acute brain injury. N Engl J Med 2001; 344:556–563.

Gibbs MA, Jones AE: Cervical spine injury: A state-of-the-art approach to assessment and management. Emerg Med Pract 2001; 3(10): 1–24.

Greenes DS, Schutzman SA: Occult intracranial injury in infants. Ann Emerg Med 1998; 32:680–686.

Hanson J, Blackmore C, Mann F, Wilson A: Cervical spine injury: Accuracy of helical CT used as a screening technique. Emerg Radiol 2000; 7:31–35.

Haydel MJ, Preston CA, Mills TJ, et al: Indications for computed tomography in patients with minor head injury. N Engl J Med 2000; 343:100–105.

Hendey GW, Wolfson AB, Mower WR, et al: Spinal cord injury without radiographic abnormality: Results of the National Emergency X-Radiography Utilization in Blunt Cervical Trauma. J Trauma 2002; 53: 1–14.

Hoffman JR, Mower WR, Wolfson AB, et al, The National Emergency X-Radiography Utilization Study Group: Validity of a set of clinical criteria to rule out injury to the cervical spine in patients with blunt trauma. N Engl J Med 2000; 343:94–99.

Jager TE, Weiss HB, Coben JH, et al: Traumatic brain injuries evaluated in U.S. emergency departments, 1992–1994. Acad Emerg Med 2000; 7:134–140.

Jagoda AS, Cantrill SV, Wearo RL, et al: Clinical policy: Neuroimaging and decisionmaking in adult mild traumatic brain injury in the acute setting. Ann Emerg Med 2002; 40: 231–249.

Jennett B, Teasdale G: Aspects of coma after severe head injury. Lancet 1977; 1:878–881.

Mandavia DP, Qualls S, Rokos I: Emergency airway management in penetrating neck injury. Ann Emerg Med 2000; 35:221–225.

Marx JA, Biros MH: Who is at low risk after head or neck trauma? N Engl J Med 2000; 343:138–140.

Mower WR, Hoffman JR, Pollack CV, et al: Use of plain radiography to screen for cervical spine injuries. Ann Emerg Med 2001; 38:1–7.

Perkin RM, Moynihan JA, McLeary M: Current concepts in the emergency management of severe traumatic brain injury in children. Trauma Rep 2000; 1:1–16.

Shaw GJ, Jauch EL, Zemlan EP: Serum cleaned tau protein levels and clinical outcome in adult patients with closed head injury. Ann Emerg Med 2002: 39:254–257.

Stiell IG, Wells GA, Vandemheem KL, et al: The Canadian C-spine rule for radiography in alert and stable trauma patients. JAMA 2001; 286:1841–1848.

Stiell IG, Wells GA, Vandemheen KL, et al: The Canadian CT Head Rule for patients with minor head injury. Lancet 2001; 357:1391–1396.

Williams J, Jehle D, Cottington E, Shufflebarger C: Head, facial, and clavicular trauma as a predictor of cervical-spine injury. Ann Emerg Med 1992; 21:719–722.

Zink BJ: Traumatic brain injury outcome: Concepts for emergency care. Ann Emerg Med 2001; 37:318–332.

CHAPTER 49

Wound Care

SCOTT A. DOAK

CASE *Study*

A 28-year-old man was caught breaking into a store by police and was attacked by a police dog. The dog bit him on the head, the left shoulder, and the back. He was escorted to the emergency department.

CASE *Study*

A 54-year-old woman stumbled and fell while raking leaves. Her right lower leg was impaled on a broken stick. She pulled the stick out and came to the hospital 6 hours later.

INTRODUCTION

Wounds of all types rival upper respiratory tract infections as the most common reason for seeking medical care. In emergency departments, minor wounds may comprise 5% to 40% of all diagnoses, depending on the clinical milieu. Minor wounds are more common in children, during warmer months, in laborers, and in those who work and play outdoors. The most common wounds are hand lacerations, minor burns, and puncture wounds.

Skin Anatomy

The major components of the skin are the epidermis, dermis, superficial fascia, and deep fascia.

Epidermis. The epidermis is the thick, totally cellular outer segment that does not contain blood, lymphatic vessels, or connective tissue. It serves as a watertight seal with its tight junctions and prevents bacterial invasion. Wounds that violate only the epidermis, such as first-degree burns or superficial scratches, are usually minor.

Dermis. The dermis is the deeper layer of the skin containing vascular, nervous, and structural connective tissues. It also houses the four skin appendages derived from the epidermis: hair follicles, eccrine and apocrine sweat glands, and seba-

ceous glands. It is a thick, strong, elastic layer that serves, with its excellent blood supply, as the primary site of the inflammatory response and skin defense once the epithelium has been breached by bacteria. The dermis is readily visible in wounds that require closure, and its proper approximation is essential to good wound healing and final cosmetic appearance.

Subcutaneous Tissue. The superficial fascia is a web of connective tissue interspersed with fat. Visualizing fat within a wound confirms the fact that the dermis has been penetrated. It is a weaker, lesser elastic layer than the dermis and serves primarily by insulating the body from thermal and mechanical forces. This is the usual space where infection occurs, leading to cellulitis, and also the space where anesthetic is infiltrated.

Deep Fascia. The deep fascia is a thin, but very strong, avascular layer that lies just deep to the superficial fascia. It generally incorporates deeper, more vital structures such as muscle, affording them both mechanical protection and a barrier to the spread of infection from the superficial fascia down into the deeper structures.

There are many regional differences of these various layers throughout the body. The scalp has an extremely rich blood supply and has a specialized fibrous layer, the galea aponeurotica. The palms and soles are known to have a very thick epidermis. The eyelids have a very thin dermis. These variations must be considered during wound exploration and repair.

Mechanisms of Injury

Lacerations are often described as resulting from shearing, tension, or compression forces. A shearing-type laceration is the simple dissection of the skin by a sharp object, such as a cut from a razor blade or knife. Little physical force is imparted to the tissue adjacent to the laceration. For this reason there is less necrosis, inflammation, and edema in simple shear lacerations. They usually heal without complication or severe scarring. Tension lacerations result when the skin is ripped apart by the application of blunt force at an angle to the skin. The force is transmitted to adjacent tissue, and considerable injury is typical. The wound tends to be irregular and jagged. Often a triangular flap of skin is created. Compression lacerations occur when a blunt opposing force presses the skin against bone, causing the skin to burst (e.g., a cut over the supraorbital ridge in a boxer who is struck by his opponent's glove). These lacerations are irregular, are often stellate, and are associated with significant damage in the adjoining skin and soft tissues. This type of injury requires far less bacterial contamination to become infected. *Many lacerations have components from each of these types of forces.*

Abrasions are wounds produced by the forcible avulsion of skin layers to a certain depth. The forces causing abrasions are usually applied horizontally to the skin. For example, "road rash" is a type of abrasion seen in motorcycle accident victims who have slid along asphalt. Such abrasions may be extensive and are often contaminated with soil, gravel, or tar. Depending on their thickness, abrasions may require the same treatment as burns.

Puncture wounds are much deeper than they are wide, which makes them difficult to explore and decontaminate. They have a greater risk of inoculation of bacteria or foreign material into the wound. In some cases, penetration to bone may occur, with a resulting risk of osteomyelitis.

Burns result from thermal injury to the skin and are typically described as first-, second-, and third-degree burns. Although this grading has historical importance, it may be clinically inaccurate. The critical factor guiding the treatment approach to burns relies on whether any dermis remains that would allow spontaneous coverage. A more clinically useful and practical classification scheme is to consider burns to be either partial thickness or full thickness. Partial-thickness burns are those that include the epidermis and only part of the dermis. Full-thickness burns involve the entire epithelium and the entire dermis.

Another type of injury to the skin is a local hypothermic injury or *frostbite*. After prolonged exposure to cold temperatures, the skin cells may freeze. Intense vasoconstriction causes hypoperfusion and occlusion of small blood vessels. Like burns, frostbite can be graded as partial or full thickness, depending on the depth of injury.

Wound Healing

Wound healing is a dynamic process initiated at the time of the insult to the skin. It does not complete itself for many months. It is a natural, predictable process, but it can be affected by a number of outside factors. The phases of wound healing are overlapping and summarized here.

Immediate Response Phase (Seconds to Hours). The immediate response phase includes initial tissue retraction and microvessel and macrovessel compression. This is followed by vasoconstriction and activation of both platelets and the coagulation cascade. Clot formation occurs, followed by secondary vasodilation and exudation of intravascular material into the wound. The function of the immediate response phase is to achieve hemostasis and then to increase blood and nutrient supply into the wound.

Inflammatory Phase (Hours to Days). With this vasodilation, complement and chemotactic factors are activated that lead to a pronounced exudation of neutrophils, macrophages, lymphocytes, and immunoglobulins into the wound. This phase serves primarily to combat contamination and control infection. Toward the end of this phase the predominant activity is phagocytosis of wound debris.

Epithelialization Phase (Hours to Weeks). Within 12 hours of injury, epithelial cells on the wound margin undergo morphologic change and begin to migrate in from the periphery of the wound to achieve coverage. This epithelialization occurs at a rate of approximately 1 mm per day. Therefore, a well-sutured wound should be completely epithelialized in 1, or at most, 2 days. Shortly after this coverage, tight junctions occur that allow the wound to become watertight.

Neovascularization Phase (Days to Weeks). Around the time the inflammatory phase is ending and macrophages are débriding the wound, new capillaries begin to grow in from the periphery of the wound at the level of the dermis. This increases nutrient and oxygen delivery within the healing wound and contributes to fibroblast stimulation. This phase is at its peak at 7 to 10 days, resulting in an erythematous blush around the wound margin at the time of suture removal. These new capillaries combine with fibroblasts from the following phase to create granulation tissue.

Collagen Synthesis Phase (Days to Months). With the wound now débrided and its vascularity restored, the milieu is right for fibroblast stimulation and proliferation. This phase actually occurs in two parts. Initially, fibroblasts proliferate and collagen is laid down in a haphazard fashion. This matrix affords some degree of tensile strength; however, a significant degree of wound strength does not occur until much later as the collagen is gradually and systematically lysed and remodeled in a more organized and stronger pattern. At 2 weeks, the wound has only

5% of its tensile strength, at 1 month it has about 35%, and it takes up to 6 to 12 months before maximum tensile strength is achieved. The tensile strength of the wound actually declines from day 7 to 10, as a consequence of the early collagen lytic phase. This illustrates that the purpose of the percutaneous sutures is not to add strength to the wound because they are often removed as the tensile strength of the wound is declining during days 7 to 10. For these reasons, a wound may need protection even after it appears well healed.

The outer appearance of the scar passes through several stages. In the first month, the scar is weak, soft, and undeveloped. In the next 2 months it becomes redder, firmer, and stronger. After 3 months the scar gradually softens and becomes more pliable, elastic, and paler. The scar continues to contract over time.

There are numerous factors that affect the efficiency of these phases of wound healing. These are summarized in Table 49–1. Patients with chronic diseases such as diabetes or lung, liver, or kidney disease, vascular impairment, or alcoholism have poorer wound healing and a higher rate of infection. Malnutrition also impairs wound healing. Corticosteroids are the most widely implicated drugs that impair wound healing, but cytotoxic agents, antibiotics, and even nonsteroidal anti-inflammatory agents also have an effect.

The most important negative influence on wound healing is wound infection. It occurs in about 5% of wounds treated in the emergency department, although each specific wound carries its own risk. For example, a relatively clean laceration on the scalp carries a risk of infection of far less than 1%, whereas a cat bite to the finger may have an infection rate as high as 80%. It is sometimes difficult to tell clinically whether a wound is infected, because the normal inflammatory response in wounded tissues may simulate infection. A pure definition of wound infection is the presence of greater than 100,000 colony-forming units of bacteria per gram of tissue. By far the most common organism implicated in wound infections is *Staphylococcus aureus*.

Blood supply also plays a critical role in wound healing and wound infection rate. The most vascular areas of the body are the scalp and face. Therefore, the infection rate in these areas is very low, and one may be more aggressive about placing deep sutures and using epinephrine. Vascularity of the skin within the body then gradually declines from the head down, with the feet being the least vascular and thus carrying the highest infection rate potential.

TABLE 49–1. Factors Associated with Impaired Wound Healing and Increased Infection

Wound Characteristics

Age of wound greater than 6 hr when treated
Wound location in an area with poor blood supply
Crushing, macerating mechanism of injury
Contamination with soil, foreign material
Puncture wounds
Bite wounds

Technical Characteristics

Use of tissue-toxic wound preparation solutions
Use of detergent scrub solutions
Inadequate cleansing and irrigation
Anesthetics containing epinephrine
Inadequate hemostasis, wound hematoma
Reactive suture material
Excessive suture tension
Tincture of benzoin
More concentrated anesthetics (2%)

Anatomic Factors

Static skin tension
Dynamic skin tension

Patient Characteristics

Advanced age
Malnourished
Poor hygiene
Alcoholism
Diabetes mellitus
Peripheral vascular disease
Uremia
Liver disease
Connective tissue diseases
Hypoxia
Anemia
Multiple trauma

Drugs

Corticosteroids
Nonsteroidal anti-inflammatory agents
Colchicine
Anticoagulants
Antineoplastic agents
Penicillamine
Pigmented skin
Oily skin

Modified from Trott A: Wounds and Lacerations: Emergency Care and Closure, 2nd ed. St Louis, CV Mosby, 1997, p.30; with permission.

All wounds are contaminated no matter how clean they may appear. The less contaminated the wound, the more efficient the inflammatory phase can be in quelling a subclinical infection and progressing to the other phases of wound healing. If a wound has a high bacterial count that is not high enough to cause a clinical infection, it may delay the various healing phases and result in a poor cosmetic outcome even though no clinical infection was evident. This underlines the importance of meticulous wound care because excellent preparation of the tissue will result in lower bacterial counts and, ultimately, in a superior cosmetic result.

Some people have problems with excessive scar formation. Hypertrophic scars are common in children, in patients with dark skin, and in burns. A hypertrophic scar is raised and may be more sensitive than a normal scar but does not extend past the original wound margins. A keloid represents the extreme of excessive scar formation. In this case, a disorder in collagen deposition produces a large, fibrous growth that extends beyond the limits of the original scar. Keloids are most common in patients with dark skin or oily skin or in wounds with retained foreign bodies.

The vast majority of wounds can be closed by primary union. *Primary union*, or healing by first intention, refers to closure of the wound by sutures, staples, or adhesives during the patient's initial visit. Wounds on the extremities may be closed primarily within the first 6 hours, wounds on the torso may be closed within the first 12 hours, and wounds on the face and scalp may be closed within the first 24 hours. These time frames all assume ideal wound, patient, and practitioner characteristics (see Table 49–1). If these characteristics are not ideal, then the more conservative times of 4, 8, and 12 hours for extremities, torso, and face/scalp wounds are recommended.

The term *secondary union* is used to describe a wound that is left open and allowed to granulate in from the bottom up. This strategy is preferred if a wound is considered too high risk for primary closure or if there is significant tissue loss during the injury, precluding initial percutaneous closure. Examples of wounds commonly allowed to heal by secondary intention are deep abrasions and ulcers.

Tertiary union, or delayed closure, is a technique in which ordinary wound care is applied to a wound and then it is left open for approximately 4 days. If a wound remains uninfected at 4 days its risk of infection thereafter is extremely low and it may be sutured together secondarily. Wounds that are candidates for tertiary union are generally wounds in which no significant tissue loss is present so they may be physically sutured; however, there is a high degree of contamination or there are wound characteristics, such as age of the wound, that make them too risky to close primarily.

INITIAL APPROACH AND STABILIZATION

Patients with wounds are usually anxious and frightened about their impending treatment and are in some degree of pain. They perceive their wounds as real emergencies, no matter how minor the injury, and dislike waiting for treatment. They often are concerned about the cosmetic appearance of the wound. Many wounds result from assaults, fights, robberies, animal bites, or careless mistakes or accidents. Patients bring the stresses from these events with them to the emergency department.

The initial management of wounded patients is aimed at reducing anxiety, relieving pain, and moving the patient quickly through the emergency care system. The exception to this goal is the intoxicated patient, who initially may be impossible to assess. In such a case, after initial examination for life- or limb-threatening injuries, it is best to wait until the effect of alcohol or drugs is reduced to the point where the patient can be evaluated and treated properly. However, the time since injury must be monitored because that may impact treatment options.

Rapid Assessment

1. A primary survey of the patient is carried out; priority is given to the patency of the airway and adequacy of the respiratory effort.
2. The circulatory system is evaluated, paying particular attention to blood pressure, heart rate, and peripheral circulation distal to the wound. Scalp lacerations are notorious for bleeding vigorously and hypotension can occur after seemingly minor wounds. Early hemorrhagic shock may present only as an elevation of the heart rate or narrowing of the pulse pressure. If active hemorrhage is seen during the initial assessment, it should be controlled with elevation and direct pressure.
3. Initial vital signs must be recorded in all wounded patients and repeated at regular intervals.
4. The time from injury and the mechanism of injury are carefully determined. This information will have a significant impact on the timing and choices made in wound care.
5. Because there are many medications that potentially could be administered, it is important to establish an allergy history.
6. In extremities, a careful neurovascular examination is performed distal to the wound to ensure proper function before anesthetics or other treatments are administered.
7. Early surgical consultation is obtained in any case of life- or limb-threatening injury.

Early Intervention

1. Clothing is removed to permit a complete examination depending on the location of the wound.
2. Rings, watches, jewelry, and other objects or apparel are also removed if they will interfere with the examination and treatment. Rings or watches must be removed early from an injured extremity before edema makes removal impossible.
3. Once initially assessed, the wound is covered and protected with a temporary dressing such as a moistened saline gauze pad.
4. Unless significant pain is present (e.g., a burn or wound with fracture), analgesia is usually not given until after a more complete examination has been done.

CASE *Study*

In the patient in Case 1, multiple dog bite wounds were noted about the head, back, and left shoulder. The injuries had occurred 1 hour before admission. The patient was alert and talking. Vital signs were unremarkable. He had a recent tetanus immunization. A brief examination revealed that the airway was intact and there was no evident neurovascular injury to the left arm. Moistened saline gauze pads were applied to the wounds, and preparations were made to evaluate and repair the wounds further.

In spite of the dramatic appearance of the patient's lacerations, attention is paid first to potential life- or limb-threatening injuries. An appropriate evaluation of the areas of most concern is carried out. Once the basic evaluation is completed and serious problems have been addressed, the individual wounds are managed.

CLINICAL ASSESSMENT

Obtaining a history from a patient with a wound is not usually a time-consuming task. The standard format for taking a wound history and examining a wound is outlined here.

History

1. *When* did the wound occur? The longer the lapse of time between the injury and the repair, the greater the chance for infection.
2. *How* did it occur, that is, what was the *mechanism of injury?* As discussed previously, the mechanism of injury has a significant impact on the degree of injury to surrounding tissue and the choices in wound treatment.
3. Is there *pain* or *numbness?* Both can be indicative of neurovascular compromise in injuries of an extremity.
4. Was there significant *bleeding?* Both the amount and intensity are noted, and an anatomic explanation must be sought.
5. Is there a sensation of a *foreign body?* Is there the possibility of a foreign body being present? A reported sensation of a foreign body by the patient is very accurate. Penetrating wounds or those associated with broken glass or fragment penetration are at high risk for a retained foreign body.
6. When dealing with a bite wound, *what kind of animal* inflicted the wound, *what is the* rabies status of the animal, and is the animal in custody or retrievable?
7. In *older* or *infected* wounds, is there *local warmth* or *exudate?* These are indicators of infection.
8. Was any *prior treatment* given, such as cleansing or application of agents to the wound?
9. Depending on the region of the wound, specific questions are directed to *functional status* of the injured area. For example, evaluation of head wounds includes questioning about loss of consciousness, headache, vomiting, visual changes, and gait abnormalities. With hand wounds, the patient's occupation, handedness, and present impairment are assessed.
10. Past *medical* history
    a. The patient's history of *tetanus immunization* is most important. In some cases, vaccination against hepatitis B virus may also be important.
    b. Are there *underlying medical diseases?* Specifically, diabetes mellitus, peripheral vascular disease, or bleeding disorders are important.
    c. *Habits* such as smoking, alcohol abuse, and drug use history are ascertained.
    d. What are the patient's *current medications?* Include potential platelet inhibitors, aspirin, and nonsteroidal anti-inflammatory agents. What is the patient's compliance with medication?
    e. Patients with *acquired immune deficiency syndrome* (AIDS) or with positive blood tests for *human immunodeficiency virus* must be identified. This knowledge is important for predicting wound infection and for the safety of staff working with the patient.

Physical Examination

With the exception of the severely injured patient, the physical examination of the patient with a wound begins with a survey of the vital signs and an assessment of the patient's general appearance and state of health. A young, previously healthy woman who hit her thumbnail with a hammer does not need a general examination in the emergency department. An elderly alcoholic who fell down some stairs and has a scalp laceration does need a full, systematic, and documented examination.

The examination of a wound includes the following observations:

1. Measurement or estimation of wound length, width, and depth.
2. Identification of all skin layers involved.
3. Degree of contamination and presence of foreign bodies.
4. Assessment of vascularity and amount and type of bleeding.
5. Identification of maceration or necrosis of tissues.
6. If the wound is in a cosmetically important area, its anatomic position in relation to skin tension lines is important in predicting whether the scar will widen as it matures. This is valuable to discuss with the patient at the time of initial repair.
7. Anatomic position of the wound in reference to joints, capsules, and skin creases. This is especially valuable in hand injuries.
8. A functional examination of the neuromuscular and vascular system distal to the injured area is performed. This examination is extremely important in forearm and hand injuries, in which tendon, nerve, and vascular damage is common. Sensation, motor function, tendon integrity, and capillary refill are tested in all extremity injuries. In children, this part of the assessment is best done before examining the wound, because better cooperation is obtained.

CASE *Study*

In Case 2, the patient stated the wound had occurred 6 hours before, when she fell against a broken stick that was part of her compost pile. The stick impaled her lower leg, but she pulled it out. Because she experienced minimal pain and bleeding, she continued with her yard work. Before coming to the hospital, she applied a warm tea bag to the wound. Further questioning about her past history revealed that she was a heavy cigarette smoker, had adult-onset diabetes mellitus, and was taking a pill for high blood pressure. She complained of having "poor circulation." She could not remember the time of her last tetanus immunization. On examination, a jagged, macerated 6-cm flap laceration containing dirt and bark fragments was found over the lateral midtibial surface.

There are several elements of the history that will influence the decision about the care of this wound. The wound is "old," is tetanus prone, and may contain foreign material. It occurred in a dirty environment. The lower leg is not a highly vascular area, and the blood supply of this patient may be more limited than normal, because the wound did not bleed. Other factors that may impair the blood supply and wound healing are heavy smoking, diabetes, high blood pressure, and a possible history of peripheral vascular disease. Clearly, this woman is not the average patient with a leg wound.

CLINICAL REASONING

Once the history has been taken and the wound explored, it is useful to ask a series of questions that may influence decisions about management.

Are the Anatomic Boundaries of the Wound Understood?

This question directs the examiner to two areas. First, the physician should understand the normal anatomy in the area of the wound and anticipate the structures that might be injured. Second, knowledge of the full extent of the wound is necessary to decide whether the wound should be closed and, if so, how many layers are involved.

Is there a Potential for a Foreign Body in the Wound?

A foreign body markedly increases the risk of infection and may impair healing and the cosmetic result. Also, it can cause pain and internal damage after wound closure. Puncture wounds, falls onto gravel or glass, and injuries from explosions are notorious for involving hidden foreign bodies. Every effort is made to find and remove them.

Are the Distal Neurovascular, Muscle, and Tendon Functions Consistent with the Anatomic Location of the Wound and the Findings on Exploration?

Any discrepancy between function and wound location needs an explanation. This usually requires a reexamination of both the distal functions and the anatomic structures involved in the wound.

Are There Factors That May Promote Infection or Impair Wound Healing?

These factors (see Table 49–1) are reviewed while care of the wound is planned. Decisions about closure, type of suture, number of layers, necessity of drainage, use of antibiotics, types of dressing, need for hospitalization, and timing of follow-up are influenced by these factors.

Does the Emergency Physician Have the Skill and the Time to Care for This Wound Properly?

Although it is expected that a trained emergency physician will be able to care for a wide variety of wounds, it is wise to know when an injury repair is beyond one's skill or, more often, beyond the time available to do it right. A wound closure that might require 30 minutes is appropriate and satisfying on a quiet Sunday morning but may need to be referred on a busy Saturday night. Both the emergency physician and the surgical consultant must be aware of the balance between skills and the available time in deciding which cases are cared for by whom.

DIAGNOSTIC ADJUNCTS

Laboratory tests and diagnostic imaging procedures, other than plain radiographs, are rarely helpful in the management of wounds.

Laboratory Studies

Blood tests are of minimal use in treating wounds. The hemoglobin and hematocrit may help in assessing blood loss but may not change from baseline for several hours. Serologic tests for hepatitis and human immunodeficiency virus are obtained in patients injured by a potentially contaminated source (e.g., needle or scalpel).

Radiologic Imaging

Plain radiographs are useful in detecting bony abnormalities and joint involvement in wounds. They are commonly used in high-risk situations to identify and localize foreign bodies and to show soft tissue changes, such as edema or gas in the tissues. Contrary to common opinion, glass foreign bodies will show up on radiographs about 90% of the time, even if the glass does not contain lead. Metal foreign bodies are almost always visible on radiographs. Less dense substances such as plastic and wood usually are not visible on plain radiographs but may be visualized by computed tomography. They may show as a "filling defect" on plain films. If there are questions about the best imaging technique to use to identify a foreign body, a discussion with the radiologist may be helpful. Alternate modalities include computed tomography, magnetic resonance imaging, and ultrasound.

PRINCIPLES OF MANAGEMENT

Once the wound and its impact on the patient have been assessed, management includes wound preparation, closure techniques, and wound aftercare.

Wound Preparation

Wound preparation is divided into five areas of concern: anesthesia, cleansing, irrigation, débridement, and hemostasis.

Anesthesia. Adequate pain relief before closure is foremost in the minds of most injured patients. It has been well shown, even in highly contaminated wounds, that infiltration of local anesthetic does not increase infection rate or decrease cosmetic result. Therefore, it is the responsibility of the clinician to achieve adequate anesthesia before any cleansing efforts to maximize patient comfort during the procedure.

A number of local anesthetic agents are available. The properties, onset, and duration of action and the maximum doses of the three most commonly used agents are summarized in Table 49–2. Lidocaine and mepivacaine are used most often. If a longer duration of anesthesia is desired, bupivacaine is favored. The addition of epinephrine to an anesthetic agent causes vasoconstriction in the wound field and prolongs the action of the anesthetic. Its use is limited to well-vascularized tissues. Fingers, toes, the penis, and the nose, as well as the ears and distal parts of flap lacerations, may suffer ischemic necrosis if epinephrine is used with the anesthetic agent because these structures are perfused by terminal arterioles.

If a patient has a number of lacerations or very large lacerations, the amount of local anesthetic agent administered must be tallied. As a benchmark, no more than 35 mL of 1% lidocaine

TABLE 49–2. Anesthetic Agents in Wound Care

Agent	Concentration	Onset of Action Infiltration/Block	Maximum Dosage (70 kg)
Lidocaine (Xylocaine)	1% or 2%	Fastest/4–10 min Duration: 1–2 hr	5 mg/kg = 35 mL of 1% solution
Mepivacaine (Carbocaine)	1% or 2%	Fast/6–10 min Duration: 1.5–2.5 hr	5 mg/kg = 35 mL of 1% solution
Bupivacaine	0.25% or 0.5%	Slower/8–12 min Duration: 4–8 hr	3 mg/kg = 70 mL of 0.25% solution

Modified from Trott A: Wounds and Lacerations: Emergency Care and Closure, 2nd ed. St Louis, CV Mosby, 1997, p.60; with permission.

(350 mg because 1% = 10 mg/mL) in a 70-kg person (5 mg/kg) may be used. If the anticipated local anesthetic requirement is greater than 35 mL, consideration should be given to using bupivacaine because its 0.25% preparation allows identical anesthesia with a larger volume of anesthetic. Seizures, hypotension, or even cardiac arrest may result from acute overdose of lidocaine and related agents.

Anesthetic allergies may occur among patients presenting for emergency wound care treatment. Adequate anesthesia is recommended even in the stoic patient who may tolerate suturing adequately. This is because proper wound preparation, irrigation, and débridement generally involve more discomfort than the suturing itself. Moderate anesthesia may be achieved by the application of sterile ice or the injection of normal saline alone. Diphenhydramine (Benadryl) is superior to these but does not achieve the level of anesthesia of the usual local anesthetics. Usually, an anesthetic allergy leads the physician to simply select another local anesthetic.

There are two classes of local anesthetics: amides and esters. Patients allergic to a local anesthetic in one of the groups are at risk to being allergic to all of the anesthetics within that class. Usually, they can be safely administered anesthetics from the alternate group without risk. Table 49–3 lists the common anesthetics by chemical group. All of the anesthetics that are amides (a word with the letter "i") will have an "i" in the prefix of their drug name (not the trade name). Anesthetics that belong to the ester group contain no "i" in their drug name prefix.

In anatomic areas that are highly vascular, such as the face, topical anesthesia can be considered. *When used properly,* TAC (tetracaine, epinephrine, cocaine) is a safe, effective alternative to injectable anesthesia. It is primarily used in children, in whom 2 to 5 mL is applied to a cotton ball or sponge and held over the facial laceration for 10 minutes. The vast majority of complications related to TAC are caused by improper use, pri-

TABLE 49–3. Common Local Anesthetics by Chemical Group

Amides

Lidocaine (Xylocaine)
Mepivacaine (Carbocaine)
Bupivacaine (Marcaine)

Esters

Procaine (Novocaine)
Chloroprocaine (Nesacaine)
Benzocaine
Cocaine

marily by applying it onto mucous membranes where the cocaine is readily and systemically absorbed. Because TAC can cause significant vasoconstriction, it does slightly increase the risk of wound infection. This is a less important concern in the generally low-risk facial area. Another preparation substituting lidocaine for cocaine, which is termed TAL or LET, has been studied and is found to be equivalent to TAC. Thus, there is no longer a need to expose these patients to the risk or expense of cocaine.

The pain of injection is most related to the rate of injection of the anesthetic. A 30-gauge needle is ideal because the small diameter limits the clinician's rate of injection. Additionally, because all anesthetics are acidic, a significant portion of the pain is caused by chemoreceptor stimulation. Therefore, it is reasonable to bring them to physiologic pH before injection. The technique to buffer these anesthetics is to add 1 mL of a 1 mEq/mL of sodium bicarbonate solution to 10 mL of a 1% anesthetic solution. This has been shown to significantly decrease the pain of injection. Warming the anesthetic to body temperature before injection does not have a clearly documented benefit. Additionally, a gentle distracting pinch and soothing discussion may provide a modicum of "vocal anesthesia."

Techniques of wound anesthesia are closely related to the type of wound repair used. Local anesthesia is obtained by local infiltration into and around the wound or by a regional block. Local infiltration into the subcutaneous tissue is used for most simple, common wounds and when some distortion of the wound by an anesthetic agent is not a problem. The anesthetic is injected either adjacent and parallel to the wound edge in a sequential fashion or directly into the subcutaneous tissue through the open wound edge. It is important to aspirate for blood before the injection to avoid injecting the anesthetic into a vein or artery. Enough anesthetic agent is infiltrated to cause a wheal or elevation of the wound margins.

Regional anesthesia (nerve block) is provided by injecting the agent at a site distant from the wound that blocks sensation in the area. It is imperative to know the anatomy of the nerves and the area they supply for regional anesthesia to be effective. Regional anesthesia usually requires less anesthetic agent, does not distort the appearance of the wound, and may be less painful than local anesthesia. However, the techniques may be difficult to master, the anesthesia may take a longer time to work, and the area anesthetized is usually larger than the wound.

Many techniques have been described for blocking various nerves, including digital, supraorbital, infraorbital, mental, median, ulnar, radial, sural, and posterior tibial nerve blocks. The basic technique used in all these blocks is locating the nerve first by identifying reliable local landmarks. A 25-gauge needle is inserted to the approximate level of the nerve. If paresthesias are produced, the needle is withdrawn slightly, then 1 to 3 mL of a high percentage anesthetic agent is infiltrated on either side of the nerve. The amount depends on the size of the nerve to be blocked. A digital nerve block is shown in Figure 49–1.

Cleansing. Wound cleansing is an unglamorous, but extremely important part of preventing wound infection. After local anesthesia, normal saline is poured over and into the wound to remove gross debris. The skin surface is further cleansed by applying an antibacterial solution. This serves to decrease the bacterial counts on the skin's surface and, thus, decreases secondary contamination during further wound care. Hydrogen peroxide, Hibiclens, pHisoHex, and even dilute povidone-iodine (Betadine) all cause significant tissue toxicity when allowed within the wound and may increase the infection rate and decrease cosmetic result. Normal saline and poloxamer 188 (Shur-Clens) are both devoid of antibacterial activity; however, they also cause no tissue toxic-

ity. It should be noted that povidone-iodine scrub, which is intended for surgical scrubbing of intact skin, should never be introduced to a wound because its detergent activity will dissolve cellular membranes and may cause considerable tissue damage. A combination of *gentle* scrubbing with normal saline or poloxamer 188 and delicate removal of foreign material with forceps causes the least tissue damage and maximizes the healing potential of the wound.

Hair rarely needs to be shaved. If an eyebrow is shaved, it may grow back a different color or curly instead of straight, or it may not grow back at all. If hair precludes good exposure and wound care in the scalp, it can be clipped with nonsterile scissors to a length of about 0.5 cm. If the scalp is shaved, the surface of the scalp becomes abraded, bacterial colonization around the wound increases, and the infection rate will actually increase.

The hair can alternatively be parted along the laceration and taped down with paper tape or held in place with an ointment such as bacitracin or water-soluble gel.

Irrigation. *The solution to pollution is dilution.* Copious irrigation does more to decrease infection rate and improve cosmetic result than any other component of wound care, including proper suture technique. Any form of irrigation will remove nonadherent foreign material and nonadherent bacteria from within the wound. To remove foreign material and especially bacteria that is adherent to the tissue within the wound, high-pressure irrigation is required. However, if the pressure is too high, the irrigation jet can cause direct tissue damage or dissect into fascial planes within the wound. The best way to achieve appropriate irrigation is to attach a 30-mL syringe to an 18-gauge needle or Angiocath and systematically irrigate all surfaces within the wound. Isotonic solution such as normal saline is used, and the volume is determined by the degree of contamination of the wound. For small, clean wounds, 250 mL may be adequate. However, for most outpatient wounds, 500 mL of irrigation is considered a bare minimum. It cannot be emphasized enough that sufficient pressure and volume of irrigant are crucial.

Débridement. After cleansing and irrigation, the wound is inspected for adherent foreign material and nonvital or tenuous tissue. Because the wound essentially becomes a Petri dish after closure, it is important to remove any tissue that is dead or may die and contribute to the theoretic "agar" within the wound. Adherent foreign material is removed with forceps and tissue scissors, as is any dead tissue. Additionally, any tissue that is purplish and ischemic should be resected in a

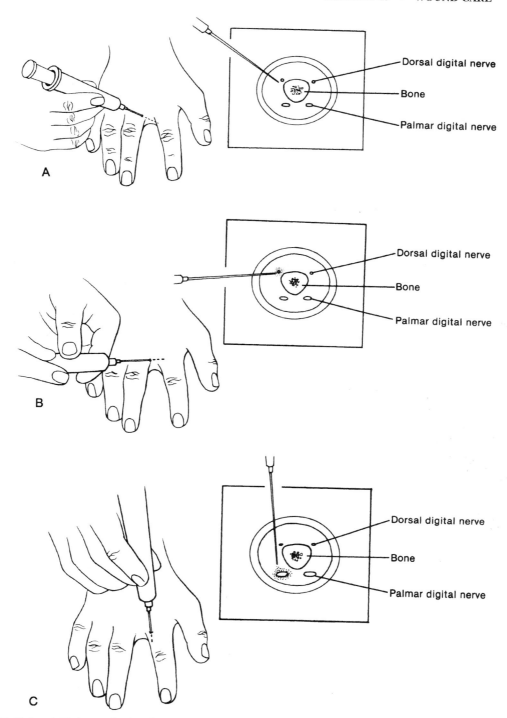

FIGURE 49–1 • *A,* Technique for digital nerve block. The needle is introduced at the proximal portion of the proximal phalanx well back into the web space. It is advanced until it touches bone. *B,* The needle is slightly withdrawn, and 1 mL of anesthetic solution is delivered to the dorsal digital nerve. *C,* Without exiting the skin, the needle is then passed along the shaft of the proximal phalanx to the palmar surface of the digit and 1 mL of anesthetic solution is delivered to the palmar digital nerve. This technique is repeated on the opposite side.

similar manner. If adequate tissue redundancy allows, irregular or "ratty" borders of the wound can be excised as well. To excise tissue margins, a No. 15 blade is used to score the epidermis just outside the irregular border. Then tissue scissors are used to cut the dermis. If epinephrine was not used in the anesthetic, capillary refill at the wound margins can be used to assess tenuous tissue (another reason to try to avoid using epinephrine). Ideally, the result of débridement will produce clean, straight, bleeding, completely viable wound margins suitable for closure. One must be extremely careful not to "burn one's bridges" by removing so much tissue that the wound must be closed under too much tension. If this is anticipated, secondary closure, tertiary closure, or leaving tenuous tissue in place to bring the wound together under appropriate tension should be considered.

Hemostasis. Once a wound has been cleansed and prepared for treatment, the amount of bleeding is assessed. In many cases, manipulation of the wound during cleansing and anesthesia opens up previously coagulated blood vessels, and fresh bleeding occurs. Bleeding is usually controlled by elevation of the part, direct pressure, and patience. If bleeding is not controlled by these measures, the next alternatives depend on the location of the wound. In facial and scalp lacerations, it is reasonable to use an anesthetic with epinephrine to aid in hemostasis. In head, scalp, and truncal wounds, the placement of deep sutures and fascial closure can tamponade bleeding vessels. It is very important to have a bloodless field when evaluating extremity injuries for nerve, artery, and tendon injury. In digit injuries, ideal hemostasis can be achieved by using a Tournicot, which is rolled over the finger from distal to proximal just after anesthesia. Specialized pneumatic arm cuffs are also available in many emergency departments. Using rubber bands, Penrose drains, gauze, or regular blood pressure cuffs should be avoided because they have all been associated with neurovascular injury when left in place for even short periods of time.

Equipment and Supplies

Good wound care can be obtained with a limited amount of materials and equipment. A standard suture tray containing a needle driver, toothed forceps, tissue scissors, and suture scissors can be prepared and sterilized. Additional instruments may include skin hooks, hemostats, and scalpels. Sterile accessory materials placed on the opened tray include gauze sponges, a basin or cups, and towels for draping.

The most practical needle holder for emergency use is the 4-inch variety with serrated carbide-tipped jaws. This has the strength to hold large needles in larger lacerations but is small enough to be used with more delicate closures. Forceps with teeth aid in manipulating and exposing underlying tissue. They should not be clamped on the external skin surface but used to grasp superficial and deep fascia only. Skin hooks, or a substitute, are used to provide better exposure in deep wounds. Tissue scissors are usually curved and are much sharper than suture scissors. They should be used only to cut tissue. If used to cut suture repeatedly, they will become dull and will no longer be adequate for débriding tissue. Suture scissors are used to cut suture only, because they are much duller than tissue scissors and will macerate tissue if used in débridement.

Suture is either monofilament or braided. Monofilament sutures have similar strength and lower tissue reactivity and infection rate, rendering braided suture nearly obsolete in outpatient wound care. The monofilament sutures are divided into absorbable and nonabsorbable types. Absorbable sutures are intended primarily for placement beneath the skin and are biodegraded and absorbed over a varying period of time, depending on the particular suture and location in the body. Although many absorbable sutures are available, polyglycolic acid (PGA) is easier to manipulate and tie. Monofilament nonabsorbable sutures, intended for percutaneous closure, are numerous as well. Polypropylene (Prolene) and nylon (Ethilon, Dermalon) constitute the majority of those in emergency settings. Prolene is somewhat stronger and has better knot security than nylon. However, it is somewhat more difficult to work with because it has a greater tendency to return to its packaged shape than nylon.

Suture size and the type of suture needle used depend on the type of laceration. Table 49–4 provides guidelines for selecting suture materials in different areas of the body. Needles are either of the tapered or cutting variety. A tapered needle is round in cross-section. A cutting needle has an edge and is triangular in cross-section. Most emergency wound care is done with a cutting needle. The smallest size appropriate for the job is chosen.

Not all wounds require sutures. Small, nongaping lacerations often can be closed with wound tapes (e.g., Steri-Strips). These are also used as adjuncts to suturing. For example, they can be placed between widely spaced sutures to help keep the skin edges together. Some emergency physicians routinely use a stapling device to close straight, uncomplicated wounds of the arms, legs,

TABLE 49–4. Suggested Guidelines for Suture Materials and Size for Body Area

Body Area	Deep Closure	Superficial Closure
Scalp	4-0°	4-0[†]
Facial structures	5-0°	6-0[†]
Trunk	4-0°	5-0, 4-0[†]
Hand		5-0[†]
Extremities	4-0°	5-0, 4-0[†]
Foot	4-0°	4-0[†]
Oral mucosa	4-0°	5-0, 4-0[†]
Deep fascia	4-0[†]	

° PGA, polyglycolic acid (Dexon) or PG 910, polyglactin 910.
[†] Polypropylene (Prolene) or nylon (Ethilon, Dermalon).

trunk, and scalp. The metal staples can be placed more quickly than sutures and provide good wound edge eversion. They are not effective in jagged, irregular lacerations or with thin, delicate skin.

Wounds closed with staples provide equivalent cosmetic result and wound infection rate. In fact, one relatively large study showed equivalent cosmetic results even when facial wounds were stapled. However, recommendations clearly state that facial wounds should be sutured in the routine fashion.

Cyanoacrylate adhesives are the newest of all techniques of wound closure. They have been found to cause less pain for the patient, require less time for the caregiver, are less expensive, and produce cosmetic results equivalent to more traditional wound closure methods. The technique involves routine wound preparation followed by application of the adhesive. The adhesive is intended to bond only with the surface of the skin and every attempt is made to keep it out of the wound itself. Forceps are used to control and approximate the wound margins, whereas the adhesive is applied to the skin surface by either a supplied applicator or a 25-gauge needle with syringe. The adhesive will polymerize within 5 seconds, joining the wound margins. Adhesive is then sequentially applied in layers to cover the wound and reinforce the first application. Considerable care must be taken that the ease of this new wound-closure technique does not distract from indicated wound anesthesia, cleansing, irrigation, débridement, and hemostasis.

Wound Closure

Simple Interrupted Closure. Placing a simple suture starts with the proper loading of the needle into the needle holder. The needle is clamped in the tips of the needle holder at a right angle to

the needle holder about one third of the way between its connection to the suture (swedge) and its point. The needle point is then placed at a 90-degree angle to the skin. The skin is punctured; and with a smooth rolling motion of the wrist, the needle is advanced (Fig. 49–2). In a straight, non-beveled laceration, the needle should emerge from the skin equidistant to the wound edge. The path of the needle should be as wide (or wider) at its base as it is near the surface (Fig. 49–3). This will evert the wound edges and result in a flatter, less noticeable scar after the wound contracts inward. In a beveled laceration, a larger "bite" of

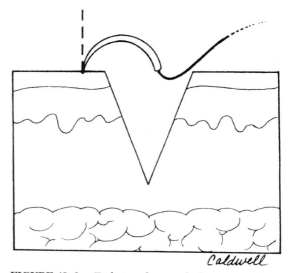

FIGURE 49–2 • Technique for wound edge eversion. The needle is introduced at a 90-degree angle to the skin.

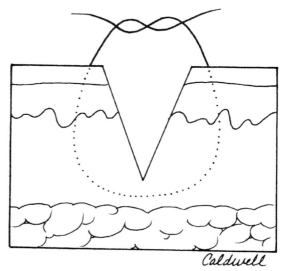

FIGURE 49–3 • By using proper needle placement technique, as illustrated in Figure 49–2, the correct suture configuration will be achieved.

tissue is taken on the thin side of the bevel to ensure the skin layers are appropriately matched. The number of skin sutures placed in a laceration and the distance between sutures depend on the location of the laceration and the skin tension in the area. In general, the fewest number of sutures that will close the laceration with minimal wound edge tension and no gaping between sutures is the appropriate number.

Deep Closure. A simple deep suture is used to approximate the subcutaneous tissues and dermis. By rejoining tissue, pockets of "dead space" are eliminated. This technique is thought to help reduce hematoma collection within the "Petri dish" and, hence, the threat of infection. Also, the tension on skin sutures is reduced, and fewer or smaller skin sutures are necessary. The most important element in this type of suture is identifying and matching the layers of tissue to avoid buckling or an uneven closure. A skin hook is helpful to lift the dermis and better observe the juxtaposition of the opposite sides. The deep suture knot is buried in the wound as shown in Figure 49–4. If deep sutures are being placed to reduce the wound tension before percutaneous closure, it is important to include the dermis in the superficial loop of the deep suture because this is the skin level with the most elasticity and its contraction contributes the most to the gapping and wound tension. The knot is inverted deeply into the superficial fascia so that it does not abrade and irritate the healing dermal margins. The need for deep sutures depends on the location of the wound and is a controversial topic. The risk of promoting infection by introducing foreign material into the wound must be weighed against any benefits in wound approximation and cosmetic appearance. In hand wounds, deep sutures are never placed. In the face, trunk, and extremities, deep sutures are more commonly used in larger lacerations. The rich vascularity of the face and head makes infection less likely, even when deep sutures are used. In general, a wound is closed with as few deep sutures as possible.

Mattress Technique. The simple interrupted skin suture and deep suture described earlier can be used to close most lacerations. In some cases special techniques or suture methods are needed. For widely gaping wounds, vertical and horizontal mattress sutures provide extra strength and good wound edge eversion (Fig. 49–5).

Running. In straight, long lacerations, such as those made by a knife or razor blade, a running suture may give a better cosmetic result and is faster to place than interrupted sutures. The disadvantages are that if the suture breaks, the entire wound is disrupted. Also, if infection develops, it

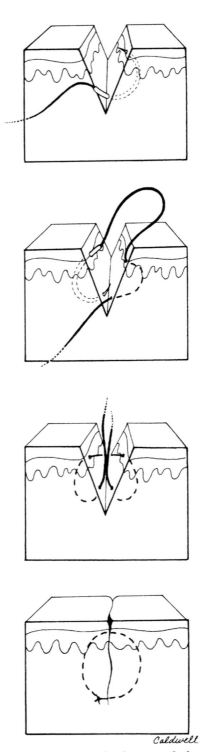

FIGURE 49–4 • Technique for placement of a deep suture closure. The needle is introduced in the subcutaneous tissue and brought upwards through the dermis. The needle is rearmed with the needle holder and introduced into the dermis on the direct opposite wound surface. The needle is exited from the superficial fascia close to the original entry point. The knot is tied deep within the wound.

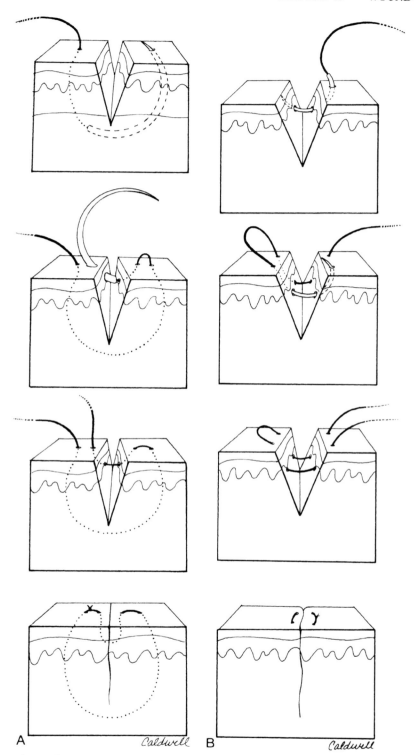

FIGURE 49–5 • Technique for mattress sutures. *A,* Vertical mattress. A deep bite, followed by a superficial bite to the dermis, completes the vertical mattress suture. *B,* Horizontal mattress. Two bites through the dermis, placed at the same level, form a horizontal mattress suture.

is not possible to open part of the wound selectively for drainage as it is with interrupted sutures (Fig. 49–6).

Corner Stitch. With irregular, jagged lacerations, flaps of tissue are often produced. The tips of these flaps are often contused and partially necrotic and may have a compromised blood supply. Securing a suture in this friable tissue is difficult and may further impair blood flow. A flap or corner stitch is used in these situations (Fig. 49–7). If the edges of a flap laceration are necrotic and require débridement, a simple flap suture will not suffice. In this case, the "V" shape of the flap is converted into a "Y" shape by using a flap (corner) stitch and simple interrupted sutures (Fig. 49–8).

CASE *Study*

In Case 2, the wound was a 6-cm jagged flap laceration at the midtibial level of the lateral aspect of the right leg. The edges of the wound and the flap were macerated and necrotic. There was contamination of the wound by dirt particles and bark fragments. On exploration there was no evident damage to muscle tissue or bone. The wound was anesthetized, prepared with Shur-Clens solution, and irrigated using a 30-mL syringe and a 18-gauge needle to produce a medium-pressure jet. A total of 2000 mL of normal saline was combined with a thorough exploration to remove all of the foreign material.

Because of the poor vascularity of this patient's leg, deep sutures were not considered for closing the wound. The irregular flap presented a problem, which was addressed first by débriding the necrotic wound edges. Next, a flap suture was placed using 4-0 nylon, which converted the wound to a "Y" shape. Seven simple interrupted sutures of 4-0 nylon were used to close the remainder of the "Y."

Before an anesthetic was administered, the maximum total dosage was calculated. For plain 1% lidocaine, the maximum dose is 5 mg/kg (375 mg for this patient) or 37.5 mL of a 1% solution. Care is taken to properly anesthetize the wounds while not exceeding this limit. Cleansing with povidone-iodine and thorough irrigation were carried out, and débridement of devitalized wound margins was performed. Nylon nonabsorbable external sutures were chosen for repair. Deep, absorbable sutures were not needed and in this situation could increase the likelihood of wound infection.

Wound Aftercare

Tetanus Prophylaxis. Before a wounded patient leaves the emergency department, the matter of tetanus prophylaxis is addressed. The patient's immunization history is obtained. The risk of tetanus is highest in people who have never been fully immunized. The elderly and people not native to the United States are at highest risk. The decision to provide tetanus prophylaxis is based on the patient's immunization history and the assessment of the wound. Table 49–5 lists current tetanus immunization recommendations.

Rabies Prophylaxis. The rabies virus is easily killed by any of the common wound care preparatory agents, including simple soap and water. For this reason, rabies-prone wounds should be treated directly with povidone-iodine, or similar agent, coupled with vigorous, rather than the usual gentle, scrubbing. Guidelines for rabies prophylaxis are listed in Table 49–6.

Bandaging. Dressings or bandages are used on wounds to provide protection, prevent contamination, and absorb wound drainage. A standard dressing may be as simple as a Band-Aid or more involved, such as an occlusive, nonadherent pad placed next to the skin covered by thicker layers of gauze that can absorb wound drainage. Tape is used to secure the bandage to the skin. An occlusive layer is used over the wound because it is easier and less painful to change because it does not adhere to the wound. There are a variety of materials for bandaging wounds and many ways of applying bandages. Even occlusion from regular petroleum-based antibiotic ointment (bacitracin and polymyxin B [Polysporin]) has demonstrated benefit. Most physicians do not bandage small face or scalp lacerations, preferring to apply an antibiotic ointment and leave the wound uncovered. If a bandage is applied circumferentially, as on an extremity, care must be taken to make it loose enough so that distal perfusion is not impaired. The timing of bandage changes depends on the nature of the wound and patient activity. If the wound has little drainage and little chance of infection and if the patient can keep it clean and dry, the bandage can be left on for several days. If there is significant drainage or if the bandage becomes soiled or wet, it should be changed daily or more frequently.

To maximize cosmetic result, it is important to prevent a dry crust from forming within a laceration or other wound. To avoid this, an ointment is commonly used to keep the evolving crust moist, and cleansing twice or three times a day with simple soap and water or dilute peroxide is prescribed. In simple sutured lacerations, dressings

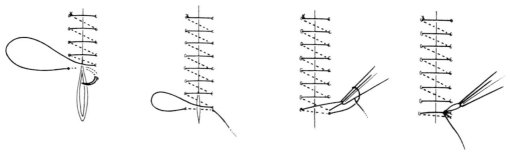

FIGURE 49–6 • Technique for running suture closure. This suture is started by placing a standard tie at the extreme right-hand portion of the laceration (left side for left-handed operators). The suture material is not cut, and tissue bites are taken at a 45-degree angle to the wound direction. The superficial portions lie at a 90-degree angle. The securing knot is fashioned, as illustrated, by using the final loop as the anchor for the needle holder. Several throws are made in the standard manner.

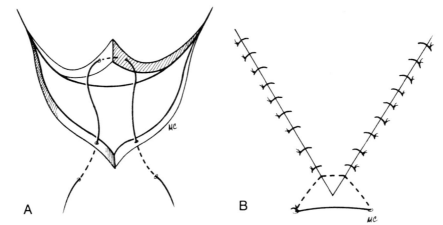

FIGURE 49–7 • Technique for corner closure. *A*, The corner stitch is fashioned as illustrated with one suture passing through all wound surfaces at the same level. *B*, The flap is secured with small-bite superficial closures to "tack" down the flap. Within the wound the suture exits and enters the side of the dermis and at no time does this stitch extend through the dermis, thus taking advantage of the strongest skin layer, the dermis, in this tenuous, friable flap.

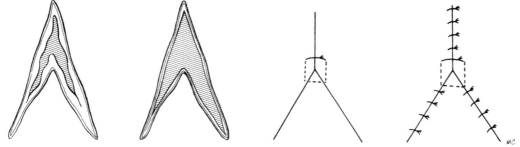

FIGURE 49–8 • Technique for V-Y closure of a flap with irregular edges. All devitalized edges of the flap are trimmed back with tissue scissors. This débridement often leaves a flap that is inadequate to close the resulting defect. A modified corner suture is placed as illustrated to convert the wound to a "Y" shape. The remainder of the wound is closed with simple interrupted sutures.

need to remain in place for only 1 to 2 days because the wound becomes watertight thereafter.

Antibiotics

For simple, uncomplicated minor wounds and lacerations, there is no good clinical evidence that systemic antibiotics provide protection against the development of wound infection. On the other hand, clinical and empirical experience suggests there are certain wounds and clinical circumstances that warrant antibiotic use. If the decision is made to initiate antibiotic therapy, evidence indicates the initial dose has to be administered as soon as possible. Antibiotics may lose

TABLE 49–5. Summary Guide to Tetanus Prophylaxis

History of Absorbed Tetanus Toxoid (Dose)	Clean, Minor Wounds		All Other Wounds°	
	Td[†]	**TIG**	**Td**[†]	**TIG**
Unknown or <three	Yes	No	Yes	Yes
≤ Three[‡]	No[§]	No	No[‖]	No

°Such as, but not limited to, wounds contaminated with dirt, feces, soil, saliva, etc., puncture wounds, avulsions, and wounds resulting from missiles, crushing, burns, and frostbite (nearly all emergency department patients).

[†]For children younger than 7 years old: DTP (DT, if pertussis vaccine is contraindicated) is preferred to tetanus toxoid alone. For persons 7 years old and older, Td is preferred to tetanus toxoid alone.

[‡]If only three doses of *fluid* toxoid have been received, a fourth dose of toxoid, preferably an absorbed toxoid, should be given.

[§]Yes, if more than 10 years since last dose.

[‖]Yes, if more than 5 years since last dose. (More frequent boosters are not needed and can accentuate side effects.)

From Advisory Committee on Immunization Practices: Diptheria, tetanus, and pertussis: Guidelines for vaccine prophylaxis and other preventive measures.

TABLE 49–6. A Guide to Rabies Postexposure Prophylaxis

Animal Species	Condition of Animal at Time of Attack	Treatment of Exposed Person°
Domestic: dog or cat	Healthy and available for 10 days of observation Rabid or suspected rabid Unknown (escaped)	None[†] HRIG and HDCV Consult public health officials; if treatment is indicated, give HRIG and HDCV
Wild: skunk, bat, fox, coyote, raccoon, bobcat, and other carnivores	Regard as rabid unless proven negative by laboratory tests[‡]	HRIG and HDCV
Other: livestock, rodents, and lagomorphs (rabbits and hares)	Consider individually. Local and state public health officials should be consulted on questions about the need for rabies prophylaxis. Bites of squirrels, hamsters, guinea pigs, gerbils, chipmunks, rats, mice, other rodents, rabbits, and hares almost never call for *antirabies* prophylaxis.	

°All bites and wounds should immediately be cleansed thoroughly with soap and water. If antirabies treatment is indicated, both human rabies immune globulin (HRIG) and human diploid cell rabies vaccine (HDCV) should be given as soon as possible, regardless of the interval from exposure. Local reactions to vaccines are common but do not contraindicate continuing treatment. Discontinue vaccine treatment if fluorescent-antibody tests of the animal are negative for rabies.

[†]During the usual holding period of 10 days, begin treatment with RIG and vaccine (preferably with HDCV) at the first sign of rabies in a dog or cat that has bitten someone. The symptomatic animal should be killed immediately and tested.

[‡]The animal should be killed and tested as soon as possible. Holding for observation is not recommended.

Center for Disease Control: Rabies Prevention—United States 1991. MMWR Morbid Mortal Wkly Rep 1991; 40:1–18.

their protective effect when given more than 3 to 5 hours after injury and bacterial contamination. The following guidelines indicate wounds for which oral antibiotics on an outpatient basis are considered:

- Wounds more than 8 to 12 hours old, especially of the hands and lower extremities
- Wounds due to a crushing (compression) mechanism, with significant devitalization, or requiring extensive revision
- Significantly contaminated wounds requiring extensive cleansing and débridement
- Wounds involving violation of the ear or nose cartilage
- Wounds involving a joint space, tendon, or bone

- Mammalian bites, particularly human and cat bites
- Extensive or contaminated wounds in patients with preexisting valvular heart disease
- Wounds in persons with conditions of immunosuppression or impaired host defenses (e.g., diabetes mellitus)

The choice of systemic prophylactic antibiotic should take into account the fact that the most common infecting agent is *Staphylococcus aureus*. However, gram-negative organisms occur with significant frequency and need to be considered as well. Because of their broad activity against gram-positive and gram-negative organisms, including penicillinase-producing *S. aureus*, first-generation cephalosporins are a reasonable choice when prophylaxis is advisable. Examples include cephalexin (Keflex) and cefadroxil (Duricef). Some authorities comment that coverage for gram-positive organisms alone is sufficient and recommend using the less-expensive dicloxacillin. For penicillin-allergic patients, erythromycin or ciprofloxacin can be used. In most situations requiring prophylaxis, 3 days of therapy should suffice. Early intravenous administration in the emergency department of the initial dose is recommended by some authorities.

SPECIAL CONSIDERATIONS

Anatomic Areas

Scalp Wounds

The scalp is anatomically different from other areas of skin. Hair usually obscures a wound, making it difficult to evaluate. The dermis of the scalp is quite thick, and it sits on a very dense layer of connective tissue (superficial fascia), which contains a rich network of arterial and venous vessels. This abundant vascular supply can lead to brisk bleeding when the scalp is lacerated, which can result in substantial blood loss. This bleeding is made worse by the stiffness of the connective tissue, which prevents the normal skin retraction and constriction of injured blood vessels. Beneath the thick connective tissue layer is the galea aponeurotica. The galea is composed of dense, fibrous tissue that attaches to the frontalis muscle anteriorly and the occipitalis muscle posteriorly. Under the galea aponeurotica is a thin layer of loose connective tissue that overlies the periosteum. It is important to identify and close lacerations in the galea aponeurotica for two reasons: First, a large defect in this layer may lead to abnormal contraction of the frontalis muscle and affect the forehead, appearance, and expression. Also, there is potential for extension of hematoma and infection in the loose connective tissue layer deep to the galea. Closure can prevent hematoma formation and reduce the chance of infection.

Facial Wounds

Facial injuries are of special concern to the physician as well as the patient. The challenge is to maintain the cosmetic appearance of the face. In general, deep sutures are placed in the dermis to close the wound and keep the tension off the skin sutures. Skin sutures are placed to align the superficial tissues. Débridement may be used to delineate the wound edges, but the amount of tissue removed is kept small. Smaller suture material is used, and greater attention is paid to skin tension lines. In some cases, definitive repair cannot be done in the emergency department. In these cases the wound is closed to align the tissues, and the patient is referred for further care.

Eyelid lacerations are explored for involvement of the globe, lacrimal gland, nasolacrimal duct, lacrimal canaliculi, palpebral ligaments, and facial muscles surrounding the orbit. Simple 6-0 suture closure is usually used. Injuries to the medial one third of either lid are at risk to involve the superior or inferior lacrimal canaliculi. Similarly, injuries to the margin of either lid can also have significant functional implications because proper repair is required to preserve adequate function of the tear film. For these reasons, these two injuries should be referred to an ophthalmologist or a plastic surgeon.

Nasal injuries require internal as well as external exploration. Trauma to the nose may produce a septal hematoma, which is a collection of blood under pressure between the mucosa and the septal cartilage. If left unevacuated, a septal hematoma can lead to necrosis of part of the septum.

Intraoral lacerations as a rule heal quickly with minimal repair. For large, gaping intraoral lacerations, a few absorbable sutures are placed to approximate the irregular mucosal edges. Lacerations of less than 2 cm in the mouth do not usually require repair unless they are actively bleeding.

Lip lacerations are challenging to repair because of the importance of exactly readjoining the disrupted tissue. If lacerated, the cosmetically important vermilion border (the thin line of transition between the lip and the facial skin) must be properly realigned. Failure to do this results in a very noticeable scar on the lip. Anesthetic blocks for the lip are ideal in this situation because they do not distort the anatomy in the area. It is helpful to realign the vermilion border with the initial suture when closing lip lacerations.

The ear has a thin layer of skin over its cartilage foundation. When traumatized, a collection of blood adjacent to the cartilage (perichondral hematoma) may exert pressure on the cartilage, causing impaired healing and necrosis. A grossly disfigured ear can result. Perichondral hematomas should be incised and drained and then covered with a pressure dressing. If extensive underlying damage to the cartilage is found, an otolaryngologist should be consulted. For uncomplicated ear lacerations, closure with 6-0 nylon simple interrupted sutures is sufficient. It is not necessary and may be harmful to suture the cartilage.

Foreign Bodies

In almost all wounds a foreign body must be suspected. Common foreign bodies are glass and metal fragments, wood chips, gravel, and dirt particles. Radiographs may be helpful, as noted in "Diagnostic Adjuncts." Some foreign bodies are superficial and easy to remove, but deeper ones, particularly those penetrating the sole of the foot, are often very difficult to find. When normal wound cleansing and exploration do not reveal a foreign body that is suspected by the history or identified on radiographs, a decision must be made about removal. In some cases the removal attempt may cause more damage than leaving the foreign body in place. If composed of an inert substance such as glass, metal, or plastic, a foreign body is less likely to cause tissue reaction and infection. Removal of inert foreign bodies is advisable but not at the expense of major tissue damage. Noninert foreign bodies are composed of organic material such as wood or vegetable matter, which may decay in the body and cause marked tissue reaction and infection. All noninert foreign bodies are removed from a wound. Foreign bodies requiring removal are best approached by extending the original wound. When extending a wound, it is important to incise along skin tension lines whenever possible. One should also keep in mind, when extending lacerations in extremities, that it is safest to extend them either proximally or distally because all neurovascular bundles run longitudinally in the extremities. Splinter forceps may make it easier to pull thin, sharp foreign bodies out of the wound. If exploration involves dissection along nerves, tendons, large blood vessels, or into joints, it is carried out in the operating room.

Puncture Wounds

Puncture wounds, although externally appearing benign, can be extremely serious injuries. The infection risk after a puncture wound may be five times greater than the infection risk of an open laceration at a similar anatomic site. This occurs for two reasons. First, the mechanism of a penetrating puncture wound, which commonly occurs through clothing or least contaminated skin, is such that bacteria and foreign material are generally deposited deep within the poorly vascular superficial fascia. Also, the superficial layers of the skin generally close over after the puncture, sealing off this deep contamination. It is a well-known surgical dictum that infection occurs much more often in wounds that do not have the ability to drain (pus under pressure). The treatment for all but the most minor puncture wounds is incision followed by routine cleansing, irrigation, débridement, and closure. If adequate preparation of the wound is not possible because of the depth of injury, the wound should be incised and remain open. Antibiotic use either with incision and wound care or without has no impact on infection rate. One of the more common puncture wounds seen in the emergency department is a fishhook injury. It is recommended that no matter what "trick" may be used to remove the hook, this contaminated puncture wound should be incised and treated as mentioned earlier.

Burns

Many burns seen in the emergency setting can be handled on an outpatient basis. Those burns usually requiring admission to hospital are summarized in Table 49–7. These are more serious burns, such as full-thickness burns with all but very small body surface areas, partial-thickness burns larger than 15% surface area, burns in patients in the extremes of age, and burns caused by nonthermal insults. Additionally, burns in particular anatomic areas such as the hands, face, perineum, or feet and burns that are suspected to have been inflicted on children require hospitalization.

Burns that do not fit criteria in Table 49–7 can be considered more minor burns and can be treated with routine outpatient burn care. This care includes adequate oral or, more likely, parenteral analgesia followed by thorough cleansing with isotonic saline or poloxamer 188 (ShurClens). Partial-thickness burns will generally have blisters. If blisters are intact, they are to be left alone. However, tissue from ruptured blisters should be débrided with forceps and tissue scissors. The burn is then covered by silver sulfadiazine (Silvadene), followed by a petroleum-impregnated gauze pad such as Adaptic. A bulky gauze wrap is then applied circumferentially. Because silver sulfadiazine can permanently discolor the skin of the head and neck, burns in this area are best dressed with bacitracin and left open to air.

A special case of very superficial partial-thickness burns commonly seen in the emergency department is sunburn. Because this primarily involves the epidermis and disrupts its tight junctions, patients become dehydrated very easily. Oral, or sometimes intravenous, hydration is a key part of the treatment, coupled with comfort measures such as nonsteroidal anti-inflammatory agents and topical relief with an aloe vera preparation or any of the numerous topical, over-the-counter anesthetics.

TABLE 49–7. Guidelines for Hospital Admission of Burn Victims

Partial-thickness burns > 15% surface area
Full-thickness burns > 5% surface area
Suspected inhalation injury
Age < 5 or > 65 years
Partial- or full-thickness burns of hands, face, perineum, or feet
Electrical burns
Chemical burns
Suspected child abuse

Bites

Animal and human bites usually occur on the extremities, where a less generous vascular supply predisposes to infection. Cat bites are most likely (40% to 80% incidence) to become infected. A rare bacteria commonly responsible for infection from a cat bite is *Pasteurella multocida*. It usually causes redness, warmth, and pain in and around the bite within 24 hours. Dog bites have a 4% to 6% incidence of infection, which is no higher than that of a nonbite wound. Human bites become infected in up to 30% of cases. One particularly aggressive bacterium resident in the oral flora of humans, *Eikenella corrodens*, can lead to rapid and severe wound infection. It can destroy a joint in a matter of hours. Thus, any human bite near a joint should be treated with the utmost of respect. Extensive irrigation and débridement of devitalized tissue can reduce the chances of infection in animal bites. Dog bites, if seen within 6 hours, can be closed primarily. Because of the low incidence of infection, dog bites to the face may be sutured even up to 24 hours after the injury if wound and patient characteristics allow. In the hands and feet, dog bites are usually left to heal by secondary union. Cat bites are often puncture wounds and are not closed unless the cosmetic concerns of scarring outweigh the risk of infection. Prophylactic antibiotics are used in all animal bites. The penicillinase-resistant penicillins have good activity against *P. multocida*, *Eikenella*, *Staphylococcus*, and *Streptococcus* species. All are common in bite infections.

The risk of rabies in animal bites is very low, but, given the lethality of the disease, all bites are considered for rabies prophylaxis. Guidelines are available for rabies prophylaxis and are summarized in Table 49–6.

DISPOSITION AND FOLLOW-UP

Outpatient Management

A large component of the eventual outcome of a wound is the care and treatment given after the

CASE *Study*

In Case 1, because the wounds were not too old, were in well-vascularized areas, and could be cleansed well, the head and shoulder wounds were judged to be acceptable for primary closure. The back wounds were small puncture wounds that were not in a cosmetically significant area. They were left open to heal by secondary intention.

Rabies is always a consideration in dog bites, but in the setting of a provoked attack, and with documentation of the dog's rabies vaccination, there was no need to provide rabies prophylaxis.

patient leaves the emergency department. It is essential to educate patients about their wounds and to give them specific instructions about aftercare.

The timing and number of follow-up visits depend on patient compliance and reliability as well as the perceived risk of wound complications. Some wounds need one-time follow-up. Examples of these are first-degree burns and clean lacerations or abrasions. Some wounds, such as hand injuries, need to be checked every 24 to 48 hours for infection and to be rebandaged. Second-degree burns and extensive animal bites also belong in this category. Suture removal is also done according to the individual needs of each wound. Guidelines are given in Table 49–8. Generally, sutures are removed from facial wounds in 3 to 5 days. Timing of suture removal from other wounds depends primarily on two factors: stress on the wound and cosmetic importance. Lacerations in anatomic areas of high stress such as extensor surfaces and the anterior leg will likely need to remain in place from 10 to 14 days to decrease the risk of wound dehiscence. Most other wounds of low or moderate stress can safely undergo suture removal at 7 to 10 days. Cosmetic importance also plays a role in suture removal timing, because the longer the sutures remain in place, the more likely "train tracks" will result and decrease the cosmetic result of the procedure. Wounds of more cosmetic importance such as

TABLE 49–8. Suture Removal Intervals

Face	3–5 days
Areas of low stress or more cosmetically important	7–10 days
Areas of high stress or less cosmetically important	10–14 days

those in the neck may be removed as early as 5 days. However, sutures in the sole of the foot should probably remain in place for 2 weeks. The key element in follow-up is making clear to the patient, in writing, the time and place of the follow-up appointment.

Pain relief once the patient leaves the emergency department is accomplished in a number of ways. For most wounds, immobilization, elevation, and ice application are adequate. Some people will require systemic analgesic medications. For musculoskeletal injuries a nonsteroidal anti-inflammatory agent such as ibuprofen provides good analgesia. Some wounds are extremely painful, and some patients have a lower tolerance for pain. In these cases, an oral narcotic medication (e.g., hydrocodone) may be necessary. Examples of injuries that might need narcotics are extensive burns or abrasions and crush injuries of the digits. Extensive sun exposure of healing scars, during the first 12 months, can lead to an exaggerated or discolored scar. Patients should be advised to use a sunblock with a sun protective factor of 15 on all scars for a year.

Inpatient Management

Certain wounds are considered for inpatient management. The general principles behind inpatient management include the possible need for surgical intervention, the need for intravenous antibiotic prophylaxis, complicating secondary illnesses, the need for extensive nursing care, and an inability to care for oneself. Specific indications include the following:

- Complex, contaminated lacerations, particularly of the face or distal extremities
- Suspected penetration of bone, tendon, or joint space
- Extensive animal or human bite wounds, particularly of the hand or foot
- Serious underlying illness such as diabetes mellitus

CASE *Study*

In Case 1, the patient had wounds that required close follow-up. The chance of an infection of his macerated dog bites is great enough to warrant a follow-up check at 48 hours. If the wound looks good at 48 hours, further follow-up can be scheduled as needed. The patient was given written instructions to return for follow-up in 2 days. He was instructed to watch for signs of infection, to keep the bandages in place, and keep the wound clean and dry. He was placed on amoxicillin-clavulanate (Augmentin), 500 mg every 8 hours for 4 days.

In Case 2, the patient was given tetanus toxoid, 0.5 mL intramuscularly, after it was determined that she had received tetanus immunization 15 years earlier. Several factors, noted earlier, increased the risk for infection of the patient's wound. Given the patient's diabetes, poor vasculature, and the degree of contamination of the wound, the emergency physician elected to give the patient prophylactic antibiotics. Cephalexin, 500 mg every 6 hours for 3 days, was prescribed. She also received 1 g of cefazolin (Ancef) intravenously before her discharge to ensure rapid establishment of first-generation cephalosporin serum concentration.

Because antibiotics do not obviate the need for close follow-up, the physician arranged a follow-up appointment in 24 hours with her primary physician for a wound check. The patient also received written instructions on recognizing signs of infection and keeping the wound bandaged, clean, and dry.

FINAL POINTS

- The mechanism of injury is an important clinical factor because it can have a significant impact on wound healing and risk of infection.
- After 2 weeks, repaired wounds have recovered only 5% of the original tensile strength of the skin. They are susceptible to reopening for a short period of time after suture removal.
- Wound infections are uncommon but occur in 5% of patients. *Staphylococcus aureus* is the most common infecting organism.
- Determining the elapsed time since injury is important because the chance of wound infection increases with each passing hour before repair.
- In evaluating patients with wounds and lacerations, it is important to determine whether a serious underlying condition caused the wound (e.g., syncope, seizures) and whether the actual surface injury is accompanied by a functional deficit (e.g., neurovascular or tendon injury).
- Inert foreign bodies, such as glass, metal, or gravel, are almost always visible on radiographs and carry a relatively low infection risk. Noninert objects, such as wood, thorns, and dirt, may not be radiopaque and need to be identified and removed because they carry a relatively high infection risk.

- Wound cleansing and irrigation are the cornerstones of wound care. Neither good wound closure techniques nor antibiotics can overcome superficial or inadequate wound preparation.
- Although deep closures with absorbable suture material are important to reduce wound tension and close deep dead spaces, they act like foreign bodies. As few as possible are used to accomplish the task.
- All but the most minor puncture wounds should be incised and undergo the same meticulous wound treatment that contaminated lacerations do.
- Tetanus remains an important worldwide disease. Proper tetanus prophylaxis must be ensured for every patient, particularly those from foreign countries or individuals older than the age of 50 who might not have been properly immunized as children.
- Most wounds heal better with frequent application of a petroleum-based ointment (containing an antibiotic or not) and frequent, gentle washing with soap and water or dilute peroxide to keep a hard crust from forming in the wound.
- During the early follow-up period, pain that results from most wounds is successfully managed with nonnarcotic analgesia, appropriate dressings, immobilization, and elevation of the area.

Bibliography

TEXT

Trott A: Wounds and Lacerations: Emergency Care and Closure, 2nd ed. St. Louis, Mosby—Year Book, 1997.

JOURNAL ARTICLES

Bello YM, Phillips TJ: Recent advances in wound healing. JAMA 2000; 283:716–718.

Berk WA, Welch RD, Bock BF: Controversial issues in clinical management of the simple wound. Ann Emerg Med 1992; 21:72–80.

Berkowitz J: Tissue adhesives. Ann Emerg Med 1999; 34:116–117.

Bruns TB, Worthington JM: Using tissue adhesive for wound repair: A practical guide to dermabond. Am Fam Physician 2000; 61:1383–1388.

Dire DJ: Emergency management of dog and cat bite wounds. Emerg Med Clin North Am 1992; 10:719–736.

Griego RD, Rosen T, Orengo IF, Wolf JE: Dog, cat, and human bites: A review. J Am Acad Dermatol 1995; 33:1019–1029.

Hollander JE, Singer AJ: Laceration management. Ann Emerg Med 1999; 34:256–267.

Hollander JE, Singer AJ, Valentine SM: Risk factors for infection in patients with traumatic lacerations. Acad Emerg Med 2001; 8:716–720.

Howell JM, Chisholm CD: Wound Care. Emerg Med Clin North Am 1997; 15:417–425.

Leaper DJ: Prophylactic and therapeutic role of antibiotics in wound care. Am J Surg 1994; 167:15S–19S.

Richardson JP, Knight AL: The management and prevention of tetanus. J Emerg Med 1993; 11:737–742.

Robson MC: Wound infection: A failure of wound healing caused by an imbalance of bacteria. Surg Clin North Am 1997; 77:637–650.

Steward GM, Simpson P, Rosenberg NM: Use of topical lidocaine in pediatric laceration repair: A review of topical anesthetics. Pediatr Emerg Care 1998; 14:419–423.

Stewart C: Skin and soft tissue infection update. Emerg Med Rep 2000; 21(4):35–44.

Stewart GM, Quan L, Horton A: Laceration management. Pediatr Emerg Care 1993; 9:247–250.

Trott AT: Cyanoacrylate tissue adhesives: An advance in wound care. JAMA 1997; 277:1559–1560.

Wijetunge DB: Management of acute and traumatic wounds: Main aspects of care in adults and children. Am J Surg 1994; 167:56S–60S.

Zempsky WT: Use of topical lidocaine in pediatric laceration repair. Pediatr Emerg Care 1999; 15:239.

Index

Note: Page numbers followed by the letter f refer to figures; those followed by t refer to tables.

EMERGENCY MEDICINE

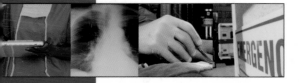

An Approach to Clinical Problem-Solving
Second Edition

Glenn C. Hamilton, MD, MSM; Arthur B. Sanders, MD; Gary R. Strange, MD, FACEP; and Alexander T. Trott, MD

On-the-go guidance when you need it!

This clinically focused resource considers the most common ED problems as they present in practice—by symptom orientation. It provides just the information you need, when you need it!

Perfect for your busy practice!

- Covers the 65 most common presentations.
- Provides case studies throughout the chapters.
- Considers pediatric and geriatric populations.

The Second Edition...

- delivers new chapters on shock, penetrating trauma, HIV patients, and domestic violence.
- incorporates current clinical guidelines.
- presents thorough updates throughout, including coverage of female patients and evidence-based medicine.
- more!

Emergency Medicine: An Approach to Clinical Problem-Solving, Second Edition is compact and concise. See how much time it can save you in the ED!

SAUNDERS
An Imprint of Elsevier Science

www.elsevierhealth.com

ISBN 0–7216–9278–8

9 780721 692784